Wallach's Interpretation *of* Diagnostic Tests

NINTH EDITION

Wallach's
Interpretation *of*
Diagnostic Tests

NINTH EDITION

Edited by

Mary A. Williamson, MT(ASCP), PhD
Director, Laboratory Operations
ACM Medical Laboratory
Rochester, New York
former Assistant Professor
Department of Pathology
University of Massachusetts Medical School
Worcester, Massachusetts

L. Michael Snyder, MD
Professor
Department of Medicine & Pathology
University of Massachusetts
Chair, Department of Hospital Laboratories
Department of Hospital Laboratories
UMass Memorial Medical Center
Worcester, Massachusetts

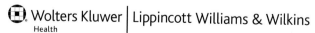
Wolters Kluwer | Lippincott Williams & Wilkins
Health
Philadelphia · Baltimore · New York · London
Buenos Aires · Hong Kong · Sydney · Tokyo

Acquisitions Editor: Sonya Seigafuse
Product Manager: Kerry Barrett
Production Manager: Alicia Jackson
Senior Manufacturing Manager: Benjamin Rivera
Marketing Manager: Kim Schonberger
Design Coordinator: Joan Wendt
Production Service: Aptara, Inc.

Library of Congress Cataloging-in-Publication Data

Wallach's interpretation of diagnostic tests. – 9th ed. / edited by
Mary A. Williamson and L. Michael Snyder.
  p. ; cm.
  Interpretation of diagnostic tests
  Rev. ed. of: Interpretation of diagnostic tests / Jacques Wallach. 8th
ed. c2007.
  Includes bibliographical references and index.
  ISBN 978-1-60547-667-4
  1. Diagnosis, Laboratory–Handbooks, manuals, etc.   I. Williamson,
Mary A.   II. Snyder, L. Michael.   III. Wallach, Jacques B. (Jacques
Burton), 1926 – Interpretation of diagnostic tests.   IV. Title:
Interpretation of diagnostic tests.
  [DNLM: 1. Laboratory Techniques and Procedures.   2. Diagnostic
Techniques and Procedures.   QY 25]
  RB38.2.W35 2011
  616.07′56–dc22   2011003431

DISCLAIMER
    Care has been taken to confirm the accuracy of the information presented and to describe generally accepted practices. However, the authors, editors, and publisher are not responsible for errors or omissions or for any consequences from application of the information in this book and make no warranty, expressed or implied, with respect to the currency, completeness, or accuracy of the contents of the publication. Application of the information in a particular situation remains the professional responsibility of the practitioner.
    The authors, editors, and publisher have exerted every effort to ensure that drug selection and dosage set forth in this text are in accordance with current recommendations and practice at the time of publication. However, in view of ongoing research, changes in government regulations, and the constant flow of information relating to drug therapy and drug reactions, the reader is urged to check the package insert for each drug for any change in indications and dosage and for added warnings and precautions. This is particularly important when the recommended agent is a new or infrequently employed drug.
    Some drugs and medical devices presented in the publication have Food and Drug Administration (FDA) clearance for limited use in restricted research settings. It is the responsibility of the health care provider to ascertain the FDA status of each drug or device planned for use in their clinical practice.

To purchase additional copies of this book, call our customer service department at (800) 638-3030 or fax orders to (301) 223-2320. International customers should call (301) 223-2300.

Visit Lippincott Williams & Wilkins on the Internet: at LWW.com. Lippincott Williams & Wilkins customer service representatives are available from 8:30 am to 6 pm, EST.

10 9 8 7 6 5 4 3 2

Special thanks to Dr. Michael Snyder for providing the opportunity to be part of this project. I would like to express my deepest gratitude for his mentorship and support over the past 3 years. I would also like to acknowledge the efforts of all the authors for their hard work and commitment to complete this book while continuing to support the laboratory operation including Drs. Michael Snyder, Guy Vallaro, Amanda Jenkins, Patricia Miron, Edward I. Ginns, Marzena Galdzicka, Charles Kiefer, Hongbo Yu, Juliana Szakacs and especially L. V. Rao, Liberto Pechet, and Michael Mitchell. I would also like to thank Suzanne O'Brien for her administrative support as well as Martha Cushman for her invaluable input and superb editing skills. Furthermore, I am grateful to my family and friends for their patience and support over the past 2 years.

Mary A. Williamson, MT(ASCP), PhD

To my wife Barbara, and children Cathe, Lizzy, and John for their tireless understanding and support throughout the years.
My assistant Suzanne O'Brien for her dedication and help with the textbook

L. Michael Snyder, MD

Marzena Galdzicka, PhD
Associate Director, Molecular Diagnostics
  Laboratory
Department of Hospital Laboratories
UMass Memorial Medical Center
Clinical Assistant Professor of Pathology
Department of Pathology
University of Massachusetts Medical School
Shrewsbury, Massachusetts

Edward I. Ginns, MD, PhD
Director, Molecular Diagnostics Laboratory
Director, Lysosomal Disorders Treatment
  and Research Program
Department of Hospital Laboratories
UMass Memorial Medical Center
Professor, Clinical Pathology, Neurology,
  Pediatrics and Psychiatry
University of Massachusetts Medical School
Shrewsbury, Massachusetts

Amanda Jenkins, PhD
Director, Toxicology Laboratory
Department of Hospital Laboratories
UMass Memorial Medical Center
Clinical Associate Professor of Pathology
Department of Pathology
University of Massachusetts Medical School
Worcester, Massachusetts

Charles Kiefer, PhD
Director, Andrology, Lyme Western Blot &
  Clinical Assay Research
Department of Hospital Laboratories
UMass Memorial Medical Center
Associate Professor
Department of Pathology
University of Massachusetts Medical School
Worcester, Massachusetts

Gary Lapidas
Senior Vice President
UMass Memorial Health Care
President, UMass Memorial Laboratories,
  Inc.
Worcester, Massachusetts

Patricia Minehart Miron, PhD
Director, Cytogenetics Laboratory
Department of Hospital Laboratories
UMass Memorial Medical Center
Clinical Associate Professor of Pathology
Department of Pathology
University of Massachusetts Medical School
Worcester, Massachusetts

Michael Mitchell, MD, FCAP
Director, Microbiology Laboratory
Department of Hospital Laboratories
UMass Memorial Medical Center
Clinical Associate Professor of Pathology
Department of Pathology
University of Massachusetts Medical School
Worcester, Massachusetts

Liberto Pechet, MD, FACP
Senior Consultant, Department of Hospital
  Laboratories
UMass Memorial Medical Center
Professor Emeritus, Medicine and
  Pathology
University of Massachusetts Medical School
Worcester, Massachusetts

L.V. Rao, PhD, FACB
Senior Director, Clinical Lab Operations
Director, Core Laboratories & Immunology
Department of Hospital Laboratories
UMass Memorial Medical Center
Clinical Associate Professor
Department of Pathology
University of Massachusetts Medical School
Worcester, Massachusetts

L. Michael Snyder, MD
Chairman, Department of Hospital
  Laboratories
UMass Memorial Medical Center
Professor of Medicine and Pathology
University of Massachusetts Medical School
Worcester, Massachusetts

Juliana Szakacs, MD
Director of Pathology and Laboratory
  Medicine
Harvard Vanguard Medical Associates
Boston, Massachusetts

Guy Vallaro, PhD
Chief Science Officer and Director
Massachusetts State Police
Forensic Service Group
Maynard, Massachusetts

Mary A. Williamson, MT(ASCP), PhD
Director, Laboratory Operations
ACM Medical Laboratory
Rochester, New York

Hongbo Yu, MD, PhD
Director, Hematology Laboratory
Department of Hospital Laboratories
Hematopathologist
Division of Anatomic Pathology
UMass Memorial Medical Center
Assistant Professor
Department of Pathology
University of Massachusetts Medical School
Worcester, Massachusetts

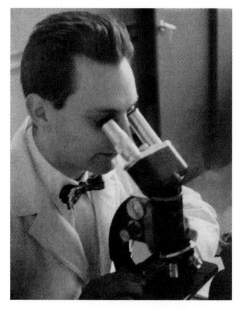

Jacques Wallach, pathologist, educator, and author of this book left us on August 10, 2010. He was 84. Forty years before that, he wrote the first edition, widely recognized as a necessary resource for both busy house staff and seasoned clinicians alike. It was the product of his vast experience as a clinical pathologist, his unquenchable thirst for medical knowledge, and his passion for teaching. He devoted tireless hours of research toward updating this book seven times since then. Several hundreds of thousands of copies have been distributed in numerous translations throughout the world.

As a resident in Internal Medicine in the mid-1980s, my first encounter with this book came in the early hours before our daily morning report, as my fellow house officers scurried to review the overnight admissions prior to presenting these cases to the Department Chief. The ensuing hour was usually punctuated by moments when one or more of us incurred the Chief's wrath for failure to accurately appreciate the patient's disorder or appropriately intervene. In an effort to avoid a similar fate, each of us would keep a copy of the book in an overfilled pocket of our lab coat to review quickly prior to this daily inquisition. Years later, I witnessed many students and house officers under my supervision do same, often secretly racing each other to the passage contained therein that would earn them the sought after recognition of their peers.

In the years that followed, I saw the third edition of the book become the fourth, fifth, and so on, never really appreciating the work that Jacques put into each update. Like many of us, however, I did appreciate the place that each update had amongst my collection of those clinical books which were always kept within easy reach and never seemed to collect any dust in my personal medical library.

When I first met Jacques, I was impressed by his dedication and commitment to medical education. He taught pathology at Albert Einstein, Rutgers, and SUNY Downstate, and consulted for Children's Specialized Hospital in Mountainside, South Amboy Memorial Hospital, Kings County Hospital in Brooklyn, and for the Bronx Zoo. He also wrote *Rheumatic Heart Disease* (1962) and *Interpretation of Pediatric Tests* (1983) as well as over 40 articles for peer review medical journals. He was a Fellow of the American College of Physicians, the American Society of Clinical Pathologists, the College of American Pathologists and the New York Academy of Medicine. From 1975 to 1985, he donated his time and expertise in pathology to laboratories around the world. His office was crammed with countless notes he made while researching, scrolled on small pieces of paper and filed between the pages of dozens of medical books and journals, waiting their turn to adorn the pages of his next book. It was like he realized that clinicians and patients around the world depended on him to unlock the keys to their own medical mysteries, and he did not take that responsibility lightly. More recently, Jacques asked me to join his small list of distinguished contributors and lend some assistance in my own area of expertise. To contribute in some small way to his labor of love was truly an honor.

As the devoted teacher, nothing was more rewarding to Jacques than being able to impart the wisdom he had worked hard to accumulate to the pupil looking for guidance. This ninth edition and all subsequent editions, now entitled *Wallach's Interpretation of Diagnostic Tests* represents his legacy, his ongoing gift to physicians around the world who continue to use his guidance every day to care for their patients. I have no doubt that nothing would have made him happier.

Anthony G. Auteri, MD

PREFACE

The faculty of the Department of Hospital Laboratories at UMass Memorial Medical Center is grateful for the opportunity to edit the 9th edition of Wallach's textbook on laboratory medicine. We realize this textbook is considered one of the leading resources for clinical laboratory medicine. We hope that the modifications we have instituted will carry on the tradition of Wallach's textbook. We have reorganized the 9th edition into two sections.

• The first section is devoted to the listing of laboratory tests in alphabetical order while stressing the integration of the clinical laboratory in the clinical decision making process. When appropriate, tests include their sensitivity, specificity, and positive and negative probabilities. Microbiology tests are listed separately.

• The second section is devoted to disease states. This section is also reorganized and, where appropriate, the patient's chief complaint and/or physical findings will initially be presented. Subsequent discussions then concentrate on discrete disease states as they relate to the patient's chief complaint. For example, in the gastrointestinal (GI) section, broad symptomatic categories such as diarrhea, jaundice, abdominal pain, GI bleeding, ascites, and hepatomegaly are presented and the disease states relating to each complaint are discussed. In addition we have integrated current molecular diagnostic testing as well as cytogenetics within the various disease states.

We hope that the reorganization will facilitate access to appropriate information.

This textbook does not include references to pathophysiology or therapy. However, common pitfalls and limitations of testing as well as identifying appropriate tests for specific clinical presentations are addressed.

As in previous editions, this textbook is geared for the primary care physician, physician's assistant, nurse practitioner, and medical and nursing students. The 9th edition is not an exhaustive catalogue of disease states, but a practical guide. We would appreciate feedback about the changes we have instituted.

L. Michael Snyder, MD
Gary Lapidas
Mary A. Williamson, MT(ASCP), PhD

Results of laboratory tests may aid in
Discovering occult disease
Preventing irreparable damage (e.g., phenylketonuria)
Early diagnosis after onset of signs or symptoms
Differential diagnosis of various possible diseases
Determining the stage of the disease
Estimating the activity of the disease
Detecting the recurrence of disease
Monitoring the effect of therapy
Genetic counseling in familial conditions
Medicolegal problems, such as paternity suits

This book is written to help the physician achieve these purposes the least amount of
Duplication of tests
Waste of patient's money
Overtaxing of laboratory facilities and personnel
Loss of physician's time
Confusion caused by the increasing number, variety, and complexity of tests currently available. Some of these tests may be unrequested but performed as part of routine surveys or hospital admission multitest screening.

In order to provide quick reference and maximum availability and usefulness, this handy-sized book features
Tabular and graphic style of concise presentation
Emphasis on serial time changes in laboratory findings in various stages of disease
Omission of rarely performed, irrelevant, esoteric, and outmoded laboratory tests
Exclusion of discussion of physiologic mechanisms, metabolic pathways, clinical features, and nonlaboratory aspects of disease
Discussion of only the more important diseases that the physician encounters and should be able to diagnose

This book is not
An encyclopedic compendium of clinical pathology
A technical manual
A substitute for good clinical judgment and basic knowledge of medicine

Deliberately omitted are
Technical procedures and directions
Photographs and illustrations of anatomic changes (e.g., blood cells, karyo-types, isotope scans)
Discussions of quality control
Selection of a referral laboratory
Performance of laboratory tests in the clinician's own office
Bibliographic references, except for the most general reference texts in medicine, hematology, and clinical pathology and for some recent references to specific conditions

The usefulness and need for a book of this style, organization, and contents have been increased by such current trends as

The frequent lack of personal assistance, advice, and consultation in large commercial laboratories and hospital departments of clinical pathology, which are often specialized and fragmented as well as impersonal

Greater demand for the physician's time

The development of many new tests

Faculty and administrators still assume that this essential area of medicine can be learned "intuitively" as it was 20 years ago and that it therefore requires little formal training. This attitude ignores changes in the number and variety of tests now available as well as their increased sophistication and basic value in establishing a diagnosis.

The contents of this book are organized to answer the questions most often posed by physicians when they require assistance from the pathologist. There is no other single adequate source of information presented in this fashion. It appears from numerous comments I have received that this book has succeeded in meeting the needs not only of practicing physicians and medical students but also of pathologists, technologists, and other medical personnel. It has been adopted by many schools of nursing and of medical technology, physicians assistant training programs, and medical schools. Such widespread acceptance confirms my original premise in writing this book and is most gratifying.

A perusal of the table of contents and index will quickly show the general organization of the material by type of laboratory test or organ system or certain other categories. In order to maintain a concise format, separate chapters have not been organized for such categories as newborn, pediatric, and geriatric periods or for primary psychiatric or dermatologic diseases. A complete index provides maximum access to this information.

Obviously these data are not original but have been adapted from many sources over the years. Only the selection, organization, manner of presentation, and emphasis are original. I have formulated this point of view during 40 years as a clinician and pathologist, viewing with pride the important and growing role of the laboratory but deeply regretting its inappropriate utilization.

This book was written to improve laboratory utilization by making it simpler for the physician to select and interpret the most useful laboratory tests for his clinical problems.

J.W.

CONTENTS

Introduction to Laboratory Medicine

L. V. Rao

Laboratory testing is an integral part of modern medical practice. Although clinical laboratory testing accounts for only 2.3% of annual health care costs in the United States, it plays a major role in the clinical decisions made by physicians, nurses, and other health care providers for the overall management of disease. More than 4000 laboratory tests are available for clinical use, and about 500 of them are performed regularly. The number of Clinical Laboratory Improvement Amendments (CLIA)–certified laboratories has grown to exceed more than 200,000. The laboratory medicine workforce comprises pathologists, doctoral level laboratory scientists, technologists, and technicians, who play a vital role in the health care system.

The health care system is increasingly dependent on reliable clinical laboratory services; however, as part of the overall health care system, these laboratory evaluations are prone to errors. Laboratory medicine comprises more than just the use of chemicals and reagents for the measurement of various analytes for clinical diagnosis purposes. Interference by both endogenous and exogenous substances is a common problem for the test analysis. These substances play a significant role in the proper interpretation of results, and such interference is adverse to patient care and adds to the cost of health care. It would be an oversimplification to conclude that each variable will always produce a specific effect; it depends on the person, the duration of exposure to that variable, the time between initial stress, the sample collection, and the degree of exposure. Awareness that many factors occurring outside the laboratory in and around the patient may affect the test result before the sample reaches the laboratory or even before the sample is collected is very important. These factors can be minimized when the clinician takes a good history and when there is a good communication of such information between the laboratory and the physician.

➤ Factors Affecting Laboratory Tests (FALTs)

The total testing process defines the preanalytic, analytic, and postanalytic phases of laboratory testing, and serves as the basis for designing and implementing interventions, restrictions, or limits that can reduce or remove the likelihood of errors. Over the last several years, there has

1

been a remarkable decrease in error rates, especially analytic errors. Evidence from recent studies demonstrate that a large percentage of laboratory errors occur in preanalytic and post-analytic steps. Errors in the preanalytic (61.9%) and postanalytic (23.1%) processes occurred much more frequently than occurrences of analytic errors (15%).

Sources of Preanalytic Error

Preanalytic factors act on both the patient and the specimen before analyses. These factors may be divided further into those acting in vivo (biologic or physiologic) and those acting in vitro (specimen handling and interference factors). Some physiologic factors are beyond our control. They include age, sex, and race, and so on, and can be managed by placing appropriate reference limits. Others factors such as diet, starvation, exercise, posture, diurnal and seasonal variations, menstrual cycle, and pregnancy must be considered in the interpretation of the test results.

The age, sex, and race of the patient influence the results of various laboratory tests. Age has noticeable effect on reference intervals. In newborns, the composition of blood is affected by the maturity of the infant at birth. Adult values are usually taken as the reference for comparison with those of the young and the elderly. The concentration of most test constituents remains constant between puberty and menopause in women and between puberty and middle age in men. The plasma concentrations of many constituents increase in women after menopause. Hormone levels are affected by aging. However, changes in concentrations are much less pronounced than an endocrine organ's response to stimuli. Until puberty, there are few differences in laboratory data between boys and girls. After puberty, the characteristic changes in the levels of sex hormones become apparent.

The dietary effect of laboratory test results is complex, and simply cannot be separated into the categories of "fasting" and "nonfasting" status of the patient. The type of diet (high fat, low fat, vegetarian, malnutrition), length of time since last meal, and test-specific dietary concerns can affect some tests. Consumption of caffeine, bran, serotonin (consumption of fruits and vegetables such as bananas, avocados, and onions), herbal preparations (e.g., aloe vera, Chinese rhubarb, senna, quinine, and quinidine), recreational drug use, ethanol, and smoking can induce both short- and long-term effects that alter the results of several analytes. Differentiations of the effects of race from those of socioeconomic conditions are difficult. Carbohydrate and lipid metabolism differ in black and whites. Glucose tolerance is less in blacks, Polynesians, and Native Americans in comparison to whites.

In addition to the commonly known hormonal changes during the menstrual cycle, there is a preovulatory increase in the concentrations of aldosterone and renin. Coincident with the ovulation, serum cholesterol levels are lower than at any other phase of the menstrual cycle. In pregnancy, a dilutional effect is observed due to the increase in mean plasma volume, which in turn causes hemodilution. Normal pregnancy is characterized by major physiologic adaptations that alter maternal blood chemistry and hematology laboratory values. In addition, there are time-related fluctuations in the levels of certain analytes. Many analytes—such as cortisol, Thyrotropin (TSH), growth hormone, potassium, glucose, iron, and proinflammatory cytokines exhibit diurnal variation. Hormones such as luteinizing hormone (LH), follicle-stimulating hormone (FSH), and testosterone released in short bursts lasting barely 2 minutes make accurate measurements problematic. Seasonal changes also affect certain analytes like vitamin D (higher during summer), cholesterol, and thyroid hormones (higher during winter). Changes in the levels of some of the constituents in blood occur when measured at sea level as opposed to measurement at a higher altitude. Hematocrit, hemoglobin, C-reactive protein (CRP) can be higher at high altitude. Levels of plasma renin, transferrin, urinary creatinine, creatinine clearance, and estriol decrease with increasing altitude.

Physical stress and mental stress influence the concentrations of many plasma constituents, including cortisol, aldosterone, prolactin, TSH, aldosterone, cholesterol, glucose, insulin, and lactate. With blindness, the normal stimulation of the hypothalamic-pituitary axis is reduced. Consequently, certain features of hypopituitarism and hypoadrenalism may be observed. In some blind individuals, the normal diurnal variations of cortisol may persist; in others it does not. Fever provokes many hormonal responses as does shock and trauma. The stress of surgery has been shown to reduce the serum triiodothyronine (T_3) levels by 50% in patients without thyroid disease.

Transfusions and infusions can also significantly affect the concentration of certain laboratory values. For persons receiving an infusion, blood should not be obtained proximal to the infusion site. Blood should be obtained from the opposite arm. A minimum of 8 hours must elapse before blood is obtained from a subject who has received fat emulsion. For patients receiving blood transfusions, the extent of hemolysis and with it, increased levels of potassium, lactate dehydrogenase (LDH), and free hemoglobin, are released progressively to the age of the transfused blood.

Exercise such as running up and down several flights of stairs or strenuous activity such as working out in a gymnasium or marathon running the night before the specimen collection can affect the results obtained for several analytes. To minimize preanalytic variables introduced by exercise, subjects should be instructed to refrain from strenuous activity on the night before testing and not to exert themselves by walking a long distance, running, or climbing stairs before blood specimen collection. In addition, the muscle damage associated with trauma of surgery will increase the serum activity of enzymes originating in skeletal muscles, and this activity may persist for several days.

The plasma and extracellular volumes decrease within a few days of the start of bed rest. With prolonged bed rest, fluid retention occurs and plasma protein and albumin levels may be decreased by an average of 0.5 and 0.3 g/dL, respectively. As a result, concentrations of bound protein are also reduced. Changes in posture during blood sampling can affect the concentrations of several analytes measured in serum or plasma. Change in posture from a supine to an erect or sitting position can result in a shift in body water from intravascular to interstitial compartments. As a result, the concentrations of larger molecules that are not filterable are increased. These effects are accentuated in patients with a tendency for edema, such as in cardiovascular insufficiency and cirrhosis of liver.

Among controllable preanalytic variables, specimen collection is most critical. Unacceptable specimen collection due to misidentification, insufficient volume to perform test, incorrect whole blood to anticoagulant ratio, and specimen quality (hemolysis, clots, contaminated, collected in wrong container) accounts for the majority of preanalytic errors. Hemolysis, lipemia, and icteric samples have variable effects on assays and depend upon testing method and analyte. The time and temperature for storage of the specimen and the processing steps in the preparation of serum or plasma or cell separation can introduce preanalytic variables.

The application of a tourniquet, by reducing the pressure below the systolic pressure, maintains the effective filtration pressure within the capillaries. As a result, small molecules and fluid are transferred from the intravasal space to the interstitium. Application of tourniquet for longer than 1 minute can result in hemoconcentration of large molecules that are unable to penetrate the capillary wall. To minimize the preanalytic effects of tourniquet application time, the tourniquet should be released as soon as the needle enters the vein. Avoidance of excessive fist clenching during phlebotomy and maintaining tourniquet application time to no more than 1 minute can minimize preanalytic errors.

Various salts of heparin, ethylenediaminetetraacetic acid (EDTA) and sodium citrate are used widely in the clinical laboratory. Heparin is the preferred anticoagulant for blood specimens for electrolyte levels and other routine chemistry tests. Obvious differences in the results of certain analytes between serum and heparinized plasma are related to the consumption of fibrinogen and the lysis of cellular elements during the process of clotting. EDTA is the commonly used anticoagulant for routine hematologic determinations. It functions as anticoagulant by chelating calcium ions, which are required for the clotting process. Citrate has been used as an anticoagulant for collection of blood specimens intended for global coagulation tests such as prothrombin time (PT) and partial thromboplastin time (PTT). A laboratory that has been using one of the concentrations (3.2% or 3.8%) to perform PT determination for patients receiving oral anticoagulant therapy should not interchange the formulations. Doing so will affect the international normalized ratios (INRs) that are used to report the results of PT. Sodium fluoride and lithium iodoacetate have been used alone or in combination with anticoagulants such as potassium oxalate, EDTA, citrate, or lithium heparin for blood collection. In the absence of glycolytic inhibitors, a decrease in the glucose level of as much as 24% can occur in one hour after blood collection in neonates, in contrast to a 5% decrease in healthy individuals when specimen is stored at room temperature. The anticoagulant-to-blood ratio is critical for some laboratory tests. In general, collecting of blood specimens to less than nominal volume increases the effective molarity of the anticoagulant and induces osmotic changes affecting cell morphologic features. Furthermore, the binding of analytes such as ionic calcium or magnesium to heparin can be enhanced when the effective concentration of unfractionated heparin increased beyond the normal 14.3 U/mL of blood.

In coagulation, testing knowledge or access to the patient history may be necessary, as many medications such as anticoagulant therapies (warfarin, heparin, and direct thrombin inhibitors), blood product, and component transfusion and coagulation factor replacement therapies all impact coagulation test results. Over-the-counter drugs (aspirin) have prolonged effect on platelet function studies. In addition, the patient's physiologic state plays a role.

The quality of the specimens submitted to the microbiology laboratory is critical for optimal specimen evaluation. The general techniques of specimen collection and handling that have been established both to maximize the yield of organisms and isolate relevant pathogens from specimens obtained from different body sites should be reviewed with clinical laboratory prior to obtaining the specimen. In addition, valid interpretation of the results of culture can be achieved only if the specimen obtained is appropriate for processing. As a result, care must be taken to collect only those specimens that may yield pathogens, rather than colonizing flora or contaminants. Specific rules for the collection of material vary, depending on the source of the specimen, but several general principles apply. Prompt transport of specimens to the microbiology laboratory is essential to optimize the yield of cultures and the interpretation of results. Delays in processing may result in the overgrowth of some microorganisms or the death of more fastidious ones. Samples for bacterial culture should ideally arrive in the microbiology laboratory within 1 to 2 hours of collection. If a delay is unavoidable, most specimens (with the exception of blood, cerebrospinal fluid, joint fluid, and cultures for *Neisseria gonorrhoeae*) should be refrigerated until transported.

Analytic Errors

Clinical laboratories have long focused their attention on quality control methods and quality assessment programs dealing with analytic aspects of testing. Total analytic error (or measurement error) refers to assay errors from all sources arising from the data collection experiment. Some error is expected, because not all components of measuring are the same. There are four major types of experimental error: random (not predictable), systematic (one direction), total (random and systematic), and idiosyncratic (nonmethodologic).

Errors due to analytic problems have been significantly reduced over time, but there is evidence that, particularly for immunoassays, interference may have a serious impact on patients. Paraproteins can interfere in chemical measurements when they form precipitates during the testing procedure. Heterophilic antibodies are human antibodies that can bind animal antibodies. They can cause problems in immunoassays, particularly immunometric assays, where they can form a bridge between the capture and detection antibodies, leading to false-positive results in the absence of analyte or if analyte is also present, a false increase in measured concentrations. Very rarely, heterophilic antibodies can also lead to false-negative or falsely low results.

Very high hormone levels can interfere with immunoassay systems resulting in falsely low analyte determinations. This is attributable to the "hook effect," which describes the inhibition of immune complex formation by excess antigen concentration. There are proteins that are well known to form aggregates with immunoglobulins or high-molecular-weight proteins. Clinically relevant proteins that can have "macro" forms—including amylase, creatinine kinase, LDH, and prolactin—can elevate the results when using certain laboratory tests, yet the patient lacks clinical disease related to elevated analyte concentration.

Immunoassay interference is *not* analyte specific and is variable with respect to time. In some patients this interference can lost for a long time and in some for only a short time. This interference affects lots of assays, but not all of them.

Incorrect results can also occur as a result of a large number of biologically common phenomena causing analytic variation. These include cold agglutinins, rouleaux, osmotic matrix effects, platelet agglutination, giant platelets, unlysed erythrocytes, nucleated erythrocytes, megakaryocytes, red cell inclusions, cryoproteins, circulating mucin, leukocytosis, in vitro hemolysis, extreme microcytosis, bilirubinemia, lipemia, and so on.

Diagnostic Test Values

Before a method is used routinely, method evaluation protocols must ensure that the measurement procedure meets defined criteria, for example, the accuracy, precision, and stability required in meeting the laboratory's patient population needs. Four indicators are most commonly used to determine the reliability of a clinical laboratory test. Two of these, accuracy and precision, reflect how well the test method performs day to day in a laboratory. The other two, sensitivity and specificity, deal with how well the test is able to distinguish disease from absence of disease.

The accuracy and precision of each test method are established and are frequently monitored by the clinical laboratory. Sensitivity and specificity data are determined by research studies and clinical trials. Although each test has its own performance measures and appropriate uses, laboratory tests are designed to be as precise, accurate, specific, and sensitive as possible.

Accuracy and Precision

"Accuracy" (trueness) refers to the ability of the test to actually measure what it claims to measure, and is defined as the proportion of all test results (both positive and negative) that are correct. **Precision (repeatability)** refers to the ability of the test to reproduce the same result when repeated on the same patient or sample. The two concepts are related, but different. For example, a test could be precise, but not accurate if on three occasions it produced roughly the same result, but that result differed greatly from the actual value determined by a reference standard.

Sensitivity is defined as the ability of the test to identify correctly those who have the disease. It is the number of subjects with a positive test who have the disease divided by all subjects who have the disease. A test with high sensitivity has few false-negative results. **Specificity** is defined as the ability of the test to identify correctly those who do not have the disease. It is the number of subjects who have a negative test and do not have the disease divided by all subjects who do not have the disease. A test with high specificity has few false-positive results. Sensitivity and specificity are most useful when assessing a test used to screen a free-living population. These test characteristics are also interdependent (Figure 1-1): an increase in sensitivity is accompanied by a decrease in specificity and vice versa.

Predictive values are important for assessing how useful a test will be in the clinical setting at the individual patient level. The **positive predictive value** (PPV) is the probability of disease in a patient with a positive test. Conversely, the **negative predictive value** (NPV) is the probability that the patient does not have disease if he has a negative test result.

PPV and sensitivity of tests are complementary in their examination of true positives. Given that the test is positive, PPV is the probability that the disease is present, in contrast to sensitivity, which is given the disease is present, the probability that test is positive. Likewise, NPV and specificity are complementary in their examination of true negatives. Given that the test is negative; NPV is the probability that the disease is absent. This is in contrast to specificity, which is given the disease is absent; the probability that test is negative. (See Figure 1-1 for more information.) Predictive values depend on the prevalence of a disease in a population. A test with a given sensitivity and specificity can have different predictive values in different patient populations. If the test is used in a population with high disease prevalence, it will have a high PPV; the same test will have a low PPV when used in a population with low disease prevalence.

Likelihood ratios (LRs) are another way of assessing the accuracy of a test in the clinical setting. They are also independent of disease prevalence. LR indicates how much a given diagnostic test result will raise or lower the odds of having a disease relative to the probability of the disease. Each test is characterized by two LRs: positive LR (PLR) and negative LR (NLR). PLR tells us the odds of the disease if the test result is positive and NLR tells the odds of disease if the test result is negative.

$$PLR = \text{Sensitivity} / (1 - \text{Specificity})$$
$$NLR = (1 - \text{Sensitivity}) / \text{Specificity}.$$

An LR greater than 1 increases the odds that the person has the target disease, and the higher the LR the greater this increase in odds. Conversely, an LR ratio less than 1 diminishes the odds that the patient has the target disease.

Receiver-operating Characteristic (ROC) Curves

ROC curves allow one to identify the cut-off value that minimizes both false positives and false negatives. An ROC curve plots sensitivity on the y axis and 1—specificity on the x axis. Applying a variety of cut-off values to the same reference population allows one to generate the curve. The perfect test would have a cut-off value that allowed an exact split of diseased and nondiseased populations (i.e., a cut-off that gave both 100 percent sensitivity and 100 percent specificity). It would plot as a right angle with the fulcrum in the far upper left corner ($x = 0$, $y = 1$). This case, however, is very rare. For most cases, as one moves from left to right on the ROC curve the sensitivity increases and the specificity decreases.

Calculation of the area under the ROC curve allows comparison of different tests. A perfect test has an area under the curve (AUC) equal to one. Therefore, the closer the AUC is to 1, the better the test. Similarly, if one wants to know the cut-off value for a test that minimizes both false positives and false negatives (and hence maximizes both sensitivity and specificity), one would select the point on the ROC curve closest to the far upper left corner ($x = 0$, $y = 1$).

However, finding the right balance between optimal sensitivity and specificity may not involve simultaneously minimizing false positives and false negatives in all situations. For example, when screening for a deadly disease that is curable, it may be desirable to accept more false positives (lower specificity) in return for fewer false negatives (higher sensitivity). ROC curves allow a more thorough evaluation of a test and potential cut-off values, but are not the ultimate arbiters of how to set sensitivity and specificity.

Postanalytic Errors

Approximately 70–80% of the patient chart or medical record is composed of laboratory test results. Postanalytic errors are dependent on the design and development of those processes and procedures that will ensure correct and timely notification of these test results to the patient's medical record with right reference range and appropriate interpretation of the test result. Manual and telephone reporting should be discouraged as this reporting is subject to transcription errors at the receiver end. The introduction of a hospitalized computer order entry system has eliminated some errors, but it has not eliminated the risk of mismatching the patients.

➤ Reference Intervals

The term "reference values" has essentially replaced the obsolete term "normal values." Laboratory tests are commonly compared to a reference interval before health care providers make physiologic assessments, medical diagnosis, or management decisions. These comparisons may be cross-sectional or longitudinal. A cross-sectional comparison is comparison of an analyte result for a single patient with the interval of results for that analyte obtained from a group of apparently healthy individuals. This is referred to as the "population based" reference interval. Another example of a cross-sectional comparison is when a single patient result is compared with a fixed value or cut-off value. There are two types of population-based reference intervals. The most common type is derived from a reference sample of persons who are in good health (health associated). The other type of reference interval has been termed "decision based" and defines specific medical decision limits that clinicians use to diagnose or manage patients. Longitudinal comparisons are when a patient's most recent value is compared with previous values for the same analyte. This may help detect a change in health status.

Comparison of patient results with a population-based reference interval or with the cut-off values is used for diagnostic or screening purposes. The reference value change over a period of time is used for monitoring patients. Both healthy reference limits and disease-associated reference limits are important for the clinical interpretation of the laboratory test results and vary from laboratory to laboratory. These variations may be caused by preanalytic processing procedures, populations of healthy individuals, inherent random biologic variations, analytic platforms, or analytic imprecision that was present when reference intervals were determined.

Decision limits for optimally classifying patients into "disease" versus "healthy" categories are difficult to define. Most diseases are not homogenous distributions but represent a continuum of mild and severe forms. Various statistical tools and models have been developed to formalize the medical decision process, but most of the models do not include the methodologic differences in laboratory test values. The major utility of healthy reference intervals for clinicians is to provide a rough assessment of the possibility that a test value on a specific patient is difficult for the values normally found in similar healthy subjects. The guidelines for medical decision making use a standard 95% reference interval. By defining the healthy reference interval to include central 95% of matched healthy subjects, there is less than a 1 in 20 chance for a value outside the reference interval to be found in a matched healthy subject. Conventionally, a common limit of acceptability is based on the mean of population data ± 2 standard deviation (SD), because this encompassed roughly 95% of the observations expected to be "normal." With this convention it must be remembered that 5% (usually 2.5% on the low side and 2.5% on the high side) of results can be expected to fall outside the ± 2 SD limit, even in a "normal" healthy population. This is best illustrated in the use of multitest chemistry profiles for screening of persons known to be free of disease. The probability of any given test being abnormal is about 2–5%, and the probability of disease if a screening test is abnormal is generally low (0–15%). The frequency of abnormal single tests is 1.5% (albumin) to 5.9% (glucose) and up to 16.6% for sodium. Based on statistical expectations, when a panel of eight tests is performed in a multiphasic health program, 25% of the patients have one or more abnormal results; when the panel includes 20 tests, 55% have one or more test abnormalities.

In terms of qualitative test reports (e.g., positive, negative) optimal decision limits (cutoff) can be determined with ROC curve analyses. If false-positive labeling leads to a more harmful outcome, the decision limits should be moved away from the ROC optimum in a direction to minimize false-positive diagnoses. Likewise, if false-negative labeling is more dangerous, the decision limits should be moved to minimize the false-negative diagnoses. Although decision limits are better tools than reference values for deriving diagnostic value from laboratory tests, they have some drawbacks. First, decision limits will not address the degree of deviation of a test result above or below the decision limit. A test result slightly above the limit will be regarded as positive the same as a result far above the decision limit, and a test result slightly below the cut-off limit will be reported as negative.

Performing the Right Test at the Right Time for the Right Reason

As with the absolute value of a result, a test result or change in sequential results must be interpreted in the context of the clinical situation, recent changes in patient management, and historical results. Excessive repetition of tests is wasteful, and the excess burden increases the possibility of laboratory errors. Appropriate intervals between tests should be dictated by the patient's clinical condition. Negative laboratory values (or any other type of tests) do not necessarily rule out a clinical diagnosis. Tests should be performed only if they will alter the patient's diagnosis, prognosis, treatment, or management. Incorrect test values or isolated individual variation in results may cause Ulysses syndrome and result in loss of time, money, and peace of mind.

Is disease actually present?

		Yes	No
		True Positive	**False Positive**
	Yes	A	B
Does my test indicate		**False Negative**	**True Negative**
that disease is present?	*No*	C	D

Sensitivity = A/(A+C)

Specificity = D/(B+D)

PPV   = A/(A+B)

NPV   = D/(C+D)

Figure 1-1. Sensitivity, specificity, and predictive values in laboratory testing. NPV, negative predictive value; PPV, positive predictive value.

CHAPTER 2

Laboratory Tests

**L.V. Rao, Liberto Pechet,
Amanda Jenkins, Edward I. Ginns, Marzena
Galdzicka, Guy Vallaro, Charles Kiefer, and
Patricia Minehart Miron**

This chapter presents the most commonly ordered serum, plasma, and whole blood laboratory tests arranged in alphabetical order. Each entry is titled using the most common naming convention existing in the United States. When appropriate, alternate name(s), definition, reference ranges, clinical use, interpretation, limitations, and suggested readings are given. Microbiology tests such as laboratory cultures have been organized into a separate chapter, Infectious Disease Assays (p. 396). The basis of current molecular assays is reviewed in the chapter on Hereditary and Genetic Diseases (p. 900).

It is important to note that many of these tests are available by point-of-care testing (POCT). The main advantage of POCT is immediate turnaround time. However, it is also necessary to consider the disadvantages of POCT, such as reliability of interpretation due to lower assay sensitivity and susceptibility to interfering substances. Other issues include ensuring personnel proficiency, quality assurance, data management, and cost.

1,5-ANHYDROGLUCITOL (1,5-AG)

➤ Definition
* 1,5-AG, sometimes known as GlycoMark, is a monosaccharide that shows a structural similarity to glucose.
* Its main source in humans is dietary ingestion, particularly meats and cereals. In addition, 10% of 1,5-AG is derived from endogenous synthesis. It is generally not metabolized, and in healthy subjects it achieves a stable plasma concentration that reflects a steady balance between ingestion and urinary excretion.
* **Normal range:** 10.7–32.0 μg/mL in males; 6.8–29.3 μg/mL in females

➤ Use
* Used clinically to monitor short-term glycemic control in patients with diabetes
* Useful marker for postprandial hyperglycemia
* Whether it is a complementary marker to HbA_{1c} is still being evaluated.

➤ Interpretation
Increased In
* 1,5-AG may be increased during IV hyperalimentation.

Decreased In
* Individuals with renal glucose thresholds that are markedly different from 180 mg/dL (e.g., chronic renal failure, pregnancy, and dialysis) and in those undergoing steroid therapy.
* α-glucosidase inhibitors can decrease 1,5-AG by interfering with its intestinal absorption.

➤ Limitations
* In patients with poorly controlled DM, 1,5-AG is less sensitive to modest changes in glycemic control because of continuous glycosuria.

11-DEOXYCORTISOL

➤ Definition
* 11-Deoxycortisol, also known as cortodoxone, corticosterone, and compound S, is a steroid and an immediate precursor to the production of cortisol. It can be synthesized from 17-hydroxyprogesterone.
* Excretion in urine is included in 17-ketogenic steroid (17-KS) and Porter-Silber 17-OHKS measurements, which were originally used to provide some measure of cortisol production. The direct measurement of cortisol has replaced determinations of 17-KS and 17-OHKS.
* **Normal range:** <50 ng/dL in males; <33 ng/dL in females

➤ Use
* Diagnosis of and monitoring therapeutic response in CAH due to 11β-hydroxylase deficiency
* Assessment of adrenal response in the metyrapone test; result after metyrapone stimulation is greater than 8000 ng/dL

➤ Interpretation
Increased In
• Values are increased in CAH (P450cII deficiency) and following metyrapone administration in normal persons.

Decreased In
• Values are decreased in adrenal insufficiency.

➤ Limitations
• Patients with myxedema, some pregnant patients, and those on oral contraceptives respond poorly during the test.

17α-HYDROXYPROGESTERONE

➤ Definition
• 17α-Hydroxyprogesterone, also known as hydroxyprogesterone, is a 21-carbon steroid produced in the adrenals—and also in the ovaries, testes, and placenta—that serves as a biosynthetic precursor to cortisol.
• **Normal range:** 18–469 ng/dL (see Table 2-1)

➤ Use
• Diagnosis and management of congenital adrenal hyperplasia, hirsutism, and infertility

➤ Interpretation
Increased In
• The luteal phase of menstruating women and pregnancy, during which it rises
• The most common form of CAH, where deficiency of the enzyme 21-hydroxylase blocks normal synthesis of cortisol, leading to a compensatory increase of ACTH secretion; this results in increased levels.

➤ Limitations
• Circulating normally exhibits a diurnal pattern similar to that of cortisol, with higher values in the early morning than in the late afternoon. Hence, the time of collection should be standardized.
• Spuriously elevated levels are sometimes seen in premature and sick newborns due to interference with other steroid metabolites. 17α-Hydroxypregnenolone sulfate (percent cross reactivity: 3.8%) has been identified as the most significant interferent in direct assays.
• 17α-Hydroxyprogesterone values for women with late-onset CAH have been found to overlap with those encountered in hirsute, oligomenorrheic women who do not have the disorder.

TABLE 2-1. Range of Normal Values for 17α-Hydroxyprogesterone		
Patient Group	Median (ng/dL)	Range (ng/dL)
Male (20–59 years)	143	60–342
Female		
Follicular phase	67	19–182
Luteal phase	210	22–469
Taking oral contraceptives	79	18–251
Postmenopausal	46	20–172

Accordingly, it is important to determine ACTH-stimulated 17α-hydroxyprogesterone levels in women suspected of having late-onset CAH.

17-KETOSTEROIDS, URINE (17-KS)

➤ Definition
- 17-Ketosteroids, urine (17-KS) is an adrenal function test.
- An alternative and more specific test for adrenal androgen function is dehydroepiandrosterone sulfate in serum.
- **Normal range:** depends on sex and age (Table 2-2)

➤ Use
- Evaluation of glucocorticoid production and neuroendocrine function
- Evaluation of androgenic adrenal and testicular function in normal male individuals and primarily adrenal androgenic secretion in normal female individuals.

➤ Interpretation
Increased In
- Adrenal tumor
- Congenital adrenal hyperplasia (very rare)
- Cushing syndrome
- Ovarian cancer
- Testicular cancer
- Ovarian dysfunction (polycystic ovarian disease)

Decreased In
- Addison disease
- Castration

TABLE 2-2. Normal Ranges for 17-Ketosteroids in the Urine	
Age	Value (mg/day)
Male	
0–11 months	0.0–1.0
1–5 years	1.0–2.0
6–10 years	1.0–4.4
11–12 years	1.3–8.5
13–16 years	3.4–9.8
17–50 years	5.3–17.6
≥51 years	4.1–12.1
Female	
0–11 months	0.0–1.0
1–5 years	1.0–2.0
6–10 years	1.4–3.9
11–12 years	3.8–9.5
13–16 years	4.5–17.1
17–50 years	4.4–14.2
≥51 years	3.2–10.6

* Hypopituitarism
* Myxedema
* Nephrosis

➤ Limitations

* A large number of substances may interfere with this test.
* Decreases may be caused by carbamazepine, cephaloridine, cephalothin, chlormerodrin, digoxin, glucose, metyrapone, promazine, propoxyphene, reserpine, and others.
* Increases may be caused by acetone, acetophenide, ascorbic acid, chloramphenicol, chloro-thiazide, chlorpromazine, cloxacillin, dexamethasone, erythromycin, ethinamate, etryptam-ine, methicillin, methyprylon, morphine, oleandomycin, oxacillin, penicillin, phenaglycodol, phenazopyridine, phenothiazine, piperidine, quinidine, secobarbital, spironolactone, and others.

5,10-METHYLENETETRAHYDROFOLATE REDUCTASE (MTHFR) MOLECULAR ASSAY

➤ Definition

* Mutations, *C677T* and *A1298C*, in the 5,10-methylenetetrahydrofolate reductase (*MTHFR*) gene increase the risk of thrombosis and other cardiovascular diseases as a result of an ele-vated plasma homocysteine concentration.
* **Normal values:** negative or no mutations are found.

➤ Use

* Suspected CAD, homocystinuria, neural tube defects, spontaneous abortion, or MTHFR deficiency

➤ Limitations

* The results of a genetic test may be affected by DNA rearrangements, blood transfusion, bone marrow transplantation, or other rare events.

5-HYDROXYINDOLEACETIC ACID (5-HIAA) URINE

➤ Definition

* 5-Hydroxyindoleacetic acid (5-HIAA), also known serotonin metabolite, is the major uri-nary metabolite of serotonin.
* **Normal range:** 0.0–15.0 mg/day (24-hour urine); 0.0–14.0 mg/g creatinine

➤ Use

* Helps diagnose and monitor treatment for serotonin-secreting carcinoid tumors

➤ Interpretation
Increased In

* Whipple disease
* Nontropical sprue
* Small increases possible in pregnancy, ovulation, and postsurgical stress
* Various food ingestions (e.g., pineapples, kiwi, bananas, eggplant, plums, tomatoes, avoca-dos, plantains, walnuts, pecans, hickory nuts, coffee)

- Use of certain drugs (e.g., acetanilid, acetaminophen, acetophenetidin, caffeine, coumaric acid, diazepam (Valium), ephedrine, fluorouracil, glyceryl guaiacolate (guaifenesin), heparin, melphalan (Alkeran), mephenesin, methamphetamine, methocarbamol, naproxen, nicotine, Lugol's solution, reserpine

Decreased In
- Use of certain drugs (e.g., chlorpromazine, promazine, imipramine, isoniazid, monoamine oxidase inhibitors, methenamine, methyldopa, phenothiazines, promethazine)
- Renal insufficiency (possible)

➤ Limitations
- Foods rich in serotonin and medications that may affect metabolism of serotonin must be avoided at least 72 hours before and during collection of urine for 5-HIAA.
- Patients should abstain, if possible, from medications, over-the-counter drugs, and herbal remedies for at least 72 hours prior to the test.
- Twenty-four-hour collections are generally recommended, but random collections may be used. Refrigeration is the most important aspect of specimen preservation.
- Urinary 5-HIAA is increased with malabsorption, in 75% of cases, usually when a carcinoid tumor is far advanced (with large liver metastases, often 300–1000 mg/day), but may not be increased despite massive metastases.
  - Sensitivity is 73%.
  - The test is useful in the diagnosis of only 5–7% of patients with carcinoid tumors but in approximately 45% of those with liver metastases.
- Disease extent and prognosis correlate generally with urine 5-HIAA excretion and the level becomes normal after successful surgery. If urine HIAA is normal, the blood level of serotonin or a precursor, 5-hydroxytryptophan should be checked.

5′-NUCLEOTIDASE (5′-RIBONUCLEOTIDEPHOSPHOHYDROLASE, 5′-NT)

➤ Definition
- This membrane-bound enzyme of liver is increased in diseases of the liver, particularly if the hepatobiliary tract is involved.
- The appearance of 5′-NT in serum is due to cholestasis and its significance is similar to that of ALP and GGT. However, 5′-NT is not as subject to drug induction as GGT and ALP, and it is not subject to confusion with alternate sources of the enzyme, as is seen with ALP.
- **Normal range:** 2.0–8.0 U/L

➤ Use
- Determining cholestatic liver disease, particularly when GGT and ALP could be falsely elevated due to drug induction
- Better test for secondary tumors and lymphomas of liver than ALP

➤ Interpretation
Increased In
- 5′-NT is increased in the following conditions:
  - Hepatobiliary disease with intrahepatic or extrahepatic biliary obstruction

- Hepatic carcinoma
- Early biliary cirrhosis
- Pregnancy (third semester)
- Inflammatory arthritis

➤ Limitations
- 5′-NT can be elevated in hyperammonemia due to analytical interference.
- Normal in pregnancy and postpartum period (in contrast to serum leucine aminopeptidase [LAP] and ALP)

ACETAMINOPHEN (N-ACETYL-P-AMINOPHENOL; APAP)

➤ Definition
- Nonopioid analgesic, antipyretic
- **Normal range:** 5–20 µg/mL serum
- **Potentially toxic:** >150 µg/mL measured 4 hour post dose.

➤ Use
- Relief of pain, such as headaches and toothaches
- Reduction of fever

➤ Interpretation
- Screen of urine: indication of exposure
- Screen of serum: used to assess potential toxicity

➤ Limitations
- Screening
  - Serum/urine: colorimetric or immunoassay on automated chemistry analyzers
  - Based on:
    - Conversion of free APAP by aryl acrylamide amidohydrolase to p-aminophenol, which is then oxidized or reacted with a dye to form a color conjugate the absorbance of which is measured spectrophotometrically OR
    - Competition between enzyme-labeled APAP (enzyme = glucose-6-phosphate dehydrogenase) and APAP in serum sample for specific antibody binding sites. If the drug is present in the sample, it binds to the specific antibody, which results in enzyme activity. If no drug is present, the drug–enzyme conjugate binds to antibody, resulting in enzyme inhibition. Therefore, there is a direct relationship between drug concentration in the sample and enzyme activity. Enzyme activity is determined by measuring the conversion of nicotinamide adenine dinucleotide (NAD) to NADH spectrophotometrically at 340 nm.
    - High bilirubin concentrations [>50 µg/mL] may cause false-positive results with immunoassay-based tests.
    - Plasma may be tested in place of serum. Anticoagulants such as EDTA and heparin do not generally interfere with the assay.
    - Do not use whole blood.

- Confirmation:
  - Serum/urine–HPLC or GC/MC
  - APAP is highly conjugated by glucuronidation and sulfation.
  - An assay that includes a hydrolysis step provides total APAP levels, which are not useful for assessing toxicity.

ACETYLSALICYLIC ACID

See Salicylates (Aspirin)

ACID PHOSPHATASE

➤ Definition
- Acid phosphatase is a hydrolytic enzyme secreted by various cells, and it has five isoenzymes. The greatest amount per gram of tissue is found in semen (prostate); it is also detectable in bone, liver, spleen, kidney, RBCs, and platelets.
- The acid phosphatase test is also known as prostatic acid phosphatase (PAP), the serum acid phosphatase test, and the tartrate-resistant acid phosphatase (TRAP) test.
- **Normal range:** 0–0.8 U/L

➤ Use
- Predicts recurrence after radical prostatectomy for clinically localized prostate cancer and following response to androgen ablation therapy, when used in conjunction with PSA

➤ Interpretation
Increased In
- Acid phosphatase is increased in the following conditions:
  - Prostate cancer
  - Gaucher's disease and Niemann-Pick disease
  - One day to 2 days after prostatic surgery or biopsy
  - Prostatic manipulation or catheterization
  - Benign prostatic hyperplasia, prostatitis, prostate infarct
  - Vaginal swabs from rape victims.

➤ Limitations
- PAP is no longer used to screen for or stage prostate cancer. In most instances, serum PSA is used instead.
- PAP measurement must not be regarded as an absolute test for malignancy, since other factors including benign prostatic hyperplasia, prostatic infarction, and manipulation of the prostate gland may result in elevated serum PAP concentrations.
- PAP measurements provide little additional information beyond that provided by PSA measurements.

➤ Suggested Reading
Moul JW, Connelly RR, Perahia B, McLeod DG. The contemporary value of pretreatment prostatic acid phosphatase to predict pathological stage and recurrence in radical prostatectomy cases. *J Urol.* 1998;159: 935–940.

ACTH STIMULATION (COSYNTROPIN) TEST

➤ Definition
- Cosyntropin is synthetic ACTH (1–24), which has the full biologic potency of native ACTH (1–39).
- It is a rapid stimulator of cortisol and aldosterone secretion.

➤ Use
- This is the initial test used to distinguish primary from secondary adrenal insufficiency.
- It is not helpful in the diagnosis of Cushing syndrome. Several protocols are used to assess the response to exogenous ACTH administration (see below).

Low-Dose ACTH Stimulation Test
- This test involves physiologic plasma concentrations of ACTH and provides a more sensitive index of adrenocortical responsiveness.
- It is performed by measuring serum cortisol immediately before and 30 minutes after IV injection of Cosyntropin in a dose of either 1 µg/1.73 m^2 or 0.5 µg/1.73 m^2.
- There is no commercially available preparation of "low-dose" Cosyntropin. The vials of Cosyntropin currently available contain 250 µg and come with sterile normal saline solution to be used as diluent. One prepares the low-dose solution of Cosyntropin locally.

High-Dose ACTH Stimulation Test
- This test consists of measuring serum cortisol immediately before and 30 and 60 minutes after IV injection of 250 µg of Cosyntropin. This dose of Cosyntropin results in pharmacologic plasma ACTH concentrations for the 60-minute duration of the test.
- The advantage of the high-dose test is that the Cosyntropin can be injected using the IM route, because pharmacologic plasma ACTH concentrations are still achieved.
- Salivary cortisol can also be measured during this test. Salivary cortisol increases to 19 ± 0.8 ng/mL (range: 8.7 to 36 ng/mL) 1 hour after injection.

Eight-Hour ACTH Stimulation Test
- The 8-hour test, which is now rarely performed, consists of infusing 250 µg of Cosyntropin continuously over 8 hours in 500 mL of isotonic saline. A 24-hour urine specimen is collected the day before and the day of the infusion for cortisol or 17-hydroxycorticoid and creatinine determination, and serum cortisol is determined at the end of the infusion. Plasma ACTH concentrations are supraphysiologic throughout the infusion.
- The 24-hour urinary excretion of 17-hydroxycorticoid should increase three- to fivefold over baseline on the day of ACTH infusion.

Two-Day ACTH Infusion Test
- The 2-day ACTH infusion test is similar to the 8-hour infusion test, except that the same dose of ACTH is infused for 8 hours on two consecutive days.
- This test may be helpful in distinguishing secondary from tertiary adrenal insufficiency. The one-day 8-hour test is too short for this purpose, whereas longer tests add little further useful information.
- Urinary excretion of 17-hydroxycorticoid should exceed 27 mg during the first 24 hours of infusion and 47 mg during the second 48 hours.

➤ Interpretation

* Low-dose stimulation test: A value of 18 μg/dL or more, before or after ACTH injection, is indicative of normal adrenal function.
* High-dose stimulation test: A serum cortisol value of 20 μg/dL or more at any time during the test, including before injection, is indicative of normal adrenal function.
* Eight-hour stimulation test: Serum cortisol should reach 20 μg/dL in 30–60 minutes after the infusion is begun and exceed 25 μg/mL after 6–8 hours.
* Two-day infusion test: Serum cortisol should reach 20 μg/mL in 30–60 minutes after the ACTH infusion is begun and exceed 25 μg/mL after 6–8 hours. Both serum and urinary steroid values increase progressively thereafter, but the ranges of normal are not well defined.

➤ Limitations

* In healthy individuals, cortisol responses are greatest in the morning, but in patients with adrenal insufficiency, the response to Cosyntropin is the same in the morning and afternoon. Therefore, ACTH stimulation tests should be done in the morning to minimize the risk of misdiagnosis in a normal individual.
* The criteria for a minimal normal cortisol response of 18–20 μg/dL are derived from the responses of healthy volunteers. However, in some studies, higher cut-off points for the diagnosis of adrenal insufficiency are based on the ACTH test responses of patients known to have an abnormal response to insulin.
* Variability in cortisol assays creates an additional problem with setting criteria for a normal response to ACTH that apply to all centers. Studies comparing cortisol results obtained with different assays showed a positive bias of RIAs and EIAs of 10–50% compared to a reference value obtained using isotope dilution GC/MS.
* In women, the response to ACTH is affected by the use of oral contraceptives, which increase cortisol-binding globulin levels.
* The response to ACTH varies with the underlying disorder. If the patient has hypopituitarism with deficient ACTH secretion and secondary adrenal insufficiency, then the intrinsically normal adrenal gland should respond to maximally stimulating concentrations of exogenous ACTH if given for a sufficiently long time. The response may be less than that in normal subjects and initially sluggish due to adrenal atrophy resulting from chronically low stimulation by endogenous ACTH. If, on the other hand, the patient has primary adrenal insufficiency, endogenous ACTH secretion is already elevated and there should be little or no adrenal response to exogenous ACTH.
* Therefore, a clearly subnormal response to the low-dose or high-dose ACTH stimulation test is diagnostic of primary or secondary adrenal insufficiency, whereas a normal response excludes both disorders.
* Cortisol values between 18.0 and 25.4 μg/dL represent a range of uncertainty in which patients may have discordant responses to ACTH, insulin, and/or metyrapone. Higher concentrations represent a normal response in the non-ICU setting.
* The low-dose test is not valid if there has been recent pituitary injury, and it supports the conclusion that a 30-minute serum cortisol concentration <18 μg/dL indicates impaired adrenocortical reserve. In addition, the low-dose test does not reliably indicate hypothalamic-pituitary-adrenal axis suppression in preterm infants whose mothers received dexamethasone for <2 weeks before delivery to hasten fetal lung development. The CRH test should be used in this situation.

ACTIVATED CLOTTING TIME (ACT)

➤ Definition
- ACT is a rapid POC standardized, clotting time. It is performed by automated, well-calibrated instruments, such as the Medtronic Automated Coagulation Timer (ACT).
- ACT has to be established in each POC testing area after induction of anesthesia and opening the chest for cardiopulmonary bypass surgery, because surgery and anesthesia reduce it. The ACT may also vary slightly with the lot number of the control cartridge.
- **Normal range in the absence of heparin (with Medtronic coagulometer):** 74–125 seconds

➤ Use
- ACT is the most widely used measure of anticoagulation with heparin (and neutralization of heparin with protamine) during extracorporeal circulation. After the initial dose of heparin, the ACT is maintained at >275 seconds for off-pump coronary procedures and >350 seconds for on-pump procedures by periodic administration of heparin.

➤ Interpretation
- There is some controversy concerning whether monitoring heparinization by ACT alone ensures optimal heparin and protamine doses. A poor correlation was found between ACT and heparin measurements using anti-Xa assays. Nevertheless, experience has shown that institution of anticoagulation under ACT guidance and monitoring and reversal user guidelines as described above improves hemostasis, limits blood loss, and reduces the need for transfusions.

➤ Limitations
- The response of ACT to heparin varies from individual to individual and with heparin potency.
- Underlying coagulopathies (antithrombin III deficiency, clotting factor deficiencies, DIC) must be excluded.
- Medications that inhibit platelet function (aspirin, NSAIDs) may affect ACT.
- Preanalytical errors (sample dilution or contamination with heparin, blood activation) must be avoided. It is particularly important to avoid the use of samples contaminated by heparin flushes.

ACTIVATED PROTEIN C RESISTANCE (APCR)

➤ Definition
- APCR reflects resistance of activated protein C (APC) substrate factor V to proteolysis. Most cases (95%) of APCR are due to factor V Leiden, a genetic mutation in factor V that predisposes to venous thromboembolism (5- to 10-times greater risk in heterozygotes and 50- to 100-times greater risk in homozygote carriers). The remaining 5% are found in pregnancy, malignancy, and the antiphospholipid antibody syndrome.
- Ratios are generated either from a modified PTT, or, more recently, by activating protein C with southern copperhead venom, using dilute Russell viper venom as the clotting reagent. The test is performed in the presence of added APC, where, in normal individuals, there is an elongation due to delayed generation of fibrin when factor V is lysed; in the absence of APC, where factor V remains intact, there is no elongation. Patients with APCR have a lower prolongation of clotting in the presence of APC than controls.
- **Normal value:** >1.8

➤ Use

- APCR is one of the assays recommended to investigate the etiology of venous thrombophilia (see p. 888). The congenital form, factor V Leiden, is present in 5% of individuals of European descent and in a high proportion of patients with unprovoked venous thromboembolism. It is virtually absent in patients of pure African ancestry.

➤ Limitations

- Protein C levels <50% and initial anticoagulation with vitamin K antagonists may give falsely low ratios. In these situations, the genetic test for factor V Leiden is recommended. The APCR assay is valid in patients stabilized on vitamin K antagonists or heparin.
- The assay is invalid in clotted specimens, as well as in lipemic, hemolyzed, or icteric samples.
- The assay is also invalid if blood is drawn with the wrong anticoagulant or the tubes are not filled appropriately.

ADIPONECTIN

➤ Definition

- Adiponectin, a hormone secreted exclusively by adipose tissue, has an important role in the regulation of tissue inflammation and insulin sensitivity.
- Perturbations in adiponectin concentration have been associated with obesity and the metabolic syndrome. Levels of the hormone are inversely correlated with body fat percentage in adults, whereas the association in infants and young children is more unclear.
- **Normal range:** See Table 2-3.

➤ Use

- Higher adiponectin levels are associated with a lower risk of type 2 diabetes across diverse populations, consistent with a dose–response relationship.

➤ Interpretation

- Adiponectin increases two-fold before a meal and decreases to trough levels within 1 hour after eating.
- It is decreased in:
  - Type 2 diabetes mellitus
  - Obesity and metabolic syndrome

➤ Limitations

- Adiponectin exerts some of its weight reduction effects via the brain. This is similar to the action of leptin, but the two hormones perform complementary actions and can have additive effects.
- Due to its important cardiometabolic actions, adiponectin represents a biologic molecule worth being studied as a new emerging biomarker of disease and also as a target for pharmacologic treatments.

TABLE 2-3. Normal Range of Adiponectin

Body Mass Index (kg/m^2)	Male (µg/mL)	Female (µg/mL)
<25	4–26	5–37
25–30	4–20	5–28
>30	2–20	4–22

➤ Suggested Reading

Li S, Shin HJ, Ding EL, van Dam RM. Adiponectin levels and risk of type 2 diabetes: a systematic review and meta-analysis. *JAMA*. 2009;302(2):179–188.

ADRENOCORTICOTROPIC HORMONE (ACTH)

➤ Definition

- ACTH, also known as adrenocorticotropin and corticotropin, is a polypeptide hormone that exists principally as a chain of 39 amino acids, with a molecular mass of approximately 4500 daltons. It is produced by the anterior pituitary gland.
- Its biologic function is to stimulate cortisol secretion by the adrenal cortex. ACTH secretion is in turn controlled by the hypothalamic hormone CRF and by negative feedback from cortisol.
- **Normal range:** <46 pg/mL

➤ Use

- Diagnosis of Addison disease, CAH, and Cushing syndrome

➤ Interpretation
Increased In

- Addison disease
- CAH
- Pituitary-dependent Cushing disease
- Ectopic ACTH-producing tumors
- Nelson syndrome

Decreased In

- Secondary adrenocortical insufficiency
- Adrenal carcinoma
- Adenoma
- Hypopituitarism

➤ Limitations

- Plasma levels of ACTH exhibit a significant diurnal variation. ACTH is normally highest in the early morning (6–8 a.m.) and lowest in the evening (6–11 p.m.). Cortisol levels are frequently measured at the same time as ACTH.
- Because ACTH is released in bursts, its levels in the blood can vary from minute to minute.
- ACTH is unstable in blood, and proper handling of specimen is important.
- Most commercial RIAs are insensitive and nonspecific, measuring intact ACTH as well as precursors and fragments. Highly sensitive IRMAs measure intact ACTH only.
- RIAs are recommended for investigating ectopic ACTH-producing tumors, because some of the tumors secrete ACTH precursors and fragments. IRMAs are more sensitive than RIAs and are useful for investigating disorders of the hypothalamic-pituitary-adrenal system.
- Patients taking glucocorticoids may have suppressed levels of ACTH with an apparent high level of cortisol.
- Pregnancy, menstruation, and stress increase secretion.

ALBUMIN, SERUM

➤ Definition
- Albumin is the most important protein and constitutes 55–65% of total plasma protein. Approximately 300–500 g of albumin is distributed in the body fluids, and the average adult liver synthesizes approximately 15 g per day. Albumin's half-life is approximately 20 days, with 4% of the total albumin pool being degraded daily.
- The serum albumin concentration reflects the rate of synthesis, the degradation, and the volume of distribution. Albumin synthesis is regulated by a variety of influences, including nutritional status, serum oncotic pressure, cytokines, and hormones.
- **Normal range:**
  - 0–4 month: 2.0 to 4.5 g/dL
  - 4 month –16 years: 3.2 to 5.2 g/dL
  - >16 years: 3.5 to 4.8 g/dL

➤ Use
- Assess nutritional status.
- Evaluate chronic illness
- Evaluate liver disease

➤ Interpretation
Increased In
- Dehydration

Decreased In
- Decreased synthesis by the liver:
  - Acute and chronic liver disease (e.g., alcoholism, cirrhosis, hepatitis)
  - Malabsorption and malnutrition
  - Fasting, protein calorie malnutrition
  - Amyloidosis
  - Chronic illness
  - DM
  - Decreased growth hormone levels
  - Hypothyroidism
  - Hypoadrenalism
  - Genetic analbuminemia
- Acute phase reaction, inflammation, and chronic diseases:
  - Bacterial infections
  - Monoclonal gammopathies and other neoplasms
  - Parasitic infestations
  - Peptic ulcer
  - Prolonged immobilization
  - Rheumatic diseases
  - Severe skin disease
- Increased loss over body surface:
  - Burns

- Enteropathies related to sensitivity to ingested substances (e.g., gluten sensitivity, Crohn disease, ulcerative colitis)
- Fistula (gastrointestinal or lymphatic)
- Hemorrhage
- Kidney disease
- Rapid hydration or overhydration
- Repeated thoracentesis or paracentesis
- Trauma and crush injuries
- Increased catabolism:
  - Fever
  - Cushing disease
  - Preeclampsia
  - Thyroid dysfunction
- Plasma volume expansion:
  - CHF
  - Oral contraceptives
  - Pregnancy

➤ Limitations
- In clinical practice, one of two dye-binding assays—bromcresol green (BCG) and bromcresol purple (BCP)—is used for measuring albumin levels, and systematic differences between these methods have long been recognized.
- BCG methods are subject to nonspecific interference from binding to nonalbumin proteins, whereas BCP is more specific. BCP has been shown to underestimate serum albumin in pediatric patients on hemodialysis and patients in chronic renal failure. Chronic dialysis units often have little influence over the method.
- Antialbumin antibodies are commonly found with hepatic dysfunction and are typically of IgA type.
- Ischemia modified albumin, in which the metal binding capacity of albumin has decreased due to exposure to ischemic events, is a biologic marker of myocardial ischemia.

ALCOHOLS (VOLATILES, SOLVENTS)

➤ Definition
- Alcohols are organic compounds that contain the $-OH$ group, including methanol (CH_3OH), ethanol (ethyl alcohol; C_2H_5OH), isopropanol (rubbing alcohol), and methanol (wood alcohol). Although acetone (CH_3COCH_3) is a ketone, not an alcohol, it is included in this group, because it is often detected in the same testing methodology.
- **Normal range:**
  - Ethanol: <10 mg/dL
    - 50 mg/dL: decreased inhibition, slight incoordination
    - 100 mg/dL: slow reaction time; altered sensory ability
    - 150 mg/dL: altered thought processes; personality, behavior changes
    - 200 mg/dL: staggering gait, nausea, vomiting, mental confusion
    - 300 mg/dL: slurred speech, sensory loss, visual disturbance
    - 400 mg/dL: hypothermia, hypoglycemia, poor muscle control, seizures

- 700 mg/dL: unconsciousness, decreased reflexes, respiratory failure (may also occur at lower concentrations)
- Isopropanol alcohol: <10 mg/dL (normal); toxic effects generally seen at 50–100 mg/dL.
- Methanol: <10 mg/dL (normal); levels >25 mg/dL are generally considered toxic.
- Acetone: <10 mg/dL; effects are said to be similar to ethanol for similar blood levels, but the anesthetic potency is greater.

➤ Use
- Beverage (ethanol)
- Solvent and reagent
- Vehicle in chemical and pharmaceutical industries
- Antiseptic (isopropyl alcohol)

➤ Limitations
- Testing
  - Immunoassay testing for ethanol:
    - Urine
    - Serum/plasma
    - Whole blood
    - Qualitative cut-off concentration 40 or 50 mg/dL
    - Semiquantitative limit of quantitation 10 mg/dL
    - Cross reactivity: <1% with isopropanol alcohol, methanol, ethylene glycol, acetaldehyde; <15% with n-propanol
  - Gas chromatographic testing for ethanol, isopropanol alcohol, methanol, acetone
    - Urine
    - Serum/plasma
    - Whole blood
    - Minimal sample pretreatment (direct injection, headspace)
    - Limit of quantitation
      - Ethanol: 10 mg/dL
      - Isopropanol: 10 mg/dL
      - Methanol: 10 mg/dL
      - Acetone: 10 mg/dL. Elevated concentrations are detected in specimens during diabetic ketoacidosis and fasting ketoacidosis and may range from 10–70 mg/dL.
- In many headspace gas chromatographic methods, acetonitrile co-elutes with acetone, leading to a false-positive result. Acetonitrile may be a component in cosmetic nail remover.
- A positive urine ethanol due to the presence of yeast in the patient's urine has been described. In these cases, glucose was also present in the urine.

ALDOSTERONE

➤ Definition
- Primary mineralocorticoid secreted by adrenal zona glomerulosa.
- The role of aldosterone in metabolism is the control of sodium and potassium.
  - Regulating sodium ion concentration, in turn regulates fluid volume.
  - Aldosterone acts to decrease excretion of sodium and increase the excretion of potassium at the kidney, sweat glands, and salivary glands.

* **Normal range:**
  * 8:00–10:00 a.m. (sitting): 3–34 ng/dL
  * 8:00–10:00 a.m. (supine): 2–19 ng/dL
  * 4:00–6:00 p.m. (sitting): 2–23 ng/dL

➤ Use

* Diagnosis of primary hyperaldosteronism
* Differential diagnosis of fluid and electrolyte disorders
* Assessment of adrenal aldosterone production

➤ Interpretation
Increased In

* Primary aldosteronism
* Secondary aldosteronism
* Barter syndrome
* Pregnancy
* Very low sodium diet
* Urine aldosterone is also increased in nephrosis.

Decreased In

* Hyporeninemic hypoaldosteronism
* CAH
* Congenital deficiency of aldosterone synthetase
* Addison disease
* Very high sodium diet

➤ Limitations

* Many physiologic factors affect plasma aldosterone. Posture, salt intake, use of antihypertensive drugs, use of steroids, oral contraceptives, age, menstrual cycle, and pregnancy can all have a strong influence on aldosterone results.

ALKALINE PHOSPHATASE (ALP)

➤ Definition

* ALP refers to a family of enzymes that catalyze hydrolysis of phosphate esters at an alkaline pH. There are at least five isoenzymes derived from liver (sinusoidal and bile canalicular surface of hepatocytes), bone, intestine (brush border of mucosal cells), placenta, and tumor-associated tissues separated by electrophoresis. Placenta and tumor-associated ALP are the most heat resistant to inactivation.
* More than 95% of total ALP activity comes from bone and liver (~1:1 ratio).
* The half-life of ALP is 7–10 days.
* **Normal range:**
  * 0–1 year: 150–350 IU/L
  * 1–16 years: 30–300 IU/L
  * >16 years: 30–115 IU/L

➤ Use

* Diagnosis and treatment of liver, bone, intestinal, and parathyroid diseases.

➤ Interpretation
Increased In

* Increased bone formation
* Bone diseases (metastatic carcinoma of the bone, myeloma, Paget disease)
* Renal disease (renal rickets due to vitamin D–resistant rickets associated with secondary hyperparathyroidism)
* Liver disease (e.g., infectious mononucleosis, uncomplicated extra hepatic biliary obstruction, liver abscess)
* Miscellaneous (extrahepatic sepsis, ulcerative colitis, pancreatitis, phenytoin and alcohol use)
* Bone origin—increased deposition of calcium
  * Hyperparathyroidism
  * Paget disease (osteitis deformans) (highest reported values 10–20 times normal). Marked elevation in absence of liver disease is most suggestive of Paget disease of bone or metastatic carcinoma from prostate.
  * Increase in cases of metastases to bone is marked only in prostate carcinoma.
  * Osteoblastic bone tumors (osteogenic sarcoma, metastatic carcinoma).
  * Osteogenesis imperfecta (due to healing fractures)
  * Familial osteoectasia
  * Osteomalacia, rickets
  * Polyostotic fibrous dysplasia
  * Osteomyelitis
  * Late pregnancy; reverts to normal level by 20th day postpartum.
  * Children <10 years of age and again during prepubertal growth spurt may have 3–4 times adult values; adult values are attained by age 20.
  * Administration of ergosterol
  * Hyperthyroidism
  * Transient hyperphosphatasemia of infancy
  * Hodgkin disease
  * Healing of extensive fractures (slightly)
* Liver disease
  * Any obstruction of biliary system (e.g., stone, carcinoma, primary biliary cirrhosis) is a sensitive indicator of intrahepatic or extrahepatic cholestasis. Whenever the ALP is elevated, a simultaneous elevation of 5′-nucleotidase (5′-N) establishes biliary disease as the cause of the elevated ALP. If the 5′-N is not increased, the cause of the elevated ALP must be found elsewhere (e.g., bone disease).
  * Liver infiltrates (e.g., amyloid, or leukemia)
  * Cholangiolar obstruction in hepatitis (e.g., infectious, toxic)
  * Hepatic congestion due to heart disease
  * Adverse reaction to therapeutic drug (e.g., chlorpropamide) (progressive elevation of serum ALP may be first indication that drug therapy should be halted); may be 2–20 times normal
  * Increased synthesis of ALP in liver
  * Diabetes mellitus—44% of diabetic patients have 40% increase of ALP
  * Parenteral hyperalimentation of glucose
* Liver diseases with increased ALP
  * <3–4 times increase lacks specificity and may be present in all forms of liver disease.
  * 2 times increase: acute hepatitis (viral, toxic, alcoholic), acute fatty liver, cirrhosis.

- 2–10 times increase: nodules in liver (metastatic or primary tumor, abscess, cyst, parasite, TB, sarcoid); is a sensitive indicator of a hepatic infiltrate.
- Increase >2 times upper limit of normal in patients with primary breast or lung tumor with osteolytic metastases is more likely caused by liver than bone metastases.
- 5 times increase: infectious mononucleosis, postnecrotic cirrhosis.
- 10 times increase: carcinoma of head of pancreas, choledocholithiasis, and drug cholestatic hepatitis.
- 15–20 times increase: primary biliary cirrhosis, primary or metastatic carcinoma. The GGT-to-ALP ratio >2.5 is highly suggestive of alcohol abuse.
- Chronic therapeutic use of anticonvulsant drugs (e.g., phenobarbital, phenytoin).
- Placental origin: appears 16th to 20th week of normal pregnancy, increases progressively to 2 times normal up to onset of labor, and disappears 3–6 days after delivery of placenta. ALP may be increased during complications of pregnancy (e.g., hypertension, preeclampsia, eclampsia, threatened abortion) but is difficult to interpret without serial determinations. It is lower in diabetic than nondiabetic pregnancy.
- Intestinal origin: is a component in ~25% of normal sera; increases 2 hours after eating in persons with blood type B or O who are secretors of H-blood group. ALP has been reported to be increased in cirrhosis, various ulcerative diseases of the GI tract, severe malabsorption, chronic hemodialysis, and acute infarction of intestine.
  - Benign familial hyperphosphatasemia
  - Ectopic production by neoplasm (Regan isoenzyme) without involvement of liver or bone (e.g., Hodgkin disease; cancer of lung, breast, colon, or pancreas; highest incidence in ovary and cervical cancer)
  - Vascular endothelium origin—some patients with myocardial, pulmonary, renal (one third of cases), or splenic infarction, usually after 7 days during phase of organization
  - Hyperphosphatasia (liver and bone isoenzymes)
  - Hyperthyroidism (liver and bone isoenzymes). Increased ALP alone in a chemical profile, especially with a decreased serum cholesterol and lymphocytosis, should suggest excess thyroid medication or hyperthyroidism.
  - Primary hypophosphatemia (often increased)
  - ALP isoenzyme determinations are not widely used clinically; heat inactivation may be more useful to distinguish bone from liver source of increased ALP (extremely 90% heat-labile: bone, vascular endothelium, reticuloendothelial system; extremely 90% heat-stable: placenta, neoplasms; intermediate 60–80% heat-stable: liver, intestine). Also differentiate by chemical inhibition (e.g., L-phenylalanine) or use serum GGT, leucine aminopeptidase.
  - Children—mostly bone; little or no liver or intestine.
  - Adults—liver with little or no bone or intestine; after age 50, increasing amounts of bone.

Decreased In

- Hypothyroidism
- Gross anemia
- Hypophosphatemia
- Vitamin B_{12} deficiency
- Nutritional deficiency of zinc or magnesium
- Excess vitamin D ingestion
- Milk-alkali (Burnett) syndrome
- Congenital hypophosphatasia (enzymopathy of liver, bone, kidney isoenzymes)
- Achondroplasia

- Hypothyroidism, cretinism
- Pernicious anemia (one third of patients)
- Celiac disease
- Malnutrition
- Scurvy
- Postmenopausal women with osteoporosis taking estrogen replacement therapy
- Therapeutic agents (e.g., corticosteroids, trifluoperazine, antilipemic agents, some hyperalimentation)
- Cardiac surgery with cardiopulmonary bypass pump

Normal In
- Inherited metabolic diseases (Dubin-Johnson, Rotor, Gilbert, Crigler-Najjar syndromes; types I–V glycogenoses, mucopolysaccharidoses; increased in Wilson disease and hemochromatosis related to hepatic fibrosis)
- Consumption of alcohol by healthy persons (in contrast to GGT); may be normal even in alcoholic hepatitis.
- In acute icteric viral hepatitis, the increase is <2 times normal in 90% of cases, but when ALP is high and serum bilirubin is normal, infectious mononucleosis should be ruled out as cause of hepatitis.

➤ Limitations
- The elevation in ALP tends to be more marked (more than threefold) in extrahepatic biliary obstruction (e.g., by stone or by cancer of the head of the pancreas) than in intrahepatic obstruction, and it is greater the more complete the obstruction. Serum enzyme activities may reach 10–12 times the upper limit of normal, returning to normal on surgical removal of the obstruction.
- Day to day variation is 5–10%.
- Recent food ingestion can increase as much as 30 U/L.
- ALP is 15% and 10% higher in African American men and women, respectively, compared to other racial/ethnic groups.
- 25% higher with increased body mass index, 10% higher with smoking, 20% lower with the use of oral contraceptives.

ALPHA₁-ANTITRYPSIN (AAT, ALPHA-1 TRYPSIN INHIBITOR, ALPHA-1 PROTEINASE INHIBITOR)

➤ Definition
- AAT is a member of the serpin family of protease inhibitors. It protects the lower airways from damage caused by the proteolytic enzyme, elastase. The normal AAT allele is the M allele. Over 100 allelic variants have been described, of which the most common severely deficient variant is the Z allele. It is normally the major constituent of the alpha-1 band on routine serum electrophoresis.
- AAT deficiency is severely under recognized, with long intervals between the first symptom and diagnosis. Clinical manifestations of severe deficiency of AAT typically involve the lung (e.g., early onset emphysema with a basilar predominant pattern on imaging), liver (e.g., cirrhosis), and, rarely, the skin (e.g., panniculitis).
- **Normal range:** 88–174 mg/dL

➤ Use
- Work-up of individuals with suspected disorders such as familial chronic obstructive lung disease
- Diagnosis of AAT deficiency
- Diagnosis of juvenile and adult cirrhosis of the liver.

➤ Interpretation
Increased In
- Inflammation (acute phase reacting protein)
- Infection, tissue injury or necrosis, rheumatic disease, and some malignancies
- Estrogen administration (oral contraceptives, pregnancy, especially third semester)

Decreased In
- Deficiency states (hereditary)
- Hepatic disease (hepatitis, cholestasis, cirrhosis, or hepatic cancer)
- Pulmonary emphysema, COPD

➤ Limitations
- Phenotypic studies are recommended to confirm a suspected hereditary deficiency.
- False-positive results can occur if rheumatoid factor present.

α-FETOPROTEIN (AFP) TUMOR MARKER, SERUM

➤ Definition
- AFP is a glycoprotein that is normally produced during gestation by the fetal liver and yolk sac, the serum concentration of which is often elevated in patients with hepatocellular carcinoma (HCC). It is also found in some patients with cancer of the testes and ovaries.
- **Normal range:** 0.6–6.60 ng/mL

➤ Use
- Marker for hepatocellular and germ cell (nonseminoma) carcinoma
- Follow-up management of patients undergoing cancer therapy, especially for testicular and ovarian tumors and for hepatocellular carcinoma. The measurement of AFP in serum, in conjunction with serum human chorionic gonadotropin, is an established regimen for monitoring patients with nonseminomatous testicular cancer. In addition, monitoring the rate of AFP clearance from serum after treatment is an indicator of the effectiveness of therapy. Conversely, the growth rate of progressive cancer can be monitored by serially measuring serum AFP concentration over time.
- Serial serum AFP testing is a useful adjunctive test for managing nonseminomatous testicular cancer.

➤ Interpretation
- AFP is increased in the following disorders:
  - Ataxia telangiectasia
  - Hereditary tyrosinemia
  - Primary hepatocellular carcinoma
  - Teratocarcinoma
  - Gastrointestinal tract cancers with and without liver metastases

- Benign hepatic conditions such as acute viral hepatitis, chronic active hepatitis, and cirrhosis

➤ Limitations
- AFP is not recommended as a screening procedure to detect cancer in the general population. This assay is intended only as an adjunct in the diagnosis and monitoring of AFP-producing tumors. The diagnosis should be confirmed by other tests or procedures.
- Serum levels of AFP do not correlate well with other clinical features of HCC, such as size, stage, or prognosis.
- A case–control study evaluated the diagnostic characteristics of the serum AFP in screening for HCC in patients with different types of chronic liver disease. The following sensitivities and specificities were observed:
  - AFP cut-off 16 µg/L (sensitivity 62%, specificity 89%)
  - AFP cut-off 20 µg/L (sensitivity 60%, specificity 91%)
  - AFP cut-off 100 µg/L (sensitivity 31%, specificity 99%)
  - AFP cut-off 200 µg/L (sensitivity 22%, specificity 99%)
- False-positive elevations can occur with tumors of the GI tract or with liver damage (e.g., cirrhosis, hepatitis, or drug or alcohol abuse)
- Failure of the AFP value to return to normal by approximately 1 month after surgery suggests the presence of residual tumor.
- Elevation of AFP after remission suggests tumor recurrence; however, tumors originally producing AFP may recur without an increase in AFP.

➤ Suggested Reading
Trevisani F, D'Intino PE, Morselli-Labate AM, et al. Serum alpha-fetoprotein for diagnosis of hepatocellular carcinoma in patients with chronic liver disease: influence of HBsAg and anti-HCV status. *J Hepatol.* 2001;34(4): 570–575.

AMINOTRANSFERASES (AST, ALT)

➤ Definition
- AST and ALT are members of transaminase family of enzymes, widely distributed in cells throughout the body. AST is primarily found in heart, liver, skeletal muscle, and kidney, whereas ALT is found primarily in liver and kidney, with lesser amounts in heart and skeletal muscle.
- AST and ALT activity in liver are about 7000 and 3000 times serum activities, respectively.
- **Normal range:**
  - AST:
    - Less than or Equal to 1 year: 30–80 U/L
    - Greater than 1 year: 10–40 U/L
  - ALT:
    - Less than or Equal to 1 year: 5–50 U/L
    - Greater than 1 year: 10–40 U/L

➤ Use
- Most sensitive tests for acute hepatocellular injury (e.g., viral, drug); precedes increase in serum bilirubin by ~1 week

➤ Interpretation
Increased In
* Hepatocellular damage, liver cell necrosis, or injury of any cause
* Alcoholic hepatitis (AST > ALT)
* Viral and chronic hepatitis (ALT > AST)
* Early acute hepatitis: AST is usually higher initially, but by 48 hours, ALT is usually higher
* AST levels of 500 U/L suggest acute hepatocellular injury; seldom >500 U/L in obstructive jaundice, cirrhosis, viral hepatitis, AIDS, alcoholic liver disease
* Acute fulminant viral hepatitis. Abrupt AST rise may be seen (rarely >4000 IU/L) and declines more slowly; positive serologic tests and acute chemical injury.
* Congestive heart failure, arrhythmia, sepsis, GI hemorrhage AST levels reach to a peak of 1000–9000 U/L, declining by 50% within 3 days and to <100 U/L within a week, suggesting shock liver with centrolobular necrosis. Serum bilirubin and ALP reflect underlying disease.
* Trauma to skeletal or heart muscle
* Acute heart failure (AST > ALT)
* Severe exercise, burns, heat stroke
* Hypothyroidism
* Drug induced injury to liver
* Acute bile duct obstruction due to a stone. Rapid rise of AST and ALT to very high levels (e.g., >600 U/L and often >2000 U/L) followed by a sharp fall in 12–72 hours is said to be typical.

Decreased In
* Azotemia
* Chronic renal dialysis
* Pyridoxal phosphate deficiency states (e.g., malnutrition, pregnancy, alcoholic liver disease)

➤ Limitations
* Half-life of AST is 18 hours and that of ALT is 48 hours.
* Patient is rarely asymptomatic with ALT and AST levels >1000 U/L.
* AST >10 times normal indicates acute hepatocellular injury but lesser increases are nonspecific and may occur with virtually any form of liver injury.
* Increases ≤8 times upper limit of normal are nonspecific; may be found in any liver disorder.
* Rarely increased >500 U/L (usually <200 U/L) in posthepatic jaundice, AIDS, cirrhosis, and viral hepatitis
* Usually <50 U/L in fatty liver
* <100 U/L in alcoholic cirrhosis; ALT is normal in 50% and AST is normal in 25% of these cases.
* <150 U/L in alcoholic hepatitis (may be higher if patient has delirium tremens)
* <200 U/L in ~50% of patients with cirrhosis, metastatic liver disease, lymphoma, and leukemia.
* Normal values may not rule out liver disease: ALT is normal in 50%, and AST is normal in 25% of cases of alcoholic cirrhosis.
* Degree of increase has poor prognostic value.
* Serial determinations reflect clinical activity of liver disease. Persistent increase may indicate chronic hepatitis.

- Mild increase of AST and ALT (usually <500 U/L) with ALP increased >3 times normal indicates cholestatic jaundice, but more marked increase of AST and ALT (especially >1000 U/L) with ALP increased <3 times normal indicates hepatocellular jaundice.
- Rapid decline in AST and ALT is sign of recovery from disease but in acute fulminant hepatitis may represent loss of hepatocytes and poor prognosis.
- Poor correlation of increased concentration with extent of liver cell necrosis and has little prognostic value.
- Although AST, ALT, and bilirubin are most characteristic of acute hepatitis, they are unreliable markers of severity of injury.
- ALT has 45% variation during the day; highest in afternoon and lowest at night. Both AST and ALT exhibit 10–30% variation from one day to next. AST levels are 15% higher in African American men.

AMMONIA (BLOOD NH3, NH3, NH4)

➤ Definition
- Ammonia is derived mostly from amino acid metabolism in the liver via the urea cycle. *Helicobacter pylori* in the stomach appears to be an important source of ammonia in patients with cirrhosis.
- **Normal range:** <50 µmol/L

➤ Use
- In the diagnosis of hepatic encephalopathy and hepatic coma in the terminal stages of liver cirrhosis, hepatic failure, acute and subacute necrosis, and Reye syndrome. Hyperammonemia in infants may be an indicator of inherited deficiencies of the urea cycle metabolic pathway.
- Should be measured in cases of unexplained lethargy and vomiting, encephalopathy, or any neonate with unexplained neurologic deterioration.
- Not useful to assess degree of dysfunction (e.g., in Reye syndrome, hepatic function improves and the ammonia level falls, even in patients who finally die of these disorders).

➤ Interpretation
Increased In
- Certain inborn errors of metabolism (e.g., defects in urea cycle, organic acid defects)
- Transient hyperammonemia in newborn; unknown etiology; may be life-threatening in first 48 hours.
- May occur in any patient with severe liver disease (e.g., acute hepatic necrosis, terminal cirrhosis, and after portacaval anastomosis). Increased in most cases of hepatic coma but correlates poorly with degree of encephalopathy. Not useful in known liver disease but may be useful in encephalopathy of unknown cause.
- Moribund children. Moderate increases (≤300 µmol/L) without being diagnostic of a specific disease.
- GU tract infection with distention and stasis
- Ureterosigmoidostomy
- Some hematologic disorders, including acute leukemia and after bone marrow transplantation
- Total parenteral nutrition
- Smoking, exercise, valproic acid therapy

Decreased In
- Hyperornithinemia (deficiency of ornithine aminotransaminase activity) with gyrate atrophy of choroid and retina

> ## Limitations
- Atmospheric ammonia may cause falsely elevated results.
- The presence of ammonium ions in anticoagulants may produce falsely elevated results.
- Ammonia levels are not always high in all patients with urea cycle disorders.
- High protein diet may cause increased levels.
- Ammonia levels may also be elevated with GI hemorrhage.
- Ammonia increases due to cellular metabolism: 20% in 1 hour and 100% by 2 hours.

AMNIOCENTESIS

> ## Definition
- Invasive procedure to obtain amniotic fluid that contains cells sloughed from the fetus. Some biochemical tests can be performed directly on the fluid; most tests first require cell culture.
- It is generally not performed until 15 weeks of gestation; recent estimates of procedural risk of fetal loss are as low as 0.06%.
- Cell culture for chromosome analysis takes 5–7 days; slightly longer culture times are required to obtain material for biochemical or molecular genetic tests.

> ## Use
- Provides fetal material for chromosome (cytogenetic) testing, biochemical testing (metabolic disorders/inborn errors of metabolism), and molecular DNA-based testing for inherited disease (e.g., CF, fragile X).

> ## Limitations
- Not performed until second trimester, which delays decisions regarding pregnancy termination.

AMPHETAMINES

> ## Definition
- Sympathomimetic amines with central nervous system stimulant activity
- Other names: amphetamine (Adderall, Dexedrine, Benzedrine, "bennies"), methamphetamine (Desoxyn, "ice," "speed," "meth"), ecstasy (3,4-methylenedioxymethamphetamine; MDMA), 3,4-methylenedioxyamphetamine (MDA), 3,4-methylenedioxyethylamphetamine (MDEA, MDE, "Eve"), pseudoephedrine (Sudafed), ephedrine, phentermine (Adipex), methylphenidate (Ritalin)
- Other psychotropic amines include 4-bromo-2,5-dimethoxyamphetamine, p-methoxyamphetamine (PMA), p-methoxymethamphetamine (PMMA). These are not generally detected in screening tests and may not be reported in confirmation tests unless specifically requested.
- Other drugs that are metabolized to methamphetamine/amphetamine: benzphetamine, clobenzorex, famprofazone, fenethylline, fenproporex

➤ Use
* Appetite suppressants
* Mood enhancers (psychotropics)
* Treatment of attention deficit/hyperactivity disorder
* Nasal decongestants, bronchodilators

➤ Limitations
* Screen [urine]: immunoassay on automated chemistry analyzers
  * Amphetamine
    * Target analyte: varies by vendor
      * d-amphetamine/d-methamphetamine
      * d-amphetamine
    * Generally do NOT give positive results for l-amphetamine, MDA, MDMA, ephedrine, phentermine
    * Cut-off concentrations
      * 500 ng/mL
      * 1000 ng/mL
  * Ecstasy
    * Target analyte: MDMA
    * Will not give positive results with d/l-amphetamine, d/l-methamphetamine, phentermine, ephedrine, pseudoephedrine, PMA, PMMA
    * Assays capable of detecting ecstasy may have other names such as amphetamine/methamphetamine. Refer to laboratory's specific protocol.
      * Cut-off concentration: 500 ng/mL
* Screen [serum]: ELISA
  * Target analyte: d-amphetamine
  * Cut-off concentration: 10-100 ng/mL [assay and laboratory dependent]
  * Will not give positive results with l-amphetamine, l-methamphetamine, phenylpropanolamine, MDMA, MDE
  * May produce positive results with MDA
* Confirmation [serum/urine]: extraction followed by chromatography based analytical technology such as GC/MS or LC/MS. Confirmation techniques do not typically differentiate between d and l forms of amphetamine and methamphetamine

AMYLASE

➤ Definition
* Amylases are a group of hydrolases that degrade complex carbohydrates into fragments.
* Amylase is produced by the exocrine pancreas and the salivary glands to aid in the digestion of starch. It is also produced by the small intestine mucosa, ovaries, placenta, liver, and fallopian tubes.
* **Normal range:** 5–125 U/L

➤ Use
* To diagnose and monitor pancreatitis or other pancreatic diseases.
* In the work-up of any intraabdominal inflammatory event.

➤ Interpretation
Increased In
* Acute pancreatitis (e.g., alcoholic, autoimmune). Urine levels reflect serum changes by a time lag of 6–10 hours.
* Acute exacerbation of chronic pancreatitis
* Drug-induced acute pancreatitis (e.g., aminosalicylic acid, azathioprine, corticosteroids, dexamethasone, ethacrynic acid, ethanol, furosemide, thiazides, mercaptopurine, phenformin, triamcinolone)
* Drug-induced methodologic interference (e.g., pancreozymin [contains amylase], chloride and fluoride salts [enhance amylase activity], lipemic serum [turbidimetric methods])
* Obstruction of pancreatic duct by:
  * Stone or carcinoma
    * Drug-induced spasm of sphincter of Oddi (e.g., opiates, codeine, methyl choline, cholinergics, chlorothiazide) to levels 2–15 times normal
    * Partial obstruction + drug stimulation
* Biliary tract disease
  * Common bile duct obstruction
  * Acute cholecystitis
* Complications of pancreatitis (pseudocyst, ascites, abscess)
* Pancreatic trauma (abdominal injury; following ERCP)
* Altered GI tract permeability
  * Ischemic bowel disease or frank perforation
  * Esophageal rupture
  * Perforated or penetrating peptic ulcer
  * Postoperative upper abdominal surgery, especially partial gastrectomy ($\leq$2 times normal in one third of patients)
* Acute alcohol ingestion or poisoning
* Salivary gland disease (mumps, suppurative inflammation, duct obstruction due to calculus, radiation)
* Malignant tumors (especially pancreas, lung, ovary, esophagus; also breast, colon); usually >25 times upper reference limit, which is rarely seen in pancreatitis
* Advanced renal insufficiency; often increased even without pancreatitis
* Macroamylasemia
* Others, such as chronic liver disease (e.g., cirrhosis; $\leq$2 times normal), burns, pregnancy (including ruptured tubal pregnancy), ovarian cyst, diabetic ketoacidosis, recent thoracic surgery, myoglobinuria, presence of myeloma proteins, some cases of intracranial bleeding (unknown mechanism), splenic rupture, dissecting aneurysm
* It has been suggested that a level >1000 Somogyi units is usually due to surgically correctable lesions (most frequently stones in biliary tree), the pancreas being negative or showing only edema; but 200–500 units is usually associated with pancreatic lesions that are not surgically correctable (e.g., hemorrhagic pancreatitis, necrosis of pancreas).
* Increased serum amylase with low urine amylase may be seen in renal insufficiency and macroamylasemia. Serum amylase $\leq$4 times normal in renal disease only when creatinine clearance is <50 mL/min due to pancreatic or salivary isoamylase; but rarely >4 times normal in absence of acute pancreatitis.

Decreased In
- Extensive marked destruction of pancreas (e.g., acute fulminant pancreatitis, advanced chronic pancreatitis, advanced cystic fibrosis). Decreased levels are clinically significant only in occasional cases of fulminant pancreatitis.
- Severe liver damage (e.g., hepatitis, poisoning, toxemia of pregnancy, severe thyrotoxicosis, severe burns)
- Methodologic interference by drugs (e.g., citrate and oxalate decrease activity by binding calcium ions)
  - Normal: 1–5%
  - Macroamylasemia: <1%; very useful for this diagnosis
  - Acute pancreatitis: >5%; use is presently discouraged for this diagnosis
- Amylase-to-creatinine clearance ratio = (urine amylase/serum amylase) (serum creatinine/urine creatinine) times 100

Normal In
- Relapsing chronic pancreatitis
- Patients with hypertriglyceridemia (technical interference with test)
- Frequently normal in acute alcoholic pancreatitis

➤ Limitations
- Composed of pancreatic and salivary types of isoamylases distinguished by various methodologies; nonpancreatic etiologies are almost always salivary; both types may be increased in renal insufficiency.
- An elevation of total serum α-amylase does not specifically indicate a pancreatic disorder, since the enzyme is produced by the salivary glands, mucosa of the small intestine, ovaries, placenta, liver, and the lining of the fallopian tubes.
- Pancreatic amylase results may be elevated in patients with macro-amylase. This elevated pancreatic amylase is not diagnostic for pancreatitis. By utilizing serum lipase and urinary amylase values, the presence or absence of macro-amylase may be determined.

AMYLASE, URINE (AMYLASE/CREATININE CLEARANCE RATIO [ALCR])

➤ Definition
- Amylase is an enzyme that helps digest glycogen and starch. It is produced mainly in the pancreas and salivary glands. Amylase is normally secreted from the pancreas through the pancreatic duct into the small intestine.
- ALCR is calculated as:
  Urine amylase/Serum amylase × Serum creatinine/Urine creatinine × 100
- **Normal range:**
  - Amylase Urine: 1–17 U/hour
  - ALCR: 1–4%

➤ Use
- Differential diagnosis of pancreatitis
- Diagnosis of pseudocyst of the pancreas, where the urine amylase may remain elevated for weeks after the serum amylase has returned to normal, after a bout of acute pancreatitis.

➤ Interpretation
Increased In
* Pancreatitis (>6%)
* DKA
* Renal insufficiency
* Duodenal perforation
* Large doses of corticosteroids
* Pancreatic cancer
* Myeloma and light chain disease

Decreased In
* Macroamylasemia

➤ Limitations
* Macroamylasemia is characterized by high serum amylase but normal urine amylase. The ALCR remains useful for the diagnosis of macroamylasemia. In macroamylasemia, the clearance is very low.

ANDROSTENEDIONE, SERUM

➤ Definition
* Androstenedione, also known as 4-androstenedione, is a 19-carbon steroid hormone produced in the adrenal glands and the gonads (testes as well as ovaries) as an intermediate step in the biochemical pathway that produces the androgen testosterone and the estrogens estrone and estradiol. It is a major adrenal androgen in serum.
* **Normal range:** 0.0–4.4 ng/mL (see Table 2-4)

➤ Use
* Diagnosis of virilism and hirsutism

TABLE 2-4. Normal Ranges for Serum Androstenedione

Age/Tanner Stage	Female (ng/mL)	Male (ng/mL)
7–9 years	0.0–0.9	0.0–0.8
10–11 years	0.0–3.0	0.0–1.3
12–13 years	0.4–3.4	0.0–1.6
14–15 years	0.7–4.3	0.4–2.9
16–17 years	0.9–4.1	1.1–3.1
18–40 years	0.5–4.3	0.9–2.9
≥41 years	0.4–2.7	0.8–2.2
Postmenopausal women	<1.0	
Tanner stage I	<1.6	<0.9
Tanner stage II	<2.2	<1.4
Tanner stage III	0.6–4.4	<2.6
Tanner stage IV–V	0.9–3.8	1.0–3.0

➤ Interpretation
Increased In
- CAH caused by 21-hydroxylase deficiency; marked increase is suppressed to normal levels by adequate glucocorticoid therapy.
  - Suppressed level reflects adequacy of therapeutic control.
  - Androstenedione may be better than 17-hydroxyprogesterone for monitoring therapy because it shows minimal diurnal variation, better correlation with urinary 17-KS excretion, and plasma levels that are not immediately affected by a dose of glucocorticoid.
- Adrenal tumors
- Cushing disease
- Polycystic ovarian disease

Decreased In
- Addison disease

ANGIOTENSIN II

➤ Definition
- Angiotensin II is an oligopeptide of eight amino acids, formed from its original precursor, angiotensinogen, by a series of two enzymatic cleavages. Angiotensinogen is released into the circulation by the liver. Renin, produced by the kidney, in response to glomerular hypoperfusion, catalyzes cleavage of angiotensinogen to angiotensin I, a decapeptide. Angiotensin I is in turn cleaved by ACE to produce the octapeptide angiotensin II.
- The concentration of ACE is highest in the lung, and it had been thought that most angiotensin II formation occurred in the pulmonary circulation. It is now clear, however, that ACE is produced in the vascular endothelium of many tissues; therefore, angiotensin II can be synthesized at a variety of sites, including the kidney, vascular endothelium, adrenal gland, and brain.
- In addition, alternative enzymatic pathways not involving ACE may contribute to angiotensin II production. Angiotensin II binds to its specific receptors and exerts its effects in the brain, kidney, adrenal, vascular wall, and the heart.
- The actions of circulating angiotensin II contribute to hypertension. This may indirectly influence cardiac function, irrespective of any direct effect on the heart and myocardium.
  - Circulating angiotensin II promotes sodium and water reabsorption, increasing intravascular fluid volume, which in turn increases cardiac preload and, therefore, stroke volume.
  - Circulating angiotensin II causes systemic arteriolar vasoconstriction, thereby increasing vascular resistance and cardiac afterload.
  - Angiotensin II also affects the autonomic nervous system, stimulating the sympathetic nervous system and reducing vagal activity.
- These actions are oriented toward maintaining the blood pressure when the renin–angiotensin system is activated by effective volume depletion.
- **Normal range:** 10–60 pg/mL

➤ Use
* Evaluating hypertension

➤ Interpretation
Increased In
* Hypertension
* Renin-secreting juxtaglomerular renal tumor
* Volume depletion
* CHF

Decreased In
* Anephric patients
* Primary aldosteronism
* Cushing syndrome

➤ Limitations
* Patient should be on normal sodium diet and be recumbent for 30 minutes before specimen collection.
* Due to stability issues, plasma should be separated and frozen immediately.

ANGIOTENSIN-CONVERTING ENZYME (ACE, KINASE II)

➤ Definition
* ACE production occurs mainly in the epithelial cells of the pulmonary bed. Smaller amounts are found in blood vessels and renal tissue, where ACE converts angiotensin I to angiotensin II; this conversion helps regulate arterial blood pressure.
* Angiotensin II stimulates the adrenal cortex to produce aldosterone. Aldosterone helps the kidneys maintains water balance by retaining sodium and promoting the excretion of potassium.
* **Normal range:** 8–53 U/L

➤ Use
* Evaluation of patients with suspected sarcoidosis
* Evaluate the severity and activity of sarcoidosis
* Evaluation of hypertension
* Evaluation of Gaucher disease

➤ Interpretation
Increased In
* Active pulmonary sarcoidosis (50–75% of patients but only 11% with inactive disease
* Gaucher disease (100%)
* DM ($>$24%)
* Hyperthyroidism (81%)
* Leprosy (53%)
* Chronic renal disease
* Cirrhosis (25%)
* Silicosis ($>$20%)

- Berylliosis (75%)
- Amyloidosis
- TB infection
- Connective tissue diseases
- Untreated hyperthyroidism
- Fungal disease, histoplasmosis

Decreased In
- Far advanced lung neoplasms
- Anorexia nervosa associated with hypothyroidism

➤ Limitations
- False-positive rate equals 2–4%.
- Levels may be normal in lymphoma and lung cancer.
- Serum ACE is significantly reduced in patients on ACE inhibitors (e.g., Enalapril and captopril).
- The reference interval for children and adolescents may be as much as 50% higher than specimens from adults.
- Serum ACE abnormality has been reported in 20–30% of $\alpha1$-antitrypsin variants (MZ, ZZ, and MS Pi types) but in only about 1% of individuals with normal MM Pi type. There is evidence that paraquat poisoning (because of its effect on pulmonary capillary endothelium) is associated with elevated serum ACE.

ANION GAP (AG)

➤ Definition
- The AG is an arithmetic approximation of difference between routinely measured serum anions (23) and cations (11) = 12 mmol/L.
- Unmeasured ions include proteins (mostly albumin) = 15 mmol/L, organic acids = 5 mmol/L, phosphates = 2 mmol/L, sulfates = 1 mmol/L; total = 23 mmol/L.
- Unmeasured cations include calcium = 5 mmol/L, potassium = 4.5 mmol/L, magnesium = 1.5 mmol/L; total = 11 mmol/L.
- Calculated as $Na^+ - (Cl^- + HCO_3^-)$; **typical normal values** = 8–16 mmol/L; **if K^+ is included, normal** = 10–20 mmol/L; reference interval varies considerably depending on instrumentation and between individuals. Increased AG reflects amount of organic (e.g., lactic acid, ketoacids) and fixed acids present.
- AG initially began as a measure of quality assurance.

➤ Use
- Identify cause of a metabolic acidosis
- Supplement to laboratory quality control, along with its components

➤ Interpretation
Increased In
- Organic (e.g., lactic acidosis, ketoacidosis)
- Inorganic (e.g., administration of phosphate, sulfate)
- Protein (e.g., hyperalbuminemia, transient)

- Exogenous (e.g., salicylate, formate, paraldehyde, nitrate, penicillin, carbenicillin)
- Not completely identified (e.g., hyperosmolar hyperglycemic nonketotic coma, uremia, poisoning by ethylene glycol, methanol)
- Artifactual
  - Falsely increased serum sodium
  - Falsely decreased serum chloride or bicarbonate
- When AG >12–14 mmol/L, diabetic ketoacidosis is the most common cause, uremic acidosis is the second most common cause, and drug ingestion (e.g., salicylates, methyl alcohol, ethylene glycol, ethyl alcohol) is the third most common cause; lactic acidosis should always be considered when these three causes are ruled out. In small children, rule out inborn errors of metabolism.

Decreased In
- Hypoalbuminemia (most common cause), hypocalcemia, hypomagnesemia
- Artifactual
- "Hyperchloremia" in bromide intoxication (if chloride determination by colorimetric method)
- False increase in serum chloride or HCO_3^-
- False decrease in serum sodium (e.g., hyperlipidemia, hyperviscosity)
  - Increased unmeasured cations
  - Hyperkalemia, hypercalcemia, hypermagnesemia
- Increased proteins in multiple myeloma, paraproteinemias, polyclonal gammopathies (these abnormal proteins are positively charged and lower the AG)
- Increased lithium, tris buffer (tromethamine)
  - AG >30 mmol/L almost always indicates organic acidosis, even in the presence of uremia.
  - AG of 20–29 mmol/L occurs in absence of identified organic acidosis in 25% of patients.
  - AG is rarely >23 mmol/L in chronic renal failure.
- Simultaneous changes in ions may cancel each other out, leaving AG unchanged (e.g., increased Cl^- and decreased HCO_3^-). The change in AG should equal change in HCO_3^-; otherwise a mixed, rather than simple, acid–base disturbance is present.

ANTIARRHYTHMIC DRUGS

See Cardiovascular Drugs

ANTIBIOTICS

➤ Definition
- Antibiotics are substances that destroy or inhibit the growth of microorganisms.
- Antibiotics consist of chemical groups such as β-lactams, polyenes, macrolides, tetracyclines, aminoglycosides, and sulfonamides. Names include amikacin, chloramphenicol, gentamicin, kanamycin, streptomycin, tobramycin, and vancomycin.
- **Normal therapeutic (and toxic) levels:** see Table 2-5

➤ Use
- Prevention and treatment of infections caused by bacteria

TABLE 2-5. Therapeutic and Toxic Serum Concentrations for Antibiotics	Therapeutic Concentration (μg/mL)	Potentially Toxic Level (μg/mL)
Amikacin		
Peak	15–25	>30
Trough	2–5	>8
Chloramphenicol		
Peak	10–20	25
Trough	5–10	15
Gentamicin		
Peak	5–10	12
Trough	0.5–2	>2
Kanamycin		
Peak	20–25	
Trough	5–10	
Netilmicin		
Peak	4–8	8
Trough	1–2	2
Streptomycin		
Peak	5–20	40
Trough	<5	40
Tobramycin		
Peak	5–10	12
Trough	0.5–2	>2
Trimethoprim/sulfamethoxazole		
Peak (trimethoprim)	4–8	8
Peak (sulfamethoxazole)	1–2	>2
Vancomycin		
Peak (not recommended)	30–40	>80
Trough	5–10	>20

➤ **Limitations**

• Testing must be performed on serum or plasma.
• Peak concentrations: collect specimen 30–120 minutes after completion of infusion (drug and route dependent).
• Trough concentrations: collect specimen 5–90 minutes before next infusion (drug dependent).
• Testing methodologies: immunoassay (e.g., fluorescence polarization) or HPLC
• *Specimens must be frozen* for streptomycin and amphotericin B.
• Specimens must be protected from light for trimethoprim and amphotericin.
• Unacceptable specimens:
  • Hemolyzed
  • Collection tubes with additives such as serum separator, citrate, oxalate, or fluoride
• Trimethoprim may be detected in urine in general toxicology screens utilizing GC/MS.

ANTICARDIOLIPIN ANTIBODIES (ACAs)

➤ Definition

- Cardiolipins, and other related phospholipids, are lipid molecules found in cell membranes and platelets. They play an important role in the blood clotting process. When antibodies are formed against cardiolipins (ACAs against IgG, IgM, and IgA), they increase an affected patient's risk of developing recurrent inappropriate blood clots (thrombi) in both arteries and veins.
- Other names include anti-phospholipid antibodies.
- **Normal range:** see Table 2-6

➤ Use

- Evaluation of suspected cases of antiphospholipid antibody syndrome (APS)
- ACAs are present in APS, SLE, acute infections, HIV, certain cancers, and with some drug (e.g., phenytoin, penicillin, procainamide). They occur in the general population, with the prevalence increasing with age.

➤ Interpretation

- APS is present if at least one of the clinical criteria and one of the laboratory criteria that follow are met
  - **Clinical criteria**
    - **Vascular thrombosis**
      - One or more clinical episodes of arterial, venous, or small vessel thrombosis, in any tissue or organ. Thrombosis must be confirmed by objective validated criteria (i.e., unequivocal findings of appropriate imaging studies or histopathology). For histopathologic confirmation, thrombosis should be present without significant evidence of inflammation in the vessel wall.
  - **Pregnancy morbidity**
    a) One or more unexplained deaths of a morphologically normal fetus at or beyond the 10th week of gestation, with normal fetal morphology documented by ultrasound or by direct examination of the fetus, or
    b) One or more premature births of a morphologically normal neonate before the 34th week of gestation because of: (i) eclampsia or severe preeclampsia defined according to standard definitions, or (ii) recognized features of placental insufficiency, or
    c) Three or more unexplained consecutive spontaneous abortions before the 10th week of gestation, with maternal anatomic or hormonal abnormalities and paternal and maternal chromosomal causes excluded.
    d) In studies of populations of patients who have more than one type of pregnancy morbidity, investigators are strongly encouraged to stratify groups of subjects according to a, b, or c above.

TABLE 2-6. Normal Levels of Anticardiolipin Antibodies

	Negative	Indeterminate	Positive	Strong Positive
IgG antibody	<15 GPL	15–19 GPL	20–80 GPL	>80 GPL
IgM antibody	<15 MPL	17–19 MPL	20–80 MPL	>80 MPL
IgA antibody	<12 APL	12–19 APL	20–80 APL	>80 APL

- **Laboratory criteria.** (Investigators are strongly advised to classify APS patients in studies into one of the following categories: I, more than one laboratory criteria present (any combination); IIa, LA present alone; IIb, aCL antibody present alone; IIc, anti-β2 glycoprotein-I antibody present alone.)
  - LAs present in plasma, on two or more occasions at least 12 weeks apart, detected according to the guidelines of the International Society on Thrombosis and Haemostasis (Scientific Subcommittee on LAs/phospholipid-dependent antibodies).
  - ACA of IgG and/or IgM isotype in serum or plasma, present in medium or high titer (i.e., >40 GPL or MPL, or >the 99th percentile), on two or more occasions, at least 12 weeks apart, measured by a standardized ELISA.
  - Anti-β2 glycoprotein-I antibody of IgG and/or IgM isotype in serum or plasma (in titer >99th percentile), present on two or more occasions, at least 12 weeks apart, measured by a standardized ELISA, according to recommended procedures.

➤ Limitations

- The cardiolipin IgA isotype is usually detected with either IgG or IgM isotypes in patients with APS; however, agreement among patients grouped according to cardiolipin titers for IgA seems lower than those for the other types. In patients with collagen disease, IgA associates with thrombocytopenia, skin ulcers, and vasculitis, indicating a patient subgroup at risk for specific clinical manifestations, and it is highly prevalent in African American patients with SLE. Hence, this isotype appears to identify patient subgroups rather than adding diagnostic power.
- A negative result means only that the cardiolipin antibody class tested (IgG, IgM, and/or IgA) is not present at this time. Because cardiolipin antibodies are the most common of the antiphospholipid antibodies, it is not unusual to find them emerging, temporarily due to an infection or drug, or asymptomatically as a person ages. The low to moderate concentrations of antibody seen in these situations are frequently not significant, but they must be examined in conjunction with a patient's symptoms and other clinical information.

➤ Suggested Reading

Miyakis S, Lockshin MD, Atsumi T, et al. International consensus statement on an update of the classification criteria for definite antiphospholipid syndrome (APS). *J Thromb Haemost.* 2006;4:295–306.

ANTICOAGULANTS, CIRCULATING

➤ Definition

- Circulating anticoagulants are antibodies that inhibit the function of specific coagulation factors, most commonly factors VIII or IX. They may be acquired following multiple transfusions in hemophiliacs (alloantibodies) or spontaneous (autoantibodies)—again, most commonly against factor VIII.
- Lupus Anticoagulants (LA) is sometimes clinically associated with circulating anticoagulants

➤ Use

- A circulating anticoagulant is suspected under two conditions:
  - A patient with hemophilia A or B who has had multiple transfusions and whose bleeding does not stop on infusion of the missing factor

* A middle-aged person, especially with lymphoma, or a postpartum patient who develops unprovoked hemorrhages

➤ Interpretation

* In a patient with hemophilia, serial determinations of the missing factor show no elevations following infusions.
* In a patient with no previous bleeding history, the finding of a prolonged PTT should raise the suspicion of an acquired circulating anticoagulant. If incubation at 37°C of half the normal plasma with half the patient's plasma for 1–2 hours does not correct the prolonged PTT, a circulating anticoagulant is present.
* Specific titration of the inhibitor's potency is performed either for factor VIII or IX inhibitors, and the results are reported in Bethesda Inhibitor Units.

ANTICOAGULATION DNA PANEL

➤ Definition

* The anticoagulation DNA panel tests for genetic variants in the *CYP2C9* and *VKORC1* genes, which account for >50% of variation in warfarin response. Genotyping may reduce the need for INR surveillance as genotype-based dosing regimens are established.
* Variants tested by the anticoagulation panel include:
  * *CYP2C9* (alleles: *1 (normal)
  * *2 (430C>T; Arg144Cys)
  * *3 (1075A>C; Ile359Leu))
  * *VKORC1* (alleles*1 (normal)
  * *2 promoter variant (−1639G>A)
* **Normal values:**
  * *CYP2C9* *1/*1
  * *VKORC1* *1/*1

➤ Use

* Initiating warfarin (Coumadin) therapy
* Optimizing dosing for warfarin

➤ Limitations

* The results of a genetic test may be affected by DNA rearrangements, blood transfusion, bone marrow transplantation, or other rare events.

ANTICONVULSANTS

➤ Definition

* A compound used to prevent or treat seizures.
* Classic agents: carbamazepine [Tegretol], phenobarbital [Luminal], phenytoin [Dilantin], ethosuximide [Zarontin], valproic acid [Depakene, Depakote]
* Newer agents gabapentin [Neurontin], lamotrigine [Lamictal], oxcarbazepine [Trileptal], vigabatrin [Sabril], topiramate [Topamax], zonisamide [Zonegran]
* **Normal therapeutic levels:** see Table 2-7

TABLE 2-7. Normal Therapeutic Levels of Anticonvulsants	
Drug	Level (µg/L serum/plasma)
Carbamazepine	6.0–12
10,11-epoxide	0.2–2.0
Phenobarbital	15–40
Phenytoin	10–20
Ethosuximide	40–100
Valproic acid	50–100
Gabapentin	2.2–6.1
Lamotrigine	0.4–9.0
Oxcarbazepine	0.5–1.2
10-hydroxy-carbazepine	3.7–37
Vigabatrin	18–77
Topiramate	1.7–8.0
Zonisamide	2.9–28

➤ Use
- Treatment of seizure disorders

➤ Limitations
- Phenobarbital may be detected by immunoassay-based screening tests for barbiturates in urine and serum.
- Immunoassay tests are available for semiquantitative analysis in serum of topiramate, valproic acid, phenytoin, phenobarbital (may demonstrate significant cross reactivity with other barbiturates), and zonisamide.
- Lamotrigine, breakdown products or artifacts of topiramate, carbamazepine, 10-OH-carbazepine, and phenytoin may be detected in general drug screens in urine or serum that utilize alkaline or weakly acidic liquid or solid phase extractions followed by gas chromatography or GC/MS analysis.
- For the majority of anticonvulsants, specific tests are required.
- Quantitative and confirmation tests: sample pretreatment followed by:
  - Gas chromatography
  - HPLC
  - GC/MS
  - LC/MS (mass spectrometry)
  - Target analyte-parent drug except oxcarbazepine
  - Limit of quantitation: drug dependent—typically 1–5 µg/mL

ANTIDEPRESSANTS

➤ Definition
- Multicyclic compounds that inhibit the reuptake of neurotransmitters or block their metabolism, resulting in an increase concentration of monamines in the synapse

TABLE 2-8. Normal Therapeutic Levels for Antidepressants*

Drug/Drug Combination	Normal Level (ng/ml)	Potentially Toxic Level (ng/ml)
Amitriptyline + nortriptyline	95–250	>500
Nortriptyline	50–150	> 500
Imipramine + desipramine	150–300	>500
Desipramine	100–300	>500
Doxepin + nordoxepin	100–300	>400
Protriptyline	70–240	>400
Bupropion	50–100	
Trazodone	800–1600	
Fluoxetine	50–480, with 20–60 mg/day	
Norfluoxetine	50–450, with 20–60 mg/day	
Clomipramine + norclomipramine	220–500	>900#

*Not established for all drugs in this class.
#When used as an antidepressant, therapeutic range not well established when prescribed for obsessive compulsive disorder.

- Tricyclic antidepressants [TCAs]: amitriptyline [Elavil®], nortriptyline, doxepin, imipramine [Tofranil®], desipramine, trimipramine, protriptyline, clomipramine [Anafranil®]
- Selective serotonin reuptake inhibitors [SSRIs]: fluoxetine [Prozac®], sertraline [Zoloft®], fluvoxamine [Luvox®], citalopram [Celexa®], paroxetine [Paxil®]
- Other agents:
  - Amoxapine [Moxadil®], maprotiline, trazodone [Desyrel®], bupropion [Wellbutrin®]
  - Venlafaxine [Effexor®], mirtazapine [Remeron®], nefazodone [Serzone®], duloxetine [Cymbalta®]
- **Normal range:** see Table 2-8; not established for all drugs in this class

➤ Use

- Treatment of mood disorders and depression

➤ Limitations

- Immunoassay screening of serum/plasma/urine for TCAs does not detect other antidepressants (e.g., SSRIs)
- Available immunoassays: EIA, EMIT, ELISA, FPIA
- Target analytes: imipramine, nortriptyline
- Cut-off concentrations:
  - 10–50 ng/mL ELISA
  - 300 or 500 ng/mL EIA qualitative
  - 150 ng/mL EIA semiquantitative
- Variable cross-reactivity with other TCAs, metabolites: consult manufacturer's package insert
- Will not detect SSRIs and newer antidepressants
- No SSRI–specific immunoassays are currently available.

- General drug screens comprising alkaline liquid–liquid extraction or solid-phase extraction followed by GC/MS or gas chromatography analysis detect TCAs, SSRIs, trazodone, bupropion, venlafaxine, mirtazapine, and amoxapine with limit of detection ranging from 20–250 ng/mL
- Confirmation and quantitative analysis
  - Gas chromatography
  - HPLC
  - GC/MS
  - LC/MSn (multiple MS)
  - Measures drug and metabolites
  - Limit of quantitation: approximately 10 ng/mL

ANTIDIURETIC HORMONE

➤ Definition
- Antidiuretic hormone (ADH), also known as vasopressin or arginine vasopressin, is a hormone secreted by the posterior pituitary.
- It regulates the water permeability of renal collecting ducts and urine concentrating ability by increasing water reabsorption, which is mediated by transcellular water channels (aquaporins).
- **Normal range:** <1.5 pg/mL (see Table 2-9 for effect of plasma osmolality on ADH levels)

➤ Use
- Diagnosis and differential diagnosis of DI and psychogenic polyuria
- Diagnosis of SIADH
- Differential diagnosis of hyponatremias

➤ Interpretation
Increased In
- Nephrogenic DI (partial or complete): high ADH and low osmolality
- Primary psychogenic polydipsia
- SIADH inappropriately increased for degree of plasma osmolality (i.e., normal ADH relative to osmolality)
- Ectopic ADH syndrome
- Certain drugs (e.g., chlorpropamide, phenothiazine, Tegretol)

TABLE 2-9. Plasma Osmolality Influences on ADH Levels	
Values in mOsm/kg	Values in pg/mL
270–280	<1.5
280–285	<2.5
285–290	1–5
290–295	2–7
295–300	4–12

Decreased In
- Central DI (partial or complete): decreased for level of plasma osmolality
- Psychogenic polydipsia
- Nephrotic syndrome

➤ Limitations
- Higher secretion occurs at night, in erect posture, with pain, stress, or exercise, and with increased plasma osmolality.
- Lower secretion occurs in recumbency, hypoosmolality, volume expansion, and hypertension.
- Plasma sample should not be left at room temperature.

ANTIHYPERTENSIVES

See Cardiovascular Drugs

ANTI-INFLAMMATORIES

See Acetaminophen, Salicylates

ANTINEOPLASTICS

See Methotrexate

ANTINEUTROPHIL CYTOPLASMIC ANTIBODY (ANCA)

➤ Definition
- ANCA testing plays a critical role in the diagnosis and classification of vasculitides. It is associated with a number of vasculitides, including Wegener granulomatosis (WG), Churg-Strauss syndrome (CSS), microscopic polyangiitis (MPA), and idiopathic necrotizing and crescentic glomerulonephritis.
- Two types of ANCA assays are currently in wide use: IFA and ELISA. Of these two techniques, IFA is more sensitive and ELISA is more specific. The optimal approach to clinical testing for ANCA is, therefore, to screen with IFA and confirm all positive results with ELISAs directed against the vasculitis-specific target antigens proteinase 3 (PR3) and myeloperoxidase antibodies (MPOs).
- When the sera of patients with ANCA-associated vasculitis are incubated with ethanol-fixed human neutrophils, two major IFA patterns are observed: the cytoplasmic neutrophil antibody (cANCA) and perinuclear anti-neutrophil cytoplasmic antibody (pANCA) patterns. Other staining patterns have been described and are generally noted as "atypical."
- Specific immunochemical assays demonstrate that cANCAs comprise mainly antibodies to PR3 and pANCA antibodies to MPO.
- PR3-ANCA pattern has been predominantly associated with cases of active WG and CSS, but many also be seen in MPA.

- MPO-ANCA has been primarily in MPA, CSS, and rarely in WG.
- pANCA pattern variations not associated with MPO (atypical) patterns may be observed on IFA testing in patients with immune-mediated conditions other than systemic vasculitis (e.g., connective tissue disorders, inflammatory bowel disease, infections, and autoimmune hepatitis).
- **Normal value:** negative

➤ Use
- Evaluation of patients suspected of having WG or systemic vasculitis, especially patients with renal disease, pulmonary disease, or unexplained multiorgan disease possibly due to vasculitis.

➤ Interpretation
Increased In
- c-ANCA (PR3-positive):
  - Systemic necrotizing vasculitis
    - Common: WG
    - CSS
    - May also be seen in systemic necrotizing vasculitis of polyarteritis group, pauci-immune type of idiopathic crescentic glomerulonephritis.
  - Propylthiouracil drug
- pANCA (MPO +ve):
  - Systemic necrotizing vasculitis
    - Common: microscopic polyarteritis
    - CSS
    - Uncommon in WG
  - Hydralazine, minocycline, propylthiouracil
- pANCA (to various antigens, MPO-negative):
  - Connective tissue disease
    - Antiphospholipid antibody syndrome
    - Juvenile chronic arthritis
    - Polymyositis/dermatomyositis
    - Relapsing polychondritis
    - RA
    - Sjögren syndrome
    - SLE
  - Inflammatory bowel disease
    - Ulcerative colitis (60–85%)
    - Crohn's disease (10–40%)
    - Bacterial enteritis (rare)
  - Autoimmune liver diseases
    - Primary sclerosing cholangitis
    - Autoimmune hepatitis
  - Infections
    - Chromomycosis
    - HIV-1
    - Acute malaria
  - 5% healthy controls

➤ Limitations

- There is a subjective component to the interpretation of IFA, because the tests are based on visual interpretation of the IF pattern, which is not straightforward. It depends on the experience of the individual who performs the assay.
- ANCA testing is not standardized; the sensitivity and specificity will vary with the laboratory. The cANCA pattern has a greater specificity than the pANCA pattern for vasculitis. However, even positive cANCA IFA results were associated with vasculitis in only 50% of patients.
- Antibodies to a host of azurophilic granule proteins can cause a pANCA staining pattern; these include antibodies directed against lactoferrin, elastase, cathepsin G, bactericidal permeability inhibitor, catalase, lysozyme, β-glucuronidase, and others. A positive pANCA IFA staining pattern may also be detected in a wide variety of inflammatory illnesses and has a low specificity for vasculitis.
- Individuals with ANA frequently have "false-positive" results on ANCA testing by IFA.
- Certain medications may induce forms of vasculitis associated with ANCA. The strongest links between medications and ANCA-associated vasculitis are with drugs employed in the treatment of hyperthyroidism: propylthiouracil, methimazole, and carbimazole. Hydralazine and minocycline are less commonly associated with the induction of ANCA-associated vasculitis. Other implicated drugs include penicillamine, allopurinol, procainamide, thiamazole, clozapine, phenytoin, rifampicin, cefotaxime, isoniazid, and indomethacin.
- Using IFA and ELISA testing in a sequential fashion substantially increases the positive predictive value of an ANCA assay.
- Elevations in the titers of ANCA do *not* predict disease flares in a timely manner. If a patient was ANCA-positive during a period of active disease, a persistently ANCA-negative status is consistent with, but not absolutely proof of, remission.
- ANCA testing should not be used to screen nonselected patient groups where the prevalence of vasculitis is low. These tests are most valuable when selectively ordered in clinical situations where some forms of ANCA-associated vasculitis are seriously considered.
- A negative ANCA result should not be used to exclude disease.

ANTINUCLEAR ANTIBODY (ANA)

➤ Definition

- ANAs refer to a diverse group of antibodies that target nuclear and cytoplasmic antigens. ANAs have been detected in the serum of patients with many rheumatic and nonrheumatic diseases as well as in patients with no definable clinical syndrome. The strong association of ANA with SLE is well established, and this finding satisfies the 1 of 11 criteria available for diagnosis.
- These autoantibodies may be useful as an aid in the diagnosis of systemic rheumatic diseases such as SLE, mixed connective tissue disease (MCTD), undifferentiated connective tissue disease, Sjögren syndrome, scleroderma (systemic sclerosis), polymyositis, and others.
- The diagnosis of a systemic rheumatic disease is based primarily on the presence of compatible clinical signs and symptoms. The results of tests for autoantibodies, including ANA and specific autoantibodies, are ancillary.
- **Normal range:** Negative

➤ Use
• Evaluating patients suspected of having a systemic rheumatic disease

➤ Interpretation
Increased In
• SLE
• Drug-induced SLE
• Lupoid hepatitis
• MCTD
• Polymyositis
• Progressive systemic sclerosis
• RA
• Sjögren syndrome

➤ Limitations
• Some patients without clinical evidence of an autoimmune disease or a systemic rheumatic disease may have a detectable level of ANA. This finding is more common in women than men, and the frequency of a detectable ANA in healthy women >40 years old may approach 15–20%. ANA may also be detectable following viral illnesses, in chronic infections, or in patients treated with many different medications.
• The traditional tool used to detect ANAs is IFA, which is a labor intensive microscopic technique. Test interpretation is operator dependent. This assay is considered the gold standard for ANA testing with greater sensitivity. The IFA testing currently performed using Hep-2 cells, and they contain approximately 100–150 possible antigens and most of them are not well defined and or characterized. When performed with a history and physical examination, it identifies almost all patients with SLE (95% sensitivity), although the specificity of this assay is only 57%. In addition, ANA by IFA has the sensitivity of 85% for systemic sclerosis, 61% for polymyositis/dermatomyositis (PM-DM), 48% for Sjögren syndrome, 57% for juvenile idiopathic arthritis, 100% for drug-induced lupus, 100% for MCTD, and autoimmune hepatitis (60%), as well as being important in monitoring and assessing prognosis in individuals with Raynaud's phenomenon.
• Multiplex immunoassay (MIA) tests have been recently developed for use in clinical laboratory. They utilize individually identifiable, fluorescence microspheres (beads), each coupled with a different antigen or antigen mixture to test for multiple antibodies simultaneously in the same tube. This Multiplex ANA screen is intended for qualitative screening of specific ANAs, the quantitative detection of dsDNA antibodies, and semiquantitative detection of 10 separate antibody assays (chromatin, ribosomal-P, SSA, SSB, Sm, SmRNP, RNP (Ribonucleoprotein), Scl-70 (topoisomerase I), Jo-1 and centromere-B). This ANA by MIA screen detects the presence of clinically relevant circulating autoantibodies in serum. These assays are specific compared to IFA, and they are not as sensitive as IFA, because it is not looking at 100–150 possible antigens in the Hep-2 cells, rather specifically looking at 11 specific targeted antibodies. These assays have typical sensitivities of 66–94% for SLE, 94% Sjögren, 68% for systemic sclerosis, and 48% for PM-DM. They are specific compared to IFA for detecting specific targeted connective tissue disorders. In persons with no connective disease the specificity of MIA ranged from 77–91% and in apparently healthy individuals it is at 93%.

- Disorders associated with a positive ANA titer include chronic infectious diseases, such as mononucleosis, hepatitis C infection, subacute bacterial endocarditis, TB, and HIV, and some lymphoproliferative diseases.
- The presence of ANAs is rarely associated with malignancy, with the exception of dermatomyositis, in which both may be present. ANAs have also been identified in up to 50% of patients taking certain drugs; however, most of these patients do not develop drug-induced lupus.

  Drugs that may cause positive results include carbamazepine, chlorpromazine, ethosuximide, hydralazine, isoniazid, mephenytoin, methyldopa, penicillins, phenytoin, primidone, procainamide, and quinidine.

- **Antibodies to double-stranded DNA (dsDNA)**
  - Moderate to high titers of antibodies directed against dsDNA are very specific (97%) for SLE, making them very useful for diagnosis. Anti-dsDNA have also been found at low frequency (<5 %), and usually in low titer and with low avidity, in patients with RA, Sjögren syndrome, scleroderma, Raynaud phenomenon, MCTD, discoid lupus, myositis, uveitis, juvenile arthritis, antiphospholipid syndrome, Grave disease, Alzheimer disease, and autoimmune hepatitis.
  - Titers of anti-dsDNA antibodies often fluctuate with disease activity and are, therefore, useful in many patients for following the course of SLE.
  - There is a well-recognized association of high titers of IgG anti-dsDNA titers, especially for high avidity antibodies, with active GN; there also appear to be highly enriched amounts of anti-dsDNA antibodies in the glomerular deposits of immune complexes found in patients with lupus nephritis. These observations have led many investigators to believe that anti-dsDNA antibodies are of primary importance in the pathogenesis of lupus nephritis.
  - Anti-dsDNA antibodies have also been reported in patients receiving minocycline, etanercept, infliximab, and penicillamine.
  - An increased frequency of these antibodies has also been noted in some otherwise normal individuals, particularly first-degree relatives of patients with lupus and some laboratory workers.
- **Antibodies to chromatin**
  - Chromatin refers to the complex of histones and DNA. Assaying for the presence of antichromatin (antinucleosome) antibodies may be more clinically relevant than testing for individual antihistone antibodies. Antichromatin antibodies are present in 69% of those with SLE but in 10% or less of patients with Sjögren syndrome, scleroderma, or antiphospholipid syndrome. Among those with SLE, the prevalence of antichromatin antibodies is twofold higher in those with renal disease (58% versus 29%).
- **Anti-Smith antibodies and anti-RNP antibodies**
  - The anti-Smith (anti-Sm) and anti-ribonucleoprotein (anti-RNP) systems are considered together, since they coexist in many patients with SLE and bind to related but distinct antigens.
  - Anti-Sm antibodies occur more frequently in African Americans and Asians than in Caucasians with SLE.
  - Anti-Sm antibodies generally remain positive when titers of anti-DNA antibodies have fallen into the normal range and clinical activity of SLE has waned. Therefore, measurement of anti-Sm titers may be useful diagnostically, particularly at a time when DNA antibodies are undetectable.

- Anti-RNP antibodies bind to antigens that are different from but related to Sm antigens. These antibodies bind to proteins containing only U1-RNA. Anti-RNP antibodies are found in 3–69% of patients with SLE, but are a defining feature in the related syndrome, MCTD. The antibody is present in lower titers in several other rheumatic diseases, including primary Raynaud phenomenon, RA, and scleroderma.
- **Ro/SSA and La/SSB Antibodies**
  - Anti-Ro/SSA and anti-La/SSB antibodies have been detected with high frequency in patients with Sjögren syndrome. They also have diagnostic usefulness in patients with SLE. They are infrequently seen in other connective tissue diseases such as scleroderma, polymyositis, MCTD, and RA.
  - Anti-Ro/SSA antibodies have been associated with photosensitivity, a rash known as subacute cutaneous lupus, cutaneous vasculitis (palpable purpura), interstitial lung disease, neonatal lupus, and congenital heart block connective tissue disease. A minority evolve into a well-defined disorder.
  - Anti-La/SSB antibodies are found in the following circumstances:
    - It is very unusual to encounter sera that contain anti-La/SSB activity without demonstrable antibodies to Ro/SSA in patients with SLE or Sjögren syndrome.
    - Isolated anti-La/SSB antibody activity has been seen in some patients with primary biliary cirrhosis and autoimmune hepatitis.
    - Antibodies to the La/SSB antigen are present in 70–95% of patients with primary Sjögren syndrome, and in 10–35% of patients with SLE, and are occasionally seen in patients with cutaneous LE, scleroderma disorders, and RA.
  - Antibodies to topoisomerase I (Scl-70)
- Antibodies to Scl-70, proteins associated with the centromere (CEN-A, CEN-B), U3-ribonucleoprotein (U-3 RNP), and RNA polymerases I and III. These antibodies are highly specific for systemic sclerosis, and are associated with a higher risk of interstitial lung disease. When present in high titers, they are associated with more extensive skin involvement and disease activity.
- **Antibodies to Ribo-P**
  - The reported incidence of antiribosomal P protein antibodies among patients with SLE is variable. These antibodies were initially detected in 10–20% of patients with SLE; however, several authors (particularly those studying Asian populations and children) have reported higher incidence rates (40–50%). Some clinical data suggest that the presence of antiribosomal P protein antibodies among patients with lupus is associated with lupus cerebritis. The presence of antibodies to ribosomal P protein has an overall sensitivity and specificity for neuropsychiatric lupus of 26 and 80%, respectively. The test characteristics were similar for psychosis, mood disorder, or both (sensitivity 27%, specificity 80%). These antibodies may also be found among patients with lupus hepatitis and/or nephritis.
- **Antibodies to Jo-1**
  - Antibodies to the Jo-1 antigen (histidyl-tRNA synthetase) are found in approximately 30% of adult patients with myositis (including polymyositis, dermatomyositis, and overlap syndromes) and are particularly common (~60%) in patients with both myositis and interstitial lung disease (cryptogenic fibrosing alveolitis or pulmonary interstitial fibrosis). Jo-1 antibodies are most commonly found in patients with the anti-synthetase syndrome, which is characterized by acute onset, steroid-responsive myositis with interstitial lung disease, fever, symmetrical arthritis, Raynaud phenomenon, and mechanic's hands. The presence

of Jo-1 antibodies in idiopathic polymyositis patients is usually accompanied by severe disease, tendency to relapse, and poor prognosis.

ANTIPSYCHOTICS

➤ Definition
- Antipsychotics are neuroleptic drugs in the following groups: phenothiazines, thioxanthenes, dibenzoxazepines, dihydro indoles, butyrophenones, and diphenylbutylpiperidine and alkali metal • Typical antipsychotics: chlorpromazine [Thorazine], fluphenazine [Permitil], thioridazine [Mellaril], thioxanthene, haloperidol [Haldol], loxapine [Loxitane]
- Atypical antipsychotics: clozapine [Clozaril], olanzapine [Zyprexa], quetiapine [Seroquel], risperidone [Risperdal]
- Other agent: lithium [Lithobid]
- **Normal range:** see Table 2-10

➤ Use
- Treatment of psychoses, schizophrenia, mania, Tourette syndrome (haloperidol)

➤ Limitations
- Suitable for serum, urine
- Immunoassay: RIA—nonspecific, semiquantitative due to varying cross reactivity with parent drug and metabolites
- Fluorometry: nonspecific, semiquantitative due to interferences from metabolites
- Extraction followed by:
  - Gas chromatography: fluphenazine and haloperidol may require derivatization
  - HPLC
  - GC/MS
  - LC/MS
  - Suitable for serum, urine
  - Chromatographic methods are not appropriate for lithium
  - Limit of quantitation: drug dependent (e.g., 1–2 ng/mL for haloperidol, 25 ng/mL clozapine)
- Lithium:
  - Measured by flame emission or atomic absorption spectrophotometry, inductively coupled plasma-mass spectrometry, ion selective electrode

TABLE 2-10. Normal Levels of Antidepressants

	Normal Range	Toxic Level
Lithium	0.4–1.0 mEq/L [serum trough—12 h post dose]	>1.5 mEq/L
Haloperidol	2.0–15.0 ng/mL	
Olanzapine	5–75 ng/mL	
Clozapine	100–700 ng/mL	
Fluphenazine	0.2–2.0 ng/mL	
Chlorpromazine	Adult therapeutic: 50–300 ng/mL	Adult: >500 ng/mL
	Child therapeutic: 30–80 ng/mL	Child: >200 ng/mL

* Suitable for serum, urine
* Erythrocytes possible
* Remove serum from clot as soon as possible
* Collect in serum separator tubes or sodium heparin
* Lithium heparin and sodium fluoride/potassium oxalate tubes are unacceptable
* Hemolyzed specimens are unacceptable

ANTI-SPERM ANTIBODIES (DIRECT)

➤ Definition
* The immunobead binding test for anti-sperm antibodies identifies antibodies on sperm cells by Ig class and general specificity (head, mid-piece, tail) by means of their ability to agglutinate polyacrylamide beads coated with anti-Ig class-specific antibodies.

➤ Use
* Detection of agglutinated sperm and/or reduced motility in a semen analysis might suggest the presence of anti-sperm antibodies on the cells, which could be associated with impaired fertility. Only the IgG and IgA classes of such antibodies are clinically significant.

➤ Interpretation
Increased In
* >20% of sperm cells bound to immunobeads: presence of clinically significant levels of anti-sperm antibodies on the cells

Decreased In
* No lower limit defined

Normal In
* ≤20% of sperm cells bound to immunobeads

➤ Limitations
* Minimum specimen volume for analysis is 0.1 mL

ANTITHROMBIN (AT)

➤ Definition
* AT, also known as antithrombin III, is a natural inhibitor of thrombin and of other clotting factors essential in the coagulation cascade. It is synthesized in the liver.
* In the presence of heparin, the activity of AT is enhanced approximately 1000 times.
* **Normal range (for functional activity):** 75–125%. The functional assay can be performed in a clot detection system or in a chromogenic one. The antigen normal range is the same as for the functional assay, but the assay is rarely necessary in clinical practice.

➤ Use
* Because deficiency of AT may result in a thrombophilic syndrome (see p. 887), determination of AT is indicated in cases suspected of congenital thrombophilia. It is also of help in determining the prognosis in DIC because levels become markedly decreased in severe cases.

➤ Interpretation

* Acquired deficiencies have been reported in severe liver disease, some malignancies, use of oral contraceptives, nephrotic syndrome, and severe infections, especially if associated with DIC (the assay is useful in determining the severity of DIC: it decreases in parallel with increasing severity of the syndrome).
* AT is not affected by deficiency in vitamin K or by vitamin K antagonists.
* It decreases during heparin therapy.
* Severe deficiency may result in diminished anticoagulant effect of heparin.

➤ Limitations

* Clotted specimen, incomplete filling of test tubes, severe lipemia, icteric samples, and hemolysis produce unreliable results.
* Heparin therapy interferes with the coagulant assay but not with the chromogenic one.
* AT results are affected by the use of thrombin inhibitors such as hirudin (or its congeners) or argatroban and the newer antithrombin drugs.

APOLIPOPROTEINS (APO) A-1 AND B

➤ Definition

* An apolipoprotein is a protein component of lipoprotein that regulates their metabolism and each of four major groups consists of a family of two or more immunologically distinct proteins.
* Apolipoprotein A (apo-A; also known as Apo A-1) is the major protein (90%) of HDL.
* Apolipoprotein B (apo B) is major protein component of low-density lipoprotein and is important in regulating cholesterol synthesis and metabolism.
* **Normal range:**
  * Apo A-1
    * Male: 94–178 mg/dL
    * Female: 101–199 mg/dL
  * Apo B
    * Male: 55–140 mg/dL
    * Female: 55–125 mg/dL
  * Apo B/A-1 ratio
    * One half risk
      * Male: 0.4
      * Female: 0.3
  * Average risk
    * Male: 1.0
    * Female: 0.9
  * Twice average risk
    * Male: 1.6
    * Female: 1.5

➤ Use

* To evaluate the risk of CAD. Levels of apo A-1 are inversely associated with premature cardiovascular disease and peripheral vascular disease. The ratio of apo A to apo B has greater sensitivity and specificity for CAD than individual lipid or lipoproteins.

➤ Interpretation
Apo A-1 Increased In
* Familial hyperalphalipoproteinemia (rare genetic disorder)

Apo A-1 Decreased In
* Nephrosis and chronic renal failure
* Familial hypoalphalipoproteinemia (rare genetic disorder)
* Uncontrolled diabetes
* Apo C-II deficiency
* Apo A-1 melano disease
* Apo A-1-C-III deficiency
* Hepatocellular disease

Apo Disorders Increased In
* Hepatic disease
* Hyperlipoproteinemia IIa, IIb, and V
* Cushing syndrome
* Porphyria
* Werner syndrome
* Diabetes
* Familial combined hyperlipidemia
* Hypothyroidism
* Nephrotic syndrome, renal failure

Apo B Decreased In
* Tangier disease
* Hyperthyroidism
* Hypo-beta-lipoproteinemia
* Apo C-II deficiency
* Malnutrition
* Reye syndrome
* Severe illness
* Surgery
* Abetalipoproteinemia
* Cirrhosis

➤ Limitations
* Drugs that affect apo A-1
  * Increased: carbamazepine, estrogens, ethanol, lovastatin, niacin, oral contraceptives, phenobarbital, pravastatin, simvastatin
  * Decreased: androgens, beta blockers, diuretics, and progestins
* Other factors that affect apo A-1
  * Increased: exercise
  * Decreased: smoking, pregnancy, diet high in polyunsaturated fats, weight reduction
* Drugs that affect apo B
  * Increased: androgens, beta blockers, diuretics, progestins
  * Decreased: estrogen, lovastatin, simvastatin, niacin, and thyroxine

* Other factors that affect apo B
  * Increased: pregnancy
  * Decreased: diet high in polyunsaturated fats and low cholesterol, weight reduction
* Other: apo A-1 and apo B are acute phase reactants and thus should not measured in sick patients.

ARRAY COMPARATIVE GENOMIC HYBRIDIZATION (aCGH) (GENOMIC MICROARRAY ANALYSIS)

➤ Definition
* This technology uses probes covering the entire genome and can detect chromosome abnormalities up to 10 times smaller than those detectable by conventional chromosome analysis.

➤ Use
* Detection of chromosome abnormalities (copy number changes; e.g., deletion, duplication) up to 10 times smaller than can be detected by conventional chromosome analysis
* Detection of abnormalities that may be causal for developmental delay, autism, and congenital anomalies. Some laboratories are offering aCGH for prenatal diagnosis.
* Cancer-appropriate arrays are in initial development.

➤ Interpretation
* **Normal:** Two copies for all tested sequences in diploid cells
* **Abnormal:** Copy number less than or greater than two

➤ Limitations
* aCGH *cannot* detect balanced rearrangements that may play a role in repeat pregnancy loss and cancer.
* Interpretation of results is not always straightforward; some detected imbalances may be of no clinical significance. Variant databases are in development.

BENZODIAZEPINES

➤ Definition
* A class of drugs with a three-ringed chemical structure consisting of a benzene ring, a seven-member diazepine ring, and a phenyl ring attached to the 5 position of the diazepine ring. The CNS depressant activity of these drugs is mediated through the neurotransmitter, GABA.
* Specific agents: alprazolam [Xanax], chlordiazepoxide [Librium], diazepam [Valium], temazepam [Restoril], oxazepam [Serax], flunitrazepam [Rohypnol], lorazepam [Ativan], midazolam [Versed], clonazepam [Klonopin], triazolam [Halcion]
* **Normal range:** see Table 2-11

➤ Use
* Assistance in the treatment of panic attacks, panic disorders, and agoraphobia (alprazolam, clonazepam)
* Treatment of anxiety (diazepam, lorazepam)

TABLE 2-11. Reference Ranges of Benzodiazepines	
	Normal Range (serum/plasma; (ng/mL)
Alprazolam	10–100
Chlordiazepoxide	500–2500
Clonazepam	5–75
Diazepam	100–1500 (may be higher to control alcohol withdrawal and in schizophrenic patients)
Flunitrazepam	10–20
Lorazepam	5–240
Midazolam	8–150 (higher for surgical anesthesia; may be >1000)
Oxazepam	300–1500
Temazepam	200–1200
Triazolam	2–10

- Treatment of seizures (diazepam, clonazepam)
- Treatment of insomnia (temazepam, triazolam)
- Preoperative sedation and to assist in induction of surgical anesthesia (midazolam, diazepam, lorazepam)
- Muscle relaxant (diazepam)
- Treatment of alcohol dependence (chlordiazepoxide, diazepam)

➤ Interpretation

- When evaluating concentrations in plasma/serum, effect of multiple active moieties must be considered. When evaluating concentrations in urine, metabolite rather than parent may be detected. Active metabolites are:
  - Alprazolam: alpha-hydroxy alprazolam
  - Flunitrazepam: 7-aminoflunitrazepam
  - Midazolam: alphahydroxy and 4-hydroxy midazolam
  - Triazolam: alphahydroxy and 4-hydroxy triazolam
  - Diazepam: nordazepam, temazepam, oxazepam
  - Chlordiazepoxide: demoxepam, norchlordiazepoxide, nordiazepam, oxazepam
  - Temazepam: oxazepam

➤ Limitations

- Testing: screening by immunoassay for urine and serum
  - ELISA (serum)
    - Target analyte: temazepam
    - Cut-off concentration: 10 ng/mL
    - No cross-reactivity with clonazepam, flunitrazepam, lorazepam and metabolites, and oxazepam
  - EMIT (serum/urine)
    - Target analyte: nitrazepam (urine), diazepam (serum)
    - Cutoff concentration: 200 or 300 ng/mL urine, 50 ng/mL serum
    - Due to low cross-reactivity, will *not* detect flunitrazepam, clonazepam, lorazepam (urine); low cross-reactivity with chlordiazepoxide and demoxepam (serum)
    - Cross-reactivity with alprazolam manufacturer (vendor) dependent

* Confirmation for urine and serum
  * Sample pretreatment necessary
  * Derivatization may be necessary for metabolite detection
  * Hydrolysis of urine samples increases detectability
  * Gas chromatography (GC)
  * HPLC
  * Low-dose benzodiazepines may not be measurable by GC and HPLC (triazolam, flunitrazepam)
  * GC/MS
  * LC/MS/mass spectrometry
  * Target drug: parent drug and metabolites
  * Limit of quantitation: typically 5–20 ng/mL

BETA-2 MICROGLOBULIN, SERUM, URINE, CEREBROSPINAL FLUID

➤ Definition

* β_2-Microglobulin is a cell membrane–associated 100 amino acid peptide, a component of the lymphocyte HLA complex. Because it is present on all nucleated cells and is almost totally reabsorbed and catabolized by the proximal tubules, it serves as a marker of immune activation and proximal tubular function. It is found in nearly all body fluids.
* **Normal range:**
  * Serum: males: 0.60–2.28 mg/L; females: 0.60–2.45 mg/L
  * Urine: 0–300 μg/L
  * CSF: 1.5 + 0.2 mg/L

➤ Use

* Prognostic marker for some lymphoproliferative disorders (adult acute lymphocytic leukemia, AIDS).
* Prognosis assessment of multiple myeloma (as a tumor marker, it reflects burden of tumor cells)
* Evaluation of renal tubular disorders, index of GFR
* CSF β_2-microglobulin levels have been used as a disease indicator of a variety of conditions, including multiple sclerosis, neuro-Behçet disease, sarcoidosis, AIDS-dementia complex, and meningeal metastases, especially meningeal dissemination of acute leukemia and malignant lymphoma.

➤ Interpretation
Increased In

* AIDS
* Aminoglycoside toxicity
* Amyloidosis
* Autoimmune disorders
* Breast cancer
* Crohn disease
* Felty syndrome
* Hepatitis

- Hepatoma
- Hyperthyroidism
- Inflammation of all types
- Leukemia (chronic lymphocytic)
- Lung cancer
- Lymphoma
- Multiple myeloma
- Poisoning with heavy metals, such as mercury or cadmium
- Renal dialysis
- Renal disease (glomerular): serum only; renal disease (tubular): urine only
- Sarcoidosis
- SLE
- Vasculitis
- Viral infections (e.g., CMV)

Decreased In
- Renal disease (glomerular): urine only; renal disease (tubular): serum only
- Response to zidovudine (AZT)

➤ Limitations
- Drugs and proteins that may increase serum β_2-microglobulin levels include cefuroxime, cyclosporin A, gentamicin, interferon-α, pentoxifylline, tumor necrosis factor, lithium, and radiographic contrast media.
- Drugs that may decrease serum β_2-microglobulin levels include zidovudine.
- Drugs that may increase urine β_2-microglobulin levels include azathioprine, cisplatin, cyclosporin A, furosemide, gentamicin, mannitol, nifedipine, sisomicin, and tobramycin.
- Drugs that may decrease urine β_2-microglobulin levels include cilostazol.

BICARBONATE (HCO₃), BLOOD

➤ Definition
- Bicarbonate is an indicator of the buffering capacity of the blood. Low bicarbonate indicates that a larger pH change will occur for a given amount of acid or base produced.
- Bicarbonate in the blood is calculated from the pH and PCO_2 using the Henderson-Hasselbalch equation.
- **Normal range:**
  - Arterial: 21–28 mEq/L
  - Venous: 22–29 mEq/L

➤ Use
- Significant indicator of electrolyte dispersion and anion deficit.
- Together with pH determination, bicarbonate measurements are used in the diagnosis and treatment of numerous potentially serious disorders associated with acid–base imbalance in the respiratory and metabolic systems. Some of these conditions are diarrhea, renal tubular acidosis, carbonic anhydrase inhibitors, hyperkalemic acidosis, renal failure, and ketoacidosis.

➤ Interpretation
Increased In
- Primary metabolic alkalosis
- Primary respiratory acidosis

Decreased In
- Primary metabolic acidosis
- Primary respiratory alkalosis

➤ Limitations
- Bicarbonate can be determined by titration, but this is rarely done.
- HCO_3 is the largest fraction contributing to the total CO_2. Therefore, both parameters usually change in the same direction.
- The standard HCO_3 is the concentration of HCO_3 in whole blood at 38°C equilibrated at a PCO_2 of 40 mm Hg with the blood Hb fully oxygenated.

BILIRUBIN; TOTAL, DIRECT, AND INDIRECT

➤ Definition
- These assays are commonly used tests to assess liver function. Daily production of unconjugated bilirubin is mainly from senescent erythrocytes. The half-life of unconjugated bilirubin is <5 minutes. UDP-Glucuronyl transferase catalyzes rapid conjugation of bilirubin to liver; conjugated bilirubin is excreted in bile and is essentially absent from the blood of the normal individuals. Delta bilirubin (bili protein) is produced by reaction of conjugated bilirubin with albumin, and its half–life is 17–20 days.
- Bilirubin is typically measured in two assays for "total" and "direct"; subtracting direct from total gives "indirect bilirubin." The direct bilirubin measures the majority of delta and conjugated bilirubin and a small percentage of unconjugated bilirubin.
- **Normal range:** Age dependent (see Table 2-12)

➤ Use
- Assessing liver function
- Evaluating a wide range of diseases affecting the production, uptake, storage, metabolism, or excretion of bilirubin
- Monitoring the efficacy of neonatal phototherapy

TABLE 2-12. Normal Range of Bilirubin

	Total Bilirubin	
From Age	Reference Range	Critical Range
0–1 day	0.0–6.0 mg/dL	>15 mg/dL
1–2 day	0.0–8.0 mg/dL	>15 mg/dL
2–5 day	0.0–12.0 mg/dL	>15 mg/dL
5 day–4 month	0.3–1.2 mg/dL	>15 mg/dL
Greater than 4 months –	0.3–1.2 mg/dL	none
Direct Bilirubin	0.0–0.4 mg/dL	none

➤ Interpretation
Increased In
• Hepatocellular damage
• Biliary obstruction
• Hemolytic diseases
• Neonatal physiologic jaundice
• Gilbert disease, Crigler-Najjar syndrome
• Hypothyroidism
• Dubin-Johnson syndrome
• Increased conjugated (direct) bilirubin in:
  • Hereditary disorders (e.g., Dubin-Johnson syndrome, rotor syndrome)
  • Hepatic cellular damage (e.g., viral, toxic, alcohol, drugs). Increased conjugated bilirubin may be associated with normal total bilirubin in up to one third of patients with liver diseases.
  • Biliary duct obstruction (extrahepatic or intrahepatic)
  • Infiltrations, space-occupying lesions (e.g., metastases, abscess, granulomas, amyloidosis)
  • Direct bilirubin:
    • 20–40% of total: more suggestive of hepatic than posthepatic jaundice
    • 40–60% of 1: occurs in either hepatic or posthepatic jaundice
    • >50% of total: more suggestive of posthepatic than hepatic jaundice
  • Total serum bilirubin >40 mg/dL indicates hepatocellular rather than extrahepatic obstruction.
• Increased unconjugated (indirect) bilirubin in (conjugated, 20% of total)
  • Increased bilirubin production
  • Hemolytic diseases (e.g., hemoglobinopathies, RBC enzyme deficiencies, DIC, autoimmune hemolysis)
  • Ineffective erythropoiesis (e.g., pernicious anemia)
  • Blood transfusions
  • Hematomas
  • Hereditary disorders (e.g., Gilbert disease, Crigler-Najjar syndrome)
  • Drugs (e.g., causing hemolysis)

Decreased In
• Drugs (e.g., barbiturates)

➤ Limitations
• Specimens should be protected from light and analyzed as soon as possible.
• Compounds that compete for binding sites on serum albumin contribute to lower serum bilirubin levels (e.g., penicillin, sulfisoxazole, acetylsalicylic acid).
• Day to day variations are 15–30% and increase an average of one- to twofold with fasting up to 48 hours.
• Total bilirubin is 33% and 15% lower in African American men and women, respectively, compared to other racial/ethnic groups.
• Light exposure can decrease total bilirubin up to 50% per hour.
• Total serum bilirubin not a sensitive indicator of hepatic dysfunction; it may not reflect degree of liver damage. Must exceed 2.5 mg/dL to produce clinical jaundice; >5 mg/dL seldom occurs in uncomplicated hemolysis unless hepatobiliary disease is also present.

- Total bilirubin is generally less markedly increased in hepatocellular jaundice ($<$10 mg/dL) than in neoplastic obstructions ($\leq$20 mg/dL) or intrahepatic cholestasis.
- In extrahepatic biliary obstruction, bilirubin may rise progressively to a plateau of 30–40 mg/dL (due in part to balance between renal excretion and diversion of bilirubin to other metabolites). Such a plateau tends not to occur in hepatocellular jaundice, and bilirubin may exceed 50 mg/dL (partly due to concomitant renal insufficiency and hemolysis).
- Concentrations are generally higher in obstruction due to carcinoma than due to stones.
- In viral hepatitis, higher serum bilirubin suggests more liver damage and longer clinical course.
- In acute alcoholic hepatitis, $>$5 mg/dL suggests a poor prognosis.
- Increased serum bilirubin with normal ALP suggests constitutional hyperbilirubinemias or hemolytic states.
- Due to renal excretion, maximum bilirubin is 10–35 mg/dL; if renal disease is present, it may reach 75 mg/dL.
- Conjugated bilirubin $>$1.0 mg/dL in an infant always indicates disease.
- Serum bilirubin (conjugated-to-total)
  - $<$20% conjugated: constitutional (e.g., Gilbert disease, Crigler-Najjar syndrome)
- Hemolytic states
  - 20–40% conjugated: favors hepatocellular disease rather than extrahepatic obstruction; disorders of bilirubin metabolism (e.g., Dubin-Johnson, Rotor syndromes)
  - 40–60% conjugated: occurs in either hepatocellular or extrahepatic type
  - $>$50% conjugated: favors extrahepatic obstruction rather than hepatocellular disease

➤ Suggested Readings

Dufour DR, Lott JA, Nolte FS, et al. Diagnosis and monitoring of hepatic injury. I. Performance characteristics of laboratory tests. *Clin Chem.* 2000;46:2027–2049.

Stevenson DK, Wong RJ, Vreman HJ. Reduction in hospital readmission rates for hyperbilirubinemia is associated with use of transcutaneous bilirubin measurements. *Clin Chem.* 2005;51:481–482.

BLEEDING TIME (BT)

➤ Definition

- BT is a functional test for primary hemostasis (platelets and small vessels), infrequently performed nowadays (see below under limitations).
- **Normal range:** 4–7 minutes (slightly longer in women)

➤ Use

- The method of Ivy as modified by Mielke, using a commercially available template, is the best standardized way to perform BT. A blood pressure cuff on the upper arm is inflated to 40 mm Hg, two small skin incisions are made through the template on the volar surface of the forearm, and cessation of bleeding is counted every 30 seconds.
- BT may be used when better standardized equipment is not available for:
  - Work-up of patients with the suspected diagnosis of a platelet defect or von Willebrand disease (see p. 879). Note the extreme variability of BT in patients with von Willebrand disease.
  - Monitoring hemostatic therapy for patients diagnosed with bleeding associated with von Willebrand disease, a thrombocytopathy, or uremia (creatinine $>$1.1 mg/L impairs hemostasis)
  - Prior to kidney biopsy in patients with uremia

➤ Interpretation
* BT is not proven to be of value in the following conditions:
  * Patients with liver disease
  * Patients prior to general surgery, coronary bypass, or coronary stent insertion
  * Patients prior to orthopedic, ear-nose-throat, or neurosurgery
  * In the follow-up of patients receiving ASA, NSAIDs, or antiplatelet drugs (clopidogrel, prasugrel)
  * Patients with myeloproliferative neoplasms or myelodysplastic syndromes
* BT is contraindicated when platelet counts are <50,000 cells/μL because it may be difficult to arrest bleeding at the incision site and the test may be noncontributory.
* BT is not prolonged in coagulation disorders such as the hemophilias.

➤ Limitations
* These include operator's variability in technique, limited precision, accuracy, reproducibility, and also variability in the same patients at different times. "*In vitro*" BT equipment, such as platelet function analyzer (PFA 100) (see p. 293) is better standardized and has better reproducibility.
* Many healthcare organizations have discontinued the use of BT entirely.

BLOOD GAS, pH

➤ Definition
* pH is the negative logarithm of the hydrogen ion concentration and is an index of acidity and alkalinity of the blood. It changes nonlinearly masking magnitude of acid–base disorders.
* The hydrogen ion concentration is dictated by the ratio of two quantities: the HCO_3^- concentration, which is regulated by the kidneys, and the PCO_2, which is controlled by the lungs.
* **Normal range:**
  * Arterial: 7.35–7.45
  * Venous: 7.31–7.41

➤ Use
* To evaluate acid–base disorders

➤ Interpretation
Increased In
* Metabolic alkalosis (plasma bicarbonate excess)
* Excessive alkali administration
* Potassium depletion (GI loss, lack of potassium intake, diuresis)
  * Excess adrenal steroids (Cushing disease, primary aldosteronism)
  * Chronic alkalosis
  * Potassium-losing nephropathy
* Respiratory alkalosis (decreased dissolved CO_2)
  * Hysteria
  * Stimulation of respiratory center by increased intracranial pressure

- Hypoxia with normal overall alveolar diffusion of CO_2
- Fever
- Salicylate poisoning (early)
- Excessive artificial ventilation

Decreased In
- Metabolic acidosis (bicarbonate deficit)
- Increased formation of acids
  - Ketosis (DM, starvation, hyperthyroidism, high fat low carbohydrate diet, after trauma)
  - Cellular hypoxia including lactic acidosis
- Decreased excretion of H^+
  - Renal failure (prerenal, renal, and postrenal)
  - Renal tubular acidosis
  - Fanconi syndrome
  - Acquired (drugs, hypercalcemia)
  - Inherited (cystinosis, Wilson disease)
  - Addison disease
- Respiratory acidosis
  - Emphysema, pneumonia, pulmonary edema
  - Bronchoconstriction, plugs, drugs depressing the respiratory center
  - Obstructive or restrictive pulmonary disease

➤ Limitations
The pH of freshly drawn blood decreases on standing at a rate of 0.04 to 0.08 pH unit/hour at 37°C, by ~0.03 units/hour at 25°C, but only 0.008 units/hour at 4°C.

BLOOD UREA NITROGEN (BUN)

➤ Definition
- Protein and nucleic acid catabolism results in the formation of urea and ammonia. Urea is synthesized mainly in the liver and >90% is excreted through the kidneys.
- **Normal range:** 7–23 mg/dL

➤ Use
- Most widely used screening test for the evaluation of kidney function
- Along with the serum creatinine, BUN levels aid in the differential diagnosis of prerenal, renal, and postrenal hyperuremia.
- Diagnosis of renal insufficiency: filtered freely in glomerulus; ≤50% is reabsorbed.
- Assessment of glomerular function: A BUN of 10–20 mg/dL almost always indicates normal glomerular function.
- In chronic renal disease, BUN correlates better with symptoms of uremia than does serum creatinine.
- Provides evidence of hemorrhage into upper GI tract.
- Assessment of patients requiring nutritional support for excess catabolism, for example, burns, cancer

➤ Interpretation
Increased In
- Impaired kidney function. A BUN of 50–150 mg/dL implies serious impairment of renal function. A markedly increased BUN (150–250 mg/dL) is virtually conclusive evidence of severely impaired glomerular function.
- Prerenal azotemia—any cause of reduced renal blood flow
  - CHF
  - Salt and water depletion (vomiting, diarrhea, diuresis, sweating)
  - Shock
- Postrenal azotemia—any obstruction of urinary tract (increased BUN-to-creatinine ratio)
- Increased protein catabolism (serum creatinine remains normal)
  - Hemorrhage into GI tract
  - AMI
  - Stress

Decreased In
- Diuresis (e.g., with overhydration, often associated with low protein catabolism)
- Severe liver damage (e.g., drugs, poisoning, hepatitis). A low BUN of 6–8 mg/dL is frequently associated with states of overhydration or liver disease.
  - Increased utilization of protein for synthesis (e.g., late pregnancy, infancy, acromegaly, malnutrition, anabolic hormones)
  - Diet (e.g., low-protein and high-carbohydrate, IV feedings only, impaired absorption [celiac disease], malnutrition)
  - Nephrotic syndrome (some patients)
  - SIADH
  - Inherited hyperammonemias (urea is virtually absent in blood)

➤ Limitations
- Urea levels increase with age and protein content of the diet.
- Corticosteroids, tetracyclines, and drugs causing nephrotoxicity frequently increase BUN.
- The presence of ammonium ions in anticoagulants may produce falsely elevated results.

BONE MARROW ANALYSIS

➤ Definition
- Bone marrow analysis refers to studies of an *aspirate* or/and a *biopsy* with the objective of obtaining marrow samples. The bone marrow is usually obtained from the posterior iliac crest. The test is indicated when abnormalities in the peripheral blood that require additional etiologic studies are found. The procedure can be performed at the bedside or in the office.
- **Normal Range:** Cellularity-to-fat ratio is 100% at birth and declines ≈10% each decade; 9:1 in young children; 2:1 in young adults; 1:1 in middle-aged adults; gradually decreases to 1:9 in the elderly. Differential distribution tables of the various hematopoietic lineages can be found in hematology and pathology textbooks.

➤ Use

* Bone marrow aspirates are used for their excellent cellular morphologic definition and maturation of cellular abnormalities, cytochemistry, cytogenetic studies, molecular studies, flow cytometry, microbial culture and identification, electron microscopic studies, and tissue culture. Aspirates can also be used for bone marrow transplantation, where large amounts of marrow need to be collected. (However, concentrated peripheral blood stem cells are now used in most cases for this purpose.)
* Bone marrow biopsies are useful for examination of intact marrow tissue and overall cellularity, histochemistry, and immunohistochemistry, as well as for certain molecular diagnostic tests. Biopsies are excellent for evaluating iron stores, fibrosis, granulomas, abscesses, metastases, and vascular lesions.
* Bone marrow is studied to diagnose or follow-up various conditions that may affect it or infiltrate it.
  * Diagnosis of anemia of iron deficiency (see p.788): bone marrow iron stains are the gold standard; also helpful in some cases of iron overload
  * Neoplasms that originate in or infiltrate the marrow: leukemias, myeloproliferative neoplasms, myelodysplastic syndromes, plasmacytic neoplasms, metastases; amyloidosis
  * Staging of Hodgkin and other lymphomas
  * Tumors and infections (e.g., TB) that invade the marrow and result in leukoerythoblastic peripheral blood picture (myelophistic anemia);
  * Aplastic anemia, agranulocytosis, cytopenias;
  * Unexplained anemia, splenomegaly, lymphadenopathy;
  * Megaloblastic anemias (rarely necessary)
  * Exposure to drugs resulting in bone marrow damage;
  * Follow-up therapy for leukemias, lymphoma (in cases that present with bone marrow infiltration), myelodysplastic and myeloproliferative neoplasms
  * Monitoring recovery following stem cell transplantation and marrow-ablative therapy
  * Infectious diseases and fever of unknown etiology (cultures, organism identification)

➤ Limitations

* Bone marrow aspirate may be diluted with peripheral blood and contain too few cellular elements
* Bone marrow biopsy may have insufficient tissue for accurate diagnosis; the underlying condition may result in patchy infiltrations of the marrow (e.g., myelomas), and the pathology be missed

BRAIN NATRIURETIC PEPTIDE (BNP)

➤ Definition

* Other names include B-type natriuretic peptide, N-terminal pro b-type natriuretic peptide, and NT-proBNP.
* BNP is a hormone secreted by myocytes in the ventricles (left ventricle) in response to pressure overload/myocyte stretch, with potent diuretic, natriuretic, and vascular smooth muscle relaxing effects. The heart normally produces low levels of a precursor protein, pro-BNP, which is cleaved to release the active hormone BNP and an inactive fragment, NT-proBNP.

- **Normal range:**
  - BNP: <100 pg/mL
  - NT proBNP: 0–74 years of age: ≤124 pg/mL; 75 years of age and older: ≤449 pg/mL

➤ Use

- Screening and diagnosis of CHF: BNP and NT-proBNP levels in the blood may be useful to establish prognosis in heart failure because both markers are typically higher in patients with worse outcome.
- Reading >480 pg/mL = 51% chance of cardiac/noncardiac events in next 6 months.
- Reading <230 pg/mL = 2.5% chance of cardiac/noncardiac events in next 6 months.
- Reading >130 pg/mL = 19% chance of sudden death.
- Reading <130 pg/mL = 1% chance of sudden death.
- Differential diagnosis of dyspnea: Readings <100 pg/mL rule out CHF as cause of dyspnea, and readings >400 pg/mL indicate a 95% likelihood of CHF. Readings between 100 and 400 pg/mL warrant further work-up.
- Determination of severity of CHF: Higher values correlate with increasing New York Heart Association classes I–IV. BNP is a prognostic tool for classes III and IV.
- Diagnosis of left ventricular dysfunction: Routine testing is not recommended for screening asymptomatic patient populations for left ventricular dysfunction. Increase in BNP in right heart failure is less than in left ventricular dysfunction.
- At appropriate cut-off values, BNP and NT-proBNP have similar S/S = 70%/70% and NPV = 80%.
- Greater increases predict worse adverse outcomes in patients with CHF.
- Increased values after acute myocardial infarction predict poorer prognosis.
- BNP increases with arrhythmias that are less marked.
- BNP and NT-proBNP can be increased in renal failure, especially if dialysis is needed.
- Abnormal echocardiogram without symptoms: mean value = 300 pg/mL.

➤ Interpretation
Increased In
- Heart failure
- Left ventricular dysfunction
- Renal impairment
- Coronary artery disease
- Valvular disease
- Arrhythmias
- Brain injury
- Anemia (BNP)
- Sepsis and shock (NT proBNP)

➤ Limitations
- Routine blood BNP or NT-proBNP testing is not justified for determining specific therapy for patients with chronic or acute heart failure.
- Nesiritide (human recombinant BNP) increases BNP. Studies indicate a minimal effect on NT-proBNP.
- Age and exercise also increase BNP.
- Obesity decreases BNP.

- Intraindividual variation (approximately 50% and 60%, respectively, for BNP and NTproBNP from week to week) indicates altered cardiac status.

➤ **Suggested Readings**

Apple FS, Wu HB, Jaffe AS, et al. National Academy of Clinical Biochemistry and IFCC Committee for Standardization of Markers of Cardiac Damage Laboratory Medicine Practice Guidelines: Analytical Issues for Biomarkers of Heart Failure. *Circulation*. 2007;226:e95–e98.

Steiner J, Guglin M. BNP or NTproBNP? A clinician's perspective. *Int J Cardiol*. 2008;129(1m):5–14.

Tang WH, Francis GS, Morrow DA, et al. National Academy of Clinical Biochemistry Laboratory Medicine. National Academy of Clinical Biochemistry Laboratory Medicine practice guidelines: clinical utilization of cardiac biomarker testing in heart failure. *Circulation*. 2007;116(5):e99–109.

BRONCHODILATORS

See Theophylline (1,3-Dimethylxanthine)

β-TRACE PROTEIN

➤ **Definition**

- β-Trace protein is also known as BTP or Lipocalin-type prostaglandin D synthase
- This test is currently not widely available in commercial laboratories.
- BTP, a low–molecular-weight glycoprotein freely filtered through the glomerular basement membrane and with minimal nonrenal elimination, is an ideal marker for GFR. BTP has been shown to be a more sensitive marker of GFR than creatinine in patients with chronic kidney disease, in kidney transplant recipients, and in children.
- **Normal range:** 0.40–0.74 mg/L

➤ **Use**

- Alternative marker for GFR in children as well as in DM and various renal diseases
- The early diagnosis of fistulas leaking CSF is an accurate marker of CSF leakage.

➤ **Suggested Reading**

Pöge U, et al. β-trace protein is an alternative marker for GFR in renal transplantation patients. *Clin Chem*. 2005;51:1531.

BUN-TO-CREATININE RATIO

➤ **Definition and Use**

- The BUN-to-creatinine ratio is used to differentiate prerenal and postrenal azotemia from renal azotemia.
- Because of considerable variability, it should be used only as a rough guide.
- **Normal range** (usual range for most people on normal diet: 12–16)

➤ **Interpretation**
Increased Ratio (> 10:1) with Normal Creatinine In

- Prerenal azotemia (e.g., heart failure, salt depletion, dehydration, blood loss) due to decreased GFR

- Catabolic states with increased tissue breakdown
- GI hemorrhage; a ratio ≥36 is reported to distinguish upper from lower GI hemorrhage in patients with negative gastric aspirate.
- High protein intake
- Impaired renal function plus
  - Excess protein intake or production or tissue breakdown (e.g., GI bleeding, thyrotoxicosis, infection, Cushing syndrome, high-protein diet, surgery, burns, cachexia, high fever)
  - Urine reabsorption (e.g., ureterocolostomy)
  - Patients with reduced muscle mass (subnormal creatinine production)
- Certain drugs (e.g., tetracycline, glucocorticoids)
- Selective increase in plasma urea (diuretic-induced azotemia) during use of loop diuretics

Increased Ratio (>10:1) with Elevated Creatinine In
- Postrenal azotemia (BUN rises disproportionately more than creatinine) (e.g., obstructive uropathy)
- Prerenal azotemia superimposed on renal disease

Decreased Ratio (<10:1) with Decreased BUN In
- Acute tubular necrosis
- Low-protein diet, starvation, severe liver disease, and other causes of decreased urea synthesis
- Repeated dialysis (urea rather than creatinine diffuses out of extracellular fluid)
- Inherited deficiency of urea cycle enzymes (e.g., hyperammonemias—urea is virtually absent in blood)
- SIADH (due to tubular secretion of urea)
- Pregnancy

Decreased Ratio (<10:1) with Increased Creatinine In
- Phenacemide therapy (accelerates conversion of creatine to creatinine)
- Rhabdomyolysis (releases muscle creatinine)
- Muscular patients who develop renal failure

➤ Limitations
- DKA (acetoacetate causes false increase in creatinine with certain methodologies, resulting in normal or decreased ratio when dehydration should produce an increased ratio)
- Cephalosporin therapy (interferes with creatinine measurement)

CALCITONIN

➤ Definition
- Calcitonin, also known as thyrocalcitonin, is a polypeptide hormone secreted by parafollicular C cells of thyroid.
- It acts directly on osteoclasts to decrease bone-resorbing activity and cause decreased serum calcium.
- **Normal range:**
  - Older children and adults: <12 pg/mL in males; <5 pg/mL in females
  - Infants and young children: <40 pg/mL in children <6 months; <15 pg/mL in children 6 months to 3 years (Basuyau)

➤ Use
- Serum calcitonin is determined to diagnose recurrence of medullary carcinoma or metastases after the primary tumor has been removed or to confirm complete removal of the tumor if basal calcitonin has been previously increased.
- Measurement of serum calcitonin has not been a part of the routine evaluation of patients with thyroid nodules in the United States. The high frequency of falsely high serum calcitonin values and the accuracy of fine needle aspiration biopsy argue against a change in this recommendation. Furthermore, occasional patients with locoregional metastases or locally invasive medullary thyroid carcinoma (MTC) have normal unstimulated serum calcitonin concentrations.

➤ Interpretation
Increased Values
- Carcinoma of lung, breast, islet cell, or ovary and carcinoid due to ectopic production and in myeloproliferative disorders
- Hypercalcemia of any etiology, stimulating calcitonin production
- Zollinger-Ellison syndrome
- C-cell hyperplasia
- Pernicious anemia
- Acute or chronic thyroiditis
- Chronic renal failure

Decreased Values
- Following surgical therapy for MTC
  - In cases of complete cures, serum calcitonin levels fall into the undetectable range over a variable period of several weeks.
  - A rise in previously undetectable or very low postoperative serum calcitonin levels is highly suggestive of disease recurrence or spread and should trigger further diagnostic evaluations.

➤ Limitations
- Basal fasting level may be increased in patients with MTC, even when there is no palpable mass in the thyroid.
  - Values follow a circadian pattern, with a peak after lunchtime.
  - Basal level is normal in approximately one third of cases of MTC.
- Levels of >2000 pg/mL are almost always associated with MTC, with rare cases due to obvious renal failure or ectopic production of calcitonin.
- Levels of 500–2000 pg/mL generally indicate medullary carcinoma, renal failure, or ectopic production of calcitonin.
- Levels of 100–500 pg/mL should be interpreted cautiously with repeat assays and provocative tests. If repeat tests in 1–2 months are still abnormal, some authors recommend total thyroidectomy.
- This test is not useful for evaluating calcium metabolic diseases.
- Falsely elevated values may occur in serum from patients who have developed human anti-mouse antibodies or heterophilic antibodies.

➤ Suggested Readings
Basuyau JP, Mallet E, Leroy M, Brunelle P. Reference intervals for serum calcitonin in men, women, and children. *Clin Chem.* 2004;50:1828–1830.

Saad MF, Ordonez NG, Rashid RK, et al. Medullary carcinoma of the thyroid. A study of the clinical features and prognostic factors in 161 patients. *Medicine (Baltimore).* 1984;63:319–342.

CALCIUM, IONIZED

➤ Definition
- Ionized calcium is the physiologically active form of calcium. Ionized calcium homeostasis is regulated by the parathyroid glands, bone, kidney, and intestine. It is most frequently used in ICUs and operating rooms.
- **Normal range:** 4.6–5.3 mg/dL
- **Critical range:** <4.1 or >5.9 mg/dL

➤ Use
- In patients with hypocalcemia or hypercalcemia with borderline serum calcium and altered serum proteins
- ~50% of calcium is ionized; 40–45% is bound to albumin; 5–10% is bound to other anions (e.g., sulfate, phosphate, lactate, and citrate); only the ionized fraction is physiologically active. Total calcium values may be deceiving, because they may be unchanged even if ionized calcium values are changed; (e.g., increased blood pH increases protein-bound calcium and decreases ionized calcium and PTH has the opposite effect) (blood pH should always be performed with ionized calcium, which is increased in acidosis and decreased in alkalosis). However, in critically ill patients, elevated total serum calcium usually indicates ionized hypercalcemia, and normal total serum calcium is evidence against ionized hypocalcemia.
- Ionized calcium is the preferred measurement rather than total calcium, because it is physiologically active and can be rapidly measured, which may be essential in certain situations (e.g., liver transplantation and rapid or large transfusion of citrated blood make interpretation of total calcium nearly impossible).
- Life-threatening complications are frequent when serum ionized calcium <2 mg/dL.
- With multiple blood transfusions, ionized calcium <3 mg/dL may be an indication to administer calcium.

➤ Interpretation
Increased In
- Normal total serum calcium associated with hypoalbuminemia may indicate ionized hypercalcemia.
- About 25% of patients with hyperparathyroidism have normal total but increased ionized calcium levels.
- Acidosis
- Metastatic bone tumor
- Milk-alkali syndrome
- Multiple myeloma
- Paget disease
- Sarcoidosis
- Tumors producing a PTH-like substance
- Vitamin D intoxication

Decreased In
- Alkalosis, (e.g., hyperventilation, to control increased intracranial pressure) (total serum calcium may be normal), administration of bicarbonate to control metabolic acidosis

- Increased serum free fatty acids (increased calcium binding to albumin) due to:
  - Certain drugs (e.g., heparin, IV lipids, epinephrine, norepinephrine, isoproterenol, alcohol)
  - Severe stress (e.g., acute pancreatitis, DKA, sepsis, AMI)
  - Hemodialysis
- Hypoparathyroidism (primary, secondary)
- Vitamin D deficiency
- Toxic shock syndrome
- Fat embolism
- Hypokalemia protects patient from hypocalcemic tetany; correction of hypokalemia without correction of hypocalcemia may provoke tetany.
- Malabsorption
- Osteomalacia
- Pancreatitis
- Renal failure
- Rickets

➤ **Limitations**
- Differences in specimen preparation and electrode selectivity are probably responsible for differences in reported reference ranges. Heparin itself cause 0.04 mg/dL decrease for each unit added per milliliter of blood.
- Adjusting the pH of the specimen to 7.4 at the time of measurement is not necessary if the specimen is collected anaerobically
- Various formulas are available for calculating CAI using total calcium, albumin, and total protein. However these formulas may not apply in some situations; their use is discouraged.
- Hypomagnesemia or hypermagnesemia; patients respond to serum magnesium that becomes normal but not to calcium therapy. Serum magnesium should always be measured in any patient with hypocalcemia.
- Increase of ions to which calcium is bound:
  - Phosphate (e.g., phosphorus administration in treatment of DKA, chemotherapy causing tumor lysis syndrome, rhabdomyolysis)
  - Bicarbonate
  - Citrate (e.g., during blood transfusion)
  - Radiographic contrast media containing calcium chelators

CALCIUM, TOTAL

➤ **Definition**
- Ninety-nine percent of the body's calcium is in bone. Of the remainder (of 1%) in blood about 50% is ionized (free), about 10% is bound to anions (e.g., phosphate, bicarbonate), about 40% (of 1%) in blood, is bound to plasma proteins, (80–40%) of that to albumin.
- **Normal range:** 8.7–10.7 mg/dL
- **Critical Values** <6.6 or >12.9 mg/dL

➤ **Use**
- Diagnosis and monitoring of a wide range of disorders, including disorders of protein and vitamin D, and diseases of bone, kidney, parathyroid gland, or GI tract.

➤ Interpretation
Increased In
* Hyperparathyroidism, primary and secondary
* Acute and chronic renal failure
* Following renal transplantation
* Osteomalacia with malabsorption
* Aluminum-associated osteomalacia
* Malignant tumors (especially breast, lung, kidney; 2% of patients with Hodgkin or non-Hodgkin lymphoma)
    * Direct bone metastases (up to 30% of these patients) (e.g., breast cancer, Hodgkin and non-Hodgkin lymphoma, leukemia, pancreatic cancer, lung cancer)
    * Osteoclastic activating factor (e.g., multiple myeloma, Burkitt lymphoma; may be markedly increased in human T-cell leukemia virus-I–associated lymphoma
    * Humoral hypercalcemia of malignancy
    * Ectopic production of 1,25-dihydroxy-vitamin D_3 (e.g., Hodgkin and non-Hodgkin lymphoma)
* Granulomatous disease (e.g., uncommon in sarcoidosis, TB, leprosy; more uncommon in mycoses, berylliosis, silicone granulomas, Crohn disease, eosinophilic granuloma, cat-scratch fever)
* Effect of drugs
    * Vitamin D and A intoxication
    * Milk-alkali (Burnett) syndrome (rare)
    * Diuretics (e.g., thiazides)
    * Others (estrogens, androgens, progestins, tamoxifen, lithium, thyroid hormone, parenteral nutrition)
* Renal failure, acute or chronic
* Other endocrine conditions
    * Thyrotoxicosis (in 20–40% of patients; usually <14 mg/dL)
    * More uncommon: Some patients with hypothyroidism, Cushing syndrome, adrenal insufficiency, acromegaly, pheochromocytoma (rare), VIPoma syndrome
    * Multiple endocrine neoplasia
* Acute osteoporosis (e.g., immobilization of young patients or in Paget disease)
* Miscellaneous
    * Familial hypocalciuric hypercalcemia
    * Rhabdomyolysis causing acute renal failure
    * Porphyria
    * Dehydration with hyperproteinemia
    * Hypophosphatasia
    * Idiopathic hypercalcemia of infancy
* Concomitant hypokalemia is not infrequent in hypercalcemia. Concomitant dehydration is almost always present because hypercalcemia causes nephrogenic diabetes insipidus.

Decreased In (Tables 2-13, 2-14)
* Hypoparathyroidism
    * Surgical
    * Idiopathic infiltration of parathyroids (e.g., sarcoid, amyloid, hemochromatosis, tumor)
    * Hereditary (e.g., DiGeorge syndrome)

TABLE 2-13. Serum phosphate, PTH, and Vitamin D Levels in Various Hypocalcemic Disorders

Hypocalcemic Disorders	Serum PO$_4$	PTH	25(OH)D	1,25(OH)$_2$D
Hypoparathyroidism	I	D	N	D
Pseudohypoparathyroidism	I	I	N	D
Vitamin D deficiency	D	I	D	Low N
1α-Hydroxylase deficiency	D	I	N	D
1,25(OH)$_2$D resistance	D	I	N	I

PO$_4$, phosphate; N, normal; I, increased; D, decreased.

* Pseudohypoparathyroidism
* Chronic renal disease with uremia and phosphate retention, Fanconi syndromes, renal tubular acidosis
* Malabsorption of calcium and vitamin D, obstructive jaundice
* Insufficient calcium, phosphorus, and vitamin D ingestion

TABLE 2-14. Variations of Various Serum and Urine Analytes in Association with Hypocalcemic Disorders

Hypocalcemia Associated With	Increased	Decreased
Serum PTH	Pseudohypoparathyroidism Renal failure, acute/chronic Malabsorption Vitamin D deficiency Phosphate administration	Hypoparathyroidism Acute pancreatitis Magnesium deficiency
Serum phosphorus	Hypoparathyroidism Pseudohypoparathyroidism Renal failure, acute (oliguric phase)/chronic Phosphate administration	Vitamin D deficiency Acute pancreatitis Renal failure, acute (diuretic phase) Malabsorption
Serum bicarbonate and pH	Hypoparathyroidism	
Serum Mg	Renal failure, acute/chronic	Magnesium deficiency Acute pancreatitis Renal failure, acute (diuretic phase)
Urine calcium	Hypoparathyroidism	Other causes of hypocalcemia
Urine phosphate	Renal failure, chronic Vitamin D deficiency Malabsorption Phosphate administration	Hypoparathyroidism Pseudohypoparathyroidism Magnesium deficiency
Urine cAMP	Renal failure, chronic Vitamin D deficiency Malabsorption	Hypoparathyroidism Pseudohypoparathyroidism

- Bone disease (osteomalacia, rickets)
- Starvation
- Late pregnancy
- Altered bound calcium citrate
  - Multiple citrated blood transfusions
  - Dialysis with citrate anticoagulation
- Hyperphosphatemia (e.g., phosphate enema/infusion)
- Rhabdomyolysis
- Tumor lysis syndrome
- Acute severe illness (e.g., pancreatitis with extensive fat necrosis, sepsis, burns)
- Respiratory alkalosis
- Certain drugs
  - Cancer chemotherapy drugs (e.g., cisplatin, mithramycin, cytosine arabinoside)
  - Fluoride intoxication
  - Antibiotics (e.g., gentamicin, pentamidine, ketoconazole)
  - Chronic therapeutic use of anticonvulsant drugs (e.g., phenobarbital, phenytoin)
  - Loop-active diuretics
  - Calcitonin
- Osteoblastic tumor metastases
- Neonates born of complicated pregnancies
  - Hyperbilirubinemia
  - Respiratory distress, asphyxia
  - Cerebral injuries
  - Infants of diabetic mothers
  - Prematurity
  - Maternal hypoparathyroidism
- Hypermagnesemia (e.g., magnesium for treatment of toxemia of pregnancy)
- Magnesium deficiency
- Toxic shock syndrome

Temporary hypocalcemia after subtotal thyroidectomy in >40% of patients; >20% are symptomatic.

➤ Limitations

- Total serum protein and albumin should always be measured simultaneously for proper interpretation of serum calcium levels, since 0.8 mg of calcium is bound to 1.0 g of albumin in serum; to correct, add 0.8 mg/dL for every 1.0 g/dL that serum albumin falls below 4.0 g/dL; binding to globulin only affects total calcium if globulin >6 g/dL.
- Serum levels increased by:
  - Hyperalbuminemia (e.g., multiple myeloma, Waldenström macroglobulinemia)
  - Dehydration
  - Venous stasis during blood collection by prolonged application of tourniquet
  - Use of cork-stoppered test tubes
  - Hyponatremia (<120 mEq/L), which increases the protein-bound fraction of calcium, thereby slightly increasing the total calcium (opposite effect in hypernatremia)
- Serum levels decreased by:
  - Hypomagnesemia (e.g., due to cisplatin chemotherapy)

* Hyperphosphatemia (e.g., laxatives, phosphate enemas, chemotherapy of leukemia or lymphoma, rhabdomyolysis)
* Hypoalbuminemia
* Hemodilution

CALCIUM, URINE

➤ Definition
* Urinary calcium levels reflects intake, rates of intestinal calcium absorption, bone resorption, and renal loss. Hypercalcemia of any cause raises urinary calcium excretion, and its measurement adds little to the differential diagnosis of hypercalcemia. Fasting calcium excretion is useful when assessing the contribution of abnormal renal tubular handling of calcium to disorders of calcium homeostasis.
* **Normal range:**
  * 24 hour urine: 100–300 mg/day
  * Random urine:
    * Males: 12–244 mg/g creatinine
    * Females: 9–328 mg/g creatinine

➤ Use
* Evaluation of patients with disorders of bone disease, calcium metabolism, and renal stones
* Follow-up of patients on calcium therapy for osteopenia
* Best test of calcium excretion in the investigation of possible familial benign hypocalciuric hypercalcemia

➤ Interpretation
Increased In
* Primary hyperparathyroidism
* Humoral hypercalcemia of malignancy
* Vitamin D excess
* Sarcoidosis
* Fanconi syndrome
* Osteolytic bone metastases
* Myeloma
* Osteoporosis
* Distal renal tubular acidosis
* Idiopathic hypercalciuria
* Thyrotoxicosis
* Paget disease
* Malignant neoplasm of breast or bladder

Decreased In
* Familial hypocalciuric hypercalcemia
* Hypoparathyroidism

- Pseudohypoparathyroidism
- Rickets and osteomalacia
- Hypothyroidism
- Celiac sprue
- Steatorrhea

➤ Limitations
- Calcium and protein intake and phosphorus excretion alter urinary calcium excretion.
- Decreases late in normal pregnancy
- About one third of hyperparathyroid patients have normal urine output.

CANCER ANTIGEN 15-3 (CA 15-3)

➤ Definition
- This glycoprotein is expressed on various adenocarcinomas, especially breast. It is a high–molecular-weight (300–450 kDa)1 polymorphic epithelial mucin.
- **Normal value:** <38 U/mL

➤ Use
- Marker for breast carcinoma. FDA approval is only for detection of breast carcinoma recurrence before symptoms and to monitor response to treatment. Significant change is ±25%.
- Not approved for screening, although increased values may occur ≤9 months before clinical evidence of disease.

➤ Interpretation
Increased In
- ~80% metastatic breast cancer
- Pancreas, lung, ovarian, colorectal, and liver cancers with less specificity

➤ Limitations
- CA 15-3 should not be used to diagnose breast cancer.
- Clinical sensitivity is 0.60, the specificity is 0.87, and the PPV is 0.91.
- It is considered equivalent to cancer antigen 27.29 mucin marker.

➤ Suggested Reading
Duffy MJ, Duggan C, Keane R, et al. High preoperative CA 15-3 concentrations predict adverse outcome in node-negative and node-positive breast cancer: Study of 600 patients with histologically confirmed breast cancer. *Clin Chem.* 2004; 50:559–563.

CANCER ANTIGEN 19-9 (CA 19-9)

➤ Definition
- CA 19-9 is a modified Lewis(a) blood group antigen and has been used as a tumor marker. It is shown to be elevated in sera of some patients with GI tumors.
- **Normal value:** <35 U/mL

➤ Use

* Detection, diagnosis, and prognosis of pancreatic cancer
* Monitor response to therapy (e.g., postsurgical recurrence correlates with increased concentrations)
* May be a useful adjunct to CEA for diagnosis and to detect early recurrence of certain cancers
* May indicate development of cholangiocarcinoma in patients with primary sclerosing cholangitis

➤ Interpretation
Increased In

* Carcinoma of pancreas (80%)
* Pancreatitis—concentrations are usually <75 U/mL, but are much higher in pancreatic cancer.
* Hepatobiliary cancer (22–51%)
* Gastric cancer (42%)
* Colon cancer (20%) is associated with very poor prognosis.
* Noncancerous conditions that may elevate include cirrhosis, cholangitis, hepatitis, pancreatitis, and nonmalignant GI diseases.

Decreased In
* Effective therapy or removal of the tumor

➤ Limitations

* Individuals with blood group antigen Le a-b- do not synthesize CA 19-9 (5–10% of population).
* No value in screening because its PPV <1%. However, levels of >1000 U/mL have 97% PPV.
* The CA 19-9 levels in a given specimen determined with assays from different manufacturers can vary due to differences in assay methods and reagent specificity and cannot be used interchangeably. If, in the course of monitoring a patient, the assay method used is changed, additional sequential testing should be carried out to confirm baseline values.

CANCER ANTIGEN 27.29 (CA 27.29)

➤ Definition
* Monoclonal antibody to a glycoprotein (Muc-1) that is present on the apical surface of normal epithelial cells.
* Tumor marker similar to cancer antigen 15-3
* **Normal value:** <38.6 U/mL

➤ Use
* As an aid in monitoring patients previously treated for stage II or III breast cancer.

➤ Interpretation
Increased In
* One third of early stage I and II breast cancers and two thirds of later stage III and IV breast cancers.
* Associated malignancies: colon, gastric, hepatic, lung, pancreatic, ovarian, and prostate cancers
* Benign conditions: breast, liver, and kidney disorders; ovarian cysts

➤ Limitations

- Lacks predictive value in early stage breast cancer and thus has no role in screening for or diagnosis of the malignancy.
- The concentration of CA 27.29 in a given specimen can vary because of differences in assay methods and reagent specificity. Values obtained with different assay methods should not be used interchangeably.
- Levels of CA 27.29 should not be interpreted as absolute evidence of the presence or the absence of malignant disease. Measurements of CA 27.29 should always be used in conjunction with other diagnostic procedures.

CANCER ANTIGEN-125 (CA-125), SERUM

➤ Definition

- CA-125 is a large glycoprotein (200–1000 kDa) found on the surface of many ovarian cancer cells and in some normal tissues. It is a product of the *MUC16* gene.
- **Normal range:** 0–35 U/mL

➤ Use

- CA-125 is recommended, together with transvaginal ultrasound, for early detection of ovarian cancer in women with hereditary syndromes because early intervention may be beneficial in these women. It is also recommended as an adjunct in distinguishing benign from malignant suspicious pelvic masses, particularly in postmenopausal women.
- It is not suggested for screening asymptomatic women.
- Measurements may also be used to monitor response to chemotherapeutic response.

➤ Interpretation
Increased Values

- Malignant disease
  - Fallopian tube tumors (100%), nonmucinous epithelial ovarian carcinoma (85%), cervical adenocarcinoma (83%), endometrial adenocarcinoma (50%), and squamous cell carcinomas of vulva or cervix (<15%)
  - Trophoblastic tumors (45%)
  - Non-Hodgkin lymphoma (40%) with pleuropericardial or peritoneal involvement
  - Cancers of pancreas, liver, and lung
- Conditions that affect the endometrium
  - Pregnancy (27%)
  - Menstruation, endometriosis
- Pleural effusion or inflammation (e.g., cancer, congestive heart failure)
- Peritoneal effusion or inflammation (e.g., pelvic inflammatory disease) and especially in bacterial peritonitis in which the ascitic concentration is greater than the serum concentration
- Some nonmalignant conditions
  - Cirrhosis, severe liver necrosis (66%)
  - Other diseases and disorders of the GI tract, liver, and pancreas
  - Renal failure
- Healthy persons (1%)

Decreased Values

* Postmenopausal women
* African American and Asian women, for whom normal values are lower

➤ Limitations

* Human antimurine or heterophile antibodies
* The CA-125 level is not increased in mucinous adenocarcinoma.
* Different assays do not produce equivalent values and should not be used interchangeably.
* Most of the commercially available assays quote the upper reference limit of 35 IU/mL; some studies have shown that the detection of disease can be significantly improved by lowering the cut-off value.
* Normal concentration of CA-125 does not exclude tumor.
* CA-125 is not useful for distinguishing benign from malignant pelvic masses, even at high concentrations.
* Although CA-125 may be increased $\leq$12 months before clinical evidence of disease, it is not recommended for screening women for serous carcinoma of ovary because it is not increased in 20% of cases at the time of diagnosis and in <10% of stage I and II cases (low sensitivity and specificity; high false-positive rate).
  * There is little benefit to early detection of late-stage cancers.
* Postoperative monitoring for persistent or recurrent disease; poorer prognosis if elevated 3–6 weeks after surgery.
  * Lower levels in patients with no residual tumor or <2 cm of residual tumor.
  * Concentration >35 U/mL detects residual cancer in 95% of patients, but a negative test does not exclude residual disease.
* Rising level of CA-125 during chemotherapy is associated with tumor progression, and fall to normal is associated with response. It remains elevated in stable or progressive serous carcinoma of ovary.
* Rising concentrations may precede clinical recurrence by many months and may be indication for second-look operation, but lack of increased values does not indicate absence of persistent or recurrent tumor.
* Greater concentration is roughly related to poorer survival; >35 U/mL is highly predictive of tumor recurrence.
  * With values >65 U/mL, 90% of women have cancer involving peritoneum.
  * Higher levels are also seen in serous cystadenocarcinoma.
* Sequential determinations are more useful than a single test, because levels in benign disease do not show significant change but progressive rise occurs in malignant disease.
* CA-125 is positive in 80% of cases of common epithelial tumors (50% of early stage disease) It should be noted that 0.6% of normal women older than 50 years of age have increased levels of CA-125.
* Prognosis may be better if:
  * There is a 50% decline in concentration within 5 days after surgery.
  * A postoperative-to-preoperative concentration ratio of 0.1 generally occurs within 4 weeks.
  * People with a postoperative-to-preoperative concentration ratio of >0.1 to <0.5 may benefit from chemotherapy, but the recurrence rate is high.
  * Patients with a postoperative-to-preoperative concentration ratio >0.8 should consider alternative therapy (e.g., radiation, different chemotherapy combinations).

➤ **Suggested Reading**

Fritsche HA, Bast RC. CA 125 in ovarian cancer: advances and controversy. *Clin Chem.* 1998;44:1379–1380.

CANNABIS SATIVA

➤ **Definition**

* An aromatic annual plant with origins in central Asia. The plant is known to contain 61 cannabinoids, including delta-9-tetrahydrocannabinol (delta-9-THC) and cannabidiol.
* Other names: marijuana, hashish, hash, sinsemilla, pot, grass

➤ **Use**

* No federally recognized medical use (schedule I, Controlled Substances Act).
* Self administered for its mood altering properties-stimulant/depressant at low doses; CNS depressant at high doses.

➤ **Limitations**

* Screening assays are commonly immunoassay based
  * ELISA for blood, serum, plasma
    * Target analyte: delta-9-THC
    * Cut-off concentration-variable 2–5 ng/mL
    * May exhibit significant cross-reactivity with 11-hydroxy-THC, carboxy-THC [THC-COOH]
    * Low cross-reactivity with cannabidiol, cannabinol, delta-8-THC
  * EIA for urine
    * Target analyte: THC-COOH (metabolite)
    * Cut-off concentration:
      * 20 ng/mL
      * 50 ng/mL
    * Approximately 50% cross-reactivity with cannabinol, 11-OH-THC
* Confirmation assays are commonly chromatography based regardless of specimen
  * Highly glucuronidated-hydrolysis recommended for analysis of urine
  * Urine confirmation assays typically target *only* THC-COOH; limit of detection/quantitation is 5–15 ng/mL
  * GC/MS: selected ion monitoring mode for quantitative analysis of serum, plasma for THC, 11-OH-THC, THC-COOH; limits of quantitation: 1–5 ng/mL
  * LC/MSn (multiple MS)
    * Multiple reaction monitoring mode for qualitative or quantitative analysis of THC, 11-OH-THC, THC-COOH
    * Limits of detection/quantitation: 0.5–5 ng/mL

CARBON DIOXIDE, TOTAL

➤ **Definition**

* Total carbon dioxide consists of carbon dioxide (CO_2) in solution or bound to proteins, bicarbonate (HCO_3^-), carbonate (CO_3^{2-}), and carbonic acid (H_2CO_3). In practice, 80–90% is present as HCO_3^- and is a general guide to the body's buffering capacity.
* It is usually measured with electrolytes as a panel.

* **Normal range:**
  0–2 years: 20–25 mmol/L
  2–16 years: 22–28 mmol/L
  >16 years: 24–32 mmol/L

Use
* To evaluate the total CO_3^{2-} buffering system in the body as well as the acid–base balance

➤ **Interpretation**
Increased In
* Respiratory acidosis with CO_2 retention
* Metabolic alkalosis (e.g., prolonged vomiting)
* Airway obstruction
* Alcoholism
* Aldosteronism
* Cardiac disorders
* Emphysema
* Fat embolism
* Pulmonary dysfunction
* Renal disorders

Decreased In
* Respiratory alkalosis, as in hyperventilation
* Metabolic acidosis (e.g., diabetes with ketoacidosis).
* Alcoholic ketosis
* Dehydration
* Diarrhea
* Head trauma
* High fever
* Hepatic disorders
* Hyperventilation
* Malabsorption syndromes
* Starvation and uremia

➤ **Limitations**
* Antacids, corticotrophin, mercurial and thiazide diuretics, sodium bicarbonate increase blood levels.
* Acetazolamide, ammonium chloride, aspirin, chlorothiazide diuretics, methicillin, paraldehyde, and tetracycline decrease blood levels.
* High altitudes decrease values.
* Hyperthermia increases blood levels.

CARBOXYHEMOGLOBIN (CARBON MONOXIDE, COHB, HBCO)

➤ **Definition**
* COHB is Hb with carbon monoxide (CO) instead of the normal oxygen bound to it. CO has a much great affinity than oxygen for Hb. The source of the CO may be exhaust (such as from a car, truck, boat or generator), smoke from a fire, or tobacco smoke.

- COHB is formed in CO poisoning. The COHB level is useful in judging the extent of CO toxicity and in considering the effect of smoking on the patient. A direct correlation has been claimed between CO level and symptoms of atherosclerotic diseases, angina, and MI.
- **Normal range:**
  - Nonsmokers: 0.5–1.5 % saturation of Hgb
  - Smokers (1–2 packs/day): 4–5%
  - Heavy smokers (>2 packs/day): 8–9%

➤ Use
- Verifying CO toxicity in cases of suspected exposure

➤ Interpretation
Increased In
- CO poisoning
- Hemolytic disease
- Blood in intestine
- Reactions of intestinal bacteria
- Calorie reduction
- Following exercise

➤ Limitations
- COHB diminishes at a rate of about 15% per hour when the patient is removed from the contaminated environment.
- The most common cause of CO toxicity is exposure to automobile exhaust fumes. Significant levels of COHB can also be observed in heavy smokers. Victims of fires often show elevated levels from inhaling CO generated during combustion.
- Susceptibility to CO poisoning is increased in anemic persons

CARCINOEMBRYONIC ANTIGEN (CEA)

➤ Definition
- CEA is a glycoprotein normally produced only during early fetal life and rapid multiplication of epithelial cells, especially those of the digestive system. CEA also appears in the blood of chronic smokers. Less than 25% of patients with disease confined to the colon have elevated CEA. Sensitivity is increased with advancing tumor stage.
- CEA levels should be ordered only after malignancy has been confirmed. CEA levels typically return to normal within 4–6 weeks after surgical resection. Major role is in following patients for relapse after intended curative treatment. The American Society of Clinical Oncology recommends monitoring CEA levels every 2–3 months for at least 2 years in patients with stage II and III disease.
- **Normal values:** <2.5 ng/mL in nonsmokers; <5 ng/mL in smokers

➤ Use
- Monitoring colorectal cancer and selected other cancers such as medullary thyroid carcinoma
- May be useful in assessing the effectiveness of chemotherapy or radiation treatment

- Diagnosis of malignant pleural effusion
- Not useful in screening the general population for undetected cancers

➤ Interpretation
Increased In
- Cancer. There is a wide overlap in values between benign and malignant disease. Increased concentrations are suggestive but not diagnostic of cancer.
  - Seventy-five percent of patients with carcinoma of endodermal origin (colon, stomach, pancreas, lung) have CEA titers >2.5 ng/mL, and two thirds of these titers are >5 ng/mL. CEA is increased in about one third of patients with small cell carcinoma of lung and in about two thirds with non–small cell carcinoma of lung.
  - Fifty percent of patients with carcinoma of nonentodermal origin (especially cancer of the breast, head and neck, ovary) have CEA titers >2.5 ng/mL, and 50% of the titers are >5 ng/mL. Titers are increased in >50% of cases of breast cancer with metastases and 25% without metastases, but they are not associated with benign lesions.
  - Forty percent of patients with noncarcinomatous malignant disease have increased CEA concentrations, usually 2.5–5.0 ng/mL.
  - Increased in 90% of all patients with solid-tissue tumors, especially with metastases to liver or lung, but they are increased in only 50% of patients with local disease or only intra-abdominal metastases.
  - May be increased in effusion fluid due to these cancers. Active nonmalignant inflammatory diseases (especially of the GI tract [e.g., ulcerative colitis, regional enteritis, diverticulitis, peptic ulcer, chronic pancreatitis]) frequently have elevated concentrations that decline when the disease is in remission.
- Liver disease (alcoholic, cirrhosis, chronic active hepatitis, obstructive jaundice) because metabolized by liver.
- Others disorders:
  - Renal failure
  - Fibrocystic disease of breast

➤ Limitations
- When an abnormal level is found, the test should be repeated. If confirmed, patient should undergo imaging of potential reoccurrence sites.
- Same methodology should be used to monitor an individual patient. A significant change in plasma concentration is +25%.
- After complete removal of colon cancer, CEA should fall to normal in 6–12 weeks. Failure to decline to normal concentrations postoperatively suggests incomplete resection. Immunohistochemistry of resected specimen is used to identify 20% of these cancers that do not express CEA for whom monitoring is misleading. In such cases, may use serum ALP and diagnostic imaging.
- Prognosis is related to serum concentration at time of diagnosis (stage of disease and likelihood of recurrence). CEA concentrations <5 ng/mL before therapy suggest localized disease and a favorable prognosis, but a concentration >10 ng/mL suggests extensive disease and a poor prognosis; >80% of colon carcinoma patients with values >20 ng/mL have recurrence within 14 months after surgery. Plasma CEA >20 ng/mL correlates with tumor volume in breast and colon cancer and is usually associated with metastatic disease or with a few types of cancer (e.g., cancer of the colon or pancreas); however, metastases may occur

with concentrations <20 ng/mL. Values <2.5 ng/mL do not rule out primary, metastatic, or recurrent cancer. Increased values in node-negative colon cancer may identify poorer-risk patients who may benefit from chemotherapy.

- Patterns of CEA change during chemotherapy
  - Uninterrupted increase indicating failure to respond
  - Decrease indicating response to therapy.
  - Surge in CEA for weeks followed by a decrease indicating response
  - Immediate, sustained decrease followed by an increase indicating lack of response to therapy
  - Significant is 25–35% change from baseline of equal or increased values during first 2 months of therapy
  - Survival is significantly longer if titer decreases below this baseline.

CARDIOVASCULAR DRUGS (SEE DIGOXIN)

➤ Definition
- Cardiovascular drugs include the antiarrhythmics, the anticoagulant warfarin, and antihypertensives, as well as the β-adrenergic antagonist propranolol and the drug digoxin (see p. 158).
- **Normal therapeutic values:** see Table 2-15

➤ Use
- To treat arrhythmia, hypertension, blood clotting, and angina
- The majority of these drugs are not routinely monitored as clinical effects do not generally correlate with serum or plasma levels. Notable exceptions are digoxin and procainamide.
- Where concentrations are required, specific gas chromatography and HPLC procedures have been developed (e.g. procainamide/N-acetylprocainamide [NAPA], quinidine, mexiletine, diltiazem, verapamil, amiodarone, and metabolite, warfarin). Limits of quantitation vary according to the drug and methodology.
- Immunoassay tests (e.g., FPIA) are available for procainamide, quinidine.
- In addition, lidocaine, diltiazem, verapamil, and quinidine are qualitatively detectable in urine with a simple alkaline liquid–liquid or solid-phase extraction followed by GC/MS analysis. Limits of detection range from 50–250 ng/mL.

➤ Interpretation
- Rifampin may decrease verapamil serum concentrations.

➤ Limitations
- With procainamide, separate cells from plasma as soon as possible to prevent loss of drug during storage.
- Hemolyzed samples are unacceptable.

CATECHOLAMINES, SERUM

➤ Definition
- The catecholamines (epinephrine, norepinephrine, and dopamine) are found in the adrenal medulla, neurons, and brain. All three catecholamines are derived from tyrosine and are

TABLE 2-15. Cardiovascular Drugs

Generic	Brand	Used to Treat	Therapeutic Level	Potential Toxic Level[†]
ANTIARRHYTHMICS				
Amiodarone	Cordarone	Supraventricular and ventricular arrhythmias*	1.5–2.5 µg/mL	≥3.0 µg/mL
Flecainide	Tambocor	Ventricular arrhythmias	0.2–1.0 µg/mL [trough]	>1.0 µg/mL
Lidocaine	Xylocaine	Ventricular arrhythmias (also prevention)	1.4–6.0 µg/mL	>6.0 µg/mL
Mexiletine	Mexitil	Arrhythmias	0.5–2.0 µg/mL [trough]	>1.5 µg/mL
Procainamide (active metabolite: N-acetylprocainamide [NAPA])	Pronestyl	Supraventricular and ventricular arrhythmias	Procainamide: 4–10 µg/mL NAPA: 6–20 µg/mL	Procainamide: ≥12 µg/mL NAPA: >30 µg/mL
Quinidine	Duraquin	Supraventricular and ventricular arrhythmias	1.5–4.5 µg/mL	>10.0 µg/mL
Verapamil (calcium channel blocker)	Calan	Supraventricular dysrhythmias, angina pectoris, and hypertension	50–200 ng/mL [peak serum]	≥400 ng/ mL [peak serum]

(Continued)

TABLE 2-15. Cardiovascular Drugs (*Continued*)

Drug Name				
Generic	Brand	Used to Treat	Therapeutic Level	Potential Toxic Level[†]
ANTICOAGULANT				
Warfarin	Coumadin	Blood clotting; drug, a synthetic vitamin K antagonist, is an anticoagulant**	7 mg/L	10 mg/L
ANTIHYPERTENSIVES				
Diltiazem (calcium channel blocker)	Cardizem	Angina pectoris and hypertension***	40–200 ng/mL	
Nifedipine	Procardia	Angina pectoris and hypertension****	25–100 ng/mL	>100 ng/mL
BETA–ADRENERGIC ANTAGONIST				
Propranolol	Inderal	Arrhythmias and hypertension	30–250 ng/mL	

*Monitor TSH and T$_4$ values during therapy.
**Prothrombin time is used to assess efficacy as target INR: 2.0–3.0. Consider long–term low–intensity (INR 1.5–2.0) or standard intensity (INR 2–3) warfarin therapy for patients with idiopathic events.
***Effect on platelets may increase bleeding time.
****Decreased glucose tolerance.
[†]Toxic concentrations have not been established.

TABLE 2-16. Normal Range for Catecholamines

Age	Value in pg/mL
EPINEPHRINE	
2–10 days	36–400
11 days to 3 months	55–200
4–11 months	55–440
12–23 months	36–640
24–35 months	18–440
3–17 years	18–460
≥18 years	10–200
NOREPINEPHRINE	
2–10 days	170–1180
11 days to 3 months	370–2080
4–11 months	270–1120
12–23 months	68–1810
24–35 months	170–1470
3–17 years	85–1250
≥18 years	80–520
DOPAMINE	
≥2 days	0–20

important neurotransmitters in the CNS and also play a crucial role in the autonomic regulation of many homeostatic functions.

* Other names: adrenaline, catecholamine fractionation, unconjugated dopamine, epinephrine, noradrenaline, norepinephrine
* **Normal range:** see Table 2-16

➤ Use

* Diagnosis of pheochromocytoma and paraganglioma, as an auxiliary test to fractionated plasma and urine metanephrine measurements.
* Diagnosis and follow-up of patients with neuroblastoma and related tumors, as an auxiliary test to urine VMA and homovanillic acid (HVA) measurements.
* Evaluation of patients with autonomic dysfunction/failure or autonomic neuropathy.

➤ Interpretation
Increased In (Epinephrine)

* Anger, exercise, fear, burns
* Ganglioblastoma and ganglioneuroma
* Hypoglycemia
* Hypotension
* Hypothyroidism
* DKA
* Neuroblastoma
* Paragangliomas
* Pheochromocytoma

Decreased In
* Norepinephrine: anorexia nervosa
* Autonomous nervous system dysfunction
* Orthostatic hypotension
* Dopamine: possibly decreased in Parkinson disease

➤ Limitations
* Most assays measure only free catecholamines, but a few measure both free and conjugated types. Free amines are more closely associated with tumor load than conjugated ones.
* Physiologic stimuli, drugs, or improper specimen collection slightly increases the levels. Patients should not eat, use tobacco, or drink caffeinated beverages for at least 4 hours before collection. Measurement of plasma or urine fractionated metanephrines provides better diagnostic sensitivity than measurement of catecholamines.
* Plasma levels drop quickly within 5 minutes if RBCs are not separated from plasma once collected.
* Amphetamines and amphetamine-like compounds, appetite suppressants, bromocriptine, buspirone, caffeine, carbidopa-levodopa, clonidine, dexamethasone, diuretics (in doses sufficient to deplete sodium), ethanol, isoproterenol, labetalol, methyldopa, MAO inhibitors, nicotine, nose drops, propafenone (Rythmol), reserpine, theophylline, tricyclic antidepressants, and vasodilators may interfere with this test and the results may not be predictable.

CELL COUNT, BODY FLUID ANALYSIS

Fluids are found in body cavities. This chapter discussion focuses on the microscopic evaluation of fluids accumulated in body cavities: cerebrospinal, pleural, pericardial, and peritoneal (ascites). Synovial fluids are described below under Other Body Fluids. Aspiration followed by chemical, microscopic, cytologic, microbiologic, and, if indicated, flow cytometry examinations should help determine the etiology of accumulated pathologic fluids by providing important information regarding infection, hemorrhage, inflammation, or malignant infiltration. Total cell counts are performed using undiluted (or in the case of very high counts, diluted) body fluids with a hemocytometer. Differential counts are done using a smear following centrifugation (Cytospin) and staining with Wright-Giemsa stain. Bacterial identification and cultures are described separately. The chemistry of body fluids is described separately.

CEREBROSPINAL FLUID (CSF)

➤ Definition
* CSF is produced by the choroid plexus in the lateral third and fourth ventricles of the brain. In normal adults the total CSF volume is 90–150 mL. Eighty percent of the CSF is contained in the arachnoid space in the cranium and spinal cord, where a small amount can be extracted for examination, most commonly through a lumbar puncture.
* CSF pressure is measured by a manometer.
* **Normal values:**
  * Appearance: clear, colorless
  * Normal opening adult pressure: 90–180 mL of water in an adult in the lateral decubitus position with the legs and neck in a neutral position

TABLE 2-17. Differential Counts for Cerebrospinal Fluid (Mean + or − SD)		
Type of Cells	Adults	Neonates
Lymphocytes	62% ± 34	20% ± 18
Mononuclear cells and Monocytes	36% ± 20	72% ± 22
Neutrophils	2% ± 5	3% ± 5
Histiocytes	rare	rare
Eosinophils	rare	rare

- Cell count and differential (Table 2-17):
  Adults: WBC 0–5 cells/mm^3, RBC 0/mm^3
  Newborns: WBC 0–30/mm^3, RBC 0/mm^3

➤ Use
- Examination of CSF is required when its involvement by inflammatory, infectious, neoplastic, or neurologic complications are suspected. Up to 20 mL of fluid can be removed
- CSF is divided into three sterile tubes:
  1. Chemistry and immunology studies
  2. Microbiology examinations
  3. Cell count, differential, and cytology (if indicated)

➤ Interpretation
- Increased number of neutrophils: bacterial or early viral CNS infection, early CNS TB, CNS syphilis, fungal infection, contamination with peripheral blood through traumatic tap, CNS hemorrhage
- Increased number of lymphocytes: viral infection of CNS, CNS TB, acute lymphocytic leukemia or lymphoma of CNS, cryptococcal infection of CNS, fungal infection of CNS, CNS syphilis, parasitic disease infecting the CNS, Guillain-Barré syndrome
- Increased eosinophils: parasitic infection of CNS, fungal infection of CNS, viral infection of CNS, CNS syphilis, allergic reaction
- Increased basophils: chronic myelogenous leukemia
- Tumor cells: primary or metastatic tumors of the CNS
- Xanthochromia (yellowish discoloration): marker of previous intracerebral bleeding

OTHER BODY FLUIDS: PLEURAL, PERICARDIAL, AND PERITONEAL SPACES

➤ Definition
- Under normal conditions, a very small amount of fluid (up to 50 mL) is present. This facilitates movement of membranes against each other.
- Abnormal fluid accumulation is called a serous effusion. In the presence of effusions, fluid can be aspirated from the affected cavity, either for diagnosis, or for relief of pressure, commonly both. Finding substantial amounts of fluid always reflects a pathologic process.

➤ Interpretation
- Pleural fluid
  - Appearance

- Cloudiness: neutrophils present indicating infection
- Milkiness: chylous effusion
- Bloody: traumatic tap, malignancy, pneumonia, trauma, status postmyocardial infarction or pulmonary infarction
- Cell counts and differentials
  - WBC count $>1 \times 10^9$/L with lymphocytes $>50\%$: TB, cancer, lymphoma, CLL
  - WBC count $>1 \times 10^{10}$/L with ~80% neutrophils: effusions associated with bacterial pneumonia
  - WBC with eosinophilia: postpneumothorax, trauma, hypersensitivity reactions, CHF, fungal and parasitic infections, SLE, Hodgkin lymphoma
- Pericardial fluid
  - Appearance
    - Bloody: pericarditis, status post myocardial infarction, TB, RA, SLE, carcinoma, aspiration of blood from cardiac cavity
  - Cell counts and differential
    - WBC count 1×10^9/L with increased lymphocytes: pericardial tuberculosis
    - WBC count 1×10^9/L with increased neutrophils: bacterial or viral pericarditis
- Peritoneal fluid
  - Appearance
    - Cloudy or turbid: appendicitis, pancreatitis, intestinal volvulus, ruptured bowel, sepsis
    - Bile-stained: perforated duodenal ulcer, perforated intestine, gallbladder disease or perforation, acute pancreatitis
    - Milky: chylous effusion
    - Bloody: traumatic tap, intra-abdominal injury
  - Cell counts and differential on lavage fluid
    - RBC count $>1 \times 10^{11}$/L: intra-abdominal injury
    - WBC count 0.5×10^9/L: possible peritonitis
  - Cell counts and differential on undiluted ascetic fluid
    - WBC count 0.3×10^9/L: bacterial peritonitis if $>50\%$ neutrophils, cirrhosis of liver if $<25\%$ neutrophils
      - Increased lymphocytes: tuberculous peritonitis
      - Increased eosinophils: CHF, hypereosinophilic syndrome, eosinophilic gastroenteritis, chronic peritoneal dialysis, abdominal lymphoma, ruptured hydatid cyst, vasculitis

➤ Limitations
- All cell counts should be performed promptly to prevent cell deterioration; distorted or degenerated cells should not be counted.
- Specimens with large clots cannot be processed.

CERULOPLASMIN

➤ Definition
- Major copper-carrying protein in the blood. An α-2 globulin, it plays a role in both iron and copper metabolism.
- Other names: CP, ferroxidase, iron(II):oxygen oxidoreductase
- **Normal range:** 22–58 mg/dL

➤ Use
* Evaluation of acute phase response
* Assessment of possible Wilson disease.
* Assessment of Menkes kinky hair syndrome, aceruloplasminemia

➤ Interpretation
Increased In
* Inflammation, infection, tissue injury
* Cardiovascular disease
* Pregnancy (double the baseline values in third trimester)
* Cancer
* Cirrhosis
* Estrogen supplementation and oral contraceptives.
* RA
* Primary sclerosing cholangitis

Decreased In
* Hepatolenticular degeneration (Wilson disease)
* Autosomal recessive disease involving copper metabolism
* Kwashiorkor, malabsorption
* Nephrosis, nephritic syndrome
* Menkes kinky hair syndrome
* Aceruloplasminea

➤ Limitations
* Anticonvulsant therapy, methadone, tamoxifen, oral contraceptives, and smoking increase serum levels.

CHLORIDE

➤ Definition
* Chloride is the major extracellular anion; it is not actively regulated normally. It reflects changes in sodium; if it changes independent of sodium, this is usually due to an acid–base disorder.
* **Normal range:** 97–110 mmol/L

➤ Use
* With sodium, potassium, and carbon dioxide to assess electrolyte, acid–base, and water balance. Chloride usually changes in the same direction as sodium except in metabolic acidosis with bicarbonate depletion and metabolic alkalosis with bicarbonate excess, when serum sodium levels may be normal.

➤ Interpretation
Increased In
* Metabolic acidosis associated with prolonged diarrhea with loss of sodium bicarbonate
* Renal tubular diseases with decreased excretion of hydrogen ions and decreased reabsorption of bicarbonate ("hyperchloremic metabolic acidosis")

- Respiratory alkalosis (e.g., hyperventilation, severe CNS damage)
- Drugs
- Excessive administration of certain drugs (e.g., ammonium chloride, IV saline, salicylate intoxication, acetazolamide therapy)
- False (methodologic) increase due to bromides or other halogens
- Retention of salt and water (e.g., corticosteroids, guanethidine, phenylbutazone)
- Some cases of hyperparathyroidism
- Diabetes insipidus, dehydration
- Sodium loss > chloride loss (e.g., diarrhea, intestinal fistulas)
- Ureterosigmoidostomy

Decreased In
- Prolonged vomiting or suction (loss of hydrochloric acid)
- Metabolic acidosis with accumulation of organic anions
- Chronic respiratory acidosis
- Salt-losing renal diseases
- Adrenocortical insufficiency
- Primary aldosteronism
- Expansion of extracellular fluid (e.g., SIADH, hyponatremia, water intoxication, CHF)
- Burns
- Drugs
- Alkalosis (e.g., bicarbonates, aldosterone, corticosteroids)
- Diuretic effect (e.g., ethacrynic acid, furosemide, thiazides)
- Other loss (e.g., chronic laxative abuse)

➤ Limitations
- Direct ISE (Ion Selective Electrode) measurements do not give the volume displacement error in specimens with high lipid or protein content, as indirect ISE and flame measurements do.
- May be slightly decreased after meals; fasting specimen collection is recommended.

CHLORIDE, URINE

➤ Definition
- Chloride is reabsorbed with sodium throughout the nephron. Because of its relationship with other electrolytes, urinary chloride results can be used to help assess volume status, salt intake, causes of hypokalemia, and to aid in the diagnosis of renal tubular acidosis (RTA).
- Approximately 30% of hypovolemic patients have >15 mmol/L difference between urine sodium and chloride concentrations. This is due to the excretion of sodium with another anion (such as bicarbonate, HCO_3^-) or to the excretion of chloride with another cation (such as ammonium, NH_4^+).
- The normal response to acidemia is to increase urinary acid excretion, primarily NH_4^+. When urine NH_4^+ levels are high, the urine anion gap [(Na + K) – Cl] will have a negative value, since chloride levels will exceed that of Na and K by the approximate amount of

TABLE 2-18. Normal Values for Urine Chloride	
24-Hour Urine	mmol/day
Male:	
<10 years	36–110
10–14 years	64–176
>14 years	110–250
>60 years	95–195
Female:	
<10 years	18–74
10–14 years	36–173
>14 years	110–250
>60 years	95–195
Random urine	mmol/g creatinine
Male	25–253
Female	39–348

NH_4^+ in the urine. Therefore, the urine chloride concentration may be inappropriately high in diarrhea induced hypovolemia because of the need to maintain the electroneutrality as NH_4^+ excretion is enhanced.

- **Normal range:** see Table 2-18

➤ Use

- Assess volume status, salt intake, and causes of hypokalemia. It is helpful to measure urine chloride concentration in a patient who seems to be volume depleted but has a somewhat elevated urine sodium concentration.
- Aid in the diagnosis of RTA
- Evaluate electrolyte composition of urine and acid–base balance studies. It is helpful to measure urine chloride in patients with a normal anion gap metabolic acidosis. In the absence of renal failure, this may be due to diarrhea or one of the forms of RTA.

➤ Interpretation
Increased In

- Postmenstrual diuresis
- Massive diuresis from any cause
- Salt-losing nephritis
- Potassium depletion
- Adrenocortical insufficiency
- Tubulointerstitial disease
- Batter syndrome

Decreased In

- Premenstrual salt and water retention
- Excessive extrarenal chloride loss
- Adrenocortical hyperfunction
- Postoperative chloride retention

➤ Limitations
- Urine chloride excretion approximates the dietary intake.
- Bromides can cause falsely elevated results.

CHOLESTEROL, HIGH-DENSITY LIPOPROTEIN (HDL)

➤ Definition
- HDL, also known as HDL-C, is produced by the liver and consists of mostly cholesterol, protein, and phospholipid. It carries cholesterol in the bloodstream from the tissues to the liver (reverse cholesterol transport).
- HDL is termed the "good cholesterol," because its levels are inversely related to CHD, and it is an independent risk factor.
- **Normal range:** see Table 2-19

➤ Use
- Assessment of risk of heart disease and atherosclerosis
- Ordered in combination with total cholesterol, LDL, and triglycerides as a lipid profile

➤ Interpretation
Increased In
- Hyperalphalipoproteinemia
- Regular physical activity or exercise
- Weight loss
- Chronic liver disease

Decreased In
- Uncontrolled diabetes
- Hepatocellular disease
- Chronic renal failure, nephrosis, uremia
- Cholestasis
- Abetalipoproteinemia
- Familial hyper-α-lipoproteinemia (Tangier disease)
- Deficiency of apo A-I and apo C-III

➤ Limitations
- HDL is increased due to moderate ethanol consumption, estrogens, and insulin.
- HDL is decreased due to starvation; stress and recent illness; smoking; obesity and lack of exercise; and drugs such as steroids, thiazide diuretics, and beta blockers; hypertriglyceridemia (>1700 mg/dL); and elevated serum immunoglobulin levels.

TABLE 2-19. Reference Values for High-Density Lipoprotein (HDL) Cholesterol	
HDL Cholesterol Level	Comments
<40 mg/dL	Major risk factor for heart disease
40–59 mg/dL	"The higher, the better"
≥60 mg/dL	Considered protective against heart disease

- Other factors that may also increase cholesterol include cigarette smoking, age, hypertension, family history of premature heart disease, preexisting heart disease, and DM.

➤ **Suggested Reading**

National Institutes of Health, National Heart Lung and Blood Institute's National Cholesterol Education Program. http://www.nhlbi.nih.gov/about/ncep/ Accessed Nov. 18, 2010.

CHOLESTEROL, LOW-DENSITY LIPOPROTEIN (LDL)

➤ **Definition**

- LDL cholesterol, also known as LDL-C, is produced by the metabolism of VLDL cholesterol and consists of mostly cholesterol, protein, and phospholipids that carry cholesterol in the bloodstream from the liver to the peripheral tissues.
- LDL-C is termed the "bad cholesterol," and LDL-C levels are associated with atherosclerosis and coronary heart disease.
- **Normal range:** see Table 2-20

➤ **Use**

- To determine risk of heart disease and atherosclerosis. LDL-C is calculated when ordered in combination with total cholesterol, HDL cholesterol, and triglycerides as a lipid profile.

➤ **Interpretation**
Increased In

- Familial hypercholesterolemia
- Nephrotic syndrome
- Hepatic disease
- Hepatic obstruction
- Chronic renal failure
- Hyperlipidemia types II and III
- DM

Decreased In

- Abetalipoproteinemia
- Hyperthyroidism
- Tangier disease
- Hypolipoproteinemia
- Chronic anemia

TABLE 2-20. Reference Intervals for Low-Density Lipoprotein (LDL) Cholesterol	
LDL Cholesterol Level	Category
<100 mg/dL	Optimal
100–129 mg/dL	Near optimal/above optimal
130–159 mg/dL	Borderline high
160–189 mg/dL	High
≥190 mg/dL	Very high

- Lecithin cholesterol acyltransferase deficiency
- Apo C-II deficiency
- Hyperlipidemia type I

➤ Limitations

- LDL-C values may be high because of a diet high in saturated fats and cholesterol, pregnancy, or use of steroids.
- LDL values should be measured only on fasting samples.
- LDL cholesterol may be decreased because of acute stress, recent illness, and estrogens.
- Other factors that may affect LDL-C values: cigarette smoking, hypertension (blood pressure >140/90 mm Hg or taking antihypertensive medication), family history of premature CHD (CHD in male first-degree relative <55 years; CHD in female first-degree relative <65 years), and age (men >45 years; women >55 years). See Table 2-21 for additional information.

➤ Other Considerations

- The lipid profile does not measure LDL level directly but rather estimates it using the Friedewald equation:

$$LDL\text{-}C \ (mg/dL) = Total\ cholesterol - HDL\ cholesterol - (0.20 \times triglycerides)$$

- Note: the formula is only valid from a fasting specimen and triglycerides must be <400 mg/dL.
- LDL-C can be measured directly when the triglycerides are elevated.

➤ Suggested Reading

National Institutes of Health, National Heart Lung and Blood Institute's National Cholesterol Education Program http://www.nhlbi.nih.gov/about/ncep/ Accessed Nov. 18, 2010.

CHOLESTEROL, TOTAL, SERUM

➤ Definition

- A steroid, carried in the bloodstream as a lipoprotein. It is necessary for cell membrane functioning and as a precursor to bile acids, progesterone, vitamin D, estrogens, glucocorticoids, and mineralocorticoids.
- **Normal range:** See Table 2-22. (See p. 110)

➤ Use

- Assessment of risk of heart disease and atherosclerosis
- Ordered in combination with HDL, LDL, and triglycerides as a lipid profile

➤ Interpretation
Increased In

- Pregnancy
- Drugs: beta blockers, anabolic steroids, vitamin D, oral contraceptives, and epinephrine
- Obesity
- Smoking
- Alcohol
- Diet high in cholesterol and fats
- Renal failure
- Hypothyroidism

TABLE 2-21. Adult Treatment Panel III LDL-C Goals and Cut-off Points for Therapy

Risk Category	LDL-C Goal	Initiate TLC	Consider Drug Therapy[9]
High risk: CHD[1] or CHD risk equivalents[2] (10-year risk >20%)	<100 mg/dL (optional goal: <70 mg/dL)[6]	≥100 mg/dL[8]	≥100 mg/dL[10] (<100 mg/dL: consider drug options)[9]
Moderately high risk: 2+ risk factors[3] (10-year risk 10–20%)[4]	<130 mg/dL[7]	≥130 mg/dL[8]	≥130 mg/dL (100–129 mg/dL; consider drug options)[11]
Moderate risk: 2+ risk factors[3] (10-year risk <10%)[4]	<130 mg/dL	≥130 mg/dL	≥160 mg/dL
Lower risk: 0–1 risk factor[5]	<160 mg/dL	≥160 mg/dL	≥190 mg/dL (160–189 mg/dL: LDL-C-lowering drug optional)

[1]Coronary heart disease (CHD) includes history of myocardial infarction, unstable angina, stable angina, coronary artery procedures (angioplasty or bypass surgery), or evidence of clinically significant myocardial ischemia.

[2]CHD risk equivalents include clinical manifestations of noncoronary forms of atherosclerotic disease (peripheral arterial disease, abdominal aortic aneurysm, and carotid artery disease [transient ischemic attacks or stroke of carotid origin or >50% obstruction of a carotid artery]), diabetes, and 2+ risk factors with 10-year risk for hard CHD >20%.

[3]Risk factors include cigarette smoking, hypertension (BP >140/90 mm Hg or on antihypertensive medication), low HDL-C (<40 mg/dL), family history of premature CHD (CHD in male first-degree relative <55 years of age; CHD in female first-degree relative <65 years of age), and age (men ≥45 years; women ≥55 years).

[4]Electronic 10-year risk calculators are available at www.nhlbi.nih.gov/guidelines/cholesterol.

[5]Almost all people with zero or 1 risk factor have a 10-year risk <10%, and 10-year risk assessment in people with zero or 1 risk factor is thus not necessary.

[6]Very high risk favors the optional LDL-C goal of <70 mg/dL, and in patients with high triglycerides, non-HDL-C <100 mg/dL.

[7]Optional LDL-C goal <100 mg/dL.

[8]Any person at high risk or moderately high risk who has lifestyle-related risk factors (e.g., obesity, physical inactivity, elevated triglyceride, low HDL-C, or metabolic syndrome) is a candidate for therapeutic lifestyle changes to modify these risk factors regardless of LDL-C level.

[9]When LDL-lowering drug therapy is employed, it is advised that intensity of therapy be sufficient to achieve at least a 30–40% reduction in LDL-C levels.

[10]If baseline LDL-C is <100 mg/dL, institution of an LDL-lowering drug is a therapeutic option on the basis of available clinical trial results. If a high-risk person has high triglycerides or low HDL-C, combining a fibrate or nicotinic acid with an LDL-lowering drug can be considered.

[11]For moderately high-risk persons, when LDL-C level is 100–129 mg/dL, at baseline or on lifestyle therapy, initiation of an LDL-lowering drug to achieve an LDL-C level <100 mg/dL is a therapeutic option on the basis of available clinical trial results.

TABLE 2-22. Initial classification based on total cholesterol and HDL cholesterol

Total Cholesterol Level	Category
<200 mg/dL	Desirable level that puts a person at a lower risk of coronary heart disease. A cholesterol level of ≥200 mg/dL raises the risk.
200–239 mg/dL	Borderline high
≥240 mg/dL	High blood cholesterol. A person with this level has more than twice the risk of CHD as someone whose cholesterol is <200 mg/dL.

- Glycogen storage disease (i.e., von Gierke and Werner diseases)
- Familial hypercholesterolemia
- DM
- Biliary cirrhosis, hepatocellular disease
- Hyperlipoproteinemia types I, IV, V
- Prostate and pancreatic neoplasms

Decreased In
- Acute illness such as a heart attack
- Malnutrition
- Liver disease
- Myeloproliferative diseases
- Chronic anemias
- Infection
- Hyperthyroidism
- Stress
- Primary lipoproteinemias
- Tangier disease (familial alpha-lipoprotein deficiency)

Limitations
- Intraindividual variation may be up to 10%.
- Seasonal variation is 8% higher in the winter than in summer.
- Positional variation is 5% and 10–15% lower when phlebotomized sitting or recumbent, respectively, as opposed to standing.
- Other factors that may also increase cholesterol include cigarette smoking, age, hypertension, family history of premature heart disease, preexisting heart disease, and DM.

➤ Suggested Reading
American Heart Association. Cholesterol. http://www.heart.org/HEARTORG/Conditions/Cholesterol/CholestrolATH_UCM_001089_SubHomePage.jsp Accessed Nov. 18, 2010.

CHOLINESTERASE (PSEUDOCHOLINESTERASE)

➤ Definition
- Cholinesterase is an enzyme that catalyzes the hydrolysis of the neurotransmitter Ach into choline and acetic acid, a reaction necessary to allow a cholinergic neuron to return to its resting state after activation.

* Serum cholinesterase, often called pseudocholinesterase or PChE, is distinguished from acetylcholinesterase (AChE or "true cholinesterase") by both location and substrate.
  * PChE is found primarily in the liver.
  * AChE, also known as RBC cholinesterase, erythrocyte cholinesterase, or Ach acetylhydrolase, is found primarily in the blood and neural synapses.
* The difference between the two types of cholinesterase has to do with their respective preferences for substrates: AChE hydrolyzes Ach more quickly, and PChE hydrolyzes butyrylcholine more quickly.
* Phenotype interpretation is based on the total PChE activity and the percent of inhibition caused by dibucaine. Although there are >25 different phenotypes, most are extremely rare. Patients with unusual phenotypes cannot metabolize succinylcholine or mivacurium in the normal fashion; therefore, these patients can have prolonged paralysis following the use of these drugs.
* Other names: choline esterase II, serum cholinesterase (SChE), Ach acylhydrolase, butyrylcholinesterase (BChE), dibucaine inhibition, plasma cholinesterase
* **Normal range:** 2900–7100 U/L

➤ Use
* Monitoring exposure to organophosphorus insecticides
* Monitoring patients with liver disease, particularly those undergoing liver transplantation
* Identifying patients who are homozygous for the atypical gene, and have low levels of PChE that are not inhibited by dibucaine
* Identifying patients, who are heterozygous for the atypical gene; have lower than normal levels of PChE and varying levels of inhibition with dibucaine

➤ Interpretation
Increased In
* Type IV hyperlipoproteinemia
* DM
* Hyperthyroidism
* Insecticide exposure (organophosphates)
* Nephritic syndrome
* Psychosis
* Breast cancer

Decreased In
* Genetic PChE variants
* Severe PA, aplastic anemia
* Cirrhosis
* CHF (causing liver disease)
* Hepatic carcinoma
* Malnutrition
* Acute infections and burns
* AMI, pulmonary embolism
* Muscular dystrophy
* After surgery
* Chronic renal disease

➤ Limitations

- PChE levels is not to be confused with AChE levels. PChE levels are earlier indicators than AChE levels of organophosphate exposure.
- Patients with normal PChE activity show 70–90% inhibition by dibucaine, whereas patients homozygous for the abnormal allele show little or no inhibition (0–20%) and usually low levels of enzyme. Heterozygous patients have intermediate PChE levels and response to inhibitors.
- Anabolic steroids, carbamates, cyclophosphamide, estrogens, glucocorticoids, lithium, neuromuscular relaxants, oral contraceptives, organophosphorus insecticides, and radiographic agents decrease the circulating levels.
- Serum separator tubes, citrate anticoagulants, detergents, and heavy metals also decrease the serum levels.

CHORIONIC VILLUS SAMPLING

➤ Definition

- Invasive procedure to obtain chorionic villus tissue generally performed between 10 and 12 weeks of gestation
- Procedural risk of fetal loss (higher than for amniocentesis): ~1%.

➤ Use

- Provides placental material for chromosome (cytogenetic) testing, biochemical testing (metabolic disorders/inborn errors of metabolism), and molecular DNA-based testing for inherited disease (e.g., cystic fibrosis, fragile X)
- Primary advantage over amniocentesis is earlier time frame, allowing pregnancy termination in first trimester or earlier relief of anxiety.

➤ Limitations

- Chromosome results may be ambiguous due to confined placental mosaicism (abnormal chromosome line limited to placental tissue) in ~2% of cases, requiring follow-up by amniocentesis
- Maternal cell contamination must be avoided for accurate diagnosis based on fetal chromosomes, enzyme assay, or DNA analysis
- Does not provide material to screen for neural tube defects,

CHROMOGRANIN A, PLASMA

➤ Definition

- Chromogranin, also known as CGA and parathyroid secretory protein 1, is a member of the chromogranin/secretogranin (granins) family of neuroendocrine secretory proteins. It is a precursor to several functional peptides, including vasostatin, pancreastatin, catestatin, and parastatin. These peptides negatively modulate the neuroendocrine function of the releasing cell (autocrine) or nearby cells (paracrine).
- Chromogranin A is cleaved by an endogenous prohormone convertase to produce several peptide fragments. Peptides derived from chromogranin A with uncertain function include chromostatin, WE-14, and GE-25.

- The method of measurement is EIA.
- **Normal range:** 0–50 ng/mL

➤ Use
- As an indicator for pancreas and prostate cancer
- Aid in diagnosis of functioning neuroendocrine tumors; predicts response to treatment
- Aid in diagnosis of nonfunctioning neuroendocrine tumors (e.g., thyroid carcinoma, small cell lung cancer, anterior pituitary adenoma).

➤ Interpretation
Disorders with Increased Values
- Functioning neuroendocrine tumors and hyperplasia
- Pheochromocytoma, aortic, and carotid body tumors
- Neural tumors (e.g., neuroblastoma, ganglioneuroma, paraganglioma, medulloblastoma)
- Carcinoid tumors in various locations
- Gastroenteropancreatic tumors (e.g., gastinoma, insulinoma, VIPoma)
- Parathyroid adneoma, carcinoma, hyperplasia
- Thyroid medullary carcinoma, hyperplasia
- Tumors with variable neuroendocrine differentiation (e.g., breast, prostate)—low sensitivity
- DM, kidney, liver, or heart failure; correlates with severity of the CHF

Disorders without Increased Values
- Tumors with possible neuroendocrine lineage (e.g., choriocarcinoma, thymoma, malignant melanoma, renal cell carcinoma)
- After adrenal-to-caudate autografting and schizophrenia

Disorders with Decreased Values
- CSF in Parkinson disease

➤ Limitations
- Chromogranin A may not distinguish neuroendocrine hyperplasia from tumor.
- EIA may have lower limit of detection than RIA. Results obtained with different assay methods or kits cannot be used interchangeably.

CLOT RETRACTION

Clot retraction does not take place in the absence of functional platelets or of fibrinogen. Historically, it was the earliest test used in the discovery of thrombasthenia, but it is no longer in use.

CLOTTING FACTORS

➤ Definition
- Clotting factors are circulating plasma proteins. The final product, a clot, results from their interaction through an enzymatic cascade. *In vivo*, many of these interactions take place on lipid surfaces, the most abundant of which are provided by platelets. In contrast, *in vitro*, the cascade can be dissected into three pathways: intrinsic, extrinsic, and common. Although to

some extent artificial, this distinction remains useful for performing and understanding the tests of coagulation. For instance, PT reflects the extrinsic and common pathway, whereas PTT reflects the intrinsic and common pathway. Fibrinogen, the penultimate step in the generation of clots, is the target of the common pathway, being changed by thrombin into fibrin; finally, fibrin is consolidated by factor XIII to generate a stable clot, essential for achieving hemostasis through clotting. (Primary hemostasis through activation of platelets and the von Willebrand factor are discussed separately.)

- Properties of individual clotting factors
  - **Factor II** (prothrombin): synthesized in the liver; becomes active only after carboxylation by vitamin K. It is converted to thrombin (factor IIa). Its deficiency results in prolonged PT (INR) and PTT.
  - **Thrombin** (factor IIa): major coagulant that converts fibrinogen into fibrin. Has multiple functions, including as an anticoagulant, by binding to thrombomodulin on endothelial cell surfaces to convert protein C into its active form.
  - **Factor V** (the term factor VI, used in the past to refer to activated factor V, is no longer in use): synthesized in the liver; 20% is released from platelets. Cofactor in the conversion of factor II to IIa. Vitamin K has no effect on its activity. Proteolyzed by the protein C/S complex.
  - **Factor VII:** Synthesized in the liver. Becomes activated in a complex with tissue factor (previously known as factor III, term no longer used). To become active (VIIa) factor VII requires carboxylation by vitamin K. Shortest half-life of all clotting factors (4 hours) reflected in the initial rapid elongation in PT (elevation of INR) in patients started on vitamin K antagonists. Recombinant factor VIIa is used therapeutically.
  - **Factor VIII** (antihemophilic factor): Synthesized in the liver and endothelial cells of others organs (principally the spleen). It is unaffected by liver failure or vitamin K deficiency. Principal cofactor in the intrinsic pathway of coagulation. PT (INR) not affected by deficiency of factor VIII. PTT becomes prolonged when factor VIII decreases to <40%. Serves as substrate for proteolysis by the protein C/S complex. Purified or recombinant factor VIII preparations are used therapeutically.
  - **Factor IX** (previously also known as Christmas factor): Synthesized in the liver. Requires vitamin K to become active in coagulation. Principal factor in the intrinsic pathway of coagulation. PT (INR) not affected by deficiency of factor IX. PTT becomes prolonged when factor IX decreases to <40%. Purified and recombinant factor IX are used therapeutically
  - **Factor X** (previously also known as Stuart-Prower factor): synthesized in the liver. Requires vitamin K to become active in coagulation. Principal factor in the common pathway of coagulation where it converts factor II into IIA (thrombin). Both PT (INR) and PTT affected in marked deficiencies.
  - **Factor XI** (previously also known as plasma thromboplastin antecedent, PTA): Synthesized in the liver and megakaryocytes. Activates factors XII and IX in the intrinsic pathway. If markedly decreased it may prolong PTT, but not PT.
  - **Factor XII** (Hageman factor): Synthesized in the liver. Activated by collagen, disrupted basement membranes, activated platelets, and high–molecular-weight kininogen and prekallikrein in conjunction with factor XI. PTT (but not PT) is prolonged in severe deficiency. No bleeding diathesis associated with its congenital deficiency.
  - **High–Molecular-Weight Kininogen and Prekallikrein** (Fletcher factor): Clotting factors that activate the early phase of the intrinsic pathway and the complement system. May prolong PTT (not PT) when decreased. No bleeding diathesis associated with their congenital deficiencies.

- **Factor XIII** (fibrin stabilizing factor): Synthesized in the liver; also present in platelets. Stabilizes polymerized fibrin in the presence of calcium. Its deficiency does not affect PT (INR) or PTT. Clots are soluble in 5 molar urea.
- **Normal ranges:**
  - *Factors based on PT reagent*:
    - Factor II: 70–120%
    - Factor V: 70–150%
    - Factor VII: 70–150%
    - Factor X: 70–150%
  - *Factors based on PTT reagent*
    - Factor VIII: 70–150%
    - Factor IX: 70–120%
    - Factor XI: 60–120%
    - Factor XII: 60–150%
    - Prekallikrein: 55–207%
    - High–Molecular-Weight Kininogen: 59–135%

➤ Use

- Quantitation of clotting factors can be achieved through assays specific for each factor, whether chromogenic or, more commonly, automated clotting tests. A plasma deficient in each factor is purchased and used to find out to what extent it corrects the patient's plasma. The resulting clotting time is quantitated using a reference curve obtained with dilutions of normal pooled plasmas.
- A plasma deficient in any factor(s) active in the extrinsic and common pathway (VII, V, X, and II) results in a prolonged PT. These four factors are quantitated in assays that use PT reagents as activators. Plasma deficient in factors active in the intrinsic (and common) pathway (high–molecular-weight kininogen, prekallikrein, and factors XII, XI, IX, and VIII) prolong the PTT and are assayed with PTT reagents.
- When to use clotting factor tests:
  - When a discrete congenital clotting deficiency (most commonly factors VIII and IX) is suspected
  - Occasionally, to separate the effect of oral anticoagulants (decrease in factors II, VII, IX and II, but not V or VIII), from liver disease (deficiencies of all these clotting factors, including factor V, but not factor VIII)
  - To measure blood heparin (factor Xa inhibition) and possibly when therapeutic inhibitors of factor X are used therapeutically

➤ Interpretation
Increased

- **Factor II:** genetic mutation *G20210A* that predisposes to thromboembolism
- **Factor VII:** pregnancy and oral contraceptive use. An increase in factor VII has been linked to thrombophilia in some studies.
- **Factor VIII:** acute phase reactant (acute inflammatory conditions), pregnancy, and the use of oral contraceptives. If markedly increased, it may predispose to thromboembolism.
- **Factor IX:** pregnancy and use of oral contraceptives. Very elevated values have been associated with a tendency to thromboembolism.
- **Factor X:** pregnancy and use of oral contraceptives

Decreased

- **Factor II**
  - Congenital deficiency (recessive inheritance): bleeding of various severities in homozygotes
  - Acquired deficiency: liver disease, DIC, pathologic fibrinolysis
- **Factor V**
  - Congenital: inherited autosomal deficiency; bleeding in homozygotes
  - Acquired: liver disease, DIC, or pathologic fibrinolysis
- **Factor VII**
  - Congenital deficiency: manifested by variable bleeding in homozygotes
  - Acquired: liver disease, vitamin K deficiency, vitamin K antagonist therapy
- **Factor VIII**
  - Congenital: hemophilia A in male patients and in some female carriers of the hemophilia gene (usually mild decrease); Von Willebrand disease, especially if moderate to severe
  - Acquired: Acquired anti-factor VIII autoantibodies in previously unaffected individuals; acquired anti-factor VIII alloantibodies in multiply transfused hemophilia A patients; DIC and pathologic fibrinolysis
- **Factor IX**
  - Congenital: hemophilia B
  - Acquired: liver disease, vitamin K deficiency or use of vitamin K antagonists, nephrotic syndrome, amyloidosis, autoantibodies to factor IX in previously healthy individuals (extremely rare), alloantibodies in hemophilia B patients treated with factor IX infusions
- **Factor X**
  - Congenital: rare autosomal recessive defect. Homozygotes may have a bleeding diathesis.
  - Acquired: severe liver disease; vitamin K deficiency or use of vitamin K antagonists, DIC, amyloidosis
- **Factor XI**
  - Congenital: autosomal recessive inheritance; mild bleeding diathesis if markedly decreased
- **Factor XIII**
  - Congenital: severe bleeding in homozygous deficiency; impaired wound healing
  - Acquired: liver disease; acute promyelocytic leukemia; autoantibodies against factor XIII

➤ Limitations

- Improperly filled test tubes, or the use of different anticoagulants than recommended (3.2% sodium citrate as provided in blue top tubes)
- Improperly stored plasma
- Hyperlipidemic, hemolyzed, or icteric blood may affect the results.
- Contamination with heparin or dilution of the collected blood if indwelling catheters are used

CLOTTING TIME (LEE-WHITE CLOTTING TIME)

The clotting time is characterized by low sensitivity and poor standardization. It is of only historical interest and is no longer in use.

COCAINE

➤ Definition
• This drug is an ester of benzoic acid and amino alcohol.
• Other names: benzoylmethylecgonine, ecgonine methyl ester benzoate
• A therapeutic range has not been established when cocaine is used clinically as a local anesthetic in ophthalmic and otolaryngologic procedures. Cocaine is considered to be a drug of abuse and is controlled in schedule II of the U.S. Controlled Substances Act of 1970.

➤ Use
• Local anesthetic due to blockade of sodium channel conductance
• CNS stimulant: blocks reuptake of neurotransmitters norepinephrine, serotonin, dopamine

➤ Interpretation
• Cocaine is metabolized primarily to benzoylecgonine and ecgonine methyl ester. Further metabolism produces ecgonine and additional compounds. Coingestion of ethanol results in the formation of cocaethylene. Presence of these compounds is indicative of exposure but does not provide guidance as to the degree of intoxication or impairment. Clinical signs and symptoms must be used.
• The clinician should be aware of testing performed in the laboratory, especially the target analyte and whether the test is a screen or confirmation. The analyte present or absent may provide guidance to the time of exposure.

➤ Limitations
• Screening assays are commonly immunoassay based
  • ELISA for blood, serum, plasma
    • Target analyte: cocaine
    • Cut-off concentration: variable—20–50 ng/mL
    • Significant cross-reactivity with cocaethylene
    • Low cross-reactivity with ecgonine methyl ester, norcocaine, ecgonine
  • EIA for urine
    • Target analyte: benzoylecgonine (metabolite)
    • Cut-off concentration:
      • 150 ng/mL
      • 300 ng/mL
    • Approximately 50–60% cross-reactivity with cocaine and cocaethylene
    • Low cross-reactivity with EME, ecgonine
• Confirmation assays are commonly chromatography based regardless of specimen
  • GC/MS
    • Full scan mode for qualitative identification of cocaine, cocaethylene and metabolites: limits of detection—20–50 ng/mL
    • Selected ion monitoring mode for quantitative analysis of serum, plasma for cocaine, cocaethylene, and metabolites: limits of quantitation—5–20 ng/mL
  • LC/MSn (multiple MS)
    • Multiple reactions monitoring mode for qualitative or quantitative analysis of cocaine, cocaethylene, and metabolites: limits of detection/quantitation—20–50 ng/mL

COLD AGGLUTININS

➤ Definition
- Autoantibodies with specificity against RBC determinants that react at low temperature but not at body temperature. (Reactions against i determinants are less common.) The cold-reactive agglutinins are of the IgM class immunoglobulins; very rarely IgG. The IgM autoantibodies bind at low temperature to complement on the RBC membrane.
- **Normal titer:** <1:32 (negative result)

➤ Use
- Blood must be collected, clotted, and the serum separated at 37°C, and in addition, the sample must be maintained at 37°C. Alternatively, it can be collected on EDTA at room temperature, but then it must be warmed for at least 15 minutes at 37°C.
- The direct (Coombs) antiglobulin test is positive against C3d and C4d components of complement.
- Testing for cold agglutinins is recommended when the clinical symptomatology suggests cold agglutinin disease.

➤ Interpretation
- Cold agglutinin titers above 1:32 are diagnostic for the presence of cold agglutinin disease. The titer in affected patients may be >1000.

➤ Limitations
- Refrigeration of blood at any time adversely affects the results, as does severely hemolyzed or lipemic specimens.

COMBINED FIRST-TRIMESTER AND SECOND-TRIMESTER SCREENING (INTEGRATED/SEQUENTIAL SCREENING)

➤ Definition
- Integrated screening combines first-semester and second-trimester screening to give one result after the second-trimester screen is completed.
- Sequential screening gives the risk after the first trimester if risk is higher than a specific cut-off and gives the combined risk after the second trimester if first trimester risk was not higher than the cut-off. It can be further divided into stepwise and contingent.
  - Stepwise screening: women with risk above a certain cut-off following the first trimester screen are offered invasive diagnostic testing directly, whereas women below cut-off are offered second trimester screening.
  - Contingent screening: women with high risk are offered diagnostic testing, women with intermediate risk are offered second trimester screening, and women with low risk have no further testing.
  - Some centers prefer to divide patients into two groups only: those with high risk who will be offered invasive testing directing and those who will proceed to second trimester testing.

➤ Use
- Risk assessment for trisomy 18, trisomy 21, and neural tube defects
- Ultrasound in the first-trimester screen also contributes to detection of other chromosome abnormalities.

➤ Interpretation
• ~95% detection of trisomy 21 with 5% screen-positive rate

➤ Limitations
• Noncompliant patients may not return for the second-semester screen.

➤ Suggested Readings
American College of Obstetrics and Gynecology. Practice Bulletin, Clinical Management Guidelines for Obstetrician-Gynecologists #77, Screening for Fetal Chromosomal Abnormalities. 2007;109:217–227.
Driscoll DA and Gross S. Prenatal screening for aneuploidy, *N Engl J Med.* 2009;360:2556–2562.

COMPLETE BLOOD COUNT (CBC)

➤ Definition
• CBC is a numerical report of all blood elements, as well as a description of some of their major characteristics. Most laboratories use automated counters. The CBC reports include RBC count, WBC count, platelet count, Hb, Hct (volume of packed red cells), mean platelet volume, and other parameters (described under individual tests).
• The CBC may be ordered as a simple count of blood elements and RBC indices or as a test that includes a WBC differential.

➤ Use
• CBC is used for screening whenever abnormalities in RBCs, WBCs, or platelets are suspected.
• New analyzers may separate reticulocytes and platelets into young and mature populations that help detect bone marrow regeneration. Automated counters flag abnormalities in RBCs, WBCs, and platelets, triggering examination of the peripheral blood smear.

➤ Limitation
• Proper specimen collection is required for reliable and accurate reporting of the CBC. Misleading results occur if the specimens contain clots, if the blood is not properly mixed, or in the presence of agglutinated RBCs. Specific pitfalls are described under each lineage.

COOMBS (ANTIGLOBULIN) TEST

DIRECT COOMBS TEST (DAT)

➤ Definition
• The DAT is used to detect IgG antibodies or complement components that bind to antigens on the RBC surface membrane. The assay uses Coombs (antihuman globulin) reagent incubated with the patient's washed RBCs.

➤ Use
• DAT is useful in diagnosing autoimmune hemolysis (see p. 809), hemolytic diseases of the newborn (see p. 809), drug-induced hemolysis, and transfusion reactions (see p. 894).

➤ Interpretation
Positive DAT
* Hemolytic disease of the newborn (erythroblastosis fetalis)
* Warm autoimmune hemolytic anemias
  * Idiopathic
  * SLE
  * Evan's syndrome (ITP and hemolytic anemia)
  * Infrequently positive in cold antibody autoimmune hemolytic anemias
* Alloimmune (delayed) hemolytic transfusion reactions
* Drug-induced reactions, such as:
  * Alpha-methyldopa
  * L-Dopa
  * High doses of penicillin
  * Quinidine

Negative DAT
* Hemolytic anemias caused by an intrinsic RBC defect (e.g., G6PD [see p. 197], hemoglobin-opathies [see p. 796])

➤ Limitations
* False-positive results may occur in plasma cell myeloma and lymphoplasmacytic lymphoma.
* 1:10,000 normal blood donors have a positive DAT.
* Negative DAT is a rare occurrence in patients with autoimmune hemolytic anemia (provided erythrocyte-bound C3b had been excluded). It may be due to a too small amount of IgG bound to RBC membrane.

INDIRECT COOMBS TEST (IAT)

➤ Definition
* The IAT uses patient's serum, which is incubated with RBC of known antigenicity. It is positive if the patient's serum contains antibodies against RBC. In about 80% of patients with autoimmune hemolytic anemia, the autoantibodies are also present in serum.
* In addition, alloantibodies induced by previous blood transfusions or fetal–maternal incompatibility are also detected by this assay. Alloantibodies present only in serum have specificity for RBC antigens not present on the patient's own RBCs (DAT is negative in such cases).

➤ Use
* Antibody screening and cross-matching prior to blood transfusions
* Prenatal testing of pregnant women
* To detect and identify autoantibodies in acquired hemolytic anemia
* RBC phenotyping
  * In genetic and forensic medicine
  * To identify syngeneic twins for stem cell transplantation

➤ Limitations
* The Coombs tests may miss low titer antibodies

CO-OXIMETRY

➤ Definition
- Co-oximetry refers to the measurement of various forms of hemoglobin by dedicated multi-wavelength spectrophotometry.

➤ Use
- It usually measures concentrations of oxygenated hemoglobin (oxyHb), deoxygenated hemoglobin (deoxyHb or reduced Hb), carboxyhemoglobin (COHb), and methemoglobin (MetHb) as a percentage of the total hemoglobin concentration in the blood sample.

➤ Indications
- History consistent with toxin exposure
- Hypoxia fails to improve with the administration of oxygen,
- Existence of a discrepancy between the PaO_2 on a blood gas determination and the oxygen saturation on pulse oximetry (SpO_2)
- Suspected other dyshemoglobinemias such as methemoglobinemia or carboxyhemoglobinemia.

Oxygen Saturation (SO₂)
- Calculated as O_2 Hgb/O_2 Hb+HHB*100%
- The availability of oxygen to tissues is dependent not only on SO_2 but also on the affinity of O_2 to Hb. It is clinically useful in cyanosis and erythrocytosis. It may differentiate between diminished oxygenation of blood, as in pulmonary diseases and admixture of venous blood, as in an AV shunt.
- Percent saturation in newborns is 40–90% and thereafter 94–98%; values decrease with age.

Oxyhemoglobin
- This represents the fraction of oxygenated Hb in relation to the total Hb present, including non–oxygen-binding Hb. In healthy individuals, oxyhemoglobin and oxygen saturation are approximately equal. In the presence of dyshemoglobins, oxyhemoglobin can be considerably lower than oxygen saturation. Although the oxygen saturation often remains within the reference limits, the oxygen-carrying capacity of the blood may be severely decreased.
- **Normal range:** 94–100%

Carboxyhemoglobin
- This is Hb that has carbon monoxide instead of the normal oxygen bound to it. Carbon monoxide (CO) has a much great affinity than oxygen for hemoglobin.
- Carboxyhemoglobin is formed in carbon monoxide poisoning. The source of the carbon monoxide may be exhaust (such as from a car, truck, boat, or generator), smoke from a fire, or tobacco smoke. The carboxyhemoglobin level is useful in judging the extent of CO toxicity and in considering the effect of smoking on the patient. A direct correlation has been claimed between CO level and symptoms of atherosclerotic diseases, angina, and MI.
  - Nonsmokers: 0.5–1.5% saturation of HgB
  - Smokers: 1–2 packs/day: 4–5%
  - Heavy smokers: >2 packs/day: 8–9%

Methemoglobin
* This is produced by the oxidation of the normal ferrous iron of Hg to ferric iron, making it chemically useless for respiration.
* A small amount of methemoglobin is normally present in blood, but the conversion of a larger fraction of hemoglobin into methemoglobin, results in perceptible cyanosis. Methemoglobinemia may be acquired anytime in life by exposure to a number of different chemical agents, such as nitrites or it may be congenital due a genetic condition
* **Normal:** 0.06–0.24 g/dL

COPPER

➤ Definition
* Copper is a metal component of various enzymes (e.g., cytochrome oxidase, superoxide dismutase, tyrosinase) involved in Hb synthesis, bone and elastic tissue development, and CNS function.
* **Normal range:** see Table 2-23

➤ Use
* Aids in the diagnosis of Wilson disease
* Assessment of primary biliary cirrhosis
* Assessment of primary sclerosing cholangitis

➤ Interpretation
Increased In
* Wilson disease
* Anemias
  * PA
  * Megaloblastic anemia of pregnancy
  * Iron-deficiency anemia
  * Aplastic anemia
* Leukemia and lymphoma
* Infection, acute and chronic
* Biliary cirrhosis and sclerosing cholangitis
* Hemochromatosis
* Collagen diseases (including SLE, RA, acute RF, GN)
* Hypothyroidism
* Hyperthyroidism
* Frequently associated with increased CRP

TABLE 2-23. Normal Levels of Serum Copper

Age	Male (µg/dL)	Female (µg/dL)
≤6 months	20–70	20–70
7 months to 18 years	90–190	90–190
≥19 years	70–140	80–155

* Ingestion of oral contraceptives and estrogens
* Pregnancy

Decreased In
* Wilson disease: mutation interferes with copper transport from intestinal mucosal cytoplasm to Golgi apparatus, where it becomes bound to protein
* Menkes kinky hair syndrome
* Nephrosis (ceruloplasmin lost in urine)
* Acute leukemia in remission
* Some iron-deficiency anemias of childhood (that require copper as well as iron therapy)
* Kwashiorkor, chronic diarrhea
* ACTH and corticosteroids

➤ Limitations
* Serum copper may be elevated with infection, inflammation, stress, copper supplementation, oral contraceptives, and pregnancy.
* Concentrations are 2–3 × normal in the third trimester of pregnancy.
* Copper may be lowered with corticosteroids, zinc, malnutrition, and malabsorption.
* Serum specimen should be collected in a trace element-free tube, such as royal blue sterile tube, to avoid contamination.
* High urinary copper levels support the diagnosis but are not unique to Wilson disease, as they can be sometimes observed in autoimmune hepatitis and cholestasis.

CORTICOTROPIN-RELEASING HORMONE (CRH)

➤ Definition
* CRH is a 41 amino acid peptide hypothalamic factor that increases ACTH release from pituitary cells. CRH is synthesized by neurons in the parvocellular division of the hypothalamic paraventricular nuclei. The axons of the nuclei project to the median eminence, where CRH is secreted into the hypophysial portal blood. The ACTH released by CRH stimulates the secretion of cortisol and other adrenal steroids, such as DHEA and, transiently, aldosterone.
* CRH circulates in human plasma bound to a high-affinity binding protein, which reduces its bioactivity and increases its clearance.
* In addition to being produced in the hypothalamus, CRH is also synthesized in peripheral tissues, such as T lymphocytes, and is highly expressed in the placenta. In the placenta, CRH is a marker that determines the length of gestation and the timing of parturition and delivery.
* Other names: corticoliberin, corticotropin-releasing factor (CRF)
* **Normal range:** up to 10 pg/mL

➤ Use
* The contribution of hypothalamic CRH to peripheral plasma CRH concentrations is small; most of the plasma CRH presumably comes from nonhypothalamic sources.
* However, under certain circumstances, such as insulin-induced hypoglycemia or during major surgery, small increments in plasma CRH concentrations may reflect hypothalamic CRH release.

➤ Interpretation
Increased In
* Cushing syndrome
* Ectopic tumors producing ACTH
* Third trimester of pregnancy

Decreased In
* Alzheimer disease
* Autosomal recessive hypothalamic corticotropin deficiency

➤ Limitations
* Patient should be fasting 10–12 hours and should not take any corticosteroid, ACTH, or estrogen medications, if possible, for at least 48 hours prior to collection of specimen. An a.m. specimen is preferred.
* A rapid increase in circulating levels of CRH occurs at the onset of parturition.
* Plasma CRH concentrations do not correlate with plasma ACTH or serum cortisol concentrations or with altered hypothalamic-pituitary-adrenal axis function (e.g., in primary adrenal insufficiency or Cushing syndrome, or during insulin-induced hypoglycemia or metyrapone administration). Some investigators have reported a correlation between plasma CRH and plasma ACTH or serum cortisol in pregnancy, but others have not.

CORTICOTROPIN-RELEASING HORMONE (CRH) STIMULATION TEST

➤ Definition
* CRH is a 41 amino acid peptide, secreted by the paraventricular nucleus of the hypothalamus in response to stress. It acts on the anterior lobes of pituitary to release ACTH. There is considerable sequence homology of CRH among species; as a result both ovine and human CRH can be used in testing.
* Also known as: CRH after low-dose dexamethasone test
* **Normal range:**
  * CRH stimulation test:
    * Most patients with Cushing disease respond with ACTH and cortisol increases within 45 minutes after CRH. However, the criteria for interpretation have varied at different centers.
    * Basal plasma ACTH concentrations increase 35–9005 (mean 400%) in normal subjects and reach a peak of 10–120 pg/mL, 10–30 minutes after CRH injection; serum cortisol concentrations increase 20–600% (mean 250%) to 13–36 µg/dL (mean 25 µg/dL), reaching a peak 30–60 minutes after CRH injection.
  * CRH after low-dose dexamethasone test:
    * Cortisol 1.4 µg/L is virtually 100% specific and 100% diagnostic for Cushing syndrome.

➤ Use
* Objectives
  * To evaluate the cause of ACTH-dependent Cushing syndrome (with or without vasopressin analogs)

* To discriminate between pseudo-Cushing and Cushing syndrome
* To discriminate between primary and central adrenal insufficiency
* CRH stimulation test: The patient fasts for 4 hours or more, after which an intravenous access line is established and synthetic ovine CRH (1 μg per kg body weight or 100 μg total dose) is injected as an intravenous bolus. Blood samples for ACTH and cortisol are drawn 15 (or 5) and 0 minutes before and as often as 5, 10, 15, 30, 45, 60, 90, and 120 minutes after CRH injection. However, in Cushing syndrome, if one measures only the plasma ACTH response, the samples at -5, -0, 15, and 30 minutes are sufficient, and if one measures only the serum cortisol response, the samples at -15, 0, 45, and 60 minutes are sufficient. Normally both hormones should be measured, since the criteria for a positive response may include increases in either plasma ACTH or serum cortisol concentrations.
* CRH test after low-dose dexamethasone procedure: The patient takes 0.5 mg of dexamethasone every 6 hours for 2 days (a total of eight doses); 2 hours after the last dexamethasone dose is taken, 1 μg/kg of CRH is administered intravenously. Blood for a plasma cortisol measurement is drawn 15 minutes after the CRH injection.

➤ Interpretation
* Normal or exaggerated response: pituitary Cushing disease
* No response: ectopic ACTH secreting tumor

➤ Limitations
* Responses to CRH are variable among subjects and from one time to another in the same subject.
* The increment in plasma ACTH is the same in the morning and evening; however, the peak value is greater in the morning in normal subjects when the basal plasma ACTH concentration is higher. In contrast, the peak serum cortisol value is similar at both times of day, but the increment is smaller in the morning when the basal value is higher. In patients with Cushing syndrome, in whom the normal circadian rhythm in ACTH secretion is absent, the CRH test can be performed at any time of day with similar results.
* The response to CRH depends on the cause of the hypoadrenalism.
  * Patients with primary pituitary ACTH deficiency (secondary adrenal insufficiency) have decreased plasma ACTH and serum cortisol responses to CRH.
  * Patients with hypothalamic disease (i.e., CRH deficiency) usually have exaggerated and prolonged plasma ACTH responses; the plasma cortisol responses are subnormal.
  * The CRH stimulation test is more reliable than the ACTH stimulation test in detecting pituitary-adrenal suppression in preterm infants whose mothers received a short course of dexamethasone before delivery to hasten fetal lung development.

CORTISOL FREE URINE, 24-HOUR

➤ Definition
* Cortisol free urine, 24-hour, or urinary free cortisol, provides a direct and reliable practical index of cortisol secretion. It is an integrated measure of serum free cortisol level that is not affected by body weight.

- **Normal range:**
  - Males: <60 µg/day; <32 µg/g creatinine
  - Females: <45 µg/day; <45 µg/g creatinine

➤ Use

- Cushing syndrome (screening). The patient can be assumed to have Cushing syndrome if basal urinary cortisol excretion is more than 3 × the upper limit of normal and one other test is abnormal.
- Adrenal insufficiency (limited usefulness)
- Assisting in diagnosing acquired or inherited abnormalities of 11β-hydroxy steroid dehydrogenase (cortisol-to-cortisone ratio)
- Diagnosis of pseudo-hyperaldosteronism due to excessive licorice consumption

➤ Interpretation

- Cortisol free urine, 24-hour, is increased in Cushing syndrome. This result is found in 95% of cases of Cushing syndrome. Values <100 µg per 24 hours exclude the diagnosis, and values >300 µg per 24 hours confirm the diagnosis. If values are intermediate, a dexamethasone suppression test is indicated.
- It is decreased in adrenal insufficiency.

➤ Limitations

- Urinary cortisol may be detected by antibody-based (immunoassays) or structurally based (HPLC-MS) tests, and the immunoassays may be less specific because antibodies may cross-react with similar steroids.
- An increase is the most useful screening test (best expressed as per gram creatine, which should vary by <10% daily; if variation is >10%, two more 24-hour specimens should be collected). Values should be measured in three consecutive 24-hour specimens to ensure proper collection and account for daily variability, even in Cushing syndrome.
- Increased values may occur in depression, chronic alcoholism, eating disorders, and polycystic ovary syndrome but do not exceed 300 µg per 24 hours.
- Various drugs (e.g., carbamazepine, phenytoin, phenobarbital, primidone) will falsely elevate free cortisol levels
- Acute and chronic illnesses can increase free cortisol levels
- Renal disease due to decreased excretion may falsely lower the levels of free cortisol.

CORTISOL, SALIVA

➤ Definition

- Serum free cortisol freely diffuses into saliva. Therefore, measurements of salivary cortisol (hydrocortisone) more accurately reflect the serum free cortisol. The salivary cortisol concentration is independent of salivary flow rate.
- **Normal range:** varies diurnally, with concentrations about 5.6 ng/mL at 8:00 to 9:00 a.m. and about 1 ng/mL at 11:00 p.m.

➤ Use

* Screening for Cushing syndrome
* Diagnosis of Cushing syndrome in patients presenting with symptoms or signs suggestive of the disease
* Assessing cortisol secretion serially in ambulatory patients. Measurements are helpful in patients with cyclical Cushing syndrome.

➤ Interpretation

* Late evening levels are increased in Cushing syndrome.
* Morning levels are decreased in adrenal insufficiency.

➤ Limitations

* The assay methodology affects normal range.
* Changes in cortisol-binding globulin and albumin affect total cortisol levels but not free levels in serum and saliva.

CORTISOL, SERUM

➤ Definition

* Cortisol (hydrocortisone) is the major glucocorticoid produced and secreted by the adrenal cortex. It affects the
  * Metabolism of protein, fat, and carbohydrates
  * Maintenance of muscle and myocardial integrity
  * Suppression of inflammatory and allergic activities
* **Normal range:**
  * AM cortisol: 8.7–22.4 µg/dL
  * PM cortisol: <10 µg/dL

➤ Use

* Discrimination between primary and secondary adrenal insufficiency
* Differential diagnosis of Cushing syndrome

➤ Interpretation

* The most common cause of increased plasma cortisol levels in women is a high circulating concentration of estrogen (e.g., estrogen therapy, pregnancy), resulting in increased concentration of cortisol-binding globulin.
* Patients with severe illness and sepsis have reduced cortisol-binding globulin and albumin levels, resulting in lowered cortisol levels.

➤ Limitations

* Bound cortisol circulates in an available but temporarily inactive state. The physiologic activity of cortisol depends on levels of the small fraction of circulating unbound cortisol.
* Acute stress (including hospitalization and surgery), alcoholism, depression, and many drugs (e.g., exogenous cortisones, anticonvulsants) can obliterate normal diurnal variation, affect response to suppression/stimulation tests, and cause elevated baseline levels.

- Patients taking prednisone may have falsely increased cortisol levels because prednisone is converted to prednisolone after ingestion and prednisolone has a 41% cross-reactivity.
- Cortisol levels may be increased in pregnancy and with exogenous estrogens.
- Some patients with depressive disorders have a hyperactive hypothalamic-pituitary-adrenal axis, similar to Cushing syndrome.

C-PEPTIDE

➤ Definition
- Human C-peptide is a 31 amino acid chain with a molecular mass of approximately 3020 daltons. Metabolically inert, it originates in the pancreatic B cells as a byproduct of the enzymatic cleavage of proinsulin to insulin. In this process, insulin and C-peptide are split from the prohormone and secreted into the portal circulation in equimolar concentrations.
- Within limits, C-peptide levels can serve as a valuable index to insulin secretion. Therefore, low C-peptide levels are to be expected where insulin secretion is diminished, as in insulin-dependent diabetes, or suppressed, as a normal response to exogenous insulin, whereas elevated C-peptide levels may result from the increased B-cell activity observed in insulinomas.
- **Normal range:** 0.9–7.1 ng/mL

➤ Use
- For estimating insulin levels in the presence of antibodies to exogenous insulin
- Diagnosis of factitious hypoglycemia due to surreptitious administration of insulin in which high serum insulin levels occur with low C-peptide levels

➤ Interpretation
Increased In
- Insulinoma
- Type 2 DM

Decreased In
- Exogenous insulin administration (e.g., factitious hypoglycemia)
- Type 1 DM

➤ Limitations
- C-peptide serum levels correlate with insulin levels in blood, except in islet cell tumors and possibly in obese patients.

C-REACTIVE PROTEIN, HIGH-SENSITIVITY

➤ Definition
- High-sensitivity C-reactive protein (hs-CRP, or cardiac CRP) is an acute-phase reactant produced by hepatocytes and induced by the release of interleukin 1 and 6.
- It reflects activation of systemic inflammation. Blood levels of CRP are known to rise rapidly from normal baseline levels to as high as 50 mg/dL as part of the body's nonspecific inflammatory response to infection or injury.
- The hs-CRP test is more sensitive than the standard CRP test.
- **Normal range:** <0.3 mg/dL (see Table 2-24)

TABLE 2-24. Cardiovascular Risk Classification By C-Reactive Protein (CRP)*

Risk Level	CRP (mg/L)
Low	<1.0
Average	1.0–3.0
High	>3.0

*Cardiovascular disease risk assessment guidelines for CRP recommended by the CDC and the American Heart Association (CDC/AHA).
Source: Pearson TA, Mensah GA, Alexander RW, et al. Markers of inflammation and cardiovascular disease. Application to clinical and public health practice. A Statement for Healthcare Professionals From the Centers for Disease Control and Prevention and the American Heart Association. *Circulation.* 2003;107:499–511.

➤ Use

• Performing risk assessment for cardiovascular disease: Cardiac disease is believed to be the end result of interplay between minor changes in the cardiovascular endothelium and the corresponding inflammatory response to these changes.
  • hs-CRP is an independent risk factor for cardiovascular disease, stroke, and peripheral vascular disease. It adds to the predictive value of total cholesterol and HDL cholesterol for future events.
  • hs-CRP may be useful as an independent marker of prognosis for recurrent events in patients with stable coronary disease or acute coronary syndrome. Recent evidence supporting this potential application has shown that high baseline values of CRP in individuals without a history of cardiac disease were associated with an increased incidence of subsequent cardiac events.
• Determining risk of hypotension: hs-CRP has been reported as a risk factor for hypotension.

➤ Interpretation

• hs-CRP appears within 24–48 hours, peaks at 72 hours, and becomes negative after 7 days; it correlates with peak CK-MB levels, but the CRP peak occurs 1–3 days later.
• Failure of CRP to return to normal indicates tissue damage in the heart or elsewhere. The absence of a CRP increase raises the question of necrosis in prior 2–10 days. CRP is usually normal in patients with unstable angina in the absence of tissue necrosis and a normal troponin T (<0.1 ng/mL).
• Peak hs-CRP correlates with peak CK-MB following AMI. CRP may remain increased for at least 3 months following AMI.

Increased In

• Acute or chronic inflammatory change
• Tissue injury or necrosis
• Ischemia or infarction of other tissues
• Infections, inflammation, tissue injury, or necrosis (possible)
• Metabolic syndrome
• Elevated blood pressure
• Malignant (but not benign) tumors, especially breast, lung, and GI tract

- Pancreatitis
- Postsurgery
- Burns, trauma
- Leukemia: fever, blast crisis, or cytotoxic drugs
- Cigarette smoking
- Hormone therapy, estrogen, and progesterone

Decreased In
- Exercise and weight loss
- Moderate alcohol consumption
- Drugs (e.g., statins, fibrates, niacin)

➤ Limitations
- Race and gender differences affect CRP levels. One study indicates that black patients have higher levels than white patients and women have higher levels than men.

➤ Suggested Readings

Khera A, McGuire DK., Murphy, et al. Race and gender differences in C-reactive protein levels. *J Am Coll Cardiol.* 2005;46: 464–469.

Pearson TA, George A, Mensah R, et al. Markers of inflammation and cardiovascular disease. Application to clinical and public health practice. A Statement for healthcare professionals from the Centers for Disease Control and Prevention and the American Heart Association. *Circulation.* 2003;107:499–511.

CREATINE

➤ Definition
- Creatine is synthesized in the liver, taken up by muscle for stored energy as creatine phosphate, and broken down to creatinine; it then enters the circulation and is excreted by the kidneys.
- **Normal range:**
  - Male: 0.2–0.7 mg/dL
  - Female: 0.3–0.9 mg/dL

➤ Use
- Serum creatine levels may be significantly increased in amyotrophic lateral sclerosis, dermatomyositis, myasthenia gravis, starvation, muscular dystrophies, and trauma. Creatine synthesis is stimulated by methyltestosterone and may also be increased in hyperthyroidism, diabetic acidosis, and puerperium.
- This test is rarely used clinically.

➤ Interpretation
Increased In
- High dietary intake (meat)
- Destruction of muscle
- Hyperthyroidism (this diagnosis is almost excluded by normal serum creatine)
- Active RA
- Testosterone therapy

Decreased In
* Not clinically significant
* Drugs (e.g., TMP/SMX, cimetidine, cefoxitin)

➤ Limitations
* Artifactual decrease in DKA

CREATINE KINASE (CK), TOTAL

➤ Definition
* CK is an enzyme that catalyzes the interconversion of ATP and creatine phosphate, control-ling energy flow within cells, principally muscle. Its activity is greatest in striated muscle, heart tissue, and brain. The determination of CK activity is a proven tool in the investiga-tion of skeletal muscle disease (muscular dystrophy) and is also useful in the diagnosis of MI and CVAs.
* **Normal range:**
  * Male: 49–348 IU/L
  * Female: 38–206 IU/L

➤ Use
* Marker for injury or diseases of cardiac muscle with good specificity
* Measurement of choice for striated muscle disorders

➤ Interpretation
Increased In
* Necrosis or inflammation of cardiac muscle: disorders listed under CK-MB (CK index usually >4%)
* Necrosis, inflammation, or acute atrophy of striated muscle
  * Disorders listed under CK-MB (CK index usually <4%)
  * Muscular dystrophy
  * Myotonic dystrophy
  * Amyotrophic lateral sclerosis (>40% of cases)
  * Polymyositis (70% of cases; average 20 × ULN)
  * Thermal and electrical burns (values usually higher than in AMI)
  * Rhabdomyolysis (especially with trauma and severe exertion); marked increase may be 1000 times ULN
  * Severe or prolonged exercise as in marathon running (begins 3 hours after start of exercise; peaks after 8–16 hours; usually normal by 48 hours); smaller increases in well-conditioned athletes
  * Status epilepticus
  * Parturition and frequently the last few weeks of pregnancy
  * Malignant hyperthermia
  * Hypothermia
  * Familial hypokalemic periodic paralysis
  * McArdle disease

* Drugs and chemicals
  * Cocaine
  * Alcohol
  * Emetine (ipecac)—(e.g., bulimia)
  * Chemical toxicity; benzene ring compounds (e.g., xylene) depolarize the surface membrane and leach out low–molecular-weight enzymes, producing very high levels of total CK (100% fraction muscle [MM]) with increased LD) (3–5 × normal)
* Half of patients with extensive brain infarction. Maximum levels are reached in 3 days; the increase may not appear before 2 days; levels are usually lower than in AMI and remain increased for a longer time; levels return to normal within 14 days; high mortality is associated with levels >300 IU. Elevated serum CK in brain infarction may obscure diagnosis of concomitant AMI.
* Some persons with large muscle mass (≤2 times normal) (e.g., football players)
* **Slight increase** (occasionally) in
  * Variable increase after IM injection to 2–6 times normal level; returns to normal 48 hours after cessation of injections; rarely affects CK-MB, LD-1 (Lactate dehydrogenase-1), AST
  * Muscle spasms or convulsions in children
* Moderate hemolysis

Decreased In
* Decreased muscle mass (e.g., elderly, malnutrition, alcoholism)
* RA (about two thirds of patients)
* Untreated hyperthyroidism
* Cushing disease
* Connective tissue disease not associated with decreased physical activity
* Pregnancy level (8th to 12th week) is said to be ~75% of nonpregnant level
* Various drugs (e.g., phenothiazine, prednisone, estrogens, tamoxifen, ethanol), toxins, and insecticides (e.g., aldrin, dieldrin)
* Metastatic tumor in liver
* Multiple organ failure
* Intensive care patients with severe infection or septicemia

Normal In
* Pulmonary infarction
* Renal infarction
* Liver disease
* Biliary obstruction
* Some muscle disorders
  * Thyrotoxicosis myopathy
  * Steroid myopathy
  * Muscle atrophy of neurologic origin (e.g., old poliomyelitis, polyneuritis)
* PA
* Most malignancies
* Scleroderma
* Acrosclerosis
* Discoid lupus erythematosus

➤ Limitations

* Following MI, CK activity increases 4–8 hour after acute onset, activities peak at 12–36 hours, and usually returns to normal activities in 3–4 days. Although total CK has been used as a diagnostic tool for MI detection, along with CK-MB, it has been predominantly replaced with troponin I or T due to lack of myocardial specificity.
* Exercise and muscle trauma (contact sports, traffic accidents, IM injections, surgery, convulsions, wasp or bee stings, and burns) can elevate serum CK values.
* To distinguish myoglobinuria from hemoglobinuria, serum CK and LD may be helpful. CK is normal with uncomplicated hemolysis but LD and LD-1 usually are increased.

CREATINE KINASE ISOENZYMES (CK-BB, CK-MM, CK-MB)

➤ Definition

* Creatine kinase is an enzyme consisting of three major isoenzymes, CK-BB (brain), CK-MB (heart) (see p. 134), and CK-MM (skeletal muscle).
  * CK-BB is rarely present. It has been described as a marker for adenocarcinoma of the prostate, breast, ovary, colon, and GI tract, and for small cell anaplastic carcinoma of lung. CK-BB has been reported with severe shock and/or hypothermia, infarction of bowel, brain injury, stroke, as a genetic marker in some families with malignant pyrexia, and with MB in alcoholic myopathy.
  * CK-MM is found in normal serum.

➤ Use

* Detection of macro forms of creatine kinase (CK)
  * Diagnosing skeletal muscle disease, in conjunction with aldolase
  * CK isoenzymes are not widely used in clinical practice today due to the use of troponin and CK-MB mass assays.
* *The CK-BB isozyme is rarely encountered clinically.*

➤ Interpretation
Increased In

Malignant hyperthermia, uremia, brain infarction or anoxia, Reyes syndrome, necrosis of intestine, various metastatic neoplasms (especially prostate), biliary atresia

MACRO CK ISOENZYME

➤ Definition

* This isoenzyme is a high-molecular mass complex of a CK isoenzyme and immunoglobulin, most often CK-BB and monoclonal IgG and a kappa light chain.
* Macro CK type 2 is an oligomeric mitochondrial CK complex that migrates cathodically, or close to CK-MM. It is found primarily in adults who are severely ill with malignancies or liver disease, or in children who have myocardial disease. It occurs transiently in about 1% of hospitalized patients and indicates a poor prognosis, except in children.

➤ Use

* Macroenzymes should be suspected when enzyme levels are persistently raised with relatively constant levels and there is no obvious clinical explanation or other laboratory abnormality

➤ Interpretation

- The clinical relevance of macro CK type 1 is not clearly established. It is not associated with a particular type of disease and has been observed in patients with various diseases, as well as in apparently healthy individuals. There are several reported disease associations, including hypothyroidism, neoplasia, autoimmune disease, myositis, and cardiovascular disease. The last two have the strongest reported associations and may support the diagnosis of an autoimmune process, but this may in part be explained by a higher frequency of requests for CK levels in these groups of patients. Myositis, including autoimmune myositis, polymyositis, malignancy-associated dermatomyositis, and drug-induced myositis, has been diagnosed in >50% of the patients with macro CK type.
- Atypical macro isoenzyme is found primarily in adults who are severely ill with malignancies or liver disease or in children who have myocardial disease. It occurs transiently in about 1% of hospitalized patients and indicates a poor prognosis, except in children.

➤ Limitations

- *Atypical macro isoenzyme may cause falsely high or low CK-MB results (depending on type of assay), resulting in an incorrect diagnosis of myocardial infarction (MI) or delayed recognition of an actual MI.* The atypical macro isoenzyme is discovered in <2% of all CK isoenzyme electrophoresis studies.

CREATINE KINASE MB (CK-MB)

➤ Definition

- CK-MB is the myocardial fraction associated with MI and occurs in certain other states. MB can be used in estimation of infarct size.
- CK-MB, or CK-MB fraction, is an 84 kDa molecular weight enzyme that represents 40% of the CK present in myocardial tissue. As with total CK, CK-MB typically begins to rise 4–6 hours after the onset of infarction but is not elevated in all patients until about 12 hours. Elevations return to baseline within 36–48 hours, in contrast to elevations in serum troponin, which can persist for as long as 10–14 days. This means that CK-MB, unlike troponins, cannot be used for the late diagnosis of an acute MI but can be used to suggest infarct extension if levels rise again after declining.
- CK-MB generally comprises a lower fraction of total CK in skeletal muscle than in the heart. As a result, percentage criteria (4%) have been proposed to distinguish skeletal muscle damage from cardiac damage. However, these criteria are not recommended. They improve specificity, but do so at the cost of sensitivity in patients who have both skeletal and cardiac injury.
- **Normal range:**

	Reference Interval	
Analyte	Male	Female
CK-MB	<4.4 ng/mL	<4.4 ng/mL
CK-MB Index	0.0–4.0	0.0–4.0

➤ Use

- CK-MB is a widely used early marker for myocardial injury.

➤ Interpretation
Increased In

* Necrosis or inflammation of cardiac muscle (CK index ~2.5%; in all other causes, CK index usually <2.5%):
  * AMI
  * Cardiac contusion
  * After thoracic/open heart surgery, values return to baseline in 24–48 hours. AMI is difficult to diagnose in the first 24 postoperative hours.
  * Resuscitation for cardiac arrest may increase CK and CK-MB in ~50% of patients, with peak at 24 hours, due to defibrillation (>400 J) and chest compression, but CK-MB/CK total ratio may not be increased, even with AMI.
  * Percutaneous transluminal coronary angioplasty
  * Myocarditis
  * Prolonged supraventricular tachycardia
  * Cardiomyopathies (e.g., hypothyroid, alcohol)
  * Collagen diseases involving the myocardium
  * Coronary angiography (transient)
* Necrosis, inflammation, or acute atrophy of striated muscle:
  * Exercise myopathy; slight to significant increases in 14–100% of persons after extreme exercise (e.g., marathons); smaller increases in well-conditioned athletes
  * Skeletal muscle trauma with rhabdomyolysis, myoglobinuria
  * Skeletal muscle diseases (e.g., myositis, muscular dystrophies, polymyositis, collagen vascular diseases [especially SLE])
  * Familial hypokalemic periodic paralysis
  * Electrical and thermal burns and trauma (~50% of patients; but not supported by LD-1 > LD-2)
  * Drugs (e.g., alcohol, cocaine, halothane [malignant hyperthermia], ipecac)
* Endocrine disorders (e.g., hypoparathyroid, acromegaly, DKA; hypothyroidism—total CK 4–8 times ULN in 60–80% of cases; becomes normal within 6 weeks of replacement therapy)
* Some infections:
  * Viral (e.g., HIV, EBV, influenza, picornaviruses, coxsackievirus, echovirus, adenoviruses)
  * Bacterial (e.g., *Staphylococcus, Streptococcus, Clostridium, Borrelia*)
  * Rocky Mountain spotted fever
  * Fungal
  * Parasitic (e.g., trichinosis, toxoplasmosis, schistosomiasis, cysticercosis)
* Others:
  * Malignant hyperthermia; hypothermia
  * Reye syndrome
  * Peripartum period for first day beginning within 30 minutes
  * Acute cholecystitis
  * Hyperthyroidism and chronic renal failure, which may cause persistent increase although the proportion of CK-MB remains low
  * Acute exacerbation of obstructive lung disease
  * Drugs (e.g., aspirin, tranquilizers)
  * Carbon monoxide poisoning

- Some neoplasms:
  - For example, prostate, breast
  - 90% of patients following cryotherapy for prostate carcinoma with peak at 16 hours to about 5 times ULN; similar increase in total CK
- % activity distribution of CK isoenzymes in tissue

	CK-MB
Skeletal muscle	1
Myocardium	22
Brain	0

- A CK-MB >15–20% should raise the possibility of an atypical macro CK-MB.

Not Increased In
- Increase in angina pectoris, coronary insufficiency, exercise testing for CAD, or pericarditis implies some necrosis of cardiac muscle, even if a discrete infarct is not identified.
- Following cardiopulmonary bypass, cardiac catheterization (including Swan-Ganz), cardiac pacemaker, and coronary arteriography, unless the myocardium has been injured by a catheter
- IM injections (total CK may be slightly increased)
- Seizures (total CK may be markedly increased)
- Brain infarction or injury (total CK may be increased)

➤ Limitations
- The presence of CK-MB is not unequivocally specific for myocardium, because it is found in patients with muscular dystrophies, polymyositis, hypothermia and hyperthermia, uremia, DKA, and septic shock. Renal failure, tissue damage following surgery, and cardiac contusion may also cause an elevation of CK-MB.
- Cardiac troponin is the preferred marker for the diagnosis of MI. CK-MB by mass assay is an acceptable alternative when cardiac troponin is not available.

➤ Suggested Readings
Apple FS, Preese LM. Creatine kinase-MB: detection of myocardial infarction and monitoring reperfusion. *J Clin Immunoassay.* 1994;17:24–29.

Gibler WB, Lewis LM, Erb RE, et al. Early detection of acute myocardial infarction in patients presenting with chest pain and nondiagnostic ECGs: serial CK-MB sampling in the emergency department. *Ann Emerg Med.* 1990;19(12):1359–1366.

CREATININE CLEARANCE (CrCl)

➤ Definition
- This test compares the creatinine in a 24-hour sample of urine to the creatinine level in the blood to show how much blood the kidneys are filtering out each minute. It is calculated by the formula:

$$\frac{U_{Cr} \times 24\text{-hour volume}}{P_{Cr} \times 24 \times 60 \text{ minutes}}$$

where U_{Cr} is urine creatinine, P_{Cr} is plasma creatinine

* **Normal range:**
  * Male: 90–139 mL/min
  * Female: 80–125 mL/min

➤ Use
* Evaluate glomerular function
* Monitor effectiveness of treatment in renal disease

➤ Interpretation
Increased In
* Acromegaly
* Acute tubular necrosis
* Carnivorous diets
* CHF
* Dehydration
* Diabetes
* Exercise
* Exposure to nephrotoxic drugs and chemicals
* Gigantism
* GN
* Hypothyroidism
* Infections
* Neoplasms (bilateral renal)
* Nephrosclerosis
* Polycystic kidney disease
* Pyelonephritis
* Renal artery atherosclerosis and obstruction
* Renal disease
* Renal vein thrombosis
* Shock and hypovolemia
* TB

Decreased In
* Acute or chronic GN
* Anemia
* Chronic bilateral pyelonephritis
* Hyperthyroidism
* Leukemia
* Muscle wasting diseases
* Paralysis
* Polycystic kidney disease
* Shock
* Urinary tract obstruction (e.g., from calculi)
* Vegetarian diets

➤ Limitations
* CrCl approximates GFR but overestimates it due to the fact that creatinine is secreted by the proximal tubule as well as filtered by the glomerulus.

- Measurement of CrCl should be considered in circumstances when the estimating equation based on serum creatinine is suspected to be inaccurate or for patients with estimated GFR >60 mL/min/1.73 m^2 when a more accurate clearance measure is required for clinical decision making. Such circumstance may occur in people who are undergoing evaluation for kidney donation, treatment with drugs with significant toxicity that are excreted by the kidneys (e.g., high-dose methotrexate), or consideration for participation in research protocols.
- Indications for a clearance measurement because estimates based on serum creatinine may be inaccurate because of extremes of age and body size, severe malnutrition or obesity, disease of skeletal muscle, paraplegia or quadriplegia, a vegetarian diet, rapidly changing kidney function, or pregnancy
- Drugs that may increase urine CrCl include enalapril, oral contraceptives, prednisone, and ramipril.
- Drugs that may decrease the urine CrCl include acetylsalicylic acid, amphotericin B, carbenoxolone, chlorthalidone, cimetidine, cisplatin, cyclosporine, guancydine, ibuprofen, indomethacin, mitomycin, oxyphenbutazone, paromomycin, probenecid (coadministered with digoxin), and thiazides.
- Excessive ketones in urine may cause falsely decreased values.
- Failure to follow proper technique in collecting 24-hour specimen may invalidate test results.
- Failure to refrigerate the specimen throughout the urine collection period allows decomposition of creatinine, causing falsely decreased values.
- Consumption of large amounts of meat, excessive exercise, and stress should be avoided for 24 hours before the test.

➤ Suggested Reading
National Kidney Foundation KDOQI Clinical Practice Guidelines for Chronic Kidney Disease: Evaluation, Classification, and Stratification http://www.kidney.org/professionals/kdoqi/guidelines_ckd/p5_lab_g4.htm Accessed Nov. 18, 2010.

CREATININE WITH ESTIMATED GLOMERULAR FILTRATION RATE (eGFR)

➤ Definition
- Creatinine is formed by the hydrolysis of creatine and phosphocreatine in muscle and by ingestion of meat. It is freely filtered at the glomerulus and secreted at the proximal tubule; some is resorbed.
- **Normal range:**
  - **Creatinine**
    - 0–1 month: 0.00 to 1.00 mg/dL
    - 1 month to 1 year: 0.10 to 0.80 mg/dL
    - 1–16 years: 0.20 to 1.00 mg/dL
    - >16 years, female: 0.50 to 1.20 mg/dL
    - >16 years, male: 0.60 to 1.30 mg/dL
  - **eGFR**
    - >16 years: >60 mL/min/1.73 m^2
    - IDMS-Traceable MDRD Study Equation for the calculation of GFR:

- GFR (mL/min/1.73 m^2) = **175** $\times$ (S$_{cr}$)$^{-1.154}$ $\times$ (Age)$^{-0.203}$ $\times$ (0.742 if female) $\times$ (1.212 if African American) (conventional units); where Scr is serum creatinine.
- (The equation has not been validated in children and will only be reported for patients >16 years of age. The equation is normalized for an average adult body surface area of 1.73 m^2; weight and height adjustment is not necessary.)

➤ Use

- To diagnose renal insufficiency; more specific and sensitive indicator of renal disease than BUN. Use of simultaneous BUN and creatinine determinations provides more information in conditions.
- Serum creatinine and BUN are not useful in discovering early renal insufficiency, because they do not become abnormal until 50% of renal function has been lost. Serum creatinine shows poor sensitivity but very good specificity.
- Adjusting dosage of renally excreted medications
- Monitoring renal transplant recipients
- Serum creatinine levels are a proxy for reduced skeletal muscle mass.
- eGFR: Serum creatinine measurement is used in estimating GFR for people with chronic kidney disease (CKD) and those with risk factors for CKD (DM, hypertension, cardiovascular disease, and family history of kidney disease).

➤ Interpretation
Increased In

- Diet: ingestion of creatinine (roast meat)
- Muscle disease: gigantism, acromegaly
- Prerenal azotemia
- Postrenal azotemia
- Impaired kidney function; 50% loss of renal function is needed to increase serum creatinine from 1.0–2.0 mg/dL. Therefore. the test is not sensitive for mild to moderate renal injury
- An increase in serum creatinine occurs in 10–20% of patients taking aminoglycosides and ≤20% of patients taking penicillins (especially methicillin).

Decreased In

- Pregnancy: normal value is 0.4–0.6 mg/dL. A value >0.8 mg/dL is abnormal and should alert the clinician to further diagnostic evaluation.
- Creatinine secretion is inhibited by certain drugs (e.g., cimetidine, trimethoprim).
- Proxy for reduced skeletal muscle mass

➤ Limitations*

- Artifactual decrease by:
  - Marked increase of serum bilirubin
  - Enzymatic reaction (glucose >100 mg/dL)
- Artifactual increase due to:
  - Reduction of alkaline picrate (e.g., glucose, ascorbate, uric acid). Ketoacidosis may substantially increase serum creatinine results with alkaline picrate reaction.

---

*Depending on methodology; can be avoided by measuring rate of color development.

- Formation of colored complexes (e.g., acetoacetate, pyruvate, other ketoacids, certain cephalosporins).
- Enzymatic reaction: 5-fluorocytosine may increase serum creatinine ≤0.6 mg/dL.
- Other methodologic interference (e.g., ascorbic acid, phenolsulfonphthalein, L-dopa,)

CREATININE, URINE

➤ Definition
- Creatine is synthesized from amino acids in the kidney, liver, and pancreas. The creatine is then transported in the blood to other organs where it is synthesized into creatinine. In the absence of kidney disease, the urinary creatinine is excreted in rather constant amounts and represents glomerular filtration and active tubular excretion of the kidney.
- Because the creatinine is excreted from the body at a constant rate, there are expected values for creatinine in normal human urine. Specimen validity testing is the evaluation of the specimen to determine if it is consistent with normal human urine (creatinine values >20 mg/dL). Creatinine is made at a steady rate and is not affected by diet or by normal physical activities.
- **Normal range:** see Table 2-25

➤ Use
- Urinary creatinine, in conjunction with serum creatinine, is used to calculate the creatinine clearance, a measure of renal function

➤ Interpretation
Increased In
- Exercise
- Acromegaly
- Gigantism
- DM
- Infections
- Hypothyroidism
- Animal meat diet

TABLE 2-25. Normal Values for Urine Creatinine	
By Sex	Value
24-hour urine	mg/day
Male	800–2000
Female	600–1800
Random urine	mg/dL
Male	
<40 years	24–392
>40 years	22–328
Female	
<40 years	16–327
>40 years	15–278

Decreased In
- Hyperthyroidism
- Anemia
- Muscular dystrophy
- Decreased muscle mass
- Advances renal disease
- Leukemia
- Vegetarian diets

➤ Limitations
- Urine creatinine is not ordered alone. Creatinine clearance, which requires a serum creatinine, offers useful renal function data. Serum creatinine alone is not an adequate index of glomerular filtration rate.
- 24-hour urine creatinine levels are used as an approximate check on the completeness of 24-hour urine collection.

CRYOFIBRINOGEN

➤ Definition
- Cryofibrinogen is an abnormal complex of proteins that precipitate out of plasma as it is cooled. These cold, insoluble protein complexes can be composed of fibrin, fibrinogen, fibrin split products, and other plasma proteins.
- If refrigerated serum and plasma both form a precipitate, then the precipitated proteins are referred to as cryoglobulins. If, however, precipitation develops after refrigeration of plasma but does not occur in cold serum, the plasma precipitate is referred to as cryofibrinogen.
- Cryofibrinogen can occur spontaneously or in association with other inflammatory conditions. Secondary cryofibrinogenemia has been reported in patients with malignancy, DM, collagen vascular disease, and active infection. Most individuals with cryofibrinogenemia are asymptomatic.
- Morbidity associated with cryofibrinogenemia occurs as the result of thrombotic occlusion of the small to medium arteries by insoluble protein complexes.
- **Normal range:**
  - Negative at 72 hours, quantitation, and immunotyping is not generally performed on positive cryofibrinogen.

➤ Use
- Patients with unexplained cutaneous ulcers, ischemia, or necrosis on cold-exposed areas
- Evaluating patients with vasculitis, GN, and lymphoproliferative diseases

➤ Interpretation
Increased In
- Vasculitis
- Hematologic and solid neoplasms
- Thromboembolic conditions
- Multiple myeloma

- Scleroderma
- Transient benign condition associated with infection
- Oral contraceptives

➤ Limitations

- If heparin is used as an anticoagulant in blood collection tubes, it may complex with fibrinogen, fibrin, and fibronectin, and leads to falsely positive results. Therapeutically administered heparin may also produce false-positive results. Therefore, collected blood should be anticoagulated with EDTA, citrate, or oxalate, and maintained at 37°C until the plasma is collected.
- Fasting specimen recommended. Proper collection and transport of specimen is critical to the outcome of the assay.
- Cryofibrinogenemia can be a primary (essential) condition or it may arise in association with an underlying condition, such as malignancy, infection, inflammation, diabetes, pregnancy, scleroderma, or oral contraceptives. A few familial cases have been reported. Skin biopsies may show leukocytoclastic vasculitis.
- May cause erroneous WBC count when performed on electronic cell counter.

➤ Suggested Reading

Nash JW, Ross P Jr, Neil Crowson A, et al. The histopathologic spectrum of cryofibrinogenemia in four anatomic sites. Skin, lung, muscle, and kidney. *Am J Clin Pathol.* 2003;119:114–122.

CRYOGLOBULINS

➤ Definition

- Cryoglobulins are abnormal serum proteins that precipitate at low temperatures and dissolve at some point when temperature is raised. They cannot be identified by serum protein electrophoresis. Cryoglobulins are made up of monoclonal antibodies IgM or IgG, rarely IgA. IgM tends to precipitate at lower temperatures than does IgG cryoglobulin.
- Other names: cryocrit, cryoprotein
- Cryoglobulins are classified as follows:
  - **Type I** (monoclonal immunoglobulin, especially IgM κ type)
    - Causes 25% of cases
    - Most commonly associated with multiple myeloma and Waldenström macroglobulinemia; other lymphoproliferative diseases with M components; may be idiopathic
    - Often present in large amounts (>5 mg/dL serum); blood may gel when drawn
    - Severe symptoms (e.g., Raynaud syndrome, gangrene without other causes)
  - **Type II** (monoclonal immunoglobulin mixed with at least one other type of polyclonal immunoglobulin, most commonly IgM and polyclonal IgG; always with RF)
    - Causes up to 25% of cases
    - Associated most often with chronic HCV infection; less often with HBV, EBV, bacterial and parasitic infections, autoimmune disorders, Sjögren syndrome, syndrome of essential mixed cryoglobulinemia, immune-complex nephritis (e.g., membranoproliferative GN, vasculitis)
    - High titer RF without definite rheumatic disease
    - C4 levels decreased

- **Type III** (mixed polyclonal immunoglobulin, most commonly IgM–IgG combinations, usually with RF)
  - Causes ~50% of cases
  - Usually present in small amounts (<1 mg/dL serum) in normal persons
  - Most commonly associated with lymphoproliferative disorders, connective tissue diseases (e.g., SLE), persistent infections (e.g., HCV)
- **Normal range:**
  - Negative (positives reported as percent)
  - If positive, immunotyping of the cryoprecipitate is performed

➤ Use
- Assist in diagnosis of neoplastic diseases, acute and chronic infections, and collagen diseases
- Detect cryoglobulinemia in patients with symptoms indicating or mimicking Raynaud disease, cyanosis, skin ulceration
- Monitor course of collagen and rheumatic disorders

➤ Interpretation
- Cryoglobulins with a detected monoclonal protein normally prompt a clinical investigation to determine if an underlying disease exists

➤ Limitations
- Cryoglobulins are not to be confused with cryofibrinogen, which precipitates in plasma, rather than serum in cold conditions. Cryofibrinogens are rare and can be associated with vasculitis.
- Failure to maintain sample at normal body temperature or warm before centrifugation can affect results.
- A recent fatty meal can increase turbidity of the blood, decreasing visibility.

➤ Suggested Readings
Coblyn JS, McCluskey RT. Case records of the Massachusetts General Hospital. Weekly clinicopathological exercises. Case 3-2003: A 36-year-old man with renal failure, hypertension and neurologic abnormalities. *N Engl J Med.* 2003;348:333–342.
Kallemuchikkal U, Gorevic PD. Evaluation of cryoglobulins. *Arch Pathol Lab Med.* 1999;123:119–125.

CRYSTAL IDENTIFICATION, SYNOVIAL FLUID

➤ Definition
- Synovial fluid, often referred to as "joint fluid," is a viscous liquid found in the joint cavities. Synovial membranes line the joints, bursae, and tendon sheaths. The function of the synovial fluid is to lubricate the joint space and transport nutrients to the articular cartilage.
- The aspiration and analysis of synovial fluid may be done to determine the cause of joint disease, especially when accompanied by an abnormal accumulation of fluid in the joint (effusion). The joint disease may be crystal-induced, degenerative, inflammatory, or infectious. Morphologic analysis for cells and crystals, together with Gram stain and culture, help in the differentiation.

- Normal synovial fluid is a clear, pale yellow, viscous liquid that does not clot. When a synovial membrane is inflamed for any reason, the WBC count in the synovial fluid increases.
- In a rough fashion, one can classify this fluid into four groups.
  - Noninflammatory effusions (group I) occur when the WBC count is normal or minimally increased, as in traumatic arthritis or degenerative joint disease. Only rarely will such fluid have WBC counts of >2000 cells/mm^3.
  - Noninfectious mildly inflammatory effusions (group II) with WBC counts rarely >5000 cells/mm^3 occur in SLE and scleroderma
  - In noninfectious acute inflammatory effusions (group III) characteristic of classic rheumatoid arthritis, gout, pseudogout, and rheumatic fever, the WBC count varies from 5000–25,000 cells/mm^3 but may exceed 50,000 or even 100,000 cells/mm^3.
  - In the inflammatory effusions caused by infection (group IV) the WBC count commonly varies from 25,000 to >100,000 cells/mm^3. As the WBC count becomes elevated, the percentage of polymorphonuclear leukocytes generally increases, the hyaluronate becomes degraded, and the synovial fluid sugar falls.
- Examination of synovial fluid for crystals is facilitated by having a microscope with polarizing filters and a quarter wave plate (also known as a "red compensator"). Birefringence is a term used to describe the optical property associated with certain transparent crystals in which the speed of propagation of light along the major and minor axes of the crystal differs, causing the plane of polarized light to be rotated.
- Detection of birefringent crystals is facilitated by use of two plane polarizing filters, one between the light source and the sample, the other between the sample and the observer's eye. When the polarized filters are crossed, the background appears dark, and birefringent material, including a variety of crystals, appears brighter than the background.
- Several types of crystals have been found in synovial fluids (Table 2-26). The two most important are monosodium urate (MSU), characteristic of gouty effusions, and calcium pyrophosphate dihydrate (CPPD), characteristic of the effusions of pseudogout (crystal deposition disease). Other crystals such as calcium hydroxyapatite, calcium oxalate, cholesterol, and corticosteroid esters may also be associated with inflammatory effusions.
- Crystals that cause inflammation are usually 0.5 to ~20 μm in length, sparingly soluble in water, and capable of being phagocytized. At the peak of inflammation, most are intracellular.
- **Normal range:** absent (no crystals present)

➤ Use

- According to the American College of Radiology, synovial fluid analysis should be undertaken in the febrile patient with an acute flare of established arthritis (e.g., RA, osteoarthritis) to rule out superimposed septic arthritis.
- Repeated aspiration and synovial fluid analysis may be used to monitor the response of septic arthritis to treatment and may also be valuable for diagnosis of some cases of gout in which the initial aspirate does not have detectable crystals.

➤ Interpretation

- Positive identification of crystals provides a definitive diagnosis of joint disease

TABLE 2-26. Birefringent Materials in Synovial Fluid

Material	Usual Shape, Size	Birefringence	Cause	Location within or Outside of PMNs, Macrophages
Crystals				
Monosodium urate	Needle, rod, parallel edges; 8–10 μm long	Strongly –	Gout	Within or outside
Calcium pyrophosphate dihydrate	Rhomboid; may be rod, diamond, square, needle; <10 μm long	Weakly +	Pseudogout	Only within
Calcium oxalate	Bipyramidal	Strong; 0	Long-term renal dialysis	Within or outside
Hydroxyapatite, other basic calcium phosphates	Aggregates only; small, (<1 μm), round, irregular	Weak; 0	Degenerating, calcifying joint (e.g., acute or chronic arthritis)	
Cholesterol	Flat, plate, corner notch; may be needle, rectangle; often >100 μm	Variable		
Cartilage, collagen	Irregular, rodlike	Strong; +		
Charcot-Leyden	Spindle; crystalloids of eosinophil membrane protein	Variable	Eosinophilic synovitis	
Steroids				
Betamethasone acetate	Rods; blunt ends; 10–20 μm	Strong; –	Injection into joint	
Cortisone acetate	Large rods	Strong; +		
Methyl prednisone acetate	Small, pleomorphic; tend to clump	Strong; 0		
Prednisone tebutate	Small, pleomorphic, branched, irregular	Strong; +		
Triamcinolone acetonide	Small, pleomorphic fragments; tend to clump	Strong; 0		
Triamcinolone hexacetonide	Large rods, blunt ends; 15–60 μm	Strong; 0		

(Continued)

TABLE 2-26. Birefringent Materials in Synovial Fluid (*Continued*)

Material	Usual Shape, Size	Birefringence	Cause	Location within or Outside of PMNs, Macrophages
Anticoagulants				
EDTA (dry)	Small, amorphous	Weak		
Lithium heparin (not sodium)	May resemble pseudogout	Weak; +	Injection into joint	
Other Materials				
Debris	Small, irregular, nonparallel	Variable edges		
Fat (cholesterol esters)	Globules	Strong; Maltese cross		
Starch granules	Round; size varies	Strong; Maltese cross		

+, positive birefringence; –, negative birefringence; 0, no axis
EDTA, ethylenediaminetetraacetic acid; PMN, polymorphonuclear neutrophil.
Crystals are best seen in fresh, wet-mount preparations examined with polarizing light.
Hydroxyapatite complexes (diagnostic of apatite disease) and basic calcium phosphate complexes can be identified only by EM; most cases are suspected clinically but never confirmed.
(Source: Judkins SW, Cornbleet PJ. Synovial fluid crystal analysis. *Lab Med.* 1997;28:774. With permission from American Society for Clinical Pathology and ASCP Press.)

➤ Limitations

- Powdered anticoagulants such as oxalate are themselves crystalline; their use may cause confusion, masking the presence of synovial fluid crystals definitive for the disease.
- Substantial variability has been noted among hospital laboratories in the ability to properly identify the presence or absence of MSU and CPPD crystals in synovial fluids. Studies of the performance of different hospital laboratories on the same synovial fluids suggest that MSU crystals are more easily detected than CPPD crystals.
- MSU crystals: reported sensitivity ranges from 63–78%; specificity, from 93–100 percent (positive likelihood ratio of 14 for a diagnosis of gout).
- CPPD crystals: reported sensitivity ranges from 12–83 percent; specificity 78–96 percent (positive likelihood ratio of 2.9 for a diagnosis of CPPD-associated arthritis)
- The stability of crystals in synovial fluids is studied by many at different temperatures. CPPD crystals dissolved significantly and MSU crystals were detectable up to weeks but became smaller and less numerous. As storage time increased, new artificial crystals developed in the form of star-shaped arrays, plate-like structures, and positive birefringent Maltese crosses. Synovial fluid should be evaluated within 1 hour of collection.

CYCLIC CITRULLINATED PEPTIDE ANTIBODY, IgG

➤ Definition

- Antibodies to citrullinated proteins are markers of RA, especially for early diagnosis of the disease. In some cases these antibodies may be detected many years before the onset of the first symptoms.
- Other names: CCP-IgG, citrullinated antibody, anticitrullinated antibody, anticitrullinated protein antibody (ACPA)
- **Normal range:**
  - <20 units: negative
  - 20–39 units: weak positive
  - 40–59 units: moderate positive
  - ≥60 units: strong positive

➤ Use

- Evaluating patients suspected of having RA. 2010 American College of Rheumatology guidelines (recommends performing at least one serologic test (RF or CCP-IgG) and one acute-phase response measure (ESR or CRP) to classify a patient as having or not having definite RA in addition to a history of symptom duration and a thorough joint evaluation.
- Differentiating RA from other connective tissue diseases that may present with arthritis and may be positive for RF, such as HCV-associated cryoglobulinemia, undifferentiated polyarthritis, and Sjögren syndrome
- Differential diagnosis of early polyarthritis

➤ Interpretation

- Increased in RA (a positive result for CCP antibodies indicates a high likelihood of RA)

➤ Limitations

- The sensitivity of CCP-IgG for RA varies from about 50–75%, depending on the assay and study population, whereas specificity for RA is relatively high, usually >90%

- Not all individuals with RA will have detectable anti-CCP antibodies, and elevated anti-CCP antibodies may be seen in individuals with no evidence of clinical disease.
- The use of anti-CCP antibody levels for monitoring the progression and/or remission of RA has not been established.
- The diagnostic value of anti-CCP antibodies has not been determined for juvenile arthritis.

➤ Suggested Reading
Aletaha D, Neogi T, Silman A, et al. 2010 Rheumatoid arthritis classification criteria: an American College of Rheumatology/European League Against Rheumatism collaborative initiative. *Ann Rheum Dis.* 2010;69(9): 1580–1588.

CYSTATIN C (CysC)

➤ Definition
- Low–molecular-weight cysteine protease inhibitor. It is a nonglycosylated peptide consisting of 120 amino acids and is produced by virtually all nucleated cells. Cystatin C is present in all investigated body fluids and is not affected by age, gender, muscle mass, or the inflammatory process.
- Cystatin C is removed from circulation by glomerular filtration and is completely reabsorbed and degraded in the tubules. Therefore, the plasma concentration of cystatin C is almost exclusively determined by the GFR, making cystatin C an excellent indicator of GFR.
- **Normal range:**
  - 0–3 months: 0.8–2.3 mg/L
  - 4–11 months: 0.7–1.5 mg/L
  - 1–3 years: 0.5–1.3 mg/L
  - 4–8 years: 0.5–1.3 mg/L
  - 9–17 years: 0.5–1.3 mg/L
  - ≥18 years: 0.5–1.0 mg/L

➤ Use
- New marker to estimate GFR independent of gender, age, and muscle mass, and cirrhosis; does not need to be corrected for height or weight. It is superior to serum creatinine.
- Sensitive marker of allograft function (although it may not be an optimal marker in patients receiving glucocorticoids).
- In the assessment of adverse cardiovascular events (CHF, ischemia, death) because kidney dysfunction is associated with such events

➤ Interpretation
Increased In
- Glucocorticoid treatment
- May also be affected by thyroid disorders

➤ Limitations
- Due to immaturity of renal function in neonates, cystatin C levels are higher in those <3 months of age.

CYSTIC FIBROSIS (CF) MUTATION ASSAY

➤ Definition
* CF testing identifies mutations in the cystic fibrosis transmembrane conductance regulator (*CFTR*) gene.
* **Normal values:** negative or no mutations are found

➤ Use
* There are three groups of tests:
  * Targeted mutation analysis tests
    * 23 mutation panel recommended by the American College of Medical Genetics in 2004, or other panels testing for more mutations
    * Reflex testing for the poly T variant (5T/7T/9T), a string of thymidine bases located in intron 8, is recommended for individuals having the *R117H* mutation or an adult male patients who is being evaluated for congenital absence of the vas deferens (CAVD). The 5T variant is thought to decrease the efficiency of intron 8 splicing.
  * Sequence analysis: analysis of the entire coding region, promoter exon–intron boundaries, and specific intronic regions—testing to identify rare mutant alleles.
  * Deletion analysis: by MLPA (multiplex ligation-dependent probe amplification) or other molecular method
* CFTR testing is performed as:
  * Confirmatory diagnostic testing
  * Carrier testing (for the identification of heterozygotes)
  * Prenatal diagnosis

➤ Limitations
* The results of a genetic test may be affected by DNA rearrangements, blood transfusion, bone marrow transplantation, or other rare events.

CYSTINE, URINE (CYSTINURIA PANEL)

➤ Definition
* Cystinuria is an autosomal recessive defect in reabsorptive transport of cystine and the dibasic amino acids ornithine, arginine, and lysine from the luminal fluid of the renal proximal tubule and small intestine. The only phenotypic manifestation of cystinuria is cystine urolithiasis, which often recurs throughout an affected individual's lifetime.
* The disorder is divided into three subtypes: Rosenberg I, II, and III. Cystinuria type I is the most common variant. Type I heterozygotes show normal aminoaciduria. Heterozygotes of types II and III often manifest cystinuria without cystine calculi and may be at increased risk for other types of urolithiasis. Type I heterozygotes are distinguished by normal levels of urinary cystine.
* Unlike type I and type II homozygotes, type III homozygotes show an increase in plasma cystine concentration after oral cystine administration.
* To classify cystinuria clinically, urinary cystine can be measured in each parent of a proband as phenotype I (recessive, urinary cystine level <100 μmol/g of creatinine), phenotype II

TABLE 2-27. Age Based Reference Range for Cystine, Arginine, Lysine and Ornithine

	0–5 Months µmol/g of Creatinine	6–11 Months µmol/g of Creatinine	1–3 Years µmol/g of Creatinine	4–12 Years µmol/g of Creatinine	13 Years and older µmol/g of Creatinine
Arginine	0–124	0–97	0–80	0–62	0–44
Cystine	62–345	53–133	53–186	35–106	27–151
Lysine	133–1761	115–699	89–611	89–602	62–513
Ornithine	0–168	0–71	0–71	0–62	0–44

(dominant, urinary cystine level >1000 µmol/g of creatinine), and phenotype III (partially dominant, urinary cystine level 100–1000 µmol/g of creatinine). Cystinuria can also be classified based on the age at which symptoms first appear (i.e., infantile, juvenile, adolescent).

* **Normal range:** see Table 2-27

➤ Use
* Diagnosis of cystinuria.
* Monitoring of patients with cystinuria on therapy.

➤ Interpretation
Increased In
* Cystinosis
* Cystinurias
* Cystinlysinuria
* Nephrolithiasis
* Nephrotoxicity due to heavy metals
* Renal tubular acidosis
* Wilson disease
* First semester of pregnancy

Decreased In
* Severely burned patients

➤ Limitations
* Urinary excretion is age dependent
* Cystine excretion is normal in dibasic aminoaciduria.

CYTOGENETICS: FLUORESCENCE IN SITU HYBRIDIZATION (FISH), CHROMOSOME ANALYSIS, AND KARYOTYPING

➤ Definition
* **FISH:** Molecular hybridization of a fluorescently labeled, cloned sequence of interest to a mitotic chromosome or interphase nucleus.

- **Chromosome analysis:** Microscopic visual inspection of banded mitotic chromosomes that assess the entire genome with the ability to detect chromosome aberrations larger than ~5–10 megabases.
- **Karyotyping:** An ordered pairing of chromosomes that aids in detecting chromosome anomalies.

➤ Use
- **FISH**
  - Assessment of a specific region of the genome; allows detection of abnormalities that are too small to be visualized by conventional cytogenetics (e.g., microdeletions, microduplications)
  - Also may be performed on interphase (nondividing) cells, eliminating the necessity of cell culture and thereby allowing rapid turnaround times, and assessment of specimens that contain few or no dividing cells
- **Chromosome analysis:** used to identify abnormalities of chromosome number and structure that may be causal for mental retardation, congenital anomalies, pregnancy loss, infertility, and cancer.
- **Karyotyping**
  - A tool in chromosome analysis
  - Sometimes used (incorrectly) to mean chromosome analysis; a karyotype is not a standalone test

➤ Interpretation
- **FISH**
  - **Normal** (two intact copies of sequence in a diploid cell)
  - **Abnormal:** examples include deletion of the genomic region, additional copies of region, and positional rearrangement of region
- **Chromosome analysis**
  - **Normal:** 46,XY (male) or 46,XX (female)
  - **Abnormal:**
    - Numeric: incorrect chromosome number (e.g., +21 in Down syndrome)
    - Structural: abnormal chromosome structure (e.g., deletion of the chromosome 5 short arm (5p–) in Wolf-Hirschhorn syndrome, translocation such as t(9;22) in CML)

➤ Limitations
- **FISH:** A targeted test, it cannot provide the total genomic assessment provided by conventional chromosome analysis.
- **Chromosome analysis:** requires *dividing cells*; therefore, all submitted specimens must contain viable cells that can be cultured in the laboratory.

CYTOMEGALOVIRUS (CMV) QUANTITATIVE MOLECULAR ASSAY

➤ Definition
- The CMV quantitative assay uses real-time PCR to quantitate CMV DNA extracted from plasma of CMV-infected individuals. The test quantifies CMV DNA over different ranges depending on the laboratory and assay methodology—for example 50–4,200,000 copies/mL.
- **Normal values:** not detected when the result is below the level of detection of the assay.

➤ Use

- Management of CMV-infected individuals undergoing antiviral therapy
- Individuals at risk of severe CMV infection
- Confirmation of the presence CMV infection

➤ Limitations

- Currently, there is no international standard available for calibration of this assay. Therefore, caution should be taken when interpreting results obtained by different laboratories or assay methodologies.
- PCR inhibitors in the patient specimen may lead to underestimation of viral quantitation or in rare cases, false-negative results.

D-DIMERS

➤ Definition

- Plasma D-dimers are fibrin products generated by the action of plasmin on cross-linked fibrin fragments D, indicating that the clotting mechanism had been activated and thrombin generated. Although it is a direct marker of active fibrinolysis, it is an indirect, but very useful, marker of ongoing coagulation.
- **Normal range:** <0.2 µg/mL for the latex assay; <1.1 mg/L for the ultrasensitive immunoturbidimetric test

➤ Use

- Two D-dimer assays are available, each with a different use.
  - The latex agglutination D-dimer has relatively low sensitivity, hence it is not positive in single clots but elevated when multiple clots are generated. For this reason, it had been proven to be the most specific and sensitive test in the diagnosis of DIC.
  - The ultrasensitive D-dimer is performed by ELISA or immunoturbidimetric techniques that allow its precise quantitation. Because of its exquisite sensitivity, it becomes elevated in the presence of single clots.
    - Its main value is its high negative predictive ability, because a negative ultrasensitive D-dimer excludes thromboembolic events, with approaching 100% certitude (depending on methodology and equipment used). Although POC methods are available, they have slightly lower negative predictive values.
    - Elevated values are less useful, although persistent elevations after 3–6 months of anticoagulation following a thromboembolic event suggest, a high probability of recurrent events.

➤ Interpretation

- The cut-off value for the ultrasensitive D-dimer is <1.1 mg/L (it varies with methods and equipment used). Any values below 1.1 mg/L are considered negative and are used in most diagnostic algorithms for the exclusion of deep vein thrombosis (DVT) or pulmonary embolism (PE).
- The latex D-dimer is elevated in all situations with multiple clots, the prototype being DIC. The higher the titer, the more severe the DIC may be (see disseminated intravascular coagulation discussion, p. 883).

- The ultrasensitive D-dimer is elevated in the following conditions:
  - DVT and PE
  - DIC
  - Renal, liver, or cardiac failure
  - Disseminated cancer and monoclonal gammopathies
  - Pregnancy
  - Major injury and surgery
  - Increasing age
  - Inflammatory conditions

➤ Limitations
- The ultrasensitive D-dimer may be falsely elevated or decreased in hyperlipidemic or very turbid blood samples and in patients treated with mouse monoclonal antibodies.
- RF may give false-positive results.

DEHYDROEPIANDROSTERONE SULFATE, SERUM (DHEA-SULFATE)

➤ Definition
- DHEA-S is produced by androgenic zone of adrenal cortex. DHEA is the principal human C-19 steroid and has very low androgenic potency but serves as the major direct or indirect precursor for most sex steroids. The bulk of DHEA is secreted as a 3-sulfo-conjugate (DHEA-S). Both hormones are albumin bound, but binding of DHEA-S is much tighter.
- In gonads and several other tissues, most notably skin, steroid sulfatases can convert DHEA-S back to DHEA, which can then be metabolized to stronger androgens and to estrogens. During pregnancy, DHEA-S and its 16-hydroxylated metabolites are secreted by the fetal adrenal gland in large quantities. They serve as precursors for placental production of the dominant pregnancy estrogen, estriol.
- **Normal range:** see Table 2-28

➤ Use
- Indicator of adrenal cortical function, especially for differential diagnosis of virilization, and investigations of hirsutism and alopecia in women. It is also of value in the assessment of adrenarche and delayed puberty.
- Differential diagnosis of Cushing syndrome
- Replaces 17-KS urine excretion with which it correlates; shows no significant diurnal variation, thereby providing rapid test for abnormal androgen secretion

TABLE 2-28. Normal Ranges of DHES-S

Sex	Median (µg/dL)	(Central 95%) (µg/dL)
Female	170	35–430
Male	280	80–560

➤ Interpretation
Increased In
* CAH: markedly increased values can be suppressed by dexamethasone. Highest values occur in CAH due to deficiency of 3β-hydroxysteroid dehydrogenase.
* Adrenal carcinoma: markedly increased levels cannot be suppressed by dexamethasone.
* Cushing syndrome caused by bilateral adrenal hyperplasia: shows higher values than Cushing syndrome due to benign cortical adenoma, in which values may be normal or low.
* Cushing disease (pituitary etiology): moderate increase in hypogonadotropic hypogonadism; DHEA-S is usually normal for chronologic age and high for bone age in contrast with idiopathic delayed puberty, in which DHEA-S is low relative to chronologic age and normal relative to bone age.
* First few days of life, especially in sick or premature infants.
* Polycystic ovary syndrome: adrenal hyperandrogenism is a fairly typical facet of this syndrome.

Decreased In
* Addison disease
* Adrenal hypoplasia

➤ Limitations
* Extremely high levels (>700 or 800 μg/dL) in women are suggestive of a hormone-secreting adrenal tumor. By contrast, DHEA-SO$_4$ levels are typically normal in the presence of ovarian tumors.
* There are currently no established guidelines for DHEA-S replacement/supplementation therapy or its biochemical monitoring.
* Many drugs and hormones can result in changes in DHEA-S levels. In most cases, the drug-induced changes are not large enough to cause diagnostic confusion, but when interpreting mild abnormalities in DHEA-S levels, drug and hormone interactions should be taken into account. Examples of drugs/hormones that can reduce DHEA-S levels include insulin, oral contraceptive drugs, corticosteroids, CNS agents that induce hepatic enzymes (e.g., carbamazepine, clomipramine, imipramine, phenytoin), many antilipemic drugs (e.g., statins, cholestyramine), dopaminergic drugs (e.g., levodopa/dopamine, bromocriptine), fish oil, and vitamin E.
* Drugs that may increase DHEA-S levels include metformin, troglitazone, prolactin, danazol, calcium channel blockers (e.g., diltiazem, amlodipine), and nicotine.

DEHYDROEPIANDROSTERONE, SERUM (DHEA, DHEA UNCONJUGATED)

➤ Definition
* DHEA has very low androgenic potency but serves as the major direct or indirect precursor for most sex steroids. DHEA is secreted by the adrenal gland and production is at least partly controlled by ACTH; the bulk of DHEA is secreted as a 3-sulfoconjugate DHEAS. Both hormones are albumin bound, but DHEAS binding is much tighter. As a result, circulating concentrations of DHEAS are much higher (greater than 100-fold) compared to DHEA.

- In most clinical situations, DHEA and DHEAS results can be used interchangeably. In gonads and several other tissues, most notably skin, steroid sulfatases can convert DHEAS back to DHEA, which can then be metabolized to stronger androgens and to estrogens. During pregnancy, DHEA/DHEAS and their 16-hydroxylated metabolites are secreted by the fetal adrenal gland in large quantities. They serve as precursors for placental production of the dominant pregnancy estrogen, estriol. Within weeks after birth, DHEA/DHEAS levels fall by 80% or more and remain low until the onset of adrenarche at age 7 or 8 in girls and age 8 or 9 in boys.
- **Normal range** (adults): male: 180–1250 ng/dL; female: 130–980 ng/dL

➤ Use
- Diagnosing and differential diagnosis of hyperandrogenism (in conjunction with measurements of other sex steroids)
- An adjunct in the diagnosis of CAH; DHEA/DHEAS measurements play a secondary role to the measurements of cortisol/cortisone, 17 alpha-hydroxyprogesterone, and androstenedione.
- Diagnosing and differential diagnosis of premature adrenarche.

➤ Interpretation
Increased In
- Hyperandrogenism
- Androgen-producing adrenal tumors
- CAH due to 3 beta-hydroxysteroid dehydrogenase deficiency

Decreased In
- With age in men and women, hyperlipidemia, psychosis, psoriasis

➤ Limitations
- DHEA levels increase until the age of 20 to a maximum roughly comparable to that observed at birth. Levels then decline over the next 40–60 years to around 20% of peak levels.
- Currently the correlation of serum DHEA/DHEAS level with disease risk factors has not been completely established. There are currently no established guidelines for DHEA replacement/supplementation therapy or its biochemical monitoring.

DEXAMETHASONE SUPPRESSION OF PITUITARY ACTH SECRETION TEST (DST)

➤ Definition
- Dexamethasone is a potent synthetic glucocorticoid not detected by serum, urine, and salivary cortisol assays. Dexamethasone should not fully suppress ACTH and, therefore, should not decrease adrenal secretion of cortisol.
- Dexamethasone suppression tests are used to assess the status of the HPA axis and for the differential diagnosis of adrenal hyperfunction.
- **Low-dose dexamethasone suppression tests** are good standard screening tests to differentiate patients with Cushing syndrome of any cause from patients who do not have Cushing syndrome.
  - Principle: If the hypothalamic-pituitary axis is normal, any supraphysiologic dose of dexamethasone is sufficient to suppress pituitary ACTH secretion. This should lead to reductions

in cortisol secretion and its concentration in serum and saliva, as well as in the 24-hour urine excretion.

- Two main protocols are used: overnight 1 mg screening test and standard 2 day, 2 mg test
- High-dose suppression tests are based on the fact that ACTH secretion in Cushing disease is only relatively resistant to glucocorticoid negative feedback inhibition and does not suppress normally with either the overnight 1 mg or the 2-day low-dose test. By increasing the dose of dexamethasone four- to eightfold, ACTH secretion can be suppressed in most patients with Cushing disease.
- Therefore, this test is used to distinguish patients with Cushing disease (Cushing syndrome caused by pituitary hypersecretion of ACTH) from most patients with ectopic ACTH syndrome (Cushing syndrome caused by nonpituitary ACTH-secreting tumors).

LOW-DOSE TEST: OVERNIGHT 1 mg SCREENING TEST

➤ Definition

- Overnight screening test is a quick screening test for nonsuppressible cortisol production and subclinical or clinical Cushing syndrome and should not be used as the sole criterion for excluding the diagnosis of Cushing syndrome.

➤ Use

- Dexamethasone (1 mg) is taken orally between 11 p.m. and midnight, and a single blood sample is drawn at 8 a.m. the next morning for assay of serum cortisol.

➤ Interpretation

- The 2008 Endocrine Society Guidelines suggest a diagnostic serum cortisol criterion of 1.8 µg/dL.
- This test has a significant false-positive rate when sensitivity is maximized. Using a serum cortisol criterion of <3.6 µg/dL, the test has a 12–15% false-positive rate. If, however, the criterion for suppression of serum cortisol is increased to <7.2 µg/dL, the false-positive rate falls to 7%. This suggests that the multiple criteria may be useful in interpreting the test
- The salivary cortisol concentration at 8 a.m. after 1 mg dexamethasone given at midnight was 0.8 ± 0.4 ng/mL (range 0.6 to 1.1 ng/mL) in 101 normal subjects, a sensitivity and specificity of 100%.

LOW-DOSE TEST: STANDARD TWO-DAY (2-mg) TEST

➤ Use

- The 2-day test is used to assess suppressibility in patients with an equivocal overnight test or in patients who have not had an overnight test.
- Dexamethasone, 0.5 mg, is taken orally every 6 hours, usually at 8 a.m., 2 p.m., 8 p.m., and 2 a.m., for a total of eight doses.
- Blood is drawn 2 or 6 hours after the last dose for measurement of cortisol.

Interpretation

- The normal response to the 2-day test consists of the following:
  - Urinary cortisol excretion should fall to <10 µg per 24 hours on the second day of dexamethasone administration.
  - Serum cortisol concentration is <5 µg/dL, a plasma ACTH concentration is <5 pg/mL, and a serum dexamethasone concentration is between 2.0 and 6.5 ng/mL.
  - In a recent meta-analysis, the 1 mg test and the 2-day 2 mg test were both accurate, but the 2 mg test had slightly less diagnostic accuracy.

HIGH-DOSE TEST: OVERNIGHT (8-mg) TEST

➤ Use

- Dexamethasone (8 mg) is taken orally between 11 p.m. and midnight, and a single blood sample is drawn at 8 a.m. the next day for measurement of serum cortisol.
- With this protocol, the 8 a.m. serum cortisol concentration is <5 µg/dL in most patients with Cushing disease (i.e., a pituitary tumor), and is usually undetectable in normals.

HIGH-DOSE TEST: STANDARD TWO-DAY (8-mg) TEST

➤ Use

- The patient collects at least one baseline 24-hour urine, at 8 a.m.
- The patient begins taking 2 mg of dexamethasone orally every 6 hours for a total of 8 doses, usually at 8 a.m., 2 p.m., 8 p.m., and 2 a.m., and the urine collections are continued.
- In practice, this test is often performed immediately after completing the low-dose dexamethasone suppression test (if the test is positive).
- The urine collections are assayed for urinary free cortisol and creatinine. In addition, a blood specimen can be collected 6 hours after the last dose of dexamethasone for measurement of cortisol, dexamethasone, and ACTH.
- This protocol leads to the following values in normal subjects:
  - Urinary free cortisol excretion is <5 µg per 24 hours.
  - Serum cortisol and plasma ACTH are low and usually undetectable.
  - Serum dexamethasone range from about 8–20 ng/mL.

➤ Limitations of All Tests

- False-positive results may occur in acute and chronic illness, alcoholism, depression, and due to certain drugs (e.g., phenytoin, phenobarbital, primidone, carbamazepine, rifampicin, and spironolactone);
- Atypical or false-positive responses may occur also due to alcohol, estrogens, birth-control pills, pregnancy, obesity, acute illness and stress, and severe depression.
- Not a good choice for patients in whom CBG levels may be abnormal
- Noncompliance (check by measuring plasma dexamethasone)
- Some patients with large ACTH-producing pituitary adenomas have marked resistance to high-dose dexamethasone suppression. In longstanding cases, nodular hyperplasia of adrenal may develop causing autonomous cortisol production and resistance to dexamethasone test.

- No suppression in 80% of cases in ectopic ACTH syndrome or nodular adrenal hyperplasia
- Urine and plasma cortisol are not decreased after high or low doses of dexamethasone in adrenal adenoma or carcinoma or ectopic ACTH syndrome.
- Patients with psychiatric illness may be resistant and do not reproducibly suppress.

DIGOXIN

➤ Definition
- A cardiac glycoside derived from *Digitalis lanata* consisting of a steroid nucleus and a lactone coupled with sugar moieties.
- Other name: Lanoxin®
- **Normal therapeutic range:** 0.8–2.0 ng/mL (1.2–2.6 nmol/L)

➤ Use
- Treatment of CHF and atrial fibrillation/flutter

➤ Interpretation
- **Toxic range:** >2.5 ng/mL, but 10% of patients may show toxicity at <2 ng/mL
- Toxicity may be observed at a lower serum concentration in presence of hypokalemia, hypercalcemia, hypomagnesemia, hypoxia, and heart disease.
- Increased with coadministration of:
  - Quinidine
  - Verapamil
  - Amiodarone
  - Indomethacin
  - Cyclosporin A

➤ Limitations
- Draw blood 6–8 hours (or 8–24 hours) after last oral dose after steady state has been achieved in 1–2 weeks.
- Pediatric toxic concentration may be higher; therapeutic index is very low (i.e., small difference between therapeutic and toxic blood concentration). However, ~10% of patients have serum concentration of 2–4 ng/mL without evidence of toxicity. On a dose of 0.25 mg/day, mean serum concentration is 1.2 ± 0.4 ng/mL; on a dose of 0.5 mg/day, mean serum concentration is 1.5 ± 0.4 ng/mL; and on a dose of 0.1 mg/day, mean serum concentration is 17 ± 6 ng/mL. A digitalis leaf dose of 0.1 g/day produces the same serum concentration as 0.1 mg/day of crystalline digitoxin. There is ECG evidence of toxicity in one third to two thirds of patients, with no symptoms or signs.
- False low results may be due to spironolactone.
- Endogenous digoxin-like substances may produce positive test results in persons who have not received the drug, especially in:
  - Uremia
  - Severe agonal states and postmortem—therefore, a high postmortem concentration may not have been high before death and a normal postmortem concentration suggests that the antemortem concentration was not toxic.

- Because most methods measure both endogenous digoxin-like substances and inactive metabolites of digoxin, therapeutic monitoring should mostly be used to assess patient compliance and to confirm drug toxicity.
- Tests: bioassay, Na^+K^+-ATPase receptor assay, colorimetry, fluorometry, HPLC, gas chromatography, enzyme assay, immunoassay, LC/MS
- Immunoassay is the most widely used methodology: RIA, FPIA, EIA, chemiluminescence
  - Confounders in analysis-low concentrations, steroid-like nucleus, endogenous digoxin-like immunoreactive factors (observed in patients with renal failure, liver disease, myocardial infarction, newborns, pregnancy, hypertension, strenuous exercise, volume expansion), digoxin metabolites, presence of antidote (Fab)
  - Immunoassays exhibit <5% cross-reactivity with digitoxin and digoxigenin, and 80–100% with the metabolites digoxigenin bis- and mono-digitoxoside.
- Hb, lipid, and bilirubin do not typically interfere.

DILUTE RUSSELL VIPER VENOM (dRVVT) ASSAY

➤ Definition
- The dRVVT assay detects the presence of LA. This test is helpful for the diagnosis of the antiphospholipid antibody syndrome (see p. 510) and acquired thrombophilia (see p. 887).

➤ Use
- The dRVVT assay consists of three stages:
  1. The screening reagent initiates plasma clotting by directly activating factor X, thereby bypassing both the intrinsic and extrinsic pathways of coagulation. LA antibodies prolong the clotting time. If the clotting time is not prolonged in the presence of the dilute venom, LA is not present, and the second stage of the assay is omitted.
  2. If the clotting time is prolonged (>20% of the control), a PTT analysis on a 1:1 incubation of normal plasma with the patient's plasma to discriminate between an inhibitor or a clotting factor deficiency (correction of the clotting time to <44 seconds) is routinely done. If there is no correction, and the clotting time remains prolonged, an inhibitor has been demonstrated, and the laboratory proceeds with the next step.
  3. A reagent containing a high concentration of phospholipid is added to the plasma under study, a confirmation reagent. If the clotting time in the first phase has been prolonged by LA antibodies, the reagent neutralizes the antibodies and the clotting time becomes shorter, similar to that of the control. If the clotting time elongation in the first stage is not due to LA but a different inhibitor, the clotting time with the confirmation reagent remains elongated. Additional studies to rule out other etiologies for the initially prolonged clotting time are then indicated.
- Results are expressed as a ratio; the clotting time of the screening reagent is divided by the clotting time of the confirmation tests.

➤ Interpretation
- Ratio greater than 2.0: LA strongly present
- Ratio of 1.6 to 2.0: LA moderately present
- Ratio between 1.2 and 1.6: LA may be present, but in a low titer.

➤ Limitations
- LA antibodies may vary in their properties and the results may be positive in the dRVVT assay, but not in other type assays. Because of that, at least two type assays have been recommended for each patient (see Lupus anticoagulant algorithm, p. 250).
- Heparin levels >1 unit/mL prolong the first-stage assay.

➤ Suggested Reading
Lambert M, Ferrard-Sasson G, Dubucquoi S, et al. Dilute Russell viper-venom time improves identification of antiphospholipid syndrome in a lupus anticoagulant-positive patient population. *Thromb Haemost.* 2009;101:577–581.

DIRECT AND INDIRECT ANTIGLOBULIN TESTS (DAT AND IAT)

➤ Definition
- Previously known as the direct and indirect Coombs tests, these assays play a major role in transfusion medicine as well as in the diagnosis of immune hemolytic anemias (see p. 804), because they detect either antibodies bound to RBCs (the DAT), or in serum (the indirect antiglobulin test, IAT). In patients that have not been transfused within the preceding 3 months, a positive DAT almost always reveals autoimmune antibodies.
- The IAT is used to demonstrate *in vitro* reactions between RBCs and antibodies that sensitize red cells that express the corresponding antigen. Patient's serum or plasma is incubated with red cells, which are then washed to remove unbound globulins. Agglutination that develops when the antiglobulin reagent is added indicates a reaction between serum antibodies (usually the result of immunization from previous transfusions) and red cells.
- The antiglobulin reagent consists in most cases of rabbit antibodies directed against human IgG. Other reagents used in the DAT assay are anticomplement (anti-C3dg), or a mixture of anti-IgG and anti-C3dg. If the DAT is positive following recent transfusions, the antibodies can be eluted from RBCs and the eluted antibodies must be identified.

➤ Use
- The DAT is used whenever hemolysis of red cells is suspected as being caused by autoantibodies. The assay determines if red cells have been coated *in vivo* with immunoglobulins, complement, or both.
- The utility of the IAT in blood banking stems from its great sensitivity in detecting various IgG antibodies in the recipient's serum prior to transfusions. It is part of the antibody screening test. It is used to detect the presence of alloantibodies directed against non-ABO blood group antigens.
- In cases of severe autoimmune hemolytic anemia, both the DAT and the IAT may be positive because the excess antibodies elute from the red cell membranes and spill out into serum.

➤ Interpretation
- Both the DAT and the IAT are reported and interpreted as either positive or negative
- The DAT is positive whenever the patient's red cells are coated with autoantibodies that developed against the patient's own red cells. It is also positive when alloantibodies in a recipient's circulation react with antigens on recently transfused red cells, as well as alloantibodies in maternal circulation, which cross the placenta and coat fetal red cells. Antibodies directed against certain drugs may also bind to red cell membranes and result in a positive test.

* The IAT is positive in the presence of serum alloantibodies in patients previously transfused and immunized against non-self red cell antigens.

➤ Limitations

* Finding of a positive DAT indicates the presence of red cell autoantibodies, alloantibodies following transfusions, or of coating of red cells with excess immunoglobulins. It requires additional work-up to elucidate the etiology of the immunoglobulins by performing tests for antibody specificity: cold agglutinins (see p. 809 under hemolytic anemias), Donath-Landsteiner antibody (see p. 812), and also serum protein electrophoresis or immunofixation when a plasmacytic disease (see p. 859) is suspected. The administration of certain drugs (α-methyldopa, IV penicillin, or procainamide) and recent transfusions must also be excluded.
* A negative DAT does not rule out hemolysis but only hemolysis of autoimmune etiology. For instance, DAT is negative in some cases of drug-induced hemolytic anemias, hemoglobinopathies, hereditary spherocytosis, and other hereditary hemolytic anemias.
* A positive IAT requires further investigation to identify more precisely the offending antigen(s).

ENZYME TESTS THAT DETECT CHOLESTASIS (ALP, 5'-NUCLEOTIDASE, GGT, LAP)

* Increased ALP in liver diseases (due to increased synthesis from proliferating bile duct epithelium) is the best indicator of biliary obstruction but does not differentiate intrahepatic cholestasis from extrahepatic obstruction. In cholestasis ALP level is increased out of proportion to other liver function tests.
* Increases before jaundice occurs
* High values (>5 time normal) favor obstruction and normal levels virtually exclude this diagnosis.
* Markedly increased in infants with congenital intrahepatic bile duct atresia but is much lower in extrahepatic atresia
* **Increased 10 times normal:** carcinoma of head of pancreas, choledocholithiasis, drug cholestatic hepatitis
* **15–20 times increase:** primary biliary cirrhosis, primary or metastatic carcinoma
* Increase (3–10 times normal) with only slightly increased transaminases may be seen in biliary obstruction and converse in liver parenchymal disease (e.g., cirrhosis, hepatitis); increased >3 times normal in <5% of acute hepatitis.
* Increased (2–10 times normal; usually 1.5–3 times increase) serum ALP and LD in early infiltrative (e.g., amyloid) and space-occupying diseases of the liver (e.g., tumor, granuloma, abscess)
* Increase <3 to 4 times normal is nonspecific and may occur in all types of liver diseases (e.g., congestive heart failure, infiltrative liver diseases, cirrhosis, acute [viral, toxic, alcoholic] or chronic hepatitis, acute fatty liver).
* **Increased 5 times normal:** infectious mononucleosis, postnecrotic cirrhosis
* Increased ALP (of liver origin) and LD with normal serum bilirubin, AST, ALT, suggests obstruction of one hepatic duct, or metastatic or infiltrative disease of liver.
* GGT/ALP ratio >5 favors alcoholic liver disease.

- Isolated increase of GGT is a sensitive screening and monitoring test for alcoholism. Increased GGT due to alcohol or anticonvulsant drugs is not accompanied by increased ALP.
- Serum 5′-nucleotidase (5′-N) and LAP parallel the increase in ALP in obstructive type of hepatobiliary disease, but the 5′-N is increased only in the latter and is normal in pregnancy and bone disease, whereas the LAP is increased in pregnancy but is usually normal in bone disease. GGT is normal in bone disease and pregnancy. Therefore, these enzymes are useful in determining the source of increased serum ALP. Although serum 5′-N usually parallels ALP in liver disease, it may not increase proportionately in individual patients.

Serum Enzyme	Biliary Obstruction	Pregnancy	Childhood; Bone Disease
ALP	Increased	Increased	Increased
GGT	Increased	Normal	Normal
5′-N	Increased	Normal	Normal
LAP	Increased	Increased	Normal

Bilirubin ("bile") in urine implies increased serum conjugated bilirubin and excludes hemolysis as the cause. Often precedes clinical icterus. May occur without jaundice in anicteric or early hepatitis, early obstruction, or liver metastases. (Tablets detect 0.05–0.1 mg/dL; dipsticks are less sensitive; test is negative in normal persons.)
- Complete absence of urine urobilinogen strongly suggests complete bile duct obstruction; is normal in incomplete obstruction and decreased in some phases of hepatic jaundice. Increased in hemolytic jaundice and subsiding hepatitis. Increase may evidence hepatic damage even without clinical jaundice (e.g., some patients with cirrhosis, metastatic liver disease, congestive heart failure). Presence in viral hepatitis depends on phase of disease (normal is <1 mg or 1 Ehrlich unit/2 hour specimen).

ERYTHROCYTE SEDIMENTATION RATE (ESR)

➤ Definition
- ESR is the distance in millimeters that erythrocytes fall during one hour in a sample of venous blood (Westergren principle). Newer techniques allow the test to be performed in 30 minutes, resulting in improved turnaround time.
- **Normal range:** 0–15 mm/hour in men and 0–20 mm/hour in women

➤ Use
- ESR is not a good screening test because of its low sensitivity. CRP is superior to ESR; CRP is more sensitive and reflects a more rapid change in the patient's condition. ESR is used as a screening test to detect the presence of a systemic disease; however, a normal test does not exclude malignancy or other serious disease, although it does rule out temporal arteritis or polymyalgia rheumatica.
- Finding a much accelerated ESR (>100 mm/hour) in patients with ill-defined symptoms directs the physician to search for a severe systemic disease, especially paraproteinemias,

disseminated malignancies, connective tissue diseases, and severe infections such as bacterial endocarditis.
* Finding a normal ESR in patients with paraproteinemia suggests the development of hyperviscosity syndrome.
* ESR is also used to monitor the course or response to therapy of diseases if greatly accelerated initially.

➤ Interpretation
Increased In
* Infections
* Vasculitis, including temporal arteritis
* Inflammatory arthritis
* Renal disease
* Anemia
* Malignancies and plasma cell dyscrasias
* Acute allergy
* Tissue injury, including myocardial infarction
* Pregnancy (but not first trimester)
* Estrogen administration
* Aging

Decreased In
* Polycythemia vera
* Sickle cell anemia
* CHF
* Typhoid and undulant fever, malarial paroxysm, trichinosis, pertussis, infectious mononucleosis, uncomplicated viral diseases
* Peptic ulcer
* Acute allergy

➤ Limitations
Causes of a Falsely Increased ESR
* Increased fibrinogen; increased gamma and beta globulins
* Drugs (dextran, penicillamine, theophylline, vitamin A, methyldopa, methysergide)
* Technical factors (e.g., hemolyzed sample, high temperature in the laboratory)
* Hypercholesterolemia

Causes of a Falsely Decreased ESR
* Abnormally shaped RBCs (sickle cells, spherocytes, acanthocytes)
* Microcytosis
* HbC disease
* Hypofibrinogenemia
* Technical factors (low temperature in the laboratory, clotted blood)
* Extreme leukocytosis
* Drugs (quinine, salicylates, high steroid levels, drugs that cause high glucose levels)

TABLE 2-29. Normal Range of Values for Estradiol, Unconjugated

Sex and Condition	Reference Range (pg/mL)
Males	<20–47
Postmenopausal females	<20–40
Nonpregnant females:	
Midfollicular	27–122
Periovulatory	95–433
Midluteal	49–291

ESTRADIOL, UNCONJUGATED

➤ Definition
• Most active of endogenous estrogens
• Other names: estradiol 17 beta, E2
• **Normal range:** see Table 2-29

➤ Use
• Of value, together with gonadotropins, in evaluating menstrual and fertility problems in women
• In the evaluation of gynecomastia or feminization states due to estrogen-producing tumors, menstrual cycle irregularities, and sexual maturity in female patients and in monitoring of human menopausal gonadotropin (Pergonal) therapy

➤ Interpretation
Increased In
• Feminization in children
• Estrogen-producing tumors
• Gynecomastia
• Hepatic cirrhosis
• Hyperthyroidism

Decreased In
• Primary and secondary hypogonadism

➤ Limitations
• Oral contraceptives inhibit physiologic increase.
• Estradiol values from pregnant females may be affected by high levels of estriol such as those present in the second and third trimesters of pregnancy.

ESTROGEN/PROGESTERONE RECEPTOR ASSAY

➤ Definition
• Estrogen and progesterone receptors play a role in hormone-directed transcriptional activation.
• Other names: estrogen receptor assay (ERA), progesterone receptor assay (PGRA), progesterone receptor protein (PRP), estrogen receptor protein (ERP)

TABLE 2-30. Percentage of Patients Who Respond to Hormone Therapy Based on the Test Results of Estrogen and Progesterone Receptor Assay		
Percent Response to Hormone Therapy	Estrogen Receptor Protein (ERP)	Progesterone Receptor Protein (PRP)
75–80	Positive	Positive
40–50	Positive	Negative
25–30	Negative	Positive
10	Negative	Negative

* **Normal range:** (ERP, PRP)
  * Negative: <5% of nuclei staining
  * Borderline: 5–19% of nuclei staining
  * Positive: 20% of nuclei staining

➤ **Use**
* To identify patients with breast cancers likely to respond to either additive or ablative hormone therapies.

➤ **Interpretation (Table 2-30)**

➤ **Limitations**
* Assay is performed on paraffin-embedded, formalin-fixed tissue.
* Receptor status is influenced by age.
* The definition of positive and negative may vary from laboratory to laboratory due to tissue and antibody treatment and antibody specificity.

➤ **Suggested Reading**
Ogawa Y, Moriya T, Kato Y, et al. Immunohistochemical assessment for estrogen receptor and progesterone receptor status in breast cancer: analysis for a cut-off point as the predictor for endocrine therapy. *Breast Cancer.* 2004;11(3):267–275.

ESTROGENS (TOTAL), SERUM

➤ **Definition**
* Estrogens are involved in development and maintenance of the female phenotype, germ cell maturation, and pregnancy. They also are important for many other, nongender-specific processes, including growth, nervous system maturation, bone metabolism/remodeling, and endothelial responsiveness.
* The two major biologically active estrogens in nonpregnant humans are estrone (E1) and estradiol (E2). A third bioactive estrogen, estriol (E3), is the main pregnancy estrogen but plays no significant role in nonpregnant women or men.
* **Normal range:** See Table 2-31

➤ **Use**
* Overall status of estrogens in females or males
* Must be interpreted according to phase of menstrual cycle

TABLE 2-31. Normal Ranges of Estrogens

Estradiol (Tandem mass spectrometry)

Reference Intervals: Children (pg/mL)

Tanner Stage	Male	Female
I	<8	<56
II	<10	2–133
III	1–35	12–277
IV and V	3–35	2–259

Age (years)	Male	Female
7–9	<7	<36
10–12	<11	1–87
13–15	1–36	9–249
16–17	3–34	2–266

Reference Intervals: Adults (pg/mL)

≥18 years	Male	Female
	10–42	**Premenopausal:**
		Early Follicular: 30–100
		Late Follicular: 100–400
		Luteal: 50–150
		Postmenopausal:
		2–21

Estrone (tandem mass spectrometry)

Reference Intervals: Children (pg/mL)

Tanner Stage	Male	Female
I	<7	<27
II	<11	1–39
III	1–31	8–117
IV and V	2–30	4–109

Age (years)	Male	Female
7–9	<7	<20
10–12	<11	1–40
13–15	1–30	8–105
16–17	1–32	4–133

Reference Intervals: Adults (pg/mL)

≥18 Years	Male	Female
	9–36	**Premenopausal:**
		Early Follicular: <150
		Late Follicular: 100–250
		Luteal: <200
		Postmenopausal:
		3–32 pg/mL

TABLE 2-31. (*Continued*)		
Estrogens, Total (By Calculation)		
Reference Intervals: Children (pg/mL)		
Tanner Stages:	Male	Female
I	1–11	1–86
II	1–19	3–169
III	3–61	23–351
IV and V	4–62	8–341
Age (years)	Male	Female
7–9	<10	1–48
10–12	1–19	2–116
13–15	3–62	15–333
16–17	4–64	6–354
Reference Intervals: Adults (pg/mL)		
18 years	Male	Female
	19–69	**Premenopausal:**
		Early Follicular: 30–250
		Late Follicular: 200–650
		Luteal: 50–350
		Postmenopausal:
		5–52

➤ Interpretation

Increased In

* Estrogen-producing tumors (e.g., granulosa cell tumor, theca-cell tumor, luteoma), secondary to stimulation by hCG-producing tumors (e.g., teratoma, teratocarcinoma)
* Pregnancy
* Gynecomastia

Decreased In

* Ovarian failure
* Primary hypofunction of ovary:
  * Autoimmune oophoritis is the most common cause; usually associated with other autoimmune endocrinopathies (e.g., Hashimoto thyroiditis, Addison disease, type 1 DM); may cause premature menopause
  * Resistant ovary syndrome
  * Toxic (e.g., irradiation, chemotherapy)
  * Infection (e.g., mumps)
  * Tumor (primary or secondary)
  * Mechanical (e.g., trauma, torsion, surgical excision)
  * Genetic (e.g., Turner syndrome)
  * Menopause
* Secondary hypofunction of ovary: disorders of hypothalamic-pituitary axis

ESTRONE

➤ Definition
- Estrone (E1) is more potent than estriol (E3) but is less potent than estradiol (E2).
- Estrone is converted to estrone sulfate, and it acts as a reservoir that can be converted as needed to the more active estradiol.
- Estrone is the major circulating estrogen in postmenopausal women.
- In premenopausal women, estrone levels generally parallel those of estradiol, rising gradually during the follicular phase and peaking just prior to ovulation, with a secondary and smaller increase during the luteal phase. After menopause, estrone levels do not decline as dramatically as estradiol levels, possibly due to increased conversion of androstenedione to estrone.
- **Normal range:**
  - Children: see Table 2-32
  - Adults: see Table 2-33

➤ Use
- Diagnosis of precocious and delayed puberty
- Work-up of suspected disorders of sex steroid metabolism
- In the fracture risk assessment of postmenopausal women

➤ Interpretation
Increased In
- Possibly in polycystic ovarian syndrome, androgen-producing tumors, or estrogen-producing tumors
- Possibly increased in postmenopausal vaginal bleeding due to peripheral conversion of androgenic steroids. Increased estrone levels may be associated with increased levels of circulating androgens and their subsequent peripheral conversion.

Decreased In
- Inherited disorders of sex steroid metabolism
- Testicular feminization

TABLE 2-32. Reference Intervals for Estrone in Children

	Boys (pg/mL)	Girls (pg/mL)
Tanner Stage		
I	<7	<27
II	<11	1–39
III	1–31	8–117
IV and V	2–30	4–109
Age (years)		
7–9	<7	<20
10–12	<11	1–40
13–15	1–30	8–105
16–17	1–32	4–133

TABLE 2-33. Reference Intervals for Estrone in Adults*	
Female	Male
Premenopausal: Early follicular: <150 pg/mL Late follicular: 100–250 pg/mL Luteal: <200 pg/mL Postmenopausal: 3–32 pg/mL	9–36 pg/mL
*18 years of age and older.	

➤ Limitations
• Significant diurnal variations in plasma levels
• Digoxin and estrogens increase plasma levels

ETHYLENE GLYCOL

➤ Definition
• A colorless odorless sweet tasting nonvolatile liquid found in antifreeze, coolants, deicers, brake fluids, detergents, paints, and inks.
• Other name: 1,2-ethanediol
• **Normal range:** none; threshold limit value for occupational exposure: 100 mg/m^3

➤ Use
• Antifreeze
• Softening agent and stabilizer
• Solvent

➤ Interpretation
• Minimum lethal oral dose for adults is approximately 100 mL; toxicity possible at serum concentrations >250 mg/L

➤ Limitations
• Propylene glycol, a similar compound used in pharmaceutical preparations is less toxic.
• Ethylene glycol can cause severe metabolic acidosis with increased anion gap and osmolal gap.
• Ethylene glycol is metabolized to glycoaldehyde, glycolic acid, glyoxylic acid, oxalic acid, formic acid, and carbon dioxide. These acids may interfere with testing of ethylene glycol and cause elevation of some immunoassay tests for lactate/lactic acid, triglycerides.
• Testing
  • Serum osmolality
  • Specimen—serum or plasma; avoid serum separator tubes and gels
  • Ethylene glycol
    • Gas chromatography
    • GC/MS
    • Liquid chromatography

- "Home brew" enzymatic assays developed for chemistry analyzers
- Limit of quantitation: 50–100 mg/L
- Methods must be extensively validated to assess potentially coeluting (interfering) substances such as propionic acid, propylene glycol
- Glycolic acid
  - Because toxicity of ethylene glycol is due to metabolites, gas chromatography and HPLC methods have been developed for these organic acids. Typically, separate procedures are required for the acids compared with ethylene glycol.

FACTOR V LEIDEN MOLECULAR ASSAY

➤ Definition
- Factor V Leiden results from a *R506Q* mutation in the *F5* gene encoding factor V, and is associated with increased risk of thrombophilia. Heterozygosity for the factor V Leiden *R506Q* mutation is associated with resistance to activated protein C (APC see p. 27) and a five- to tenfold increased risk of venous thrombosis. Homozygosity for this mutation is associated with resistance to APC and an approximately 80-fold increased risk of venous thrombosis. Other factors can further increase the risk of thrombosis.
- **Normal values:** negative or no mutations are found

➤ Use
- Factor V Leiden testing should be performed in the following cases:
  - A first occurrence of a venous thrombotic embolism (VTE) before age 50 years
  - A first unprovoked VTE at any age
  - A history of recurrent VTE
  - Venous thrombosis at unusual sites (e.g., cerebral, mesenteric, portal, and hepatic veins)
  - VTE during pregnancy or the puerperium
  - VTE associated with use of oral contraceptives or hormone replacement therapy
  - A first VTE in an individual with a first-degree family member with VTE before age 50 years
  - Women with unexplained fetal loss occurring after 10 weeks of gestation
- Factor V Leiden testing may be considered in the following cases:
  - In women with unexplained severe preeclampsia, placental abruption, or a fetus with intrauterine growth retardation
  - A first VTE related to the use of tamoxifen or other selective estrogen receptor modulators
  - Female smokers younger than age 50 years with a myocardial infarction or stroke
  - Individuals older than age 50 years with a first provoked VTE in the absence of malignancy or an intravascular device
  - Asymptomatic adult family members of a known factor V Leiden proband, especially those with a strong family history of VTE at a young age
  - Asymptomatic female family members of probands with known factor V Leiden thrombophilia who are pregnant or who are considering oral contraceptive use or pregnancy
  - Women with recurrent unexplained first-trimester pregnancy loss with or without second- or third-trimester pregnancy loss
  - Children with arterial thrombosis

➤ Limitations
- The results of a genetic test may be affected by DNA rearrangements, blood transfusion, bone marrow transplantation, or other rare events.

FACTOR VIII (ANTIHEMOPHILIC FACTOR)*

➤ Definition
- Factor VIII is synthesized in the liver and endothelial cells of other organs, including the spleen, which plays an important role in the synthesis of factor VIII. It is unaffected by liver failure or vitamin K deficiency.
- It is the principal cofactor in the intrinsic pathway of coagulation and serves as a substrate for proteolysis by the proteins C/protein S complex.
- PT (INR) is not affected by deficiency of factor VIII.
- Most laboratories use a specific coagulant assay to measure factor VIII.
  - Chromogenic assays are also available.
  - Immunologic assays determine factor VIII antigen. The antigen is concordant to activity in most cases but may be normal occasionally in patients with a functional defect in the molecule.
- **Normal range:** 70–150%

➤ Use
- Purified or recombinant factor VIII is used therapeutically for patients with hemophilia A.
- Immunologic assays for factor VIII may be useful in the diagnosis of von Willebrand disease but are not necessary in the diagnosis of most cases of hemophilia.

➤ Interpretation
Decreased In
- If factor VIII decreases below 40%, PTT becomes prolonged. In the presence of an inhibitor to factor VIII, PTT remains prolonged even after therapeutic infusions of factor VIII; mixing the patient's plasma with normal plasma in a 1:1 proportion does not correct the prolonged PTT and does not increase the original low factor VIII. Specific methodology can report the titer of the inhibitor in Bethesda Inhibitory Units.
- **Congenital disorders**
  - Hemophilia A (see p. 878): usually severe deficiency in male carriers and usually mild decrease in some female carriers of the hemophilia gene
  - Von Willebrand disease (see p. 879): especially if moderate to severe; more so in individuals with blood type B
- **Acquired disorders**
  - Acquired anti-factor VIII autoantibodies in previously unaffected individuals (see p. 887)
  - Acquired anti-factor VIII alloantibodies in hemophilia A patients treated with infusions of factor VIII
  - DIC and pathologic fibrinolysis

---

*Note: similar concepts apply to the quantitation of factor IX (see p. 887) and its inhibitors.

Increased In
* Acute-phase reactant (acute inflammatory conditions)
* Pregnancy and the use of oral contraceptives
* If markedly increased, it may predispose to thromboembolism.

FACTOR XI

➤ Definition
* Factor XI (previously known as plasma thromboplastin antecedent) is synthesized in the liver and megakaryocytes.
* Factor XI is activated by factor XIIa and by thrombin, the preferred activator on platelet surface. In turn, factor XI activates factors XII and IX in the intrinsic pathway.
* Factor XI is not affected by vitamin K antagonists.
* **Normal range:** 60–120%

➤ Use
* For the diagnosis of factor XI deficiency, a specific functional assay to quantitate the factor has to be performed.

➤ Interpretation
* If factor XI is decreased to less than 20–25%, PTT, but not PT, is prolonged. A normal PTT does not rule out a mild factor XI deficiency.
* Antibody inhibitors develop relatively often as a consequence of replacement therapy in factor XI deficient patients.
* Decreased values, if congenital, are characteristic for patients with factor XI deficiency (see p. 882). Acquired low values occur in severe liver disease and DIC.
* High levels of factor XI have been recently shown to be a risk factor for venous thromboembolism.

FACTOR XII (HAGEMAN FACTOR)

➤ Definition
* Factor XII is synthesized in the liver. It circulates in an active form.
* It is activated by collagen, disrupted basement membranes, and activated platelets, as well as high–molecular-weight kininogen and prekallikrein in conjunction with factor XI.
* It is unaffected by vitamin K antagonists.
* **Normal range:** 60–150%

➤ Use
* Specific factor assay is needed for the diagnosis of factor XII deficiency and to distinguish the anomaly from factor XI or other intrinsic pathway initiating factors deficiencies.

➤ Interpretation
* PTT, but not PT, is prolonged in severe deficiency.
* Asian population has lower factor XII levels than Caucasians (average, 44%).

* Factor XII levels are decreased in the neonate; they reach adult values at 2 weeks of age.
* Factor XII levels are increased in pregnancy.

➤ Limitation
* Factor XII may be artifactually decreased by the presence of LA (see p. 249).

FACTOR XIII

➤ Definition
* Factor XIII, formerly known as fibrin-stabilizing factor, is synthesized in the liver and also present in high concentrations in platelets.
* Factor XIII is a proenzyme activated by thrombin in the presence of calcium. It is a plasma transglutaminase that promotes clot stability by forming intermolecular covalent bonds between fibrin monomers.
* **Normal range:** reported qualitatively as normal or decreased; quantitation performed in research laboratories

➤ Use
* Factor XIII values are decreased in factor XIII deficiency, which can be either inherited or acquired (see p. 882).

➤ Interpretation
Decreased In (Acquired Type)
* AML
* Liver disease
* Association with hypofibrinogenemia in obstetric complications
* Presence of circulating inhibitors

FATTY ACIDS, FREE

➤ Definition
* Free fatty acids are formed by the breakdown of lipoprotein and triglycerides.
* All but 2–5% of the serum fatty acids are esterified. The "nonesterified" or "free" fatty acids are protein bound.
* Epinephrine, norepinephrine, glucagon, TSH, and ACTH release free fatty acids. Tumors producing such hormones cause release of excessive quantities of free fatty acids.
* Other names: nonesterified fatty acids (NEFA), FFA
* **Normal range:**
  * Adults: 8–25 mg/dL or 0.28–0.89 mmol/L
  * Children (or obese adults): <31 mg/dL or <1.0 mmol/L

➤ Use
* Monitoring nutritional status in the presence of malabsorption, starvation, and long-term parenteral nutrition
* Valuable for the differential diagnosis of polyneuropathy when Refsum disease is suspected. In this disease, the enzyme that degrades phytanic acid is lacking.

- Detection of pheochromocytoma and glucagon thyrotropin and adrenocorticotropin-secreting tumors
- Diabetes management

➤ Interpretation
Increased In
- Poorly controlled DM
- Pheochromocytoma
- Hyperthyroidism
- Huntington chorea
- Von Gierke disease
- Alcoholism
- Acute myocardial infarction
- Reye syndrome
- Phytanic acid increased in:
  - Refsum disease
  - Zellweger syndrome
  - Neonatal adrenoleukodystrophy
  - β-Lipoproteinemia

Decreased In
- CF
- Malabsorption (acrodermatitis enteropathica)
- Zinc deficiency (arachidonic acid and Linoleic acid low)

➤ Limitations
- Free fatty acids increase by 12–25% in 24 hour in refrigerated plasma.
- Strenuous exercise, anxiety, hypothermia, and long-term fasting elevate the levels.
- Long-term IV or parenteral nutrition therapy decrease the levels.
- Prolonged fasting or starvation affects levels (rise as much as 3 times normal).

FERRITIN

➤ Definition
- Ferritin is the cellular storage protein for iron, with 1 ng of ferritin per mL indicating 10 mg of total iron stores. It is a huge (440 kDa), 24-subunit protein consisting of light and heavy chains, which can store up to 4500 atoms of iron. Ferritin is an acute-phase reactant, and, along with transferrin and its receptor, coordinates cellular defense against oxidative stress and inflammation.
- Ferritin measured clinically in plasma is usually apoferritin, a non–iron-containing molecule.
- **Normal range:**
  - Male: 23–336 ng/mL (in patients with normal iron stores it should be >30 ng/mL)
  - Females: 11–306 ng/mL

➤ Use
- Predict and monitor iron deficiency
- Determine response to iron therapy or compliance with treatment

- Differentiate iron deficiency from chronic disease as cause of anemia
- Monitor iron status in patients with chronic renal disease with or without dialysis
- Detect iron overload states and monitor rate of iron accumulation and response to iron-depletion therapy
- Population studies of iron levels and response to iron supplement

➤ Interpretation
Increased In
- Acute and chronic liver disease
- Alcoholism (declines during abstinence)
- Malignancies (e.g., leukemia, Hodgkin disease)
- Infection and inflammation (e.g., arthritis)
- Hyperthyroidism, Gaucher disease, acute myocardial infarction
- Iron overload (e.g., hemosiderosis, idiopathic hemochromatosis).
- Anemias other than iron deficiency (e.g., megaloblastic, hemolytic, sideroblastic, thalassemia major and minor, spherocytosis, porphyria cutanea tarda)
- Renal cell carcinoma due to hemorrhage within tumor
- End-stage renal disease; values ≥ 1000 µg/L are not uncommon. Values <200 µg/L are specific for iron deficiency in these patients.

Decreased In
- Iron deficiency
- Hemodialysis

➤ Limitations
- In hepatic, malignant and inflammatory conditions, ferritin levels can be normal. In such cases bone marrow stain of iron may be used to exclude iron deficiency.
- Transferrin saturation is more sensitive to detect early iron overload in hemochromatosis; serum ferritin is used to confirm diagnosis and as an indication to proceed with liver biopsy. Ratio of serum ferritin (in ng/mL) to ALT (in IU/L) >10 in iron-overloaded thalassemic patients but averages ≤ 2 in viral hepatitis; ratio decreases with successful iron chelation therapy.
- Increases with age, is higher in men than women, in women who use oral contraceptives, and in persons who eat red meat compared with vegetarians.

FETAL BIOPSY

➤ Definition
- Invasive procedure to obtain fetal tissue such as skin, muscle, or liver

➤ Use
- Diagnosis of specific inherited disorders when gene mutation is unknown
  - Liver biopsy for specific inherited metabolic disorders (e.g., ornithine transcarbamylase deficiency, carbamoyl phosphate synthetase deficiency, G6PD (type 1a)
  - Skin biopsy for specific genetic skin disorders (e.g., epidermolysis bullosa)
  - Muscle biopsy for Duchenne muscular dystrophy

➤ **Limitations**
- High-risk procedures with value for a limited number of disorders

FETAL BLOOD SAMPLING (PERCUTANEOUS UMBILICAL BLOOD SAMPLING [PUB], CORDOCENTESIS)

➤ **Definition**
- Invasive procedure to obtain fetal blood generally performed after 18 weeks of gestation.
- Procedural risk of fetal loss is ~1–2%.

➤ **Use**
- Usually performed when diagnostic information cannot be obtained through amniocentesis, chorionic villus sampling (CVS), ultrasound examination, or following an inconclusive result from one of these tests.
- Provides fetal material for chromosome (cytogenetic) testing, biochemical testing, and molecular DNA-based testing for inherited disease
- Chromosome analysis faster than with either amniocentesis or CVS because less culture time required; therefore, useful for late presentations
- Used to assess fetal isoimmunization (e.g., Rhesus factor, Kell), anemia, platelet count, hemolytic disease, and infection (e.g., toxoplasmosis, rubella, or CMV)
- May also be used to administer medication to the fetus

➤ **Limitations**
- Riskier procedure than either amniocentesis of CVS performed late in pregnancy, limiting pregnancy termination options
- Does not assess neural tube defects

FETAL LUNG MATURITY (FLM) FLUORESCENCE POLARIZATION TEST

➤ **Definition**
- Uses polarized light to quantitate the competitive binding of a probe to both albumin and surfactant in amniotic fluid.
- It is a true direct measurement of pulmonary surfactant concentration.
- It reflects the ratio of surfactant to albumin and is measured by an automatic analyzer, such as the TDx-FLM.
- An elevated ratio has been correlated with the presence of fetal lung maturity; the threshold for maturity is 55 mg of surfactant per gram albumin.
- **Normal range:**
  - Mature fetal lungs: >55 mg/g albumin
  - Borderline: 35–55 mg/g albumin
  - Immature fetal lungs: <35 mg/g albumin

➤ **Use**
- Biophysical test to assess fetal lung maturity

➤ Interpretation
* Increased in mature fetal lungs
* Decreased in immature fetal lungs

➤ Limitations
* Study published by Fantz et al. (see Suggested Reading) has indicated that optimal cut-point to differentiate FLM from respiratory distress syndrome (RDS) for the TDx-FLMII assay is 45 mg/g albumin. At this cut-point, the sensitivity of the assay is 100% (82–100%) and specificity 84% (78–89%). The predictive value for immature result is 36% and predictive value for mature result is 100%. A result of ≥45 mg/g (albumin) indicates maturity and a result of <45 mg/g indicates immaturity and increased risk of RDS.
* Blood and meconium contamination interfere with interpretation, although the degree and direction of the interference are not well defined.
* Extreme caution should be used in the evaluation of fetal lung maturity in cases of multiple births (e.g., twins, triplets)

➤ Suggested Reading
Fantz CR, Powell C, Karon B, et al. Assessment of the diagnostic accuracy of the TDx-FLM II to predict fetal lung maturity. *Clin Chem.* 2002;48:761–765.

FIBRINOGEN (FACTOR I)

➤ Definition
* Fibrinogen is a glycoprotein synthesized in the liver. It is modified by thrombin to become fibrin, a visible clot.
* It is also an acute-phase reactant.
* **Normal range:** 150–400 mg/dL (most abundant circulating clotting factor)

➤ Use
* This test detects decreased or abnormal fibrinogen.
* It may be used to determine the severity and evolution of DIC by performing serial determinations.
* Because of the initial elevation of fibrinogen, its determination is not useful in the diagnosis of DIC.

➤ Interpretation
* Severe fibrinogen deficiency may prolong PT, PTT, and TT.

*Increased In**
* Acute inflammatory/infectious processes
* Cancer
* Pregnancy and use of oral contraceptives
* Older age
* Early DIC

---

*Increased fibrinogen may contribute to thrombophilia; however, this is not well documented (see p. 887)

Decreased In
- Afibrinogenemia (congenital) or hypofibrinogenemia (congenital)
- Dysfibrinogenemia (congenital or acquired)
- DIC and pathologic fibrinolysis. Fibrinogen is consumed after initial elevation as an acute-phase reactant.
- Very advanced liver disease

➤ Limitations
Preanalytic
- Clotted specimens or those obtained with the wrong anticoagulant.
- Inappropriately filled test tubes
- Inappropriately stored blood
- Hyperlipidemic, icteric, or hemolyzed blood
- Hct >55%

FIBRINOGEN DEGRADATION PRODUCTS (FDPs)

➤ Definition
- FDPs represent fragments D and E, major breakdown products of fibrinogen and fibrin. FDPs do not distinguish between fibrinolysis, fibrinogenolysis (the effect of pathologic or therapeutic fibrinolysis), or the combined effect of fibrinolysis plus thrombin generation, as seen in DIC.
- **Normal range:** <10 µg/mL

➤ Use
- FDP, as performed in most laboratories, is a simple and rapid semi-quantitative, latex-based test.
- It is used, in conjunction with other assays, to diagnose activated fibrinolysis or DIC in suspected patients.

➤ Interpretation
- Causes of increased results:
  - Pathologic and therapeutic fibrinolysis
  - DIC
  - Venous thromboembolism and pulmonary embolism
  - Myocardial infarction
  - Following trauma and surgery
  - Disseminated cancer
  - Complications of pregnancy
  - Small increase with exercise, severe liver disease

Limitations
- Because of its rather limited sensitivity, FDP may not be elevated in single, discrete clots, as seen in isolated deep vein thrombosis or in pulmonary embolism. In such situations a sensitive D-dimer assay is recommended.
- The assay itself, if performed on serum obtained from firmly clotted blood (the designated test tubes contain a potent coagulant venom). If blood is drawn on tubes containing anticoagulant, the assay is invalid (newer tests that use plasma have been developed).
- In the presence of rheumatoid factor the results may be falsely elevated.

FIBRONECTIN, FETAL (fFN)

➤ Definition
- This protein is located at the choriodecidual interface, between fetal membranes and the lining of the uterus. It acts as a kind of "glue" that binds the fetus to the mother.
- The fFN test measures the protein "leaked" through the cervix in to vagina in pregnancy's final stages, as the fetus prepares for the birth process.
- **Normal range:** negative

➤ Use
- To predict the risk of preterm delivery in symptomatic patients, since identifying women with preterm contractions who will go on to deliver prematurely is an inexact process.
- To identify asymptomatic women, usually in a high-risk group (e.g., previous preterm delivery, multiple gestation), who are most likely to deliver preterm.

➤ Interpretation
Increased (Positive) In
- Up to 40% of women with signs and symptoms deliver within the next 7 days.
- A woman tested at 24 weeks is nearly 60 times more likely to deliver within the next 4 weeks compared with a woman with a normal fetal fibronectin test when taken between weeks 22 and 24. The test detects nearly two thirds of the preterm births that occur prior to 28 weeks.

Decreased (Negative) In
- 99.5% of women with signs and symptoms will not deliver within the next 7 days.
- Less than 1% of women with identified risk factors will deliver before 28 weeks if they have a normal fetal fibronectin test result at 22–24 weeks.

➤ Limitations
- fFN results should not be interpreted as absolute evidence for the presence or absence of a process that will result in delivery in <14 days from specimen collection in symptomatic women or delivery in ≤34 weeks, 6 days in asymptomatic women evaluated between 22 weeks, 0 days and 30 weeks, 6 days of gestation.
- A positive rapid fFN result may be observed for patients who have experienced cervical disruption caused by, but not limited to, events such as sexual intercourse, digital cervical examination, or vaginal probe ultrasound.
- The rapid fFN result should always be used in conjunction with information available from the clinical evaluation of the patient and other diagnostic procedures such as cervical examination of a cervical microbiologic culture, assessment of uterine activity, and evaluation of other risk factors.
- The assay has been optimized with specimens taken from the posterior fornix of the vagina or the ectocervical region of the external cervical os. Samples obtained from other locations should not be used.
- Assay interference from the douches, white blood cells, red blood cells, bacteria. and bilirubin has not been ruled out.
- Manipulation of the cervix may lead to false positive results. Specimens should be obtained prior to digital examination or manipulation of the cervix.

- Care must be taken not to contaminate the swab or cervicovaginal secretions with lubricants, soaps, or disinfectants (e.g., K-Y® Jelly lubricant, Betadine® disinfectant, Monistat® cream). These substances may interfere with absorption of the specimen by the swab.
- Patients with suspected or known placental abruption, placenta previa, or moderate or gross vaginal bleeding should not be tested for fFN.

FIRST-TRIMESTER SCREENING

➤ Definition
- Performed between 11 and 13 weeks of gestation, first-trimester screening combines maternal age plus two serum biochemical markers: pregnancy-associated plasma protein A (PAPP-A) and β-hCG. It also includes fetal nuchal translucency (NT) measurement.

➤ Use
- Risk assessment for trisomy 21

➤ Interpretation
- Increased NT associated with trisomy 13, trisomy 18, trisomy 21, 45,X, triploidy, and other chromosome aberrations
- Trisomy 21 biochemical profile typically has increased β-hCG and decreased PAPP-A
- Trisomy 18 has decreased β-hCG and decreased PAPP-A
- Combining NT and maternal serum profile detects ~85% of affected trisomy 21 pregnancies with a 5% positive screening rate.

➤ Limitations
- Does not detect neural tube defects
- Detects fewer affected pregnancies than combined first-semester plus second-trimester screening modalities
- NT measurement requires experienced ultrasonographers.

FOLATE, SERUM AND ERYTHROCYTES (RBCs)

➤ Definition
- Folate refers to all derivatives of folic acid. Folate is an essential vitamin present in a wide variety of foods such as dark leafy vegetables, citrus fruits, yeast, beans, eggs, and milk. Folate is vital to normal cell growth and DNA synthesis. A folate deficiency can lead to megaloblastic anemia and ultimately to severe neurologic problems.
- Folate levels in both serum and RBCs are used to assess folate status. The serum folate level is an indicator of recent folate intake. RBC folate is the best indicator of long-term folate stores. A low RBC folate value may indicate a prolonged folate deficiency.
- Other names: vitamin B_9
- **Normal range:**
  - Serum folate: >6.5 ng/mL
  - RBC folate: 280–903 ng/mL

* Use
  * Evaluation of folate deficiency

➤ Interpretation

Increased In

* Blind loop syndrome
* Vegetarian diet
* Distal and small bowel disease
* PA

Decreased In

* Untreated folate deficiency, associated with megaloblastic anemia
* Infantile hyperthyroidism
* Alcoholism
* Malnutrition
* Scurvy
* Liver disease
* Vitamin B_{12} deficiency
* Dietary amino acid excess
* Chronic hemodialysis
* Celiac disease
* Disorders of glutathione metabolism
* Sideroblastic anemia
* Pregnancy
* Whipple disease
* Amyloidosis

➤ Limitations

* Serum folate is a relatively nonspecific test. Low serum folate levels may be seen in the absence of deficiency, and normal levels may be seen in patients with macrocytic anemia, dementia, neuropsychiatric disorders, and pregnancy disorders.
* Patients with low RBC folate or megaloblastic anemia should be evaluated for vitamin B_{12} deficiency. To distinguish between vitamin B_{12} and folate deficiency, determination of homocysteine (HCS) and methylmalonic acid (MMA) will help. In vitamin B_{12} deficiency both HCS and MMA are elevated, where as in folate deficiency only HCS levels are elevated.

FOLLICULAR-STIMULATING HORMONE (FSH) AND LUTEINIZING HORMONE (LH), SERUM

➤ Definition

* These glycoproteins are produced by the anterior pituitary gland, regulated by hypothalamic gonadotropin-releasing hormone (GnRH) and feedback by gonadal steroid hormones.
* FSH stimulates follicular growth and stimulates seminiferous tubules and testicular growth.
* LH stimulates ovulation and production of estrogen and progesterone. LH controls production of testosterone by Leydig cells.
* **Normal range:** See Table 2-34

TABLE 2-34. Normal Ranges of Human FSH and LH

		FSH			
		Females (mIU/mL)			
	Males (mIU/mL)	Mid-Follicular Phase	Mid-Cycle Peak	Mid-Luteal Phase	Postmenopausal
Number	65	29	26	27	50
Mean	5.88	6.43	12.27	3.45	60.76
Range	1.27–19.26	3.85–8.78	4.54–22.51	1.79–5.12	16.74–113.59
		LH			
		Females (mIU/mL)			
	Males (mIU/mL)	Mid-Follicular Phase	Mid-Cycle Peak	Mid-Luteal Phase	Postmenopausal
Number	50	29	26	27	50
Mean	3.75	5.88	52.84	4.84	30.55
Range	1.24–8.62	2.12–10.89	19.18–103.03	1.20–12.86	10.87–58.64

➤ **Use**
• Diagnosis of gonadal, pituitary, hypothalamic disorders
• Diagnosis and management of infertility

➤ **Interpretation**
Increased In
• Primary hypogonadism (anorchia, testicular failure, menopause)
• Gonadotropin-secreting pituitary tumors
• Precocious puberty (secondary to a CNS lesion or idiopathic)
• Complete testicular feminization syndrome
• Luteal phase of menstrual cycle

Decreased In
• Secondary hypogonadism
• Kallmann syndrome (inherited X-linked or autosomal isolated deficiency of GnRH; occurs in both sexes); Found in ~5% of patients with primary amenorrhea. Causes failure of both gametogenic function and sex steroid production (LH and FSH are "normal" or undetectable but rise in response to prolonged GnRH stimulation).
• Pituitary LH or FSH deficiency
• Gonadotropin deficiency

➤ **Limitations**
• Because of the episodic, circadian, and cyclic nature of its secretion, clinical evaluations may require determinations in pooled multiple serial specimens.

FRUCTOSAMINE, SERUM

➤ **Definition**
• Fructosamine describes serum proteins that have been glycated (i.e., derivatives of nonenzymatic reaction product of a sugar [glucose] with serum protein [albumin]). It reflects the

mean glucose concentration in blood over recent period (2–3 weeks), whereas glycated Hb (HbA1c) is indicative of blood glucose over intermediate to long term (4–8 weeks).

- **Normal range** (nondiabetic individuals): 170–285 μmol/L

➤ Use

- To assess short-term glycemic control in diabetic patients
- When glycated Hb cannot be used due to interferences (e.g., abnormal Hb), which invalidate HbA1c
- It should be compared with previous values in same patient rather than reference range.

➤ Interpretation
Increased In
Hyperglycemia in patients with poorly controlled DM

➤ Limitations

- Because the assay is nonspecific, color may be generated by compounds other than glycated proteins. Interferences are seen from ascorbic acid (vitamin C) and elevated bilirubin values. However, the second-generation assays have been shown to be highly specific for glycated proteins.
- Fasting blood glucose and HbA_{1c} are the usual and preferred means of monitoring glycemic control.
- Changes in fructosamine values correlate with significant changes in serum protein concentrations (e.g., liver disease, acute systemic illness). Abnormal values also occur during abnormal protein turnover (e.g., thyroid disease), even though patients are normoglycemic. It may be obviated by using fructose: albumin ratio.
- The within-subject variation for serum fructosamine is higher than that for HbA_{1c}; as a result, serum fructosamine concentrations must change more before a significant change can be said to have occurred.

GALACTOSE-1-PHOSPHATE URIDYLTRANSFERASE (GALT)

➤ Definition

- GALT is an enzyme responsible for converting ingested galactose to glucose. This measurement is used to identify in born errors of galactose metabolism, which can result in widespread tissue damage and abnormalities such as cataracts, liver disease, and renal disease. It also causes failure to thrive and mental retardation. The screening test should be done immediately to enable diet treatment if testing is positive.
- The deficiency of three enzymes, galactokinase (GALK); GALT, or UDP; and galactose-4-epimerase (GALE) are clinically important and result in inborn errors of galactose metabolism.
  - GALT deficiency, referred to as classical galactosemia or GG genotype, is the most commonly occurring of the three disorders.
  - GALK deficiency is the second most common cause of galactosemia and results in a milder variant of galactosemia. GALK deficiency is very rare and usually is expressed by occurrence of juvenile cataracts in the absence of mental retardation (which occurs in transferase deficiency).
  - GALE deficiency is an extremely rare cause of galactosemia.
- Other names: GPT, galactokinase; galactose-1-phosphate
- **Normal range:** 14.7–25.4 U/g Hb

➤ Use
* Diagnosis of GALT deficiency, the most common cause of galactosemia.
* Confirmation of abnormal state newborn screening results

➤ Interpretation
* Decreased in galactosemia

➤ Limitations
* Enzyme activity only may not differentiate variant form of galactosemia or carriers. For a more accurate evaluation of patients suspected to have galactosemia, the preferred test is a genetic test to identify mutation.

GAMMA GLUTAMYL TRANSFERASE (GGT)

➤ Definition
* The activity of this membrane-bound enzyme comes primarily from liver. GGT is responsible for the extracellular metabolism of glutathione, the main antioxidant in cells.
* It is slightly more sensitive than ALP in obstructive liver disease.
* **Normal range:**
  * 0–3 months: 4–120 IU/L
  * 3 months to 1 year: 2–35 IU/L
  * 1–16 years: 2–25 IU/L
  * ≥16 years: 7–50 IU/L

➤ Use
* To diagnose and monitor hepatobiliary disease; most sensitive enzymatic indicator of liver disease
* To ascertain whether observed elevations of ALP are due to skeletal disease (normal GGT) or reflect the presence of hepatobiliary disease (elevated GGT).
* As a screening test for occult alcoholism
* To aid in diagnosis of liver disease in the presence of bone disease, pregnancy, or childhood, which increase serum ALP and LAP but not GGT

➤ Interpretation
Increased In
* DM, hyperthyroidism, RA, COPD
* Drugs (phenytoin, carbamazepine, cimetidine, furosemide, heparin, methotrexate, oral contraceptives, and valproic acid)
* Liver disease—generally parallels changes in serum ALP, LAP, and 5'-NT but is more sensitive
* Acute hepatitis. Elevation is less marked than that of other liver enzymes, but it is the last to return to normal and, therefore, is useful to indicate recovery.
* Chronic active hepatitis; increased (average >7 times ULN) more than in acute hepatitis; more elevated than AST and ALT. In dormant stage, it may be the only enzyme elevated.
* Alcoholic hepatitis; average increase >3.5 times ULN.
* Alcohol abuse; a GGT/ALP ratio >2.5 is highly suggestive.

- Cirrhosis. In inactive cases, average values are lower (4 times ULN) than in chronic hepatitis. Increases of more than 10–20 times normal in cirrhotic patients suggest superimposed primary carcinoma of the liver (average increase >21 times ULN).
- Primary biliary cirrhosis. Elevation is marked: average >13 times ULN.
- Fatty liver. Elevation parallels that of AST and ALT but is greater.
- Obstructive jaundice. Increase is faster and greater than that of serum ALP and LAP; average increase >5 times ULN.
- Liver metastases; parallels ALP; elevation precedes positive liver scans. Average increase >14 times ULN.
- Cholestasis. In mechanical and viral cholestasis, GGT and LAP are increased about equally, but in drug-induced cholestasis, GGT is much more increased than LAP. Average increase >6 times ULN.
- Children; much more increased in biliary atresia than in neonatal hepatitis (300 IU/L is useful differentiating level). Children with α1-antitrypsin deficiency have higher levels than other patients with biliary atresia.
- Pancreatitis. The GGT level is always elevated in acute pancreatitis. In chronic pancreatitis, it is increased when there is involvement of the biliary tract or active inflammation.
- AMI; increased in 50% of patients. Elevation begins on the fourth to the fifth day, reaching a maximum at 8–12 days. With shock or acute right heart failure, an early peak may appear within 48 hours, with a rapid decline followed by a later rise.
- When increased, it is a risk factor for myocardial infarction and cardiac death.
- Heavy use of alcohol; the most sensitive indicator and a good screening test for alcoholism, because elevation exceeds that of other commonly assayed liver enzymes
- Some cases of carcinoma of prostate
- Neoplasms, even in absence of liver metastases; especially malignant melanoma, carcinoma of breast and lung; highest levels seen in hypernephroma
- Others (e.g., gross obesity [slight increase], renal disease, cardiac disease, postoperative state)

Decreased In
- Hypothyroidism

Normal In
- Pregnancy (in contrast to serum ALP, LAP) and children older than 3 months of age; therefore, may aid in differential diagnosis of hepatobiliary disease occurring during pregnancy and childhood
- Bone disease or patients with increased bone growth (children and adolescents); therefore, useful in distinguishing bone disease from liver disease as a cause of increased serum ALP
- Renal failure
- Strenuous exercise

➤ Limitations
- Half-life is about 7–10 days; in alcohol-associated liver injury, the half-life is increased to as much as 28 days, suggesting impaired clearance.
- Day to day variations are 10–15%; approximately double in African Americans
- There is a 25–50% increase with higher body mass index.
- Values are 25% lower during early pregnancy.

GASTRIN

➤ Definition

* Gastrin is a hormone secreted by the G-cells of the antrum of the stomach and the pancreatic islet of Langerhans. Its secretion is stimulated by alkalinity; by distention of the stomach by the antrum; by vagal stimulation; and by the presence of peptides, amino acids, alcohol, or calcium in the stomach. Its secretion is inhibited by gastric acidity via negative feedback system.
* Principal forms of gastrin in the blood are G-34 (big gastrin), G-17 (little gastrin), and G-14 (mini gastrin). Each of these circulates in nonsulfated and sulfated forms.
* The gastric stimulation test after calcium infusion (15 mg of Ca/kg in 500 mL normal saline over 4 hour) is useful in patients with marked elevation of gastrin levels. This test should be reserved for patients with a negative secretin test, gastric acid hypersecretion, and a strong suspicion of Z-E syndrome.
* **Normal range:**
  * Gastrin: 0–100 pg/mL
  * Gastrin stimulation test (after secretin): no response or slight suppression
  * Gastrin stimulation test (after calcium infusion): little or no increase over baseline

➤ Use

* Diagnosis of Z-E syndrome. The gastrin test after secretin (2–3 U/kg injected over 30 seconds) is preferred provocative test for patients suspected of having Z-E syndrome.
* Diagnosis of gastrinoma. Basal and secretin-stimulated serum gastrin measurements are the best laboratory tests for gastrinoma.
* Investigation of patients with achlorhydria or pernicious anemia

➤ Interpretation
Increased In

* Increased serum gastrin without gastric acid hypersecretion
  * Atrophic gastritis, especially when associated with circulating parietal cell antibodies
  * PA in ~75% of patients
  * Some cases of carcinoma of body of stomach, a reflection of the atrophic gastritis that is present
  * Gastric acid inhibitor therapy
  * After vagotomy
* Increased serum gastrin with gastric acid hypersecretion
  * Z-E syndrome
  * Hyperplasia of antral gastrin cells
  * Isolated retained antrum (a condition of gastric acid hypersecretion and recurrent ulceration after antrectomy and gastrojejunostomy that occurs when the duodenal stump contains antral mucosa)
* Increased serum gastrin with gastric acid normal or slight hypersecretion
  * RA
  * DM
  * Pheochromocytoma
  * Vitiligo
  * Chronic renal failure with serum creatinine >3 mg/dL; occurs in 50% of patients

* Pyloric obstruction with gastric distention
* Short-bowel syndrome due to massive resection or extensive regional enteritis
* Incomplete vagotomy

Decreased In
* Antrectomy with vagotomy
* Hypothyroidism
* Drugs, including anticholinergics and tricyclic antidepressants

➤ Limitations
* Gastrin levels follow circadian rhythms (lowest in early morning and highest during day).
* No consistent relationship has been established between *H. pylori* and gastric acid secretion or serum gastrin levels.

GAUCHER DISEASE MOLECULAR DNA ASSAY

➤ Definition
* Gaucher disease (GD) molecular DNA testing identifies mutations in the β-glucosylceramidase (*GBA*) gene in carriers and affected individuals. Glucosylceramidase enzyme activity is very low in affected individuals, but is not recommended for detection of *GBA* gene mutation carriers. Carrier testing should be accomplished through DNA testing of the *GBA* gene.
* **Normal values:** negative or no mutations are found

➤ Use
* There are two groups of tests:
  * **Targeted mutation analysis:**
    * A panel of four common mutations comprising *N370S, L444P, 84GG, IVS2+1*
    * More extended panels include rare mutations such as:
    * *V394L, D409H, D409V, R463C, R463H, R496H,* 55-bp deletion (exon 9)
  * **Sequence analysis:** analysis of the entire coding region and exon–intron boundaries is useful for identifying rare mutant alleles associated with GD.
* GBA molecular genetic testing is performed as:
  * Confirmatory diagnosis in symptomatic individuals
  * Carrier testing for Ashkenazi Jewish individuals
  * Carrier testing for at-risk family members of affected individuals
  * Prenatal diagnosis—when both parental mutations are known

➤ Limitations
* The results of a genetic test may be affected by DNA rearrangements, blood transfusion, bone marrow transplantation, or other rare events.

GENETIC CARRIER TESTING

➤ Definition
* Parental testing performed to assess carrier status for a specific genetic abnormality.
* Typically performed on DNA from a blood specimen to test for targeted mutations, but testing also can include other modalities such as enzymatic testing and gel electrophoresis.

➤ Use
* Carrier testing for autosomal recessive disease (may be targeted to specific ethnic groups). Examples:
  * CF: DNA testing for common mutations
  * Spinal muscular atrophy: DNA testing for common mutation
  * Sickle cell anemia: presence of sickling; confirmed by Hb electrophoresis
  * Tay-Sachs disease: enzyme activity
  * α- and β-thalassemia: decreased mean corpuscular volume; confirmed by Hb electrophoresis
* Carrier testing for X-linked disease. Example:
  * Fragile X (DNA testing for premutation); not currently offered to general population

➤ Limitations
* DNA testing for common mutations does not eliminate the possibility that an individual carries a rare mutation not included in the screening panel. Therefore, even if testing is negative, a residual carrier risk remains. Residual risk depends on many factors, including disease prevalence, patient ethnicity, family history, and the number of mutations included in the screen.

GHRELIN

➤ Definition and Use
* Ghrelin is a 28 amino acid peptide that is the natural ligand for the growth hormone secretagogue receptor. Based on its structure, it is a member of the motilin family of peptides. When administered peripherally or into the CNS, ghrelin stimulates secretion of growth hormone, increases food intake, and produces weight gain.
* Ghrelin, which is produced by the stomach, increases during periods of fasting or under conditions associated with negative energy balance such as starvation or anorexia. In contrast, ghrelin levels are low after eating or with hyperglycemia and in obesity. Accumulating evidence indicates that ghrelin plays a central role in the neurohormonal regulation of food intake and energy homeostasis.
* **Normal range** (fasting plasma levels): approximately 550–650 pg/mL

➤ Interpretation
Increased In
* Fasting
* Cachexia and anorexia

Decreased In
* After eating

➤ Limitations
* This test is not available routinely in many commercial clinical laboratories.

GLIADIN (DEAMIDATED) ANTIBODIES, IgG AND IgA

➤ Definition
* ELISA-based deamidated gliadin (DGP) antibody assay is a more useful test in the diagnosis of celiac disease than the native gliadin antibody assays. DGP assays seems to be equivalent

to, but not better than, tissue transglutaminase–IgA (TTG-IgA); however, DGP assays may have additive benefits in celiac screening because the combination of the two tests can increase the sensitivity without actually lowering the specificity.
* The DGP test also may be beneficial in circumstances when the TTG results are indeterminate. In addition, among young children it seems to appear before TTG and to resolve faster in the context of gluten withdrawal.
* Other names: DGP, gliadin IgA and IgG
* **Normal range:**
  * Negative: ≤19 units
  * Weak positive: 20–30 units
  * Positive: ≥31 units

➤ Use
* For initial evaluation for celiac disease in IgA-deficient population
* Monitoring response to dietary therapy
* When TTG-IgA is normal in patients with villous atrophy
* Patients with a high pretest probability of celiac disease but a negative TTG-IgA: guiding a decision regarding the need for endoscopy and biopsy

➤ Interpretation
Increased In
* Celiac disease
* Dermatitis herpetiformis

➤ Limitations
* Biopsy of the proximal small intestine is indicated to confirm the diagnosis of celiac disease in a patient with positive serologic test(s) for antibodies to TTG or deamidated gliadin. It is recommended that multiple tissue specimens be taken at biopsy to avoid false-negative histology in patients with focal disease.
* The levels of antibodies to TTG and deamidated gliadin peptides decline slowly in patients treated with a gluten-free diet, and serologic testing may be repeated to assess the response to treatment. In a typical patient, it may take up to 1 year for results to normalize. Persistently elevated results suggest poor adherence to the gluten-free diet.

GLUCAGON

➤ Definition
* Polypeptide hormone secreted by the islet alpha cells in the pancreas
* Stimulates the production of glucose in the liver and the oxidation of fatty acids
* **Normal range** (by age):
  * Newborn (1–3 days): 0–1750 pg/mL
  * Child (4–14 years): 0–148 pg/mL
  * Adult: 20–100 pg/mL

➤ Interpretation
Increased In
* Glucagonoma
* Diabetes mellitus

- Chronic renal failure
- Hyperlipoproteinemia types III and IV
- Severe stress, infections, trauma, burns, surgery, and acute hypoglycemia

Decreased In
- Cystic fibrosis
- Chronic pancreatitis

GLUCAGON STIMULATION TEST

➤ Definition and Use
- Failure of glucagon to increase after arginine stimulation is seen in glucagon deficiencies such as cystic fibrosis and chronic pancreatitis.
- This test is of rare clinical utility.
- After fasting overnight, an IV infusion of 0.5 g arginine/kg (not >30 g) should be given over 30 minutes. Fasting samples at should be drawn at 15, 30, 45, and 60 minutes.
- **Normal range:** Peak glucagon concentration at 30 min: 100–1500 pg/mL

➤ Limitations
- Arginine also stimulates insulin.
- There is an exaggerated response in diabetes, chronic renal failure, and liver failure.

GLUCOSE TOLERANCE TEST, ORAL (OGTT)

➤ Definition and Use
- OGTT should be reserved principally for patients with "borderline" fasting plasma glucose levels (i.e., fasting range 110–140 mg/dL). It is necessary for the diagnosis of impaired fasting glucose and impaired glucose tolerance.
- All pregnant women should be tested for gestational DM with a 50-g dose at 24–28 weeks of pregnancy; if that is abnormal, OGTT should be performed for confirmation. OGTT is the gold standard, and currently, its chief use is in the diagnosis of gestational DM (GDM).
- **Normal range:** see Tables 2-35, 2-36

➤ Interpretation
- Criteria for the diagnosis of DM (males and nonpregnant females) (ONE of the following):
  - Symptoms of DM plus casual (random) plasma/serum glucose concentration ≥200 mg/ dL Casual is defined as any time of day without regard to time since the last meal.

TABLE 2-35. Screening and Diagnostic Scheme for GDM

	Plasma Glucose (mg/dL)	
State	50-g (GCT) Screening Test	100-g (OGTT) Diagnostic Test
Fasting	—	95
1-hour	140	180
2-hour	—	155
3-hour	—	140

TABLE 2-36. Diagnosis of GDM Using the 75-g OGTT	
State	Plasma Glucose (mg/dL)
Fasting	95
1-hour	180
2-hour	155

- Fasting plasma glucose (FPG) ≥126 mg/dL. Fasting is defined as no caloric intake for at least 8 hours.
- Two-hour post load glucose (PG) ≥200 mg/dL during an OGTT. The test should be performed using a 75-g glucose load.
  - In the absence of unequivocal hyperglycemia with acute metabolic decompensation, these criteria should be confirmed by repeat testing on a separate day. The third measure (OGTT) is not recommended for routine clinical use.
  - For diagnosis of DM in nonpregnant adults, at least two values of OGTT should be increased (or fasting serum glucose ≥140 mg/dL on more than one occasion) and other causes of transient glucose intolerance must be ruled out.
- Criteria for the diagnosis of GDM (any degree of glucose intolerance with onset or first recognition during pregnancy), with the screening test for GDM:
  - A fasting serum glucose level >126 mg/dL or a casual plasma glucose >200 mg/dL meets the threshold for the diagnosis of DM if confirmed on a subsequent day, and it precludes the need for any glucose challenge.
  - In the absence of this degree of hyperglycemia, evaluation for GDM in women with average or high-risk characteristics should follow one of two approaches.
    - ONE STEP APPROACH:
      - Perform a diagnostic oral glucose tolerance test (OGTT) without prior plasma/serum glucose screening.
      - This approach may be cost-effective in high-risk patients or populations.
    - TWO-STEP APPROACH:
      - Perform an initial screening by measuring the plasma or serum glucose concentrations one hour after a 50-g oral glucose load (GCT) and perform a subsequent diagnostic OGTT on those women exceeding the glucose threshold value on the GCT.
      - A value of ≥140 mg/dL one (1) hour after the 50-g load indicates the need for a full diagnostic, 100-g, three (3) hour OGTT performed in the fasting state. (Table 2-35)
      - Two or more of the venous plasma concentrations must be met or exceeded for a positive diagnosis. The test should be done in the morning after an overnight fast of between 8 and 14 hours and after at least 3 days of unrestricted diet (≥150 g carbohydrate per day) and unlimited physical activity. The subject should remain seated and should not smoke throughout the test.
    - With either approach the diagnosis of GDM is based on OGTT.
- Alternatively, the diagnosis can be made using 75-g glucose load and the glucose threshold values listed for fasting, 1 hour, and 2 hours (Table 2-36). However, this test is not well validated as the 100-g OGTT for detection of at-risk infants or mothers.
- Two or more of the venous plasma concentrations must be met or exceeded for a positive diagnosis. The test should be done in morning after an overnight fast of between 8 and

14 hours and after at least 3 days of unrestricted diet (>150 g carbohydrate per day) and unlimited physical activity. The subject should remain seated and should not smoke throughout the test.

➤ Limitations

* Prior diet of >150 g of carbohydrate daily, no alcohol, and unrestricted activity for 3 days before test.
* Test in morning after 10–16 hours of fasting. No medication, smoking, or exercise (remain seated) during test.
* Not to be done during recovery from acute illness, emotional stress, surgery, trauma, pregnancy, inactivity due to chronic illness; therefore, is of limited or no value in hospitalized patients.
* Certain drugs should be stopped several weeks before the test (e.g., oral diuretics, oral contraceptives, and phenytoin). Loading dose of glucose consumed within 5 minutes:
* OGTT is not indicated in:
  * Persistent fasting hyperglycemia (>140 mg/dL)
  * Persistent fasting normoglycemia (<110 mg/dL)
  * Patients with typical clinical findings of DM and random plasma glucose >200 mg/dL
  * Secondary diabetes (e.g., genetic hyperglycemic syndromes, following administration of certain hormones)
  * OGTT should never be used for the evaluation of reactive hypoglycemia.
  * OGTT is of limited value for the diagnosis of DM in children.

GLUCOSE, CEREBROSPINAL FLUID (CSF)

➤ Definition

* Glucose in the CSF is about two thirds of the serum glucose measured during the preceding 2–4 hours in normal adults. This ratio decreases with increasing serum glucose levels. CSF glucose levels generally do not go above 300 mg per dL regardless of serum levels. Critical values are <30 mg/dL.
* Glucose in the CSF of neonates varies much more than that in adults, and the CSF-to-serum ratio is generally higher than in adults.
* **Normal range:** 50–80 mg/dL

➤ Use

* Diagnosis of tumors, infections, inflammation of the CNS, and other neurologic and medical conditions

➤ Interpretation

Increased In

* Elevated levels of glucose in the blood
* CNS syphilis

Decreased In

* CNS infections (glucose levels are usually normal in viral infections)
* Chemical meningitis
* TB meningitis

* Cryptococcal meningitis
* Mumps
* Primary and metastatic tumors of meninges
* Sarcoidosis
* Inflammatory conditions
* Subarachnoid hemorrhage
* Hypoglycemia

➤ Limitations
* Normal glucose levels do not rule out infection because up to 50% of patients who have bacterial meningitis have normal CSF glucose levels

GLUCOSE, URINE

➤ Definition
* Detection of glucose on a semiquantitative urine dipstick or Clinitest tablets is an insensitive means of screening for type 2 diabetes. The high rate of false-negative results suggests that the urine dipstick is not adequate as a screening test. In addition, not all patients with glucosuria have diabetes. Glucosuria can occur with defects in renal tubular function, as seen in type 2 (proximal) renal tubular acidosis and in familial renal glucosuria, a genetic disorder associated with salt-wasting, polyuria, and volume depletion.
* **Normal range:** see Table 2-37

➤ Use
* Aiding the evaluation of glucosuria and renal tubular defects
* Management of DM

➤ Interpretation
Increased In
* Any cause of increased blood glucose
* Endocrine disorders (DM, thyrotoxicosis, gigantism, acromegaly, Cushing syndrome)
* Major trauma
* Stroke
* Myocardial infarction

TABLE 2-37. Normal Values for Urine Glucose	
Specimen Type	Value
24-hour urine	0.04–0.21 g/day
Random urine	In mg/g creatinine
Male	
<40 years	3–181
>40 years	19–339
Female	
<40 years	5–203
>40 years	8–331

* Oral steroid therapy
* Burns, infections
* Pheochromocytoma

Decreased In
* Treatment with ascorbic acid, levodopa, or mercurial diuretics

➤ Limitations
* Prolonged exposure of urine sample to room temperature lower glucose results due microbial contamination and glycolysis.
* Specific gravity >1.020 and increased pH causes reduced sensitivity and falsely low glucose levels.

GLUCOSE, WHOLE BLOOD, SERUM, PLASMA

➤ Definition
* A blood glucose test measures the amount of a type of sugar, called glucose. Glucose comes from carbohydrate foods and is the main source of energy used by the body. Glucose levels are regulated by insulin and glucagon.
  Normal ranges: see Table 2-38

➤ Use
* Diagnosis of DM
* Control of DM
* Diagnosis of hypoglycemia
* Other carbohydrate metabolism disorders including gestational diabetes, neonatal hypoglycemia, idiopathic hypoglycemia, and pancreatic islet cell carcinoma
* Criteria for the diagnosis of DM (American Diabetes Association Expert Committee)
  * Four ways to diagnose diabetes are possible. Each must be confirmed on a subsequent day by any one of the four methods given above.
    1. Symptoms of diabetes plus casual (random) plasma/serum glucose concentration ≥ 200 mg/dL (11.1 mmol/L). Casual is defined as any time of day without regard to time since the last meal.
    2. FPG (fasting plasma glucose) ≥ 126 mg/dL (7.0 mmol/L). Fasting is defined as no caloric intake for at least 8 hours.
    3. Two-hour PG (post load glucose) ≥ 200 mg/dL (11.1 mmol/L) during an OGTT. The test should be performed using a 75-g glucose load.
    4. HbA_{1c} of >6.5%

TABLE 2-38. Normal Ranges for Glucose

Age	Reference Range	Critical Range
0–4 months	50–80 mg/dL	<35, >325 mg/dL
4 months to 1 year	50–80 mg/dL	<35, >325 mg/dL
>1 year	70–99 mg/dL	<45, >500 mg/dL

* In the absence of unequivocal hyperglycemia with acute metabolic decompensation, these criteria should be confirmed by repeat testing on a separate day. The third measure (OGTT) is not recommended for routine clinical use.
* The Expert Committee recognizes an intermediate group of subjects whose glucose levels, although not meeting the criteria for diabetes, are nevertheless too high to be considered altogether normal. This group is defined as having FPG levels >110 mg/dL but <126 mg/dL or 2-hour values in OGTT of >140 mg/dL but <200 mg/dL.

➤ Interpretation
Increased In
* DM, including:
  * Hemochromatosis
  * Cushing syndrome (with insulin-resistant diabetes)
  * Acromegaly and gigantism (with insulin-resistant diabetes in early stages; hypopituitarism later)
* Increased circulating epinephrine
  * Adrenalin injection
  * Pheochromocytoma
  * Stress (e.g., emotion, burns, shock, anesthesia)
* Acute pancreatitis
* Chronic pancreatitis (some patients)
* Wernicke encephalopathy (vitamin B_1 deficiency)
* Some CNS lesions (subarachnoid hemorrhage, convulsive states)
* Effect of drugs (e.g., corticosteroids, estrogens, alcohol, phenytoin, thiazides, propranolol, chronic hypervitaminosis A)

Decreased In
* Pancreatic disorders
  * Islet cell tumor, hyperplasia
  * Pancreatitis
  * Glucagon deficiency
* Extrapancreatic tumors
  * Carcinoma of adrenal gland
  * Carcinoma of stomach
  * Fibrosarcoma
  * Other
* Hepatic disease
  * Diffuse severe disease (e.g., poisoning, hepatitis, cirrhosis, primary or metastatic tumor)
* Endocrine disorders
  * Hypopituitarism*
  * Addison disease
  * Hypothyroidism
  * Adrenal medulla unresponsiveness
  * Early DM
* Functional disturbances
  * Postgastrectomy

- Gastroenterostomy
- Autonomic nervous system disorders
- Pediatric anomalies
  - Prematurity*
  - Infant of diabetic mother
  - Ketotic hypoglycemia
  - Zetterström syndrome
  - Idiopathic leucine sensitivity
  - Spontaneous hypoglycemia in infants
- Enzyme diseases
  - von Gierke disease*
  - Galactosemia*
  - Fructose intolerance*
  - Amino acid and organic acid defects*
- Methylmalonic acidemia*
- Glutaric acidemia, type II*
- Maple syrup urine disease*
- 3-hydroxy, 3-methyl glutaric acidemia*
  - Fatty acid metabolism defects*
- Acyl CoA dehydrogenase defects*
- Carnitine deficiencies*
- Other
  - Exogenous insulin (factitious)
  - Oral hypoglycemic medications (factitious)
  - Leucine sensitivity
  - Malnutrition
  - Hypothalamic lesions
  - Alcoholism

➤ Limitations

- Most glucose strips and meters quantify whole blood glucose, whereas most laboratories use plasma or serum, which reads 10–15% higher.
- In whole blood glucose determinations, hematocrit of >55% causes decreased result. Hematocrit of <35% causes increased result.
- Blood samples in which serum is not separated from blood cells shows glucose values decreasing at rate of 3–5% per hour at room temperature.
- Postprandial capillary glucose is ≤36 mg/dL higher than venous glucose at peak of 1 hour postprandial; usually returns to negligible fasting difference within 4 hours but in ~15% of patients, there may still be >20 mg/dL difference.
- Low oxygen content (e.g., venous blood, high altitudes >3000 meters) gives falsely increased values.
- Strenuous exercise, strong emotions, shock, burns, and infections can increase glucose physiologically.

---

*May cause neonatal hypoglycemia.

➤ Suggested Readings

American Diabetes Association Clinical Practice Recommendations: Executive Summary. *Standards of Medical Care in Diabetes* – 2010. *Diabetes Care.* 2010;33(suppl 1):S11–S69.

Sacks D, Bruns DE, Goldstein DE, et al. Guidelines and recommendations for laboratory analysis in the diagnosis and management of diabetes mellitus. *Clin Chem.* 2002;48(3):436–472.

GLUCOSE-6-PHOSPHATE DEHYDROGENASE (G6PD)

➤ Definition

- G6PD catalyzes the initial step in the hexose monophosphate shunt and is critical in protecting RBCs from oxidant injury.
- Deficiency of G6PD results in rigidity and lysis of RBCs, preferentially affecting older cells.
- **Screening assay:** reported as normal or deficient
- **Normal range (quantitative assay):** 7.0–20.5 units/g Hb

➤ Use

- The G6PD assay is used when G6PD deficiency is suspected (see G6PD Deficiency, p. 805).

➤ Interpretation
Decreased In

- Hemolytic anemia
- All persons with favism (but not all persons with decreased G6PD have favism)

➤ Limitation

- This assay should not be used following a hemolytic crisis in African Americans who carry the A⁻ variant, because reticulocytes (elevated after acute hemolysis) may have sufficient enzyme to give erroneous normal results.

GROWTH HORMONE (GH)

➤ Definition

- GH is a polypeptide (191 amino acids) originating in the anterior pituitary. Its metabolic effects are primarily anabolic. It promotes protein conservation and engages a wide range of mechanisms for protein synthesis. It also enhances glucose transport and facilitates the buildup of glycogen stores.
- Testing is used in the diagnosis and treatment of various forms of inappropriate growth hormone secretion.
- **Normal range:**
  - 0–7 years: 1–13.6 ng/mL
  - 7–11 years: 1–16.4 ng/mL
  - 11–15 years: 1–14.4 ng/mL
  - 15–19 years: 1–13.4 ng/mL

- Adult male: 0–4 ng/mL
- Adult female: 0–18 ng/mL

➤ Interpretation
Increased In
- Pituitary gigantism
- Acromegaly
- Laron dwarfism (defective GH receptor)
- Ectopic GH secretion (neoplasm of stomach and lung)
- Malnutrition
- Renal failure
- Cirrhosis
- Stress, exercise, prolonged fasting
- Uncontrolled diabetes mellitus
- Anorexia nervosa

Decreased In
- Pituitary dwarfism
- Hypopituitarism
- Adrenocortical hyperfunction

➤ Limitations
- Random levels provide little diagnostic information.
- GH levels vary throughout the day, making it difficult to define a reference range or to judge an individual's status based on single determination.
- Periods of sleep and wakefulness, exercise, stress, hypoglycemia, estrogens, corticosteroids, L-dopa, and factors influence the rate of growth hormone secretion.
- Because of its similarity to prolactin and placental lactogen, earlier GH immunoassays were often plagued with falsely high values in pregnant and lactating women.

GROWTH HORMONE–RELEASING HORMONE (GHRH, SOMATOCRININ)

➤ Definition and Use
- A 44 amino acid peptide, secreted by hypothalamus, stimulates pituitary to release growth hormone.
- Useful in differentiating between a pituitary tumor and ectopic GHRH hypersecretion.
- **Normal range:** <50 pg/mL

➤ Interpretation
Increased In
1% of cases of acromegaly caused by GHRH by hypothalamus or ectopic secretion by neoplasms (e.g., pancreatic islet, carcinoid of thymus or bronchus, neuroendocrine tumors)

Normal In
Most cases of acromegaly due to pituitary tumors

HALLUCINOGENS

See Amphetamines, *Cannabis sativa*

➤ Definition

* Drugs that are capable of altering perception of reality; also known as psychotomimetic drugs. Although many drugs (e.g. anticholinergics, cocaine) can induce delusions and/or hallucinations, this class has the capacity to reliably induce states of altered perception, feeling, and thought.
* Other names:
  * Ketamine: 2-(2-chlorophenyl)-2-(methyl-amino) cyclohexanone
  * Phencyclidine: PCP, 1-(1-phenylcyclohexyl) piperidine, angel dust, elephant tranquilizer, peace pill, Sherman, T
  * D-lysergic acid diethylamide (LSD): 9,10-d-N,N-diethyl-6-methylergoline-8b-carboxamide, microdots, window pane
* **Normal range:** ketamine: 500–2000 ng/mL plasma [IV administration]; PCP/LSD: not available

➤ Use

* Ketamine: induction of anesthesia
* Phencyclidine: no current medical use in the United States; abused as a hallucinogen
* LSD: no current medical use in the United States; abused as a hallucinogen

➤ Limitations

* LSD unstable in light, elevated temperature, and alkaline conditions and may irreversibly adsorb to containers.
* **Screening:** individual drug-specific tests required; immunoassay based on automated chemistry analyzers using blood/serum/urine.
  * **Ketamine**
    * No tests currently available by immunoassay
    * TLC procedures have a high limit of detection of approximately 1000 ng/mL.
    * See confirmation: readily detected with alkaline liquid–liquid or solid-phase extraction followed by gas chromatography or GC/MS analysis
  * **PCP**
    * Tests available from multiple manufacturers
    * Target; PCP
    * Limit of quantitation: 25 ng/mL [urine]; 2–10 ng/mL [blood/serum]
    * Little to no cross-reactivity with PCP metabolites and varying cross reactivity (20–90%) with PCP analogs [e.g. TCP-1-(1-thiophenecyclohexyl) piperidine]
    * May cross react with dextromethorphan
  * **LSD**
    * Target: d-LSD
    * Limit of quantitation: 0.5 ng/mL
    * Low (<20%) cross-reactivity with metabolites, no cross-reactivity with lysergic acid
* **Confirmation:** chromatography based; sample pretreatment/extraction procedure often required
  * **Ketamine** [blood/serum/urine]
    * Gas chromatography
    * HPLC

- GC/MS
- Target analyte: ketamine
- Limit of quantitation: 25–50 ng/mL
- **PCP** [blood/serum/urine]
  - Gas chromatography
  - HPLC
  - GC/MS
  - Target analyte: PCP
  - Limit of quantitation: 10–50 ng/mL
- **LSD** [blood/serum/urine]
  - LC/MS
  - LC/MS/MS
  - Target analytes; d-LSD, hydroxy-LSD, 2-oxo-LSD, 2-oxo-3-hydroxy-LSD, N-desmethyl-LSD
  - Limit of quantitation: 0.5–2 ng/mL
  - Multiple identified and unidentified metabolites formed, resulting in a low confirmation rate for LSD of positive-screened specimens

HAPTOGLOBIN

➤ Definition
- Haptoglobin is a glycoprotein synthesized mainly in liver. It sequesters free Hb released from hemolyzed RBCs, which is transported by macrophages to liver where the heme is broken down to bilirubin. The same function is served by hemopexin and especially albumin. Haptoglobin is also an acute-phase reactant.
- **Normal range:** 36–195 mg/dL

➤ Use
- Most sensitive test for RBC destruction; absent when rate of destruction is double that of normal
- Indicator of chronic hemolysis (e.g., hereditary spherocytosis, PK deficiency, sickle cell disease, thalassemia major, untreated PA)
- In the diagnosis of transfusion reaction by comparison of concentrations in pretransfusion and posttransfusion samples. In a posttransfusion reaction, the serum haptoglobin level decreases in 6–8 hours; at 24 hours it is <40 mg/dL or <40% of pretransfusion level.
- In paternity studies, may aid by determination of haptoglobin phenotypes.
- Evaluate known or suspected disorders involving a diffuse inflammatory process or tissue destruction, as indicated by elevated levels.

➤ Interpretation
Increased In
- Conditions associated with increased ESR and α-2 globulin (infections, inflammation, trauma, necrosis of tissue, hepatitis, scurvy, amyloidosis, nephrotic syndrome, disseminated neoplasms such as lymphomas and leukemias, collagen diseases such as rheumatic fever, RA, and dermatomyositis). Therefore, these conditions may mask presence of concomitant hemolysis.
- One third of patients with obstructive biliary disease
- Therapy with steroids or androgens

- Aplastic anemia (normal to very high)
- DM
- Smoking
- Aging
- Red cell membrane or metabolic defects (G6PD deficiency, hereditary spherocytosis, paroxysmal nocturnal hemoglobinuria)

Decreased In
- Hemoglobinemia (related to the duration and severity of hemolysis) due to:
  - Intravascular hemolysis (e.g., hereditary spherocytosis with marked hemolysis, PK deficiency, autoimmune hemolytic anemia, some transfusion reactions)
  - Extravascular hemolysis (e.g., large retroperitoneal hemorrhage)
  - Intramedullary hemolysis (e.g., thalassemia, megaloblastic anemias, sideroblastic anemias)
  - Genetically absent in 1% of white population and 4–10% of U.S. blacks.
  - Parenchymatous liver disease (especially cirrhosis)
  - Protein loss via kidney, GI tract, skin
  - Infancy, pregnancy
  - Malnutrition

➤ Limitations
- Low haptoglobin is normal for the first 3–6 months of life. Haptoglobin is an acute-phase reactant and increases with inflammation or tissue necrosis.
- Three main phenotypes of haptoglobin are known: Hp 1-1, 2-1, and 2-2. Hp 1-1 circulates as a monomer, and Hp 2-1 and 2-2 are polymers.
- Significant interlaboratory variations are observed from the sera of healthy individuals.

HEAVY METALS

➤ Definition
- Elements in the periodic table that form cations due to electron loss when ionized.
- Metals with a high relative atomic mass and a density >5 g/cm^3, which include aluminum, arsenic, lead (see p. 1094), mercury, cadmium, copper, selenium, thallium, and zinc
- **Normal range:**
  - Aluminum: <10 ng/mL (serum)
  - Arsenic: <13 ng/mL (blood)
  - Cadmium: <5 ng/mL (blood)
  - Copper: <10 ng/mL (serum/plasma)
  - Lead: <10 μg/dL (blood)
  - Mercury: <10 ng/mL blood
  - Selenium: 58–234 ng/mL blood
  - Thallium: <10 ng/mL serum
  - Zinc: 0.6–1.2 μg/mL plasma

➤ Use
- Many are naturally occurring in the environment (soil, air, water) and human body.
- Depending on the metal, heavy metals have widespread use in consumer products such as cooking utensils, cosmetics, pharmaceutical products, packing materials, insecticides, wood

products, batteries, computer chips, semiconductor industry, military, barometers, gauges, wiring, paint, fungicides, preservatives, canning industry, glass, plastic, ceramics, smelting, and refining and construction industries.

➤ **Limitations**
• Typically whole blood, free of clots, is tested. (Note exceptions above under normal range.)
• Specimen must be collected using a procedure that minimizes environmental contamination.
• Specimen container must be trace-element free (e.g., royal blue sodium EDTA tube).
• Laboratory-based instrumentation
  • Atomic absorption
  • Inductively coupled plasma mass spectrometry
  • Limit of quantitation (metal dependent): 1–10 ng/mL
  • Sample pretreatment may be necessary

HEMATOCRIT (Hct)

➤ **Definition and Use**
• Hct is the ratio of spun RBCs to plasma, reflecting the volume of packed RBCs.
• It may be performed manually following centrifugation or calculated in automated counters as the product of MCV and the RBC count. It is expressed as a percentage.
• **Normal range** (adults): 37–47% for women and 42–52% for men

➤ **Interpretation**
• Abnormalities in Hct levels parallel those for Hb.

➤ **Limitations**
• Errors may occur in patients with polycythemia vera, as well as in those with very high WBC counts because of an elevated buffy coat, with RBC agglutination, and with large platelets. These errors are more marked in the manual methods.
• Errors in both methodologies may also occur in patients with abnormal plasma osmotic pressure. Such errors are minimized with the current generation machines.
• Technical errors in blood preparation may also result in false values (see Hemoglobin, p. 203). In blood kept at room temperature for more than 6 hours, the Hct and MCV are elevated due to swelling of RBCs, whereas cell counts and indices are stable for 24 hours.

HEMOGLOBIN (Hb)

➤ **Definition**
• Hb is the respiratory protein of RBCs, consisting of 3.8% heme and 96.2% globin. There are more than 800 variants due to mutations in the globin molecule.
• **Normal range** (adults): 12–16 g/dL in women and 14–18 g/dL in men

➤ **Use**
• Hb is of great utility in detecting anemias or erythrocytosis.

➤ Interpretation
Decreased In
• Hb is reduced in all anemias, in most cases as a consequence of another underlying disease or a deficiency (iron, folate, vitamin B_{12}).

Increased In
• Hb is higher as a physiologic response to high altitude due to low oxygen tension or in advanced lung or cardiac disease.
• Certain myeloproliferative neoplasms, especially polycythemia vera (see p. 839), present with inappropriate elevation of Hb.

➤ Limitations
• Errors arise from improper venipuncture technique, which may introduce hemoconcentration.
• Dilution mistakes during sample preparation for manual methods or increased sample turbidity due to improperly lysed RBCs during processing by automated counters affect the accuracy of results.
• Marked leukocytosis, hyperlipidemia, dehydration, or high plasma proteins result in erroneous results and may be flagged by automated counters.

HEMOGLOBIN (Hb) VARIANT ANALYSIS

➤ Definition
• Hb variant analysis is a separation process used to identify normal and abnormal forms of Hb. HbA is the main form of Hb in the normal adult. HbF (fetal) is the major Hb in the fetus, and the remainder is HbA_2. Approximately 400 mutant forms of hemoglobin have been identified. Some are asymptomatic, especially in heterozygotes. Some may cause major morbid effects, especially in homozygotes.
• Globins found in different hemoglobins during fetal and adult life are indicated by Greek characters: α, β, γ, and δ.
• Variations in the amino acid composition of the globin chains cause the hemoglobinopathies.
• **Normal range:** In healthy adults, 95–98% of the total Hb is HbA ($\alpha 2 \beta 2$), 2–3% is HbA_2 ($\alpha 2 \delta 2$), and 0.8–2.0 % is fetal Hb (HbF) ($\alpha 2 \gamma 2$). Note that the reference range is different in individuals younger than age 1. See Table 2-39.

➤ Use
• Once there is a high clinical suspicion and the preliminary hematologic and genetic information point toward a hemoglobinopathy, an investigation for definitive diagnosis of an abnormal Hb is warranted. Such a diagnosis will:
  • Assist in the diagnosis of thalassemia, especially in patients with a family history positive for the disorder
  • Evaluate hemolytic anemia of unknown cause
  • Evaluate a positive sickle cell screening test to differentiate sickle cell trait from sickle cell disease
• Measurement of HbA_2 and HbF has great clinical value in the diagnosis as well as in characterization of some Hb structural variants and other hemoglobinopathies.

TABLE 2-39. Normal Values for Hemoglobin Variants by Age

Age	HbF (%)	HbA₂ (%)	HbA (%)
0–30 days	61–81	<1.3	19–39
1 month	46–67	<1.3	33–54
2 months	29–61	<1.9	39–71
3 months	15–56	<3.0	44–85
4 months	9.4–29	2.0–2.8	68–89
5 months	2.3–22	2.1–3.1	75–96
6 months	2.7–13	2.1–3.1	84–96
8 months	2.3–12	1.9–3.5	84–96
10 months	1.5–5.0	2.0–3.3	92–97
12 months	1.3–5.0	2.0–3.3	92–97
>1 year	<2%	1.5–3.5	96–100

- Increase in the HbA$_2$ level is considered the most characteristic diagnostic feature of β thalassemia trait and represents an essential test in the screening programs for β thalassemia prevention.
- There are two methods in use to screen for Hb variants:
  - HPLC is used as the primary screening tool because it readily quantitates HbA, HbA$_2$, and HbF; in addition, it presumptively identifies three of the most common Hb variants seen in North America: HbS, HbC, and HbD. All other abnormal variants will be flagged and need to be identified by HE.
  - Alkaline and acid hemoglobin electrophoresis (HE) is used to investigate the whole array of Hb variants. A practical method for HE is cellulose acetate at alkaline pH. Hb molecules in an alkaline solution have a net negative charge and move toward the anode. The method separates HbA, HbA$_2$, HbS, HbF, and HbC. Citrate agar gel electrophoresis at an acid pH separates hemoglobin variants that migrate together on cellulose acetate: HbS from HbD and HbG, HbC from HbE and HbO. Many of the hemoglobin forms that are difficult to differentiate by gel HE can be differentiated by HPLC. For instance, on gel electrophoresis, HbA$_2$ is difficult to distinguish from HbC because they migrate together. Testing by HPLC allows the quantification of HbA$_2$ in the presence of HbC. The two methods complement each other.
  - All Hb variants that are not diagnosed by these two methods require further testing with mass spectroscopy, capillary isoelectric focusing, or sequencing of DNA fragments generated by PCR.

➤ Interpretation
Increased In
- HbA$_2$: megaloblastic anemia, β thalassemias
- HbF: acquired aplastic anemia, hereditary persistence of fetal Hb, hyperthyroidism, leakage of fetal blood into maternal circulation, leukemia (acute or chronic), myeloproliferative neoplasms, sickle cell disease, thalassemias, β chain substitutions
- HbC (second most common variant in the United States; has a higher prevalence among African Americans)
- HbD (hemoglobinopathy that may also be found in combination with HbS or thalassemia)

- HbE
- HbS (sickle trait or disease)

Decreased In
- HbA_2
- Erythroleukemia
- α Thalassemia
- Iron-deficiency anemia (untreated)
- Sideroblastic anemia

➤ Limitations
- HbA_2 and HbF levels should be considered in conjunction with family history plus laboratory data, including serum iron, TIBC, ferritin, red cell morphology, hemoglobin, Hct, and MCV.
- Blood transfusions may obscure or dilute abnormal Hb for 3–4 months.
- In HPLC, when HbA_2 exceeds 10%, the presence of HbE or other Hb with similar resolution should be investigated.
- Quantitation of hemoglobins is performed optimally after one year of age
- HbLepore arises from an unequal crossing over and recombination event between adjacent δ and β globin genes. The resulting Hb has the mobility of HbS on alkaline electrophoresis and HbA on acid electrophoresis.
- HbH is composed of a tetramer of normal β chains, resulting in a markedly reduced production of α chains. HbH has mobility at alkaline pH much faster than that of HbA. (HbH disease is a severe form of α thalassemia with only one α chain).

HEMOGLOBIN A1c

➤ Definition
- Glucose combines with Hb continuously and nearly irreversibly during the lifespan of RBC (120 days). Therefore, glycosylated Hb (GHb) will be proportional to mean plasma glucose level during previous 6–12 weeks.
- May be reported as Hb A1c or as total of A1b, A1a, or A1c.
- Values may not be comparable with different methodologies and even different laboratories using same methodology.
- **Normal range** (ADA 2010 Recommendations):
  - <5.6%
  - 5.7–6.4% increased risk for Diabetes
  - >6.5% Diabetic range
- The interpretation of $HgbA_{1c}$ levels is not intuitively obvious to many patients with DM, who are accustomed to thinking in terms of blood glucose levels. The American Diabetes Association (ADA) has called for laboratories to express $HgbA_{1c}$ results as estimated average blood glucose (eAG). ADA believes that eAG will be easier for patients to understand and will lead to improved management of DM.
- The formula recommended to calculate eAG is:

$$eAG\ (mg/dL) = 28.7 \times Hemoglobin\ A1c - 46.7$$

➤ Use

* Monitoring compliance and long-term blood glucose level control in patients with diabetes
* Index of diabetic control (direct relationship between poor control and development of complications)
* Predicting development and progression of diabetic microvascular complications
* Possibly for diagnosis of DM. Usefulness is still to be determined.

➤ Interpretation

* A1C test should be performed at least 2 times a year in patients who are meeting treatment goals (and who have stable glycemic control).
* A1C test should be performed quarterly in patients whose therapy has changed or who are not meeting glycemic goals.
* Lowering A1C to below or around 7% has been shown to reduce microvascular and neuropathic complications of type 1 and type 2 diabetes. Therefore, for microvascular disease prevention, the A1c goal for nonpregnant adults in general is <7%.
* Dietary preparation or fasting is not required.
* An increase almost certainly means DM if other factors (see below) are absent (>3 SD above the mean has S/S = 99%/48%), but a normal value does not rule out impaired glucose tolerance. Values less than the normal mean are not seen in untreated DM.
* May rise within one week after rise in blood glucose due to stopping therapy but may not fall for 2–4 weeks after blood glucose decrease when therapy is resumed.
* Mean blood glucose in first 30 days (days 0–30) before sampling GHb contributes ~50% to final GHb value, whereas days 90–120 contribute only ~10%. Time to reach a new steady state is ~30–35 days.
* When fasting blood glucose is <110 mg/dL, HbA_{1c} is normal in >96% of cases.
* When fasting blood glucose is 110–125 mg/dL, HbA_{1c} is normal in >80% of cases.
* When fasting blood glucose is >126 mg/dL, HbA_{1c} is normal in >60% of cases.
* 1% increase in GHb is related to ~30 mg/dL increase in glucose.
* When mean annual HbA_{1c} is <1.1 times ULN, renal and retinal complications are rare, but complications occur in >70% of cases when HbA_{1c} is >1.7 times ULN.

Increased In

* Fetal Hb above normal or 0.5% (e.g., heterozygous or homozygous persistence of HbF, fetomaternal transfusion during pregnancy)
* Chronic renal failure with or without hemodialysis
* Iron deficiency anemia
* Splenectomy
* Increased serum triglycerides
* Alcohol ingestion
* Lead and opiate toxicity
* Salicylate treatment

Decreased In

* Shortened RBC lifespan (e.g., hemolytic anemias, blood loss)
* Following transfusions
* Pregnancy
* Ingestion of large amounts (>1 g/day) of vitamin C or vitamin E

- Hemoglobinopathies (e.g., spherocytes), which produce variable increase or decrease depending on assay method.

HEPARIN-INDUCED THROMBOCYTOPENIA (HIT) ASSAYS

➤ Definition

- HIT refers to thrombocytopenia that develops during or following the administration of heparin. There are various assays in use, none entirely satisfactory.
- There are two groups of assays:
  - Immunologic: two assays are available:
    - PIFA Heparin/PF4 Rapid Assay: the assay has a high negative predictive value but low specificity. Whenever the assay is positive, it requires confirmation
    - ELISA assays: use specific IgG antibodies; these assays have a high negative and positive predictive value
  - Functional: serotonin release assay, the gold standard for diagnosing HIT. An alternative functional assay is platelet aggregation standardized to use heparin as the aggregating agent. This method is laborious and has poor sensitivity.
- **Normal values**
  - PIFA: negative in the absence of heparin/platelet factor 4 antibodies
  - ELISA: negative if <0.4 optical density
  - Serotonin release assay (depends on the laboratory's own methodology): negative or positive

➤ Use

- An HIT assay should be performed whenever HIT is clinically suspected

➤ Limitations

- The PIFA assay, although easy to perform, has low specificity when positive; hence it requires confirmation by one of the two other assays as described. It is also operator dependent for interpretation
- ELISA is laborious and requires well-trained, experienced technologists for accurate performance
- Serotonin release requires the use of radioactive materials. It is performed in only a few specialized laboratories.

HEREDITARY HEMOCHROMATOSIS MUTATION ASSAY

➤ Definition

- Hereditary hemochromatosis (HH) testing identifies mutations in the *HFE* gene. *HFE* mutations exhibit incomplete penetrance; therefore, the HFE genotype cannot be used as the sole diagnostic criterion for disease. The majority (approximately 80–90%) of HH patients are homozygous for the *C282Y* mutation. Less than 2% of all *C282Y/H63D* compound heterozygotes will develop HH. Other reported genotypes associated with a clinical diagnosis of HH include compound heterozygosity for *C282Y/S65C* and homozygosity for *H63D*.
- **Normal values:** negative or no mutations are found

➤ Use
- HFE testing is performed as:
  - Confirmatory diagnostic testing
  - Predictive testing for at-risk relatives
  - Carrier testing (for the identification of heterozygotes)
  - Prenatal diagnosis (rarely performed)
- There are two groups of tests:
  - Targeted mutation analysis tests for only two (*C282Y, H63D*) or three (*C282Y, H63D,* and *S65C*) mutations in the *HFE* gene.
  - Sequence analysis: analysis of the entire coding region—testing to identify rare mutant alleles.

➤ Limitations
- The results of a genetic test may be affected by DNA rearrangements, blood transfusion, bone marrow transplantation, or other rare events.

HIGH–MOLECULAR-WEIGHT KININOGEN AND PREKALLIKREIN (FLETCHER FACTOR)

➤ Definition
- These clotting factors activate the early phase of the intrinsic pathway and the complement system. When decreased they may prolong PTT, but not PT. They do not depend on vitamin K carboxylation.
- **Normal ranges:**
  - High–molecular-weight kininogen: 59–135%*
  - Prekallikrein: 55–207%*

➤ Interpretation
Decreased In
- Extremely rare congenital deficiencies
- No bleeding diathesis associated with deficiencies; reflected in prolonged PTT

HOMOCYSTEINE (Hcy)

➤ Definition
- Total Hcy is a thiol-containing amino acid, produced by the intracellular demethylation of methionine to cysteine. Elevated tHcy has primary atherogenic and prothrombotic properties. Elevations in plasma homocysteine may be the result of genetic defects, nutritional deficiencies of vitamin B_6 (pyridoxine), vitamin B_{12}, and folic acid, some chronic medical conditions such as chronic renal insufficiency, and certain drugs. The most common form of genetic hyperhomocysteinemia results from the production of a thermolabile variant of methylene tetrahydrofolate reductase (MTHFR). Homozygosity for this form of MTHFR is a relatively common cause of elevated total Hcy (tHcy) in the general population.
- Highly elevated levels of tHcy are found in patients with homocystinuria (hyperhomocysteinemia), a rare genetic disorder of enzymes involved in homocysteine metabolism.

These patients exhibit arterial and venous thromboembolism, severe early arteriosclerosis, mental retardation, osteoporosis, and ocular abnormalities. Moderately elevated levels of tHcy are associated with less severe genetic defects. Moderate hyperhomocysteinemia is an independent risk factor for venous and arterial thromboembolism but less profound than the other well-established risk factors. Because of that, population screening for total Hcy level is not recommended.

- **Normal range:** 5.0–15 μmol/L.

➤ Use

- Elevated levels of tHcy may be used to exclude or confirm deficiencies of vitamin B_{12} or folate.
- Elevations in tHcy levels have also been used as an independent risk factor of coronary or cerebral vascular disease.

➤ Interpretation

- Hyperhomocystinemia has been classified as follows:
  - Moderate: 15–30 μmol/L
  - Intermediate: 30–100 μmol/L
  - Severe: >100 μmol/L

Increased In

- Vitamin B_{12}, vitamin B_6, or folate deficiency
- Hypothyroidism
- Chronic renal failure
- Coronary heart disease

Decreased In

- Down syndrome
- Pregnancy
- Hyperthyroidism
- Early diabetes

➤ Limitations

- The plasma (or serum) must be separated immediately on collection to avoid continuous synthesis of Hcy by red cells.
- Samples must be immediately stored on ice and serum centrifuged immediately, before a complete clot is formed, to prevent erroneous results due to the presence of fibrin.
- Certain drugs, such as anticonvulsants, methotrexate, or nitrous oxide may interfere with the assay.
- Cigarette smoking and coffee consumption increase tHcy levels.
- Intraindividual variability is approximately 8%; it can be as much as 25% in patients with hyperhomocystinemia.
- Generally, a single measurement of tHcy is considered adequate.

➤ Suggested Readings

Clarke R, Daly L, Robinson K, et al. Hyperhomocysteinemia: an independent risk factor for vascular disease. *N Engl J Med.* 1991;324:1149–1155.

Kluijtmans LA, Young IS, Boreham Ca, et al. Genetic and nutritional factors contributing to hyperhomocysteinemia in young adults. *Blood.* 2003;101:2483–2488.

Refsum H, Smith AD, Ueland PM, et al. Facts and recommendations about total homocysteine determinations: an expert opinion. *Clin Chem.* 2004;50:3–32.

HOMOVANILLIC ACID, URINE (HVA)

➤ Definition
- HVA is the main terminal metabolite of catecholamine neurotransmitter, dopamine.
- For the diagnosis of neuroblastoma, it is important to carry out simultaneous determinations of HVA and VMA because either or both elevated.
- **Normal range:** 0.0–15.0 mg/day

➤ Use
- Assist in the diagnosis of pheochromocytoma, neuroblastoma, and ganglioblastoma
- Monitor the course of therapy
- Screening for catecholamine-secreting tumors in children when accompanied by VMA
- Evaluating patients with possible inborn errors of catecholamine metabolism

➤ Interpretation
Increased In
- Neuroblastoma
- Pheochromocytoma
- Paraganglioma
- Riley-Day syndrome

Decreased In
- Schizotypal personality disorders

➤ Limitations
- Preferred specimen is 24-hour urine, because of intermittent excretion.
- Moderately elevated HVA may be caused by a variety of factors such as essential hypertension, intense anxiety, intense physical exercise, and numerous drug interactions (including some over-the-counter medications and herbal products).
- Medications that may interfere include amphetamines and amphetamine-like compounds, appetite suppressants, bromocriptine, buspirone, caffeine, chlorpromazine, clonidine, disulfiram, diuretics (in doses sufficient to deplete sodium), epinephrine, glucagon, guanethidine, histamine, hydrazine derivatives, imipramine, levodopa (L-dopa, Sinemet), lithium, MAO inhibitors, melatonin, methyldopa (Aldomet), morphine, nitroglycerin, nose drops, propafenone (Rythmol), radiographic agents, rauwolfia alkaloids (Reserpine), and vasodilators. The effects of some drugs on catecholamine metabolite results may not be predictable.

HUMAN CHORIONIC GONADOTROPIN (hCG)

➤ Definition
- Glycoprotein hormone, which is also known as β-hCG and chorionic gonadotropin, is produced by the placenta, with structural similarity to the pituitary hormones FSH, TSH, and LH.

TABLE 2-40. Representative Ranges in Human Chorionic Gonadotropin (hCG) During Normal Pregnancy	
Approximate Gestational Age (weeks postconception)	Approximate hCG Range (mIU/mL)
0.2–1	5–50
1–2	50–500
2–3	100–5000
3–4	500–10,000
4–5	1000–50,000
5–6	10,000–100,000
6–8	15,000–200,000
8–12	10,000–100,000

- The hCG test is widely used to detect pregnancy. It is also used as tumor marker for choriocarcinoma and some germ cell tumors.
- **Normal range:** ≥5.0 mIU/mL (generally indicative of pregnancy; Table 2-40)

➤ Use
- Diagnosis of pregnancy
- Investigation of suspected ectopic pregnancy
- Monitoring *in vitro* fertilization patients

➤ Interpretation
Increased In
- Normal pregnancy
- Recent termination of pregnancy
- Gestational trophoblastic disease
- Choriocarcinoma and some germ cell tumors
- Hydatiform mole

Decreased In
- Threatened abortion; microabortion
- Ectopic pregnancy

➤ Limitations
- False elevations (phantom hCG) may occur with patients who have human anti-animal or heterophilic antibodies.
- Patients who have been exposed to animal antigens, either in the environment or as part of treatment or an imaging procedure, may have circulating anti-animal antibodies present. These antibodies may interfere with the assay reagents to produce unreliable results.

HYDROXYBUTYRATE BETA (BHB)

➤ Definition
- In DKA, three ketone bodies are produced: BHB, acetoacetic acid, and acetone. BHB present in the greatest concentration and accounts for approximately 75% of the three ketone

bodies. During periods of ketosis, BHB increases even more than acetoacetate and acetone, and has been shown to be a better indicator of ketoacidosis including subclinical ketosis. Other names for this test include 3-hydroxybutyric acid and ketones.

- Testing for ketones is generally performed with nitroprusside (Acetest) tablets or reagent sticks. A 4+ reaction with serum-diluted 1:1 is strongly suggestive of ketoacidosis. Nitroprusside reacts with acetoacetate and acetone but not with BHB. This is important because BHB is the predominant ketone, particularly in severe DKA. It is, therefore, possible to have a negative serum nitroprusside reaction in the presence of severe ketosis.
- **Normal range:** 0.02–0.27 mmol/L

➤ Use
- Monitoring therapy for DKA
- Investigating the differential diagnosis of any patient presenting to the emergency department with hypoglycemia, acidosis, suspected alcohol ingestion, or an unexplained increase in the AG
- In pediatric patients, the presence or absence of ketonemia/urea is an essential component in the differential diagnosis of inborn errors of metabolism.
- Key parameter monitored during controlled 24-hour fasts.

➤ Interpretation
Increased In
- Alcoholic ketoacidosis
- Lactic acidosis (shock, renal failure)
- Liver disease
- Infections
- Phenformin and salicylate poisoning

➤ Limitations
- Not detectable by common tests for ketone bodies
- The nitroprusside test (Acetest) may give false-negative readings because it does not detect BHB.

IMMUNOGLOBULIN A (IgA)

➤ Definition
- IgA makes up the majority of immunoglobulin in mucosal secretions, including nasal and pulmonary secretions, saliva and intestinal fluids, tears, and secretions of the genitourinary tract. IgA is important in preventing attachment or penetration of the body surfaces by microorganisms, and in protection against respiratory, GI, and GU infections. IgA cannot cross the placenta. It can be produced by infants, and their secretions tend to be typically low.
- IgA is second most frequent type of monoclonal immunoglobulin identified in multiple myeloma.
- **Normal ranges:** see Table 2-41

➤ Use
- Detection or monitoring of monoclonal gammopathies and immune deficiencies
- Assist in the diagnosis of multiple myeloma

TABLE 2-41. Normal Ranges for IgA by Age

Age	Range (mg/dL)
0–30 days	1–7
1 month	1–53
2 months	3–47
3 months	5–46
4 months	4–72
5 months	8–83
6 months	8–67
7–8 months	11–89
9–11 months	16–83
1 year	14–105
2 years	14–122
3 years	22–157
4 years	25–152
5–7 years	33–200
8–9 years	45–234
10–17 years	68–378
≥18 years	82–453

- Monitor therapy for multiple myeloma
- Evaluate patients suspected of IgA deficiency prior to transfusion
- Evaluate anaphylaxis associated with the transfusion of blood and blood products (anti-IgA antibodies may develop in patients with low levels of IgA, possibly resulting in anaphylaxis when donated blood is transfused)

➤ Interpretation
Increased In
- Polyclonal:
  - Cirrhosis of liver
  - Chronic infections
  - Chronic inflammatory diseases
  - Inflammatory bowel disease
  - RA with high titers of RF
  - SLE (some patients)
  - Mixed connective tissue diseases
  - Sarcoidosis (some patients)
  - Wiskott-Aldrich syndrome
- Monoclonal:
  - IgA myeloma (M component)
  - Solitary plasmacytoma
  - Alpha-heavy chain disease
  - MGUS
  - Lymphoma
  - Chronic lymphocytic leukemia

Decreased In
- Normal persons (1:700)
- Hereditary telangiectasia (80% of patients)
- Type III dysgammaglobulinemia
- Malabsorption (some patients)
- SLE (occasionally)
- Cirrhosis of liver (occasionally)
- Still disease (occasionally)
- Recurrent otitis media (occasionally)
- Non-IgA myeloma
- Waldenström macroglobulinemia
- Acquired immunodeficiency
- Gastric carcinoma

➤ Limitations
- Immunochemical methods do not distinguish between polyclonal and monoclonal levels. Serum protein electrophoresis and immunofixation need to be performed for quantification of M-proteins.

IMMUNOGLOBULIN D (IgD)

➤ Definition
- IgD is mainly found on the surface of B cells and may help regulate B-cell function. IgD likely serves as an early B-cell antigen receptor; however, the function of the circulating IgD is largely unknown. IgD functions to activate some lymphocytes.
- **Normal value:** ≤ 15.3 mg/dL

➤ Use
- Diagnosis of rare IgD myelomas (greatly increased)

➤ Interpretation
Increased In
- Monoclonal
  - IgD multiple myeloma
  - MGUS
- Polyclonal
  - Chronic infection (moderately)
  - Autoimmune disease
  - Acute viral hepatitis
  - COPD
  - After allogeneic bone marrow transplantation

Decreased In
- Hereditary deficiencies
- Acquired immunodeficiency
- Non-IgD myeloma
- Infancy, early childhood

IMMUNOGLOBULIN E (IgE)

➤ Definition
- IgE mediates allergic and hypersensitivity reactions. There is a significant overlap in total IgE between allergic and nonallergic individuals. Measurement of total IgE is not very useful as a standalone screen for allergy disease.
- **Normal values:** see Table 2-42

➤ Use
- For allergy testing; IgE antibodies and skin tests are essentially interchangeable.
- Indicates various parasitic diseases
- Diagnosis of E-myeloma
- Diagnosis of bronchopulmonary aspergillosis; a normal serum IgE level excludes the diagnosis.

➤ Interpretation
Increased In
- Atopic diseases
  - Exogenous asthma in ~60% of patients
  - Hay fever in ~30% of patients
  - Atopic eczema
- Influenced by type of allergen, duration of stimulation, presence of symptoms, hyposensitization treatment
- Parasitic diseases (e.g., ascariasis, visceral larva migrans, hookworm disease, schistosomiasis, Echinococcus infestation)
- Monoclonal IgE myeloma

Decreased In
- Hereditary deficiencies
- Acquired immunodeficiency
- Ataxia-telangiectasia
- Non-IgE myeloma

TABLE 2-42. Normal Values for IgE by Age	
Age (years)	Value (kU/L)
0–2	<53
2	<93
3	<120
4	<160
5	<192
6	<224
7	<248
8	<260
9	<304
10	<328
18	<127

Normal In

- Asthma

➤ Limitations

- A normal level of IgE in serum does not eliminate the possibility of allergic disease.

IMMUNOGLOBULIN G (IgG)

➤ Definition

- IgG activates complement and fights infection. IgG represents 70–80% of the total serum immunoglobulins in the normal adults. It exists in four subclasses (IgG1, IgG2, IgG3, and IgG4). IgG1 predominates as 65% of the total IgG.
- IgG of maternal origin provides passive immunity to the neonate. It is transported across the placenta.
- **Normal ranges:** see Table 2-43

➤ Use

- Diagnosis of IgG myeloma
- Diagnosis of hereditary and acquired IgG immunodeficiencies
- Serologic diagnosis of infectious diseases and immunity

➤ Interpretation

Increased In

- Monoclonal
  - Multiple myeloma
  - Solitary plasmacytoma
  - MGUS

TABLE 2-43. Normal Ranges for IgG by Age	
Age	Range (mg/dL)
0–30 days	611–1542
1 month	241–870
2 months	198–577
3 months	169–558
4 months	188–536
5 months	165–781
6 months	206–676
7–8 months	208–868
9–11 months	282–1026
1 year	331–1164
2 years	407–1009
3 years	423–1090
4 years	444–1187
5–7 years	608–1229
8–9 years	584–1509
≥10 years	768–1632

- Lymphoma
- CLL
- Polyclonal
  - Sarcoidosis
  - Chronic liver disease (e.g., cirrhosis)
  - Autoimmune diseases
  - Parasitic diseases
  - Chronic infection
  - Intrauterine contraceptive diseases

Decreased In
- Protein-losing syndromes
- Pregnancy
- Non-IgG myeloma
- Waldenström macroglobulinemia
- Primary immunodeficiency states
- Combined with other immunoglobulin decreases:
  - Agammaglobulinemia
    - Acquired
      - Primary
      - Secondary (e.g., multiple myeloma, leukemia, nephrotic syndrome, protein-losing enteropathy)
    - Congenital
      - Hereditary thymic aplasia
      - Type I dysgammaglobulinemia (decreased IgG and IgA and increased IgM)
      - Type II dysgammaglobulinemia (absent IgA and IgM and normal levels of IgG)
      - Infancy, early childhood

IgG-TO-ALBUMIN RATIO, CSF

> ### Definition
- The two most commonly used diagnostic laboratory tests for multiple sclerosis are the CSF index and oligoclonal banding. The CSF index is the IgG-to-albumin ratio in CSF compared to the IgG-to-albumin ratio in serum. The CSF index is, therefore, an indicator of the relative amount of CSF IgG compared to serum, and any increase in the index is a reflection of IgG production in the CNS.
- The IgG synthesis rate is a mathematical manipulation of the CSF index data and can also be used as a marker for CNS inflammatory diseases. The index is independent of the activity of the demyelinating process.
- **Normal range:**
  - IgG, CSF: 0.0–6.0 mg/dL
  - Albumin, CSF: 0–35 mg/dL
  - IgG-to-Albumin Ratio, CSF: 0.09–0.25

> ### Use
- Diagnosis of individuals with multiple sclerosis

➤ **Interpretation**
Increased In
• Multiple sclerosis
• High normal values may indicate degenerative diseases such as cerebral or cerebellar atrophy, amyotrophic sclerosis, or brain tumor.

➤ **Limitations**
• The CSF index can be elevated in other inflammatory demyelinating diseases such as neurosyphilis, acute inflammatory polyradiculoneuropathy, and subacute sclerosing panencephalitis.
• Oligoclonal banding in the CSF is slightly more sensitive (85%) than the CSF index. The use of CSF index plus oligoclonal banding has been reported to increase the sensitivity to >90%.
• Normal levels can occur in incomplete obstruction of the spinal canal.
• Increase in albumin alone can be a result of a lesion in the choroid plexus or a blockage in the flow of CSF.
• Determination of myelin basic protein in CSF may be of use in diagnosis of multiple sclerosis or other active demyelinating processes.

IMMUNOGLOBULIN M (IgM)

➤ **Definition**
• IgM is the first antibody to appear in response to antigen. It can be produced by the fetus and cannot be crossed by the placenta.
• **Normal range:** see Table 2-44

➤ **Use**
• Diagnosis of hereditary and acquired IgM immunodeficiencies
• Diagnosis of Waldenström macroglobulinemia
• Earliest Ig serologic diagnosis of infectious disease

TABLE 2-44. Normal Ranges for IgM by Age	
Age	Range (mg/dL)
0–30 days	0–24
1 month	19–83
2 months	16–100
3 months	23–85
4 months	26–96
5 months	31–103
6 months	33–97
7–8 months	32–120
9–11 months	39–142
1 year	41–164
2 years	46–160
3 years	45–190
4 years	41–186
5–7 years	46–197
8–9 years	49–230
≥10 years	60–263

➤ Interpretation
Increased In
- Polyclonal:
  - Liver disease
  - Chronic infections
  - Secondary to nephritic syndrome
  - Hyper IgM syndrome
- Monoclonal:
  - Waldenström's macroglobulinemia
  - Lymphoma
  - CLL
  - Multiple myeloma (rare)
  - Schnitzler syndrome
  - Cold IgM antibody agglutinin
  - MGUS

Decreased In
- Protein-losing syndromes
- Non-IgM myeloma
- Infancy, early childhood
- See neutrophil function tests (p. 265)

IMMUNOGLOBULINS, FREE LIGHT CHAINS, SERUM

➤ Definition
- Plasma cells do not produce complete immunoglobulin molecules. Instead they produce the heavy and light chain components separately and then assemble them before secretion into the bloodstream. Because plasma cells usually make slightly more light chain components, there are usually some leftover light chains that are secreted in the blood without being bound to a heavy chain. These are known as serum free light chains (FLCs). Normally, there are only very low levels of free light chains in the blood (serum).
- The Freelite, free kappa and free lambda light chain assays, are a new, highly sensitive aid in the diagnosis and monitoring of patients with multiple myeloma and related plasma cell disorders. The Freelite serum free kappa and free lambda light chain assays are run on serum and not urine with increased sensitivity over current electrophoretic assays.
- Recent studies have shown that Freelite serum free kappa and lambda light chain assays:
  - Detect up to 82% of nonsecretory myeloma
  - Detect and monitor AL amyloid patients, including those with no monoclonal protein by immunofixation (IFE)
  - Detect and assess response to treatment in >95% of patients with light chain and intact Ig multiple myeloma
  - Detect up to 96% of intact immunoglobulin myeloma patients
  - Provide an earlier marker of therapeutic response or resistance, compared to whole immunoglobulin/M spike assays

- Evaluate risk of progression to myeloma in patients with monoclonal gammopathy of undetermined significance (MGUS)
- In combination with serum protein electrophoresis or IFE alone, provide the optimal detection rate for all paraproteins
- **Normal range:**
- Free kappa: 3.30–19.40 mg/L
- Free lambda: 5.71–26.30 mg/L
- Kappa/lambda ratio: 0.26–1.65

➤ Use

- Diagnosis and monitoring progress of patients with nonsecretory myeloma and oligosecretory (<1 g/dL monoclonal protein in the serum and <200 mg/day monoclonal protein in the urine) myeloma.
- Diagnosis and monitoring progress of patients with light chain myeloma as well as primary systemic amyloidosis, in whom the underlying clonal plasma cell disorder may otherwise be difficult to detect and monitor
- Predicting risk of progression of MGUS
- Predicting risk of progression of solitary bone plasmacytoma
- Diagnosis, monitoring during and after treatment, and perhaps prognosis of patients with multiple myeloma and an intact immunoglobulin

➤ Interpretation (Table 2-45)
Increased In (see Limitations)

- Multiple myeloma
- Lymphocytic neoplasms
- Waldenström's macroglobulinemia
- Amyloidosis
- Light chain deposition disease
- Connective tissue diseases such as SLE
- Renal impairment (common).
- Overproduction of polyclonal free light chains (FLCs) from inflammatory conditions (common)
- Biclonal gammopathies of different FLC types (rare)

Decreased In
- Bone marrow function impairment

➤ Limitations
- Elevated kappa and lambda FLC may occur due to polyclonal hypergammaglobulinemia or impaired renal clearance. A specific increase in FLC (e.g., FLC kappa/lambda ratio) must be demonstrated for diagnostic purposes.

➤ Suggested Readings
Bradwell AR. Serum free light chain analysis. 3rd ed. Birmingham, UK: The Binding Site Ltd; 2005:13–21.

Katzmann JA, Clark RJ, Abraham RS, et al. Serum reference intervals and diagnostic ranges for free κ and free λ immunoglobulin light chains: relative sensitivity for detection of monoclonal light chains. *Clin Chem.* 2002;48:1437–1444.

TABLE 2-45. Interpretation of Serum Free Light Chain Assays in Serum

Kappa	Lambda	K/L Ratio	Interpretation
N	N	N	Normal Serum
L	L	N	BM suppression without monoclonal gammopathy
L	L	H	Monoclonal Gammopathy
L	L	L	Monoclonal Gammopathy
L	N	N	Normal Serum
L	N	L	Monoclonal Gammopathy
L	H	L	Monoclonal Gammopathy
N	L	H	Monoclonal Gammopathy
N	L	N	Normal Serum
N	N	H	Monoclonal Gammopathy
N	N	L	Monoclonal Gammopathy
N	H	N	Polyclonal Ig increase or renal impairment
N	H	L	Monoclonal Gammopathy
H	L	H	Monoclonal Gammopathy
H	N	H	Monoclonal Gammopathy
H	N	N	Polyclonal Ig increase or renal impairment
H	H	N	Polyclonal Ig increase or renal impairment
H	H	H	Monoclonal Gammopathy with renal impairment
H	H	L	Monoclonal Gammopathy with renal impairment

IMMUNOSUPPRESSANTS

➤ Definition

- Cyclosporin A is a cyclic polypeptide containing 11 amino acids. It is produced by the fungus *Tolypocladium inflatum*.
- Sirolimus is a macrocyclic triene antibiotic that is produced by fermentation of *Streptomyces hygroscopicus*. Sirolimus was discovered from a soil sample collected in Rapa Nui, which is also known as Easter Island. Structurally, sirolimus resembles tacrolimus and binds to the same intracellular binding protein or immunophilin known as FKBP-12.
- Tacrolimus is a macrolide antibiotic produced by *Streptomyces tsukubaensis*.
- Other names: cyclosporine (Sandimmune, Neoral); sirolimus (rapamycin, Rapamune), tacrolimus (FK-506, Prograf)
- **Normal range:** see Table 2-46

➤ Use

- Cyclosporine is a drug that suppresses the immune system and is used to prevent organ rejection and marrow transplant. It is used in combination with other immunosuppressants or corticosteroids

TABLE 2-46. Normal Ranges of Immunosuppressants Following Transplantation

Drug	Type of Transplant	Therapeutic Concentration (ng/mL) 12-hour Postdose
Cyclosporin A		
	Renal	100–200
	Cardiac	150–250
	Hepatic	100–400
	Bone marrow	100–300
		Toxicity at >400
Sirolimus		4–20 (trough)
	Kidney	4–12
	Liver	12–20
Tacrolimus		5–20 (12-hour trough level)
	Kidney and liver	
	0–2 months post–transplant	10.0–15.0
	3 months and older	5.0–10.0
	Heart	
	0–2 months posttransplant	10.0–18.0
	3 months and older	8.0–15.0
		Toxicity at ≥26

- Although sirolimus was originally developed as an antifungal agent, it was later found to have immunosuppressive and antiproliferative properties.
- Tacrolimus is an immunosuppressive drug that has been shown to be effective for the treatment of rejection following transplantation. Tacrolimus has been used for therapy of the following disorders: adult RA, as a single agent or in combination with methotrexate, adult refractory myositis, systemic sclerosis, Crohn disease, autoimmune chronic hepatitis, pediatric autoimmune enteropathy, uveitis, steroid-resistant nephrotic syndrome, (severe) recalcitrant chronic plaque psoriasis, and atopic dermatitis (administered as ointment)

➤ Limitations

- Testing performed on whole blood samples
- Clotted specimens unacceptable
- Frozen specimens unacceptable
- Testing performed by immunoassay or LC/MSn (multiple MS) technology
  - Immunoassay (e.g., MEIA, EMIT, FPIA, RIA): FPIA demonstrates more cross-reactivity with cyclosporine metabolites than EMIT. Therefore, EMIT concentration may be 70% of FPIA concentration. Note that cross-reactivity of immunoassays may change over time, so consult the manufacturer's package insert for current information.
  - LC/MS concentrations are generally lower than immunoassay due to cross-reactivity of the immunoassay with metabolites.
  - Limit of quantitation
    - Cyclosporine: 50 ng/mL
    - Sirolimus/tacrolimus: 1.0 ng/mL

TABLE 2-47. Normal Ranges Inhibin A

Age/Phase	Inhibin A (Dimer) (pg/mL)
Normal cycling females:	*Normal cycling females:*
Early follicular phase (−14 to −10)	1.8–17.3
Mid follicular phase (−9 to −4)	3.5–31.7
Late follicular phase (−3 to −1)	9.8–90.3
Mid cycle (Day 0)	16.9–91.8
Early luteal (1–3)	16.1–97.5
Mid luteal (4–11)	3.9–87.7
Late luteal (12–14)	2.7–47.1
IVF-peak levels	354.2–1690.0
PCOS-ovulatory	5.7–16.0
Postmenopausal	<7.9
Normal males	<2.1

INHIBINS A AND B, SERUM

➤ Definition

- Polypeptide hormones that belong to transforming growth factor family; these are secreted by granulosa cells of ovary and Sertoli cells of testis. Inhibit pituitary production of FSH. Secreted by placenta during pregnancy.
- Inhibins are heterodimers and hence have two forms: alpha-beta A (inhibin A) and alpha-beta B (inhibin B).
- **Normal ranges:** see Tables 2-47, 2-48

➤ Use

- Females
  - Inhibin A is mostly produced by corpus luteum.
    - Undetectable before puberty
    - Very low levels in postmenopausal state due to absent follicular secretions
    - During pregnancy is secreted by placenta. Inhibin A peaks at 8–10 weeks, declines until 20 weeks, and then increases gradually to term.
  - Inhibin B is produced by granulosa cells of small developing antral follicles.
    - Rises to peak in early puberty; constant level thereafter.

TABLE 2-48. Normal Range for Inhibin B by Sex and Age

Male	Female
<3 years: No range established	<3 years: No range established
3–9 years: <162 pg/mL	3–9 years: <30 pg/mL
10–13 years: 42–339 pg/mL	10–13 years: < 93 pg/mL
14–17 years: 68–300 pg/mL	14–17 years: <140 pg/mL
≥18 years: <305 pg/mL	Premenopausal: <255 pg/mL
	Postmenopausal: <30 pg/mL

- Gradually declines after age 40. In early menopause, follicular phase inhibin B declines, whereas inhibin A and estradiol is still within normal range.
- May indicate low ovarian reserve in perimenopausal women and transition to menopause; useful for assisted reproduction. Measure on days 3–5 of menstrual cycle.
- After menopause, inhibin A and B fall to very low levels.
- Also used as a serum marker for detecting Down syndrome pregnancies
- May be useful to screen for preeclampsia
- Males
  - Inhibin B is predominant in males and supports spermatogenesis by negative feedback of FSH.
  - Inhibin A is not significant in males (normal values <480 pg/mL); values remain fairly constant.
  - May be decreased in male infertility.

➤ Interpretation
Increased In
- Inhibin A: elevated during normal pregnancy
- Preeclampsia, Down syndrome, and some cancers

Decreased In
- Ovarian aging

➤ Limitations
- Mainly limited to the second trimester screening for Down syndrome (inhibin A) and the detection and monitoring of ovarian granulosa cell tumors

INSULIN

➤ Definition
- This peptide hormone is enzymatically processed from proinsulin in pancreatic secretory granules of beta cells. Approximately 50% is removed from the blood during initial passage through liver. Its half-life is 4–9 minutes.
- Secretion is regulated primarily by blood glucose levels; therefore, it should always be measured with concomitant blood glucose. Insulin deficiency is the crucial factor in the pathogenesis of type 1 DM.
- **Normal range:** 6–27 μIU/mL

➤ Use
- Diagnosis of insulinoma
- Diagnosis of fasting hypoglycemia
- Not clinically useful for diagnosis of DM

➤ Interpretation
Increased In
- Insulinoma. Fasting blood insulin level >50 μU/mL in the presence of low or normal blood glucose level. Administration of tolbutamide or leucine causes a rapid rise of blood insulin to very high levels within a few minutes, with a rapid return to normal.
- Factitious hypoglycemia in presence of normal blood glucose

* Insulin autoimmune syndrome
* Untreated mild DM in obese individuals. The fasting blood level is often increased.
* Cirrhosis due to insufficient clearance from blood
* Acromegaly (especially with active disease) after ingestion of glucose
* Reactive hypoglycemia after glucose ingestion, particularly with the diabetic type of glucose tolerance curve

Decreased In
* Type 1 DM
* Hypopituitarism
* Severe DM with ketosis and weight loss, which may result in an absence of insulin. In less severe cases, insulin is frequently present but only at lower glucose concentrations.

➤ Limitations
* Insulin values are normal in:
  * Hypoglycemia associated with nonpancreatic tumors
  * Idiopathic hypoglycemia of childhood, except after administration of leucine
* Circulating anti-insulin antibodies are often found in patients who have been treated with nonhuman forms of insulin. If present, these antibodies may interfere with the assay.
* For individuals who are significantly overweight, fasting insulin levels are typically somewhat higher than for adults of normal weight.
* Heterophilic antibodies in human serum can react with the immunoglobulins included in the assay components, causing interference with *in vitro* immunoassays. Samples from patients routinely exposed to animals or animal serum products can demonstrate this type of interference, potentially causing an anomalous result.

INSULIN TOLERANCE TEST

➤ Definition
* Insulin is administered, 0.1 unit/kg body weight IV. A smaller dose should be used if hypopituitarism is suspected. IV glucose should be kept available to prevent severe reaction.
* Blood is obtained for serum glucose and cortisol assays (and for growth hormone [GH], if indicated) immediately before insulin is injected and 30 and 45 minutes thereafter. All patients, in whom adequate hypoglycemia is achieved, defined as 35 mg/dL or less should have some symptoms of hypoglycemia, either of sympathetic discharge or of CNS glucose deprivation, such as simply falling asleep.

➤ Use
* Assessing syndromes of extreme insulin resistance
* Crude classification of insulin sensitivity
* Assessing GH deficiency

➤ Interpretation
* Blood glucose normally falls to 50% of fasting level within 20–30 minutes and returns to fasting level within 90–120 minutes
* Blood glucose that falls <25% and returns rapidly to fasting level represents an increased tolerance to insulin

Increased In
* Hypothyroidism
* Acromegaly
* Cushing syndrome (peak cortisol response <18–20 μg/dL and change over baseline <7 μg/dL indicates glucocorticoid deficiency)
* DM (some patients; especially older, obese ones)

Decreased In
* Increased sensitivity to insulin (excessive fall of blood glucose)
  * Hypoglycemic nonresponsiveness (lack of response by glycogenolysis)
  * Pancreatic islet cell tumor
  * Adrenocortical insufficiency
  * Adrenocortical insufficiency secondary to hypopituitarism
  * Hypothyroidism
    * von Gierke disease (some patients)
    * Starvation (depletion of liver glycogen)

➤ Limitations
* In premenopausal women, the test can be performed at any phase of the menstrual cycle, because there are no cycle effects on the hypothalamic-pituitary-adrenal axis response to insulin-induced hypoglycemia.
* Almost all patients have some degree of perspiration. If the patient does not perspire, the adequacy of the stress stimulus must remain suspect irrespective of the serum glucose concentration.
* Most patients also have a hyperactive precordium (but not tachycardia or hypotension, because they are supine), and feelings of hunger, drowsiness, detachment, or anxiety. The last is common and sometimes severe, and many patients find this an unpleasant experience.
* Patients with primary or secondary adrenal insufficiency or long-standing DM have an impaired compensatory response to hypoglycemia.
* The criteria for a normal serum cortisol response ranged from 18 to about 22 μg/dL in multiple studies. Ideally, reference ranges would be determined locally but this is rarely done in practice. If serum cortisol reaches this level, it is unimportant whether hypoglycemia was adequate. On the other hand, failure to reach this level is indicative of an inadequate response only if the serum glucose fell to 35 mg/dL or less. If this was not achieved, the stimulus was inadequate and the test must be repeated. It is the serum cortisol concentration that is achieved rather than the increment that is important.

INSULIN-LIKE GROWTH FACTOR BINDING PROTEIN-3 (IGFBP-3)

➤ Definition
* This 264-amino acid peptide (molecular weight, 29 kDa) is produced by the liver. It is the most abundant of a group of IGFBPs that transport and control bioavailability and half-life of insulin-like growth factors (IGFs), in particular IGF-I. In addition to its IGF binding-function, IGFBP-3 also exhibits intrinsic growth-regulating effects that are not yet fully understood but have evoked interest with regard to a possible role of IGFBP-3 as a prognostic tumor marker.

TABLE 2-49. Normal Ranges for IGFBP-3

Age (in years unless otherwise specified)	Reference Range (μg/mL)
0–15 days	0.5–1.4
1	0.7–3.6
2	0.8–3.9
3	0.9–4.3
4	1.0–4.7
5	1.1–5.2
6	1.3–5.6
7	1.4–6.1
8	1.6–6.5
9	1.8–7.1
10	2.1–7.7
11	2.4–8.4
12	2.7–8.9
13	3.1–9.5
14	3.3–10
15	3.5–10
16	3.4–9.5
17	3.2–8.7
18	3.1–7.9
19	2.9–7.3
20	2.9–7.2
21–25	3.4–7.8
26–30	3.5–7.6
31–35	3.5–7.0
36–40	3.4–6.7
41–45	3.3–6.6
46–50	3.3–6.7
51–55	3.4–6.8
56–60	3.4–6.9
61–65	3.2–6.6
66–70	3.0–6.2
71–75	2.8–5.7
76–80	2.5–5.1
81–85	2.2–4.5

- Other name: somatomedin C binding protein
- **Normal range:** see Table 2-49

➤ Use

- Diagnosing growth disorders
- Diagnosing adult growth hormone deficiency
- Monitoring of recombinant human growth hormone treatment
- Possible adjunct to IGF-I and growth hormone in the diagnosis and follow-up of acromegaly and gigantism

➤ **Interpretation**
Increased in
• Overproduction of GH
• Excessive rhGH therapy
• Chronic renal failure

Decreased In
• GH deficiency
• GH resistance
• Fasting/chronic malnutrition
• Hepatic failure
• Diabetes mellitus

➤ **Limitations**
• IGF-I and IGFBP-3 reference ranges are highly age-dependent, and results must always be interpreted within the context of the patient's age.
• Discrepant IGFBP-3 and IGF-I results can sometimes occur due to liver and kidney disease; however, this is uncommon and such results should alert laboratories and physicians to the possible occurrence of a preanalytic or analytic error.
• At this time, IGFBP-3 cannot be reliably used as a prognostic marker in breast, colon, prostate, or lung cancer.
• IGFBP-3 assays exhibit significant variability among platforms and manufacturers. Direct comparison of results obtained by different assays is problematic. Re-baselining of patients is preferred if assays are changed.

INSULIN-LIKE GROWTH FACTOR-I (IGF-I)

➤ **Definition**
• IGF-I is secreted by hypothalamus; release is mediated by growth hormone (GH) in many tissues, especially hepatocytes. It is a single polypeptide chain with 70 amino acid residues with a molecular mass of 7,649 daltons. It is structurally homologous to IGF-II and insulin. IGF-I circulates primarily in a high–molecular-weight tertiary complex with IGF-binding protein-3 (IGFBP-3) and acid-labile subunit.
• Plasma IGF-I levels are barely detectable at birth, rise gradually during childhood, peak during mid-puberty until approximately 40 years of age, and then decline gradually. Maternal plasma levels increase during pregnancy.
• **Normal range:** See Table 2-50; 0–7 days: <26 ng/mL; 8–15 days: <41 ng/mL

➤ **Use**
• Diagnosis of acromegaly and pituitary deficiency; preferable to GH because it is constant after eating and during the day
• Help determine optimum dosage of GH
• Screening other growth disorders
• Assessing nutritional status
• Monitoring effectiveness of nutritional repletion; a more sensitive indicator than prealbumin, transferrin index, or retinol-binding protein

TABLE 2-50. Normal Range of IGF-I	
Age (years)	Central 95% Range
16 days to −1 year	55–327
2	51–303
3	49–289
4	49–283
5	50–286
6	52–297
7	57–316
8	64–345
9	74–388
10	88–452
11	111–551
12	143–693
13	183–850
14	220–972
15	237–996
16	226–903
17	193–731
18	163–584
19	141–483
20	127–424
21–25	116–358
26–30	117–329
31–35	115–307
36–40	109–284
41–45	101–267
46–50	94–252
51–55	87–238
56–60	81–225
61–65	75–212
66–70	69–200
71–75	64–188
76–80	59–177
81–85	55–166

➤ **Interpretation**

Increased In

• Acromegaly and gigantism
• Pregnancy (2–3 times nonpregnant values)

Decreased In

• Pituitary deficiency
• Laron dwarfism
• Anorexia or malnutrition
• Acute illness

- Hepatic failure
- Hypothyroidism
- DM
- Normal aging

INSULIN-LIKE GROWTH FACTOR-II

➤ Definition
- IGF-II is a 7.5 kDa, 67 amino acid peptide that is thought to mediate some of the actions of growth hormone (GH). IGF-II peptide is structurally homologous to IGF-I and proinsulin. IGF-II is secreted by the liver and other tissue and is postulated to have mitogenic and metabolic actions at or near the sites of synthesis. IGF-II also appears in the peripheral circulation, where it circulates primarily in a high–molecular-weight tertiary complex with IGF-binding protein-3 (IGFBP-3) and acid-labile subunit.
- The proportion of unbound IGF-II in the circulation has been estimated at >5%. Plasma levels of IGF-II are dependent on adequate levels of GH and other factors, including adequate nutrition.
- The actions of IGF-II are mediated by binding to specific cell surface receptors. Although its specific physiologic role has not been defined, it has been postulated that the interplay of IGF-I and IGF-II with the different cell surface receptors and circulating binding proteins modulates tissue growth.
- **Normal ranges:**
  - Child, prepubertal: 334–642 ng/mL
  - Child, pubertal: 245–737 ng/mL
  - Adult: 288–736 ng/mL
  - GH deficiency: 51–299 ng/mL

➤ Use
- IGF-II is an adjunct to IGF-I in the clinical evaluation of GH-related disorders

➤ Interpretation
Increased In
- Hypoglycemia associated with non-islet cell tumors
- Hepatoma
- Wilms tumor

Decreased In
- GH deficiency

INSULIN–TO–C-PEPTIDE RATIO

➤ Definition
- Insulin and C-peptide are secreted into portal vein in equimolar amounts but serum ratio = 1:5 to 1:15 due to removal of ~50% of insulin from blood during initial passage through liver. C-peptide half-life = ~30 minutes.
- **Normal range:** fasting molar ratio Insulin to C-peptide = 1.0.

➤ Use

* To differentiate insulinoma from factitious hypoglycemia due to insulin

➤ Interpretation

* **<1.0 in molarity units (or >47.17 µg/ng in conventional units)**
  * Increased endogenous insulin secretion (e.g., insulinoma, sulfonylurea administration)
  * Renal failure
* **>1.0 in molarity units (or <47.17 µg/ng in conventional units)**
  * Exogenous insulin administration
  * Cirrhosis

➤ Limitations

There are ethnic differences in insulin/C-peptide ratio in both fasting and glucose-stimulated conditions in normal young nondiabetic pregnant women. Compared with their Caucasian and Hispanic counterparts, African American women had indices suggestive of lower insulin production and greater insulin resistance (i.e., a lower C-peptide concentration, a lower C/I ratio, and elevations in insulin and the I/G ratio).

INTRINSIC FACTOR ANTIBODY

➤ Definition

* Intrinsic factor (IF), or anti-intrinsic factor, intrinsic factor blocking antibody, type 1 intrinsic factor antibody, IFAB, is a glycoprotein produced by the gastric parietal cells. It binds to, transports, and facilitates absorption from the terminal ileum of the very small amount of vitamin B_{12} in the diet. If there are antibodies to either the parietal cells, the B_{12} binding site of IF, or the binding site of IF to the ileum, the patient's ability to absorb dietary B_{12} by the IF route will be reduced.
* Over time, the presence of these antibodies leads to a reduction in B_{12} stores and ultimately to vitamin B_{12} deficiency, the consequences of which vary. The presence of circulating autoantibodies to IF is a very specific indicator of PA. Antibodies against IF are found in approximately 50% of cases but rarely in other conditions.
* **Normal range:** negative

➤ Use

* Diagnosis of PA
* Evaluation of patients with decreased vitamin B_{12} levels

➤ Interpretation

* Increased in PA

➤ Limitations

* Cyanocobalamin may give a false-positive test result.
* Methotrexate and folic acid may give false-positive test results.
* Negative or inconclusive test results do not exclude the diagnosis of PA.
* Some patients with other autoimmune diseases may have positive test results, particularly in patients with autoimmune thyroid disease or type 1 DM.

IODINE EXCRETION, URINE 24 HOUR

➤ Definition

- Iodine is an essential component of T_4 and T_3, and it must be provided in the diet. Inadequate iodine intake leads to inadequate thyroid hormone production, and all the consequences of iodine deficiency stem from the associated hypothyroidism. However, iodide excess can also cause thyroid dysfunction. Goiter is the most obvious manifestation of iodine deficiency. Low iodine intake leads to reduced T_4 and T_3 production, which results in increased thyrotropin (TSH) secretion in an attempt to restore T_4 and T_3 production to normal.
- **Normal range:**
  - International groups recommend the following median urinary iodine concentration as the best single indicator of iodine nutrition in populations:
    - Severe deficiency: 0–0.15 µmol/L (0–19 µg/L)
    - Moderate deficiency, 0.16–0.38 µmol/L (20–49 µg/L)
    - Mild deficiency, 0.40–0.78 µmol/L (50–99 µg/L)
    - Optimal iodine nutrition, 0.79–1.56 µmol/L (100–199 µg/L)
    - More than adequate iodine intake, 1.57–2.36 µmol/L (200–299 µg/L)
    - Excessive iodine intake, 2.37 µmol/L (300 µg/L)
  - The range in which the median falls is more important than the precise number.

➤ Use

- Diagnosis of transient thyroid dysfunction and iodine-induced hyperthyrosis.
- Biochemical indicator for the assessment of iodine status.
- Monitoring iodine excretion rate as an index of daily iodine replacement therapy
- Correlating total body iodine load with (131)I uptake studies in assessing thyroid function.

➤ Interpretation

Increased in

- Dietary excess
- Recent drug or contrast media exposure

Decreased In

- Dietary deficiency

➤ Limitations

- Urinary iodine levels are influenced by gender, age, sociocultural and dietary factors, drug interferences, geographic location and season.
- In most instances it provides little useful information on long-term iodine status of the individual, since the results obtained merely reflect the dietary iodine intake.
- Administration of iodine-based contrast media and drugs containing iodine, such as amiodarone, will yield elevated results.
- High concentrations of gadolinium are known to interfere with most metals tests. If gadolinium-containing contrast media has been administered, a specimen should not be collected for 48 hours.
- Frozen specimens sometimes result in falsely lowered results

➤ Suggested Reading

International Council for the Control of Iodine Deficiency Disorders. WHO. UNICEF. *Assessment of Iodine Deficiency Disorders and Monitoring their Elimination. A Guide for Programme Managers.* 2nd ed. Geneva, Switzerland: World Health Organization; 2001.

IRON (Fe)

➤ Definition

- Iron exists in the body in many forms: hemoglobin in circulating red cells and developing erythroblasts, iron-containing proteins such as myoglobin and cytochromes, and bound to transferrin and storage in the form of ferritin and hemosiderin. Iron homeostasis is regulated strictly at the level of intestinal absorption and release of iron from macrophages. The serum iron level reflects Fe^{3+} bound to transferrin, not free Hb in serum.
- **Normal range:**
  - Female: 28–170 µg/dL
  - Male: 45–182 µg/dL

➤ Use

- Diagnosis of blood loss
- Differential diagnosis of anemias
- Diagnosis of hemochromatosis and hemosiderosis
- Evaluation of iron deficiency; should always be measured with TIBC
- Diagnosis of acute iron toxicity, especially in children
- Evaluation of thalassemia and sideroblastic anemia.
- Monitor response to treatment for anemia.

Increased In

- Idiopathic hemochromatosis
- Hemosiderosis of excessive iron intake (e.g., repeated blood transfusions, iron therapy, iron-containing vitamins) (may be >300 µg/dL)
- Decreased formation of RBCs (e.g., thalassemia, pyridoxine-deficiency anemia, PA in relapse)
- Increased destruction of RBCs (e.g., hemolytic anemias)
- Acute liver damage (degree of increase parallels the amount of hepatic necrosis) (may be >1000 µg/dL); some cases of chronic liver disease
- Progesterone birth control pills (may be >200 µg/dL) and pregnancy
- Premenstrual elevation by 10–30%
- Acute iron toxicity; serum iron-to-TIBC ratio is not useful for this diagnosis
- Repeated transfusions
- Lead poisoning
- Acute hepatitis
- Vitamin B_6 deficiency

Decreased In

- Iron-deficiency anemia
- Normochromic (normocytic or microcytic) anemias of infection and chronic diseases (e.g., neoplasms, active collagen diseases)

- Acute and chronic infection
- Carcinoma
- Hypothyroidism
- Postoperative state and kwashiorkor
- Nephrosis (because of loss of iron-binding protein in urine)
- PA at onset of remission
- Menstruation (decreased by 10–30%)

➤ Limitations

- Serum iron is not reliable as the primary test to identify iron deficiency or screening for hemochromatosis and other iron overload diseases. For these conditions, a serum TIBC, percent transferrin saturation, and ferritin assay are recommended.
- Diurnal variation—normal values in mid-morning, low values in mid-afternoon, very low values ($\sim$10 µg/dL) near midnight. Diurnal variation disappears at levels <45 µg/dL.
- Iron dextran administration causes increase for several weeks (may be >1000 µg/dL)
- Ingestion of oral contraceptives will elevate iron and/or total iron binding capacity values.
- Not recommended for patients undergoing treatment with deferoxamine or other iron-chelating compounds.
- Ingestion of iron (including iron-fortified vitamins or supplements) may cause transient elevated iron levels.

IRON BINDING CAPACITY, TOTAL (TIBC)

➤ Definition

- TIBC measures the blood's capacity to bind iron with transferrin (TRF). One milligram of TRF binds to 1.25 µg of iron, and, therefore, a serum TRF level of 300 mg/dL is equal to TIBC of (300 × 1.25) 375 µg/dL. TIBC is an indirect way of assessing TRF level. TIBC correlates with serum TRF, but the relationship is not linear over the wide range of TRF values and is disrupted in diseases affecting transferring binding capacity and iron-binding proteins.
- TIBC should not be confused with unsaturated binding capacity (UIBC), where UIBC = TIBC minus serum iron (µg/dL).
- **Normal range:** 255–450 µg/dL

➤ Use

- Differential diagnosis of anemias
- Should always be performed whenever serum iron is done to calculate percent saturation for diagnosis of iron deficiency
- Screening for iron overload
- Acute hepatitis
- Late pregnancy

➤ Interpretation
Increased In

- Iron deficiency
- Acute and chronic blood loss
- Acute liver damage
- Late pregnancy
- Progesterone birth control pills

Decreased In
* Hemochromatosis
* Cirrhosis of the liver
* Thalassemia
* Anemias of infection and chronic diseases (e.g., uremia, RA, some neoplasms)
* Nephrosis
* Hyperthyroidism

➤ Limitations
* Estrogens and oral contraceptives increase TIBC levels.
* Asparaginase, chloramphenicol, corticotropin, cortisone, and testosterone decrease the TIBC levels.

IRON SATURATION

➤ Definition
* Iron saturation is a better index of iron stores than serum iron alone. Iron saturation is calculated as:
  * % Saturation = Serum iron/TIBC × 100
* This number represents the amount of iron-binding sites that are occupied.
* **Normal range:** 20–50%

➤ Use
* Differential diagnosis of anemias
* Screening for hereditary hemochromatosis

➤ Interpretation
Increased In
* Hemochromatosis
* Hemosiderosis
* Thalassemia
* Birth control pills (≤75%)
* Ingestion of iron (≤100%)
* Iron dextran administration causes increase for several weeks (may be >100%)
* Vitamin B_6 deficiency
* Aplastic anemias

Decreased In
* Iron-deficiency anemia (usually <10% in established deficiency)
* Anemias of infection and chronic diseases (e.g., uremia, RA, some neoplasms)
* Malignancy of stomach and small intestine

ISLET AUTOANTIBODIES (IAA)

➤ Definition
* Diabetes-related (islet) autoantibody testing is primarily ordered to help distinguish between autoimmune type 1 DM and DM due to other causes (e.g., diabetes resulting from obesity and insulin resistance).

TABLE 2-51. Autoimmune Antibodies in Type 1 DM	
Islet Antibody	Frequency of Occurrence
Glutamic acid decarboxylase autoantibodies*	70–80%
Islet cell cytoplasmic autoantibodies	70–80%
Insulin autoantibodies	Adults <10%; children ~50% ~60%
Insulinoma-2 associated autoantibodies (IA-2A)	(>60%)

*Recommended because it is most persistent islet autoantibody after onset of autoimmune DM.

- In conjunction with family history, HLA-typing and measurement of other islet cell autoantibodies, insulin autoantibody measurements are useful in predicting the future development of type 1 DM in asymptomatic children, adolescent, and young adults.
- If IAA, glutamic acid decarboxylase autoantibodies, or insulinoma-2 associated autoantibodies are present in an individual with DM, the diagnosis of type 1 DM has been established.
- **Normal range:** negative

➤ Use
- Differential diagnosis of type 1 versus type 2 DM
- Evaluating diabetics with insulin resistance
- Investigation of hypoglycemia in nondiabetic subjects
- Marker for type 1 DM. In 95% of cases of new onset type 1 DM, ≤1 of 4 is positive. (see Table 2-51)

➤ Limitations
- IAA testing must be performed before insulin therapy is initiated.
- Children at onset of type 1 DM are more commonly IAA positive than adults. Up to 80% of new–onset type 1 DM patients before the age of 5 years have IAA compared with only ~30% for adults.

JANUS KINASE-2 (JAK2) DNA MUTATION ASSAY

➤ Definition
- The *V617F* mutation in the *JAK-2* gene is associated with myeloproliferative disorders (MPDs). This mutation was found in more than 80% (up to 97%) of patients with polycythemia vera, in approximately 50% of patients with idiopathic myelofibrosis (IMF), 30–50% of patients with essential thrombocythemia (ET), and also in other rare MPDs.
- **Normal values:** an individual is negative for the *JAK-2* gene mutation when the frequency of wild type and mutant alleles are 100% and 0%, respectively.

➤ Use
- Suspected polycythemia vera, IMF, or ET

➤ Limitations
- The results of a genetic test may be affected by DNA rearrangements, blood transfusion, bone marrow transplantation, or other rare events.

KLEIHAUER-BETKE TEST

➤ Definition
- The Kleihauer-Betke test was developed to demonstrate fetal RBCs in maternal blood.
- The results are automatically calculated as fetal bleed (mL), which equals the number of fetal cells counted per 1000 maternal RBCs/10^5.
- **Normal range** (adult RBCs): <1% fetal Hg

➤ Interpretation
- The presence of fetal RBCs in maternal blood indicates fetal–maternal hemorrhage.

➤ Limitations
False-Positive Results
- Fetal Hb-containing RBCs may be found in approximately 50% of pregnant women, but in only 1% of pregnancies is the infant anemic.
- Certain hematologic disorders in adults, such as leukemias or myelodysplastic syndromes, may increase the level of fetal-type cells
- Lymphocytes may take up stain in varying degrees.

False-Negative Results
- A major blood group incompatibility between mother and infant because of the elimination of fetal RBCs through hemolysis.

LACTATE DEHYDROGENASE

➤ Definition
- LD occurs in the cytoplasm of all cells; there are five isoenzymes. The highest concentrations are found in heart, liver, skeletal muscle, kidney, and the RBCs, with lesser amounts in lung, smooth muscle, and brain. LD catalyzes the interconversion of lactate and pyruvate.
- **Normal range:** 110–240 IU/L

➤ Use
- To monitor tumor activity involving anemias and lung cancer
- Liver and renal disease
- After acute myocardial infarction (AMI) (The use of LDH for MI detection has been replaced by cardiac troponins.)
- Marker for hemolysis, *in vivo* (e.g., hemolytic anemias) or *in vitro* (artifactual)

➤ Interpretation
Increased In
- **Cardiac diseases**
  - AMI. Increases in 10–12 hours, peaks in 48–72 hours (~3 times normal). Prolonged elevation over 10–14 days was formerly used for late diagnosis of AMI; now replaced by

cTroponins. An LD reading >2000 IU suggests a poorer prognosis. An LD-1/LD-2 ratio >1 ("flipped" LD) may also occur in acute renal infarction, hemolysis, some muscle disorders, pregnancy, and some neoplasms.

* CHF. LD isoenzymes are normal, or LD-5 may be increased due to liver congestion.
* Insertion of intracardiac prosthetic valves consistently causes chronic hemolysis, with increase of total LD, LD-1, and LD-2. This is also often present before surgery in patients with severe hemodynamic abnormalities of cardiac valves.
* Cardiovascular surgery. LD is increased ≤2 times normal without cardiopulmonary bypass and returns to normal in 3–4 days; with extracorporeal circulation, it may increase ≤4–6 times normal; this increase is more marked when the transfused blood is older.
* Increases have been described in acute myocarditis and RF.
* **Liver diseases**
  * Cirrhosis, obstructive jaundice, and acute viral hepatitis show moderate increases.
  * Hepatitis—most marked increase is of LD-5, which occurs during prodromal stage and is greatest at time of onset of jaundice; total LD is also increased in 50% of the cases. LD increase is isomorphic in infectious mononucleosis. An ALT-to-LD or AST-to-LD ratio within 24 hours of admission ≥1.5 favors acute hepatitis over acetaminophen or ischemic injury.
  * Acute and subacute hepatic necrosis. LD-5 is also increased with other causes of liver damage (e.g., chlorpromazine hepatitis, carbon tetrachloride poisoning, exacerbation of cirrhosis, or biliary obstruction) even when total LD is normal.
  * Metastatic carcinoma to the liver may show marked increases. It has been reported that an LD-4-to-LD-5 ratio <1.05 favors diagnosis of hepatocellular carcinoma, compared to a ratio >1.05, which favors liver metastases in >90% of cases.
  * If liver disease is suspected but total LD is very high and isoenzyme pattern is isomorphic, rule out cancer.
  * Liver disease, per se, does not produce marked increase of total LD or LD-5.
  * Various inborn metabolic disorders affecting the liver (e.g., hemochromatosis, Dubin-Johnson syndrome, hepatolenticular degeneration, Gaucher disease, McArdle disease).
* **Hematologic diseases**
  * Untreated PA and folic acid deficiency show some of the greatest increases, chiefly in LD-1, which is >LD-2 ("flipped"), especially with Hb <8 g/dL.
  * Increased in all hemolytic anemias, which can probably be ruled out if LD-1 and LD-2 are not increased in an anemic patient; normal in aplastic anemia and iron deficiency anemia, even when the anemia is very severe.
* **Diseases of lung**
  * Pulmonary embolus and infarction—pattern of moderately increased LD with increased LD-3 and normal AST 24v48 hours after onset of chest pain.
  * Sarcoidosis
* **Malignant tumors**
  * Increased in ~50% of patients with various solid carcinomas, especially in advanced stages.
  * In patients with cancer, a higher LD level generally indicates a poorer prognosis. Whenever the total LD is increased and the isoenzyme pattern is nonspecific or cannot be explained by obvious clinical findings (e.g., MI, hemolytic anemia), cancer should always be ruled out. LD is moderately increased in ~60% of patients with lymphomas

and lymphocytic leukemias and ~90% of patients with acute leukemia; degree of increase is not correlated with WBC counts; levels are relatively low in lymphatic types of leukemia. LD is increased in 95% of patients with chronic myelogenous leukemia, especially LD-3.

- **Diseases of muscle**
  - Marked increase of LD-5, likely due to anoxic injury of striated muscle
  - Electrical and thermal burns and trauma; marked increase of total LD (about the same as in MI) and LD-5
- **Renal diseases**
  - Renal cortical infarction may mimic pattern of AMI. Rule out renal infarction if LD-1 (>LD-2) is increased in the absence of MI or anemia or if increased LD is out of proportion to AST and ALP levels.
  - May be slightly increased (LD-4 and LD-5) in nephrotic syndrome. LD-1 and LD-2 may be increased in nephritis.
- **Miscellaneous conditions**
- These conditions may be related to hemolysis, involvement of liver, striated muscle, or heart,
  - Various infectious and parasitic diseases
  - Hypothyroidism, subacute thyroiditis
  - Collagen vascular diseases
  - Acute pancreatitis
  - Intestinal obstruction
  - Sarcoidosis
  - Various CNS conditions (e.g., bacterial meningitis, cerebral hemorrhage, or thrombosis)
  - Drugs

Decreased In
- Irradiation
- Genetic deficiency of subunits

➤ Limitations
- RBCs contain much more LD than serum. A hemolyzed specimen is not acceptable.
- LD activity is one of the most sensitive indicators of *in vitro* hemolysis. Causes can include transportation via pneumatic tube, vigorous mixing, or traumatic venipuncture.

LACTATE DEHYDROGENASE ISOENZYMES

➤ Definition
- LD is a tetrameric cytoplasmic enzyme. The most usual designation of the isoenzyme is LD-1 (H[4]), LD-2 (H[3]M), LD-3 (H[2]M[2]), LD-4 (HM[3]), and LD-5 (M[4]).
- The tissue specificity is derived from the fact that there is tissue-specific synthesis of subunits in well-defined ratios. Most notably, heart muscle cells preferentially synthesize H subunits, whereas liver cells synthesize M subunits nearly exclusively. Skeletal muscle also synthesizes largely M subunits, so that LD(5) is both a liver and skeletal muscle form of LD. The LD-1 and LD-5 forms are ones most often used to indicate heart or liver pathology, respectively.

TABLE 2-52. Percent Activity Distribution of LD Isoenzymes in Tissue					
	LD Activity				
Organ	LD-1	LD-2	LD-3	LD-4	LD-5
Heart	60	30	5	3	2
Liver	0.2	0.8	1	4	94
Kidney	28	34	21	11	6
Cerebrum	28	32	19	16	5
Skeletal muscle	3	4	8	9	76
Lung	10	18	28	23	21
Spleen	5	15	31	31	18
RBCs	40	30	15	10	5
Skin	0	0	4	17	79

- LD isoenzyme patterns cannot be interpreted without the knowledge of clinical history. See Table 2-52.

➤ Use
- LD is useful in the investigation of a variety of diseases involving the heart, liver, muscle, kidney, lung, and blood; and differentiating heart-synthesized LD from liver and other sources of LD.
- Isoenzymes are used by many clinicians in the diagnosis of MI in combination with total CK and CK-MB.
- Investigating unexplained causes of LD elevations
- Detection of macro-LD

➤ Interpretation
See Table 2-53
- Macroenzymes, high–molecular-weight complexes, occur with LD as well as with CK and other enzymes. LD isoenzymes may complex to IgA or IgG. Such LD macroenzymes are characterized by abnormal position of isoenzyme bands, broadening or abnormal motility of a band, and otherwise unexplained increase of total serum LD. Some of these patients have abnormal ANA results and IgG complexes. Some have abnormalities of light chains but not in amounts that are useful for diagnosis. Treatment with streptokinase was found to produce a LD-streptokinase complex, which was seen as a band at the origin in electrophoresis.
- Increased total LD with normal distribution of isoenzymes may be seen in myocardial infarction, arteriosclerotic heart disease with chronic heart failure, and various combinations of acute and chronic diseases (this may represent a general stress reaction).
- About 50% of patients with malignant tumors have altered LD patterns. This change often is nonspecific and of no diagnostic value. Solid tumors, especially those of germ cell origin, may increase LD-1.
- In megaloblastic anemia, hemolysis, renal cortical infarction, and some patients with cancer, the isoenzyme pattern may mimic that of myocardial infarction, but the time to peak value and the increase help to differentiate these conditions.

TABLE 2-53. LD Isoenzyme Patterns in Various Disease Conditions

Condition	LD Isoenzyme(s) Increased
AMI	LD-1 more so than LD-2
Acute renal cortical infarction	LD-1 more so than LD-2
PA	LD-1
Sickle cell crisis	LD-1 and LD-2
Electrical and thermal burn, trauma	LD-5
Mother carrying erythroblastotic child	LD-4 and v5
AMI with acute congestion of liver	LD-1 and LD-5
Early hepatitis	LD-5 (may become normal, even when ALT is still rising)
Malignant lymphoma	LD-3 and LD-4 (LD-2 may also increase) (reflects effect of chemotherapy)
Active chronic granulocytic leukemia	LD-3 increased in >90% of cases but normal during remission
Carcinoma of prostate	5; 5:1 ratio >1
Dermatomyositis	5
SLE	3 and 4
Collagen disorders	2, 3, and 4
Pulmonary embolus and infarction	2, 3, and 4
Pulmonary embolus with acute cor pulmonale causing acute congestion of liver	3 and 5
Congestive heart failure	2, 3, and 4
Viral infections	2, 3, and 4
Various neoplasms	2, 3, and 4
Strenuous physical activity	4 and 5
Leptomeningeal carcinomatosis	5

- An isoenzyme band cathodal to LD-5 has been called LD-6. It is not an immunoglobulin complex. It has occurred in subjects with liver disease and is said to indicate a grave prognosis.

➤ Limitations

- A hemolyzed specimen is not acceptable as RBCs contain much more LD than serum. Causes can include transportation via pneumatic tube, vigorous mixing, or traumatic venipuncture. Tubes should be void of air bubbles to prevent minor hemolysis.
- LD activity is one of the most sensitive indicators of *in vitro* hemolysis.
- Hemolysis causes anomalous elevation of LD-1 such that any *ex vivo* hemolysis must be strictly avoided.
- Freezing or prolonged storage at 4°C (>12 hours) causes LD-5 to be lost.
- Elevations of intermediate forms (LD-2–LD-4) of LD are rarely used to define a tissue of origin and such reports are largely anecdotal.

- Although increases in serum LD also are seen following an MI, the test has been replaced by the determination of troponins.

LACTATE, BLOOD

➤ Definition
- Blood lactate, also known as 2-hydroxypropanoic acid, lactic acid, or L-Lactate, is an end product of anaerobic glycolysis as an alternative to pyruvate entering the Krebs cycle, enabling metabolism of glucose. Major sites of production are skeletal muscle, brain, and erythrocytes. Lactate is metabolized by the liver.
- **Normal range:** 0.3–2.4 mmol/L
- **Critical value:** >5 mmol/L

➤ Use
- Monitoring of metabolic acidosis, lactic acidosis

➤ Interpretation
Increased In
- Hypoperfusion: CHF, shock
- Decrease oxygen content: hypoxemia, severe anemia, carbon monoxide poisoning.
- Sepsis
- DKA
- Drugs and toxins (e.g., Ringer lactate solution, biguanides, retroviral therapy, isoniazid, acetaminophen, ethanol, ethylene glycol, and others)
- Strenuous exercise
- Seizures
- Liver failure
- Kidney failure
- D-lactate acidosis (due to short bowel syndrome or other forms of malabsorption)
- Inborn errors of metabolism (e.g., pyruvate dehydrogenase deficiency, glycogen storage disease)

➤ Limitations
- No identified limitation.
- Methodologic interference (e.g., ascorbic acid)
- Proper specimen collection and processing techniques are critical for reliable results. Use of tourniquet or clenching hands increases lactate.
- This test does not measure D-lactate, an uncommon, often undiagnosed cause of lactic acidosis.

LEAD (Pb)

➤ Definition
- An element with four stable isotopes (204, 206, 207, 208) found naturally in minerals; in man-made products such as paint, gasoline, cigarette smoke, solder in cans, and ceramics; and as a contaminant in soil and water.
- **Normal range:** <10 µg/dL (<0.48 mmol/L)

➤ Use
- Lead is malleable, ductile, and a poor conductor of electricity; therefore, it is used in building construction, bullets, lead acid batteries, pewter, and radiation shields

➤ Interpretation
- Refer to current local state or federal (CDC) guidelines regarding treatment at specific blood lead concentrations. Note that thresholds for treatment vary for adults, children, and pregnant women.
- See discussion of lead poisoning in Chapter 15.

➤ Limitations
- Whole blood free of clots
- Specimen must be collected using a procedure that minimizes environmental contamination.
- Specimen container must be lead free.
- POC testing devices
  - Electrochemical methodology
  - 1 step sample pretreatment
  - Limit of quantitation: 3–5 µg/dL
  - Results available in <5 minutes
  - Results may agree within +/− 20% ICP-MS
- Laboratory-based instrumentation
  - Atomic absorption
    - Target analyte: nonionized atomic lead
    - Limit of quantitation: 1 µg/dL
  - Anodic stripping
    - Target analyte: oxidized lead
    - Limit of quantitation: 1–2 µg/dL
    - Requires sample pretreatment
  - Inductively coupled plasma mass spectrometry
    - Target analyte: ions at mass/charge ratio of natural isotopes of Pb
    - Limit of quantitation: <1 µg/dL
    - Expensive technology

LECITHIN-TO-SPHINGOMYELIN (L:S) RATIO

➤ Definition
- The L:S ratio is based on the observation that there is outward flow of pulmonary secretions from the lungs into the AF, and this changes the phospholipid composition of AF, thereby enabling indirect assessment of fetal lung maturity.
- The concentrations of L and S in AF are approximately equal until 32–33 weeks of gestation, at which time the concentration of L begins to increase significantly, whereas the S concentration remains about the same.
- The measurement of S serves as a constant comparison for control of the relative increases in L because the volume of amniotic fluid cannot be accurately measured clinically.
- This technique involves TLC after organic solvent extraction. It is a difficult test to perform and interpret. The presence of blood or meconium can interfere with test interpretation.

TABLE 2-54. Values of L:S Ratio and Lung Maturity

L:S Ratio	(Values in Some Laboratories)	Lung Maturity
<1	<2.0	Very immature lungs (up to 30th week of gestation); severe RDS is expected; lung maturity may require many weeks; do not resample before 2 weeks.
1.0–1.49		Immature lungs; moderate to severe RDS is expected; lung maturity may occur in 2 weeks; resample in 1 week.
1.5–1.9	2.0–3.0	Lungs on threshold of maturity (within 14 days); mild to moderate RDS may occur. Test should be repeated in 1 week.
≥2	>3.0	Mature lungs (35th week of gestation); low incidence of RDS even if phosphatidylglycerol is absent. S/S = 80–85%.
Abundant lecithin with trace or no sphingomyelin		Postmature lungs

- Empirically, the risk of respiratory distress syndrome (RDS) is exceedingly low when the L:S ratio is greater than 2.0.
- **Normal range:** see Table 2-54

➤ **Use**
- Traditional biochemical test to measure fetal lung maturity

➤ **Interpretation**
- Increased in mature fetal lungs (see Limitations and Table 2-54 for high ratios)
- Decreased in immature fetal lungs

➤ **Limitations**
- Labor intensive test offered by few laboratories
- Offers no advantage over fluorescence polarization
- Sensitivity of >95%, specificity of 70%
- Blood and meconium contamination can affect result
- Definite exceptions to prediction of pulmonary maturity with L:S ratio >2.0
  - Infant of diabetic mother (L:S ratio >2.0 has been frequently seen in cases in which RDS developed)
  - Erythroblastosis fetalis
- Possible exceptions
  - Intrauterine growth retardation
  - Toxemia of pregnancy
  - Hydrops fetalis
  - Placental disease
  - Abruptio placentae
  - Foam (shake) test

LEPTIN

➤ Definition
- Serum leptin level is associated with appetite and energy expenditure in healthy individuals. Leptin is produced primarily in fat cells, and also in the placenta and probably in the stomach. Serum leptin concentrations are highly correlated with body fat content. These processes are stimulated by insulin, glucocorticoids, and tumor necrosis factor-alpha, another product of adipocytes. These observations suggest that leptin signals the brain about the quantity of stored fat.
- **Normal range:**
  - Male: 0.5–12.7 ng/mL
  - Female: 3.9–30.0 ng/mL

➤ Use
- Biomarker for body fat metabolism

➤ Interpretation
Increased In
- Obesity
- Pregnant women

Decreased In
- Fasting
- Very low calorie diet

➤ Limitations
- Serum leptin concentrations increase with progressive obesity. The concentrations are higher in women than in men, for any measure of obesity, and they decrease with age in both women and men.
- Pregnant women have higher serum leptin concentrations than nonpregnant women.
- Serum leptin concentrations increase during childhood, with the highest concentrations in children who gain the most weight; higher serum leptin concentrations are associated with an earlier onset of puberty.
- The concentrations are similar in normal subjects and patients of the same weight with type 2 DM.
- There is a diurnal rhythm of serum leptin concentrations, the values being 20–40% higher in the middle of the night as compared with daytime. The peak shifts in parallel with shifts in the timing of meals.
- Leptin production is strongly influenced by nutritional state. Overeating increases serum leptin concentrations by nearly 40% within 12 hours, long before any changes in body fat stores. Conversely, in both normal-weight and obese subjects, fasting reduces serum leptin concentrations by 60–70% in 48 hours.

LEUCINE AMINO PEPTIDASE (LAP)

➤ Definition
- LAP is a proteolytic enzyme widely distributed in bacteria, plants, and animals with high activity in the duodenum, kidney, and liver.
- **Normal range:** 1.0–3.3 U/mL

➤ Use

- As a marker of hepatic and pancreatic carcinoma
- As a marker of early tubular (renal) injury in diabetes and as an indicator of SLE activity
- Parallels serum ALP except that:
  - LAP is usually normal in the presence of bone disease or malabsorption syndrome.
  - LAP is a more sensitive indicator of choledocholithiasis and of liver metastases in anicteric patients.
- When serum LAP is increased, urine LAP is almost always increased, but when urine LAP is increased, serum LAP may have already returned to normal.

➤ Interpretation
Increased In

- Obstructive, space-occupying, or infiltrative lesions of the liver
- SLE, in correlation with disease activity
- Various neoplasms (even without liver metastases) (e.g., breast, endometrium, and germ cell tumors)
- Preeclampsia, between 33 and 39 weeks of pregnancy

➤ Limitations

- Testing serum LAP is generally not as sensitive or as convenient as testing other liver enzymes to detect some liver problems. ALT, AST, ALP, LDH, and GGT are more commonly measured for the same purpose. Unlike other liver enzymes, LAP can be measured in the urine.
- Elevated LAP activity in serum usually indicates diseases of liver and bile ducts, and this elevation is less affected by damage of liver parenchyma than by active participation of biliary tract in the process.

LEUKOCYTE ALKALINE PHOSPHATASE (LAP)

➤ Definition

- LAP, or neutrophil alkaline phosphatase, refers to a staining reaction of peripheral blood smears. It reflects the presence of LAP in neutrophils and their precursors.
- Normally, about 20% of mature neutrophils show stainable leukocyte LAP activity.
- **Normal range:** score of 11–95. The scoring is based on counting 100 neutrophils and grading the stained granules from 0–4 on the basis of the intensity and appearance of the precipitated dye in the cytoplasm.

➤ Use

- LAP stain helps differentiate a severe neutrophilia (leukemoid reaction) and myeloproliferative neoplasms, where it is increased, from chronic myeloid leukemia, in which case it is decreased or absent.
- With the advent of modern diagnostic technology in hematology, the use of LAP stains has diminished greatly.

➤ Interpretation
Increased In

- Leukemoid reaction
- Polycythemia vera and essential thrombocythemia (may be normal) (see p. 839 and 841)

- Idiopathic myelofibrosis (see p. 841)
- Pregnancy
- Trisomy 21 (see p. 922)
- Klinefelter syndrome

Decreased In
- Chronic myeloid leukemia (see p. 837)
- PNH (see p. 810)
- PA
- Congenital hypophosphatasia

➤ Limitations
- Old blood may cause low LAP scores.
- There is observer-dependent variability.

LIPASE

➤ Definition
- Glycoprotein enzyme filtered by glomeruli and completely reabsorbed by proximal tubules; method should always include colipase in reagent.
- **Normal range:** 0–50 U/L

➤ Use
- Investigating pancreatic disorders, usually pancreatitis
- More specific for pancreatitis than is serum amylase; diagnosis of peritonitis, strangulated or infarcted bowel, pancreatic cyst

➤ Interpretation
Increased In
- Acute pancreatitis
- Perforated or penetrating peptic ulcer, especially with involvement of pancreas
- Obstruction of pancreatic duct by:
  - Stone
  - Drug-induced spasm of sphincter of Oddi (e.g., codeine, morphine, meperidine, methacholine, cholinergics) to levels 2–15 times normal
  - Partial obstruction plus drug stimulation
- Chronic pancreatitis
- Acute cholecystitis
- Small bowel obstruction
- Intestinal infarction
- Acute and chronic renal failure (increased 2–3 times in 80% of patients and 5 times in 5% of patients)
- Organ transplant (kidney, liver, heart), especially with complications (e.g., organ rejection, CMV infection, cyclosporin toxicity)
- Alcoholism
- DKA
- After ERCP

* Some cases of intracranial bleeding (unknown mechanism)
* Macro forms in lymphoma, cirrhosis
* Drugs
  * Induced acute pancreatitis (see preceding section on serum amylase)
  * Cholestatic effect (e.g., indomethacin)
  * Methodologic interference (e.g., pancreozymin [contains lipase], deoxycholate, glyco-cholate, taurocholate [prevent inactivation of enzyme], bilirubin [turbidimetric methods])
* Chronic liver disease (e.g., cirrhosis) (usually ≤2 times normal)

Decreased In
* Methodologic interference (e.g., presence of Hb, quinine, heavy metals, calcium ions)

Normal In
* Mumps
* Macroamylasemia
* Lower value in neonates

➤ Limitations
* Certain drugs such as cholinergics and opiates may elevate serum lipase.
* Renal disease may elevate the serum lipase.

LIPOPROTEIN-ASSOCIATED PHOSPHOLIPASE A2 (Lp-PLA2)

➤ Definition
* Lipoprotein-associated phospholipase A2 (Lp-PLA2) is a 45-kDa protein enzyme produced by inflammatory cells and activated endothelial cells. It travels in the blood mainly with LDLs.
* Lp-PLA2 hydrolyzes oxidized phospholipids in LDLs, resulting in formation of oxidized free fatty acids and lysophosphatidylcholine, which is proatherogenic.
* Alternate name is platelet-activating factor acetylhydrolase (PAF-AH)

➤ Use
* Lp-PLA2 is considered a risk marker rather than a risk factor for cardiac heart disease.
  * Increased Lp-PLA2 with low LDL-C increases risk of heart disease 2 times.
  * Increased Lp-PLA2 with high CRP increases risk of heart disease 3 times.

➤ Interpretation
* Concentrations ≥235 ng/mL are associated with increased risk of cardiovascular events, including myocardial infarction and ischemic stroke.
* Elevated Lp-PLA2 has been found to be associated with ischemic stroke and may be useful in risk assessment.

➤ Limitations
* Smoking increases Lp-PLA2 measurements.

➤ Suggested Readings
Corson MA, Jones PH, Davidson MH. Review of the evidence for the clinical utility of lipoprotein-associated phospholipase A2 as a cardiovascular risk marker. *Am J Cardiol.* 2008;101(12A):41F–50F.

Davidson MH, Corson MA, Alberts MJ, et al. Consensus panel recommendation for incorporating lipoprotein-associated phospholipase A2 testing into cardiovascular disease risk assessment guidelines. *Am J Cardiol.* 2008;101(12A):51F–57F.

Nambi V, Hoogeveen RC, Chambless L, et al. Lipoprotein-associated phospholipase A2 and high-sensitivity c-reactive protein improve the stratification of ischemic stroke risk in the atherosclerosis risk in communities (ARIC) study. *Stroke.* 2009;40:376. Tselepis AD, Panagiotakos DB, Pitsavos C, et al. Smoking induces lipoprotein-associated phospholipase A2 in cardiovascular disease free adults: The ATTICA study. *Atherosclerosis.* 2009;206(1):303–308.

LUPUS ANTICOAGULANT (LA)*

► Definition
- LAs are heterogeneous IgG or IgM autoantibodies that inhibit phospholipid-dependent assays of blood coagulation.
- Because phospholipid is essential for several steps in the coagulation cascade, the presence of LAs can prolong various phospholipid-dependent clotting times, such as PTT, PT, and the dilute Russell viper venom time (dRVVT, see p. 159).

► Use
- None of the tests mentioned in the Definition discussion is sufficiently sensitive to detect all LAs; therefore, *two screening tests* are required before LA can be excluded.
- The most commonly used screening tests are PT (1:100 diluted) and dRVVT. (Kaolin or micronized silica clotting time are no longer in use). A positive screening test (prolonged dilute PT or dRVVT) requires confirmation by adding excess phospholipids in the test.

► Interpretation
- A normalization of the clotting time in either test confirms the presence of LA but requires that the tests be repeated in 12 weeks, because frequently the LA is a temporary phenomenon (Figure 2-1).

► Limitations
- There is considerable interlaboratory variation with the performance of the LA assays, especially dRVVT. In recent surveys, there was a false-positive detection of LAs in 24% of samples, and a false-negative result of 18.5% in participating centers.
  - One of the factors that may contribute to a false-positive result is contamination with heparin.
  - Preanalytical variables, such as improper plasma preparation, may lead to false-negative results because of contamination with platelets.
- It is recommended that assessment for LA not be undertaken while the patient is on oral anticoagulants, if at all possible (see Figure 2-1).

► Suggested Readings
Giannakopoulos B, Passam F, Ioannou Y, Krilis SA. How we diagnose the antiphospholipid antibody syndrome. *Blood.* 2009;113:985–994.

Moffat KA, Ledford-Kraemer MR, Plumhoff EA, et al. Are laboratories following published recommendations for lupus anticoagulant testing? *Thromb Haemost.* 2009;101:178–184.

---

*Prepared with the help of Guilin Tang, M.D., and Diane Connor, M.T.

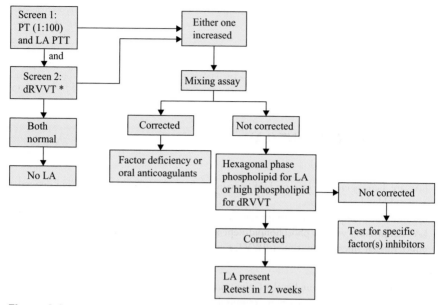

Figure 2-1. Algorithm for testing lupus anticoagulant antibodies.

LUTEINIZING HORMONE (LH)

See Follicular-Stimulating Hormone (FSH) and Luteinizing Hormone (LH), Serum

MAGNESIUM (Mg)

➤ Definition

- Mg is primarily an intracellular ion associated with GI absorption and renal excretion. At least 65–70% of Mg is in ionized state and ~35% serum Mg is protein bound.
- **Normal range:** 1.6–2.4 mg/dL
- **Critical values:** <1.0 and >4.9 mg/dL

➤ Use

- Diagnosis and monitoring of hypomagnesemia and hypermagnesemia, especially in renal failure or GI disorders
- To monitor preeclampsia patients being treated with magnesium sulfate, although in most cases monitoring clinical signs (respiratory rate and deep tendon reflexes) is adequate, and blood magnesium levels are not required

➤ Interpretation
Increased In

- Iatrogenic (is usual cause; most often with impaired renal function).
  - Diuretics (e.g., furosemide >80 mg/day, thiazides)

- Antacids or enemas containing Mg
- Laxative and cathartic abuse
- Parenteral nutrition
- Mg for eclampsia or premature labor
- Lithium carbonate intoxication
- Renal failure (when GFR approaches 30 mL/min); in chronic renal failure, hypermagnesemia is inversely related to residual renal function. Increase is rarely observed with normal renal function.
- Dehydration with diabetic coma before treatment
- Hypothyroidism
- Addison disease and after adrenalectomy
- Controlled DM in older patients
- Accidental ingestion of large amount of sea water

Decreased In

- Almost always GI or renal disturbance; chronic Mg deficiency produces hypocalcemia secondary to decreased production and effectiveness of PTH.
  - GI disease
    - Malabsorption (e.g., sprue, small bowel resection, biliary and intestinal fistulas, abdominal irradiation, celiac disease and other causes of steatorrhea; familial Mg malabsorption)
    - Abnormal loss of GI fluids (chronic ulcerative colitis, Crohn disease, villous adenoma, carcinoma of colon, laxative abuse, prolonged aspiration of GI tract contents, vomiting)
  - Renal disease: a level >2 mEq/day in urine during hypomagnesemia indicates excessive renal loss.
    - Chronic GN
    - Chronic pyelonephritis
    - Renal tubular acidosis
    - Diuretic phase of acute tubular necrosis
    - Postobstructive diuresis
    - Drug injury
- Diuretics (e.g., mercurials, ammonium chloride, thiazides, furosemide)
- Antibiotics (e.g., aminoglycosides, gentamicin, tobramycin, carbenicillin, ticarcillin, amphotericin B)
- Digitalis (in 20% of patients taking digitalis)
- Antineoplastic (e.g., cisplatin)
- Cyclosporine: tubular losses due to ions or nutrients
- Hypercalcemia
- Diuresis caused by glucose, urea, or mannitol
- Phosphate depletion
- Extracellular fluid volume expansion
- Primary renal Mg wasting
- Nutritional
  - Prolonged parenteral fluid administration without Mg (usually >3 weeks)
  - Acute and chronic alcoholism and alcoholic cirrhosis
  - Starvation with metabolic acidosis
  - Kwashiorkor, protein-calorie malnutrition

- Endocrine
  - Hyperthyroidism
  - Aldosteronism (primary and secondary)
  - Hyperparathyroidism and other causes of hypercalcemia
  - Hypoparathyroidism
  - DM (in ≤39% of patients; caused by osmotic diuresis)
- Metabolic
  - Excessive lactation
  - Third trimester of pregnancy
  - Insulin treatment of diabetic coma
- Other
  - Toxemia of pregnancy or eclampsia
  - Lytic tumors of bone
  - Active Paget disease of bone; caused by increased uptake by bone
  - Acute pancreatitis
  - Transfusion of citrated blood
  - Severe burns
  - Sweating
  - Sepsis
  - Hypothermia
- Mg deficiency frequently coexists with other electrolyte abnormalities; it may cause apparently unexplained hypocalcemia and hypokalemia and should always be measured in such cases. About 40% of patients have coexisting hypokalemia.
- About 90% of patients with high or low serum Mg levels are not clinically recognized; therefore, routine inclusion of Mg with electrolyte measurements has been suggested.
- Digitalis sensitivity and toxicity frequently occur with hypomagnesemia.
- Ionized Mg is decreased in only ~70% of critically ill patients with decreased total Mg.
- Because deficiency can exist with normal or borderline serum Mg levels, a 24-hour urine test may be indicated by frequent concomitant disorders (see previous).
- A 24-hour urine level <25 mg suggests Mg deficiency (in the absence of conditions or agents that promote magnesium excretion). If caused by renal loss, urine Mg should be >3.65 to 6 mg/day.
- If level is <2.4 mg/day, collect 24-hour urine sample during IV administration of 72 mg of MgCl. Some 60–80% of the load is excreted by patients with normal Mg stores; <50% excretion suggests nonrenal Mg depletion.

➤ Limitations

- Serum magnesium levels may remain normal even when total body stores of magnesium are depleted up to 20%.
- Phylate, fatty acids, and an excess of phosphate impair Mg absorption
- Hemolysis yields elevated results because levels in erythrocytes are 2–3 times higher than serum.

➤ Suggested Reading

Lum G. Clinical utility of magnesium measurement. *Lab Med.* 2004;35:106.

MAGNESIUM, URINE

➤ Definition

- Magnesium is an important but commonly neglected electrolyte. Magnesium deficiency is often inadequately documented by serum magnesium levels. Urinary magnesium analyses have been advocated before and after therapeutic magnesium administration to further investigate the significance of apparent low serum magnesium.
- Abnormal levels of magnesium are most frequently seen in conditions or diseases that cause impaired or excessive excretion of magnesium by the kidneys or that cause impaired absorption in the intestines. Magnesium levels may be checked as part of an evaluation of the severity of kidney problems and/or of uncontrolled diabetes and may help in the diagnosis of GI disorders. Renal magnesium wasting occurs in renal transplant recipients who are on cyclosporine and prednisone. Renal conservation of magnesium is diminished by hypercalciuria, salt-losing conditions, and the SIADH.
- **Normal range:**
  - 24 hour urine: 72–120 mg/day
  - Random urine:
    - Male: 18–110 mg/g creatinine
    - Female: 14–139 mg/g creatinine

➤ Use

- Investigate chronic pancreas inflammation
- Decreased blood magnesium

➤ Interpretation
Increased In

- Alcohol
- Diuretics
- Bartter syndrome
- Corticosteroids
- Cisplatin therapy
- Aldosterone

Decreased In

- Insufficient magnesium intake
- Extra renal loss

➤ Limitations

- Magnesium forms insoluble complexes with normal urine constituents that precipitate as soon as urine is passed. Acidification is not required.
- Urine concentration is diet dependent.
- Magnesium depletion could be common condition found in 26% of hospitalized patients.
- High concentrations of gadolinium are known to interfere with most metals tests.

MEAN CORPUSCULAR HEMOGLOBIN (MCH)

➤ Definition and Use
* MCH is the Hb concentration per RBC count.
* It has limited value in classifying anemias.
* **Normal range:** 27–34 pg per red cell

➤ Interpretation
Increased In
* Macrocytic anemias and infants as well as newborns

Decreased In
* Microcytic and normocytic anemias

MEAN CORPUSCULAR HEMOGLOBIN CONCENTRATION (MCHC)

➤ Definition and Use
* MCHC is the Hct divided by Hb
* It has limited value in classifying anemias, although it may identify hypochromasia better than MCH.
* **Normal range:** 31.5–36 g

➤ Interpretation
Decreased In
* Microcytic and normocytic anemias.

Increased In
* Macrocytic anemias and hereditary spherocytosis (see p. 807)
* Infants and newborns

MEAN CORPUSCULAR VOLUME (MCV)

➤ Definition
* MCV represents the average measurement of RBC volume. It is measured directly by automated instruments but calculated as Hct divided by RBC count with manual methods.
* **Normal range:** 82.0–101.0 fL

➤ Use
* MCV is helpful in the classification of anemias.

➤ Interpretation
Increased In
* Macrocytic anemias (see p. 791)
* Myelodysplastic syndromes (see p. 843)
* Alcoholism
* Liver disease

* Hypothyroidism
* Hemolysis with high reticulocyte count
* Infants and newborns

Decreased In
* Iron deficiency anemias
* Thalassemias (see p. 801)
* Hereditary sideroblastic anemia
* Lead poisoning
* Anemia of chronic disease (see p. 793) and other hemoglobinopathies (may be decreased or normal)

➤ Limitations
* MCV may be artificially increased with marked leukocytosis, numerous large platelets, cold agglutinins, methanol poisoning, marked hyperglycemia, and marked reticulocytosis.
* MCV may be falsely decreased with *in vitro* hemolysis or fragmentation of RBCs.

MEAN PLATELET VOLUME (MPV)

➤ Definition
* MPV reflects the frequency distribution of platelet volumes.
* **Normal range:** 7.8–11.0 fL

➤ Use
* MPV is used to evaluate variations in platelet size as related to various platelet abnormalities.

➤ Interpretation
Increased In
* Hypothyroidism
* Myeloproliferative neoplasms
* All cases of accelerated bone marrow production of platelets (immune thrombocytopenias, postchemotherapy)
* Bernard-Soulier syndrome

Decreased In
* Disorders associated with decreased platelet production
* In some patients with sepsis
* In some patients with inherited thrombocytopenias, such as Wiskott-Aldrich syndrome

➤ Limitations
* Reference values appear to vary with the platelet count. MPV is affected by numerous variables related to specimen collection, anticoagulant, temperature, and duration of storage.

METANEPHRINES, URINE

➤ Definition
* Metanephrine and normetanephrine are metabolic products of epinephrine and norepinephrine, the adrenal medullary hormones secreted by pheochromocytomas.

TABLE 2-55. Normal Range for Urine Metanephrines	
Age	Reference Interval (μg/g creatinine)
Metanephrine	
0–3 months	0–700
4–6 months	0–650
7–11 months	0–650
1 year	0–530
2–5 years	0–500
6–17 years	0–320
≧18 years	0–300
Normetanephrine	
0–3 months	0–3400
4–6 months	0–2200
7–11 months	0–1100
1 year	0–1300
2–5 years	0–610
6–17 years	0–450
≧18 years	0–400

* Fractionated tests provide higher diagnostic sensitivity than assays for total catecholamines.
* **Normal range:** see Table 2-55

➤ Use

* Confirmation of elevated plasma catecholamine levels
* Diagnosis of pheochromocytoma and paraganglioma
* Diagnosis and follow-up of patients with neuroblastoma and related tumors

➤ Interpretation

* Increases occur with catecholamine-secreting neurochromatin tumors such as pheochromocytoma, paraganglioma, and neuroblastoma

➤ Limitations

* No caffeine intake should occur before or during collection. MAO inhibitors should be discontinued at least one week prior to beginning collection.
* Methylglucamine in x-ray contrast medium can cause false-negative test results.
* False-positives can be caused by stress and drugs, which includes amphetamines and amphetamine-like compounds, appetite suppressants, bromocriptine, buspirone, caffeine, carbidopa-levodopa (Sinemet), clonidine, dexamethasone, diuretics, methyldopa (Aldomet), nose drops, propafenone (Rythmol), tricyclic antidepressants, and vasodilators. The effects of some drugs on catecholamine metabolite results may not be predictable.

METHOTREXATE

➤ Definition

* Folic acid antagonist
* Other names: Folex®, Mexate®, Trexall®

* **Normal range:** TDM generally performed to ensure plasma/serum concentration <1 micromol/L at 48 hours postinfusion and <0.1 micromol/L at 72 hours postdose

➤ Use
* Methotrexate is an antineoplastic drug used solely or in combination with other antineoplastic drugs for the treatment of leukemia and other diseases.
* Severe psoriasis, sarcoidosis, and granulomatosis have been treated with methotrexate in relatively low doses.
* High-dose methotrexate (greater than approximately 20 mg/kg body weight) with citrovorum-factor rescue have been used with favorable results in the treatment of osteogenic sarcoma, leukemia, non-Hodgkin lymphoma, lung cancer, carcinoma of the head and neck, and breast cancer.
* The efficacy of methotrexate in the treatment of other tumors such as prostate cancer is being investigated.

➤ Interpretation
* Potential toxicity: reported therapeutic and toxic ranges are dependent on dose and the time the sample is drawn post dose. Consult protocol to assess toxicity.
  * 24 hours: >10 micromol/L
  * 48 hours: >1.0 micromol/L
  * 72 hours: >0.1 micromol/L
* Refer to the manufacturer's cross-reactivity data found in the product insert for approximate concentrations of individual drugs that will give positive results against the chosen cut-off concentration. Other substances not listed in the manufacturer's package insert may produce a positive response.
* Methotrexate levels may be falsely elevated in patients receiving carboxypeptidase G2 therapy due to cross-reactivity with methotrexate metabolites.

➤ Limitations
* Immunoassay based tests (EMIT, FPIA) for serum/plasma
* Serum must be collected in tubes without serum separator gel
* Cells must be separated as soon as possible after collection
* Heparinized, EDTA, and fluoridated collection tubes for plasma are acceptable
* This assay measures the total (protein bound and free) levels of methotrexate in serum and plasma.
* It is known that aminopterin and APA (a metabolite of methotrexate) cross-react significantly with the EMIT assay and less so with the FPIA.
* Patients should be re-baselined when changing methodology.
* Samples are stable for up to 24 hours when refrigerated and protected from light.

METHYLMALONIC ACID

➤ Definition
* Methylmalonic acid (MMA) is an intermediate in the propionate degradation pathway. Deficient activity of the enzyme responsible for the conversion of methylmalonyl CoA to succinyl CoA (methylmalonyl CoA mutase) results in the organic aciduria known as methylmalonic aciduria, with a classical presentation of neonatal-onset metabolic acidosis, hyperammonemia, and poor outcome if untreated.

- The concentrations of the metabolic markers MMA and homocysteine (Hcy) are considered to be more sensitive indicators of vitamin B_{12} status. Both MMA and Hcy increase in vitamin B_{12} deficiency. However, Hcy has been shown to have low specificity, being influenced by lifestyle factors such as smoking and alcohol intake and increasing in patients with folate deficiency and renal impairment.
- **Normal range:** 0.00–0.40 μmol/L

➤ Use
- Evaluation of methylmalonic academia in children
- Evaluation of megaloblastic anemia (cobalamin deficiency). Serum MMA may be a more reliable marker of cobalamin deficiency than direct cobalamin determination.

➤ Interpretation
Increased In
- Vitamin B_{12} deficiency
- Pregnancy
- Cobalamin genetic defects
- Methylmalonic acidemia

➤ Limitations
- MMA, while considered a more sensitive indicator of vitamin B_{12} status, is an expensive assay requiring specialized instrumentation not readily available in most clinical laboratories.
- Diet, nutritional status, and age should be considered in the evaluation of serum MMA level.

METYRAPONE TEST

➤ Definition
- The metyrapone stimulation test is based on the principle that decreasing serum cortisol concentrations is expected to produce an increase in ACTH secretion.

➤ Use
- The utilization of the metyrapone test has become less frequent as a result of the larger availability of plasma ACTH assays. The limited accessibility to metyrapone in certain countries, as well as the limited number of clinical laboratories who have maintained the urinary 17-hydroxycorticosteroid (17-OHCS) and serum 11-deoxycortisol tests, have also further limited the use of the metyrapone test.
- Metyrapone blocks the conversion of 11-deoxycortisol to cortisol by CYP11B1 (11-beta-hydroxylase, P-450c11), the last step in the synthesis of cortisol. It induces a rapid fall of cortisol and an increase of 11-deoxycortisol in serum.
- The metyrapone test can be performed as an overnight single-dose test or as a 2- or 3-day test. It cannot be performed in a patient who is taking any glucocorticoid.
  - The 2-day test is used primarily in the differential diagnosis of hypercortisolism.
    - The 2-day test is a slight variation on the standard 3-day test: 24-hour urine and 8 a.m. blood specimens are collected during and at the end of a baseline day and during and at

the end of the day during which the patient takes 750 mg of metyrapone by mouth every 4 hours for six doses.

* Urinary 17-OHCS excretion and serum 11-deoxycortisol are measured.
* The 3-day test is used mainly for the evaluation of adrenal insufficiency.
  * The 3-day test is begun by obtaining a baseline 24-hour urine collection. Immediately after completing this collection, the patient begins taking metyrapone (750 mg orally every 4 hours for six doses) with a glass of milk or a small snack to minimize gastrointestinal symptoms.
  * Subsequent 24-hour urine specimens are collected the day of and the day after metyrapone administration for measurement of urinary 17-OHCS and creatinine excretion. Serum 11-deoxycortisol, cortisol, and plasma ACTH can also be measured 4 hours after the last dose of metyrapone.
* The single-dose overnight test can be used for both indications
  * The single-dose test is performed by oral administration of metyrapone (30 mg/kg body weight, or 2 g for <70 kg, 2.5 grams for 70–90 kg, and 3 g for >90 kg body weight) at midnight with a glass of milk or a small snack.
  * Serum 11-deoxycortisol and cortisol are measured between 7:30 and 9:30 a.m. the next morning; plasma ACTH can also be measured.

➤ Interpretation
Standard Three-day Metyrapone Test

* The increase in serum 11-deoxycortisol is used as a criterion of response as in the single-dose overnight test. Measuring serum cortisol and plasma ACTH is important, as a fall in serum cortisol confirms the metyrapone-induced biosynthetic blockade, and an increase in plasma ACTH confirms that the changes in steroid levels are ACTH dependent.
* A normal response is a two- to threefold increase above the baseline 24-hour urinary 17-OHCS excretion on either the day of or, more often, the day after metyrapone administration. The serum cortisol concentration should decrease to <5 µg/dL. The plasma ACTH concentration should exceed 75 pg/mL, with a mean of about 200 pg/mL 4 hours after the last metyrapone dose. An increase in serum 11-deoxycortisol to 7–22 µg/dL or more at 8 a.m., 4 hours after the last dose of metyrapone.

Two-day Metyrapone Test

* A normal response to the 2-day test has not been defined. In the differential diagnosis of ACTH-dependent Cushing syndrome, however, a clear rise in plasma ACTH concentration indicates that the ACTH-secreting tumor responds to falling serum cortisol concentrations. In one large study, as an example, a positive response was defined as a >70% increase in urinary 17-OHCS excretion and/or more than a fourfold increase in serum 11-deoxycortisol concentrations.

Overnight Single-dose Metyrapone Test

* A normal response is 8 a.m. serum 11-deoxycortisol concentration of 7–22 µg/dL. A serum cortisol concentration at 8 a.m. of <5 µg/dL confirms adequate metyrapone blockade and thereby documents compliance and normal metabolism of metyrapone. Serum 11-deoxycortisol concentrations <7 µg/dL with concomitantly suppressed cortisol values indicate adrenal insufficiency.
* The ACTH response to metyrapone can distinguish between primary and secondary insufficiency. In general, patients with secondary adrenal insufficiency have ACTH responses from

10–200 pg/mL, whereas patients with primary adrenal insufficiency have higher responses. However, healthy individuals have an ACTH response of 42–690 pg/mL. Because of this overlap, the ACTH response alone cannot be used to distinguish between healthy individuals and those with adrenal insufficiency.

➤ **Limitations**

• Adrenal tumor with excess cortisol production: no increase or fall in urinary 17-KS. The test is positive in 100% of patients with adrenal hyperplasias without tumor, 50% of those with adrenal adenomas, and 25% of those with adrenal carcinomas.

• Ectopic ACTH syndrome: it may not be accurate in this condition.

• Metyrapone administration may result in hypotension, nausea, and vomiting in patients with adrenal insufficiency; as a result, the 2- and 3-day tests should not be performed outside of the hospital in patients suspected of having this disorder.

• Acute or chronic ingestion of synthetic glucocorticoids can result in a subnormal response as a result of suppression of the corticotropes.

• One of the more common causes of a false-positive result is unusually rapid clearance of metyrapone from the plasma, resulting in inadequate blockade of cortisol biosynthesis. This is manifested by a serum cortisol concentration >7.5 μg/dL in the sample drawn at 8 a.m. in the overnight test, by a serum cortisol concentration >5 μg/dL 4 hours after the last dose of metyrapone, or by urinary cortisol excretion >20 μg per 24 hours the day metyrapone was administered in the standard 2-day test.

MICROALBUMIN, URINE

➤ **Definition**

• The urine dipstick is a relatively insensitive marker for proteinuria, not becoming positive until protein excretion exceeds 300–500 mg/day. The normal rate of albumin excretion is <20 mg/day (15 μg/min); persistent albumin excretion between 30 and 300 mg/day (20 and 200 μg/min) is called microalbuminuria. Albumin excretion >300 mg/day (200 μg/min) is considered to represent overt or dipstick positive proteinuria (also called macroalbuminuria).

• In type 1 and 2 DM, the presence of microalbuminuria on repeat specimens collected in the basal state may signify early diabetic nephropathy. It is a marker, in patients with or without diabetes, for cardiovascular mortality. For a definition of microalbuminuria, see Table 2-56.

TABLE 2-56. American Diabetes Association Definition of Microalbuminuria

Category	24-Hour Collection	Timed Collection	Spot Collection
Normal	<30 mg/24 hours	<20 μg/min	<30 μg/mg creatinine
Microalbuminuria	30–300 mg/24 hours	20–200 μg/min	30–300 μg/mg creatinine
Clinical albuminuria	>300 mg/24 hours	>200 μg/min	>300 μg/mg creatinine

- Measurement of the urine albumin-to-creatinine ratio in an untimed urinary sample is the preferred screening strategy for microalbuminuria. This test has several advantages: it does not require early morning or timed collections, it gives a quantitative result that correlates with the 24-hour urine values over a wide range of protein excretion, it is simple to perform and inexpensive, and repeat values can be easily obtained to ascertain that microalbuminuria, if present, is persistent.
- Other name: albumin/creatinine ratio
- **Normal range:**
  - Albumin/creatinine ratio (random urine): <30.0 μg/mg creatinine
  - Microalbumin excretion (24 hour urine): 0–29.9 mg/day

➤ Use
- Diagnosis of kidney dysfunction
- Recommended by the American Diabetes Association to screen for microalbuminuria.
- Medications that act on renin-angiotensin system may delay onset of renal and cardiovascular disease, making screening for microalbumin is important in the care of diabetic patients.

➤ Interpretation
- Increased excretion of albumin (microalbuminuria) is a predictor of future development of clinical renal disease in patients with hypertension or DM.

➤ Limitations
- Microalbuminuria may be seen transiently during pregnancy, after exercise, and with protein loading, hyperglycemia, fever, and urinary tract infections. There is also day-to-day, as well as diurnal, variation in albumin excretion. Hence, it is important to base treatment on the results of several tests.
- Vigorous exercise can cause a transient increase in albumin excretion. Patients should refrain from vigorous exercise in the 24 hours prior to the test.
- The optimal time to measure the urine albumin-to-creatinine ratio is not clearly defined. The first-morning void specimen is preferred.
- The accuracy of the urine albumin-to-creatinine ratio will be diminished if creatinine excretion is substantially different from the expected value; this is particularly important in patients with borderline values. Albumin excretion will be underestimated in a muscular man with a high rate of creatinine excretion and overestimated in a cachectic patient in whom muscle mass and creatinine excretion are markedly reduced.

➤ Suggested Reading
American Diabetes Association. Standards of medical care in diabetes. *Diabetes Care*. 2004;27(suppl 1):S79.

MÜLLERIAN-INHIBITING SUBSTANCE

➤ Definition
- The primary function of Müllerian-inhibiting substance (MIS) is to initiate regression of müllerian structures in males as a part of normal sexual development. Secreted by the Sertoli cells of testes during embryogenesis of the male fetus. It is also expressed by granulose cells of ovary during reproductive years and controls the primary follicles by inhibiting the excessive follicular development by FSH.

TABLE 2-57. Normal Ranges for Müllerian-Inhibiting Substance

Age	Range (ng/mL)
Male	
0–13 days	15.5–48.7
14 days to 11 months	39.1–91.1
12 months to 6 years	48.0–83.2
7–8 years	33.8–60.2
9 years to Adult	3.0–5.4
Female	
0–8 years	0.0–7.1
9 years to Adult	0.0–6.9

* Other names: anti-Müllerian hormone, müllerian inhibiting hormone
* **Normal range:** see Table 2-57

➤ Use
* Specific and sensitive marker for the presence of testicular tissue in boys with cryptorchidism.
* When measured either alone or in tandem with measurement of hCG-stimulated testosterone, MIS levels can be used to guide the treatment of these patients.
* Evaluation of presence of any functioning testicular tissue in infants and children with ambiguous genitalia.
* Early detection of recurrence in patients with granulosa cell tumors.
* Assess the condition of PCO and premature ovarian failure
* Assess ovarian reserve

➤ Interpretation
Increased In
* PCOS (polycystic ovarian syndrome)

Decreased In
* Anorchia
* Abnormal or absence of testis
* Pseudohermaphroditism
* Syndrome of persistent Müllerian ducts, despite the presence of structurally normal testes.

➤ Limitations
* Compared with white women, average MIS values were lower among black (25.2% lower) and Hispanic (24.6% lower) women.
* Not well standardized test. Interpretation needs to be in conjunction with clinical symptoms.

MYELOPEROXIDASE (MPO), PLASMA

➤ Definition
* MPO is an enzyme stored in granules of PMNs and macrophages. It is released in plasma in inflammatory conditions. It is thought to indicate atherosclerotic plaque instability.

* At the time of this writing, plasma MPO is offered by one company only, PrognostiX, Inc, as an ELISA immunoassay.
* **Normal range:** <539 pM in healthy individuals

➤ Use

* Marker of inflammation when elevated in plasma. MPO may be used for the evaluation of patients presenting with acute chest pain, in conjunction with ECG and cardiac biomarkers.

➤ Interpretation

* An initial increase independently predicts risk of myocardial infarction and adverse cardiac events and predicts sudden death in the next 1–6 months, even in the absence of signs of ischemic necrosis or of increase in other inflammatory markers, such as CRP. A low MPO improves the negative predictive value of normal troponins in unstable angina.
* Elevated plasma MPO concentration is associated with a more advanced cardiovascular risk profile; however, plasma MPO does not predict mortality independent of other cardiovascular risk factors in patients with stable coronary artery disease.

➤ Limitations

* No interference or cross-reactivity with other blood components has been reported by PrognostiX.

➤ Suggested Reading

Stefanescua A, Braun S, Ndrepepa G, et al. Prognostic value of plasma myeloperoxidase concentration in patients with stable coronary artery disease. *Am Heart J.* 2008;155(2):356–360.

MYOGLOBIN

➤ Definition

* Myoglobin is the primary oxygen-carrying protein of muscle tissues found only in skeletal and cardiac muscle.
* It is linked in a reversible manner with oxygen, playing an important part in cellular aerobic metabolism.
* **Normal range** (may be wide): 6–90 ng/mL
  * Male: 28–72 ng/mL
  * Female: 25–58 ng/mL

➤ Use

* A cardiac biomarker, myoglobin is the earliest marker for myocardial necrosis.
* Myoglobin levels start to rise within 2–3 hours of myocardial infarction, reach their highest levels within 8–12 hours, and generally fall back to normal within one day.
* A negative myoglobin result effectively rules out a heart attack, but a positive result must be confirmed by testing for troponin or another biomarker.
* Sensitivity is >95% within 6 hours of onset of symptoms.
* Myoglobin may precede release of CK-MB by 2–5 hours.

➤ Interpretation

* Within 1–3 hours in >85% of patients with AMI, myoglobin peaks in about 8–12 hours (may peak within 1 hour) to about 10 times the upper reference limit and becomes normal in about 24–36 hours or less; reperfusion causes a peak 4–6 hours earlier.

- It is also increased in:
  - Renal failure (High levels of urine myoglobin indicate an increased risk of kidney damage.)
  - Shock
  - Open heart surgery
  - Carriers of progressive muscular dystrophy
  - Extensive trauma
  - Myocarditis
  - Acute infectious diseases

➤ Limitations
- The myoglobin test is not recommended as a standalone test.
- Increased values may occur with skeletal muscle damage, exhaustive exercise, or heavy alcohol abuse.
- The myoglobin test displays a low specificity for AMI. Myoglobin may come from either heart or skeletal muscle, so an increase in serum myoglobin is not specific for damage to the heart.
- Blood samples should be drawn every 2–3 hours for the first several hours after experiencing chest pain (myoglobin may be released in multiple short bursts) for accurate measurements.
- Values are usually much higher in patients with uremia and muscle trauma compared to AMI.

➤ Suggested Reading
Ordway GA, Garry DJ. Myoglobin: an essential hemoprotein in striated muscle. *J Exp Biol.* 2004;207:3441–3446.

NEURON-SPECIFIC ENOLASE (NSE)

➤ Definition
- Specific serum marker for the family of neuroendocrine tumors of amine precursor uptake and decarboxylation series, which includes neuroblastoma, retinoblastoma, medullary carcinoma of thyroid, carcinoid, pancreatic cell carcinoma, pheochromocytoma, and small cell carcinoma of the lung (SCLC).
- **Normal range:** 3.7–8.9 µg/L

➤ Use
- A follow-up marker in patients with NSE-secreting tumors of any type
- An auxiliary test in the diagnosis of SCLC
- An auxiliary test in the diagnosis of carcinoids, islet cell tumors, and neuroblastomas
- An auxiliary tool in the assessment of comatose patients

➤ Interpretation
- NSE is increased in neuroblastoma and SCLC

➤ Limitations
- All NSE test results must be considered in the clinical context, and interferences or artifactual elevations should be suspected if the clinical NSE test results are at odds with the clinical picture or other tests.
- Hemolysis can lead to significant artifactual NSE elevations, because erythrocytes contain NSE.

- Proton pump inhibitor treatment, hemolytic anemia, hepatic failure, and end-stage renal failure can also result in artifactual NSE elevations.
- When performing NSE testing for tumor diagnosis or follow-up, epileptic seizure, brain injury, encephalitis, stroke, and rapidly progressive dementia might result in false-positive results. On the other hand, when NSE testing is performed to assist in neurologic diagnosis, NSE-secreting tumors can represent a source of false-positive results.
- NSE values can vary significantly between methods/assays. Serial follow-up should be performed with the same assay. If assays are changed, patients should be re-baselined.

NEUTROPHIL TESTS FOR DYSFUNCTION

➤ Definition
- Inherited or acquired disorders affecting neutrophils (and other leukocytes) may result in abnormal function and a predisposition to recurrent bacterial infections.
- Acquired neutrophil dysfunction may be the result of disorders of immunoglobulins, complement or T cells; in such cases the underlying disease should be characterized before specific assays for neutrophil dysfunction are undertaken.

➤ Use
Neutrophil function tests are used to evaluate neutrophil dysfunction in patients with recurrent bacterial infections, especially in patients with a family history suggestive of a neutrophil dysfunction syndrome. The functions used to investigate neutrophil dysfunction are adherence, locomotion, phagocytosis, and secretion (see Table 2-58). Morphologic studies are performed in parallel with the functional assays.
- Because of the rarity of these conditions, only a limited number are mentioned below (see Table 2-58).

TABLE 2-58. Assays for Suspected Congenital Neutrophil Dysfunction Syndromes

Assay	Abnormal in
NBT slide test: abnormal (negative test)	Chronic granulomatous disease
Decreased chemotaxis (and giant granules)	Chediak-Higashi syndrome
Mo-1, chemotaxis, and bacterial killing are markedly reduced; can be tested also by flow cytometry	Leukocyte adhesion deficiency
Myeloperoxidase (for neutrophils) and lysozyme (for monocytes)	Primary myeloperidoxidase deficiency (MYD)
Chemotaxis and antilactoferrin stain of polymorphonuclear neutrophils are markedly reduced	Specific granule deficiency
Chemotaxis and bacterial killing are markedly decreased	Neutrophil actin dysfunction, a genetic disorder

NICOTINE/COTININE

➤ Definition
- Nicotine is a hygroscopic alkaloid obtained from tobacco. Cotinine is the major metabolite of nicotine.
- **Normal range** (serum):
  - Nonsmokers: <6 ng/mL
  - Cigarette smokers: 10–50 ng/mL

➤ Use
- Insecticide and fumigant
- Constituent of tobacco products
- Constituent of smoking cessation products

➤ Interpretation
- Serum cotinine concentrations may be up to 10 times greater than corresponding nicotine level in smokers.
- Urine nicotine and cotinine concentrations in smokers are typically >1000 ng/mL.

➤ Limitations
- Screening tests are immunoassay based
  - Target analyte: cotinine
  - Cut-off concentration: 500 ng/mL (urine)
  - Cross-reactivity with 3-hydroxy cotinine
  - Little or no demonstrated cross-reactivity with nicotine, nicotinic acid, niacinamide
- Confirmation tests are chromatography based
  - HPLC, gas chromatography, GC/MS, LC/MS
  - Potentially measure nicotine and cotinine in serum or urine
  - Limit of quantitation: 1–2 ng/mL

OCCULT BLOOD, STOOL

➤ Definition
- Occult bleeding refers to the initial presentation of a positive fecal occult blood test (FOBT) result and/or iron-deficiency anemia, when there is no evidence of visible blood loss to the patient or physician. The differential diagnosis for occult GI bleeding is broad. Some of the more common causes include colon cancer, esophagitis, peptic ulcers, gastritis, inflammatory bowel disease, vascular ectasias, portal hypertensive gastropathy, and gastric antral vascular ectasias. However, less common causes such as gastroesophageal cancers, hemosuccus pancreaticus, hemobilia, and infections also need to be considered. Non-GI sources of blood loss such as hemoptysis and epistaxis can also cause a positive FOBT.
- FOBT falls into two primary categories based on the detected analyte: guaiac based (gFOBT) and immunoassay based (FIT). gFOBT are the most common stool blood tests in use for colorectal cancer screening, and they detect blood in the stool through the pseudoperoxidase activity of heme or hemoglobin, whereas immunochemical-based tests react to human globin.
- **Normal range:** negative

➤ Use
* Screens for carcinomas (particularly colon) and polyps of GI tract
* Identifies GI bleeding related to upper GI bleeding (gastric ulcer)
* Screens for diverticulitis and colitis

➤ Interpretation
Increased In
* GI malignancies (colon)
* Diverticular disease
* GI polyps
* Ischemic bowel disease
* Inflammatory lesions (ulcerative colitis, Crohn disease, shigellosis, amebiasis)
* Trauma, bleeding diatheses
* Vasculitis (polyarteriosis nodosa, Henoch purpura, Schönlein purpura)
* Amyloidosis
* Hiatal hernia
* Neurofibromatosis
* Kaposi sarcoma
* Hematobilia

➤ Limitations
* If using guaiac-based test, individuals should be instructed to avoid aspirin and other NSAIDs, vitamin C, red meat, poultry, fish, and some raw vegetables because of diet–test interactions that can increase the risk of both false-positive and false-negative (specifically, vitamin C) results.
* The sensitivity and specificity of a gFOBT has been shown to be highly variable and varies based on the brand or variant of the test; specimen collection technique; number of samples collected per test; whether or not the stool specimen is rehydrated; and variations in interpretation, screening interval, and other factors.
* A gFOBT test must be performed properly with three stool samples obtained at home. A single-stool sample FOBT collected after digital rectal examination in the office is not an acceptable screening test, and it is not recommended.
* FIT has several technologic advantages when compared with gFOBT. FIT detects Hb; therefore, it is more specific for human blood than guaiac-based tests are. In addition, because globin is degraded by digestive enzymes in the upper GI tract, FIT also are more specific for lower GI bleeding, thus improving their specificity for colorectal cancer. At this time, the optimal number of FIT stool samples is not established, but two samples may be superior to one.
* Drugs causing intestinal bleeding (e.g., aspirin, corticosteroids, and NSAIDs) and drugs causing colitis (e.g., methyldopa and a variety of antibiotics) can cause positive test results.

➤ Suggested Reading
Levin B, Lieberman DA, McFarland B, et al. Screening and Surveillance for the Early Detection of Colorectal Cancer and Adenomatous Polyps, 2008: A Joint Guideline from the American Cancer Society, the US Multi-Society Task Force on Colorectal Cancer, and the American College of Radiology. *CA Cancer J Clin.* 2008;58:130–160.

OPIATES

See Opioids

OPIOIDS

➤ Definition

- Opioids are natural and semisynthetic alkaloids prepared from opium and synthetic compounds whose pharmacologic properties, rather than structure, mimic morphine.
- Specific names: heroin, codeine, morphine, oxycodone, oxymorphone, hydrocodone, hydromorphone, buprenorphine, methadone, meperidine, propoxyphene, nalbuphine, fentanyl, levorphanol, butorphanol, pentazocine, tramadol
- There is no single test that will screen for/confirm all the opioids listed.
- **Normal range:** drug and use dependent

➤ Use

- Treatment of pain, usually moderate to severe
- Preoperative sedation
- Postoperative analgesia and surgical and medical emergencies including myocardial infarction, trauma, burns, orthopedic pain
- Management of chronic pain associated with cancer
- Antitussive and antidiarrheal agent
- Detoxification and maintenance therapy of opiate addicts

➤ Limitations

- Screening
  - Typically performed in urine
  - Immunoassay based technology performed on automated chemistry analyzers
    - EIA (KIMS, CEDIA), EMIT, RIA, FPIA
    - Qualitative
    - Target: morphine, morphine-glucuronide
      - These "opiate" assays *do not detect* the semi/synthetic opioids, which include buprenorphine, methadone, meperidine, propoxyphene, nalbuphine, fentanyl, levorphanol, butorphanol, pentazocine, and tramadol.
      - These "opiate" assays have variable cross-reactivity with oxycodone, oxymorphone, hydrocodone, and hydromorphone.
      - Cut-off concentration-user defined
        - 300 ng/mL
        - 2000 ng/mL
  - Specific immunoassays are available for individual synthetic compounds
    - **Oxycodone:** cut-off concentration 300 ng/mL; depending on manufacturer, may exhibit approximately 100% cross-reactivity with oxymorphone
    - **Methadone:** cut-off concentration 300 ng/mL; depending on manufacturer, may exhibit approximately 40% cross-reactivity with methadol
    - **Buprenorphine:** cut-off concentration 5 ng/mL; typically do not exhibit cross-reactivity with norbuprenorphine

- **Propoxyphene:** cut-off concentration 300 ng/mL; depending on manufacturer, may exhibit approximately 60% cross-reactivity with norpropoxyphene
  - Variable cross-reactivity with opioid metabolites
- Several vendors offer assays in semiquantitative mode
- Immunoassay available specifically for heroin metabolite-6-acetylmorphine: cut-off concentration 10 ng/mL; <1% cross reactivity with morphine, codeine, and synthetic opioids
- Screening in blood, serum
  - Immunoassay-based technology (FPIA, ELISA, RIA)
  - Opioid specific except for general "opiates," which targets morphine with a cut-off concentration typically of 10 ng/mL
  - Target (cutoff concentration)
    - Fentanyl <1 ng/mL
    - Methadone 10–50 ng/mL; <5% cross-reactivity with methadol
    - Oxycodone 10–50 ng/mL; >50% cross-reactivity with oxymorphone
    - D-Propoxyphene 10–50 ng/mL; >400% cross-reactivity with norpropoxyphene
- Confirmation/quantitation in serum, urine
  - Confirmation of urine samples often includes hydrolysis to cleave the glucuronide bond. In this case the concentration provided is total drug (compared with free or unbound drug)
  - Common opioid confirmation profiles will include 6-acetylmorphine, morphine, codeine, oxycodone, oxymorphone, hydrocodone, and hydromorphone with limit of quantitation drug dependent but ranging 5–25 ng/mL
  - Most synthetic opioids require individual specific tests for confirmation and quantitation; for potent low dose synthetic opioids such as buprenorphine and fentanyl, the limit of quantitation is ≤1 ng/mL
  - Sample preparation required: liquid–liquid or solid-phase extraction
  - Testing methodologies: gas chromatography, HPLC, GC/MS, LC/MSn (multiple Sn)

OSMOLAL GAP

➤ Definition
- The osmolal gap is a mathematical concept similar to the AG that is used to detect concentration changes in osmotically active solutes rather than ion changes.
  The osmolal gap is calculated by subtracting the calculated osmolality from the measured osmolality.
- **Normal range:** <10 mOsm/kg

➤ Use
- Osmolal gap has been used to estimate the blood alcohol. Serum osmolality increases 22 mOsm/kg for every 100 mg/dL of ethanol; therefore, estimated blood alcohol (mg/dL) = osmolal gap × 100 ÷ 22.

➤ Interpretation
Increased In
- Decreased serum water content
  - Hyperlipidemia (serum will appear lipemic)
  - Hyperproteinemia (total protein >10 g/dL)

- Additional low–molecular-weight substances in the serum (measured osmolality is >300 mOsm/kg water)
- Ethanol; an especially large osmolal gap with a low or only moderately elevated ethanol level should raise the possibility of another low–molecular-weight toxin (e.g., methanol).
  - Methanol
  - Isopropyl alcohol
  - Mannitol (osmolal gap can be used to detect accumulation of infused mannitol in serum)
  - Ethylene glycol, acetone, ketoacidosis, and paraldehyde result in relatively small osmolal gaps, even at lethal levels
- Severely ill patients, especially those in shock, acidosis (lactic, diabetic, alcoholic), renal failure

➤ Limitations
- Laboratory analytic error
  - Random error from all measurements could add or subtract ≤15 mOsm/kg
  - Use of incorrect blood collection tubes

OSMOLALITY, SERUM AND URINE

➤ Definition
- Osmolality refers to the osmotic concentration of a fluid. The osmolality of serum, urine, or any other body fluid depends on the number of active ions or molecules in a solution and yield important information about a patient's ability to maintain a normal fluid balance status. Osmolality is measured with an osmometer by freezing point depression or vapor pressure elevation techniques, or it can be calculated from a formula.
- Osmolarity is the osmotic concentration of solution expressed as osmoles of solute per liter of solution, or the property of solution that depends on the concentration of solute per unit of total volume of solvent.
- Serum osmolality measures the amount of chemicals dissolved in the blood. Chemicals that affect serum osmolality include sodium, chloride, bicarbonate, proteins, and glucose. A serum osmolality test is done to evaluate electrolyte and water balance. Serum osmolality is controlled partly by ADH, or vasopressin. ADH is produced by the hypothalamus and is released by the pituitary gland into the blood.
- Urine osmolality reflects the total number of osmotically active particles in the urine, without regard to the size or weight of the particles. Substances such as glucose, proteins, or dyes increase the urine specific gravity. Therefore, urine osmolality is a more accurate measurement of urine concentration than specific gravity, and urine osmolality can be compared with the serum osmolality to obtain an accurate picture of a patient's fluid balance.
- **Normal range:** See Table 2-59

TABLE 2-59. Normal Ranges for Osmolality		
	Reference Range (mOsm/kg)	Critical Range (mOsm/kg)
Serum or plasma	279–295	<250, >295
Urine	500–800	None

➤ Use
* Evaluate the balance between the water and the chemicals dissolved in blood.
* Determine whether severe dehydration or overhydration is present.
* Help determine if the hypothalamus is producing ADH normally.
* Help determine the cause of seizures or coma. In severe cases, an imbalance between water and electrolytes in the body can cause seizures or coma.
* Screen for the ingestion of certain poisons, such as isopropanol, methanol, or ethylene glycol.
* Evaluate concentrating ability of the kidneys.
* Evaluate electrolyte and water balance;
* Used in work-up for renal disease, SIADH, and diabetes insipidus.
* May be used with urinalysis when patient has had radiopaque substances, has glycosuria, or proteinuria
* Evaluate dehydration, amyloidosis. Osmolality is desirable in examination of neonatal urine when protein or glucose is present.

➤ Interpretation
Increased In
* Hyperglycemia
* DKA (osmolality should be determined routinely in grossly unbalanced diabetic patients)
* Nonketotic hyperglycemic coma
* Hypernatremia with dehydration
  * Diarrhea, vomiting, fever, hyperventilation, inadequate water intake
  * Diabetes insipidus—central
  * Nephrogenic diabetes insipidus—congenital or acquired (e.g., hypercalcemia, hypokalemia, chronic renal disease, sickle cell disease, effect of some drugs)
  * Osmotic diuresis—hyperglycemia, administration of urea or mannitol
* Hypernatremia with normal hydration—caused by hypothalamic disorders
  * Insensitivity of osmoreceptors (essential hypernatremia)—water loading does not return serum osmolality to normal; chlorpropamide may lower serum sodium toward normal
  * Defect in thirst (hypodipsia)—forced water intake returns serum osmolality to normal
* Hypernatremia with overhydration—iatrogenic or accidental (e.g., infants given feedings with high sodium concentrations or given $NaHCO_3$ for respiratory distress or cardiopulmonary arrest)
* Alcohol ingestion, which is the most common cause of hyperosmolar state and of coexisting coma and hyperosmolar state

Decreased In
* Hyponatremia with hypovolemia (urine sodium is usually >20 mmol/L)
  * Adrenal insufficiency (e.g., salt-losing form of CAH, congenital adrenal hypoplasia, hemorrhage into adrenals, inadequate replacement of corticosteroids, inappropriate tapering of steroids)
  * Renal losses, (e.g., osmotic diuresis; proximal renal tubular acidosis; salt-losing nephropathies, usually tubulointerstitial diseases such as GU tract obstruction; pyelonephritis; medullary cystic disease; polycystic kidneys)
  * GI tract loss (e.g., vomiting, diarrhea)
  * Other losses (e.g., burns, peritonitis, pancreatitis)

TABLE 2-60. The Relationship Between Serum and Urine Osmolality and the Clinical Significance of Laboratory Values

Serum Osmolality	Urine Osmolality	Clinical Significance
Normal values: 282–295 mOsm	Normal values: 500–800 mOsm	
Normal or increased	Increased	Fluid volume deficit
Decreased	Decreased	Fluid volume excess
Normal	Decreased	Increased fluid intake or diuretics
Increased or normal	Decreased (with no increase in fluid intake)	Kidneys unable to concentrate urine or lack of ADH (diabetes insipidus)
Decreased	Increased	SIADH

- Hyponatremia with normal volume or hypervolemia (dilutional syndromes)
  - CHF, cirrhosis, nephrotic syndrome
  - SIADH

➤ Limitations

- Variations in the urine osmolality play a central role in the regulation of the plasma osmolality and Na+ concentration. This response is mediated by osmoreceptors in the hypothalamus that influence both thirst and the secretion of ADH.

The relationship between serum and urine osmolality and the clinical significance of laboratory values are shown in Table 2-60.

$$(1.86 \times \text{serum Na}) + (\text{serum glucose} \div 18) + (\text{BUN} \div 28) + 9 \text{ (in mg/dL)}$$

or

in SI units: $= (1.86 \times \text{serum Na}) + \text{serum glucose (mmol/L)} + \text{BUN (mmol/L)} + 9$

- More simply: $\text{NA}^+ + \text{K}^+ + (\text{BUN} \div 28) + (\text{glucose} \div 18)$. Because K^+ is relatively small, and BUN has no influence on water distribution, the formula can be simplified to $2\text{Na}^+ + (\text{glucose} \div 18)$.

PARATHYROID HORMONE (PTH)

➤ Definition

- Peptide hormone secreted by parathyroid gland chief cells that controls ionized calcium levels in blood and body fluids by increasing 1,25 dihydroxy vitamin D_3 (by kidney), mobilizing calcium from bone (due to increased osteoclast activity), increasing renal tubular resorption of calcium, and reducing renal clearance of calcium, increasing intestinal calcium absorption.
- The half-life of PTH is <5 minutes. Ionized calcium in blood inhibits PTH secretion. Biologic activity resides in first 34 terminal amino acids. The intact hormone has 84 amino acids but can be quickly cleaved by proteolysis into smaller less-active fragments.
- Assay for the intact PTH has largely superseded tests for various PTH fragments. It is important that the PTH assay not cross-react with PTH (7-84) lacking the 6 N-terminal, which has been shown to be a weak antagonist to PTH activity and may lower serum and plasma calcium levels.
- **Normal range:** 12–65 pg/mL

➤ **Use**

- Differential diagnosis of hyperparathyroidism and hypoparathyroidism
- Very sensitive in detecting PTH suppression by 1,25-dihydroxyvitamin D; therefore, used for monitoring that treatment of chronic renal failure
- Intraoperative PTH assay to determine removal of abnormally secreting tissue; may replace routine frozen section; can replace traditional four-gland explorations and distinguishes single from multiglandular disease
- Preoperative and 10–20 minutes postresection assay; this causes 50–75% reduction indicating successful resection of parathyroid adenoma.

➤ **Interpretation**

Increased In

- Primary and secondary hyperparathyroidism
- Pseudohypoparathyroidism
- Hereditary vitamin D dependency types 1 and 2, vitamin D deficiency
- Z-E syndrome
- Familial medullary thyroid carcinoma
- MEN types I, IIa, and IIb

Decreased In

- Autoimmune hypoparathyroidism
- Sarcoidosis
- Nonparathyroid hypercalcemia in the absence of renal failure
- Hyperthyroidism
- Hypomagnesemia
- Transient neonatal hypocalcemia
- DiGeorge syndrome

➤ **Limitations**

- The finding of a persistently high-normal calcium accompanied by a high-normal PTH (alternatively, a low-normal calcium accompanied by a low-normal PTH) warrants further investigation; for the PTH, although itself within normal limits, may still be inappropriately high (or inappropriately low) relative to the circulating calcium level.
- Because of a pronounced nocturnal rise in intact PTH levels observed in a small experimental male population, sampling after 10 a.m. for optimum discrimination between normals and those with mild primary hyperparathyroidism has been suggested.
- Sedative–hypnotic drug propofol (Diprivan) may give falsely low PTH values.
- High concentrations of hemolysis, lipemia, and bilirubin should be avoided.
- Rapid intraoperative PTH that declines ≥50% from the highest baseline in 10 minutes after resection indicates successful total excision.

PARATHYROID HORMONE–RELATED PEPTIDE (PTHrP)

➤ **Definition**

- PTHrP is a protein secreted by some cancer cells leading to humeral hypercalcemia of malignancy (HHM). It shares the same 13 N-terminal amino acids as PTH; however, the remaining structure is different. PTHrP is larger than PTH and contains 139–173 amino acids compared to 84 for PTH.

TABLE 2-61. Serum Calcium and PTH in Various Conditions

	PTH Increased	PTH Not Increased
Serum calcium decreased*	Secondary hyperparathyroidism (chronic renal disease)	Hypoparathyroidism (surgical, autoimmunity, hormone resistance, magnesium deficiency)
Serum calcium increased†	Primary hyperparathyroidism Familial hypocalciuric hypercalcemia, Lithium-induced hypercalcemia, tertiary hyperparathyroidism	HHM, milk-alkali syndrome, thiazide diuretics, vitamin D or A intoxication, granulomatous diseases (sarcoidosis, TB), multiple myeloma, thyrotoxicosis, immobilization
Serum calcium normal	Pregnancy nephrolithiasis, secondary hyperparathyroidism (chronic renal disease)	Normal

HHM, humoral hypercalcemia of malignancy; PTH, parathyroid hormone.
*PTH may be normal or increased in hypocalcemic patients due to renal failure, acute pancreatitis, vitamin D deficiency.
†PTH may be normal or increased in hypercalcemic patients due to acromegaly, vitamin A intoxication, MEN type IIA, renal tubular acidosis, chronic renal failure.

- PTHrP shares many actions with PTH leading to increased calcium release from bone, reduced renal calcium excretion, and reduced renal phosphate reabsorption. However, PTHrP does not produce the normal anion gap metabolic acidosis commonly found with hyperparathyroidism.
- See Tables 2-61, 2-62, and 2-63 and Figures 2-2 and 2-3.
- **Normal value:** <1.3 pmol/L

➤ Use

- PTHrP is useful clinically in differentiating primary hyperthyroidism from HHM. Also useful as a marker in the management of patients with tumor associated hypercalcemia.
- The usual pattern of HHM is elevated total and ionized calcium, low PTH in the absence of other causes of hypercalcemia (e.g., excessive vitamin D, sarcoid, TB). If the presence of a malignancy is uncertain, or there are several possible causes for hypercalcemia, measurement of PTHrP can be of assistance.
- HHM occurs in patients with cancer (typically squamous, transitional cell, renal, ovarian), 5–20% who have no bone metastases compared to patients with widespread bone metastases (myeloma, lymphoma, breast cancer).
- HHM occurs in ~20% to 35% of patients with breast cancer, ~10% to 15% of cases of lung cancer, ~70% of cases of multiple myeloma, rare in lymphoma and leukemia.
- Rarely hypercalcemia may occur in association with benign tumors (e.g., pheochromocytoma, dermoid cyst of ovary) ("humoral hypercalcemia of benignancy").

TABLE 2-62. Laboratory Findings in Various Diseases of Calcium and Phosphorus Metabolism

Disease	Serum Calcium[a]	Serum Phosphorus	Serum ALP	Urine Calcium[b]	Urine Phosphorus	Serum PTH	Serum 1.25-Dihydroxy-Vitamin D
Primary hyperparathyroidism	I; frequently marked	D (<3 mg/dL in 50%)	I slightly in 50% (N if no bone disease)	I in two thirds	I	I	I
Humoral hypercalcemia of malignancy	I; frequently marked	D in 50%	Frequently I	I	I	D	D
Familial hypocalciuric hypercalcemia	Mild I	N or slightly D	N	D or low N		I or inappropriately N	Proportional to PTH
Hypoparathyroidism	D	I	N	D	D[c]	D	D
Pseudohypoparathyroidism	D	I	N; occasionally D	D	D[c]	N or I	D
Pseudohypoparathyroidism	N	N	N	N	N	N	
Secondary hyperparathyroidism (renal rickets)	D or N	I	I or N	D or I	D	I	D
Vitamin D excess	I	N	D	I	D	—	—
Rickets and osteomalacia	D or N	D or N	I	D	—	D	D
Osteoporosis	N	N	N	N or I	D		
Polyostotic fibrous dysplasia	N	N	N or I	N or I	N		
Paget's disease	N or I	N or I	I	N or I	N		
Metastatic neoplasm to bone	N or I	N or I	N or I	V	—		
Multiple myeloma	N or I	N or I	N or I	N or I	N or I		
Sarcoidosis	N or I	N or I	N or I	I	N		I
Fanconi syndrome or renal loss of fixed base	D or N	D	N or I	—	—		
Histiocytosis X (Letterer-Siwe disease, Hand-Schüller-Christian disease, eosinophilic granuloma)	N	N	N or I	N or I	N		
Hypercalcemia and excess intake of alkali (Burnett syndrome)	I	I or N	N	N	N		
Solitary bone cyst	N	N	N	N	N		N

D = decreased; I = increased; N = normal; V = variable.

[a] Serum calcium. Repeated determinations may be required to demonstrate abnormalities. Serum total protein level should always be known. See also response to cortisone.

[b] Urine calcium. Patient should be on a low-calcium diet (e.g., Bauer-Aub).

[c] See Ellsworth-Howard test.

TABLE 2-63. Comparison of Primary Hyperparathyroidism (HPT) and Humoral Hypercalcemia of Malignancy (HHM)

	HHM	HPT
Etiology	Squamous or large cell carcinoma of bronchus, hypernephroma of kidney, cancer of ovary, colon, others	Primary hyperplasia, adenoma, carcinoma of parathyroids
Serum calcium	Very high: >14 mg/dL in 75% of patients Suppressed by cortisone in 25–50% of patients	Moderately high: >14 mg/dL in 25% of patients Suppressed by cortisone in 50% of cases with and 23% of cases without osteitis fibrosa
Serum PTH	Decreased	Increased
Serum PTHRP	Increased	Not increased
Serum chloride	Low: <99 mEq/L	High: >102 mEq/L
Serum chloride phosphorus ratio	<30	>33
Serum bicarbonate	Increased or normal	Normal or low
pH	Alkalosis	Acidosis
Serum ALP	Increased in 50% of patients, even without bone disease	Seldom increased unless bone disease is present
Serum phosphorus	Increased, normal, or low	Normal or low
Urine calcium	Often >400 mg/24 hours	Usually <400 mg/24 hours
Serum 1,25-dihydroxy-vitamin D	Decreased	Increased
Urine cAMP	Increased in HHM but not due to bone metastases only	Increased in 90% of cases
ESR	Usually increased	Normal
Anemia	May be present	Absent
Serum albumin	Often decreased	Usually normal
Renal stones	Absent	Common
Pancreatitis	Rare	Occurs
Radiographic changes in hand bones	Absent	May be present

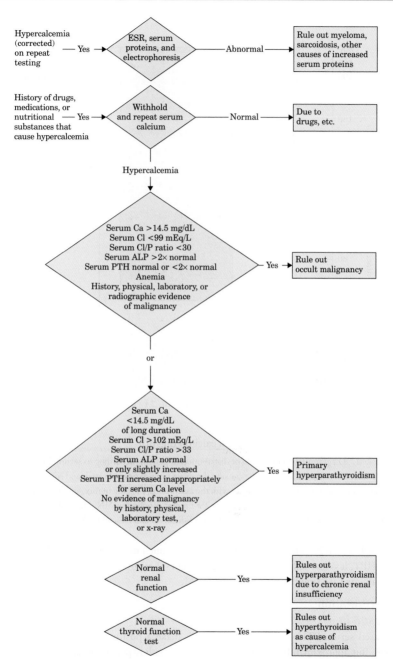

Figure 2-2. Algorithm for diagnosis of hypercalcemia. (ESR, erythrocyte sedimentation rate; PTH, parathyroid hormone.) (Data from ET Wong, Freier EF. The differential diagnosis of hypercalcemia: an algorithm for more effective use of laboratory tests. *JAMA.* 1982;247:75, and KR Johnson, Howarth AT. Differential laboratory diagnosis of hypercalcemia. *CRC Crit Rev Clin La Sci.* 1984;21:51.)

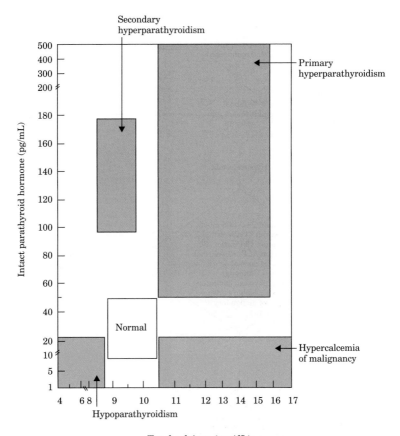

Secondary
hyperparathyroidism

Figure 2-3. Diagrammatic illustration of distribution of patients according to serum calcium and serum PTH. The values of some patients may lie outside the exact boundaries indicated, and some conditions may overlap. The exact cut-off will vary somewhat with the assays used, the patient mix, and the locally established normal reference ranges. (From *Mayo Laboratories Test Catalog*. Rochester, MN: Mayo Medical Laboratories; 1995. By permission of Mayo Foundation for Medical Education and Research. All rights reserved.)

- Very high serum calcium (e.g., >14.5 mg/dL) is much more suggestive of HHM than primary HPT; less marked increase with renal tumors. Less than or equal to 5% of hypercalcemia patients have simultaneous HPT and HHM.

➤ Interpretation

Increased In

- Increased serum PTHrP (>2.6 pmol/L) can make a positive diagnosis in most cases of HHM. But approximately 20% of cancer patients with hypercalcemia have only local osteolytic changes with no increased PTHrP.
- PTHrP is also increased in (>2.6 pmol/L):
  - >80% of hypercalcemic patients with solid tumors with or without bone metastasis
  - Some patients with hypercalcemia and hematologic cancers

- ~10% of cancers without hypercalcemia; PTHrP becomes normal when hypercalcemia is corrected by treatment of cancer
- May be increased in nonmalignant pheochromocytoma

Normal In
- Healthy persons: values <1.0 pmol/L.
- Other causes of hypercalcemia (e.g., sarcoidosis, vitamin D intoxication)
- Low-normal or suppressed intact PTH (<20 pg/mL) excludes hyperparathyroidism.
- Serum 1,25-dihydroxy vitamin D is usually decreased or low-normal in HHM but is increased in HPT.

➤ Limitations
- Production of PTHrP by the fetoplacental unit can cause transient increase during pregnancy, especially in the third semester.
- Primary hyperparathyroidism occurs in ≤10% of patients with HHM as well as in those receiving thiazides, or with other causes of hypercalcemia.

PARTIAL PRESSURE OF CARBON DIOXIDE (pCO$_2$), BLOOD

➤ Definition
- pCO$_2$ is a measure of tension or pressure of carbon dioxide dissolved in the blood. The pCO$_2$ of blood represents the balance between cellular production of CO$_2$ and ventilatory removal of CO$_2$. A normal, steady pCO$_2$ indicates that the lungs are removing CO$_2$ at about same rate as tissues producing CO$_2$. A change on pCO$_2$ indicates an alteration in this balance, usually due to the change in ventilatory status.
- **Normal range:**
  - Arterial: 35–45 mm Hg
  - Venous: 41–51 mm Hg

➤ Interpretation
Increased In
- Acute respiratory acidosis
  - Depression of respiratory center
  - Suppressed neuromuscular system
  - Pulmonary disorders
  - Inadequate mechanical ventilation
- Chronic respiratory acidosis
  - Decreased alveolar ventilation
  - Hypoventilation
- Compensation in metabolic alkalosis

Decreased In
- Respiratory alkalosis
  - Increased stimulation of respiratory center
  - Hypermetabolic states
  - Mechanical hyperventilation
- Compensation in metabolic acidosis

➤ Limitations

- Respiratory conditions will primarily affect pCO_2, whereas metabolic disturbances are first reflected in the HCO_3.
- Values are slightly lower in supine position.
- Difference between arterial blood and venous blood varies considerably, depending on the skin temperature, length of stasis, and muscular activity.

PARTIAL PRESSURE OF OXYGEN (pO_2), BLOOD

➤ Definition

- The partial pressure of oxygen (pO_2) is a measure of the tension or pressure of oxygen dissolved in the blood. The pO_2 of arterial blood is primarily related to the ability of the lungs to oxygenate blood from alveolar air.
- **Normal range:**
  - Arterial: > 80–95 mm Hg (see Table 2-64)
  - Venous: 35–40 mm Hg

➤ Use

- To evaluate patients with pulmonary or acid–base disturbances.
- To monitor patients with carbon monoxide poisoning, methemoglobinemia, or hemoglobin variant for O_2 saturation.
- To manage patients on mechanical respirators.
- Prior to thoracic or general surgery.

➤ Interpretation
Increased In

- Decreased ventilation
  - Airway obstruction
  - Drug overdose
  - Metabolic disorders (e.g., myxedema, hypokalemia)
  - Neurologic disorders (e.g., Guillain-Barré syndrome, multiple sclerosis)
  - Muscle disorders (e.g., muscular dystrophy, polymyositis)
  - Chest wall abnormalities (e.g., scoliosis)
- Increased dead space in lungs (perfusion decreased more than ventilation decreased)
  - Lung diseases (e.g., chronic obstructive pulmonary disease [COPD], asthma, pulmonary fibrosis, mucoviscidosis)

TABLE 2-64. Arterial PO$_2$	
Age (years)	Range (mm Hg)
0–14	>95
15–30	>96
31–50	>91
51–70	>85
71–110	>80

- Chest wall changes affecting lung parenchyma (e.g., scoliosis)
- Increased production (e.g., sepsis, fever, seizures, excess carbohydrate loads)

Decreased In
- Hypoventilation (e.g., chronic airflow obstruction): caused by increased alveolar CO_2 that displaces O_2.
- Alveolar hypoxia (e.g., high altitude, gaseous inhalation).
- Pulmonary diffusion abnormalities (e.g., interstitial lung disease): Supplemental oxygen usually improves pO_2.
- Right-to-left shunt: Supplemental oxygen has no effect; requires positive end-expiratory pressure.
  - Congenital anomalies of heart and great vessels
  - Acquired (e.g., ARDS)
- Ventilation–perfusion mismatch: Supplemental O_2 usually improves pO_2
  - Airflow obstruction (e.g., COPD, asthma)
  - Interstitial inflammation (e.g., pneumonia, sarcoidosis)
  - Vascular obstruction (e.g., pulmonary embolism)
- Decreased venous oxygenation (e.g., anemia)
- Cyanosis is clearly visible at pO_2 <40 mm Hg; may be seen at 50 mm Hg depending on skin pigmentation.

➤ Limitations
- Capillary blood is not suitable for estimation of high arterial pO_2 values.
- Values measured at 37°C must be corrected to the actual temperature of the patient.
- Drugs causing respiratory depression, for example, barbiturates, diazepam, heron, meperidine, and midazolam cause decrease in pO_2.

PARTIAL THROMBOPLASTIN TIME (PTT, aPTT)

➤ Definition
- The PTT assesses the coagulation activity of the intrinsic and common pathways of coagulation. It is the best screening test for the diagnosis of disorders of coagulation that do not involve factor VII (extrinsic pathway) or platelet function.
- The conventional prefix "activated" is obsolete; there is no nonactivated PTT in use. The "activation" reflects a technical aspect of the assay because the reagents contain a negatively charged surface that accelerates the rate of the reaction.
- **Normal range:** 22.3–34.0 seconds (varies slightly from lot to lot of reagent, type of the commercial reagent used, and equipment)

➤ Use
- Screening for hemophilia A and B and other possible coagulopathies (except factors VII and XIII). PTT does not detect single clotting factors defects above 40% of normal.
- Detection of clotting inhibitors. This is best performed by mixing studies once an otherwise unexplained prolonged PTT is found. Mixing equal parts of patient and normal plasma (1:1) for 1–2 hours at 37°C normalizes the prolonged PTT if it is caused by a coagulation factor deficiency but not if it is caused by an inhibitor. This inhibitor is most commonly factor VIII inhibitor, or it can be LA if sensitive reagents are used (see p. 249).

- Monitoring of therapy with unfractionated heparin it is not useful in monitoring low–molecular-weight heparins or fondaparinux; these anticoagulants can be monitored with anti-Xa assay.
- Not recommended for preoperative screening in patients without a personal or immediate family history of unprovoked bleeding

➤ Interpretation

Increased (>36 seconds) In

- Single clotting factor deficiencies
- Inhibitors
- Therapy with unfractionated heparin
- Therapy with warfarin (variable response)
- Therapy with antithrombin agents such as hirudin and its derivatives, argatroban, and newer antithrombin and anti-Xa agents
- High-titer LA
- Moderate to severe von Willebrand disease

Decreased (<22 seconds) In

- Excessive generation of thrombin. No clinical correlation with a predisposition to thromboembolism has been convincibly demonstrated.

Normal In

- Thrombocytopenias and thrombocytopathies without associated clotting defects
- Majority of cases of mild von Willebrand disease
- Isolated defects of factors VII or XIII

➤ Limitations

Preanalytic Pitfalls

- Partial clotting of sample due to insufficient mixture with anticoagulant
- Overfilling or underfilling the test tube, thereby changing the 9 (blood)-to-1 (anticoagulant) ratio
- Use of wrong anticoagulant rather than the recommended 3.2% sodium citrate (currently used in blue top tubes)

Analytic Pitfalls

- Hemolyzed, severely icteric, or hyperlipemic blood may affect results (modern equipment may override icteric or hyperlipidemic blood)

Other Limitations: Drugs

- Short values may be seen with estrogen therapy or oral contraceptives.
- Prolonged values may result from diphenylhydantoin, naloxone, and radiographic contrast agents.

PERIPHERAL BLOOD SMEARS (PBS)

➤ Definition

- The primary purpose of studying PBS is to obtain differential counts of WBC and to study blood cell morphology. They are most helpful for the rapid identification of anemias, leukemias, and platelet abnormalities.

➤ Use

- Blood collected for CBC is prepared manually (or by automated equipment), smearing a thin layer of blood on a glass slide, and then staining with special dyes for microscopic examinations. PBS is also studied for the presence of organisms. When malaria is suspected, the PBS (thin smear) is most useful in finding and identifying parasites (thick film: a concentrated technique by which a large amount of blood is placed in a small area it—is used in cases with sparse parasites).
- Special stains may be added to provide additional diagnostic information:
  - Leukocyte (neutrophil) alkaline phosphatase: normal range is 11–95. It is an absolute value derived fro counting the leukocytes granules at the microscope. It is used primarily to differentiate between CML and leukocytosis of other etiologies. It is decreased in myeloid cells of CML patients, and in some cases of myelodysplastic syndrome, as well as in pernicious anemia and PNH. It is increased in leukemoid reactions and myeloproliferative neoplasms.
  - Myeloperoxidase: stains primary granules of neutrophils and secondary granules of eosinophils, identifying myeloid lineage (helpful for blast lineage identification in leukemias)
  - Specific (naphthol AS-D chloroacetate esterase) identifies cells of myeloid series, but not monocytes or lymphocytes.
  - Nonspecific (α-naphthyl butyrate or α-naphthyl acetate) esterase identifies monocytic cells, but do not stain granulocytes or eosinophils. These two stains are used to identify leukemic lineage.
  - Iron stain (used as Prussian blue reaction). It identifies iron in nucleated red cells (either as siderocytes or ringed sideroblasts (Myelodysplastic syndromes, p. 843); it also identifies Pappenheimer bodies in erythrocytes (RBCs, Table 2-73 see p. 322)
  - Periodic acid-Schiff (PAS): detects intracellular glycogen and neutral mucosubstances, which are found in most hematopoietic cells. It is helpful in the diagnosis of erythroleukemia because of the intensity of its diffuse staining in primitive erythroid cells.

➤ Limitations

- Poorly prepared smears may be difficult to evaluate accurately.

PHOSPHATE, BLOOD

➤ Definition

- Phosphate is used in the synthesis of phosphorylated compounds. It accompanies glucose into cells. The total body content in normal adults is ~700–800 g. About 80–85% of phosphate is contained in bones; the remaining 15–20% is in ICF in tissue as organic phosphates (phospholipids, nucleic acids, NADP, ATP).
- Only 0.1% is in the ECF as inorganic phosphate and only this fraction of phosphorus is measured in routine clinical settings.
- **Normal range:** See Table 2-65

➤ Use

- Monitoring of blood phosphate level in renal, endocrine, and GI disorders

➤ Interpretation
Increased In

- Acute or chronic renal failure (most common cause) with decreased GFR
- Most causes of hypocalcemia (except vitamin D deficiency, in which it is usually decreased)

TABLE 2-65. Normal Ranges for Phosphate

Age	Reference Range	Critical Range
0–28 days	4.2 to 9.0 mg/dL	<1.2 mg/dL
28 days to 2 years	3.8 to 6.2 mg/dL	<1.2 or >8.9 mg/dL
2–16 years	3.5 to 5.9 mg/dL	<1.2 or >8.9 mg/dL
>16 years	2.5 to 4.5 mg/dL	<1.2 or >8.9 mg/dL

* Increased tubular reabsorption or decreased glomerular filtration of phosphate
  * Hypoparathyroidism (idiopathic, surgical, irradiation)
  * Secondary hyperparathyroidism (renal rickets)
  * Pseudohypoparathyroidism types I and II
  * Other endocrine disorders (e.g., Addison disease, acromegaly, hyperthyroidism)
  * Sickle cell anemia
* Increased cellular release of phosphate
  * Neoplasms (e.g., myelogenous leukemia, lymphomas)
  * Excessive breakdown of tissue (e.g., chemotherapy for neoplasms, rhabdomyolysis, malignant hyperthermia, lactic acidosis, acute yellow atrophy, thyrotoxicosis)
  * Bone disease, (e.g., healing fractures, multiple myeloma [some patients], Paget disease [some patients], osteolytic metastatic tumor in bone [some patients])
  * Childhood
* Increased phosphate load: exogenous phosphate (oral or IV) form
* Phosphate enemas, laxatives or infusions
* Excess vitamin D intake
* IV therapy for hypophosphatemia or hypercalcemia
* Milk-alkali (Burnett) syndrome (some patients)
* Massive blood transfusions
* Hemolysis of blood
* Miscellaneous
  * High intestinal obstruction
  * Sarcoidosis (some patients)

Decreased In

* Primary hypophosphatemia
* Decreased GI absorption
  * Decreased dietary intake
  * Decreased intestinal absorption, for example, malabsorption, steatorrhea, secretory diarrhea, vomiting, vitamin D deficiency, drugs (antacids, alcohol, glucocorticoids)
* Decreased renal tubular reabsorption (>100 mg/day in urine during hypophosphatemia indicates excessive renal loss)
  * Primary (e.g., Fanconi syndrome, rickets [vitamin D-deficient or dependent or familial], idiopathic hypercalciuria)
  * Secondary or acquired tubular disorders (e.g., hypercalcemia, excess PTH, primary hyperparathyroidism, hypokalemia, hypomagnesemia, diuresis, glycosuria, metabolic or respiratory acidosis, metabolic alkalosis, volume expansion, acute gout, dialysis)
* Intracellular shift of phosphate
  * Osteomalacia, steatorrhea

* Growth hormone deficiency
* Acute alcoholism
* DM
* Acidosis (especially DKA)
* Hyperalimentation
* Nutritional recovery syndrome (rapid refeeding after prolonged starvation)
* IV administration of glucose (e.g., recovery after severe burns, hyperalimentation)
* Respiratory alkalosis (e.g., gram-negative bacteremia) or metabolic
* Salicylate poisoning
* Administration of anabolic steroids, androgens, epinephrine, glucagon, insulin
* Cushing syndrome (some patients)
* Prolonged hypothermia (e.g., open heart surgery)
* TPN with inadequate phosphate supplementation
* Refeeding after prolonged starvation (e.g., anorexia nervosa)
* Thyrotoxic periodic paralysis
* Sepsis
* PTH-producing tumors
* Familial hypocalciuric hypercalcemia
* Severe malnutrition, malabsorption, severe diarrhea
* Often more than one mechanism is operative, usually associated with prior phosphorus depletion.

➤ Limitations

* Interference may occur with serum samples from patients diagnosed as having plasma cell dyscrasias and lymphoreticular malignancies associated with abnormal Ig synthesis, such as multiple myeloma, Waldenström's macroglobulinemia, and heavy chain disease.
* Should be measured in fasting morning specimens because of a diurnal variation. Phosphorus has a very strong biphasic circadian rhythm. Values are lowest in the morning, peak first in the late afternoon, and peak again in the late evening. The second peak is quite elevated and results may be outside the reference range.
* Levels are influenced by dietary intake, meals, and exercise.

PHOSPHATIDYLGLYCEROL (PG)

➤ Definition

* This minor constituent of pulmonary surfactant begins to increase appreciably in AF several weeks after the rise in lecithin.
* Because PG enhances the spread of phospholipids on the alveoli, its presence indicates an advanced state of fetal lung development and function.
* PG determination is not generally affected by blood, meconium, or other contaminants.
* PG can be performed by TLC, so it can be determined alone or in conjunction with lecithin-to-sphingomyelin testing.
* It may be reported qualitatively as positive or negative, where positive represents an exceedingly low risk of respiratory distress syndrome (RDS), or in a quantitative fashion, in which a value 0.3 is associated with a minimal rate of respiratory distress.
* AmnioStat-FLM is an immunologic qualitative agglutination test for determining the presence of PG in AF. This test is specific, sensitive, and rapid. Results are not affected by moderate

blood or meconium contamination. It requires <0.1 mL of specimen, which can be obtained by transabdominal amniocentesis or from a vaginal pool.
* **Normal range:**
  * Mature fetal lung: positive and weak positive
  * Immature fetal lung: negative

➤ Use
* Assessing fetal lung maturity
* Determining the ability of fetal lungs to produce sufficient quantities of pulmonary surfactant
* Predicting the likelihood of the development of respiratory distress syndrome if the fetus were delivered

➤ Interpretation
* Increased in mature fetal lungs
* Decreased in immature fetal lungs

➤ Limitations
* AmnioStat-FLM is not subject to artifacts associated with other lung surfactant tests.
* TLC test can produce false-positive test results with meconium contamination and vaginal fluid contamination.
* The absence of PG or low levels of PG cannot dependably predict the presence of RDS.
* Diabetes, regardless of glucose control, delays PG production.

PHOSPHOLIPIDS

➤ Definition
* Phospholipids are a class of lipids consisting of a hydrophilic polar head group and a hydrophobic tail. The polar head group contains one or more phosphate groups. The hydrophobic tail is made up of two fatty acyl chains.
* In an aqueous environment, the hydrophilic heads of the phospholipid molecules tend to face water and the hydrophobic tails bond together, forming a bilayer, which constitutes a major portion and function of cell membranes.
* Most of the phospholipids in human plasma are phosphatidyl choline (70–75%) or sphingomyelin (18–20%). The remaining phospholipids include phosphatidyl serine, phosphatidyl ethanolamine (3–6%), and lysophosphatidyl choline (4–9%).
* **Normal range:** 150–380 mg/dL

➤ Use
* There are a number of disease states for which phospholipid analysis may be desirable, including obstructive jaundice, Tangier disease, beta- or hypobetalipoproteinemia, and lecithin cholesterol acyltransferase deficiency.
* Phospholipid analysis rarely provides added beneficial information in cases of dyslipoproteinemia.

➤ Interpretation
* Phospholipids are increased in hyperlipidemias and obstructive liver disease.
* They are decreased in Tangier disease.

➤ Suggested Reading

McPherson RA, Pincus MR. Lipids and dyslipoproteinemia (estimation of plasma lipids). In: McPherson RA, Pincus MR, eds. *Henry's Clinical Diagnosis and Management by Laboratory Methods.* 21st ed. Philadelphia: Saunders Elsevier; 2007: Chapter 17: 200–218.

PHOSPHORUS, URINE

➤ Definition

- Urinary phosphorus levels are used to evaluate calcium-to-phosphorus balance. High urinary phosphorus (i.e., increased renal losses) occurs in primary hyperparathyroidism, vitamin D deficiency, renal tubular acidosis, and diuretic use. Phosphates are among the substances that may be lost in Fanconi syndrome. Renal loss of phosphate may itself lead to rickets or osteomalacia. Low levels are observed in hypoparathyroidism, pseudohypoparathyroidism, and vitamin D intoxication.
- These levels are also useful in the evaluation of nephrolithiasis. Hypophosphatemia with normal serum calcium, high alkaline phosphatase, hypercalciuria, and low urinary phosphorus occur with osteomalacia from excessive antacid ingestion. Children with thalassemia may have normal phosphorus absorption but high renal phosphaturia, leading to a deficiency of phosphorus. Increasing dietary intake of potassium has been reported to increase serum phosphate concentrations apparently by decreasing renal excretion of phosphate. During the last trimester of pregnancy there is a sixfold increase in calcium and phosphorus accumulation as the fetus triples its weight. Plasma phosphorus concentrations and increased urinary phosphate may provide a useful means to assess response to phosphate supplements in the premature infants.
- **Normal range:**
  - 24 hour urine: 0.4–1.3 g/day
  - Random urine:
    - Male:
      - <40 years: 36–1770 mg/g creatinine
      - >40 years: 54–860 mg/g creatinine
    - Female:
      - <40 years: 111–927 mg/g creatinine
      - >40 years: 105–1081 mg/g creatinine

➤ Use

- Evaluation of calcium-to-phosphorus balance
- Evaluation of nephrolithiasis

➤ Interpretation

Increased In

- Primary hyperparathyroidism
- Humoral hypercalcemia of malignancy
- Vitamin D excess
- Paget disease
- Metastatic neoplasm of the bone
- Fanconi syndrome (renal tubular damage)
- Nonrenal acidosis (increased phosphate excretion as renal buffer)

Decreased In
* Hypoparathyroidism
* Pseudohypoparathyroidism
* Secondary hyperparathyroidism (renal rickets)
* Rickets and osteomalacia
* Parathyroidectomy

➤ Limitations
* Interpretation of urinary phosphorus excretion is dependent on the clinical situation and should be interpreted in conjunction with the serum phosphorus concentration.
* There is significant diurnal variation in excretion, with values highest in the afternoon.
* Urinary excretion depends on diet.

PLASMA RENIN ACTIVITY (PRA)

➤ Definition
* Renin activity is measured indirectly by the ability of patient's plasma to generate angiotensin.
* **Normal range:**
  * **Cord blood:** 4.0–32.0 ng/mL/hour
  * **Newborn** (1–7 days): 2.0–35.0 ng/mL/hour
  * **Child, normal sodium diet, supine:**
    * 1–12 months: 2.4–37.0 ng/mL/hour
    * 1–3 years: 1.7–11.2 ng/mL/hour
    * 3–5 years: 1.0–6.5 ng/mL/hour
    * 5–10 years: 0.5–5.9 ng/mL/hour
    * 10–15 years: 05–3.3 ng/mL/hour
  * **Adult, normal sodium diet**
    * Supine: 0.2–1.6 ng/mL/hour
    * Standing: 0.7–3.3 ng/mL/hour
* Normal values depend on the laboratory and the patients prevailing Na and K, status of hydration, and posture. Only stimulated values are of practical value in evaluating hypertensive patients.

➤ Use
* Particularly useful to diagnose curable hypertension (e.g., primary aldosteronism, unilateral renal artery stenosis).
* May help differentiate patients with volume excess (e.g., primary aldosteronism) with low PRA from those with medium to high PRA; if latter group shows marked increase in PRA during captopril test, patients should be worked up for renovascular hypertension, but those with little or no increase are not likely to have curable renovascular hypertension.
* Captopril test criteria for renovascular hypertension: stimulated PRA ≥12 µg/L/hour, absolute increase PRA ≥10 µg/L/hour, increase PRA ≥150% (or ≥400% if baseline PRA <3 µg/L/hour)
* In children with salt-losing form of congenital adrenal hyperplasia due to 21-hydroxylase deficiency, severity of disease is related to degree of increase. PRA level may serve as guide to adequate mineralocorticoid replacement therapy.

TABLE 2-66. Differentiation of Primary and Secondary Aldosteronism Based on Blood tests and Clinical Symptoms

	Primary Aldosteronism		Secondary Aldosteronism	
	Adenoma	Hyperplasia	Hypertension	Edema
Aldosterone	↑	↑	↑↑	↑
PRA	↓↓	N/↑	↑↑	↑
Serum sodium	N/↑	N	N/↓	N/↓
Serum potassium	↓	N/↓	↓	N/↓
Edema	0	0	0	Present
Hypertension	↑	↑	↑↑↑↑	N/↑

↑, increased; ↓, decreased; N, normal.

➤ Interpretation
Increased In
- Secondary aldosteronism (usually very high levels), especially malignant or severe hypertension 50–80% of patients with renovascular hypertension (Table 2-66).
  - Normal or high PRA is of limited value to diagnose or rule out renal vascular hypertension.
  - Very high PRA is highly predictive but has poor sensitivity.
  - Low PRA using renin–sodium nomogram in untreated patients with normal serum creatinine is strongly against this diagnosis.
- 15% of patients with essential hypertension (high-renin hypertension)
- Renin-producing tumors of the kidney
- Reduced plasma volume due to low-sodium diet, diuretics, hemorrhage, Addison disease
- Some edematous normotensive states (e.g., cirrhosis, nephrosis, congestive heart failure)
- Sodium or potassium loss due to GI disease or in 10% of patients with chronic renal failure
- Normal pregnancy
- Pheochromocytoma
- Last half of menstrual cycle (twofold increase)
- Erect posture for 4 hours (twofold increase)
- Ambulatory patients compared to bed patients
- Bartter syndrome
- Various drugs (diuretics, ACE inhibitors, vasodilators; sometimes by calcium antagonists and alpha-blockers, e.g., diazoxide, estrogens, furosemide, guanethidine, hydralazine, minoxidil, spironolactone, thiazides)

Decreased In
- 98% of cases of primary aldosteronism. Usually absent or low and can be increased less or not at all by sodium depletion and ambulation in contrast to secondary aldosteronism. PRA may not always be suppressed in primary aldosteronism; repeated testing may be necessary to establish the diagnosis. Normal PRA does not preclude this diagnosis; it is not a reliable screening test.
- Hypertension due to unilateral renal artery stenosis or unilateral renal parenchymal disease
- Increased plasma volume due to high-sodium diet, administration of salt-retaining steroids

- 18–25% of essential hypertensives (low-renin essential hypertension) and 6% of normal controls
- Advancing age in both normal and hypertensive patients (decrease of 35% from the third to the eighth decade)
- May also be decreased in CAH secondary to 11-hydroxylase or 17-hydroxylase deficiency with oversecretion of other mineralocorticoids.
- Rarely in Liddle syndrome and excess licorice ingestion
- Use of various drugs (propranolol, clonidine, reserpine; slightly with methyldopa)
- Usually cannot be stimulated by salt restriction, diuretics, and upright posture that deplete plasma volume; therefore, measure before and after furosemide and 3–4 hours of ambulation

➤ Limitations

- The plasma renin activity cannot be interpreted if the patient is being treated with spironolactone (Aldactone). Spironolactone should be discontinued for 4–6 weeks before testing.
- ACE inhibitors have the potential to "falsely elevate" PRA. Therefore, in a patient treated with an ACE inhibitor, the findings of a detectable PRA level or a low SA-to-PRA ratio do not exclude the diagnosis of primary aldosteronism. In addition, a strong predictor for primary aldosteronism is a PRA level undetectably low in a patient taking an ACE inhibitor.
- Not useful for determination of plasma renin concentration
- This test should not be requested in patients who have recently received radioisotopes, therapeutically or diagnostically, because of potential assay interference. A recommended time period before collection cannot be made, because it depends on the isotope administered, the dose given, and the clearance rate in the individual patient.

➤ Suggested Reading

Mann SJ, Pickering TG. Detection of renovascular hypertension. State of the art. *Ann Intern Med.* 1992;117:845.

PLASMINOGEN

➤ Definition

- Plasminogen is the inactive, circulating precursor of plasmin, the final product of the fibrinolytic system. Therapy with plasminogen activators results in the generation of plasmin and intended thrombolysis.
- **Normal range:** 70–113%

➤ Interpretation
Decreased In

- Congenital: rare reported cases; may result in a predisposition to thrombosis
- Acquired: severe DIC, pathologic fibrinolysis, or as the result of thrombolytic therapy, liver disease

PLASMINOGEN ACTIVATOR INHIBITOR 1

➤ Definition

- This inhibitor of tissue plasminogen activator is synthesized in endothelial cells, in platelets, and by the liver.
- **Normal range:** 0.0–22.0 IU/mL

➤ Use
- This test is used in rare cases with a tendency to thrombosis when no other cause is identified.

➤ Interpretation
Decreased Values
- Difficult to determine because the normal range can be as low as 0.0
- Cases with an increased fibrinolytic tendency (bleeding, rapid dissolution of hemostatic clots)

Increased Values
- May result in a tendency to arterial or venous thrombosis
- Acquired: during acute thrombotic episodes; pregnancy; sepsis
- Congenital: rare congenital elevations have been described

➤ Limitations
- This test is a biologic assay that is difficult to perform reproducibly
- The inhibitor has diurnal variations, with highest levels during morning hours (blood should be drawn fasting between 8 a.m. and 12 noon)

PLATELET AGGREGATION

➤ Definition
- Platelets participate in primary hemostasis by forming aggregates at the site of injury. *In vivo* the platelets are stimulated by chemical substances called agonists or by interaction with surfaces in the presence of von Willebrand factor and collagen. These properties are used *in vitro* to study the change in optical density as the platelets aggregate under the effect of added agonists (ADP, collagen, epinephrine, arachidonic acid, thrombin). Ristocetin is used to assess binding to von Willebrand factor, as reflected in the platelets' agglutination.
- The aggregometers are photooptical instruments that require platelet-rich plasma. The more advanced equipment can use whole blood and can also assess ATP release by chemoluminescence methodology, thereby better determining platelet functionality.
- **Normal range:** decrease in optical density of ≥65% (represented by graphs waves generated by the aggregometer). The results are also interpreted in relation to the role of each agonist in platelet physiology.
- The normal response to various agonists of ATP release in chemoluminescence assays is measured in nanomoles and reported as normal or abnormal.

➤ Use
- Platelet aggregation studies are indicated in patients with a bleeding diathesis, especially mucocutaneous bleeding (but without acquired thrombocytopenia), when a platelet defect or von Willebrand disease is suspected. By varying the amount of the ristocetin reagent, subtype 2B or platelet type of von Willebrand disease can be diagnosed preliminarily (see p. 874).

➤ Interpretation
Causes of Decreased Values
- **Congenital conditions:**
  - The prototype for a severe platelet defect (thrombocytopathy) is Glanzmann thrombasthenia, where there is no aggregation with any agonists but positive agglutination with ristocetin (see p. 874)

- Storage pool disease (see p. 874)
- Bernard-Soulier syndrome (see p. 876)
- Abnormal response to ristocetin may be due to von Willebrand disease (see p. 879) or if the platelet receptors responsible for binding von Willebrand factor (see p. 880) are missing.
- **Acquired conditions:**
  - Effect of drugs. Abnormalities in response to arachidonic acid reflect, in most cases, ingestion of aspirin or other NSAIDs
  - Myeloproliferative neoplasms
  - Uremia
  - Plasmacytic neoplasms with high monoclonal globulins

➤ Limitations

- Because of the short functional viability of platelets, the assay must be initiated within 2 hours from blood collection and completed within 4 hours.
- The blood must be kept at room temperature at all times
- Platelet activation during blood drawing, such as traumatic draws with initiation of clotting, makes the assay invalid. Pneumatic tubes for delivering the blood should not be used.
- Lipemic or hemolyzed blood may affect the *in vitro* platelet response.
- Assays cannot be performed in severely thrombocytopenic patients.
- Platelet aggregation studies have not been standardized to test for aspirin or clopidogrel "resistance" or hyperaggregability.
- Platelet aggregation studies are labor intensive and require highly skilled, experienced technicians.

PLATELET ANTIBODY DETECTION

➤ Definition

- Platelet antibodies can be divided into two categories: autoimmune and alloimmune. Autoimmune antibodies are part of an autoimmune condition, such as autoimmune thrombocytopenic purpura (see p. 874) or SLE (see p. 936), or they may develop following administration of certain drugs. Alloimmune antibodies develop as the result of immunization of transfused, incompatible, platelets.
- The development of platelet antibodies may result in shortened platelet survival and refractoriness to platelet transfusions (lack of adequate and sustained increment in platelet number). Therefore, from 20–70% of multitransfused thrombocytopenic patients become refractory to transfused platelets. Platelet antibodies in pregnant women may cause neonatal alloimmune thrombocytopenia. Platelet antibodies react with several antigenic groups on the platelet surface: ABO antibodies, HLA antibodies.
- The most common platelet antigen is known as HPA-1, also known as Pl^{A1}, present in 98% of the Caucasian population. Anti HPA-1 are the most common clinically significant antibodies. The HPA-1b (Pl^{A2}) antigen occurs in 27% of the Caucasian population. Both reside on the platelet membrane protein GPIIIa.

➤ Use

- In refractory, multitransfused patients, the common approach is to determine the HLA type of the patient (ideally to be done before treatments that predictably result in the need for repeated platelet transfusions) and transfuse platelets from the best HLA matched, ABO compatible, donor. Platelet cross-matching may also be used to select the best cross-matched compatible donors. Unfortunately, cross-matched platelets are effective in only 50% of transfused patients.

* Many hematologists used the platelet antibody assays to diagnose immune thrombocytopenias (see p. 868). Because of the low specificity, this assay is presently not recommended.

➤ Limitations
* Attachment of antibodies to platelets is difficult to measure because platelets have normally cell-bound immunoglobulins attached to them. In addition, platelets do not lend themselves to agglutination methodology, as used for RBC antibody detection (see p. 119, DAT). The use of different proposed methodologies remains difficult to standardize, and practicality is limited. Solid-phase methodologies, such as those using ELISA immunoassays, are used by some laboratories to detect IgG antibodies against HLA, ABO, and HPA antigens.

➤ Suggested Reading
Roback JD, Combs MR, Grossman BJ, Hillyier CD. *AABB. Technical Manual.* 16th ed. Bethesda, Md: AABB Press; 2008.

PLATELET FUNCTION ASSAY, *IN VITRO*

➤ Definition
* Assay involves an instrument (PFA-100) that measures high shear-dependent platelet function *in vitro*. For this reason, it has been dubbed "an *in vitro* bleeding time." It requires only 0.8 mL of blood, and its results are obtained in a few minutes. Therefore, it can be used either in the laboratory or as a POC test.
* It is advantageous in pediatric practice.

➤ Use
* This platelet function assay is useful in screening for:
  * Von Willebrand disease types 1 (results may be inconclusive in mild type 1), 2A, 2B, 2M and 3
  * Severe functional platelet defects
  * Rapid preoperative evaluation of patients with a bleeding history
  * Useful in detecting the effect of therapy with DDAVP (desmopressin acetate)
  * To detect improved hemostasis after platelet transfusions
* It is abnormal in the conditions described above as well as in the use of aspirin or NSAIDs

➤ Limitations
* The *in vitro* assay does not detect mild platelet abnormalities.
* The *in vitro* results have a good negative (rule out) predictive value in cases with low or intermediate suspicion for a hemostatic defect. If, however, the results with the *in vitro* assay are negative, but the clinical suspicion of a hemostatic defect is strong, more definitive studies are recommended (platelet aggregation assays or vWF panels [see p. 880])
* If the results are positive, additional studies (platelet aggregation and/or vWF panels) are recommended for a definitive diagnosis.

PLATELETS

➤ Definition
- Platelets are small discoid blood corpuscles, the primary link in achieving hemostasis.
- They are counted by automated counters (rarely manually) that also report mean platelet volume (see p. 255). Their morphology is studied on peripheral blood smear (see p. 282). Automated counters flag abnormal platelet count or appearance.
- **Normal range:** 140–440 ($\times 10^{-6}$ cells/L). Platelets can be estimated on peripheral blood smear (number of platelets/100$\times$ oil immersion field $\times$ 10,000); for accuracy, platelets in at least 10 different fields should be counted.

➤ Interpretation
Causes of Increases
- Clonal bone marrow disorders such as myeloproliferative neoplasms
- Reactive in the following situations: after acute hemorrhage, in malignancies (about 50% of patients with "unexpected" thrombocytosis are found to have a malignancy), after splenectomy, severe trauma, infections, chronic inflammatory disorders, drug reactions, and many miscellaneous conditions

Causes of Decreases
- Immune destruction such as in ITP, reaction to certain drugs, neonatal alloimmune thrombocytopenia, aplastic anemia, leukemias, lymphoproliferative diseases, hypersplenism, extracorporeal circulation, and in DIC or TTP/HUS (see respective discussions p. 883 and 889)
- Following chemotherapy, posttransfusion thrombocytopenia (develops after 5–10 days)
- Numerous congenital conditions, which may be associated with low platelet counts (see p. 874).

➤ Limitations
- Interference and limitations of testing are more numerous with platelets than with RBC and WBC. Preanalytic errors occur if the blood was not admixed well with anticoagulant upon drawing; as soon as the clotting is activated, the platelets are consumed.
- Platelets cannot be accurately counted after being stored at 4°C for more than 24 hours. In some cases, and for no known reason, the EDTA used for anticoagulation of the CBC may clump platelets, reducing their number. In such situations the blood must be drawn with a different anticoagulant, usually 3.2% sodium citrate. A similar situation resulting in low counts is platelet satellitism (platelet adherence to neutrophils).
- Other sources of error, especially in automated counters, are giant platelet (may be counted as RBC), white cell fragments, very small red cells, or red cell fragments, thought by automated counters to be platelets.

PLEURA, NEEDLE BIOPSY (CLOSED CHEST)

➤ Definition
- A needle biopsy of the pleura is performed whenever the clinician cannot make a diagnosis otherwise.

➤ **Use** (see Chapter 14, Respiratory and Acid-Base Disorders, for more information about pleural effusions)
* Evaluation of lymphocyte-predominant pleural effusion.
* Diagnosis of an exudative pleural effusion that is undiagnosed after cytologic examination (diagnostic in 40–75% of cases).

➤ **Interpretation**
* The test is positive for tumor in ~ 6% of malignant mesotheliomas and ~ 60% of other cases of malignancy.
* The test is positive for tubercles in two thirds of cases on first biopsy, with increased yield on second and third biopsies; therefore, repeat biopsy if suspicious clinically. Acid-fast stain or granulomas can be found in 50–80% of cases, and culture of biopsy material for TB is positive in ≤75% of cases. A fluid culture alone establishes a diagnosis of TB in 25% of cases.

POTASSIUM (K)

➤ **Definition**
* Potassium is a primary intracellular ion; <2% is extracellular. High intracellular concentrations are maintained by the Na-K ATPase pump, which continuously transports potassium into the cell against a concentration gradient.
* This pump is a critical factor in maintaining and adjusting the ionic gradients, on which nerve impulse transmission and contractility of cardiac and skeletal muscle depends.
* In acidemia, potassium moves out of cells; in alkalemia, potassium moves into cells. Hypokalemia inhibits aldosterone production; hyperkalemia stimulates aldosterone production. Plasma sodium and potassium control potassium reabsorption.
* Each 1 mmol/L decrease of serum potassium reflects a total deficit of <200 to 400 mmol; a serum potassium <2 mmol/L may reflect a total deficit >1000 mmol.
* **Normal range:** see Table 2-67

➤ **Use**
* Evaluation of electrolyte balance, cardiac arrhythmia, muscular weakness, hepatic encephalopathy, and renal failure.
* Diagnosis and monitoring hyperkalemia and hypokalemia in various conditions (e.g., treatment of diabetic coma, renal failure, severe fluid and electrolyte loss, effect of certain drugs)
* Diagnosis of familial hyperkalemic periodic paralysis and hypokalemic paralysis

➤ **Interpretation**
Increased In
* Potassium retention
  * GFR <3 to 5 mL/min
    * Oliguria caused by any condition (e.g., renal failure)

TABLE 2-67. Normal Range for Potassium		
From Age	Reference Range (mmol/L)	Critical Range (mmol/L)
0–4 months	4.0 to 6.2	<2.6 >7.5
4 months to 1 year	3.7 to 5.6	<2.6 >7.5
>1 year	3.5 to 5.3	<3.0 >6.2

- Chronic nonoliguric renal failure associated with dehydration, obstruction, trauma, or excess potassium
- Drugs
- Renal toxicity (e.g., amphotericin B, methicillin, tetracycline)
- GFR >20 mL/min
  - Decreased (aldosterone) mineralocorticoid activity
  - Addison disease
  - Hypofunction of renin-angiotensin-aldosterone system
  - Hyporeninemic hypoaldosteronism with renal insufficiency (GFR, 25–75 mL/min)
  - Various drugs (e.g., NSAIDs, ACE inhibitors, cyclosporine, pentamidine)
  - Decreased aldosterone production
  - Pseudohypoaldosteronism
  - Aldosterone antagonist drugs (e.g., spironolactone, captopril, heparin)
- Inhibition of tubular secretion of potassium
  - Drugs (e.g., spironolactone, triamterene, amiloride)
  - Hyperkalemic type of distal renal tubular acidosis (e.g., sickle cell disease, obstructive uropathy)
- Mineralocorticoid-resistant syndromes
  - Primary tubular disorders
  - Hereditary
  - Acquired (e.g., SLE, amyloidosis, sickle cell nephropathy, obstructive uropathy, renal allograft transplant, chloride shift)
- Potassium redistribution
  - Familial hyperkalemic periodic paralysis (Gamstorp disease, adynamia episodica hereditaria)
  - Acute acidosis (especially hyperchloremic metabolic acidosis; less with respiratory; little with metabolic acidosis due to organic acids) (e.g., diabetic ketoacidosis, lactic acidosis, acute renal failure, acute respiratory acidosis)
    - Decreased insulin
    - Beta-adrenergic blockade
    - Drugs (e.g., succinylcholine, great excess of digitalis, arginine infusion)
    - Use of hypertonic solutions (e.g., saline, mannitol)
    - Intravascular hemolysis (e.g., transfusion reaction, hemolytic anemia), rhabdomyolysis
    - Rapid cellular release (e.g., crush injury, chemotherapy for leukemia or lymphoma, burns, major surgery)
- Urinary diversion
  - Ureteral implants into jejunum
  - In neonates—dehydration, hemolysis (e.g., cephalohematoma, intracranial hemorrhage, bruising, exchange transfusion), acute renal failure, CAH, adrenocortical insufficiency

Decreased In
- Excess renal excretion (in patients with hypokalemia, urine potassium, >25 mmol in 24 hours or >15 mmol/L implies at least a renal component)
  - Osmotic diuresis of hyperglycemia (e.g., uncontrolled diabetes)
  - Nephropathies

- Renal tubular acidosis (proximal and especially distal)
- Bartter syndrome
- Liddle syndrome
- Magnesium depletion due to any cause
- Renal vascular disease, malignant hypertension, vasculitis
- Renin-secreting tumors
- Endocrine
  - Hyperaldosteronism (primary, secondary)
  - Cushing syndrome especially caused by ectopic ACTH production
  - CAH
  - Hyperthyroidism (especially in Asian persons)
- Drugs
  - Diuretics (e.g., thiazides, ethacrynic acid, furosemide); assay for diuretics should be done if urine chloride >40 mmol/L
  - Mineralocorticoids (e.g., fluorocortisone)
  - High-dose glucocorticoids
  - High-dose antibiotics (e.g., penicillin, nafcillin, ampicillin, carbenicillin)
  - Substances with mineralocorticoid effect (e.g., glycyrrhizic acid [licorice], carbenoxolone, gossypol)
  - Drugs associated with magnesium depletion (e.g., aminoglycosides, cisplatin, amphotericin B, foscarnet)
- Acute myelogenous, monomyeloblastic, or lymphoblastic leukemia
- Nonrenal causes of excess potassium loss
- In patients with hypokalemia, urine potassium <25 mmol/24 hours <15 mmol/L implies extrarenal loss.
- GI
  - Vomiting
  - Diarrhea (e.g., infections, malabsorption, radiation)
  - Drugs (e.g., laxatives [phenolphthalein], enemas, cancer therapy)
  - Neoplasms (e.g., villous adenoma of colon, pancreatic VIPoma that produces VIP >200 pg/mL, Zollinger-Ellison syndrome)
  - Excessive spitting (sustained expectoration of all saliva in neurotic persons and to induce weight loss in professional wrestlers)
- Skin
  - Excessive sweating
  - CF
  - Extensive burns
  - Draining wounds
- Cellular shifts
  - Respiratory alkalosis
  - Classic periodic paralysis
  - Insulin
  - Drugs (e.g., bronchodilators, decongestants)
  - Accidental ingestion of barium compounds
  - Treatment of severe megaloblastic anemia with vitamin B_{12} or folic acid
  - Physiologic (e.g., highly trained athletes)

- Diet
  - Severe eating disorders (e.g., anorexia nervosa, bulimia)
  - Dietary deficiency
- Delirium tremens
- In neonates—asphyxia, alkalosis, renal tubular acidosis, iatrogenic (glucose and insulin), diuretics
- Major causes of hypokalemia with hypertension:
  - Diuretic drugs (e.g., thiazides)
  - Primary aldosteronism
  - Secondary aldosteronism (renovascular disease, renin-producing tumors)
  - Cushing syndrome
  - Malignant hypertension
  - Renal tubular acidosis

➤ Limitations

- Laboratory artifacts
  - Hemolysis during venipuncture, conditions associated with thrombocytosis or leukocytosis, incomplete separation of serum and clot, double spinning (re-spinning) of blood collection tubes.
  - Arm in upward position while collecting blood
  - Betadine application
  - Laboratory order of draw (lavender top tubes drawn before serum chemistry tubes)
  - Drawing above IV site
  - Vigorously mixed tubes
  - Collection techniques
  - Traumatic draw
  - Pneumatic tube system issues: speed too high, unpadded canisters, excessive agitation
  - Delay in processing
  - Centrifuging at too high G force
  - Increased heat exposure in centrifuge.
  - Chilling whole blood beyond 2 hours
  - Prolonged tourniquet use and hand exercise when drawing blood.
- Potassium value can be elevated ~15% in slight hemolysis (Hb ≤50 mg/dL) and elevated ~30–50% in moderate hemolysis (Hb >100 mg/dL). Therefore, potassium status can be assessed in those with slight hemolysis but not in those with moderate hemolysis.
- Excess dietary intake or rapid potassium infusion
- Drugs with high potassium content (e.g., 1 million units of penicillin G potassium contains 1.7 mmol of potassium)
- Transfusion of old blood

POTASSIUM, URINE

➤ Definition

- Urinary potassium levels are helpful in the evaluation of patients with unexplained hypokalemia, electrolyte and acid–base balance. In the presence of such hypokalemia, urine excretion is helpful to separate renal from nonrenal losses. Excretion <20 mmol/24 hours is evidence that hypokalemia is not from renal loss. Renal loss >50 mmol/L in a hypokalemic, hypertensive patient not on a diuretic may indicate primary or secondary aldosteronism.

- **Normal range:**
  - 24-hour urine:
    - Male:
      - <10 years: 17–54 mmol/day
      - 10–14 years: 22–57 mmol/day
      - >14 years: 25–125 mmol/day
    - Female:
      - 6–10 years: 8–37 mmol/day
      - 10–14 years: 18–58 mmol/day
      - >14 years: 25–125 mmol/day
  - Random urine:
    - Male: 13–116 mmol/g creatinine
    - Female: 8–129 mmol/g creatinine

➤ Use

- Evaluation of patients with unexplained hypokalemia, electrolyte and acid–base balance.

➤ Interpretation

Increased In

- Dehydration
- Primary and secondary aldosteronism
- Diabetic acidosis
- Mercurial and thiazide diuretic administration
- Ammonium chloride administration
- Renal tubular acidosis
- Chronic renal failure
- Starvation
- Cushing syndrome

Decreased In

- Acute renal failure
- Malabsorption
- Chronic potassium deficiency states
- Addison disease
- Severe GN
- Pyelonephritis
- Nephrosclerosis

➤ Limitations

- Urinary potassium may be elevated with dietary (food and/or medicinal) increase, hyperaldosteronism, renal tubular acidosis, onset of alkalosis, and with other disorders.
- Urine chloride is often ordered with sodium and potassium as timed urine. The urinary anion gap $[Na^+ - (Cl^- + HCO_3^-)]$ or $[(Na^+ + K^+) - (Cl^-)]$ is useful in the initial evaluation of hyperchloremic metabolic acidosis.

PREALBUMIN

➤ Definition
- This 54-kDa protein tetramer is synthesized in the liver, choroid plexus, CNS, placenta, intestine, pancreas, and meninges. It contains two binding sites for thyroid hormones T_3 and T_4 and two binding sites for serum retinol-binding protein. These different binding sites do not overlap.
- As a thyroid hormone transport and binding protein, transthyretin binds 10–15% of serum T_3 and T_4 for transport in the blood. In CSF, where there is typically no albumin or thyroglobulin present, transthyretin serves as the only CSF binding protein for T_3 and T_4.
- The presence of high concentrations of transthyretin in the CSF makes it a key indicator of leakage of the CSF into the sinus cavities, eyes, and ears when cranial trauma has occurred.
- Other names: prealbumin (PA), thyroxine-binding prealbumin (TBPA)
- **Normal range:** 18–40 mg/dL

➤ Use
- Evaluation of nutritional status, total parenteral nutrition
- Clinical indicator of liver status

➤ Interpretation
Increased In
- Chronic renal failure
- Hodgkin disease

Decreased In
- Inflammation
- Hepatic dysfunction
- Protein deficiency states
- Cancer
- CF
- Chronic illness

➤ Limitations
- Anabolic steroids, corticosteroids, and androgens increase prealbumin levels.
- Estrogens and oral contraceptives decrease prealbumin levels.

PRENATAL CYTOGENETICS: FLUORESCENCE IN SITU HYBRIDIZATION (FISH) AND CHROMOSOME ANALYSIS

➤ Definition and Use
- **FISH**
  - Analysis of fetal tissue to detect targeted numeric or structural chromosome aberrations.
  - Interphase FISH performed on uncultured cells is used to provide a rapid (1 day) result for targeted chromosome enumeration. Typically, chromosomes 13, 18, 21, X, and Y are assessed. Metaphase FISH performed on cultured cells is used to assess chromosome aberrations too small to be detected by conventional chromosome analysis.
  - Generally used only in cases with specific risk (specific ultrasound anomalies, family history).

- **Chromosome analysis**
  - Analysis of fetal tissue to detect numeric and structural chromosome aberrations. Most chromosome aberrations are numeric (e.g., trisomies 13, 18, 21 [Down syndrome], 45,X [Turner syndrome], 47,XXY [Klinefelter syndrome]).
  - Principle indications:
    - Increased risk determined from maternal screening
    - Ultrasound anomaly
    - Family history of chromosome anomaly (previous affect pregnancy, balanced rearrangement carrier parent)
    - Fetal sexing for history of X-linked disorders

➤ Limitations
- **FISH**
  - Targeted test that assesses only specific region on chromosome; does not ensure entire chromosome is normal and does not assess every chromosome.
  - Mosaicism may also confound results.
- **Chromosome analysis**
  - Analysis cannot detect aberrations smaller than 5–10 megabases; requires cell culture to obtain actively dividing metaphase cells.
  - Mosaicism, the presence of two cell lines, may be difficult to interpret, because chromosome anomalies can arise *in vitro* during specimen culture.

PRENATAL MOLECULAR GENETIC ANALYSIS (PRENATAL DNA ANALYSIS)

➤ Definition
- Molecular testing on fetal DNA to test directly for specific mutations or to assess closely linked markers for an unknown mutation

➤ Use
- To assess mutational status for specific inherited diseases
- Typically performed only when parents are affected or known carriers for disease.

➤ Limitations
- Direct testing assesses only particular targeted mutation(s) of interest
- Linkage analysis, testing of a nearby genetic marker used when the particular mutation is unknown, is limited by potential recombination between the tested marker and the causal mutation.
- Mitochondrial DNA testing may be problematic because the mutated mitochondrial mutation is likely to exist in combination with normal mitochondria (heteroplasmy).

PRETRANSFUSION COMPATIBILITY TESTING

➤ Definition and Use
- Demonstration of RBC antigen–antibody reactions is the foundation for pretransfusion compatibility testing and key to immunohematology. Agglutination is the endpoint for most

tests for antibody detection and cross-match. Increased genetic knowledge has added a new approach to blood antigen typing, based on DNA sequence determination. The tests described in this chapter are based on classical agglutination methodology.

* Three major requirements must be satisfied for safe RBC transfusions:
  * The RBCs to be transfused must be ABO compatible
  * RhD-positive RBCs should not be given to women of phenotype RhD-negative
  * Transfused RBCs should lack blood group antigens reactive with any preexisting clinically significant antibodies that the recipient may have.
* To achieve these objectives, pretransfusion compatibility testing begins with the type-and-screen procedure that starts with determining the recipient's major blood groups, ABO and Rh. Safe transfusion can be ensured for most recipients by the correct typing of patients and donors with respect to ABO and Rh phenotype and screening the patient's serum for the presence of clinically significant antibodies directed against antigens polymorphic in the local population (see p. 119). If an antibody is detected by the antibody screen, an antibody identification panel must be performed. Antibodies to the ABO antigens are naturally occurring and are used to determine a person's ABO blood group.

➤ ABO Typing

* Each donation intended for transfusion must be tested for ABO and D (the major Rh determinant) antigens.
* A type A individual has anti-B but not anti-A antibodies. A type B individual has anti-A but not anti-B antibodies. A type AB individual has neither anti-A nor anti-B antibodies. The serum of type O persons contains antibodies that have reactivity against both A and B antigens, so-called anti-A, anti-B antibodies. There are two ways to test the ABO phenotype:
  * Forward (or front) typing tests the RBC with commercial reagents containing anti-A_1 and anti-B antibodies. The strength of the agglutination is graded.
  * Reverse (or back) typing tests serum with commercial RBC reagents carrying various known red cell antigens.

➤ Rh Typing

* The major clinical consequence of Rh immunization is the development of hemolytic disease of the newborn (see p. 812).
* The CDE terminology is the most commonly used one. It is based on the finding of three sets of closely linked genes: D and d, C and c, and E and e. Five blood typing reagents are available: anti-D, anti-C, anti-E, anti-c, and anti-e. (Routine pretransfusion tests include only tests for D.) In practice, the terms Rh-positive and Rh-negative, respectively, refer to the presence or absence of the D antigen. The procedures are similar to those described above for ABO typing. Antibodies to Rh antigens are immune-stimulated in most cases, mostly following pregnancy or transfusion. The most potent immunogens are D, followed by C and E.
* Some patients may not show clear agglutination after centrifugation with anti-D but still have the D antigen. This is known as weak D and requires incubation or addition of antihuman globulin serum for identification of the D antigen. These patients are still considered Rh positive.
* Limitations include:
  * Acquired antigens, such as acquired A antigens in group B individuals
  * Forward and reverse typing discrepancies. When they occur, the cause must be immediately investigated. The most common cause is in a patient who belongs to a subgroup A and

who has formed anti-A_1 antibodies (80% of A patients are subgroup A_1). Most of the remainder are A_2 (or A_2B) and may develop reciprocal antibodies, especially anti A_1.
* Warm autoantibodies
* Cold autoantibodies
* Recent transfusions
* Transplant patients

➤ Antibody Screening
* Antibody screening is used to detect the presence of unexpected alloantibodies in the recipient's serum, directed against non-ABO blood group antigens, such as Kell, Duffy, and Kid. This is accomplished by using commercial panels of two or three group O RBCs of known, but varied non-ABO composition.
* Antibody screening is crucial for detecting weak antibodies that may be missed on cross-match alone. If agglutination or hemolysis is detected in the antibody screen test, the antibody must be identified and antigen-negative RBCs selected for transfusion.

➤ Cross-Matching
* The cross-match assay involves testing the patients' serum with donor RBC taken from a segment attached to the selected blood unit. Unless there is a very urgent need for blood, cross-matching is mandatory. The method used must be able to demonstrate ABO incompatibility and clinically significant antibodies to RBC antigens.
* In patients in whom no antibodies have been detected by antibody screening and have no history of RBC alloantibodies, random units of the ABO and Rh type can be selected and an abbreviated cross-match may be sufficient. When antibodies are detected, or there is a positive history of alloimmunization, antigen-negative donor units must be selected, and the crossmatch must be carried through the antiglobulin test.

➤ Suggested Readings
Anstee DJ. Red cell genotyping and the future of pretransfusion testing. *Blood*. 2009;114:248–256.
Petrides M, Stack G. *Practical Guide to Transfusion Medicine*. 2nd ed. Bethesda, Md: AABB Press; 2007.

PROGESTERONE

➤ Definition
* Hormone synthesized by ovary; low in follicular phase but increases to 10–40 mg/day during luteal phase and $\leq$300 mg/day if pregnancy occurs.
* **Normal range:** see Table 2-68

➤ Use
* Detection of ovulation in the evaluation of the function of the corpus luteum.
* Monitoring patients having ovulation during induction with hCG, human menopausal gonadotropin, FSH/LH-releasing hormone, or clomiphene
* To evaluate patients at risk for early abortion

➤ Interpretation
Increased In
* Luteal phase of menstrual cycle
* Luteal cysts of ovary; ovarian tumors (e.g., arrhenoblastoma)

TABLE 2-68. Normal Ranges of Progesterone

Reference Group	n	Mean (ng/mL)	Range (ng/mL)
Male	50	0.36	0.14–2.06
Female			
Mid-follicular phase	14	0.69	0.31–1.52
Mid-luteal phase	13	11.42	5.16–18.56
Postmenopausal	49	0.25	<0.08–0.78
Pregnancy			
First trimester	34	22.17	4.73–50.74
Second trimester	29	29.73	19.41–45.30

- Adrenal tumors
- CAH caused by 21-hydroxylase, 17-hydroxylase, and 11-beta hydroxylase
- Molar pregnancy

Decreased In
- Amenorrhea
- Threatened abortion (some patients)
- Fetal death
- Toxemia of pregnancy
- Gonadal agenesis

PROINSULIN

➤ Definition
- Enzymatic process forms insulin in pancreatic secretory granules of beta cells. Proinsulin level is normally ≤20% of total insulin.
- Proinsulin is included in the immunoassay of total insulin and separation requires special technique.
- **Normal range:** 2.0–2.6 pmol/L

➤ Use
- Proinsulin: Insulin ratio is used as an indirect marker of beta cell function.

➤ Interpretation
- Insulinoma tumor may secrete predominantly insulin or proinsulin.
- Proinsulin >30% of serum insulin after overnight fast suggests insulinoma.
- Proinsulin is increased in factitious hypoglycemia due to sulfonylurea
- Proinsulin is increased in familial hyperproinsulinemia—heterozygous mutation affecting cleavage of proinsulin leading to secretion of excess amounts of proinsulin
- Type 2 DM

➤ Limitations
- Proinsulin may also be increased in renal disease.
- Elevation of proinsulin: insulin ratio correlates with a decreased acute illness response to glucose in patients with type 2 DM.

PROLACTIN

➤ Definition
* Prolactin is a single chain polypeptide composed of 198 amino acids and is secreted by the anterior cells of the pituitary gland. Prolactin secretion is controlled by the hypothalamus primarily through the release of prolactin inhibiting factor (dopamine) and prolactin releasing factor (serotonin). TRH stimulates prolactin secretion and is useful as a provocative test to evaluate prolactin reserves and abnormal secretion of prolactin by the pituitary.
* The primary physiologic function of prolactin is to stimulate and maintain lactation in women.
* **Normal range:**
  * Males: 2.64–13.13 μg/L
  * Females <50 years (premenopausal): 3.34–26.72 μg/L
  * Females >50 years (postmenopausal): 2.74–19.64 μg/L

➤ Use
* Aiding in evaluation of pituitary tumors, amenorrhea, galactorrhea, infertility, and hypogonadism
* Monitoring therapy of prolactin-producing tumors

➤ Interpretation
Increased In
* Amenorrhea/galactorrhea
  * 10–25% of women with galactorrhea and normal menses
  * 10–15% of women with amenorrhea without galactorrhea
  * 75% of women with both galactorrhea and amenorrhea/oligomenorrhea
  * Cause of 15–30% of cases of amenorrhea in young women
* Pituitary lesions (e.g., prolactinoma, section of pituitary stalk, empty sella syndrome, 20–40% of patients with acromegaly, ≤80% of patients with chromophobe adenomas); concentrations are usually >200 ng/mL.
* Hypothalamic lesions (e.g., sarcoidosis, eosinophilic granuloma, histiocytosis X, TB, glioma, craniopharyngioma); concentrations are usually >200 ng/mL.
* Other endocrine diseases:
  * ~20% of cases of hypothyroidism (second most common cause of hyperprolactinemia). Therefore serum TSH and T-4 should always be measured.
  * Addison disease
  * Polycystic ovaries
  * Glucocorticoid excess—normal or moderately elevated prolactin
* Ectopic production of prolactin (e.g., bronchogenic carcinoma, renal cell carcinoma, ovarian teratomas, acute myeloid leukemia)
* Children with sexual precocity—may be increased into pubertal range
* Neurogenic causes (e.g., nursing and breast stimulation, spinal cord lesions, chest wall lesions such as herpes zoster)
* Stress (e.g., surgery, hypoglycemia, vigorous exercise, seizures)
* Pregnancy (increases to 8–20 times normal by delivery, returns to normal 2–4 weeks postpartum unless nursing occurs)

- Lactation
- Chronic renal failure (20–40% of cases; becomes normal after successful renal transplant but not after hemodialysis)
- Liver failure (due to decreased prolactin clearance)
- Idiopathic causes (some probably represent early cases of microadenoma too small to be detected by CT scan)
  - Drugs—most common cause; usually subsides a few weeks after cessation of using drug; these concentrations are usually 20–100 ng/mL
    - Neuroleptics (e.g., phenothiazines, thioxanthenes, butyrophenones)
    - Antipsychotic drugs (e.g., Compazine, Thorazine, Stelazine, Mellaril, Haldol)
    - Dopamine antagonists (e.g., Metoclopramide, Sulpiride)
    - Opiates (morphine, methadone)
    - Reserpine
    - Alpha-methyldopa (Aldomet)
    - Estrogens and oral contraceptives
    - Thyrotropin-releasing hormone
    - Amphetamines
    - Isoniazid

Decreased In
- Hypopituitarism: postpartum pituitary necrosis (Sheehan syndrome), idiopathic hypogo-nadotropic hypogonadism
- Drugs
  - Dopamine agonists
  - Ergot derivatives (bromocriptine mesylate, lisuride hydrogen maleate)
  - Levodopa, apomorphine, clonidine

➤ Limitations
- Normal prolactin secretion varies with time, which results in serum prolactin levels 2–3 times higher at night than during the day.
- The biologic half-life of prolactin is approximately 20–50 minutes. Serum prolactin levels during the menstrual cycle are variable and commonly exhibit slight elevations during the mid-cycle.
- Prolactin levels in normal individuals tend to rise in response to physiologic stimuli including sleep, exercise, nipple stimulation, sexual intercourse, hypoglycemia, pregnancy, and surgical stress.
- Prolactin values that exceed the reference values may be due to macroprolactin (prolactin bound to immunoglobulin). Macroprolactin should be evaluated if signs and symptoms of hyperprolactinemia are absent or pituitary imaging studies are not informative.

PROSTATE SPECIFIC ANTIGEN (PSA), TOTAL AND FREE

➤ Definition
- PSA is a glycoprotein that is expressed by both normal and neoplastic prostate tissue and is prostate tissue specific and not prostate cancer specific. PSA is consistently expressed in nearly all prostate cancers, although its level of expression on a per cell basis is lower than in normal prostate epithelium. The absolute value of serum PSA is useful for determining the

TABLE 2-69. Normal Range	
PSA Total: <4 ng/mL	
Probability of Cancer	**PSA Total Levels**
1%	0–2 ng/mL
15%	2–4 ng/mL
25%	4–10 ng/mL
>50%	>10 ng/mL
PSA Free: >25% of Total PSA	
Probability of Cancer	**Percent Free PSA**
56%	0–10%
28%	10–15%
20%	15–20%
16%	20–25%
8%	>25%

extent of prostate cancer and assessing the response to prostate cancer treatment; its use as a screening method to detect prostate cancer is also common, although controversial.

- PSA exists primarily as three forms in serum. One form of PSA is enveloped by the protease inhibitor, alpha-2 macroglobulin, and has been shown to lack immunoreactivity. A second form is complexed to another protease inhibitor, alpha-1 antichymotrypsin (ACT). The third form of PSA is not complexed to a protease inhibitor, and is termed "free PSA." The latter two forms are immunologically detectable in commercially available PSA assays and are referred to collectively as "total PSA."

- Free PSA values alone have not been shown to be effective in patient management and should not be used. Both total PSA and free PSA concentrations should be determined on the same serum specimen and used to calculate the percentage of free PSA. Percent free PSA values are then used for patient management.

$$\frac{\text{free PSA (ng/mL)}}{\text{total PSA (ng/mL)}} \times 100\% = \text{percent free PAS}$$

- **Normal range:** see Table 2-69

➤ Use
- Monitoring patients with a history of prostate cancer as an early indicator of recurrence and response to treatment
- Prostate cancer screening

➤ Interpretation
*Increased In**
- Prostate diseases
  - Cancer
  - Prostatitis, 5–7 times

---

*Transient increases return to normal in 2–6 weeks.

- Benign prostatic hyperplasia
- Prostatic ischemia
- Acute urinary retention 5–7 times
- Manipulations
  - Prostatic massage, ≤2 times
  - Cystoscopy: 4 times
  - Needle biopsy: >50 times for ≤1 month
  - Transurethral resection: >50 times
  - Digital rectal examination increases PSA significantly if initial value is >20 ng/mL and is not a confusing factor in falsely elevating PSA
  - Radiation therapy
  - Indwelling catheter
  - Vigorous bicycle exercise: ≤2–3 times several days
- Treadmill stress test: no change
- Drugs (e.g., testosterone)
- Physiologic fluctuations: ≤30%
- PSA has no circadian rhythm but 6–7% variation can occur between specimens collected on same day.
- Ambulatory values are higher than sedentary values which may decrease ≤50% (mean = 18%).
- Ejaculation causes transient increase <1.0 ng/mL for 48 hours.
- Analytic factors
  - Different assays yield different values
  - Antibody cross-reactivity
  - High titer heterophile antibodies
- Other diseases/organs
  - Also found in small amounts in other cancers (sweat and salivary glands, breast, colon, lung, ovary) and in Skene's glands of female urethra and in term placenta
  - Acute renal failure
  - Acute myocardial infarction

Decreased In
- Ejaculation within 24–48 hours
- Castration
- Antiandrogen drugs (e.g., finasteride)
- Radiation therapy
- Prostatectomy
- PSA falls 17% in 3 days after lying in hospital
- Artifactual (e.g., improper specimen collection; very high PSA levels)
- Finasteride (5-α-reductase inhibitor) reduces PSA by 50% after 6 months in men without cancer

➤ Limitations
- PSA has been recommended by the American Cancer Society for use in conjunction with a DRE for the early detection of prostate cancer starting at age 50 years for men with at least a 10 year life expectancy. Men at high risk, such as those of African descent or with a family history of the disease, may begin testing at an earlier age.

- PSA levels that are measured repeatedly over time may vary both because of imprecision in the analysis and biologic variability where the true PSA level in a given man is different on different measurements. This could potentially lead to an apparent rise in PSA level, when no actual rise had occurred.
- It is highly recommended that the same assay method be used for longitudinal monitoring.
- A change in PSA of >30% in men with a PSA initially below 2.0 ng/mL was likely to indicate a true change beyond normal random variation.
- The acceptable PSA levels are less clear after radiation therapy, where values may not reach undetectable concentrations. With a nadir of <0.5 ng/mL, relapse is not likely with 5 years of treatment. Biochemical recurrence has been defined by the ASTRO as three consecutive increases in PSA above the nadir.
- The 5-α-reductase inhibitor drugs may affect PSA levels in some patients. Other drugs used to treat benign prostatic hyperplasia may also affect PSA levels. Drugs that decrease PSA levels include buserelin, finasteride, and flutamide. Care should be taken in interpreting results from patients taking these drugs.

PROTEIN (TOTAL), SERUM

➤ Definition
- Total serum protein is the sum of the concentration of the circulating proteins. A total serum protein test is a blood test that measures the amounts of total protein, albumin, and globulin in the blood.
- The amounts of albumin and globulin also are compared (albumin/globulin ratio). Normally, there is a little more albumin than globulin, and the ratio is >1. A ratio <1 or much >1 can give clues about problems in the body.
- **Normal range:**
  - 0–7 days: 4.6–7.0 g/dL
  - 7 days to 1 year: 4.4–7.5 g/dL
  - 1–3 years: 5.5–7.5 g/dL
  - 3 years to adult: 6.0–8.0 g/dL

➤ Use
- Diagnosis and treatment of diseases involving the liver, kidney, or bone marrow, as well as other metabolic or nutritional disorders
- Screening for nutritional deficiencies and gammopathies

➤ Interpretation
Increased In
- Hypergammaglobulinemias (monoclonal or polyclonal; see following sections)
- Hypovolemic states

Decreased In
- Nutritional deficiency (e.g., malabsorption, Kwashiorkor, marasmus)
- Decreased or ineffective protein synthesis (e.g., severe liver disease, agammaglobulinemia)
- Increased loss

- Renal (e.g., nephrotic syndrome)
- GI disease (e.g., protein-losing enteropathies, surgical resection)
- Severe skin disease (e.g., burns, pemphigus vulgaris, eczema)
- Blood loss, plasmapheresis
- Increased catabolism (e.g., fever, inflammation, hyperthyroidism, malignancy, chronic diseases)
- Dilutional (e.g., IV fluids, SIADH, water intoxication)
- Third trimester of pregnancy.

➤ Limitations

- Falsely elevated proteins (pseudohyperproteinemia) can be caused by hemoconcentration due to dehydration or sample desiccation.
- Upright posture for several hours after rising increases total proteins and several other analytes

PROTEIN (TOTAL), URINE

➤ Definition

- Normal urine contains up to 150 mg (1–14 mg/dL) of protein each day. This protein originates from ultrafiltration of plasma.
- Presence of increased amounts of proteins in urine is termed as proteinuria and is the first indication of renal disease. Proteinuria can be classified into three types:
  - Prerenal: overflow proteinuria, with an increase in plasma, low–molecular-weight proteins spill into urine (normal proteins, acute phase reactants, light chain immunoglobulins)
  - Renal
    - Glomerular proteinuria: defective glomerular filtration barrier. This could be selective or nonselective to different proteins.
    - Tubular proteinuria: defective tubular reabsorption; increase in low–molecular-weight proteins.
  - Postrenal: proteins produced by the urinary tract; during inflammation, malignancy; or injury
- **Normal range:**
  - 24-hour urine: <150 mg/day
  - Random urine: <200 mg/g creatinine

➤ Use

Evaluation of proteinuria (see Table 2-70) (e.g., following urinalysis in which proteinuria is detected)

- Evaluation of renal diseases, including proteinuria complicating DM and the nephrotic syndromes.
- Work-up of other renal diseases, including malignant hypertension, GN, TTP, collagen diseases, toxemia of pregnancy, drug nephrotoxicity, hypersensitivity reactions, and allergic reactions and renal tubular lesions
- Management of myeloma and evaluation of hypoproteinemia.

➤ Interpretation
Increased In

- Nephrotic syndrome
- Diabetic neuropathy

TABLE 2-70. National Kidney Foundation Guidelines for Assessment of Proteinuria

- Guidelines for adults and children
  - Under most circumstances, untimed (spot) urine samples should be used to detect and monitor proteinuria in children and adults.
  - It is usually not necessary to obtain a timed urine collection (overnight or 24-hour) for these evaluations in either children or adults.
  - First morning specimens are preferred, but random specimens are acceptable if first morning specimens are not available.
  - In most cases, screening with urine dipsticks is acceptable for detecting proteinuria:
    - Standard urine dipsticks are acceptable for detecting increased total urine protein.
    - Albumin specific dipsticks are acceptable for detecting albuminuria.
  - Patients with a positive dipstick test (1+ or greater) should undergo confirmation of proteinuria by a quantitative measurement (protein-to-creatinine ratio or albumin-to-creatinine ratio) within 3 months.
  - Patients with two or more positive quantitative tests temporally spaced by 1–2 weeks should be diagnosed as having persistent proteinuria and undergo further evaluation and management for chronic kidney disease.
  - Monitoring proteinuria in patients with chronic kidney disease should be performed using quantitative measurements.
- Specific guidelines for adults
  - When screening adults at increased risk for chronic kidney disease, albumin should be measured in a spot urine sample using either:
    - Albumin specific dipstick
    - Albumin-to-creatinine ratio
  - When monitoring proteinuria in adults with chronic kidney disease, the protein-to-creatinine ratio in spot urine samples should be measured using:
    - Albumin-to-creatinine ratio
    - Total protein-to-creatinine ratio is acceptable if albumin-to-creatinine ratio is high (>500 to 1000 mg/g)
- Specific guidelines for children without diabetes
  - When screening children for chronic kidney disease, total urine protein should be measured in a spot urine sample using either:
    - Standard urine dipstick
    - Total protein-to-creatinine ratio
  - Orthostatic proteinuria must be excluded by repeat measurement on a first morning specimen if the initial finding of proteinuria was obtained on a random specimen.
  - When monitoring proteinuria in children with chronic kidney disease, the total protein-to-creatinine ratio should be measured in spot urine specimens.
- Specific guidelines for children with diabetes
  - Screening and monitoring of postpubertal children with diabetes of 5 or more years of duration should follow the guidelines for adults.
  - Screening and monitoring other children with diabetes should follow the guidelines for children without diabetes.

Source: http://www.kidney.org/professionals/kdoqi/guidelines_ckd/p5_lab_g5.htm

- Monoclonal gammopathies such as multiple myeloma and other myeloproliferative or lymphoproliferative disorders.
- Abnormal renal tubular absorption.
  - Fanconi syndrome
  - Heavy metal poisoning
  - Sickle cell disease
- Urinary tract malignancies
- Inflammatory, degenerative, and irritative conditions of the lower urinary tract
- After exercise

➤ **Limitations**
- Highly alkaline urine produces false-negative results.
- Not reliable to quantify urinary immunoglobulin light chains.

PROTEIN C

➤ **Definition**
- Protein C is a vitamin-K dependent coagulation inhibitor which, in its activated form, activated protein C (APC), downregulates the activity of factors V and VIII through proteolysis. It is produced mainly in the liver. Congenital deficiency leads to a high incidence of venous thrombosis. Because of its short half-life, measured in hours, initiation of vitamin K antagonist therapy results in very rapid decline in the protein C level in normal individuals. In heterozygous individuals, such therapy may lead to very low levels of protein C activity—approaching 0%, with a high risk for venous thrombosis and coumarin necrosis.
- **Normal range:** 70–140%

➤ **Use**
- Protein C functional level is examined in cases of suspected congenital thrombophilia, such as patients with unprovoked venous thromboembolism, especially when in unusual sites.
- Determination of protein C antigen discriminates between type 1 protein C deficiency (concordant decrease of functional and immunologic assays) and type II deficiency, where the antigen level is normal. This difference has no known clinical implication.

➤ **Interpretation**
Increased In
- Diabetes
- Nephrotic syndrome
- Ischemic heart disease
- Pregnancy
- Oral contraceptives
- Heparin therapy
- Increased age

Decreased In
- Congenital heterozygous deficiency of protein C, which is an autosomal trait with variable penetrance, with a prevalence of 1/500 individuals of European descent. Homozygous deficiency results in life-threatening massive thromboses in neonates (purpura fulminans).

* Acquired: liver disease; vitamin K deficiency or use of vitamin K antagonists, L-Asparaginase therapy, DIC, acute phase reaction (thrombotic, inflammatory, surgical)

➤ **Limitations**

* Highly elevated factor VIII levels falsely lower protein C measurements
* Lupus anticoagulant may falsely elevate reported protein C levels

PROTEIN S

➤ **Definition**

* Protein S is a plasma protein synthesized in the liver and dependent on vitamin K for its functionality. It has an anticoagulant function, serving as a cofactor for activated protein C. Together they inhibit the activities of activated factors V and VIII.
* Protein S circulates in a free form, free protein S (about 40% of the protein), where the major co-factor function resides, and as bound to complement C4b, bound protein S. The bound form may also play a role in the natural anticoagulation mechanism, this possibility being under active investigation.
* **Normal range:** "free" or "total"
* Free protein S (measured functionally): 60–140% in males, slightly lower in females but increases with age
* Total protein S (measured as antigen by enzyme immunoassay): 60–140%, lower in females but increases with age
* During the first year of life, the total PS is low (free PS level is identical with that of adults). Adult levels of total PS are reached by 1 year of life.

➤ **Use**

* Protein S, both free and total, should be requested in patients with unprovoked venous thrombosis (see p. 883).
* Protein S should not be performed in patients on vitamin K antagonist therapy. It is necessary to wait for 2 weeks after cessation of therapy
* It is advisable to request protein S together with protein C, because both are affected by therapy with vitamin K antagonists, but they have different half-lives. Comparing the two facilitates the interpretation.
* If the functional assay for free protein S is decreased, an immunoassay for free protein S is recommended for confirmation.

➤ **Interpretation**
Decreased In

* Congenital condition. Prevalence of the congenital deficiency of protein S is 1 in 500 for the Caucasian population. It predisposes to venous thromboembolism. The rare homozygous type may cause severe neonatal purpura fulminans.
  * Acquired: oral anticoagulants or vitamin K deficiency; pregnancy, hormone replacement therapy, oral contraceptives; young age; liver disease; acute-phase reaction situations (decreased free protein S but increased total protein S); proteinuria; DIC; L-asparaginase therapy

➤ **Limitations**

* Very elevated (>250%) factor VIII decreases the activity of protein S
* High titers of rheumatoid factor may lead to overestimation of protein S

* Heparin (up to 1 IU/mL), high bilirubin, or hemolyzed blood do not interfere with measurements, but elevated values may be seen artificially during high dose heparin therapy

PROTEIN, CEREBROSPINAL FLUID

➤ Definition
* CSF protein concentration is one of the most sensitive indicators of pathology within the CNS.
* **Normal range:** 15–45 mg/dL

➤ Use
* To detect increased permeability of the blood–brain barrier to plasma proteins
* To detect increased intrathecal production of immunoglobulins

➤ Interpretation
Increased In
* Bacterial meningitis
* Brain tumor
* Brain abscess
* Aseptic meningitis
* Multiple sclerosis
* Cerebral hemorrhage
* Epilepsy
* Acute alcoholism
* Neurosyphilis

Decreased In
* Repeated lumbar puncture or a chronic leak, in which CSF is lost at a higher than normal rate
* Some children between the ages of 6 months and 2 years
* Acute water intoxication
* Minority of patients with idiopathic intracranial hypertension

➤ Limitations
* CSF protein levels do not fall in hypoproteinemia.
* The normal reference ranges is somewhat technique-dependent and vary from laboratory to laboratory.
* Excessive amounts of CSF proteins are seen in Froin syndrome, clotted specimens, xanthochromia, or the presence of free blood.
* In premature infants, values >130 mg/dL may occasionally be observed.

PROTHROMBIN G20210A MOLECULAR MUTATION ASSAY

➤ Definition
* The prothrombin mutation *20210G>A* in the *F2* gene is associated with increased plasma prothrombin levels and an increased risk of venous thrombosis. Heterozygosity for the

prothrombin *20210G>A* mutation is associated with an approximately threefold increased risk of venous thrombosis. Homozygosity for this mutation is rare, but the associated risk of venous thrombosis is likely to be higher than the heterozygous risk.
* Other factors can further increase the risk of thrombosis.
* **Normal values:** negative or no mutations are found

➤ Use
* Prothrombin G20210A testing should be performed in the following cases:
  * A first venous thrombotic embolism (VTE) before age 50 years
  * A first unprovoked VTE at any age
  * A history of recurrent VTE
  * Venous thrombosis at unusual sites such as the cerebral, mesenteric, portal, or hepatic veins
  * VTE during pregnancy or the puerperium
  * VTE associated with the use of oral contraceptives or hormone replacement therapy
  * A first VTE at any age in an individual with a first-degree family member with a VTE before age 50 years
  * Women with unexplained fetal loss after 10 weeks of gestation
* Prothrombin G20210A testing may be considered in the following cases:
  * Women with unexplained early onset severe preeclampsia, placental abruption, or significant intrauterine growth retardation
  * A first VTE related to tamoxifen or other selective estrogen receptor modulators (SERM)
  * Female smokers younger than 50 years with a myocardial infarction
  * Individuals older than age 50 years with a first provoked VTE in the absence of malignancy or an intravascular device
  * Asymptomatic adult family members of probands with one or two known prothrombin *G20210A* alleles, especially those with a strong family history of VTE at a young age
  * Asymptomatic female family members of probands with known prothrombin thrombophilia who are pregnant or who are considering oral contraception or pregnancy
  * Women with recurrent unexplained first-trimester loss with or without second- or third-trimester loss
  * Children with arterial thrombosis

➤ Limitations
* The results of a genetic test may be affected by DNA rearrangements, blood transfusion, bone marrow transplantation, or other rare events.

PROTHROMBIN TIME (PT) AND THE INTERNATIONAL NORMALIZED RATIO (INR)

➤ Definition
* The PT assesses the coagulation activity of the extrinsic and common coagulation pathways.
* Tissue thromboplastin (tissue factor) is used as a potent activator of the coagulation system in the presence of added calcium. Currently, recombinant tissue factor is used in most commercial reagents. The potency of tissue factor explains the shortness of clotting (in seconds) in the assay.

- **Normal ranges:**
  - PT: 9.6–12.4 seconds (may vary slightly from laboratory to laboratory)
  - INR: 1.0 ratio (remains constant independent of equipment or reagent used)

➤ Use

- Evaluation of clotting disorders that may involve the extrinsic coagulation mechanism (factor VII) and the common pathway (factors II, V, X and fibrinogen). In these situations the PTT should be ordered in parallel with the PT. PT is not sensitive to clotting factors if they are modestly decreased (>30%). In addition, it is not sensitive to abnormalities in factors involved in the intrinsic coagulation pathway (factors XII, XI, IX, and VIII) or in protein C or S deficiencies.
- Evaluation of liver function reflecting abnormalities in factors VII, II, X, and V (but not VIII).
- To monitor long-term oral anticoagulant therapy with coumarin and indanedione derivatives. PT is prolonged >PTT, and more consistently so. Factor V is not affected by oral anticoagulants, whereas it may be decreased in liver disease.
  - INR is the preferred reporting to monitor patients on oral anticoagulant therapy. For all other uses, the use of PT is encouraged rather than INR. The recommended range for INR during most indications for oral anticoagulants is 2–3, or 2.5–3.5 for patients with mechanical heart valves.

➤ Interpretation

- Marked prolongation of the PT in liver disease indicates advanced disease.
- Marked elevation of INR in patients receiving oral anticoagulants is a marker of excessive anticoagulation and requires prompt action Contrariwise, an INR below 2.0 reflects insufficient anticoagulation.
- Combined abnormal PT and PTT is found under two circumstances:
  - Medical: administration of oral anticoagulants, DIC, liver disease, vitamin K deficiency, massive transfusions
  - Coagulation factor abnormalities: dysfibrinogenemias; factors V, X, and II defects

➤ Limitations

- Preanalytic errors:
  - Partially clotted specimens due to poor mixture with the anticoagulant (3.2 sodium citrate, as offered by manufacturers' blue top vacuum tubes)
  - Over- or underfilled test tubes, altering the ratio of blood (9 parts) to anticoagulant (1 part)
- Analytic errors: Hemolyzed, lipemic, or icteric plasma may interfere with photoelectric measuring instruments (assay may have to be repeated on a mechanical clot measuring instrument)

PYRUVATE KINASE (PK), RED BLOOD CELL

➤ Definition

- PK is an enzyme involved in glycolysis. Genetic defects of this enzyme cause the disease known as PK deficiency. This deficiency is one of the most common enzymatic defects of the erythrocyte.
- The disorder manifests clinically as a hemolytic anemia, and the symptomatology is less severe than hematologic indices indicate. The clinical severity of this disorder varies widely,

ranging from a mildly compensated anemia to severe anemia of childhood. Most affected individuals do not require treatment. Individuals who are most severely affected may die in utero of anemia or may require blood transfusions or splenectomy, but most of the symptomatology is limited to early life and to times of physiologic stress or infection.
* **Normal range:** 9.0–22.0 U/g Hb

➤ Use
* Evaluation of nonspherocytic hemolytic anemia
* Investigating families with PK deficiency to determine inheritance pattern and for genetic counseling

➤ Interpretation
* Increased in patients with younger erythrocyte population
* Decreased in congenital nonspherocytic hemolytic anemia

➤ Limitations
* Patients who have recently received transfusions have normal donor cells that may mask PK-deficient erythrocytes.
* Most PK deficient patients have 5–25% of normal activity.

QUANTITATIVE PILOCARPINE IONTOPHORESIS SWEAT TEST

➤ Definition
* The sweat test consists of the quantitative analyses of sweat chloride with or without sodium. This procedure, often referred to as the quantitative pilocarpine iontophoresis test, involves collection and quantification of sweat after pilocarpine iontophoresis with the use of gauze, filter paper or Macroduct coils and quantitative analyses of sweat chloride.
* The sweat test entails three consecutive procedures: sweat stimulation; sweat collection; and sweat analysis.
* **Normal range** (sweat chloride):
  * <40 mmol/L (>3 months)
  * <30 mmol/L (<3 months)
* **Borderline results:** sweat chloride 40–60 mmol/L
* A positive test is defined by sweat chloride >60 mmol/L in sweat from both arms, provided that a minimum of 15 μL of sweat is obtained from each site.

➤ Use
* Standard test for the diagnosis of CF

➤ Interpretation
Increased In
* CF (see Table 2-71)
* Endocrine disorders (e.g., untreated adrenal insufficiency, hypothyroidism, vasopressin-resistant diabetes insipidus, familial hypoparathyroidism, pseudohypoaldosteronism)
* Metabolic disorders (e.g., malnutrition, glycogen storage disease type I, MPS I H (Hurler syndrome), MPS I S, (Scheie syndrome), fucosidosis)
* GU disorders (e.g., Klinefelter syndrome, nephrosis)

TABLE 2-71. Sweat Values in Cystic Fibrosis (mEq/L)

	Chloride		Sodium		Potassium	
	Mean	Range	Mean	Range	Mean	Range
Cystic Fibrosis	115	79–148	111	75–145	23	14–30
Normal	28	8–43	28	16–46	10	6–17

* Allergic/immunologic disorders (e.g., hypogammaglobulinemia, prolonged infusion with prostaglandin E_1, atopic dermatitis)
* Neuropsychologic disorders (e.g., anorexia nervosa)
* Others (e.g., ectodermal dysplasia, G6PD deficiency)

Decreased In

* False-negative results if patient is edematous or if an inadequate quantity of sweat is collected and analyzed
* Methodologic and technical errors

➤ Limitations

* Values may be increased to CF range in healthy persons when sweat rate is rapid (e.g., exercise, high temperature) but pilocarpine test does not increase sweating rate.
* Mineralocorticoids decrease sodium concentration in sweat by ~50% in normal subjects and 10–20% in CF patients whose final sodium concentration remains abnormally high.
* Confirmation of a diagnosis of CF requires two positive sweat tests done on different days. Borderline results should be reported with the suggestion that the test be repeated if clinically indicated.
* The preferred patient age for testing is after 48 hours. During the first 24 hours after birth, sweat electrolytes are transiently elevated and rapidly decline on the second day. Therefore, sweat testing should not be performed within 48 hours after birth.

➤ Suggested Readings

Boat TF, Acton JD. Cystic fibrosis. In: Kliegman RM, Behrman RE, Jenson HB, Stanton BF, eds. *Nelson Textbook of Pediatrics.* 18th ed. Philadelphia: Saunders Elsevier; 2007;1803–1817.

Farrell PM, Rosenstein BJ, White TB, et al. Guidelines for diagnosis of cystic fibrosis in newborns through older adults: Cystic fibrosis consensus report. *J Pediatr.* 2008;153(2):S4-S14.

RED BLOOD CELLS (RBCs): COUNT AND MORPHOLOGY

➤ Definition and Use

* The RBC count is part of the CBC as obtained by automated counters.
* It is less useful than the Hb or Hct.
* **Normal range:** 4.2–5.4 cells/µL in women and 4.4–6.0 cells/µL in men (reported by automated counters in a random adult population)
  * Different values are reported for newborns, infants, and children until they reach adulthood.
  * Automated counters adjust normal values for age groups.

➤ Interpretation
• The RBC count is interpreted in conjunction with red cell indices, hemoglobin, and hematocrit.

Increased In
• Certain myeloproliferative neoplasms (e.g., polycythemia vera [see p. 836])
• Severe dehydration. RBC counts may be *appropriately* decreased or increased in certain physiologic states.

Decreased In
• Various types of anemia (See p. 788)

Abnormal RBC Morphology
• It is flagged by automated counters, triggering microscopic examination of stained peripheral blood smears (see p. 282).
• Abnormalities (see Tables 2-72, 2-73) may be specific for certain conditions (e.g., spherocytes for hemolytic anemias, sickle cells for sickle cell anemias), or may be informative but not specific. *Anisocytosis* refers to variation in RBC size, *poikilocytosis* variation in shape, and *polychromasia* refers to bluish discoloration of RBC reflecting reticulocytes (see p. 323).

Limitations
• Patient's circumstances (e.g., vomiting or diarrhea)
• Other preanalytic factors
  • Marked leukocytosis marginally increases the RBC count.
  • Inappropriate blood collection is a major source of preanalytic errors. For instance, inappropriate filling of test tube results in excess anticoagulant, thereby diluting the blood and decreasing the red cell parameters.
  • Very low temperatures may lyse the red cells. Anticoagulated blood may be stored at 4°C for 24 hours, but beyond this interval, the results become increasingly altered.

RED CELL DISTRIBUTION WIDTH (RDW)

➤ Definition
• RDW is a coefficient of variation of the distribution of individual RBC volume.
• **Normal range:** 12.1–14 fL

➤ Use
• An elevation in RDW is useful in drawing attention to anisocytosis, a marker for various anemias.

➤ Interpretation
• The RDW is particularly helpful in separating iron deficiency anemia (high RDW, normal to low MCV), from β thalassemia trait (normal RDW, low MCV).
• Increased RDW is also useful in identifying red cell fragmentation, agglutination, or dimorphic cell populations.

➤ Limitations
• Very high WBC, numerous large platelets, and autoagglutination result in falsely elevated RDW.

TABLE 2-72. Abnormal Shapes of Red Blood Cells

Shape	Description	Conditions
Acanthocytes (spur cells)	Pointed membrane spicules of uneven length	Hereditary: acanthocytosis in abetalipoproteinemia Acquired: postsplenectomy, fulminant liver disease, malabsorption
Bite cells (precipitated hemoglobin [Heinz bodies])	RBCs with a peripheral smooth semicircle fragment missing	Hemolysis due to certain drugs, with or without G6PD deficiency; unstable hemoglobin
Burr cells	Crenated RBCs with preserved central pallor	Uremia, liver disease, Rhesus factor null cells, phosphokinase deficiency, anorexia nervosa, hypophosphatemia, hypomagnesemia, hyposplenism
Echinocytes	Blunt uniform spicules	Similar to burr cells; may be artifacts
Elliptocytes/ovalocytes	Oval RBCs	Hereditary elliptocytosis, iron deficiency, sickle cell trait, thalassemias, HbC disease; megaloblastic anemias
HbC crystalloids	Rhomboid crystals inclusions in RBCs	HbC trait or disease
Leptocytes	Flat, water-like, thin, hypochromic RBCs	Obstructive liver disease, thalassemia
Macrocytes	RBCs larger than normal, well filled with hemoglobin	Oval macrocytes in megaloblastic anemias; round macrocytes in liver disease Increased erythropoiesis
Microcytes	Decreased MCV (RBC smaller than normal)	Hypochromic anemias with defective iron stores
Microspherocytes		Artifacts; severe frostbite
RBC agglutination	Grouping together of RBCs due to IgM antibodies	Cold agglutinins, most commonly *Mycoplasma pneumoniae*; infectious mononucleosis
Rouleaux formation	Stack of coins appearance	Hyperproteinemias, especially multiple myeloma and plasmacytic lymphoma of IgM type; most frequently artifact

Cell type	Morphology	Associated conditions
Schistocytes (mechanical destruction of RBC in the circulation)	Helmet-like or fragmented, distorted RBCs	Micro- or macroangiopathic (small or large arteries) hemolytic anemias, prosthetic heart valves, severe valvular disease or large atheromas, DIC, TTP, severe iron deficiency, megaloblastic anemias, severe burns, renal transplant rejection, postchemotherapy, snake bite, inherited abnormalities of RBC membrane spectrin
Sickle cells (drepanocytes)	Bipolar, spiculated RBCs, pointed at both ends (shaped like sickles)	Sickle cell anemia (absent in sickle cell trait, unless induced by oxygen reduction)
Spherocytes (loss of RBC membrane)	Increased MCHC, usually decreased MCV; spherical cells with dense appearance and without central pallor	Hereditary spherocytosis, autoimmune hemolytic anemias, recent RBC transfusion
Stomatocytes	Mouth-like deformity with slit-like central pallor	Hereditary stomatocytosis, Rhesus factor null disease, immune hemolytic anemia, acute alcoholism, certain drugs (phenothiazines); frequently artifacts
Target cells (increased ratio of RBC surface area to volume)	Target-like appearance, often hypochromic; decreased osmotic fragility	Thalassemias, HbC disease or trait, HbD and E, iron deficiency anemia, liver disease, postsplenectomy, artifacts
Teardrop cells (dacryocytes)	Distorted, teardrop-shaped RBCs	Primary myelofibrosis, myelophthisic anemia, other myeloproliferative neoplasms or myelodysplastic syndromes, β-thalassemia major, iron deficiency, conditions with Heinz bodies

TABLE 2-73. Red Blood Cell Inclusions

Red Cell Type	Description	Disease State Association
Basophilic stippling	Punctuate basophilic inclusions composed of precipitated ribosomes (RNA)	A variety of anemias, thalassemias; coarse in lead poisoning
Cabot rings	Circular, blue, threadlike inclusion with dots	Occasional in severe megaloblastic and hemolytic anemias, overwhelming infections, postsplenectomy
Heinz bodies	Precipitates of denatured hemoglobin attached to RBC membrane; require supravital stains (e.g., crystal violet) for visualization	G6PD deficiency, methemoglobin reductase, drug-induced hemolytic anemias, unstable hemoglobin (e.g., hemoglobin Zurich), postsplenectomy; can be artifactual
Howell-Jolly bodies	Nuclear remnants of DNA; one, rarely two, dark purple, nonrefractile spherical bodies located at periphery of RBCs	Postsplenectomy, megaloblastic anemias, thalassemia, myelodysplasia, lead poisoning
Organisms on smears, outside RBCs	Specific morphology	*Wuchereria bancrofti; Brugia malayi; Loa loa; Trypanosoma brucei gambiense, T. cruzi,* and *T. rhodesiense; Borrelia recurrentis*
Organisms within RBCs	Specific shapes	*Plasmodium* trophozoites, babesiosis, other organisms
Pappenheimer bodies	Siderotic, nonheme iron granules at periphery of RBC; seen best with Prussian blue stain	Sideroblastic anemias, iron load, thalassemia, lead poisoning, postsplenectomy

REPTILASE TIME

➤ Definition
- RT measures the conversion of fibrinogen to fibrin when added to plasma. The reagent is a thrombin-like enzyme derived from venom of *Bothrops atrox*. It is unaffected by heparin or hirudin.
- **Normal value:** <20 seconds

➤ Use
- An abnormal reptilase time indicates an abnormality of fibrinogen, whereas a normal RT suggests heparin or hirudin as the cause of an abnormal thrombin time (see p. 345).
- A reptilase time valuates prolonged PTT when heparin or hirudin contamination is suspected.
- It also excludes dysfibrinogenemia

➤ Interpretation
Causes of Increased Results
- Hypofibrinogenemia or dysfibrinogenemia
- Slightly prolonged in the presence of fibrin degradation products as seen in severe DIC or pathologic fibrinolysis

➤ Limitations
- Preanalytic: partially clotted blood or hemolyzed blood, improperly filled or stored test tubes, specimens collected in wrong tubes
- Lipemic or icteric samples

RETICULOCYTES

➤ Definition
- Reticulocytes are immature RBC without nuclei. To visualize the reticulum-like RNA and count reticulocytes as a separate group of RBC, a special stain is required. The reticulocytes can be counted manually (at the microscope) and reported as percent per 100 RBC, or by automated counters. The reticulocyte count provides an estimate of the rate of red cell production.
- **Normal range:** 0.3–2.3/100 RBC with automated counters. However, this varies to some extent in the manual methodology. An absolute reticulocyte count or reticulocyte production index is more helpful than the percentage, and this can be calculated from the hematologic data.

➤ Interpretation
Causes of Increased Result
- Reticulocytosis. Enhanced red cell production most marked in hemolytic anemias (see p. 804) or during bone marrow regeneration.

Causes of Decreased Result
- Conditions with inadequate or ineffective hematopoiesis, despite the presence of anemia

➤ Limitations
- The manual counts result in great variability, being operator-dependent. The automated counters provide better precision. Erythrocyte inclusions, other than the true reticulum, may falsely increase the reticulocyte count. Similar errors occur in sickle cell anemia (see p. 796) and sickle/C hemoglobinopathies.

REVERSE T₃ (rT₃), TRIIODOTHYRONINE, REVERSE

➤ Definition
- Hormonally inactive isomer of T_3.
- **Normal range:**
  - Birth to 6 days: 600–2500 pg/mL
  - ≥7 days: 90–350 pg/mL

➤ Use
- To distinguish low T_3 "sick thyroid" patients (usually increased) from true hypothyroidism

➤ Interpretation
Increased In
- Severe nonthyroidal illness except in some liver disorders, HIV, renal failure
- Usually in hyperthyroidism and increased serum TBG

Decreased In
- Often in hypothyroidism but overlaps with normal range

RHEUMATOID FACTOR (RF)

➤ Definition
- RF is an immunoglobulin present in the serum of 50–95% of adults with RA. It appears in serum and synovial fluid several months after onset of RA and is present up to years after therapy. The auto antibodies are usually of IgM class, although ~15% of RA has IgG class. Most methods detect only the IgM class.
- **Normal range:** <20 IU/mL

➤ Use
- Assisting in the diagnosis of RA, especially when clinical diagnosis is difficult

➤ Interpretation
Increased In
- Chronic hepatitis
- Chronic viral infections
- Cirrhosis
- Dermatomyositis
- Infectious mononucleosis
- Leishmaniasis
- Leprosy

* Malaria
* RA
* Sarcoidosis
* Scleroderma
* Sjögren syndrome
* SLE
* Syphilis
* TB
* Waldenström macroglobulinemia

➤ **Limitations**
* RF is not a finding isolated to RA and may be present in a number of connective tissue and inflammatory diseases, including infectious mononucleosis, SLE, scleroderma, and hepatitis.
* Older patients may have higher values.
* Recent blood transfusion, multiple vaccinations or transfusions, or an inadequately activated complement may affect results.
* Serum with cryoglobulin or high lipid levels may cause false-positive test results.

ROSETTE TEST

➤ **Definition**
* The rosette test detects D-positive red cells in the blood of a D-negative mother, whose fetus or recently delivered baby is D-positive. It can only be used in the setting of Rh incompatibility. The presence of the D-positive red cells indicates fetomaternal hemorrhage >30 mL whole blood because a positive test reflects admixture of fetal blood with maternal blood in the maternal circulation.
* **Normal value:** Absence of rosettes is considered negative for major fetomaternal hemorrhage in an Rh positive mother with an Rh-negative fetus.

➤ **Use**
* The test is used to determine the presence of marked fetomaternal hemorrhage (FMH). The assay has a sensitivity of 99–100% when FMH is 15 mL of fetal RBCs or more.
* When anti-D reagent is added to mother's blood, fetal D-positive red cells become coated with anti-D on incubation and exhibit mixed-field agglutination when antiglobulin (see p. 119) reagent is added. Because the mixed-field agglutination may be difficult to detect, D-positive RBCs are added to the mixture to demonstrate rosettes of several cells clustered against antibody-coated D-positive cells.

➤ **Interpretation**
* The presence of a positive result indicates that the fetal blood is admixed with that of the mother. This happens when the fetus has hemorrhaged into the mother's circulation and may require intrauterine transfusion or obstetric intervention.

➤ **Limitations**
* Specimens giving a positive result need to be further investigated (acid-elution procedure, Kleihauser-Betke assay (see p. 237) flow cytometry, or enzyme-linked antiglobulin test) to quantify the number of fetal cells, thus assessing the severity of the fetal hemorrhage.

SALICYLATES (ASPIRIN)

➤ Definition

- An acidic drug that is rapidly metabolized to an active metabolite, salicylate; also known as acetylsalicylic acid (ASA)
- **Normal therapeutic range (serum)**
  - Analgesic/antipyretic use: <60 µg/mL
  - Anti-inflammatory use: 150–300 µg/mL

➤ Use

- ASA and salicylate have analgesic, antipyretic, and anti-inflammatory properties; used in the treatment of RA
- ASA also inhibits platelet aggregation and, therefore, prolongs bleeding time

➤ Interpretation

- See discussion of salicylate poisoning in Chapter 15.

➤ Limitations

- Requires specific test request; not usually detected in routine screens
- Color test: Trinder reagent (hydrochloric acid + ferric nitrate + mercuric chloride) produces a violet/purple color in the presence of salicylate; the color reaction may be observed visually or spectrophotometrically by measuring absorbance at 540 nm.
  - Limit of detection: 40–50 µg/mL
  - Suitable for blood, serum, plasma, urine
  - Not recommended for quantitative purposes due to interferences from metabolites, plasma constituents, and issues with specificity outlined below
  - Specificity:
    - Specimens that are either strongly basic or acidic may produce a negative response.
    - Excessive concentrations (>1000 mg/L) of aromatic compounds with free phenolic groups and aliphatic enols will react with ferric nitrate and absorb light in the visible range.
    - Compounds such as phosphates and oxalates in high concentrations will inhibit color development and cause falsely decreased results.
    - Phenothiazines (chlorpromazine, promazine, thioridazine, prochlorperazine and promethazine), if present, may produce a purple color that fades rapidly.
    - Atypical color reactions will occur if sodium azide or thiopropazate are present.
- Immunoassay
  - Automated chemistry analyzer
  - Serum/plasma
  - Not whole blood
  - Enzyme and fluorescence methodologies
  - Measures absorbance intensity at 540 nm (color complex formed with salicylate and ferric nitrate under acid conditions)
  - Anticoagulants (heparin, citrates, oxalates, EDTA) do not interfere
  - Do not use sodium azide in collection tubes
  - Hemolysis produces false-negative results
  - Hemoglobin concentrations >100 mg/dL may interfere
  - Limit of quantitation: 50 µg/mL

- Cross reactivity:
  - Typically >90% with ASA
  - None with benzoic acid
  - Varying with salicyluric acid and salicylamide
- Confirmation
  - Sample pretreatment required
  - Gas chromatography: derivatization may be necessary
  - HPLC: preferred technique for distinguishing metabolites
  - Limit of quantitation: 50 µg/mL

SCREENING FOR FETAL CHROMOSOME ABNORMALITIES AND NEURAL TUBE DEFECTS

➤ Definition
- Noninvasive testing with goal of limiting invasive diagnostic procedures that carry risk to pregnancy

➤ Use
- Screening modalities have been developed for Down syndrome/trisomy 21 detection because trisomy 21 is the most common viable autosomal chromosome abnormality. However, screening also provides specific risk assessment for trisomy 18 and neural tube defects.
- In addition, with inclusion of early ultrasound examination, increased fetal nuchal translucency may indicate other chromosome abnormalities including Turner syndrome (45,X), trisomy 13, and triploidy.
- Second-trimester measurement of AFP is used to assess risk of fetal neural tube defects.
- Screening is offered to all women, regardless of age, to provide more accurate risk information than provided by age alone.

➤ Limitations
- Risk for trisomy 13 is *not* calculated; however, trisomy 13 pregnancies are typically associated with ultrasound anomalies detectable with second-trimester ultrasound examination. By definition, screening is not diagnostic; most screen-positive pregnancies are chromosomally normal, and some affected pregnancies will be missed.

SECOND TRIMESTER SCREENING (MATERNAL SERUM SCREENING; QUAD SCREEN)

➤ Definition
- Performed between 15 and 22 weeks of gestation, the quadruple screen combines maternal age plus four serum biochemical markers: hCG, inhibin A, AFP, and unconjugated estriol to assess the risk of trisomy 21 and trisomy 18.

➤ Use
- Risk assessment for trisomy 21 (Down syndrome), trisomy 18, and open neural tube defects.

➤ Interpretation

* Trisomy 21 profile typically has high levels of hCG and inhibin A with low levels of AFP and unconjugated estriol.
* Trisomy 18 is associated with low levels of hCG, AFP, and estriol. (Inhibin A does not contribute to trisomy 18 risk profile.)
* Different centers use different cut-offs, balancing detection rate against number of invasive procedures performed. A cut-off of 1:270 (~5% positive screening rate) detects ~80% of trisomy 21 and trisomy 18 pregnancies.

➤ Limitations

* Detects fewer affected pregnancies than combined first-semester plus second-trimester screening modalities.
* Does not permit first trimester decision-making regarding termination of affected pregnancies.

SEDATIVE-HYPNOTICS

See Alcohols (Volatiles, Solvents), Benzodiazepines

➤ Definition

* This group of drugs includes those that reduce tension and anxiety, induce calm [sedative], or induce sleep [hypnotic]. All have CNS depressant effects. Although other drugs may produce similar effects, the distinctive ability of these drugs is that they achieve their effects without altering mood or reducing sensitivity to pain.
* This class includes ethanol, chloral hydrate, glutethimide, ethchlorvynol [Placidyl], barbiturates, benzodiazepines, meprobamate [Miltown], methaqualone [Quaalude], buspirone [BuSpar], zolpidem [Ambien], zopiclone [Imovane]
* **Therapeutic range (serum)**
  * Chloral hydrate (metabolite trichloroethanol [TCE]): 2–12 µg/mL serum
  * Ethchlorvynol: 2–8 µg/mL
  * Glutethimide: 1–5 µg/mL
  * Methaqualone: 1000-4000 ng/ml
  * Meprobamate: 5–25 µg/mL
  * Buspirone: 1–10 ng/mL
  * Zolpidem: 25–300 ng/mL
  * Zopiclone: 50–150 ng/mL
* Barbiturates
  * Ultrashort acting (thiopental, methohexital) [approximate]: 40 µg/mL [thiopental]; 3–10 µg/mL [methohexital for surgical anesthesia]
  * Short acting (pentobarbital, secobarbital): 0.5–2.0 µg/mL
  * Intermediate acting (amobarbital, butalbital, butabarbital): 1.0–5.0 µg/mL
  * Long acting (phenobarbital): 5–15 µg/mL (sedative-hypnotic); 15–40 µg/mL (anticonvulsant)

➤ Use

* Treatment of sleeping disorders
* Reduction of anxiety

➤ Limitations
Specific Agents

- Chloral hydrate, ethchlorvynol, glutethimide, methaqualone (currently little used in the United States; requires specific request to test)
  - **Chloral hydrate:** measure metabolite trichloroethanol (TCE) with gas chromatography, GC/MS, LC/MS
  - **Ethchlorvynol:** color test, gas chromatography, GC/MS; measure parent
  - **Glutethimide:** gas chromatography, GC/MS, liquid chromatography, LC/MS; measure parent and active metabolite hydroxyglutethimide
  - **Methaqualone:** immunoassay screening test available for this agent
    - Target analyte—methaqualone
    - Cutoff concentration [urine]—300 ng/mL
    - Confirmation by gas chromatography, GC/MS, liquid chromatography, LC/MS: limit of quantitation: 50–200 ng/mL
- **Meprobamate**
  - Older CNS depressant
  - Metabolite of muscle relaxant carisoprodol
  - No immunoassay-based screening tests available
  - Readily extracted in acidic neutral liquid–liquid or solid-phase extraction scheme: GC, GC/MS, liquid chromatography, LC/MS; limit of quantitation: 500–1000 ng/mL
- **Buspirone**
  - Newer antianxiety drug
  - No immunoassay based screening tests available
  - Extracted in alkaline liquid–liquid or solid-phase extraction scheme
  - GC/MS (SIM) due to low concentrations difficult to observe in full scan mode; LC/MS
  - Active metabolite 1-(2-pyrimidinyl)piperazine (1-PP) may also be measured
  - Limit of quantitation: 1 ng/mL
- **Zolpidem**
  - Structurally similar to benzodiazepines
  - No specific immunoassay-based screening tests available for clinical use [recently available for forensic applications]
    - Readily extracted in alkaline liquid–liquid or solid-phase extraction scheme
    - Gas chromatography, liquid chromatography, GC/MS, LC/MS
    - Limit of quantitation: 10–50 ng/mL
- **Zopiclone**
  - Newer hypnotic
  - No immunoassay-based screening tests currently available for clinical use
  - Readily extracted in neutral liquid–liquid or SPE extraction scheme
    - Unstable in acidic and basic conditions
    - Gas chromatography, GC/MS, liquid chromatography, LC/MS; may thermally degrade depending on gas chromatography, GC/MS operating parameters
    - Limit of quantitation: 10–50 ng/mL

Barbiturates

- Older class of CNS depressants
- Largely replaced by benzodiazepines and newer hypnotics such as zolpidem

- Current main use as anticonvulsants, in treatment of migraines, and in reduction of cerebral edema and intracranial pressure resulting from head injury
- Screening
  - Immunoassays for automated chemistry analyzers
    - Urine
      - Target analyte—secobarbital
      - Cut-off concentration—200 or 300 ng/mL
      - Cross-reactivity—approximately 100% with amobarbital, 60–90% with butabarbital, butalbital, pentobarbital, and phenobarbital
    - Serum/Plasma/Blood
      - EMIT, ELISA, FPIA
      - Target analyte—secobarbital
      - Cut-off concentration—10–50 ng/mL ELISA; 1000 ng/mL EMIT
      - Cross-reactivity—manufacturer kit reagent dependent:
        - Low cross-reactivity with amobarbital, phenobarbital, butabarbital and butalbital and high cross-reactivity with thiopental and pentobarbital
        - FPIA generally demonstrates more cross-reactivity than EMIT to other barbiturates
- Confirmation: chromatography or UV-visible spectrophotometry
- Sample pretreatment required
- Gas chromatography
- HPLC
- GC/MS
  - LC/MS
  - Limit of quantitation: analyte dependent—0.5–5.0 µg/mL

SEMEN ANALYSIS

➤ Definition
- A complete semen analysis measures the sperm concentration (count), sperm motility, and sperm morphology of a semen specimen.
- **Normal ranges:**
  - Concentration: 70–80 million/mL (critical fertility level 20 million/mL)
  - Motility: >50% progressive (critical fertility level 30% progressive)
  - Morphology: >30% normal forms (WHO criteria), or >14% normal forms (Kruger strict criteria)

➤ Use
- A semen analysis is the primary test for male factor infertility in the work-up of infertility in a couple. Infertility is a rate-relative term, defined as an involuntary reduction in the ability to achieve pregnancy within one year (10–17 cycles for cycles ranging from 35–21 days), which is the 90th percentile of normal fertility.
- Sperm concentration alone is also used to confirm the effectiveness of vasectomy.

➤ Interpretation
Increased In
- No upper limit defined

Decreased In
* Anatomic problems (e.g., cryptorchidism, varicocele)
* Medical problems (e.g., postpubertal mumps, surgical procedures/bladder neck or prostate, testicular cancer, postradiation or chemotherapy, diabetes mellitus)
* Medication/environmental issues (e.g., ethanol, tobacco, anabolic steroids, drugs of abuse, and gonadotoxins such as the solvents carbon disulfide, benzene, and glycol ethers, the pesticides dibromochloropropane and chlordecone, and the heavy metals lead and methylmercury)

➤ Limitations
* Minimum specimen volume for microscopic analysis is 0.1 mL.
* Highly viscous specimens may affect accuracy of concentration results.
* A minimum of two analyses, preferably one month apart, is recommended to correct for cyclical variation in sperm concentration. Specimen collection should occur within a window of 48–72 hours abstinence to maximize average concentration of live cells.

SEMEN FRUCTOSE

➤ Definition
* The semen fructose test is a test for fructose in seminal plasma.
* **Normal range:** ≥ 13 μ moles per ejaculate

➤ Use
* Fructose, the major energy source for ejaculated spermatozoa, is produced almost entirely in the seminal vesicles, which contribute a significant amount of fluid to the total ejaculate volume via the ejaculatory duct.
* Fructose levels should be determined in any patient with azoospermia and especially in those whose ejaculate volume is <1 mL and fails to coagulate.

➤ Interpretation
Increased In
* No upper limit is defined

Decreased In
* In conjunction with low semen volume and failure to coagulate, this result is suggestive of seminal vesicle obstruction or atresia distal to the seminal vesicles.

➤ Limitations
* Minimum specimen volume for analysis is 0.1 mL.

SEROTONIN, BLOOD

➤ Definition
* Serotonin is an indole amine synthesized by the cells of the intestinal mucosa. It is stored in and transported by platelets but also found in many body tissues, including the CNS. Serotonin acts as a vasoconstrictor, neurotransmitter; stimulant of smooth muscle contraction, prolactin release, and GH release; and functions in hemocoagulation.

- Other names: 5-Hydroxytryptamine
- **Normal range:** 50–200 ng/mL

➤ Use
- Confirming the diagnosis of carcinoid tumors.
- Adjunct test for 5-HIAA and chromogranin-A test to follow-up patients with carcinoid tumors.

➤ Interpretation
Increased In
- Metastasizing abdominal carcinoid tumors
- Dumpling syndrome
- Acute intestinal obstruction
- Cystic fibrosis
- AMI and nontropical sprue
- Oat cell carcinoma of the lung
- Pancreatic islet tumor
- Thyroid medullary carcinoma

Decreased In
- Down syndrome
- Severe depression
- Parkinson disease
- Phenylketonuria (treated and untreated)
- Renal insufficiency
- Teratomas

➤ Limitations
- Blood serotonin is very unstable.
- Medications that may affect serotonin concentrations include lithium, MAO inhibitors, methyldopa, morphine, and reserpine.
- In general, foods that contain serotonin do not interfere significantly.
- Slight increases may be seen in acute intestinal obstruction, acute MI, cystic fibrosis, dumping syndromes, and nontropical sprue.

SERUM PROTEIN ELECTROPHORESIS/IMMUNOFIXATION

➤ Definition
- Serum protein electrophoresis (SPE) is a method of physical separation of protein molecules based on their charge. Changes in both quality and nature of proteins determined by SPE, allows clinicians to detect and monitor various pathophysiologic states. SPE, enhanced by follow-up procedures like protein quantification and immunofixation (IF), provides the best tools for general screening of human health state.
- The monoclonal gammopathies are a group of disorders characterized by the proliferation of a single clone of plasma cells, which produces an immunologically homogeneous protein commonly referred to as a paraprotein or monoclonal protein (M-protein).
- SPE is usually done by the agarose gel electrophoresis, or by the capillary zone electrophoretic method. It is the recommended method for the detection of an M-protein. The

resulting M-protein, if found, can then be quantitated by means of a densitometer tracing of the gel.

- In the electrophoretic methodologies (agarose or capillary zone), proteins are classified by their final position after electrophoresis is complete into five general regions: albumin, alpha-1, alpha-2, beta, and gamma. The various immunoglobulin classes (IgG, IgA, IgM, IgD, and IgE) are usually of gamma mobility and make up most of the gamma region, but they may also be found in the beta-gamma and beta regions, and may occasionally extend into the alpha-2 globulin area.
- Other names: serum protein electrophoresis (SPEP)
- **Normal range:**
  - SPE:
    - Albumin: 3.5–5.0 g/dL
    - Alpha-1 globulin: 0.1–0.3 g/dL
    - Alpha-2-globulin: 0.5–1.0 g/dL
    - Beta globulin: 0.5–0.9 g/dL
    - Gamma globulin: 0.6–1.4 g/dL
  - IF: no monoclonal protein detected.

➤ Use
- Monitoring patients with monoclonal gammopathies
- Diagnosis of monoclonal gammopathies, when used in conjunction with immunofixation.
- Assist in the diagnosis of hepatic disease, hypogammaglobulinemias and hypergammaglobulinemias, inflammatory states, neoplasms, renal disease, and GI disorders.
- SPE should also be considered in any patient with an elevated total serum protein or otherwise unexplained signs and symptoms suggestive of the presence of a plasma cell disorder. These include any one or more of the following:
  - Elevated ESR or serum viscosity
  - Unexplained anemia, back pain, weakness, or fatigue
  - Osteopenia, osteolytic lesions, or spontaneous fractures
  - Renal insufficiency with a bland urine sediment
  - Heavy proteinuria in a patient older than 40 years of age
  - Hypercalcemia
  - Hypergammaglobulinemia
  - Immunoglobulin deficiency
  - BJ proteinuria
  - Unexplained peripheral neuropathy
  - Recurrent infections

➤ Interpretation
Increased In
- **Albumin**
  - Usually in hospitalized patients, hemoconcentration, albumin perfusion
  - Normal individuals: no clinical significance
  - Bisalbuminemia (double band), permanent
  - Bisalbuminemia, acquired, transient
    - High doses of beta lactam antibiotics (complex formation).
    - Hyperbilirubinemia (jaundice, complexed with bilirubin).

- Azotemia (urea and other N-compounds in blood).
- Pancreatitis, pancreatic fistulas, or ascites (lysis of albumin by pancreatic enzymes).
- **Alpha-1 globulin**
  - Acute inflammatory disorders
  - Severe alcoholism
  - Some hepatic disorders
  - Double bands (AAT phenotypes)
- **Alpha-2 globulin**
  - Inflammatory syndromes
  - Nephrotic syndrome
  - Increased estrogen stimulation
  - Double bands in
    - Haptoglobin (Hp) phenotypes (no clinical significance)
    - Hemolysis (Hb-Hp complex)
    - Abnormal migrating beta-lipoproteins (aged samples)
- **Beta-globulin**
  - Primary and secondary hyperlipoproteinemias
  - Iron deficiency anemia
  - Estrogen, pregnancy or anabolic steroids
  - Increase co-migrates with transferrin, Hb (in excess to that bound in Hb-Hp complexes).
  - Acute inflammation (later phase)
  - Monoclonal immunoglobulins (IgA is frequent)
  - Double bands
    - Transferrin phenotypes (different degrees of sialation)
    - Alcoholics
- **Gammaglobulin**
  - Polyclonal gammopathy: chronic, subacute infections (AIDS, hepatic infections, chronic liver associated with beta-gamma bridging, autoimmune disorders).
  - Narrow band: monoclonal component, monoclonal gammopathy of undetermined significance, fibrinogen, CRP
  - Two narrow bands:
    - Biclonal or double gammopathies
    - >2 bands: oligoclonal hypergamma globulinemia (present in low concentrations, transient, results in polyclonal processes); autoimmune, viral, bacterial, parasitic infections; restoration of immunoglobulin synthesis of immunosuppressants, 15% normal (no clinical significance)

Decreased In
- **Albumin**
  - Congenital analbuminemia.
  - Nutritional deficiency
  - Decreased synthesis
  - Hepatocellular insufficiency, damaged liver (cirrhosis, hepatitis)
  - Organ, tissue loss
  - Urinary (nephrotic syndrome), cutaneous (excessive burns) urinary excretion in pregnancy
  - Hypercatabolism
  - Endocrine disorders (thyrotoxicosis, Cushing syndrome)

- **Alpha-1-globulin**
  - Hepatocellular insufficiency
  - Malnutrition, protein loss
  - Congenital deficiency of AAT
  - Tangier disease
- **Alpha-2-globulin**
  - Hereditary deficiency of Hp phenotypes
  - Nutritional deficiency, hepatocellular insufficiency, protein loss, intravascular hemolysis (decreased Hp)
  - Pancreatitis
- **Beta-globulin**
  - Chronic liver or renal disease
  - Hypo-beta-lipoproteinemias
  - Thermal injuries
  - Acute inflammation
  - IgA deficiency
  - C3 degrades and eventually disappears in aged samples
- **Gammaglobulin**
  - Physiologic (newborn)
  - Immunodeficiencies, induced (steroids, immunosuppressants, chemotherapy, radiotherapy)
  - Suppressed synthesis caused by monoclonal gammopathies (multiple myeloma, light chain disease, amyloidosis)
  - Lymphomas, leukemias

➤ Limitations

- The presence of a circulating monoclonal protein may interfere with one of more laboratory tests performed on liquid-based automated analyzers, either by precipitating during the analysis or by virtue of its specific binding properties.
- A small M-protein may be present even when quantitative immunoglobulin values, beta and gamma mobility components on SPEP, and total serum protein concentrations are all within normal limits.
- Fibrinogen (in plasma) is seen as a discrete band between the beta and gamma mobility regions. This is indistinguishable from an M-protein; the addition of thrombin to the specimen produces a clot if fibrinogen is present. The presence of fibrinogen is established if the discrete band is no longer detected when electrophoresis is repeated after the addition of thrombin.
- Hb-Hp complexes secondary to hemolysis may appear as a large band in the alpha-2-globulin region.
- High concentrations of transferrin in patients with iron deficiency anemia may produce a localized band in the beta region.
- Nephrotic syndrome is often associated with increased alpha-2 and beta bands, which can be mistaken for an M-protein. Serum albumin and gammaglobulin concentrations are usually reduced in this setting.
- Nonspecific increases in acute phase reactants or certain hyperlipoproteinemias may result in increases in alpha-1 bands.
- Serum IF is more sensitive than SPE and also determines the heavy and light chain type of the monoclonal protein. However, unlike SPE, IF does not give an estimate of the size of the

M-protein (i.e., its serum concentration) and thus should be done in conjunction with electrophoresis.

SEX HORMONE–BINDING GLOBULIN (SHBG)

➤ Definition
- A glycoprotein, synthesized in the liver, which binds testosterone and 5-dihydrotestosterone with high affinity, and estradiol with a somewhat lower affinity. SHBG typically circulates at higher concentrations in women than in men, due to the higher ratio of estrogens to androgens in women. Administration of androgens tends to be associated with decreased SHBG levels.
- Because variations in the carrier protein levels may affect the concentration of testosterone in circulation, SHBG levels are commonly measured as a supplement to total testosterone determinations. The "free androgen index" (FAI), calculated as the ratio of total testosterone to SHBG, has proved to be a useful indicator of abnormal androgen status in conditions such as hirsutism.
- **Normal range:** see Table 2-74

➤ Use
- Diagnosis and follow-up of women with symptoms or signs of androgen excess (e.g., polycystic ovarian syndrome and idiopathic hirsutism)
- As an adjunct in monitoring sex steroid and antiandrogen therapy
- As an adjunct in the diagnosis of disorders of puberty
- As an adjunct in the diagnosis and follow-up of anorexia nervosa

➤ Interpretation
Increased In
- Hyperthyroidism
- Hepatic cirrhosis
- Pregnancy
- Drugs: estrogens (e.g. certain oral contraceptives, phenytoin (hepatic enzyme induction)
- Use of dexamethasone in the treatment of women with hyperandrogenic hirsutism

Decreased In
- Hirsutism
- Acne vulgaris
- Polycystic ovary syndrome
- Hypothyroidism
- Acromegaly
- Cushing disease
- Hyperprolactinemia

TABLE 2-74. Normal Ranges of Sex Hormone–Binding Globulin		
Group	Central 95% (nmol/L)	Median (nmol/L)
Male	13–71	32
Female (nonpregnant)	18–114	51

SICKLE SOLUBILITY TEST (SST)

➤ Definition
- The SST (also called "sickle cell screen") was developed as a rapid screening for the presence of HbS.
- Red cells are lysed and the released Hg is reduced by sodium hydrosulfite.

➤ Use
- Patients with sickle cell trait are asymptomatic and do not present with sickle cells on the peripheral blood smear. The definitive diagnosis is made by hemoglobin electrophoresis. Reduced HbS is insoluble and forms a turbid suspension in the SST.
- HgA and most other hemoglobins are soluble under these conditions. Both sickle cell anemia (homozygous) and the sickle cell trait can be detected with this procedure.

➤ Limitations
- Recent transfusions may cause false-positive and false-negative results.
- False-negative results may occur with:
  - Patient's Hb $<$7 g/dL
  - Phenothiazine drugs
  - Unreliable for newborn screening because of high HbF
  - Low percentage of HbS in the first year of life
- False-positive results may occur with:
  - Increased turbidity (e.g., lipemic specimens)
  - Abnormal β globulins
  - Polycythemia
  - Increased number of Heinz bodies (e.g., postsplenectomy)
  - Increased number of nucleated RBCs
  - Some rare Hb variants, such as HbC Harlem or C Georgetown

SODIUM (NA)

➤ Definition
- Sodium is the major extracellular cation and exerts a major influence on plasma osmolality. It plays a central role in maintaining the normal distribution of water and osmotic pressure.
- Changes in serum sodium most often reflect changes in water balance rather than sodium balance. It is adjusted by ADH and the thirst receptors to maintain plasma osmolality and volume. Aldosterone causes tubular reabsorption of sodium. Atrial natriuretic peptide hormone decreases sodium reabsorption.
- **Normal range:** 136–145 mmol/L
- **Critical values:** $<$121 or $>$158 mmol/L

➤ Use
- Diagnosis and treatment of dehydration and overhydration. If a patient has not received large load of sodium, hypernatremia suggests need for water, and values $<$130 mmol/L suggest overhydration.
- Electrolyte, acid–base balance; water balance; water intoxication

➤ Interpretation

Increased In

- Conditions associated with water loss in excess of salt loss through skin, lungs, GI tract, and kidneys
- Hyperaldosteronism

➤ Limitations

- Plasma sodium levels depend greatly on the intake and excretion of water and, to a somewhat lesser degree, the renal regulation of sodium.
- Determinations of blood sodium and potassium levels are not useful in diagnosis in estimating net ion losses but are performed to monitor changes in sodium and potassium during therapy.
- Hyperglycemia: serum sodium decreases 1.7 mmol/L for every increase of serum glucose of 100 mg/dL.
- Hyperlipidemia and hyperproteinemia, which cause spurious results only with flame photometric but not with specific ion electrode techniques for measuring sodium

SODIUM, URINE

➤ Definition

- Urinary sodium determinations are usually performed to detect or confirm the presence of conditions that affect body fluids (e.g., dehydration, vomiting, and diarrhea) or disorders of the kidneys or adrenal glands.
- **Normal range:**
  - 24-hour urine:
    - Male:
      - <10 years: 41–115 mmol/day
      - 10–14 years: 63–177 mmol/day
      - >14 years: 40–120 mmol/day
    - Female:
      - <10 years: 20–69 mmol/day
      - 10–14 years: 48–168 mmol/day
      - >14 years: 27–287 mmol/day
  - Random urine
    - Male: 23–229 mmol/g creatinine
    - Female: 26–297 mmol/g creatinine

➤ Use

- Volume depletion: to determine the route of sodium loss. Low urinary sodium indicate extrarenal loss and high value indicates renal salt wasting or adrenal insufficiency.
- Differential diagnosis of acute renal failure: high values are consistent with acute tubular necrosis.
- In hyponatremia, low urinary sodium indicates avid renal sodium retention, which may be either attributable to either severe volume depletion or sodium retaining states seen in cirrhosis, the nephrotic syndrome, and CHF. When hyponatremia is associated with urinary sodium excretion that equals or exceeds the dietary sodium intake, it is likely that SIADH is present.

➤ Interpretation
Increased In
* Dehydration
* Salicylate intoxication
* Adrenocortical insufficiency
* Diabetic acidosis
* Mercurial and thiazide diuretic administration
* Ammonium chloride administration
* Renal tubular acidosis (<15 mmol/L are seen in prerenal acidosis)
* Chronic renal failure
* SIADH of different etiology
* Any form of alkalosis and alkaline urine

Decreased In
* Acute renal failure
* Pulmonary emphysema
* CHF
* Excessive sweating
* Diarrhea
* Pyloric obstruction
* Malabsorption
* Primary aldosteronism
* Premenstrual sodium and water retention
* Acute oliguria and prerenal azotemia

➤ Limitations
* Large diurnal variations exist in urine sodium levels. The rate of excretion during night is one-fifth of the peak rate during the day.
* Levels are highly dependent on dietary intake and state of hydration.

TAY-SACHS DISEASE MOLECULAR DNA ASSAY

➤ Definition
* Tay-Sachs disease (TSD) molecular DNA testing identifies mutations in the beta-hexosaminidase A gene but should be used concurrently with the hexosaminidase A (HEX A) enzyme activity assay to diagnose TSD. HEX A enzymatic activity is the primary method for diagnosing TSD or carrier identification.
* HEX A activity is determined by the ratio of HEX A to total hexosaminidase and can be measured in serum from women who are not pregnant and not using oral contraceptives, serum from male patients, or WBCs from all individuals.
* **Normal values:** negative or no mutations are found

➤ Use
* There are two groups of tests:
  * Targeted mutation analysis
    * A panel of six mutations comprising:

- 1278insTATC, IVS12+1G>C, G269S: the most common Ashkenazi mutations
- IVS9+1G−>A: non-Jewish mutation
- R247W and R249W: the two pseudodeficiency alleles that do not cause TSD, but reduce HEX A enzymatic activity as measured by the synthetic substrate
- More extended panels include ethnic specific mutations as IVS7+1G>A, del 7.6kb, R170Q, R170W, del F304/305, IVS5-2A>G.
- Sequence analysis: analysis of the entire coding region and exon–intron boundaries useful for identifying rare mutant alleles associated with TSD.
- TSD molecular genetic testing is performed for:
- Confirmation of a clinical diagnosis
- Carrier testing for Ashkenazi Jewish individuals
- Carrier testing for at-risk family members of affected individuals
- Confirmation that the reduced HEX A enzymatic activity is caused by a disease-causing allele rather than a pseudodeficiency allele, R247W or R249W. About 35% of non-Jewish individuals and 2–4% of Jewish individuals identified as heterozygotes by HEX A enzyme assay testing are carriers of a pseudodeficiency allele.
- Prenatal diagnosis: when both parental mutations are known.
- Identification for genetic counseling of specific disease-causing alleles in affected individuals and carriers

➤ Limitations
- The results of a genetic test may be affected by DNA rearrangements, blood transfusion, bone marrow transplantation, or other rare events.

TESTOSTERONE, TOTAL, FREE, BIOAVAILABLE

➤ Definition
- Testosterone circulates in the blood of men and women in several forms. In healthy adults, approximately 44% of circulating testosterone is specifically bound to sex hormone–binding globulin (SHBG), 50% is nonspecifically bound to albumin and 3–5% is bound to cortisol-binding globulin, indicating that only 2–3% is unbound and free.
- Current methods available to evaluate the androgen status include measurement of total testosterone, free testosterone by direct immunoassays, equilibrium dialysis, HPLC-MS, SHBG, calculated free (non-SHBG–nonalbumin bound) testosterone, and bioavailable (non-SHBG bound) testosterone. In most, but not all clinical conditions, a measurement of total testosterone is adequate for the evaluation of a patient.
- It is widely believed that SHBG-bound testosterone is not readily available to most tissues, whereas albumin bound and free testosterones are bioavailable. Because SHBG concentrations can be influenced by many factors (e.g., decreased by obesity, testosterone treatment, and hypoandrogenic female conditions such as polycystic ovary syndrome; increased by aging, pregnancy, and estrogen therapy), there are clinical situations in which measured concentrations of total testosterone may not reflect the bioavailable concentrations or the clinical status of the patient. In these circumstances, a supplemental test assessing bioavailable and free testosterone is helpful in clinical decision making.
- **Normal range:** see Table 2-75

TABLE 2-75. Normal Ranges of Testosterone

Age	Range
Testosterone, Total, Male	
Premature (26–28 weeks)	59–125 ng/dL
Premature (3–35 weeks)	37–198 ng/dL
Newborn	75–400 ng/dL
−7 months	Levels decrease rapidly the first week to 20–50 ng/dL, and then increase to 60–400 ng/dL between 20 and 60 days. Levels then decline to prepubertal range levels of 3–10 ng/dL by 7 months.
7–9 years	<9 ng/dL
10–11 years	2–57 ng/dL
12–13 years	7–747 ng/dL
14–15 years	33–585 ng/dL
16–17 years	185–886 ng/dL
18–39 years	400–1080 ng/dL
40–59 years	350–890 ng/dL
≥60 years	350–720 ng/dL
Tanner Stage I	<20 ng/dL
Tanner Stage II	2–149 ng/dL
Tanner Stage III	7–762 ng/dL
Tanner Stage IV	164–854 ng/dL
Tanner Stage V	194–783 ng/dL
Testosterone, Free Male	
1–6 years	<0.6 pg/mL
7–9 years	0.1–0.9 pg/mL
10–11 years	0.1–6.3 pg/mL
12–13 years	0.5–98.0 pg/mL
14–15 years	3–138.0 pg/mL
16–17 years	38.0–173.0 pg/mL
≥18 years	47–244 pg/mL
Tanner Stage I	≤3.7 pg/mL
Tanner Stage II	0.3–21 pg/mL
Tanner Stage III	1.0–98.0 pg mL
Tanner Stage IV	35.0–169.0 pg/mL
Tanner Stage V	41.0–239.0 pg/mL
Testosterone, Total, Female	
Premature (26–28 weeks)	5–16 ng/dL
Premature (31–35 weeks)	5–22 ng/dL
Newborn	20–64 ng/dL
−7 months	Levels decrease during the first month to <10 ng/dL and remain at this level until puberty
7–9 years	<15 ng/dL

(Continued)

TABLE 2-75. Normal Ranges of Testosterone (*Continued*)

Age	Range
10–11 years	2–42 ng/dL
12–13 years	6–64 ng/dL
14–15 years	9–49 ng/dL
16–17 years	8–63 ng/dL
18–30 years	11–59 ng/dL
31–40 years	11–56 ng/dL
41–51 years	9–55 ng/dL
Postmenopausal	6–25 ng/dL
Tanner Stage I	<17 ng/dL
Tanner Stage II	4–39 ng/dL
Tanner Stage III	10–60 ng/dL
Tanner Stage IV	8–63 ng/dL
Tanner Stage V	10–60 ng/dL
Testosterone, Free Females	
1–6 years	<0.6 pg/mL
7–9 years	0.6–1.8 pg/mL
10–11 years	0.1–3.5 pg/mL
12–13 years	0.9–6.8 pg/mL
14–15 years	1.2–7.5 pg/mL
16–17 years	1.2–9.9 pg/mL
18–30 years	0.8–7.4 pg/mL
31–40 years	1.3–9.2 pg/mL
41–51 years	1.1–5.8 pg/mL
Postmenopausal	0.6–3.8 pg/mL
Tanner Stage I	<2.2 pg/mL
Tanner Stage II	0.4–4.5 pg/mL
Tanner Stage III	1.3–7.5 pg mL
Tanner Stage IV	1.1–15.5 pg/mL
Tanner Stage V	0.8–9.2 pg/mL
Testosterone, Male, Bioavailable	
1–6 years	<1.3 ng/dL
7–9 years	0.3–2.8 ng/dL
10–11 years	0.1–17.9 ng/dL
12–13 years	1.4–288.0 ng/dL
14–15 years	9.5–337.0 ng/dL
16–17 years	35.0–509.0 ng/dL
≥18 years	130–680 ng/dL
Tanner Stage I	0.3–13.0 ng/dL
Tanner Stage II	0.3–59.0 ng/dL
Tanner Stage III	1.9–296.0 ng/dL
Tanner Stage IV	40.0–485.0 ng/dL
Tanner Stage V	124.0–596.0 ng/dL
Testosterone, Female, Bioavailable	
1–6 years	<1.3 ng/dL
7–9 years	0.3–5.0 ng/dL

TABLE 2-75. (*Continued*)

Age	Range
10–11 years	0.4–9.6 ng/dL
12–13 years	1.7–18.8 ng/dL
14–15 years	3.0–22.6 ng/dL
16–17 years	3.3–28.6 ng/dL
18–30 years	2.2–20.6 ng/dL
31–40 years	4.1–25.5 ng/dL
41–51 years	2.8–16.5 ng/dL
Postmenopausal	1.5–9.4 ng/dL
Tanner Stage I	0.3–5.5 ng/dL
Tanner Stage II	1.2–15.0 ng/dL
Tanner Stage III	3.8–28.0 ng/dL
Tanner Stage IV	2.8–39.0 ng/dL
Tanner Stage V	2.5–23.0 ng/dL

➤ Use
• Evaluation of gonadal hormonal function

➤ Interpretation
Increased In
• Adrenal virilizing tumor causing premature puberty in boys or masculinization in women
• CAH
• Idiopathic hirsutism (inconclusive)
• Stein-Leventhal syndrome: variable; increased when virilization is present
• Ovarian stromal hyperthecosis
• Use of certain drugs that alter thyroxine-binding globulins may also affect testosterone-binding globulins; however, the free testosterone level is not affected.

Decreased In
• Primary hypogonadism (e.g., orchiectomy)
• Secondary hypogonadism (e.g., hypopituitarism)
• Testicular feminization
• Klinefelter syndrome levels lower than in normal male individual but higher than in normal female and orchiectomized male
• Estrogen therapy
• Total (but not free) testosterone decreased due to decreased SHBG (e.g., cirrhosis, chronic renal disease)

➤ Limitations
• Due to the availability of many different forms of testosterone assays, as well as the confusion in the literature regarding their clinical relevance, there is a lack of consistency for its measurement in routine clinical situations. The earliest approaches to the measurement of free testosterone were equilibrium dialyses and ultrafiltration. These assays were very cumbersome for routine use.
• Indirect measurement of free testosterone using isotope labeled testosterone was one of the earlier methods proposed and widely used. The endocrine society recently reported a review of

the evidence that the analog-based free testosterone immunoassays should be avoided because of the problems with accuracy and sensitivity. Free testosterone measurements by calculation using algorithms based on the law of mass action, which requires total testosterone, SHBG, and albumin concentrations have excellent correlations with physical separation measures.

THEOPHYLLINE (1,3-DIMETHYLXANTHINE)

➤ Definition
- A naturally occurring (tea) xanthine derivative with diuretic, cardiac stimulant, and smooth muscle relaxant properties
- Other names: Theo-Dur®, Uniphyl®, Slo-bid®, Theolair®
- **Normal range:**
  - 0–5 months: 6–12 μg/mL
  - >6 months: 10–20 μg/mL

➤ Use
- As a bronchodilator to prevent and treat asthma

➤ Interpretation
- **Potentially toxic:** 20–25 μg/mL

➤ Limitations
- Serum: quantitative
  - Immunoassay
    - FPIA, chemiluminescence, EMIT, particle-enhanced turbidimetric inhibition immunoassay
    - No serum separator tubes or gels
    - Separate serum from cells as soon as possible
    - The incidence of patients having antibodies to *Escherichia coli* β-galactosidase is extremely low. However, some samples containing such antibodies may result in artificially high results that do not fit the clinical profile
    - Due to cross-reactivity with 1,3-dimethyluric acid (metabolite), the assay should not be used to quantitate samples from uremic patients
    - If mouse antibodies are utilized, the possibility exists for interference by human anti-mouse antibodies (HAMA) in the sample, which could cause falsely elevated results
    - Limit of quantitation: 0.5–0.8–2.5 μg/mL
  - Reflectance spectrophotometry
    - No serum separator tubes or gels
    - No EDTA, oxalate, citrate tubes
    - Heparin tubes acceptable
    - Separate serum from cells as soon as possible
- Serum/urine-qualitative
  - Extraction followed by GC/MS
  - Component of a multidrug screen
  - No serum separator tubes or gels
  - Separate serum from cells as soon as possible

THROMBIN TIME

➤ Definition
* TT measures the time of conversion of fibrinogen into fibrin once thrombin (used as a reagent) is added
* **Normal range:** 14–21 seconds (may vary depending on reagent and equipment used)

➤ Use
* Detects decreased or abnormal fibrinogen
* Detects unreported heparin use
* Detects other thrombin inhibiting drugs, for example, hirudin, argatroban, and newer agents

➤ Interpretation
Causes of Increased Result
* Very low fibrinogen ($<$80 mg/dL)
* Dysfibrinogenemia
* Interference with polymerization of fibrinogen
  * Fibrin degradation products, such as DIC and pathologic or therapeutic fibrinolysis However, thrombin time is not recommended in the diagnosis of pathologic fibrinolysis or DIC because of very low specificity and low sensitivity
  * High concentrations of monoclonal immunoglobulins
  * Uremia
* Heparin therapy

➤ Limitations
* Preanalytic conditions may interfere with this test.
  * Improper filling of blood collecting tube or use of wrong tubes (containing different anticoagulant than recommended or no anticoagulant)
  * Clots in specimen
  * Hemolysis
  * Heparin contamination of blood, such as drawings from IV lines with heparin flushes (when heparin contamination is suspected, a reptilase time can be performed instead [see p. 323])
* Hyperlipidemia may artificially prolong the thrombin time obtained by optical equipment (most modern machines). In such cases the assay can be done on equipment that uses mechanical clotting, such as the fibrometer.
* Results are unreliable in patients with high fibrinogen ($>$500 mg/dL)
* Patients previously exposed to bovine thrombin to arrest bleeding may develop thrombin antibodies.
* Use of various radiocontrast agents may affect test results.

THROMBOELASTOGRAM (TEG)

➤ Definition
* TEG uses equipment (TEG Analyser) that records the process of blood coagulation, including fibrinolysis and platelet defects.

* It measures *in vitro* the kinetics of clot formation and dissolution by a mechanical process, which monitors very low shear elasticity changes. The different parameters represent different aspects of the patient's hemostasis.

➤ Use
* The TEG is commonly used for cardiac bypass surgery, providing a rapid assessment of anti-coagulation (heparin), restoration of coagulation with the use of protamine sulfate, excess fibrinolysis, and platelet function during the procedure.
* It has been demonstrated to reduce the number of red cell or platelet transfused during open heart surgery or shortly after its termination.

THYROGLOBULIN (Tg)

➤ Definition
* Heterogeneous iodoglycoprotein secreted only by thyroid follicular cells that is involved in iodination and synthesis of thyroid hormones. It is proportional to thyroid mass.
* **Normal value:** <55 ng/mL

➤ Use
* To assess the presence and possibly the extent of residual or recurrent or metastatic follicular or papillary thyroid carcinoma after therapy. In patients with these carcinomas treated with total thyroidectomy or radioiodine and taking thyroid hormone therapy, Tg is undetectable if functional tumor is absent, but is detected by sensitive immunoassay if functional tumor is present. Tg correlates with tumor mass with highest values in patients with metastases to bones and lungs.
* To diagnose factitious hyperthyroidism: Tg is very low or not detectable in factitious hyperthyroidism and is high in all other types of hyperthyroidism (e.g., thyroiditis, Graves disease).
* To predict outcome of therapy for hyperthyroidism; higher remission rates in patients with lower Tg values. Failure to become normal after drug-induced remission suggests relapse after drugs are discontinued.
* To diagnose of thyroid agenesis in newborn

➤ Interpretation
* See Table 2-76

Increased In
* Most patients with differentiated thyroid carcinoma but not with undifferentiated or medullary thyroid carcinomas
* Hyperthyroidism—rapid decline after surgical treatment; gradual decline after radioactive iodine treatment
* Silent (painless) thyroiditis
* Endemic goiter (some patients)
* Marked liver insufficiency

Decreased In
* Thyroid agenesis in newborns
* Total thyroidectomy or destruction by radiation

TABLE 2-76. Thyroid Function Tests in Various Conditions

Condition	TSH	TT4	FT4	T3	Tg	RAIU	Comment
Hypothyroidism							
Primary	I	D	D	D	N/I	D	Increased response to TRH administration
Clinical Subclinical	I	N	N	N	N	NA	No response to TRH administration
Secondary	N/D	D	D	D			
Tertiary	N/D	D	D	D			
Nonthyroidal* illness	V	N/D	N/D	D	D		
Hyperthyroidism							
Primary							
Clinical	D	I	I	I	N	I	
Subclinical	D	N	N	N	N	NA	
T3 thyrotoxicosis	D	N	N	I	N	NA	
TSH-secreting tumor	I	I	I	I	N	NA	
TRH-secreting tumor	I	I	I	I	N	NA	
Factitious							
T4 ingestion	D	I	I	I	D/N	D	Augmented RAIU response to TSH administration
T3 ingestion	D	N	N	I	D/N		
Pregnancy							
With hyperthyroidism	N	I	N	I		X	
With hypothyroidism	N		D			X	I T4 and T3 to normal range
Hereditary increased TBG	N	I	N	I		X	
Hereditary decreased TBG	V	D	V	D	D		
Hashimoto's thyroiditis	V	V	V	V	V	V	Thyroid antibodies; biopsy

(Continued)

347

TABLE 2-76. Thyroid Function Tests in Various Conditions (*Continued*)

Condition	TSH	TT₄	FT₄	T₃	Tg	RAIU	Comment
Goiter	N	N	N	N	N	A	Biopsy
Thyroid carcinoma	N	N	N	N	I	N	Serum calcitonin I in medullary CA; Tg I in differentiated
Nephrosis	N	D	D		D	VI	
Drug effects							
Thyroxine	D	I					
Inorganic iodine	I						
Radiopaque contrast media			I				
Estrogen; birth control pills		I	N		I		
Testosterone	N	D	N	D	D		D TBH
ACTH and corticosteroids	N	D	N	D	D		D TBH
Dilantin	V/I	D	N	N	D		Tissue resistance to T₄
Pituitary only		I	I				T₄ administration does not suppress TSH
Generalized tissue	V/I	V/I	V/I				

0, absent; A, abnormal; D, decreased; I, increased; N, normal; NA, not useful; TT₄, total thyroxine; V, variable; VD, variable decrease; VI, variable increase; X, contraindicated. Underlined test indicates most useful diagnostic change.
*Forms of nonthyroidal illness (euthyroid sick syndrome).

➤ Limitations

- A Tg test is not recommended for initial diagnosis of thyroid carcinomas. The presence of Tg in pleural effusions indicates metastatic differentiated thyroid cancer.
- A Tg test should not be used in patients with preexisting thyroid disorders.
- Tg autoantibodies: patients' serum must always first be screened for these antibodies (present in <10% of persons). In such cases, Tg mRNA can be measured using RT-PCR.
- Because Tg autoantibodies can interfere with both competitive immunoassays and immunometric assays for Tg, all patients should be screened for Tg autoantibodies by a sensitive immunoassay; recovery studies are not adequate for ruling out interference by these autoantibodies.
- Tg antibodies are present in the majority of patients with Hashimoto's thyroiditis but also in approximately 3% of healthy individuals.
- At least 6 weeks should elapse after thyroidectomy or Iodine-125 treatment before a Tg test. Some reports have indicated that Tg levels may remain elevated for several weeks following successful treatment. In this case, serial determinations assessed relative to a posttreatment baseline established for the patient may still be of value in monitoring.

THYROID AUTOANTIBODY TESTS

➤ Definition

- Antithyroid peroxidase (TPO) antibodies are autoantibodies directed against the peroxidase enzyme. This enzyme catalyzes the iodination of tyrosine in thyroglobulin (Tg) during the biosynthesis of T_3 and T_4. Historically, these antibodies were referred to as antimicrosomal antibodies (AMAs) because the antibodies bind to the microsomal part of the thyroid cells. Recent research has identified thyroid peroxidase as the primary antigenic component of microsomes. Measurement of TPO antibodies has essentially replaced the measurement of antimicrosomal antibodies.
- In virtually all cases of Hashimoto disease and in the majority of cases of Graves disease cases, anti-TPO antibodies are elevated. High levels of anti-TPO antibodies, in the context of the clinical presentation of hypothyroidism, confirm the diagnosis of Hashimoto disease.
- Tg autoantibody measurements are most useful for evaluating samples submitted for Tg measurements because Tg autoantibodies can interfere with both competitive immunoassays and immunometric assays for Tg.
- **Normal range:**
  - Tg antibodies: <40 IU/mL
  - TPO antibodies: <35 IU/mL

➤ Use

- To assess the thyroid autoantibody status in patients with thyroid disease.
- To distinguish subacute thyroiditis from Hashimoto thyroiditis, as antibodies are more common in the latter
- Occasionally useful to distinguish Graves disease from toxic multinodular goiter when physical findings are not diagnostic
- Thyroid receptor antibodies mainly used in Graves disease, especially as a predictor of relapse of hyperthyroidism

➤ Interpretation

* Positive in ~95% of cases of Hashimoto disease and ~85% of Graves disease. Very high titer is suggestive of Hashimoto thyroiditis but absence does not exclude Hashimoto thyroiditis. >1:1000 occurs virtually only in Graves disease or Hashimoto thyroiditis.

Increased In

* Significant titer of microsome antibodies indicates Hashimoto thyroiditis or postpartum thyroiditis.
* Significant titer of antibodies in euthyroid patient with unilateral exophthalmos suggests the diagnosis of euthyroid Graves disease. Elevated antibody titer in a patient with Graves disease should direct a surgeon to perform a more limited thyroidectomy to avoid late post-thyroidectomy hypothyroidism.
* Occasionally positive in papillary-follicular carcinoma of thyroid, subacute thyroiditis (briefly), and lymphocytic (painless) thyroiditis (in ~60% of patients)
* Primary thyroid lymphoma often shows very high titers. This result should suggest need for biopsy in elderly patient with a firm enlarging thyroid.
* Low titers are present in >10% of normal population, increasing with age.
* Other autoimmune diseases (e.g., PA, RA, SLE, myasthenia gravis)

Decreased In

* In the absence of antibodies, Hashimoto thyroiditis is very unlikely cause of hypothyroidism.

➤ Limitations

* Tg antibodies may interfere with assay for serum Tg.

THYROID HORMONE–BINDING RATIO (THBR)

➤ Definition

* THBR values can be calculated according to the following equation proposed by the Committee on Nomenclature of the American Thyroid Association.

$$\text{THBR (FTI)} = \frac{T_4 \text{ Value } (\mu g/dL) \times \text{Thyroid Uptake } (\%)}{\text{Median of Reference Interval } (\%)^*}$$

* See Table 2-77
* **Normal range:** 5.93–13.13 μg/dL

➤ Use

* This calculated product permits correction of misleading results of T_3 and T_4 determinations caused by conditions that alter the thyroxine-binding protein concentration (e.g., pregnancy, estrogens, birth control pills).

➤ Interpretation
Increased In

* Hyperthyroidism
* States with decreased TBG (e.g., androgen treatment, chronic liver disease), protein loss, or genetically low TBG.

TABLE 2-77. Free Thyroxine Index in Various Conditions

Condition	T_3	T_4	Free Thyroxine Index (T_7) (T_3 Uptake $\times$ T_4)
Normal			
Range	24–36	4–11	96–396
Mean	31	7	217
Hypothyroid	22	3	66
Hyperthyroid	38	12	456
Pregnancy, estrogen use (especially birth control pills)	20	12	240*

*Normal even though T_3 and T_4 alone are abnormal.

Decreased In
* Hypothyroidism
* States with increased TBG (e.g., estrogen treatment, pregnancy, acute hepatitis, genetically high TBG)

➤ Limitations
* Concordance values of T_4 and THBR tests suggest altered thyroid function.
* Discordant variance suggests primary change in TBG in a euthyroid state (e.g., pregnancy)

THYROID RADIOACTIVE IODINE UPTAKE (RAIU)

➤ Definition
* A tracer dose of radioactive iodine (^{131}I or ^{123}I) is administered orally, and the radioactivity over the thyroid is measured at specific time intervals.
* **Normal range:** 10–35% in 24 hours depending on local variations in iodine intake

➤ Use
* Evaluation of hyperthyroidism associated with low RAIU (e.g., factitious hyperthyroidism, subacute thyroiditis, struma ovarii)
* Distinguish Graves disease from toxic nodular goiter
* Assess function of nodules ("hot" or "cold")
* Determine location and size of functioning thyroid tissue
* Detect metastases from differentiated thyroid cancers
* Evaluate use of radioiodine therapy
* Determine presence of an organification defect in thyroid hormone production
* In combination with T_3 suppression test: Administration of triiodothyronine suppresses RAIU by >50% in the normal person but not in patients with Graves disease or toxic nodules; shows autonomy of TSH secretion. Infrequently used.

➤ Interpretation
Increased In
* Graves disease (diffuse toxic goiter)
* Plummer disease (toxic multinodular goiter)

- Toxic adenoma (uninodular goiter)
- Thyroiditis (early Hashimoto; recovery stage of subacute thyroiditis)
- TSH excess
  - TSH administration
  - TSH production by pituitary tumor (TSH >4 μU/mL) or other neoplasm
  - Defective thyroid hormone synthesis
  - Human chorionic gonadotropin–mediated hyperthyroidism (e.g., choriocarcinoma, hydatidiform mole, embryonal carcinoma of testis, hyperemesis gravidarum)

Decreased In
- Hypothyroidism (tertiary, secondary, late primary)
- Thyroiditis (late Hashimoto; active stage of subacute thyroiditis; RAIU does not usually respond to TSH administration)
- Thyroid hormone administration (T_3 or T_4)
  - Therapeutic
  - Factitious (RAIU is augmented after TSH administration)
- Antithyroid medication
- Iodine-induced hyperthyroidism (Jodbasedow)
- X-ray contrast media, iodine-containing drugs, iodized salt
- Graves disease with iodine excess
- Ectopic hypersecreting thyroid tissue
- Metastatic functioning thyroid carcinoma
- Struma ovarii
- Drugs (e.g., calcitonin, thyroglobulin, corticosteroids, dopamine)

➤ Limitations
- Contraindications: pregnancy, lactation, childhood
- Not valid for 2–4 weeks after administration of antithyroid drugs, thyroid, or iodides; the effect of organic iodine (e.g., x-ray contrast media) may persist for a much longer period.
- Because of widespread dietary use of iodine in the United States, RAIU should not be used to evaluate euthyroid state.
- Increased by withdrawal rebound (thyroid hormones, propylthiouracil), increased iodine excretion (e.g., diuretics, nephrotic syndrome, chronic diarrhea), decreased iodine intake (salt restriction, iodine deficiency)

THYROID-STIMULATING HORMONE (TSH)

➤ Definition
- This glycoprotein hormone of 28–30 kDa is comprised of alpha and beta subunits. It is secreted by the anterior pituitary.
- TSH controls the biosynthesis and release of thyroid hormones T_4 and T_3.
- **Normal range:** 0.5–6.3 μIU/mL, depending on age and sex (Table 2-78)

➤ Use
- Sensitive measure of thyroid function
- Assessing true metabolic status

TABLE 2-78. Normal Ranges of TSH According to Age and Sex

Age	TSH (μIU/mL)	
	Male	Female
0–1 month	0.5–6.5	0.5–6.5 (same as in males)
1–11 month	0.8–6.3	0.8–6.3 (same as in males)
1 year	0.7–6.0	0.7–5.9
6 years	0.7–5.4	0.6–5.1
11 years	0.6–4.9	0.5–4.4
16 years	0.5–4.4	0.5–3.9
18 years	0.28–3.89	0.28–3.89 (same as in males)

- Screening for euthyroidism
  - Normal level in stable ambulatory patient not on interfering drugs excludes thyroid hormone excess or deficiency.
  - TSH is recommended as the initial test rather than T_4.
  - Screening is not recommended for asymptomatic persons without suspicion of thyroid disease or for hospital patients with acute medical or psychiatric illness.
- Initial screening and diagnosis for hyperthyroidism (decreased to undetectable levels except in rare TSH-secreting pituitary adenoma) and hypothyroidism
- Especially useful in early or subclinical hypothyroidism before the patient develops clinical findings, goiter, or abnormalities of other thyroid tests
  - Differentiation of primary (increased levels) from central (pituitary or hypothalamic) hypothyroidism (decreased levels)
  - Monitoring of adequate thyroid hormone replacement therapy in primary hypothyroidism, although T_4 may be mildly increased (up to 6–8 weeks before TSH becomes normal). Serum TSH suppressed to the normal level is the best monitor of dosage of thyroid hormone for treatment of hypothyroidism.
  - Monitoring adequate thyroid hormone therapy in the suppression of thyroid carcinoma (should suppress to <0.1 μIU/mL) or goiter or nodules (should suppress to subnormal levels) with third- or fourth-generation assays
- Replacement of TRH stimulation test in hyperthyroidism, because most patients with euthyroid TSH level have a normal TSH response and patients with undetectable TSH level almost never respond to TRH stimulation

➤ Interpretation
Increased In

- Primary untreated hypothyroidism. The increase is proportionate to the degree of hypofunction, varying from 3 times normal in mild cases to 100 times normal in severe myxedema. A single determination is usually sufficient to establish the diagnosis.
- Patients with hypothyroidism receiving insufficient thyroid hormone replacement therapy
- Patients with Hashimoto thyroiditis, including those with clinical hypothyroidism and about one third of those patients who are clinically euthyroid
- Use of various drugs: amphetamines (abuse), iodine-containing agents (e.g., iopanoic acid, ipodate, amiodarone), and dopamine antagonists (e.g., metoclopramide, domperidone, chlorpromazine, haloperidol)

- Other conditions (test is not clinically useful)
  - Iodide deficiency goiter or iodide-induced goiter or lithium treatment
  - External neck irradiation
  - Postsubtotal thyroidectomy
  - Neonatal period; increased in first 2–3 days of life due to postnatal TSH surge
  - Thyrotoxicosis due to pituitary thyrotroph adenoma or pituitary resistance to thyroid hormone
  - Euthyroid sick syndrome, recovery phase
  - TSH antibodies

Decreased In
- Toxic multinodular goiter
- Autonomously functioning thyroid adenoma
- Ophthalmopathy of euthyroid Graves disease; treated Graves disease
- Thyroiditis
- Extrathyroidal thyroid hormone source
- Factitious
- Overreplacement of thyroid hormone in treatment of hypothyroidism
- Secondary pituitary or hypothalamic hypothyroidism (e.g., tumor, infiltrates)
- Euthyroid sick patients (some patients)
- Acute psychiatric illness
- Severe dehydration
- Drug effect, especially large doses (use FT_4 for evaluation)
  - Glucocorticoids, dopamine, dopamine agonists (bromocriptine), levodopa, T_4 replacement therapy, apomorphine, and pyridoxine; normal or low T_4
  - Antithyroid drug for thyrotoxicosis, especially early in treatment; normal or low T_4
- Assay interference (e.g., antibodies to mouse IgG, autoimmune disease)
- First trimester of pregnancy
- Isolated deficiency (very rare)

➤ Limitations
- TSH may be normal in:
  - Central hypothyroidism. In the absence of hypothalamic or pituitary disease, normal TSH excludes primary hypothyroidism.
  - Recent rapid correction of hyperthyroidism or hypothyroidism
  - Pregnancy
  - Phenytoin therapy
- TSH may not be useful to evaluate thyroid status of hospitalized ill patients.
  - Approximately 3 months of treatment of hypo- or hyperthyroidism; FT_4 is test of choice.
  - Lag time of 6–8 weeks is required for normalization of TSH after initiation of thyroid hormone replacement therapy.
- Dopamine or high doses of glucocorticoids may cause false normal values in primary hypothyroidism and may suppress TSH in nonthyroid illness.
- Rheumatoid factor, human antimouse antibodies, heterophile antibodies, and thyroid hormone autoantibodies may produce spurious results, especially in patients with autoimmune disorders (≤10%).
- Amiodarone may interfere with TSH.

- TSH is not affected by variation in thyroid-binding proteins.
- TSH has a diurnal rhythm, with peaks at 2:00 to 4:00 a.m. and troughs at 5:00 to 6:00 p.m. with ultradian variations.

THYROTROPIN-RELEASING HORMONE (TRH) STIMULATION TEST

➤ Definition
- TRH is a hormone produced in hypothalamus; it can stimulate the release of TSH from the pituitary gland. TSH then further stimulates the production and the release of T_3 and T_4 from the thyroid gland. Therefore, the TRH stimulation test can evaluate the thyroid function status. However, TRH also stimulate the release of growth hormone (GH) as well as prolactin.
- Three blood specimens are collected for serum TSH testing: one immediately prior to TRH injection, and one 15 minutes and one 30 minutes after TRH injection. TRH is administrated IV (200–500 µg). Pharmacy consultation for TRH dosage is recommended.
- See Figure 2-4

➤ Use
- Rarely used clinically for diagnosis of the thyroid diseases. Measurements of serum TSH and T_3 and T_4 levels are informative in evaluating thyroid function in most clinical situations. However, when the diagnosis is still unclear, the TRH stimulation test can be of help.
- May be particularly useful in T_3 toxicosis in which the other test results are normal or in patients clinically suspicious for hyperthyroidism with borderline serum T_3 levels. TRH

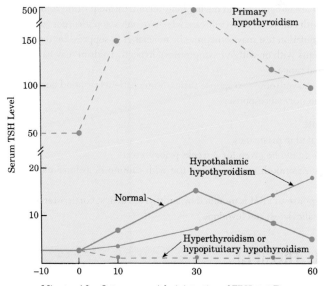

Figure 2-4. Sample curves of serum thyroid-stimulating hormone (TSH) response to administration of thyrotropin-releasing hormone (TRH) in various conditions.

stimulation test is superior to the T_3 suppression test of RAIU. Abnormal TSH response to TRH administration does not definitely establish the diagnosis of hyperthyroidism (because autonomous production of normal or slightly increased amounts of thyroid hormones causes pituitary suppression). TRH test may remain abnormal even after successful therapy of Graves disease.
- Helps differentiate two forms of thyrotropin-induced hyperthyroidism (whether or not due to tumor)
- May help differentiate hypothalamic from pituitary hypothyroidism

➤ Interpretation
- Normally, a significant rise in serum TSH occurs from a basal level of 2–3 µU/mL, and this then returns to normal by 120 minutes. Response is usually greater in women than in men. A blunted response indicates hyperthyroidism but may occur in other conditions (e.g., uremia, Cushing syndrome, starvation, elevated levels of glucocorticoids, depression, some elderly patients). Largely replaced by sensitive TSH assays.
  - Hyperthyroidism: ruled out by a normal increase of >2–3 µU/mL after TRH administration.
  - Primary hypothyroidism: an exaggerated prolonged rise of an already increased TSH level
  - Secondary (pituitary) hypothyroidism: no rise in the decreased TSH level
  - Hypothalamic hypothyroidism: low serum T_3, T_4, and TSH levels, with a TRH response that may be exaggerated or normal or (most characteristically) with a peak delay 45–60 minutes
- TSH high-sensitivity <0.1 mU/L, obviates need for TRH, except for TSH-secreting tumor and thyroid hormone resistance (in which case TSH thyroxine is high).
- Interpretation must be based on clinical studies that exclude the pituitary gland as the site of the disease.
- Lack of response shows adequate therapy in patients receiving thyroid hormones to shrink thyroid nodules and goiters and during long-term treatment of thyroid carcinoma.
- In patients with euthyroid Graves disease who have only exophthalmos (unilateral or bilateral), the TRH stimulation test may sometimes be normal. A T_3 suppression test may be required.
- Elderly patients with or without symptoms of hyperthyroidism may have serum T_4 and T_3 in upper normal range.
- Euthyroid sick syndrome—response varies. Some patients respond normally, whereas many have less than normal response.

➤ Limitations
- Contraindicated in pregnancy
- No T4 or T3 should be given for 3 weeks prior to test
- TRH can cause smooth muscle spasm; use with caution in asthma and ischemic heart disease.
- The TSH response to TRH is modified by antithyroid drugs, corticosteroids, estrogens, large amounts of salicylates, and levodopa.

THYROXINE, FREE (FT₄)

➤ Definition
- Both free and bound forms of T_4 and T_3 are present in the blood. More than 99% of the T_4 and T_3 circulates in the blood bound to carrier proteins, leaving less than 1% unbound. It is

this level of unbound or free hormone that correlates with the functional thyroid state in most individuals.

- FT_4 is usually 0.02–0.04% of total T_4.
- See Table 2-76.
- **Normal range** (adults): 0.58–1.64 ng/dL
  - Pregnant women:
    - First trimester: 0.73–1.13 ng/dL
    - Second trimester: 0.54–1.18 ng/dL
    - Third trimester: 0.56–1.09 ng/dL

➤ Use

- FT_4 gives corrected values in patients in whom the total T_4 is altered on account of changes in serum proteins or in binding sites (e.g., pregnancy, drugs [such as androgens, estrogens, birth control pills, phenytoin], altered levels of serum proteins [e.g., nephrosis])
- Monitoring restoration to normal range is the only laboratory criterion to estimate appropriate replacement dose of levothyroxine because 6–8 weeks are required before TSH reflects these changes.
- Not generally helpful unless pituitary/hypothalamic disease is suspected.

➤ Interpretation

Increased In

- Hyperthyroidism
- Hypothyroidism treated with thyroxine
- Euthyroid sick syndrome
- Occasional patients with hydatidiform mole or choriocarcinoma with marked hCG elevations may show increased FT_4, suppressed TSH, and blunted TSH response to TRH stimulation; returns to normal with effective treatment of trophoblastic disease; severe dehydration (may be >6.0 ng/dL).

Decreased In

- Hypothyroidism
- Hypothyroidism treated with triiodothyronine
- Euthyroid sick syndrome

➤ Limitations

- FT_4 assays based on direct equilibrium dialysis are considered reference methods.
- FT_4 assays are prone to inaccurate readings in pregnant women. The studies have shown that FT_4 index measurement is more reliable than free T_4 immunoassays in pregnant women.
- Anticonvulsant drug therapy (particularly phenytoin) may result in decreased FT_4 levels due to an increased hepatic metabolism and secondarily to displacement of hormone from binding sites

THYROXINE, TOTAL (T₄)

➤ Definition

- T_4 is major secretion of thyroid. Bound to TBG, prealbumin, and albumin in blood. In tissues, it is deiodinated to T_3, which causes hormonal action and is responsible for hormonal action.
- See Tables 2-76, 2-79, and Figure 2-5.

TABLE 2-79. Free Thyroxine (FT$_4$) and Thyroid-Stimulating Hormone (TSH) Levels in Various Conditions

		Sensitive TSH		
		Normal	Low	High
Normal		Euthyroid	Subclinical/early hyperthyroidism* NTI Drug effects (e.g., L-dopa, glucocorticoids) Replacement therapy or excess T$_4$ therapy for hypothyroidism Rule out thyrotoxicosis	Subclinical/early hypothyroidism[†] NTI Drug effects (e.g., iodine, lithium, antithyroid drugs, amiodarone, interferon alfa) Insufficient T$_4$ therapy for hypothyroidism First 4–6 weeks of therapy for hypothyroidism
T$_4$	**Low**	Secondary hypothyroidism Drug effects (e.g., T$_3$, phenytoin, androgens, salicylates, carbamazepine, rifampin)	Secondary hypothyroidism NTI Drug effects (e.g., dopamine, T$_3$, corticosteroids) T$_3$ hyperthyroidism (e.g., Graves disease, toxic goiter, thyroiditis, factitious/iatrogenic, hyperthyroidism, struma ovarii, thyroid carcinoma)	Primary hypothyroidism Drug effects (e.g., iodine, lithium, antithyroid drugs, amiodarone) Insufficient T$_4$ therapy for hypothyroidism
	High	NTI (e.g., psychiatric and acute illness) Abnormal binding (excess TBG, familial dysalbuminemic hyperthyroxemia, some monoclonal proteins) Thyroid hormone resistance Drug effects (e.g., estrogen, iodine drugs or contrast media, thyroxine [factitious])	NTI (e.g., psychiatric and acute illness) Primary hyperthyroidism[‡]	TSH-secreting tumor Thyroid hormone resistance

T$_3$, triiodothyronine; T$_4$, thyroxine; NTI, nonthyroid illness.
*Low TSH with normal T$_4$.
[†]High TSH with normal T$_4$.
[‡]In 95% of cases of thyrotoxicosis. Serum T$_3$ is needed for diagnosis of T$_3$-thyrotoxicosis in the other 5% of cases of thyrotoxicosis.

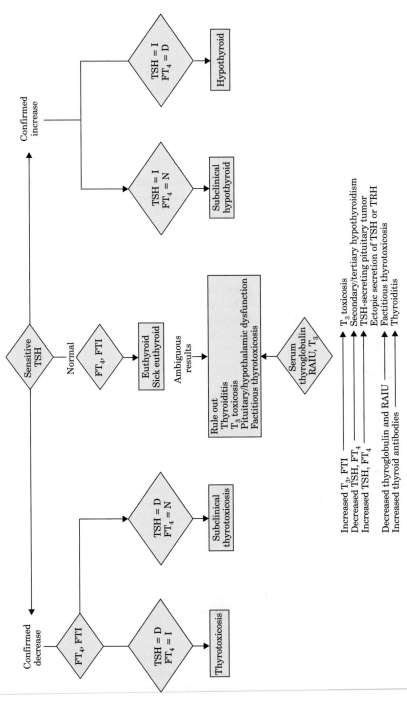

Figure 2-5. Algorithm for thyroid function testing. (D, decreased; I, increased; N, normal.)

➤ Use
- Reflects secretory activity; useful in diagnosis of hyper- and hypothyroidism, especially when overt or due to pituitary or hypothalamic disease
- **Normal range:** 6.09–12.23 μg/dL

➤ Interpretation
- Not affected by:
  - Mercurial diuretics
  - Nonthyroidal iodine

Increased In
- Hyperthyroidism
- Pregnancy
- Drugs (e.g., estrogens, birth control pills, d-thyroxine, thyroid extract, TSH, amiodarone, heroin, methadone, amphetamines, some radiopaque substances for x-ray studies [ipodate, iopanoic acid])
- Euthyroid sick syndrome
- Increase in TBG or abnormal thyroxine-binding prealbumin
- Familial dysalbuminemic hyperthyroxinemia—albumin binds T_4 but not T_3 more avidly than normal, causing changes similar to thyrotoxicosis (total T_4 ~20 μg/dL, normal thyroid hormone–binding ratio, increased free T_4 index) but patient is not clinically thyrotoxic.
- Serum T_4 >20 μg/dL usually indicates true hyperthyroidism rather than increased TBG.
- May be found in euthyroid patients with increased serum TBG
- Much higher in first 2 months of life than in normal adults

Decreased In
- Hypothyroidism
- Hypoproteinemia (e.g., nephrosis, cirrhosis)
- Certain drugs (phenytoin, triiodothyronine, testosterone, ACTH, corticosteroids)
- Euthyroid sick syndrome
- Decrease in TBG

Normal In
- Hyperthyroid patients with:
  - T_3 thyrotoxicosis
  - Factitious hyperthyroidism owing to T_3 (Cytomel)
  - Decreased binding capacity due to hypoproteinemia or ingestion of certain drugs (e.g., phenytoin, salicylates)

➤ Limitations
- Various drugs can interfere with the test result.

THYROXINE-BINDING GLOBULIN (TBG)

➤ Definition
- This glycoprotein is the principal carrier for T_3 and T_4. It declines with age in parallel with total and free T_4 and T_3. The latter changes are accompanied by an increase in rT_3 and rT_3 index, suggesting a decrease in peripheral conversion of T_4 and T_3 rather than the change in secretory behavior of thyroid gland itself.

* With the availability of better free thyroid hormone tests, the TBG test is rarely used to assess the thyroid binding hormone status.
* **Normal range:**
  * Male: 1.2–2.5 mg/dL
  * Female: 1.4–3.0 mg/dL

➤ Use
* Diagnosis of genetic or idiopathic excess TBG
* Sometimes used to detect recurrent or metastatic differentiated thyroid carcinoma, especially follicular type and where patient has had an increased level due to carcinoma.
* To distinguish increased/decreased total T_3 or total T_4 concentrations due to changes in TBG; same purpose as T_3 resin uptake and free thyroxine index.

➤ Interpretation
Increased In
* Pregnancy
* Certain drugs (e.g., estrogens, birth control pills, perphenazine, clofibrate, heroin, methadone)
* Estrogen-producing tumors
* Systemic illness is increased early
* Acute intermittent porphyria
* Acute or chronic active hepatitis
* Lymphocytic painless subacute thyroiditis
* Neonates
* Inherited
* Idiopathic
* An increased TBG is associated with increased serum T_4 and decreased T_3 resin uptake; a converse association exists for decreased TBG.

Decreased In
* Nephrosis and other causes of marked hypoproteinemia such as liver disease, severe illness (late), stress (thyroxine-binding-prealbumin [TBPA] also decreased)
* Deficiency of TBG, genetic or idiopathic
* Acromegaly (TBPA also decreased)
* Severe acidosis
* Certain drugs (e.g., androgens, anabolic steroids; glucocorticoids [TBPA is increased])
* Testosterone-producing tumors
* Major illness, surgical stress, protein malnutrition, malabsorption resulting from various causes

➤ Limitations
* Decreased binding of T_3 and T_4 due to drugs (salicylates, phenytoin, Orinase, Diabinese, penicillin, heparin, barbital)

TISSUE TRANSGLUTAMINASE IgA ANTIBODY (tTG-IgA)

➤ Definition
* Celiac disease (CD) is an immune-mediated enteropathy caused by a permanent sensitivity to gluten in genetically susceptible individuals. Testing should begin with serologic evaluation, and the most sensitive and specific tests are tissue transglutaminase

IgA antibody (tTG-IgA) and endomysial IgA antibody (EMA-IgA), which have equivalent diagnostic accuracy. Anti-tTG antibodies are highly sensitive and specific for the diagnosis of CD. The enzyme tTG is the major target antigen recognized by anti-endomysial antibodies.

- Based on the current evidence and practical considerations, including accuracy, reliability, and cost, measurement of tTG-IgA is recommended for initial testing for CD. Although as accurate as tTG, measurement of IEMA-IgA is observer dependent and, therefore, more subject to interpretation error and added cost. Because of the inferior accuracy of the antigliadin antibody tests (AGA), the use of AGA IgA and AGA IgG tests is no longer recommended for detecting CD.
- **Normal range:** <20 units (negative)

➤ Use

- Diagnosis of certain gluten-sensitive enteropathies, such as CD and dermatitis herpetiformis
- Monitoring adherence to gluten-free diet in patients with dermatitis herpetiformis and CD
- Evaluating children with failure to thrive

➤ Interpretation
Increased In

- CD (20–30 units: weak positive; >30 units: moderate to strong positive)
- Autoimmune skin disease and dermatitis herpetiformis

➤ Limitations

- All testing should be performed while patients are on a gluten-containing diet.
- IgA deficiency is more common in CD (2–5%) than in the general population (<0.5 percent). The EMA-IgA and tTG-IgA serology tests will be falsely negative in untreated CD in patients with IgA deficiency. As a result, total serum IgA can be measured in addition to EMA-IgA or tTG-IgA, especially when there is heightened clinical suspicion for CD and IgA markers are negative. If total IgA levels are abnormally low, an IgG-based assay should be used to test for CD.
- The IgG antigliadin assay has been traditionally used in this circumstance, but is not ideal, since it yields frequent false-positive results. Therefore, serum IgG-tTG or IgG deamidated gliadin peptide (DPG) tests are preferable. Negative results on testing for HLA DQ2 or DQ8 can also help exclude the diagnosis in this setting.
- If serology is negative and/or there is substantial clinical doubt remaining, then further investigation should be performed with endoscopy and bowel biopsy. This is especially important in patients with frank malabsorptive symptoms, since many syndromes can mimic CD. For the patient with frank malabsorptive symptoms, bowel biopsy should be performed regardless of serologic test results.
- False-positive tests are rare but have been reported in patients with other autoimmune syndromes. Because the tTG antigen is derived from liver cells, false-positive results may be seen in patients with autoimmune liver disease.

➤ Suggested Reading
Guideline for the diagnosis and treatment of celiac disease in children: recommendations of the North American Society for Pediatric Gastroenterology, Hepatology and Nutrition. *J Pediatr Gastroenterol Nutr.* 2005;40(1): 1–19.

TRANSFERRIN (TRF)

➤ Definition
* Transferrin transports circulating Fe^{3+} molecules. Normally only about one third of iron-binding sites are occupied (the remainder is called unsaturated iron-binding capacity).
* The half-life of transferrin is approximately 8–10 days. Plasma levels are regulated primarily by availability of iron, iron deficiency anemia. Plasma levels rise on successful treatment with iron and return to normal.
* **Normal range:** 202–336 mg/dL

➤ Use
* Differential diagnosis of anemias

➤ Interpretation
Increased In
* Iron-deficiency anemia; inversely proportional to iron stores
* Pregnancy, estrogen therapy, hyperestrogenism

Decreased In
* Hypochromic microcytic anemia of chronic disease
* Acute inflammation
* Protein deficiency or loss (e.g., burns, chronic infections, chronic diseases [e.g., various liver and kidney diseases, neoplasms]), nephrosis, malnutrition)

➤ Limitations
* Transferrin in CSF appears in its desialated form, the Tau protein (beta2-transferin). This form can be identified electrophoretically. The clinical application for identification of Tau protein is in the investigation of rhinorrhea or otorrhea, where its presence confirms the source of CSF leakage through a fracture or operative or traumatic site.
* Partly desialated transferrin is a marker for heavy alcohol ingestion.

TRIGLYCERIDES

➤ Definition
* Triglycerides are a form of fat and a major source of energy for the body. Most triglycerides are stored in adipose tissue as glycerol, monoglycerides, and fatty acids, and the liver converts these to triglycerides. Following eating, increased levels of triglycerides are found in the blood.
* Triglycerides move via the blood from the gut to adipose tissue for storage. Most triglycerides are carried in the blood by lipoproteins. Of the total triglycerides, about 80% are in VLDLs and 15% in LDLs, which play an important role in metabolism as energy sources and transporters of dietary fat.
* **Normal ranges:** see Table 2-80

➤ Use
* Elevated levels of triglycerides in the blood are associated with an increased risk of developing cardiovascular disease and arteriosclerosis.

TABLE 2-80. National Cholesterol Education Program Guidelines for Triglycerides*

Triglyceride Level (mg/dL)	Category
<150	Normal
150–199	Borderline-high
200–499	High
≥500	Very high

*These values are based on fasting plasma triglyceride levels.

➤ Interpretation

- Concentrations associated with certain disorders:
  - <150 mg/dL not associated with any disease state
  - 250–500 mg/dL associated with peripheral vascular disease; may be a marker for patients with genetic forms of hyperlipoproteinemias who need specific therapy
  - >500 mg/dL associated with high risk of pancreatitis
  - >1000 mg/dL associated with hyperlipidemia, especially type I or type V; substantial risk of pancreatitis
  - >5000 mg/dL associated with eruptive xanthoma, corneal arcus, lipemia retinalis, enlarged liver and spleen

Increased In

- Hyperlipoproteinemia types I, IIb, III, IV, and V
- Glycogen storage disease (Von Gierke disease)
- Diabetes
- Hypothyroidism
- Nephrosis, chronic renal disease
- Pancreatitis
- Liver disease, alcoholism
- Werner syndrome
- Down syndrome
- Myocardial infarction
- Gout

Decreased In

- Abetalipoproteinemia
- Malnutrition
- Hyperthyroidism
- Hyperparathyroidism
- Malabsorption syndrome

➤ Limitations

- Factors that increase triglyceride levels include food and alcohol intake (should be 12-hour fast [24 hours for alcohol]); corticosteroids, protease inhibitors for HIV, beta blockers, and estrogens; pregnancy; acute illness; smoking; and obesity
- Factors that decrease triglyceride levels include exercise and weight loss
- Diurnal variation causes triglycerides to be lowest in the morning and highest around noon

➤ Other Considerations
- Serum for triglyceride and for calculating LDL-C should follow a 12-hour fast.

➤ Suggested Reading
National Institutes of Health, National Heart Lung and Blood Institute's National Cholesterol Education Program. http://www.nhlbi.nih.gov/about/ncep/ Accessed Nov. 18, 2010.

TRIIODOTHYRONINE (T₃)

➤ Definition
- T_4 (thyroxine) is converted to T_3 in peripheral tissues; ~20% is synthesized by follicular cells. Most T_3 is transported bound to protein; only 0.3% is in free unbound state.
- See Table 2-76 and Figure 2-5.
- **Normal range:**
  - Total T_3: 87–178 ng/dL
  - Free T_3: 2.5–3.9 pg/mL

➤ Use
- Diagnosis of T_3 thyrotoxicosis (when TSH is suppressed but T_4 is normal) or cases in which FT_4 is normal in presence of symptoms of hyperthyroidism
- Evaluating cases in which FT_4 is borderline elevated
- Evaluating cases in which overlooking diagnosis of hyperthyroidism is undesirable (e.g., unexplained atrial fibrillation)
- Monitoring the course of hyperthyroidism
- Monitoring T_4 replacement therapy—is better than T_4 or FT_4, but TSH is preferred to both
- Predicting outcome of antithyroid drug therapy in patients with Graves disease
- Evaluation of amiodarone-induced thyrotoxicosis
- Good biochemical indicator of severity of thyrotoxicity in hyperthyroidism
- Free T_3 gives corrected values in patients in whom the total T_3 is altered on account of changes in serum proteins or in binding sites (e.g., pregnancy), drugs (e.g., androgens, estrogens, birth control pills, phenytoin [Dilantin]), altered levels of serum proteins (e.g., nephrosis)

➤ Interpretation
Increased In
- Elevated concentrations of T_3 occur in Graves disease and most other classical causes of hyperthyroidism.

Decreased In
- Decreased concentrations occur in primary hypothyroid diseases such as Hashimoto thyroiditis and neonatal hypothyroidism or secondary hypothyroidism due to defects at the hypothalamohypophyseal level
- May decrease by ≤25% in healthy older persons while FT_4 remains normal

➤ Limitations
- Serum T_3 parallels FT_4; is early indicator of hyperthyroidism but TSH is better
- Not recommended for diagnosis of hypothyroidism; decreased values have minimal clinical significance

- More than 99% of the total concentration of T_3 and T_4 is bound by serum proteins, which is not available to elicit biologic activity. It is only the free fraction ($<1\%$) that is readily available to bind its receptor and stimulate a response from the target organ or tissues
- Values below the lower limit of the expected values range can be caused by a number of conditions, including nonthyroidal illness, acute and chronic stress, and hypothyroidism.

TRIIODOTHYRONINE (T_3) RESIN UPTAKE (RUR)

➤ Definition
- Measures unoccupied binding sites on TBG
- Now replaced by free T_4
- Not a measure of T_3 concentration, which is assayed by other methods for diagnosis of T_3 thyrotoxicosis
- See Table 2-77.
- **Normal range:** median value of 40.0% (0.40) with a 95% nonparametric range of 32.0–48.4%

➤ Use
- Only with simultaneous measurement of serum T_4 to calculate T_7 in order to exclude the possibility that an increased Total T_4 is due to an increase in TBG
- RUR is inversely proportional to unsaturated hormone binding sites.
- Total T4 × RUR is proportional to free T_4 and inversely proportional to TSH

➤ Interpretation
- Decreases when binding protein increases (pregnancy)
- Increases when binding protein decreases (hyperthyroidism)

➤ Limitations
- Normal in pregnancy with hyperthyroidism, nontoxic goiter, and in use of certain drugs (e.g., mercurials, iodine)
- In some cases of severe nonthyroid illness, RUR does not fully compensate and does not adjust the T_4 into the normal range.

TROPONINS, CARDIAC-SPECIFIC TROPONIN I AND TROPONIN T

➤ Definition
- Cardiac troponin T and troponin I, also known as TnI, TnT, cTnI, cTnT, and cTn, are cardiac regulatory proteins specific to the myocardium that control the calcium-mediated interaction between actin and myosin.
- **Normal range:**
  - Troponin T: 0.0–0.1 ng/mL
  - Troponin I: 0.0–0.04 ng/mL

➤ Use
- Cardiac troponin is the preferred test for diagnosis of acute coronary syndrome (ACS). cTn establishes the diagnosis of irreversible myocardial necrosis (e.g., anoxia, contusion, inflam-

mation), even when ECG changes or CK-MB are nondiagnostic (which occurs in ≤50% of patients with ACS).

* Serial normal cTn rules out myocardial necrosis.
* In patients with a clinical syndrome consistent with ACS, a peak concentration exceeding the 99th percentile of values for a reference control group should be considered indicative of increased mortality, myocardial infarcts, and recurrent ischemic events.
* Patients with ACS patients and cTnI and cTnT results above the decision-limit should be labeled as having myocardial injury and a high-risk profile.
* Troponin testing on hospital presentation followed by serial sampling with timing of sampling based on the clinical circumstances. cTnI may remain increased for ≤9 days, and cTnT may remain increased for ≤14 days.
* The long duration of increased cTn provides a longer diagnostic window than CK-MB but may make it difficult to recognize reinfarction.
* cTn is as sensitive as CK-MB during the first 48 hours after an AMI (>85% concordance with CK-MB); sensitivity is 33% from 0–2 hours, 50% from 2–4 hours, 75% from 4–8 hours, and approaching 100% from 8 hours after onset of chest pain. It may take ≤12 hours for all patients to show an increase. Sensitivity remains high for 6 days. Specificity is close to 100%.
* Serial cTn values may be indicator of cardiac allograft rejection. In selecting heart donors, cTnT >1.6 ng/mL predicts early graft failure with S/S = 73%/94%; cTnT >0.1 ng/mL predicts early graft failure with S/S = 64%/>98%.
* Troponin measurements are also useful in the differential diagnosis of skeletal muscle injury. Normal cTn values exclude myocardial necrosis in patients with increased CK of skeletal muscle origin (e.g., arduous physical exercise).
* Useful for diagnosis of perioperative AMI when CK-MB may be increased by skeletal muscle injury.
* Troponin may also be increased in <50% of patients with acute pericarditis. A value <0.5 ng/mL indicates no myocardial damage. A value >2.0 ng/mL indicates some myocardial necrosis.
* Troponin is not increased by electrical cardioversion or by pulmonary or orthopedic surgery.

➤ Interpretation
Increased In
* Myocardial infarction
* Cardiac trauma, including ablation, pacing, cardioversion, cardiac surgery
* CHF (acute and chronic)
* Aortic dissection, aortic valve disease, or hypertrophic cardiomyopathy
* Tachy- or bradyarrhythmias, or heart block
* Myocarditis
* Rhabdomyolysis with cardiac injury
* Hypotension

➤ Limitations
* cTnT may be increased in some patients with skeletal muscle injury and myotonic dystrophy but not in third-generation assays. cTnI is not increased by skeletal muscle injury, making it more highly specific for myocardial injury.
* Heterophile antibodies may cause false-positive results.
* Presence of fibrin due to incomplete clot retraction can cause false-positive reactions.

➤ Suggested Readings

Apple FS, Jesse RL, Newby LK, et al. National Academy of Clinical Biochemistry. National Academy of Clinical Biochemistry and IFCC Committee for Standardization of Markers of Cardiac Damage Laboratory Medicine Practice Guidelines: Analytical issues for biochemical markers of acute coronary syndromes. *Clin Chem.* 2007;53(4):547–551.

Jaffe AS. The clinical impact of the universal diagnosis of myocardial infarction. *Clin Chem Lab Med.* 2008;46(11):1485–1488.

Morrow DA, Cannon CP, Jesse RL, et al. National Academy of Clinical Biochemistry. National Academy of Clinical Biochemistry Laboratory Medicine Practice Guidelines: Clinical characteristics and utilization of biochemical markers in acute coronary syndromes. *Circulation.* 2007;115(13):e356–375.

Roongsritong C, Warraich I, Bradley C. Common causes of troponin elevations in the absence of acute myocardial infarction incidence and clinical significance. *Chest.* 2004;125(5):1877–1884.

Starrow AB, Apple FS, Wu AH, et al. National Academy of Clinical Biochemistry Laboratory Medicine Practice Guidelines: point of care testing, oversight, and administration of cardiac biomarkers for acute coronary syndromes. *Point Care.* 2007;6(4):215–222.

Thygesen K, Alpert JS, White HD, Joint ESC/ACCF/AHA/WHF Task Force for the Redefinition of Myocardial Infarction. Universal definition of myocardial infarction. *Eur Heart J.* 2007;28:2525–2538; *Circulation.* 2007;116:2634–2653; *J Am Coll Cardiol.* 2007;50:2173–2195.

UREA NITROGEN, URINE

➤ Definition

- Urea is a low–molecular-weight substance that is freely filtered by glomeruli and the majority is excreted into the urine, although variable amounts are reabsorbed along the nephron. Urine urea nitrogen is a measure of protein breakdown in the body. Urea is excreted by the kidneys, so excretion of urea can reflect kidney function. Approximately 50% of urinary solute excretion and 90–95% of total nitrogen excretion is composed of urea under normal conditions.
- **Normal range:**
  - 24-hour urine: 2–20 g/day
  - Random urine:
    - Male: 2.8–9.8 g/g creatinine
    - Female: 3.1–11.6 g/g creatinine

➤ Use

- Determination of a person's protein balance and the amount of dietary protein needed by severely ill patients.

➤ Interpretation

Increased In

- Too much protein intake and/or increased protein breakdown in the body
- Hyperthyroidism

Decreased In

- Malnutrition
- Kidney damage and insufficiency from any cause
- Normal growing children and infants
- Pregnancy
- Low-protein and high-carbohydrate diet
- Liver disease

➤ Limitations
- Levels increase with age and protein content in the diet.
- Administration of GH, testosterone, and insulin decrease the urine levels.

URIC ACID (2,6,8 TRIOXYPURINE, URATE)

➤ Definition
- Uric acid is an end product of purine catabolism; it is released as DNA and RNA are degraded by dying cells. Most uric acid is synthesized in the liver and intestinal mucosa. Two thirds is excreted by the kidneys, and one third is excreted via the GI tract.
- **Normal range:**
  - Male: 2.5–8.0 mg/dL
  - Female: 1.9–7.5 mg/dL

➤ Use
- Monitor treatment of gout
- Monitor chemotherapeutic treatment of neoplasms to avoid renal urate deposition with possible renal failure (tumor lysis syndrome)

➤ Interpretation
Increased In
- Renal failure (does not correlate with severity of kidney damage; urea and creatinine should be used)
- Gout
- 25% of the relatives of patients with gout
- Asymptomatic hyperuricemia (e.g., incidental finding with no evidence of gout; clinical significance is not known but people so afflicted should be rechecked periodically for gout); the higher the level of serum uric acid, the greater the likelihood of an attack of acute gouty arthritis
- Increased destruction of nucleoproteins
  - Leukemia, multiple myeloma
  - Polycythemia
  - Lymphoma, especially postirradiation; other disseminated neoplasms
  - Cancer chemotherapy (e.g., nitrogen mustards, vincristine, mercaptopurine, prednisone)
  - Hemolytic anemia
  - Sickle cell anemia
  - Resolving pneumonia
  - Toxemia of pregnancy (serial determinations to follow therapeutic response and estimate prognosis)
  - Psoriasis (one third of patients)
- Drugs (examples)
  - Intoxicants (e.g., barbiturates, methyl alcohol, ammonia, carbon monoxide); some patients with alcoholism
  - Decreased renal clearance or tubular secretion (e.g., various diuretics [thiazides, furosemide, ethacrynic acid], and all diuretics except spironolactone and ticrynafen)
  - Nephrotoxic effect (e.g., mitomycin C)

- Low-dose salicylates (<4 g/day)
- Other effects (e.g., levodopa, phenytoin sodium)
- Metabolic acidosis
- Diet
  - High-protein weight-reduction diet
  - Excess nucleoprotein (e.g., sweetbreads, liver) may increase level ≤1 mg/dL
  - Alcohol consumption
- Miscellaneous
  - von Gierke disease
  - Chronic lead poisoning
  - Lesch-Nyhan syndrome
  - Maple syrup urine disease
  - Down syndrome
  - Polycystic kidneys
  - Calcinosis universalis and circumscripta
  - Hypoparathyroidism
  - Primary hyperparathyroidism
  - Hypothyroidism
  - Sarcoidosis
  - Chronic berylliosis
  - Patients with arteriosclerosis and hypertension (serum uric acid is increased in 80% of patients with elevated serum triglycerides)
  - Certain population groups (e.g., Blackfoot and Pima Indians, Filipinos, New Zealand Maoris)
- Most common causes in hospitalized men are azotemia, metabolic acidosis, diuretics, gout, myelolymphoproliferative disorders, other drugs, unknown causes
- It is difficult to justify therapy in asymptomatic persons with hyperuricemia to prevent gouty arthritis, uric acid stones, urate nephropathy, or risk of cardiovascular disease.

Decreased In

- Drugs
  - ACTH
  - Uricosuric drugs (e.g., high doses of salicylates, probenecid, cortisone, allopurinol, coumarin)
  - Various other drugs (radiographic contrast agents, glyceryl guaiacolate, estrogens, phenothiazines, indomethacin)
- Wilson disease
- Fanconi syndrome
- Acromegaly (some patients)
- Celiac disease (slightly)
- PA in relapse (some patients)
- Xanthinuria
- Neoplasms (occasional cases) (e.g., carcinomas, Hodgkin disease)
- Healthy adults with isolated defect in tubular transport of uric acid (Dalmatian dog mutation)
- Decreased in ~5% of hospitalized patients; most common causes are postoperative state (GI surgery, coronary artery bypass), DM, various drugs, and SIADH in association with hyponatremia

Unchanged In

- Colchicine administration

➤ Limitations
- Methodologic interference (e.g., ascorbic acid, levodopa, methyldopa)
- A purine rich diet (liver, kidney, sweat bread) as well as severe exercise, increases uric acid values.
- Rapid degradation of uric acid occurs at room temperature in the plasma of patients with tumor lysis syndrome who are treated with rasburicase. Blood should be collected in prechilled tubes containing heparin, immediately immersed in ice water bath, centrifuged in a precooled centrifuge, and the separated plasma maintained in an ice-water bath; and it should be analyzed within 4 hours of collection.

URIC ACID, URINE

➤ Definition
- Uric acid is produced in the liver from the degradation of dietary and endogenously synthesized purine compounds. The normal male adult has a total body urate pool of approximately 1200 mg, twice that of the female adult. This gender difference may be explained by an enhancement of renal urate excretion due to the effects of estrogenic compounds in premenopausal women.
- Under normal steady state conditions, daily turnover of 60% of the urate pool is achieved by balanced production and elimination of uric acid. Human tissues do not have the ability to metabolize urate. Therefore, to maintain homeostasis, urate must be eliminated by the gut and the kidney. The entry of urate into the intestine is most likely a passive process that varies with serum urate concentration. Intestinal tract bacteria are able to degrade uric acid. This breakdown process is responsible for approximately one third of total urate turnover, and accounts for nearly all urate disposed of by extra renal routes. Under normal conditions, uric acid is almost completely degraded by colonic bacteria, with little being found in the stool. Urinary uric acid excretion accounts for the remaining two thirds of the uric acid turned over daily.
- **Normal range:**
  - 24-hour urine: 250–750 mg/day
  - Random urine:
    - Male: 104–593 mg/g creatinine
    - Female: 95–741 mg/g creatinine

➤ Use
- Diagnosis of kidney stones
- Monitoring of people with gout, since many of these patients develop uric acid kidney stones

➤ Interpretation
Increased In
- Gout
- Renal failure
- Leukemia
- Multiple myeloma
- Lymphoma
- Toxemia of pregnancy
- Lesch-Nyhan syndrome

- Down syndrome
- Polycystic kidney disease
- Chronic lead nephropathy

Decreased In
- Wilson disease
- Fanconi syndrome
- Some malignancies
- Low purine diet
- Folic acid deficiency

➤ Limitations
- Hyperuricosuria is present in patients with renal calculus formation. Even mild renal failure decreases uric acid excretion. Uric acid excretion is decreased with hypertension
- Urine uric acid levels are elevated in states of uric acid overproduction such as in leukemia and polycythemia and after intake of food rich in nucleoproteins.
- High levels of bilirubin and ascorbic acid may interfere with measurement.
- Rasburicase (Elitek) causes enzymatic degradation of uric acid within blood samples left at room temperature resulting in spuriously low uric acid levels. To ensure accurate measurements in patients who have received rasburicase, blood must be collected into pre-chilled tubes containing heparin anticoagulant and immediately immersed and maintained in an ice bath; plasma samples must be assayed within 4 hours of sample collection.

URINALYSIS, COMPLETE

➤ Definition
- The dipstick reagent strip method is commonly used to assess the chemical evaluation of urine. The most frequently performed chemical tests using reagent test strips are specific gravity, pH, protein, glucose, ketones, blood, leukocyte esterase, nitrite, bilirubin, and urobilinogen.
- **Specific gravity:** Specific gravity is a measure of the dissolved substances present in the urine. It is a physical property of urine and an expression of concentration.
- **Color:** The color of the specimen is measured by comparison to four known wavelengths of light (red, violet, blue, and green), which are used to determine the color and hue of the sample.
- **Clarity:** The clarity or turbidity of the urine specimen is measured by passing a light beam through the sample and measuring the scattered light. The amount of scattered light increases as the specimen becomes more turbid. Clarity is reported as clear, turbid, or extremely turbid.
- **pH:** Along with the lungs, the kidneys are the major regulator of acid–base balance. pH testing provides valuable information for assessing and managing disease and determine the suitability of a specimen for chemical testing. Freshly voided urine has a pH of 5.0–6.0. The pH of urine can be controlled by dietary regulation and medication.
- **Glucose:** Glucosuria is usually indicative of hyperglycemia due to diabetes but can also be seen in patients with other causes for hyperglycemia, in patients with renal tubular dysfunction, and in pregnancy due to increased glomerular filtration. In children especially younger than 2 years of age, it is important to perform a screening test for reducing sugar.

- **Protein:** The presence of protein in urine is mostly indicative of renal disease, but its appearance in the urine does not always signify renal disease. The strip is primarily sensitive to albumin.
- **Bilirubin:** The appearance of urinary bilirubin can be a sign of liver disease or extrahepatic or intrahepatic biliary obstruction.
- **Urobilinogen:** The normal urine has a small amount of urobilinogen. Increased amounts appear in hemolytic anemias and liver dysfunction.
- **Blood:** Equally specific for RBCs, Hb, or myoglobin present in the urine. Hematuria can be seen due to bleeding as a result of trauma or irritation. Hemoglobinuria occurs when there is lysis of RBCs in the urinary tract, intravascular hemolysis, or transfusion reactions. Very dilute or extremely alkaline urine can also lyse the cells. Myoglobinuria indicates muscular destruction that may appear in hypothermia, convulsions, and extensive exertions.
- **Ketones:** Ketonuria appears when there is an increased use of fat instead of carbohydrate for metabolism. Conditions of ketonuria include DM, vomiting, and inadequate intake of carbohydrates due to starvation or weight reduction, or pregnancy.
- **Nitrite:** Bacteria, specifically gram-negative bacteria, are detected. This analysis provides a rapid and economical means of detecting significant bacteriuria caused by nitrate reducing bacteria. It is limited by various factors, including characteristics of microorganisms, dietary factors, urinary retention time, and specimen storage.
- **Leukocytes:** The presence of WBCs is an indicator of inflammation; lysed and intact WBCs are detected.
- **Normal range:** see Table 2-81

➤ Use
- Frequently performed screening test for metabolic and kidney disorders and for UTIs.

➤ Interpretation
- For specific causes of increased and decreased values of constituents, see individual tests.

TABLE 2-81. Reference Values for Urinalysis	
Test	Reference Range
Color	Yellow
Appearance	Clear
Specific gravity	1.005–1.030
pH	4.6–8.0
Protein	Negative
Glucose	Negative
Ketone	Negative
Bilirubin	Negative
Occult blood	Negative
Nitrite	Negative
Urobilinogen	Normal
Leukocyte esterase	Negative
White blood cells	0–2/HPF
Red blood cells	0–2/HPF
Hyaline casts	0–2/LPF
Bacteria	None

TABLE 2-82. Interferences Which May Cause False-Positive or False-Negative Test Results

Analyte	Causes of False-Positive Results	Causes of False-Negative Results
Specific gravity	High protein concentrations between 100 and 500 mg/dL and presence of ketoacids	Greater than 1 g/dL glucose and urea concentrations
pH	No interferences known	
Blood	Menstrual contamination, microbial peroxidases, strong oxidizing agents (soap and detergents)	Ascorbic acid, high specific gravity, captopril
	Dehydration, exercise	
Leukocyte esterase	Highly colored substances mask results, beets, drugs (phenazopyridine), vaginal contamination of urine	High specific gravity, increased glucose, protein, strong oxidizing agents, drugs such as gentamicin, cephalosporins, presence of lymphocytes
Nitrite	Highly colored substances mask results, beet ingestion, drugs (phenazopyridine), improper storage with bacterial proliferation, exposure of dipstick to air	Ascorbic acid, various factors that inhibit nitrite formation despite bacteriuria.
Protein	Alkaline urine, alkaline drugs, improperly preserved specimen, contamination with quaternary ammonium compounds; highly colored substances mask results, beet ingestion, drugs (phenazopyridine)	Presence of protein other than albumin
Glucose	Strong oxidizing agents such as bleach, peroxidase contaminants	Ascorbic acid, improperly stored specimens (glycolysis)
Ketones	Compounds containing free sulfhydryl groups such as captopril, N-acetylcysteine, highly pigmented urine, atypical colors with phenylketones and phthaleins, large amounts of levodopa metabolites, acidic urine, elevated specific gravity	Improper storage, resulting in volatilization, bacterial breakdown.
Bilirubin	Drug-induced color changes such as phenazopyridine, indicant-indoxyl sulfate, large amounts of chlorpromazine metabolites	Ascorbic acid, high nitrite concentrations, improper storage resulting in oxidation or hydrolysis to nonreactive biliverdin and free bilirubin, light exposure, chlorpromazine (Thorazine), selenium
Urobilinogen	Atypical colors caused by sulfonamides, p-aminobenzoic acid, p-aminosalicylic acid, substances that induce color mask results, beet ingestion, elevated nitrite levels	Formalin, improper storage resulting in oxidation to urobilin

➤ Limitations (See Table 2-82)
➤ Suggested Reading
Brunzel NA. *Fundamentals of Urine and Body Fluid Analyses.* 2nd ed. Philadelphia: Saunders; 2004.

URINE PROTEIN ELECTROPHORESIS/IMMUNOFIXATION

➤ Definition
* Urine protein electrophoresis (UPEP) is analogous to the serum protein electrophoresis test and is used to detect monoclonal proteins (M-proteins) in the urine by an electrophoretic method.
* A 24-hour urine collection is necessary for determination of the total amount of protein excreted in the urine per day. The quantity of M-protein excreted is determined by measuring the size (percent) of the M-spike in the densitometer tracing and multiplying it by the total 24-hour urinary protein excretion. The amount of protein can be expressed as mg/dL or mg/L, but it is much more useful to report the M-protein in g/24 hours because of wide variability in the daily urinary volume.
* On UPEP, a urinary M-protein is seen as a dense localized band on agarose or a tall narrow peak on the densitometer tracing. Generally, the amount of urinary monoclonal protein correlates directly with the size of the plasma cell burden, as long as renal function is relatively normal.
* Other names: Bence-Jones protein test
* **Normal range:** Negative or no monoclonal free light chains detected

➤ Use
* All patients with a diagnosis of a plasma cell dyscrasia should have a baseline UPEP (and immunofixation) of an aliquot from a 24-hour urine collection. This test is essential for detection of the presence of potentially nephrotoxic concentrations of urinary light chains.
* UPEP testing is subsequently required to detect progression and to monitor response to therapy in patients who have urinary monoclonal proteins at baseline.
* UPEP (and immunofixation) has been used also as a standard screening test for patients in whom there is clinical suspicion for a monoclonal plasma cell proliferative disorder such as myeloma or primary amyloidosis. The serum free light chain assay can be used as an alternative method.
* Quantitative determination of M-protein is useful in the response to chemotherapy or progression of disease.

➤ Interpretation
Increased In
* Various proteinuria states
* Monoclonal plasma cell proliferative disorders such as myeloma or primary amyloidosis

➤ Limitations
* The 24-hour urine specimen requires no preservative and may be kept at room temperature during collection.
* Immunofixation should be performed in these patients even if the routine urine analysis is negative for protein, 24-hour urine protein concentration is within normal limits, and electrophoresis of a concentrated urine specimen shows no globulin peak.

- If the patient has nephrotic syndrome, the presence of a monoclonal light chain strongly suggests either primary amyloidosis (AL) or light chain deposition disease in almost all instances.

VANILLYLMANDELIC ACID (VMA), URINE

➤ Definition
- Major metabolite of catecholamine, historically has been used to screen pheochromocytoma. The current recommended test now is fractionated plasma free metanephrines.
- Other names: 3-methoxy-4-hydroxymandelic acid; 4-hydroxy-3-methoxymandelic acid
- **Normal range:** 0–7 mg/day

➤ Use
- Screening for catecholamine-secreting tumors in children when accompanied by HVA
- Supporting a diagnosis of neuroblastoma
- Monitoring neuroblastoma treatment

➤ Interpretation
Increased In
- Pheochromocytoma
- Paraganglioma
- Neuroblastoma

➤ Limitations
- Patients should avoid salicylates, caffeine, phenothiazine, and antihypertension agents, as well as coffee, tea, chocolate, fruit (especially bananas and any vanilla-containing substances for 72 hours prior to collection).
- Some neuroblastoma patients are positive for urinary homovanillic acid abnormality but do not excrete increased VMA. Twenty percent to 32% of patients with neuroblastoma do not have elevation of VMA. Many have other laboratory abnormalities such as increased metanephrines, HVA, or dopamine.

VASOACTIVE INTESTINAL POLYPEPTIDE (VIP)

➤ Definition
- A member of the secretin-glucagon family; highest levels in the gut and nervous system
- A neuropeptide that functions as a neuromodulator and neurotransmitter
- A potent vasodilator that regulates smooth muscle activity, epithelial cell secretion, and blood flow in the gastrointestinal tract
- Functions as a neurohormone and paracrine mediator, being released from nerve terminals and acting locally on receptor bearing cells
- **Normal range:** 0–60 pg/mL

➤ Use
- Detection of VIP-secreting tumors
- To detect occult metastases
- To evaluate the success of surgical or drug therapies

➤ **Interpretation**
Increased In
- VIPomas
- Neural crest tumors in children (ganglioneuroblastoma, ganglioneuroma and neuroblastoma)
- Pancreatic islet cell hyperplasia
- Liver disease
- MEN type I, pheochromocytoma
- MTC
- Branchiogenic carcinoma
- Retroperitoneal histiocytoma
- CHF

➤ **Limitations**
- This test should not be requested in patients who have recently received radioisotopes, therapeutically or diagnostically, because of potential assay interference.

VISCOSITY, SERUM

➤ **Definition**
- Blood viscosity is a measure of the resistance of blood to flow due to any stress. Changes in the concentration of one or more blood protein fractions will result in a change in viscosity. Blood or serum viscosity can, therefore, be used both as a diagnostic tool for the presence of diseases known to alter the proteins, and as a measure of the extent of the condition.
- **Normal range:** 1.10–1.80 cP (relative to water)

➤ **Use**
- Evaluate hyperviscosity syndrome associated with monoclonal gammopathy states (myeloma, Waldenström macroglobulinemia, and other dysproteinemias), including RA, SLE, hyperfibrinogenemia.

➤ **Interpretation**
Increased In
- Increased leukocyte count
- Thrombocytosis
- Hyperlipoproteinemia
- Macroglobulinemia
- Sjögren syndrome
- SLE
- Lymphoproliferative disorders
- Hyperglobulinemia associated with cirrhosis
- Chronic active hepatitis
- Acute thermal burns

Decreased In
- No clinical significance

➤ Limitations
• Whole blood measurement is of limited use because of differences in shear rates between instrumentation and *in vivo* conditions.
• Clinical symptoms do not correlate well with test results.

VITAMIN A (RETINOL, CAROTENE)

➤ Definition
• Vitamin A is a subclass of a family of lipid-soluble compounds referred to as retinoic acids. There are essentially three forms of vitamin A: retinols, beta-carotenes, and carotenoids. Retinol, also known as preformed vitamin A, is the most active form and is mostly found in animal sources of food. Beta-carotene, also known as provitamin A, is the plant source of retinol from which mammals make two thirds of their vitamin A. Carotenoids, the largest group of the three, contain multiple conjugated double bonds and exist in a free alcohol or in a fatty acyl-ester form.
• Vitamin A promotes normal vision and prevents night blindness; contributes to growth of bone, teeth, and soft tissues; supports thyroxine formation; maintains epithelial cell membranes, skin, and mucous membranes; and acts as an anti-infection agent.
• **Normal range:** see Table 2-83

➤ Use
• Assist in the diagnosis of night blindness
• Evaluate skin disorders
• Investigate suspected vitamin A deficiency

➤ Interpretation
Increased In
• Chronic kidney disease
• Idiopathic hypercalcemia in infants
• Vitamin A toxicity

Decreased In
• Abetalipoproteinemia
• Carcinoid syndrome
• Chronic infections
• CF
• Disseminated TB
• Hypothyroidism
• Infantile blindness

TABLE 2-83. Normal Ranges for Vitamin A by Age	
Age	Reference Interval (mg/L)
0–1 month	0.18–0.50
2 months to 12 years	0.20–0.50
13–17 years	0.26–0.70
≥18 years	0.30–1.20

- Liver, GI, or pancreatic disease
- Night blindness
- Protein malnutrition
- Sterility and teratogenesis
- Zinc deficiency

➤ Limitations

- Alcohol (moderate intake), oral contraceptives, and probucol increase vitamin A levels
- Alcohol (chronic intake, alcoholism), allopurinol, cholestyramine, colestipol, mineral oil, and neomycin decrease vitamin A levels
- Serum retinol is typically maintained until hepatic stores are almost depleted. Values >0.30 mg/L represent adequate liver stores, whereas values less than 0.10 mg/L indicate deficiency.
- Samples that come in contact with plastic tubing or have been exposed to excessive light may show low results.

VITAMIN A RELATIVE DOSE RESPONSE (RDR) TEST

➤ Definition

- Retinol (vitamin A) measurements in blood has several disadvantages. It is decreased only in severe vitamin A deficiency, when liver stores are nearly exhausted. In addition, infection can decrease serum vitamin A levels in blood, leading to misclassification of individuals. Because the majority of vitamin A is stored in Liver, RDR test/calculation was developed to reliably measure vitamin A storage.
- Retinyl palmitate is given either as a water miscible solution of 1000 μg administered IV over 30 minutes or as 450 μg diluted in corn oil and administered orally. Fasting and 5 hour after-dose plasma specimens should be drawn.
- RDR is calculated as vitamin A 5 hour-vitamin A fasting (0 hr)/vitamin A 5 hour × 100
- **Normal range:** <10%

➤ Use

- Identify subjects with marginal liver vitamin A stores
- As a tool for estimation of total body stores of vitamin A

➤ Interpretation
Increased In
- RDR values of >20% indicate depleted liver vitamin A stores.

➤ Limitations

- The vitamin A RDR oral dose test has the similar limitations of other absorption tests. It decreases in malabsorption, cirrhosis, cholestasis, hepatocellular disease, protein calorie malnutrition, and zinc deficiency.

VITAMIN B₁ (THIAMINE)

➤ Definition

- Thiamine, first named "the antiberiberi factor" in 1926, has a historical value due to the very early description of beriberi in the Chinese medical texts, as far back as 2697 BC. Thiamine is found in larger quantities in food products such as yeast, legumes, pork, rice, and cereals. Milk products, fruits, and vegetables are poor sources of thiamine. The thiamine molecule is denatured at high pH and high temperatures. Hence, cooking, baking, and canning of some foods as well as pasteurization can destroy thiamine.

- Thiamine is an essential vitamin required for carbohydrate metabolism, brain function, and peripheral nerve myelination. Thiamine deficiency has been associated with three disorders:
  - Beriberi (infantile and adult)
  - Wernicke-Korsakoff syndrome
  - Leigh syndrome
- **Normal range:** 70–180 nmol/L

➤ Use

- Assessment of thiamine deficiency. Thiamine measurement is appropriate in patients with behavioral changes, eye signs, gait disturbances, delirium, and encephalopathy; or in patients with questionable nutritional status, especially those who appear at risk and who also are being given insulin for hyperglycemia.
- Investigation of suspected beriberi
- Monitoring the effects of chronic alcoholism

➤ Interpretation
Increased In
- Leukemia
- Polycythemia vera
- Hodgkin disease

Decreased In
- Alcoholism with and without liver disease
- Deficient diet
- Chronic febrile infections
- Prolonged diarrhea
- Diabetes
- Carcinoid syndrome
- Hartnup disease
- Pellagra

➤ Limitations
- Whole blood is the preferred specimen for thiamine assessment. Approximately 80% of thiamine present in whole blood is found in RBCs.
- Drugs that may decrease vitamin B_1 levels include glibenclamide, isoniazid, and valproic acid.
- Diets high in freshwater fish and tea, which are thiamine antagonists, may cause decreased vitamin B_1 levels.
- Thiamine deficiency can be assessed by measuring the blood thiamine concentration, erythrocyte thiamine transketolase (ETKA), or transketolase urinary thiamine excretion (with or without a 5-mg thiamine load). Most laboratories now measure blood thiamine concentration directly, in preference to the ETKA method. The ETKA method is a functional test and results are influenced by the hemoglobin concentration.

VITAMIN B$_{12}$ (CYANOCOBALAMIN, COBALAMIN)

➤ Definition

- Vitamin B$_{12}$ is essential in DNA synthesis, hematopoiesis, and CNS integrity. Its absorption depends on the presence of intrinsic factor (IF) and may be due to lack of IF secretion by gastric mucosa (e.g., gastrectomy, gastric atrophy) or intestinal malabsorption (e.g., ileal resection, small intestinal diseases). Vitamin B$_{12}$ deficiency frequently causes macrocytic anemia, glossitis, peripheral neuropathy, weakness, hyperreflexia, ataxia, loss of proprioception, poor coordination, and affective behavioral changes. These manifestations may occur in any combination; many patients have the neurologic defects without macrocytic anemia. PA is a macrocytic anemia caused by B$_{12}$ deficiency that is due to a lack of IF secretion by gastric mucosa.
- Serum methylmalonic acid (MMA) and homocysteine levels are also elevated in vitamin B$_{12}$ deficiency states. A significant increase in RBC MCV may be an important indicator of vitamin B$_{12}$ deficiency.
- **Normal range:** 180–914 pg/mL
  - Indeterminate range: 145–180 pg/mL
  - Deficient range: <145 pg/mL

➤ Use

- Investigation of macrocytic anemia
- Work-up of deficiencies seen in megaloblastic anemias
- Assistance in the diagnosis of CNS disorders
- Evaluation of alcoholism
- Evaluation of malabsorption syndromes

➤ Interpretation
Increased In

- Chronic granulocytic leukemia
- COPD
- Chronic renal failure
- Diabetes
- Leukocytosis
- Liver cell damage (hepatitis, cirrhosis)
- Obesity
- Polycythemia vera
- Protein malnutrition
- Severe CHF
- Some carcinomas

Decreased In

- Abnormalities of cobalamin transport or metabolism
- Bacterial overgrowth
- Crohn disease
- Dietary deficiency (e.g., in vegetarians)
- Diphyllobothrium (fish tapeworm) infestation

- Gastric or small intestine surgery
- Hypochlorhydria
- Inflammatory bowel disease
- Intestinal malabsorption
- Intrinsic factor deficiency
- Late pregnancy
- PA

➤ Limitations

- Serum samples should be protected from light at room temperature (15–30°C) for no longer than one hour. If the assay will not be completed within 2 hours, samples should be frozen and be protected from light exposure.
- Drugs such as chloral hydrate increase vitamin B_{12} levels. On the other hand, alcohol, aminosalicylic acid, anticonvulsants, ascorbic acid, cholestyramine, cimetidine, colchicine, metformin, neomycin, oral contraceptives, ranitidine, and triamterene decrease vitamin B_{12} levels.
- Many other conditions are known to cause an increase (vitamin C, vitamin A, estrogens, hepatocellular injury, myeloproliferative disorders, uremia) or decrease (pregnancy, smoking, hemodialysis, multiple myeloma) serum B_{12} levels.
- The evaluation of macrocytic anemia requires measurement of both vitamin B_{12} and folate levels; ideally they should be measured simultaneously.
- Specimen collection soon after blood transfusion can falsely increase vitamin B_{12} levels.
- Patients taking vitamin B_{12} supplementation may have misleading results
- A normal serum concentration of B_{12} does not rule out tissue deficiency of vitamin B_{12}. The most sensitive test for B_{12} deficiency at the cellular level is the assay for MMA. If clinical symptoms suggest deficiency, measurement of MMA and homocysteine should be considered, even if serum B_{12} concentrations are normal.

VITAMIN B_2 (RIBOFLAVIN)

➤ Definition

- Vitamin B_2, or riboflavin, is one of the water-soluble vitamins. It is synthesized in plants and microorganisms and occurs naturally in three forms: the physiologically inactive riboflavin and the physiologically active coenzymes flavin mononucleotide (FMN) and flavinadeninedinucleotide (FAD). The latter accounts for about 90% of the total riboflavin in whole blood. Because of their capacity to transfer electrons, FAD and FMN are essential for proton transfer in the respiratory chain, for the dehydration of fatty acids, the oxidative deamination of amino acids, and for other redox processes.
- **Normal range:** 3–15 µg/L
  - Marginally low: 2 µg/L
  - Diminished: <2 µg/L

➤ Use

- Evaluation of persons who present the signs of ariboflavinosis
- Detect riboflavin deficiency

➤ Interpretation
Decreased In
* Patients with anorexia nervosa
* Individuals who avoid dairy products (such as people with lactose intolerance) because dairy products are a good source of riboflavin
* Patients with malabsorptive syndromes such as celiac sprue, malignancies, and short bowel syndrome
* Rare inborn errors of metabolism in which there is a defect in riboflavin synthesis
* Long-term use of phenobarbital and other barbiturates, which may lead to oxidation of riboflavin and impair its function

➤ Limitations
* Testing of nonfasting specimens or the use of dietary vitamin B$_2$ supplementation can result in elevated plasma vitamin B$_2$ concentrations.
* Sample should be frozen immediately to reduce the stability of B$_2$ in serum.

➤ Suggested Reading
Russell RM, Suter PM. Vitamin and trace mineral deficiency and excess. In: *Harrison's Principles of Internal Medicine.* 17th ed. Fauci AS, Kasper DL, Braunwald E, et al., eds. New York: McGraw-Hill; 2008:441–449.

VITAMIN B$_6$ (PYRIDOXINE)

➤ Definition
* Vitamin B$_6$ is a complex of six vitamers: pyridoxal, pyridoxol, pyridoxamine (pyridoxine), and their 5′-phosphate esters. Because of its role as a cofactor in a number of enzymatic reactions, pyridoxal phosphate (PLP) has been determined to be the biologically active form of vitamin B$_6$. Vitamin B$_6$ is important in heme synthesis and functions as a coenzyme in amino acid metabolism and glycogenolysis.
* Vitamin B$_6$ deficiency is associated with symptoms of irritability, weakness, depression, dizziness, peripheral neuropathy, and seizures. In the pediatric population, deficiencies have been characterized by diarrhea, anemia, and seizures.
* **Normal range:** 5–50 µg/L

➤ Use
* Determining vitamin B$_6$ status
* Investigating suspected malabsorption or malnutrition
* Determining the overall success of a vitamin B$_6$ supplementation program
* Diagnosis and evaluation of hypophosphatasia

➤ Interpretation
Increased In
* Hypophosphatasia

Decreased In
* Alcoholism
* Asthma

- Carpal tunnel syndrome
- Gestational diabetes
- Lactation
- Malabsorption
- Malnutrition
- Neonatal seizures
- Normal pregnancies
- Occupational exposure to hydrazine compounds
- Pellagra
- Preeclamptic edema
- Renal dialysis
- Uremia

➤ Limitations
- In addition to PLP, the following methods can be used to assess for vitamin B_6 deficiency:
  - Erythrocyte transaminase activity with and without PLP added has been used as a functional test of pyridoxine status.
  - Urinary 4-pyridoxic acid excretion >3.0 mmol/day can be used as an indicator of adequate short-term vitamin B_6 status.
  - Urinary excretion of xanthurenic acid is normally <65 mmol/day following a 2-g tryptophan load.
- Drugs that may decrease vitamin B_6 levels include amiodarone, anticonvulsants, cycloserine, disulfiram, ethanol, hydralazine, isoniazid, levodopa, oral contraceptives, penicillamine, pyrazinoic acid, and theophylline.
- B_6 may be decreased with pregnancy, lactation, alcoholism, DM, and in an uncommon B_6 dependency state, vitamin B_6 responsive neonatal convulsions. There is evidence of significant neurotoxicity associated with pyridoxine megavitaminosis; tingling, numbness, clumsiness, gait disturbances, and pseudoathetosis, with doses >2 g/day.

VITAMIN C (ASCORBIC ACID)

➤ Definition
- Ascorbic acid is essential for the enzymatic amidation of neuropeptides, production of adrenal cortical steroid hormones, promotion of the conversion of tropocollagen to collagen, and metabolism of tyrosine and folate. It also plays a role in lipid and vitamin metabolism and is a powerful reducing agent or antioxidant.
- Specific actions include activation of detoxifying enzymes in the liver, antioxidation, interception and destruction of free radicals, preservation and restoration of the antioxidant potential of vitamin E, and blockage of the formation of carcinogenic nitrosamines. Vitamin C promotes collagen synthesis, maintains capillary strength, facilitates release of iron from ferritin to form hemoglobin, and functions in the stress response.
- In addition, vitamin C appears to function in a variety of other metabolic processes in which its role has not been well characterized.
- **Normal range:** 0.4–2.0 mg/dL

➤ Use
* Investigate suspected metabolic or malabsorptive disorders
* Investigate suspected scurvy

➤ Interpretation
Decreased In
* Alcoholism
* Anemia
* Cancer
* Hemodialysis
* Hyperthyroidism
* Malabsorption
* Pregnancy
* Rheumatoid disease
* Scurvy

➤ Limitations
* Drugs and substances that may decrease vitamin C levels include acetylsalicylic acid, aminopyrine, barbiturates, estrogens, heavy metals, oral contraceptives, nitrosamines, and paraldehyde.
* Chronic tobacco smoking decreases vitamin C levels.
* Testing of nonfasting specimens or the use of vitamin supplementation can result in elevated plasma vitamin concentrations. Reference values were established in patients who were fasting.
* After consuming vitamin C, plasma values rapidly rise within 1–2 hours and reach peak concentration within 3–6 hours after ingestion.

VITAMIN D, 1,25-DIHYDROXY

➤ Definition
* It is the active form of vitamin D and is produced primarily in the kidney by the hydroxylation of 25-hydroxy vitamin D.
* Other names: calcitriol; 1,25-dihydroxycholecalciferol; 1,25-OHD.
* **Normal range:** 15–75 pg/mL

➤ Use
* As a second-order test in the assessment of vitamin D status, especially in patients with renal disease
* Investigation of some patients with clinical evidence of vitamin D deficiency (e.g., vitamin D–dependent rickets due to hereditary deficiency of renal 1-alpha hydroxylase or end-organ resistance to 1,25-dihydroxy vitamin D)
* Differential diagnosis of hypercalcemia

➤ Interpretation
Increased In
* Sarcoidosis (synthesized by macrophages within granulomas)
* Non-Hodgkin lymphoma (~15% of cases). Returns to normal after therapy.

Decreased In
* Renal failure
* Hyperphosphatemia
* Vitamin D dependent rickets, types 1 and 2

Normal In
* HPT
* Humoral hypercalcemia of malignancy

➤ Limitations
* The level of 1,25 OHD is maintained despite significant vitamin D depletion, because secondary hyperparathyroidism stimulates increased conversion of 25OHD to 1,25 OHD in this situation.
* Although 1,25 OHD is the biologically active form of vitamin D, its level in the body provides *no* useful information about a patient's vitamin D status. The kidney tightly controls serum 1,25 OHD levels, which are often normal or even elevated in vitamin D deficiency. Therefore, a patient with normal or high level of 1,25 OHD levels is vitamin D deficient despite high serum levels of the active hormone. At this time, there is consensus that serum 1,25 OHD is a measure of only the endocrine function of vitamin D and not an indicator of the body stores or the ability of vitamin D to perform its pleiotropic autocrine functions.

VITAMIN D, 25 HYDROXY

* Other names: 25-Hydroxy D2; 25-hydroxy D3; 5-hydroxy vitamin D; 25-hydroxycholecalciferol; 25-hydroxyergocalciferol; 25-OH vitamin D; calcidiol

➤ Definition
* A steroid hormone that has long been known for its important role in regulating body levels of calcium and phosphorus and in the mineralization of bone.
* The term "vitamin D" specifically refers to two biologically inert precursors, vitamin D_3 (cholecalciferol) or D_2 (ergocalciferol). Neither vitamin D_3 nor vitamin D_2 have significant biologic activity; rather they must be metabolized within the body to the hormonally active form. Vitamin D_3 is generated in the skin when light energy is absorbed (UV radiation in the UVB spectrum 290–320 nm) by a precursor molecule 7-dehydrocholesterol (7-DHC; provitamin D_3). However, cutaneous vitamin D_3 production after single prolonged UVB exposure is capped at approximately 10–20% of the original epidermal 7-DHC concentration, a limit achieved with suberythemogenic UV exposures. Vitamin D_2 is plant derived, produced exogenously by irradiation of ergosterol and enters the circulation through diet. Vitamin D_3 from the skin and vitamin D_3 and D_2 from the diet enter the blood and are metabolized to their 25-hydroxy counterparts.
* Once formed, 25-hydroxy vitamin D (25-OHD) is metabolized in the kidney to 1,25 dihydroxy vitamin D (1,25 OHD)
* **Normal range:** see Table 2-84

➤ Use
* Diagnosis of vitamin D deficiency
* Differential diagnosis of causes of rickets and osteomalacia

TABLE 2-84. Normal Ranges of 25-OH Vitamin D	
Vitamin D Status	25-OH Vitamin D (ng/mL)
Deficiency	<10
Insufficiency	10–30
Sufficiency	30–100
Toxicity	>100

- Monitoring vitamin D replacement therapy
- Diagnosis of hypervitaminosis D

➤ Interpretation
Increased In
- Vitamin D intoxication
- Excessive exposure to sunlight

Decreased In
- Malabsorption
- Steatorrhea
- Dietary osteomalacia, anticonvulsant osteomalacia
- Biliary and portal cirrhosis
- Thyrotoxicosis
- Pancreatic insufficiency
- Celiac disease
- Inflammatory bowel disease
- Rickets
- Alzheimer disease

➤ Limitations
- More recently, it has become clear that receptors for vitamin D are present in a wide variety of cells and that this hormone has biologic effects extending beyond the control of mineral metabolism.
- The definition of vitamin D deficiency is changing almost every year. Levels needed to prevent rickets and osteomalacia (15 ng/mL) are lower than those that dramatically suppress parathyroid hormone levels (20–30 ng/mL). In turn those levels are lower than levels needed to optimize intestinal calcium absorption (34 ng/mL). Neuromuscular peak performance is associated with levels ~38 ng/mL. A recent study states that increasing mean baseline levels from 29–38 ng/mL was associated with a 50% lower risk for colon cancer and levels of 52 ng/mL with a 50% reduction in the incidence of breast cancer.
- Various methods for measuring circulating concentrations 25-OH D are available. Current methods include RIA, CIA, HPLC, and LCMS/MS tandem mass spectrometry. Immunoassays measure total 25-OHD, which includes levels of both 25-OH D_2 and 25-OH D_3. The antibodies cross-react 100% with both D_2 and D_3 to give the total 25-OH D. Some commercial laboratories use LCMS/MS technology and report 25-OH D_2 and 25-OH D_3 separately and add both values to get the total 25-OH D. The studies report reasonable correlations between methods, but with significant differences, the reasons for which are not well understood. There could be many reasons for these variations, including drifts in

the reagents being manufactured, and there is an urgent need for harmonization and standardization.
- The reference ranges discussed in the preceding are related to total 25-OH D; as long as the combined total is 30 ng/mL or more, the patient has sufficient vitamin D. Given the absence of assay standardization and lack of consensus regarding clinical cut-off values, vitamin D levels must be interpreted within the clinical context of each patient and one should not rely solely on cut-off values based on so-called normal values.

VITAMIN E (ALPHA-TOCOPHEROL)

➤ Definition
- Tocopherol is a fat-soluble vitamin with antioxidant properties; it protects cell membranes from oxidation and destruction. Vitamin E is found in a variety of foods, including oils, meat, eggs, and leafy vegetables. Serum vitamin E levels are strongly influenced by concentration of serum lipids and do not accurately reflect tissue vitamin levels. Effective vitamin E levels are calculated as the ratio of serum alpha-tocopherol per gram total lipids.
- Vitamin E reserves in lung tissue provide a barrier against air pollution and protect red blood cell membrane integrity from oxidation. Oxidation of fatty acids in red blood cell membranes can result in irreversible membrane damage and hemolysis. Studies are in progress to confirm the suspicion that oxidation also contributes to the formation of cataracts and macular degeneration of the retina. Because vitamin E is found in a wide variety of foods, a deficiency secondary to inadequate dietary intake is rare.
- **Normal range:** see Table 2-85

➤ Use
- Evaluate neuromuscular disorders in premature infants and adults
- Evaluate patients with malabsorption disorders
- Evaluate suspected hemolytic anemia in premature infants and adults
- Monitor patients on long-term parenteral nutrition
- Evaluation of individuals with motor and sensory neuropathies
- Monitoring vitamin E status of premature infants requiring oxygenation

➤ Interpretation
Increased In
- Obstructive liver disease
- Hyperlipidemia
- Vitamin E intoxication

TABLE 2-85. Normal Ranges for Vitamin E	
	Range (mg/L)
Age: 0–17 years	3.8–18.4
Age: ≥18 years	5.5–17.0
Significant deficiency	<3.0
Significant excess	>40

Decreased In
* Abetalipoproteinemia
* Hemolytic anemia
* Malabsorption disorders, such as biliary atresia, cirrhosis, CF, chronic pancreatitis, pancreatic carcinoma, and chronic cholestasis

➤ Limitations
* As previously stated, serum vitamin E levels are strongly influenced by concentration of serum lipids and do not accurately reflect tissue vitamin levels. Therefore, effective vitamin E levels are calculated as the following ratio:
  * Effective serum vitamin E level = Alpha-tocopherol/(cholesterol + triglycerides)
  * A normal ratio is >0.8 mg alpha-tocopherol/gram total lipids.
  * For patients with normal levels of serum lipids, serum alpha-tocopherol levels provide an adequate estimate of vitamin E sufficiency. Alpha-tocopherol levels of <0.5 mg/dL (5 µg/ml) are considered deficient
* Drugs that may increase vitamin E levels include anticonvulsants (in women).
* Drugs that may decrease vitamin E levels include anticonvulsants (in men).
* Exposure of the specimen to light decreases vitamin E levels, resulting in a falsely low result.
* Platelet tocopherol is suggested to be a better measure of vitamin E nutritional status than plasma tocopherol because it is more sensitive to vitamin E intake and is not dependent on circulating lipid levels.

WATER DEPRIVATION TEST

➤ Definition
* Normal physiologic response to the water deprivation will increase plasma osmolality, which will then lead to a progressive elevation in ADH release and an increase in urine osmolality. Once the plasma osmolality reaches 295–300 mOsm/kg (normal: 275–290 mOsm/kg), the effect of endogenous ADH on the kidney is maximal. At this point, administering ADH does not further elevate the urine osmolality unless endogenous ADH release is impaired (e.g., the patient has central diabetes insipidus [DI]).
* This test is also known as the water restriction test
* **Normal response:** Water deprivation causes kidney to increase urine osmolality to 1,000 to 1200 mmol/kg. ADH does not cause further increase in urine osmolality because endogenous ADH is already at maximum.

➤ Use
* To distinguish the major forms of DI—neurogenic, nephrogenic, and polydipsic.
* Steps:
  1. Have the patient should stop drinking 2–3 hours before coming to the office or clinic; overnight fluid restriction should be avoided, because potentially severe volume depletion and hypernatremia can be induced in patients with marked polyuria.
  2. Collect 7–10 mL of heparinized blood for immediate measurements of serum sodium concentration and osmolality. Also ask patient to void his/her bladder; record the urine volume and send urine specimen for immediate measurement of osmolality.

3. Repeat step 2 every hour until (a): plasma sodium concentration or osmolality rises above the upper limit of normal range; or (b): urine osmolality rises above 300 mOsm/kg H_2O
   - If (a) occurs before (b): primary polydipsia, partial neurogenic, and partial nephrogenic DI are excluded, and a dDAVP (synthetic analog of ADH) challenge test should be done as follows:
     - Inject 2 µg of dDAVP subcutaneously
     - Ask patient to empty bladder at 1 and 2 hours after the injection; measure the urine osmolality. Also measure patient's plasma ADH level.
       - If either urine samples has an osmolality >50% higher than the value immediately before injection, the patient probably has complete neurogenic DI.
       - If both urine samples have osmolality increase of <50% than the value immediately before injection, the patient is very likely to have complete nephrogenic DI.
   - If (b) occurs before (a): complete neurogenic and nephrogenic DI are excluded. Further differentiate among partial nephrogenic DI, partial neurogenic DI, and primary polydipsia will require trained personnel and specialized measurements.

➤ Interpretation

- **Complete DI:** Water deprivation increases plasma osmolality but urine osmolality stays <290 mmol/kg and does not increase following dDAVP challenge.
- **Partial DI:** Water deprivation causes some increase in urine osmolality to 400–500 mmol/kg (less than normal).
- **Complete or partial nephrogenic DI or psychogenic polydipsia:** Increased ADH levels. Giving ADH does not increase urine osmolality in complete nephrogenic DI.
- **Complete or partial neurogenic DI:** Low ADH relative to plasma osmolality. Giving ADH increases urine osmolality ~200 mmol/kg but not in partial nephrogenic DI.

➤ Limitations

- Some nonosmotic stimuli, such as smoking, hypotension, and nausea, can increase ADH release. If a transient episode of hypotension and nausea occurs, the entire test is invalid and it needs to be repeated in another day.
- Complete emptying of the bladder during each collection is important because incomplete emptying may dilute the urine of the next collection.
- The plasma sample for osmolality measurement should be from heparinized blood, and EDTA should be avoided because it artificially increases the osmolality by 3–10%.
- The plasma for ADH measurement should be collected without disturbing the buffy coat in order to minimize the contamination from platelets.
- The test should be performed only when the patient's basal plasma sodium concentration is within the normal range, otherwise it may cause potential harm to the patient.
- The test should not be performed in patients with renal insufficiency, uncontrolled DM, or hypovolemia of any cause or uncorrected adrenal or thyroid hormone deficiency.
- Patients should be observed for the entire duration of the test.
- For pregnant patients, the blood sample for ADH measurement should be drawn into a tube that contains 6 mg of 1,10-phenanthroline to prevent the degradation of ADH by placental vasopressinase. The results should be evaluated in the context of altered relationship between the plasma osmolality/sodium concentration and the plasma ADH concentration

WHITE BLOOD CELL: INCLUSIONS AND MORPHOLOGIC ABNORMALITIES

➤ Definition
* The WBC morphology may present with unusual inclusions (Table 2-86) or with other abnormalities in granules or morphology (Table 2-87). Some are associated with congenital syndromes; some are acquired.
* These morphologic abnormalities are not always associated with functional abnormalities.

WHITE BLOOD CELL COUNTS AND DIFFERENTIALS

➤ Definition
* WBC counts refer to numerical reporting of the total number of WBCs as well as to describing and classifying the white cell components: neutrophils (which include bands), lymphocytes, monocytes, eosinophils and basophils (Table 2-88).
* **Normal range** (adults): $4.3–10.3 \times 10^3$ cells/μL. Different values are reported for infants, and children, separated by age groups.
* Automated counters report results in percentages or as absolute counts of each WBC population. The absolute counts are considered more relevant in evaluating WBC abnormalities.

➤ Use
* Most automated WBC counters separate the white cells into the five categories. Immature white cells are flagged as abnormal, requiring direct examination of the peripheral blood smears. Recent machines do a six-part differential, the sixth parameter being "immature fraction."
* Abnormalities are discussed separately for each population (see Leukocytosis and Leukopenia p. 814, and Leukemoid Reactions p. 820).

➤ Limitations
* Poorly prepared stains (mostly the manual ones) may corrupt the ability of the technician to report accurate differentials.
* Moreover, because in most laboratories the technician examines only 100 randomly selected cells, there is an inherent bias in the report, and rare, but important, abnormal WBCs may be missed, especially in leukopenic conditions. With the recent introduction of automated equipment for reporting differential counts this bias is minimized.

ZINC (Zn)

➤ Definition
* Zinc, an essential trace element, is the intrinsic metal component or activating cofactor for more than 70 important enzyme systems, including carbonic anhydrase, the ALPs, dehydrogenases, and carboxypeptidases. It is involved in the regulation of nucleoproteins and the activity of various inflammatory cells and plays a role in growth, tissue repair and wound healing, carbohydrate tolerance, and synthesis of testicular hormones. Zinc intake is closely

TABLE 2-86. White Blood Cell Inclusions in Peripheral Blood

Inclusions	Morphology and Conditions
Howell-Jolly bodies	Cytoplasmic chromatin remnants; seen in granulocytic series in splenectomized patients
Auer rods	Linear azurophilic granules; seen in immature myeloid or monocytic cells of acute leukemias
Döhle bodies	Small, oval inclusions in the peripheral cytoplasm of neutrophils, remnants of ribosomes or endoplasmic reticulum; seen in infections, burns, aplastic anemia, following administration of toxic agents
Toxic granulation	Primary granules in bands and neutrophils; seen in infections, especially with leukemoid reactions, toxic conditions, and after therapy with granulocyte colony forming unit drugs.
Chédiak-Higashi syndrome granules	Coarse, deeply staining, peroxidase-positive fused large granulations in cytoplasm of granulocytes; characteristic of Chédiak-Higashi syndrome
May-Hegglin anomaly	Basophilic and pyroninophilic inclusions in neutrophils, eosinophils, basophils and monocytes; accompanied by variable thrombocytopenia with giant platelets containing few granules; rare, dominantly inherited anomaly, without clinical consequences in most affected subjects
Alder-Reilly anomaly bodies	Dense azurophilic granules in all WBC lines on peripheral blood smear (inconstant) and marrow (always present in white cells and macrophages); seen in genetic mucopolysaccharidoses
Jordan anomaly (familial vacuolization of leukocytes)	Presence of vacuoles in the cytoplasm of granulocytes, monocytes, and occasionally lymphocytes and plasma cells; vacuoles with lipids; familial disorder
Batten (Batten-Spielmeyer-Vogt) granules	Azurophilic hypergranulation of WBCs in patients with Batten disease (autosomal recessive type of juvenile amaurotic idiocy) and members of their families.
Organisms (especially pneumococcal sepsis), *Neisseria meningitides*, *Staphylococcus aureus*, *Ehrlichia chaffeensis*, *Histoplasma capsulatum*, candidiasis, CMV	It usually means overwhelming sepsis; frequently found in splenectomized or immunodeficient patients

TABLE 2-87. White Cell Morphologic Abnormalities

Abnormalities	Morphology and Condition
Pelger-Huet anomaly	Nuclei of >80% of granulocytes show hyposegmentation (2 pince-nez eyeglass lobes); hereditary in heterozygotes for an autosomal dominant mutation at chromosome 1q42.1 and of no clinical consequence (neutrophils are functionally normal); acquired (pseudo–Pelger-Huet anomaly) in myelodysplastic syndromes, acute and chronic myeloproliferative neoplasms, myxedema, transient in some infections or with certain drugs
Hereditary hypersegmentation of neutrophils and hereditary hypersegmentation of eosinophils	Most neutrophils (or eosinophils) have 4 or more lobes; rare, harmless autosomal dominant condition; ≥5 lobes in >10% of heterozygotes and >30% in homozygotes
Acquired hypersegmentation of neutrophils	Normally only 10–20% of neutrophils have 4 lobes, and no more than 5% have 5 lobes; increases found in patients with megaloblastic anemias and chronic renal disease with BUN >30 mg/dL for >3 months
Giant bands and metamyelocytes	Patients with megaloblastic anemias
Hereditary giant neutrophilia	1–2% of neutrophils are ≤2 times normal size and contain 6–10 nuclear lobes; innocuous dominant anomaly

related to protein intake; as a result, it is an important component of nutritionally related morbidity worldwide.

- Symptoms attributable to severe zinc depletion include growth failure, primary hypogonadism, skin disease, impaired taste and smell, and impaired immunity and resistance to infection. Subclinical zinc deficiency may significantly increase the incidence of and morbidity and mortality from diarrhea and upper respiratory tract infections. Along with iron, iodine,

TABLE 2-88. Normal Values for White Blood Cell Counts*

White cells	% of 100 White Cells	Absolute Count × 10³ cells/µL
Neutrophils	43–72	1.6–7.5
Lymphocytes	18–43	0.9–3.4
Reactive lymphocytes	0–6 (manual differentials only)	
Monocytes	4–12	0.0–1.2
Eosinophils	0–8	0.0–0.6
Basophils	0–2	0.0–0.3

*Note that the normal values described in the table do not reflect differences related to age or race.

TABLE 2-89. Normal Range for Zinc by Age	
Age	Conventional Units (µg/dL)
Newborn to 6 months	26–141
6–11 months	29–131
1–4 years	31–115
4–5 years	48–119
6–9 years	48–129
10–13 years	25–148
14–17 years	46–130
Adult	70–120

and vitamin A, zinc deficiency is one of the most important micronutrient deficiencies globally. Several studies have now demonstrated that supplementation of high risk populations can have substantial health benefits.

- **Normal range:** (see Table 2-89)

➤ Use
- Detecting zinc deficiency
- Assist in confirming acrodermatitis enteropathica
- Evaluate nutritional deficiency
- Evaluate possible toxicity
- Monitor replacement therapy in individuals with identified deficiencies
- Monitor therapy of individuals with Wilson disease

➤ Interpretation
Increased In
- Anemia
- Arteriosclerosis
- Coronary heart disease
- Primary osteosarcoma of the bone

Decreased In
- Acrodermatitis enteropathica
- AIDS
- Acute infections
- Acute stress
- Burns
- Cirrhosis
- Conditions that decrease albumin
- Diabetes
- Long-term TPN
- Malabsorption
- Myocardial infarction
- Nephrotic syndrome
- Nutritional deficiency
- Pregnancy

* Pulmonary TB
* Ulcerative colitis, Crohn disease,
* Regional enteritis, sprue, intestinal bypass, neoplastic disease
* Increased catabolism induced by anabolic steroids

➤ Limitations

* Plasma levels of zinc do not necessarily correlate with tissue levels and do not reliably identify individuals with zinc deficiency. Although plasma levels are generally a good index of zinc status in healthy individuals, these levels are depressed during inflammatory disease states.
* Erythrocyte concentrations of zinc may provide a more useful measure of zinc status during acute or chronic inflammation. Several functional indices also can be used to indirectly assess zinc status. Serum superoxide dismutase and erythrocyte alkaline phosphatase activities have been proposed as indirect markers of zinc status, but these tests are not widely available.
* The conditions of anorexia and starvation also result in low zinc levels.
* Hemolyzed specimens cause false elevation of serum zinc levels.
* Specimens should be collected in metal-free specimen containers.
* Auranofin, chlorthalidone, corticotropin, oral contraceptives, and penicillamine increase zinc levels.
* Anticonvulsants, cisplatin, citrates, corticosteroids, estrogens, interferon, and oral contraceptives decrease zinc levels.

CHAPTER 3

Infectious Diseases Assays

Michael J. Mitchell and L.V. Rao

T his chapter presents the most commonly ordered infectious diseases—related tests arranged in alphabetical order. For pathogen-specific tests, the entry is grouped under the pathogen name. The test methods in this chapter include general cultures by source, targeted cultures to rule out specific pathogens, direct antigen assays, antibody assays, macroscopic and microscopic detection, as well as molecular methods.

It is important to consider the limitations for each of these methods. In general, cultures are considered the gold standard for pathogen detection; however, testing typically takes 24–48 hours for completion. Targeted cultures are available and requested when pathogens cannot be efficiently detected by routine culture methods. Nevertheless, it is important to consider that (1) selective culture conditions may also inhibit some individual strains of the target pathogen, (2) nonselective media should also be inoculated along with selective media, and (3) cultures for specific pathogens may not detect other significant pathogens when used for evaluation of infected patient samples. Submission of routine bacterial cultures appropriate for the specimen type is usually recommended in addition to targeted cultures.

Direct antigen detection assays are widely available and provide quick turnaround time; however, they often have low sensitivity. Molecular methods are becoming common in detecting pathogens due to the high sensitivity and shorter turnaround time than conventional cultures, yet these assays are currently costly. See Chapter 13 for additional information regarding the basis of microbiology identification methods and pathogen-specific diseases.

ACID-FAST BACILLUS (AFB) SMEAR

➤ Definition and Use

* Smears of patient specimens are stained and examined for the presence of mycobacteria.
  * AFB staining should be undertaken for most specimens that are submitted for mycobacterial culture.

- Certain dyes bind to the thick, mycolic acid–rich cell walls of mycobacteria. The lipids of the cell wall make the cells resistant to decolorization with acid–alcohol solutions.
- The AFB smear may provide early evidence of TB or other mycobacterial disease.
- **Methods**
  - There are two types of AFB stains: chromogenic (carbolfuchsin stains [hot: Ziehl-Neelsen; cold: Kinyoun]) and fluorogenic (auramine O + rhodamine). After staining, the smear is destained with an acid–alcohol solution, typically HCl in ethanol. Mycobacteria retain the stain.
    - In chromogenic methods, slides are examined using a 100× oil immersion objective with light microscopy. Nonmycobacterial cells are counterstained with methylene blue. Mycobacteria appear red, whereas other bacteria and background are stained blue.
    - In fluorogenic methods, auramine-stained slides are examined by fluorescence microscopy using a 25× or 40× objective. Mycobacteria are yellow-orange against a dark background.
  - The improved signal-to-noise of auramine fluorochrome staining, allowing scanning with lower power objective, results in examination of a greater area of the slide at a given time, and therefore greater sensitivity. Any detected organisms should be confirmed by examination for typical morphology using the 100× objective. Some laboratories confirm positive fluorochrome smears with a carbolfuchsin-based stain.
- Specimens should be collected and transported to the laboratory according to recommendations for mycobacterial cultures.
- **Turnaround time:** <24 hours

➤ Interpretation

- **Expected results:** negative
- Detection of mycobacteria requires 10,000 or more organisms per milliliter or gram of sample for consistent detection.
- Sensitivity may be improved by concentration of specimen, such as by centrifugation, and by examination of multiple specimens. Rapidly growing mycobacteria, such as *Mycobacterium fortuitum*, have relatively thin layers of cell wall mycolic acid and may decolorize with acid–alcohol decolorizing solutions. These organisms may be stained using a weaker acid in aqueous solution.
- **Positive results:**
  - Positive specimens are very likely (>90%) to yield growth of mycobacteria in culture.
  - Nonviable organisms may be detected by AFB stains. *Nocardia* and related species are weakly acid fast and may give false-positive results if staining protocols are not followed closely.

➤ Limitations

- Standardized protocols, such as those published by the American Thoracic Society, should be followed carefully to ensure sensitive detection and accurate interpretation of smears.
- **Common pitfalls:**
  - Care must be taken to avoid contaminating slides with acid-fast organisms.
  - Common causes of slide contamination are use of tap water for solution preparation, carryover between slides with immersion oil, and use of common staining chambers.

ACID-FAST STAIN, MODIFIED

➤ Definition and Use
- This stain may be used for detection of *Nocardia* in patient specimens or culture isolates when nocardiosis is suspected on the basis of clinical presentation or because of typical morphology in culture isolates.
- The Gram stain is very sensitive for detection of *Nocardia* in patient specimens.
- The modified acid-fast stain is typically used to confirm nocardioform organisms detected by Gram stain. The modified acid-fast stain is useful for differentiating *Nocardia* (positive) from *Streptomyces* (negative), especially in culture isolates.
- The modified acid-fast stain is similar to the carbol-fuchsin–based acid-fast stains (Ziehl-Neelsen or Kinyoun stains) except that a less active decolorizer is used (1% H_2SO_4 or 3% HCl in aqueous solution).
- Specimens should be collected and transported as appropriate for routine bacterial cultures for the specimen type.
- **Turnaround time:** 24–72 hours

➤ Interpretation
- **Expected results:** negative. Negative stains do not rule out nocardiosis. Rapidly growing mycobacteria, such as *M. fortuitum*, may be negative by routine acid-fast staining (because of a thin mycolic acid layer in the cell wall) but positive for modified acid-fast staining.
- **Positive results with *Nocardia*:** delicate, branching filaments that retain the carbol-fuchsin stain.

➤ Limitations
- *Nocardia* may stain poorly in direct staining of patient specimens.
- Gram stains should also be examined carefully for organisms with typical nocardioform morphology.

➤ Other Considerations
Several organisms, such as *Rhodococcus equi* and occasionally coryneform bacteria, may be modified acid-fast positive.

➤ Suggested Reading
Winn Jr. WC, SD Allen, WM Janda, et al. *Koneman's Color Atlas and Textbook of Diagnostic Microbiology*. 6th ed. Lippincott Williams & Wilkins (Baltimore, MD and Philadelphia, PA). 2006.

AEROBIC CULTURE

➤ Definition and Use
- Aerobic cultures are indicated for evaluation of patient specimens taken from sites with signs and symptoms of bacterial infection (e.g., swelling, redness, heat, pus, or exudate)
- These cultures are used for the detection of common aerobic bacterial pathogens from patient specimens. Site-specific bacterial cultures (e.g., sputum culture, genital culture) are recommended, if available.

- Specimens are inoculated on several types of aerobic culture media, including supportive, differential, and selective media. Typical media for aerobic cultures include:
  - Supportive: sheep blood agar (SBA)
  - Enriched: chocolate agar
  - Selective/differential, gram-negative bacilli: MacConkey or eosin-methylene blue
  - Selective/differential, gram-positive: colistin-nalidixic acid (CNA) or phenylethyl alcohol blood agar (PEA)
  - Broth (e.g., brucella, brain-heart infusion, trypticase-soy).
    - Broth media can be inoculated with a larger volume than agar plates, which may improve detection of infections with low concentrations of pathogens. Broth media may allow detection of some relatively aerotolerant anaerobic pathogens.
    - Broth cultures, however, have been associated with an increased rate of contamination.
- **Expected results:** no pathogen isolated
- **Turnaround time:** 48–72 hours
  - Additional time is required for positive cultures for additional testing required for isolation, identification, susceptibility testing, and further characterization, as needed.

➤ Special Collection and Transport Instructions
- Standard precautions apply.
- Ensure that material from the site of infection is collected.
- Decontaminate skin or mucous membranes that must be crossed to obtain the specimen.
- Use appropriate sterile supplies to collect the specimen.
- Place the specimen in a sterile, leak-proof container for transport. Ensure that the lid is firmly tightened, but avoid over-tightening.
- Use specific transport medium and/or procedures as required for suspected pathogens (described below) or if transport to the lab will be prolonged (>2 hours).
- Apply a label to the specimen with information to identify the patient and type of specimen, as described below.
- Transport the specimen to the lab as quickly as possible, avoiding extremes of temperature.
- Note that collection protocols for some types of specimens require specific training and/or certification of the health care professional performing the collection. Examples include collection of bone marrow and CSF specimens.

➤ Limitations
- Anaerobic culture is recommended for infections at sites likely to be infected by anaerobic pathogens. Examples include pelvic infections, intra-abdominal infections, abscesses, and traumatic and surgical wounds.
- Certain aerobic pathogens, such as *Legionella* species, require special processing or culture techniques for detection.
- **Common pitfalls:**
  - Specimens may be collected from sites that are not the primary site of active infection (even though there may be signs of inflammation at the site).
  - Inadequate site preparation may result in false-positive cultures due to specimen contamination with endogenous flora. Contaminated specimens may also mask the recognition of slow-growing or fastidious pathogens in the culture.

ANAEROBIC CULTURE

➤ Definition and Use

- Anaerobic cultures are indicated for evaluation of patient specimens taken from sites with signs and symptoms of bacterial infection (e.g., swelling, redness, heat, pus, or exudate). Infections associated with anaerobic pathogens include:
  - Surgical and traumatic wounds
  - Sinusitis and para-respiratory infections
  - Pelvic and intra-abdominal infections
  - Osteomyelitis
  - Myositis, gangrene, and necrotic wounds
  - Abscesses
  - Actinomycosis and infections associated with fistula formation
- These tests are used for the detection of common anaerobic bacterial pathogens from patient specimens. Site-specific aerobic bacterial cultures (e.g., tissue culture, abscess culture, wound culture) are recommended, if available.
- Specimens are inoculated on several types of anaerobic culture media, including supportive, differential/selective, and broth media. Media should be fresh and prereduced. Typical media for aerobic cultures include:
  - Supportive: anaerobic brucella blood agar, Schaedler agar, CDC anaerobic blood agar
  - Selective/differential media:
    - Phenylethyl alcohol or CAN agar for anaerobic gram-positive pathogens
    - Kanamycin-vancomycin-laked blood agar, for anaerobic gram-negative bacilli
    - Bacteroides bile-esculin agar, for *Bacteroides fragilis* group
    - Egg yolk agar, for characterization of *Clostridium* species
    - Cycloserine-cefoxitin-egg yolk-fructose agar (CCFA), for *Clostridium difficile*
  - Broth:
    - Specimens are usually inoculated into broth media, such as enriched thioglycolate medium or chopped meat broth.
    - Broth media can be inoculated with a larger volume than agar plates, which may improve detection of infections with low concentrations of pathogens.
    - Broth cultures, however, have been associated with an increased rate of contamination.
- **Turnaround time:** typically, incubation for up to 7 days
  - Additional time is required for positive cultures for additional testing required for isolation, confirmation as anaerobic (aerotolerance testing), identification, susceptibility testing, and further characterization, as needed.
  - Anaerobic infections are frequently polymicrobial; final results may require several weeks for full laboratory evaluation, if needed.

➤ Special Collection and Transport Instructions

- Because of the anaerobic endogenous flora, specimens from the following sites should not be submitted for anaerobic culture:
  - Sputum or bronchoscopically collected lower respiratory specimens
  - Swabs from skin or mucosal surfaces
  - Specimens from the GI tract, including fistulae, stoma surfaces, and so on
  - Superficial ulcers or eschars, including decubitus ulcers
  - Vaginal or cervical swabs

- Urine (except suprapubic aspirate urine)
- Standard precautions apply.
- Ensure that material from the site of infection is collected.
- Ensure that sufficient specimen is collected for all of the diagnostic testing required (e.g., aerobic, fungal, and/or mycobacterial cultures and stains).
- Decontaminate skin or mucous membranes that must be crossed to obtain the specimen.
- Use appropriate sterile supplies to collect the specimen.
- Minimize exposure to atmospheric oxygen and transport in an anaerobic transport system.
- Apply a label to the specimen with information to identify the patient and type of specimen.
- Transport the specimen to the laboratory as quickly as possible, avoiding extremes of temperature.
- Do not refrigerate or freeze specimens for anaerobic culture.
- Note the following:
  - Specimens collected and transported for anaerobic culture are also acceptable for aerobic bacterial, fungal or mycobacterial culture, provided a sufficient volume of specimen is provided.
  - Collection protocols for some types of specimens require specific training and/or certification of the health care professional performing the collection. Examples include collection of empyema or lung abscess specimens.

➤ Interpretation
- **Expected results:** no anaerobic pathogen isolated

➤ Limitations
- Anaerobic infections are frequently polymicrobial.
  - Initial isolation and aerotolerance testing may require repeated subculture of different media.
  - In addition, many anaerobic pathogens are slow-growing and biochemically indolent, making identification, susceptibility testing, and further characterization of isolates in the laboratory much slower than most aerobic bacterial pathogens. Therefore, the extensive work-up of cultures for anaerobic isolates may be of limited value clinically. Many anaerobic infections may be treated empirically, and patient response documented before final laboratory results are available.
- **Common pitfalls**
  - Specimens are frequently not collected from the site of active infection using anaerobic techniques.
  - Anaerobic culture may be significantly compromised by transport conditions that are not strictly anaerobic or because of refrigeration during transport.
  - Inadequate site preparation may result in false-positive cultures due to specimen contamination with endogenous flora. Contaminated cultures may also mask the recognition of slow-growing or fastidious anaerobic pathogens in the culture.

BACTERIAL ANTIGEN DETECTION

➤ Definition and Use
- This test in intended for the rapid initial detection of *Streptococcus pneumoniae*, *Haemophilus influenzae* type b, group B beta-hemolytic *Streptococcus* (GBS), or *Neisseria meningitidis* in CSF.
- The indication for this test is probably limited. Published reports have demonstrated limited sensitivity for the detection of patients with meningitis caused by common pathogens, and test results rarely result in changes to the management or therapy of patients.

- There may be some utility in patients who have been treated with antibiotics prior to CSF collection.
- There is some evidence that the performance for initial detection of GBS meningitis in neonates is acceptable.
- Latex particles are coated with antibodies directed against specific antigens of the pathogens noted above. Agglutination should occur if the antigen is present in CSF, either as free antigen or intact bacterial cells.
- Specimens are collected and transported according to directions for CSF culture.
- **Turnaround time:** <4 hours

➤ Interpretation
- **Expected results:** negative; no agglutination means that a CSF infection caused by specific pathogen is less likely.
- Positive agglutination for specific Latex reagent: CSF infection caused by the specific pathogen is more likely.

➤ Limitations
- The sensitivity for detection is too low to be recommended for routine use in the evaluation of patients with suspected meningitis. False-positive reactions have been reported.

➤ Suggested Readings
Perkins MD, Mirrett S, Reller LB. Rapid bacterial antigen detection is not clinically useful. *J Clin Microbiol.* 1995; 30(06):1486–1491.
Ringelmann R, Heym B, Kniehl E. Role of immunologic tests in diagnosis of bacterial meningitis. *Antibiot Chemother.* 1992;45:68–78.

BD AFFIRM VPIII MICROBIAL IDENTIFICATION TEST

➤ Definition and Use
- Symptoms of vaginitis and vaginosis occur frequently and are a common reason for women seeking medical care. The most common causes of these symptoms are bacterial vaginosis (BV), trichomoniasis, and vulvovaginal candidiasis. Because there may be significant clinical overlap in the symptoms in these conditions, specific diagnostic testing may be required to guide appropriate antimicrobial therapy and patient management.
- The Affirm VPIII Microbial Identification Test is intended for use in the detection of common pathogens in vaginal secretions of patients with symptoms of vaginitis or vaginosis. This test is based on pathogen detection by nucleic acid probe hybridization. The testing includes probes for the detection *Gardnerella vaginalis* (a marker for the disruption of the normal vaginal flora seen in BV), *Candida* species (for candidiasis), and *Trichomonas vaginalis* (for trichomoniasis).
- The assessment of test accuracy depends on the populations studied, the comparator method, and other factors.
  - Sensitivity and specificity for detection of candidiasis in symptomatic women: 82% and 95%, respectively
  - Sensitivity and specificity for detection of BV in symptomatic women: 98% and 100%, respectively
  - Sensitivity and specificity for detection of trichomoniasis, compared to wet mount detection: 93% and 99%, respectively
- **Turnaround time:** 24 hours

➤ Specimen Collection and Transport Instructions
- Vaginal fluid specimens should be collected only from patients with symptoms compatible with vaginosis or vaginitis.
- Use only supplies provided in the Affirm VPIII transport system, sample collection set, or test kit for specimen collection.
- Samples are collected from the posterior vaginal fornix, using an unlubricated (no water or jelly) speculum to visualize the collection site, ensuring that the entire circumference of the swab has been inoculated with vaginal secretions.
- Place the swab into sample collection tube and snap on cap following the kit instructions.
- Transport specimens according to kit instructions for the kit used. Specimens may be transported at room temperature or refrigerated. The transport time to the laboratory depends on the transport temperature and the Affirm VPIII system used.

➤ Interpretation
- **Expected Results:** Negative for all three pathogens. Negative results for a specific pathogen suggest that infection with that pathogen is unlikely.
- Positive results for one or more of the pathogens tested indicate infection when consistent signs and symptoms are present. Infection with more than one of the pathogens is not uncommon.

➤ Limitations
- Specimens must be collected, transported, tested, and interpreted using protocols described in the package insert of the kit used.
- Performance of the test depends on optimal specimen collection.
- Negative results do not exclude the possibility of infection with any of the specific pathogens.
- Alternative testing, like pH, "whiff test," and microscopic examination of vaginal fluid may be considered for the evaluation of patients.
- The Affirm VPIII test does not detect infection by *Neisseria gonorrhoeae* or *Chlamydia trachomatis*; these pathogens, and other possible causes of the patient's symptoms, should be considered, and ruled out as appropriate, in women presenting with vaginal discharge or other compatible symptoms.
- The test cannot be used as a test of cure because DNA from nonviable pathogens may be detectable after resolution of infection.

BLOOD CULTURE, FUNGAL

➤ Definition and Use
- Fungal blood cultures are used for detection of bloodstream infection caused by fungi, especially when dimorphic species and uncommon pathogens are suspected. Identification, susceptibility, and further testing can be performed on culture isolates.
- The culture is indicated primarily for patients with cancer; extensive therapy with broad-spectrum antibiotics; trauma; and HIV and other immunocompromising conditions that lead to such conditions as sepsis syndrome, fever, chills, malaise, hypotension, poor perfusion, toxicity, tachycardia, and hyperventilation.
- Biphasic and lysis-centrifugation methods have demonstrated improved isolation of dimorphic and filamentous fungi.
- **Turnaround time:** 4 weeks

➤ Special Collection and Transport Instructions
- Inoculate blood culture system according to manufacturer's recommendations.
- Alert the laboratory if infection due to *Malassezia furfur* is suspected. Special culture processing is needed for isolation of this lipophilic yeast.
- Transport to the laboratory at room temperature.

➤ Interpretation
- **Expected results:** no growth
- Most commonly isolated pathogens in positive cultures:
  - Yeasts: *Candida albicans*, non-albicans *Candida* species, and *Cryptococcus neoformans*. (*Candida* and other commonly isolated yeasts may be efficiently detected using routine blood cultures.)
  - Dimorphic fungus: *Histoplasma capsulatum*
  - Mold: Fusarium species

➤ Limitation
- *Aspergillus* species are rarely isolated by blood culture even in the presence of acute systemic infection.

➤ Suggested Reading
CLSI. *Principles and Procedures for Blood Cultures; Approved Guideline.* CLSI document M47-A. Wayne, PA: Clinical and Laboratory Standards Institute; 2007.

BLOOD CULTURE, MYCOBACTERIAL

➤ Definition and Use
- The mycobacterial blood culture is used for the detection of bloodstream infection due to *Mycobacterium* species.
- Mycobacteremia is most commonly seen in patients with AIDS, although it may occur in other congenital and acquired immunocompromising conditions, including patients taking chronic corticosteroid therapy, those with malignancies, and so on.
- Growth of mycobacteria in culture requires the use of specialized, supplemented media with prolonged incubation time. Lysis of blood cells improves detection, by releasing phagocytized organisms, and is used in most methods (e.g., lysis-centrifugation methods).
- **Turnaround time:** 4–8 weeks

➤ Special Collection and Transport Instructions
- Collect 5–10 mL of blood in sodium polyanethol sulfonate (SPS) or heparin, or directly inoculate specific mycobacterial blood culture media.
- Inoculate the blood culture media or collection system according to manufacturer's instructions.
- Transport to the laboratory at room temperature.

➤ Interpretation
- **Expected results:** no growth
- **Positive results:** *Mycobacterium avium* complex (MAC) is the most commonly isolated mycobacterial pathogen.

➤ Limitations
- Some species that are uncommon causes of mycobacteremia may require additional supplementation (e.g., *Mycobacterium haemophilum*) or incubation temperature (e.g., *Mycobacterium marinum*) for optimal recovery.

- EDTA or acid citrate dextrose (ACD) anticoagulated blood should not be used for mycobacterial blood culture inoculum.
- *Mycobacterium tuberculosis* is rarely isolated by blood culture, even in disseminated disease.
- Rapidly growing mycobacteria, such as *M. fortuitum*, have been associated with chronic indwelling vascular catheters and other prosthetic material.

➤ Suggested Reading
CLSI. *Principles and Procedures for Blood Cultures; Approved Guideline*. CLSI document M47-A. Wayne, PA: Clinical and Laboratory Standards Institute; 2007.

BLOOD CULTURE, ROUTINE

➤ Definition and Use
- The routine blood culture is used for detection of bloodstream infections (BSIs) due to common aerobic and anaerobic bacterial and yeast pathogens. Potentially pathogenic isolates are identified and susceptibility testing performed, as appropriate. Special testing is required for the detection of mycobacteria, parasites, viruses, and certain fungal pathogens. (See entries for specific tests.)
- Indications
  - Sepsis syndrome, fever, chills, malaise, hypotension, poor perfusion, toxicity, tachycardia, hyperventilation
  - Evaluation of serious localized infections, such as pneumonia, UTIs, and meningitis. Classic signs and symptoms may be absent in infants, the elderly and patients with certain medical or surgical conditions.
- Methods
  - Most commercially available blood culture systems use inoculation of blood into two broth media: one aerobic and one anaerobic. Some institutions recommend inoculation of two aerobic broth media instead of the aerobic/anaerobic combination. For young children, a single, usually aerobic, medium is recommended at some institutions.
  - Lysis-centrifugation methods may be used for routine detection of BSIs due to bacteria or yeast but are more typically used for detection of mycobacteremia or fungemia. (See Blood Culture, Mycobacterial, and Blood Culture, Fungal, for more details (p. 405 and p. 406, respectively).
- **Turnaround time:** generally, incubation for 5–7 days. Most true-positive blood cultures become positive within 24–48 hours after inoculation.

➤ Special Collection and Transport Instructions
- Decontamination of the collection site is the most important factor in preventing false-positive (contaminated) blood cultures.
- Inoculate media according to manufacturer's instructions. Usually, 8–10 mL of blood is inoculated into each blood culture bottle. The greatest sensitivity is achieved when 2 or 3 blood cultures are submitted for the initial evaluation of a patient. A smaller inoculum volume is recommended for small children.
- Submission of two or three independently drawn (different venipuncture sites) blood cultures is recommended for the initial evaluation of patients with suspected BSI.
- Transport blood cultures to the laboratory at room temperature.

➤ Interpretation
- **Expected results:** no growth
- **Positive results:** see Table 3-1 for a listing of common pathogens and contaminants.

TABLE 3-1. Common Blood Culture Isolates

True-Positive Blood Cultures	Contaminated Blood Cultures
Pseudomonas aeruginosa	*Staphylococcus*, coagulase negative
Escherichia coli	*Corynebacterium* spp./diphtheroids
Klebsiella pneumoniae	*Propionibacterium acnes*
Other Enterobacteriaceae	*Neisseria* spp., saprophytic
Staphylococcus aureus	Bacillus spp., not *anthracis*
Staphylococcus, coagulase negative	Alpha-hemolytic *Streptococcus* (*viridans*)
Streptococcus pneumoniae	*Micrococcus* spp.
Beta-hemolytic *Streptococcus*	
Enterococcus spp.	
Alpha-hemolytic *Streptococcus* (*viridans*)	
Candida albicans	
Candida spp., other	

* In patients with clinically relevant BSIs (true positive), the pathogen is typically isolated from a majority of cultures/bottles.
* In patients with contaminated blood cultures (false positive), a common contaminant is typically isolated in a single culture or bottle, whereas other cultures drawn during evaluation remain negative.

➤ Limitations
* Prior antibiotic treatment may result in negative blood cultures, or delayed time to detection in positive cultures.
* Routine blood cultures are optimized for detection of the pathogens most frequently associated with BSIs. Clinically relevant BSIs may be associated with pathogens for which special blood cultures are required (e.g., mycobacteria, dimorphic fungi)
* **Common pitfalls:**
  * Decreased sensitivity because of such factors as a low volume of blood submitted for culture or prior antimicrobial therapy
  * Decreased specificity because of contamination due to poor preparation of collection site

➤ Suggested Reading
CLSI. *Principles and Procedures for Blood Cultures; Approved Guideline*. CLSI document M47-A. Wayne, PA: Clinical and Laboratory Standards Institute; 2007.

BLOOD PARASITE EXAMINATION

➤ Definition and Use
* This test is used to detect parasites circulating in peripheral blood. It should be ordered in patients when infection caused by *Plasmodium* species (malaria), *Babesia* species (babesiosis), *Trypanosoma* species (sleeping sickness, Chagas disease), certain microfilaria species, or systemic infection with *Leishmania* species is suspected.

- Thin and thick blood smears are prepared from free-flowing capillary blood or EDTA-anticoagulated blood. Smears are inspected after staining with Giemsa, Wright, or Wright-Giemsa stain. For positive smears, the level of parasitemia should be determined for each specimen.
- **Turnaround time:**
  - Preliminary examination should be performed "STAT" if malaria is suspected (turnaround time <4 hours).
  - Final report for positive smears: <24 hours

➤ Special Collection and Transport Instructions
- Preparation of smears at the bedside, from free-flowing capillary blood if possible, yields the best morphology.
- Alternatively, EDTA-anticoagulated blood may be collected.
- If trypanosomes or microfilariae are suspected, examination of buffy coat smears or other concentration technique is recommended. For microfilariae, the diurnal circulation of some species must be taken into account in timing specimen collection.
- Specimens should be transported to the laboratory as soon as possible.
- In general, specimens should be collected on each of three successive days. Specimens should be collected every 6–8 hours (until positive) for optimal detection in suspected cases. Blood should be examined in treated patients after 24, 48, and 72 hours to determine effectiveness of therapy.

➤ Interpretation
- **Expected results:** negative
- Sensitive detection of parasitemia may require the examination of several specimens, as recommended above.
- **Positive result:** disease caused by specific parasite identified.

➤ Limitations
- Low level of parasitemia may require the examination of multiple specimens for detection. Examination of smears prepared from buffy coat preparations may improve the sensitivity of detection for some parasites, like microfilaria and trypanosomes.
- The efficient detection of microfilaria requires specimen collection during the specific hours when circulation of the parasite is expected.
- **Common pitfalls** include the collection of too few specimens for examination.

➤ Other Considerations
- In effectively treated patients, the level of parasitemia should drop very quickly. In patients with drug-resistant parasites, the level may remain stable, or even increase.

➤ Suggested Readings
Garcia LS. *Diagnostic Parasitology*, 5th ed. ASM Press (Washington, DC). 2007.
NCCLS document M15-A. *Laboratory Diagnosis of Blood-borne Parasitic Diseases*; Approved Guideline. 2000. Clinical and Laboratory Standards Institute.

BODY FLUID CULTURE

➤ Definition
- Sterile fluid-filled spaces are present at a number of anatomic sites and are subject to infection. Examples of sterile fluids include peritoneal, pleural, pericardial, synovial/joint, and

others. Infections associated with CSF are life-threatening and associated with a different etiology of bacterial pathogens, so these cultures are typically processed differently from other sterile fluids. Urine is also processed with different culture techniques because of its connection with the external environment, via the urethra, and pathogenesis of infection.
* A broad etiology of bacterial pathogens may cause infections of sterile sites, and culture methods are optimized for recovery of organisms present in low concentrations. The diagnostic strategy may be influenced by the pathogenesis of infections (e.g., hematogenous, direct extension from contiguous infected site, trauma/direct inoculation).

➤ Use
* Sterile fluid cultures should be collected from sites associated with signs and symptoms of inflammation, including redness, swelling, pain, heat, fluid accumulation, pus formation, and so on.
* **Method:** Supportive and enriched solid agar (SBA and chocolate agar) and broth media (blood culture media) are typically inoculated; selective/differential agar media, such as Mac-Conkey agar (gram-negative bacilli), CNA, or phenylethyl alcohol agar (gram-positive organisms), should be inoculated for specimens likely to show polymicrobial infection (e.g., peritonitis) or contamination by endogenous flora (e.g., cul-de-sac aspirates). Anaerobic broth media should be inoculated, as well as anaerobic agar media, if there is a significant possibility of anaerobic pathogens. If infection with an uncommon, fastidious pathogen is suspected, the laboratory should be informed so that special cultures may be inoculated, as needed.
* **Turnaround time:** Cultures are incubated for up to 7 days. Additional time is required for isolation, identification, susceptibility testing, and further characterization, as needed.

➤ Special Collection and Transport Instructions
* Fluid aspiration is performed after preparation of the puncture site in a manner consistent with a surgical prep. Submission of specimens from drainage devices is discouraged because of the high incidence of contamination with endogenous flora; direct collection of the sterile fluid is recommended.
* Collection of the maximum amount of fluid from the infected site is recommended. Blood culture bottles may be inoculated and is recommended for patients with spontaneous bacterial peritonitis, but a small amount of fluid should be retained for Gram stain and special culture inoculation, if needed, in the laboratory.
* Swabs should not be used for fluid collection.
* Fluid is placed into sterile transport tubes; small volume specimen, or several milliliters from large volume specimens, should be placed into an anaerobic transport tube. Note: Specimens transported under anaerobic conditions are acceptable for inoculation of cultures for aerobic bacterial, mycobacterial, and fungal cultures.
* Submission of specimens from repeated fluid collections prior to antibiotic therapy may significantly improve sensitivity of culture detection.
* The use of anticoagulants is discouraged because of possible inhibition of some pathogens. If anticoagulation is required, heparin or SPS is recommended.
* Transport specimens at room temperature; do not refrigerate or freeze specimens.

➤ Interpretation
* **Expected results:** no growth. Infection is not excluded by a negative culture, especially after initiation antibiotic therapy. Uncommon, fastidious pathogens may not be isolated in culture without inoculation of special media.

- Positive cultures indicate infection of the sterile site, but cultures that may be contaminated with contiguous flora must be interpreted with caution in the context of quantity or bacterial growth, purity of culture, Gram stain findings, and clinical signs and symptoms.
- Infected peritoneal fluid usually yields numerous aerobic and anaerobic pathogens. Extensive identification and susceptibility testing is usually not clinically useful; final results are often not available until well into therapy, and empirical treatment regimens are usually effective.

➤ Suggested Readings

Atkins BL, Athanasou N, Deeks JJ, et al., and the Osiris Collaborative Study Group. Prospective evaluation of criteria for microbiological diagnosis of prosthetic-joint infection at revision arthroplasty. *J Clin Microbiol.* 1998;36:2932–2939.

Baselski V, Beavis KG, Bell M, et al. *Clinical Microbiology Procedures Handbook*, 3rd Edition. Editor in Chief: Lynne S. Garcia, ASM Press (Washington, DC). 2010.

Bernard L, Pron B, Vaugnat A, et al., and the Groupe d'Etude sur l'Osteite. The value of suction drainage fluid culture during aseptic and septic orthopedic surgery: a prospective study of 901 patients. *Clin Infect Dis.* 2002;34:46–49.

BORDETELLA PERTUSSIS CULTURE (RULE OUT)

➤ Definition and Use
- This test is used to detect acute infection caused by the slow-growing, fastidious pathogen *B. pertussis*.
- *B. pertussis* is the cause of pertussis, or whooping cough. A presumptive diagnosis of pertussis may be made on the basis of clinical presentation; culture should be ordered when a specific diagnosis is required.
- Specimens are typically inoculated onto Regan-Lowe or fresh Bordet-Gengou agar.
- Nasopharyngeal specimens should be submitted for *B. pertussis* culture; aspirates are preferred.
- Ideally, the sample should be inoculated onto media at the point of collection or transported quickly to the laboratory. Transport medium, such as a modified Regan-Lowe formulation, may be used if transport will be delayed.
- **Turnaround time:**
  - Most cultures are positive in 7–10 days, although some cultures are incubated for up to 14 days.
  - Additional time is required for final identification and further characterization.

➤ Interpretation
- **Expected results:** negative. A negative culture does not exclude the diagnosis of pertussis, especially when a specimen is collected after the early, acute phase of infection.
- **Positive results:** Confirm the diagnosis of pertussis

➤ Limitations
- The sensitivity of culture for *B. pertussis* falls significantly after the first 7–14 days after onset of symptoms.
- Poor specimen collection, submission of specimens other than nasopharyngeal specimens, and submission of specimens during the chronic phase of disease are associated with poor sensitivity of culture.

➤ Other Considerations

- PCR methods have been described for diagnosis of pertussis. Cross-reactions have been described (e.g., *Bordetella holmesii*) and may limit the utility of molecular diagnostic testing. The sensitivity of PCR is greatest in the early acute phase of infection, but *B. pertussis* DNA may be detectable for weeks after resolution of acute disease.
- A number of serologic assays are commercially available, including assays for IgM and IgA. Variable sensitivity and specificity has limited the clinical utility of these assays.

BORDETELLA PERTUSSIS SEROLOGY IgG

➤ Definition

- *B. pertussis* infection is an acute, highly contagious disease. It is characterized clinically by a severe and prolonged cough. Coughing fits may be paroxysmal and, usually in infants, followed by an inspirational "whoop." A clinical diagnosis will form the basis of most pertussis diagnosis and treatment decisions. The CDC provides the following clinical case definition for pertussis. A cough illness lasting at least 2 weeks with one of the following: paroxysms of coughing, inspiratory "whoop," or post-tussive vomiting, without other apparent cause.
- Because of the contagiousness of the infection, specific laboratory testing may be needed to confirm the diagnosis when pertussis is suspected clinically. Laboratory diagnosis of pertussis is complicated by the limitation of available tests. Options for diagnostic and confirmatory testing, when required, depend on the age of the patient and the phase of illness.
- **Normal range:** negative

➤ Use

- Although *B. pertussis* serology is most useful in epidemiologic investigations or vaccine trials, it does have some utility in the diagnosis of pertussis in some patients, particularly in adolescents, adults, and previously vaccinated individuals. Serologic testing may also be useful for patients with cough >2–3 weeks in duration. Antibodies can be detected against *B. pertussis* antigens 1–2 weeks after the onset of the symptoms of pertussis in nonvaccinated individuals. Both IgG and IgA isotypes are produced in response to infection, whereas IgG is the predominant isotype detected after vaccination. However, no single antigen or isotype can be used to distinguish between infection and a response to vaccination with certainty. IgM responses are usually not measured for pertussis, and have questionable diagnostic significance.
- Serologic testing for *B. pertussis* infection involves the detection of antibodies to pertussis antigens using standardized assays. Pertussis toxin (PT) and filamentous hemagglutinin (FHA) are the most widely used antigens. Only PT is specific for *B. pertussis*; FHA and pertactin antigens cross-react with antibodies arising from infection by other *Bordetella* species and possibly by other bacteria. Serum antibodies have been measured by ELISA, complement fixation, agglutination, and toxin neutralization; ELISA is the detection method of choice due to its wide availability and ease of performance.
- The most reliable serologic approach to diagnosis of pertussis is with simultaneous testing of paired acute and convalescent sera. A significant increase (fourfold or greater) in IgG or IgA antibody titers to PT or FHA, comparing convalescent to acute sample, suggests recent *B. pertussis* infection in patients with a clinical illness compatible with pertussis. Paired sera, however, are not practical in most clinical settings.

- Single-sample serology tests for antipertussis toxin IgG must be collected at least 2 weeks after symptom onset. A high antibody titer >2 years following vaccination supports the diagnosis of pertussis.
- Aids in the detection of *B. pertussis* infection

➤ Interpretation
- **Positive:** IgG antibody to *B. pertussis* detected, which may indicate a current or past exposure/immunization to *B. pertussis*.

➤ Limitations
- The CDC does not currently accept serology as laboratory verification of pertussis; cases that meet the clinical case definition with a positive serology but a negative culture or PCR are considered probable cases. Single serology tests are used for the diagnosis of pertussis by the state laboratory in Massachusetts and in selected countries in the European Union.
- The IgG serology test results are not interpretable in children younger than 11 years of age because of interference due to persistent antibody formed by childhood vaccination. The test also cannot be interpreted in older patients who have received the Tdap vaccination in the previous 3 years.

BORRELIA BURGDORFERI (LYME DISEASE)—ANTIBODY SCREEN

➤ Definition
Enzyme-Linked Immunosorbent Assay for the detection of IgG and/or IgM antibodies to *Borrelia burgdorferi*.

➤ Use
This test is used if Lyme Disease is suspected in at risk patients. Testing is not necessary if a patient presents with a tick bite and erythema migrans.

➤ Interpretation
<1.00 = negative
1.00-1.19 = equivocal
>1.19 = positive
Note: Current CDC recommendations state that equivocal and positive results should be confirmed with Western Blot prior to reporting screen results. If testing is negative, consider other tick-borne diseases (*i.e. Babesia, Ehrlichia*).

➤ Limitations
- False negative results can occur if patient is tested too early, repeat testing in 2-4 weeks. The IgG antibody response is usually not detectable until 4 to 6 weeks after infection; the IgM antibody response usually not detected during the first two weeks of infection, peaking 3 to 6 weeks following infection.
- False-positive results may occur from other spirochetal diseases, autoimmune diseases or other infections (EBV, HIV, syphilis, infectious mononucleosis, etc)
- No objective tests for Lyme borreliosis are 100% sensitive and 100% specific
- Diagnosis depends on clinical features, combined with available laboratory tests

➤ **Resources**

FDA Public Health Advisory: Assays for Antibodies to Borrelia burgdorferi; Limitations, Use, and Interpretation for Supporting a Clinical Diagnosis of Lyme Disease. July 7. 1997. http://www.fda.gov/MedicalDevices/Safety/AlertsandNotices/PublicHealthNotifications/UCM062429

BORRELIA BURGDORFERI (LYME DISEASE)—WESTERN BLOT

➤ **Definition**

• The western blot assay for antibodies to *Borrelia burgdorferi*, the etiologic agent of Lyme disease, is a qualitative method of categorizing specific immunoreactivities in serum or plasma to *B. burgdorferi* proteins that have been formatted according to molecular weight into discrete bands on nitrocellulose strips.

➤ **Use**

• The western blot assay for *B. burgdorferi* is used as a second-tier test to characterize the specificity of an individual's immune response to the component proteins of *B. burgdorferi* by identifying the presence, relative level, and pattern of reactivities to the complete set of the bacterial proteins.
• The assay is used routinely to provide supportive serologic evidence of infection following a more sensitive but less specific screening test (such as EIA) for general reactivity to *B. burgdorferi*. Both IgM and IgG reactivities to the bacterial proteins are assayed to provide information on the evolution of the immune response relative to the stage of infection (i.e., early localized, early disseminated, or late disseminated).

➤ **Interpretation**

• Reactivity scores: Specimen reactions with protein bands are first scored in terms of relative reaction intensity versus a cut-off control or minimally positive ("+") band reaction intensity by a positive control specimen.
• Test interpretation (IgM class reactivities)
  • **Positive:** Reactivity scores of "+" or greater for at least two of three clinically significant proteins at the early stage of the disease (2–3 weeks after infection): 41, 39, 23 kDa
  • **Negative:** Absence of any band reactivity on the test strip or reactivity for only one of the three clinically significant proteins
• Test interpretation (IgG class reactivities)
  • **Positive:** Reactivity scores of "+" or greater for at least five of ten clinically significant proteins at the later stages of the disease (weeks to months after infection): 93, 66, 58, 45, 41, 39, 30, 28, 23, 18 kDa
  • **Negative:** Absence of any band reactivity on the test strip or reactivity for less than five of the ten clinically significant proteins

➤ **Limitations**

• Minimum specimen volume is 40 μL (20 μL each for the IgM and IgG tests).
• Like any second-tier test, the positive predictive value for a western blot assay is a function of the a priori likelihood of the disease by clinical and epidemiologic criteria, whereas the negative predictive value is not as well defined because of the variability of the immune response among infected individuals. Cross-reactive diseases are most frequently evidenced by reactivity to the 41-kDa flagellar protein, and at much lower frequency to the 66-kDa heat shock protein. Specimens from patients diagnosed with *Ehrlichia* or *Babesia* infections can show other *Borrelia*-specific bands.

BRONCHIAL BRUSH CULTURE, QUANTITATIVE

➤ Use
- Quantitative bacterial cultures of specimens collected bronchoscopically using a protected brush are usually submitted for the evaluation for ventilator-associated pneumonia (VAP).
- The diagnosis of VAP is challenging, requiring a combination of clinical, imaging, and laboratory studies. Cultures are assessed in comparison to thresholds established by the laboratory in collaboration with clinicians. They are most useful in terms of providing information to help limit prolonged, broad-spectrum antimicrobial therapy through de-escalation of empirical treatment for suspected VAP and should be considered for the evaluation of intubated patients with pulmonary abnormalities consistent with VAP. Tissue histopathology and quantitative culture of biopsy are considered the "gold standard" for diagnosis.
- Method
  - The brush is vigorously agitated in the saline transport fluid to release trapped microorganisms. The saline is then used to inoculate media and/or prepare further dilutions for media inoculation.
  - Known volumes of the specimen (or specimen dilution) are inoculated onto sheep blood, chocolate, and MacConkey agar (and other media as required for uncommon pathogens, such as *Legionella*).
  - Media are incubated according to standard laboratory protocol.
  - The concentration of each type of organism is calculated using the colony count on the solid media, volume inoculated onto the solid media, and the dilution of the original specimen. Cultures are interpreted on the basis of the isolate identification, quantity of isolate in culture, and the presence of other flora, especially endogenous flora of low pathogenicity.
  - **Turnaround time:** incubation for 48 hours. Additional time is required for pathogen isolation, identification, susceptibility testing, and further characterization, if needed.

➤ Special Collection and Transport Instructions
- Protected brush specimens are collected by a trained physician using standard procedures. The brush is inserted through a plugged catheter via the biopsy channel of the bronchoscope. After expulsion of the plug, the brush is used to collect cells and secretions from the distal airways.
- The brush end should be removed, using sterile technique, and placed in a small volume (1 mL) of nonbacteriostatic saline for transport.
- Samples should be transported to the laboratory as quickly as possible, using standard protocols for bacterial cultures.

➤ Interpretation
- **Expected results:** A low quantity ($<10^4$ CFU/mL) of endogenous upper respiratory flora is often seen.
- **Positive results:** In patients with pneumonia, growth of a respiratory pathogen is expected at a concentration of $>10^3$ CFU/mL.
- **Negative results:**
  - False-negative cultures may be caused by prior antimicrobial therapy.
  - Detection of pneumonia caused by certain fastidious pathogens may require inoculation of special media.
  - Heavy contamination of the specimen with endogenous flora may mask the growth of the causative pathogen.

➤ Limitations

- Quantitative culture of protected brush specimens has only moderate to good performance, with the PPV and NPV of 74% and 85%, respectively. The presence of intracellular organisms in >5% of cells may be associated with higher specificities.
- **Common pitfalls:**
  - The predictive value of cultures is markedly decreased for patients with any antibiotic therapy prior to the procedure.
  - *Candida* species are common contaminants and should not routinely be identified to species level.

➤ Suggested Readings

Carroll KC. Laboratory diagnosis of lower respiratory tract infections: controversy and conundrums. *J Clin Microbiol.* 2002;40:3115–3120.

Koenig SM, Truwit JD. Ventilator-associated pneumonia: diagnosis, treatment, and prevention. *Clin Microbiol Rev.* 2006;19:637–657.

BRONCHOALVEOLAR LAVAGE (BAL) CULTURE, QUANTITATIVE

➤ Definition and Use

- Quantitative bacterial culture of BAL fluid is usually submitted for the evaluation for ventilator-associated pneumonia (VAP). These cultures should be considered for the evaluation of intubated patients with pulmonary abnormalities consistent with VAP; they are assessed in comparison to thresholds established by the laboratory in collaboration with clinicians.
- The diagnosis of VAP is challenging, requiring a combination of clinical, imaging, and laboratory studies. Cultures are most useful in terms of providing information to help limit prolonged, broad-spectrum antimicrobial therapy through de-escalation of empirical treatment for suspected VAP.
- Tissue histopathology and quantitative culture of biopsy are considered the "gold standard" for diagnosis.
- Method
  - A measured aliquot of BAL fluid is used to inoculate media and/or prepare dilutions in saline for media inoculation. Known volumes of the specimen (or specimen dilution) are inoculated onto sheep blood, chocolate, and MacConkey agar (and other media as required for uncommon pathogens, such as *Legionella*).
  - Media are incubated according to standard laboratory protocol.
- The concentration of each type of organism is calculated using the colony count on the solid media, volume inoculated onto the solid media, and the dilution of the original specimen.
- **Turnaround time:** incubation for 48 hours. Additional time is required for pathogen isolation, identification, susceptibility testing, and further characterization, if needed.

➤ Special Collection and Transport Instructions

- BAL specimens are collected by a trained physician using standard procedures. The procedure and placement of the tip may be done under direct visualization or "blindly" through an endotracheal tube (mini-BAL).
- The return from the procedure should be 10–100 mL, sampling approximately 1 mL of alveolar secretions.
- Samples should be transported to the laboratory as quickly as possible, using standard protocols for bacterial cultures.

➤ Interpretation

• Cultures are interpreted on the basis of the isolate identification, quantity of isolate in culture, and the presence of other flora, especially endogenous flora of low pathogenicity.

• A low quantity ($<10^4$ colony forming units [CFU]/mL) of endogenous upper respiratory flora is often seen.

• Positive results may be obtained. In patients with pneumonia, growth of a respiratory pathogen is expected at a concentration of $>10^4$ CFU/mL for visually guided BAL ($>10^5$ to 10^6 for blind mini-BAL).

• **Negative results:**
  • False-negative cultures may be caused by prior antimicrobial therapy.
  • Detection of pneumonia caused by certain fastidious pathogens may require inoculation of special media.
  • Heavy contamination of the specimen with endogenous flora may mask the growth of the causative pathogen.

➤ Limitations

• Quantitative culture of BAL has only moderate to good performance, with a PPV of 83–91%, and NPV of 87–89%.

• The presence of intracellular organisms in $>5\%$ of cells is associated with higher specificities.

• **Common pitfalls:**
  • The predictive value of cultures is markedly decreased for patients with any antibiotic therapy prior to the procedure.
  • Bronchial washing (BW) specimens, collected through a nonwedged bronchoscope, may be submitted instead of a BAL specimen. BW specimens are usually small volume (<10 mL) and are more likely to be contaminated with endogenous upper respiratory flora.
  • *Candida* species are common contaminants and should not routinely be identified to species level.

➤ Suggested Readings

Carroll KC. Laboratory diagnosis of lower respiratory tract infections: controversy and conundrums. *J Clin Microbiol.* 2002;40:3115–3120.

Koenig SM, Truwit JD. Ventilator-associated pneumonia: diagnosis, treatment, and prevention. *Clin Microbiol Rev.* 2006;19:637–657.

BRUCELLA CULTURE (RULE OUT)

➤ Definition

• Human infection may be caused by several species of the genus *Brucella*. These organisms are fastidious, slow-growing gram-negative bacilli capable of producing severe localized and systemic infection. Infections have typically been acquired by zoonotic transmission, primarily related to livestock and dairy industries.

• There is great concern regarding the use of this organism for a bioterror-related attack. The organism is easily transmissible, so it is critical that the laboratory be informed whenever brucellosis is suspected. The incubation period after exposure is variable, from 1–8 weeks. *Brucella* species may cause a variety of infections with acute or insidious onset and fairly nonspecific clinical presentations. Typical disease syndromes include:

- Bacteremia, fever of unknown origin, sepsis
- Hepatic and GI infection
- Bone and joint infection
- Pneumonia and pulmonary infection
- Meningoencephalitis and CNS infection

➤ Use

- This culture is used to isolate *Brucella* species from clinical specimens.
- Method: Specimens are inoculated onto a blood agar (such as *Brucella* blood agar), chocolate agar, and Thayer-Martin agar (if contamination with endogenous flora is suspected). Specimens for *Brucella* are also inoculated onto MacConkey agar.
- Because of the risk of laboratory-acquired infection and because isolation of *Brucella* species may represent a sentinel event in a bioterror attack, most clinical microbiology laboratories limit the work-up of suspected isolates to simple tests to rule out suspicious colonies, referring isolates that fail to "rule out" to their local public health laboratory for identification and further characterization. Final results for testing, therefore, may be delayed compared to common bacterial isolates.
- **Turnaround time:** Isolation and preliminary identification for routine cultures is usually available in 5–7 days. Additional time is required for transfer to the local public health laboratory, confirmation of identification, and further testing.

➤ Special Collection and Transport Instructions

- The organisms primarily infect the reticuloendothelial system, so bone marrow and blood are the specimens of choice for patient evaluation. Specimens from other infected tissue or sites should also be submitted for culture.
- Bone marrow and blood cultures are recommended for evaluation of patients with suspected brucellosis.
- Serologic testing is recommended for diagnosis in patients with suspected brucellosis.
- PCR for specific *Brucella* species may be available through local public health laboratories for evaluation of patients with a high suspicion of brucellosis.

➤ Interpretation

- **Expected results:** negative
- **Positive:** Isolation of *Brucella* in culture is diagnostic for brucellosis; positive cultures must be reported to the local department of health.

➤ Limitations

- *Brucella* may be difficult to detect by Gram stain in primary specimens.
- **Common pitfalls:**
  - Because brucellosis may present after a prolonged incubation period, or present with nonspecific symptoms and an indolent onset, the diagnosis may not be considered until progression into the chronic phase of illness.
  - Clinicians may fail to request specific cultures for brucellosis, or alert the laboratory of their clinical suspicion.

➤ Other Considerations

- Brucellosis is a reportable disease. Patients with a diagnosis of brucellosis must be reported to the local department of health.

CEREBROSPINAL FLUID (CSF) CULTURE

➤ Definition and Use
- CSF culture is used for specific diagnosis of bacterial meningitis. Patients commonly present with severe headache, fever, neck stiffness and meningeal signs, mental status changes, and signs of systemic toxicity.
- Method
  - CSF is inoculated onto sheep blood and chocolate agar, incubated aerobically. Broth media may be inoculated.
  - Special media or culture conditions may be used for non–community-acquired meningitis, such as infections associated with trauma and prosthetic implants.
- **Turnaround time:** Cultures are incubated for 96 hours. Additional time is required for isolate identification, susceptibility testing, and further characterization, as needed.

➤ Special Collection and Transport Instructions
- CSF is collected by needle aspiration after preparation of the puncture site in a manner consistent with a surgical sterilization.
- Fluid in transported in a sterile container or tube with a tight-fitting lid.
- CSF should be transported at room temperature; do not refrigerate or freeze for transport.
- Specimens submitted for bacterial culture are also acceptable for fungal or mycobacterial stains and culture, antigen testing, and VDRL, if sufficient volume of fluid is submitted.

➤ Interpretation
- **Expected results:** no growth. False-negative cultures may be caused by low pathogen concentration in CSF, especially when low-volume samples are submitted, or prior antibiotic therapy.
- **Positive results:** Positive CSF culture supports a specific diagnosis of meningitis. False-positive cultures may be caused by endogenous flora if skin puncture site is not adequately disinfected. For most bacterial pathogens, CSF samples in patients with acute bacterial meningitis usually show increased WBCs (PMNs predominate), increased protein, and decreased glucose.

➤ Limitations
- A broad etiology, which may require a number of different tests for diagnosis, is often considered for patients presenting with signs and symptoms of meningitis.
- The volume of CSF submitted is often insufficient for optimal sensitivity for the range of tests requested.

CHLAMYDIA TRACHOMATIS, AMPLIFIED NUCLEIC ACID DETECTION (URINE, CERVICAL, URETHRAL)

➤ Use
- *C. trachomatis*—amplified nucleic acid testing may be submitted for evaluation of sexually active patients with symptoms consistent with an STD.
  - Amplified nucleic acid techniques are the most sensitive for detection of *C. trachomatis* in urine and urogenital specimens.

- Commercially available amplified nucleic acid tests may be used with urine and urogenital specimens. They are not validated for use with other types of specimens and should not be used as the only method for testing in the evaluation of rape or child abuse.
- Culture techniques for detection of *C. trachomatis* require optimized cell cultures and transport conditions, which are often not available in clinical practice.
- Method
  - Several amplification techniques have been used in FDA-approved kits for diagnosis of *C. trachomatis* infection, including transcription-mediated amplification (Gen-Probe, San Diego, CA), strand displacement amplification (BD Diagnostics-GeneOhm, San Diego, CA), and PCR (Roche Molecular Diagnostics, Pleasanton, CA).
  - Combination tests for simultaneous detection of *N. gonorrhoeae* and *C. trachomatis* are also available.
- Specimens must be collected and transported according to instructions of specific kits and restricted to specimen types for which the kit is validated.
- **Turnaround time:** 24–72 hours

➤ Interpretation
- **Expected results:** negative

➤ Limitations
- **Common pitfalls** include the use of incorrect swabs for specimen collection, improper filling of urine transport tubes, and submission of inappropriate specimen types.

➤ Other Considerations
- The CDC has recommended confirmation of positive *C. trachomatis* tests in patients from low or moderate prevalence (1–7%) populations; however, recent publications have demonstrated limited clinical utility for the results of routine confirmatory testing for positive specimens. If confirmatory testing is needed, it should be performed with a different type of test or target sequence.
- Amplified nucleic acid tests should not be used for test of cure evaluations (within 4 weeks of treatment), because DNA may be detectable even after viable organisms have been eliminated.
- Laboratories that use amplified nucleic acid tests should evaluate the possibility of laboratory contamination and false-positive tests by performing "wipe tests" of surfaces in the laboratory and by monitoring their rates of *C. trachomatis* infection detected by amplified nucleic acid techniques. (Significantly increasing rates may be due to laboratory contamination and should be investigated.)

➤ Suggested Readings
Moncada J, E Donegan, J Schachter. Evaluation of CDC-Recommended Approaches for Confirmatory Testing of Positive *Neisseria gonorrhoeae* Nucleic Acid Amplification Test Results. *J Clin Microbiol* 2008; 46: 1614–19.

Schachter J, JM Chow, H Howard, G Bolan, J Moncada. Detection of *Chlamydia trachomatis* by Nucleic Acid Amplification Testing: Our Evaluation Suggests that CDC-Recommended Approaches for Confirmatory Testing Are Ill-Advised. *J Clin Microbiol* 2006; 44: 2512–17.

CHLAMYDIA TRACHOMATIS CULTURE

➤ Use
- *C. trachomatis* is an obligate intracellular pathogen, and this culture is used to diagnose *C. trachomatis* infections.

- Although tests based on nucleic acid amplification have emerged as the most sensitive methods for diagnosis of *Chlamydia* genital infections, *Chlamydia* culture is still required for specimen types for which molecular diagnostic tests have not been validated.
- *Chlamydia* cultures should also be performed in cases that may have legal implications, such as rape and child abuse.
- Method
  - Infected cells from patient specimens are inoculated onto cultured eukaryotic cells, most commonly McCoy cells.
  - Cultures are incubated for 48–72 hours.
  - Positive cultures are now most commonly detected by staining fixed monolayers with specific anti–*C. trachomatis* antibodies; positive cultures show staining of intracellular inclusions. The sensitivity of cultures for *C. trachomatis* detection is improved by blind subculture of a primary culture after the initial incubation.
- **Turnaround time:** Cultures are incubated for 72 hours. An additional 48–72 hours are required if primary cultures are subcultured prior to final examination.

➤ Special Collection and Transport Instructions

- It is critical to collect infected epithelial cells from infected sites, usually using toxicity-tested swabs. Swabs may be pre-moistened with sterile nonbacteriostatic saline before specimen collection. Scrapings or biopsy specimens may be submitted for some specimen types. (See specimens below.)
- After collection, specimens should be placed into a *Chlamydia* transport media, such as 2-SP and transported to the laboratory at 4°C (wet ice). Deliver to the laboratory as quickly as possible.
- Specimens commonly submitted for *Chlamydia* culture come from the following sites:
  - **Cervix:** Remove excess mucus from the exocervix. Insert a new swab approximately 1 cm into the cervical canal and gently rotate for 10–15 seconds. Remove and place into transport media.
  - **Urethra:** Express excess mucus from the urethra and clear from the meatus with a swab. Insert a new thin-shafted swab 2–4 cm into the urethra and gently rotate for 10–15 seconds. Remove and place into transport media.
  - **Conjunctiva:** Remove excess purulent discharge with a swab. With a new swab, gently rotate over the affected conjunctival surface.
  - **Anus:** Insert a premoistened swab into the anorectal juncture and rotate gently. The swab should not be heavily stained with feces. Remove and place into transport media.
  - **Fallopian tube or epididymis:** Place aspirate into an equal volume of *Chlamydia* transport media.
  - **Respiratory tract (neonate):** Place aspirate or wash into an equal volume of *Chlamydia* transport media.
- Biopsies (lymph node, endometrium, fallopian tube, lung) may be taken. Place the biopsy specimen in a sterile container with *Chlamydia* transport medium.

➤ Interpretation

- **Expected results:** no growth
- **Positive results:** *Chlamydia* culture is very specific for infection caused by *C. trachomatis*.
- **Negative results:** *Chlamydia* infection is not ruled out by a negative culture. Tests based on nucleic acid amplification are more sensitive and are recommended for patients with a negative culture and high suspicion for chlamydial infection.

➤ Limitations

- *Chlamydia* culture is intrinsically less sensitive than molecular diagnostic techniques.
- *Chlamydophila* species, *C. psittaci,* and *C. pneumoniae,* are not isolated by *C. trachomatis* culture.
- The following specimens are not recommended for *Chlamydia* culture:
  - Peritoneal fluid
  - Urethral discharge
  - Urine
  - Cul-de-sac fluid
  - Vagina or vaginal fluid
  - Throat
- **Common pitfalls:**
  - Poor specimen collection (sample selection or collection technique) and loss of viability during transport are associated with false-negative cultures.
  - Swabs may be toxic for *C. trachomatis.* Specific types and lots of swabs should be tested for toxicity before releasing for clinical use.
  - Urethral specimens should not be collected within 1 hour after the patient has urinated. Delay collection to improve detection.

CLOSTRIDIUM DIFFICILE DETECTION

➤ Definition and Use

- *Clostridium difficile* is a major cause of antibiotic-associated diarrhea and pseudomembranous colitis, and it represents a significant and serious agent of nosocomial infection. *C. difficile* disease may be mild and self-limited after discontinuation of antibiotics, but a significant number of patients have persistent and/or severe diarrheal illness that may progress to pseudomembranous colitis or toxic megacolon.
- *C. difficile* is an anaerobic, spore-forming, gram-positive bacillus. It forms several toxins that have been used as the basis for detection. Toxin A is an enterotoxin and toxin B is a potent cytotoxin.
- *C. difficile* detection is recommended for patients in whom diarrheal illness develops after antibiotic therapy or during hospitalization, especially when colitis (increased fecal leukocytes) is a prominent feature.
- Methods
  - **Cytotoxicity:** Initially, detection of specific cytotoxicity was the primary diagnostic method. In this method, a suspension of stool, passed through a membrane filter to remove bacteria, is inoculated on cultured eukaryotic cells (e.g., WI-38). The cell monolayer is examined for 48 hours for evidence of typical "actinomorphic" cytotoxicity (disruption of the normal cellular morphology in the monolayer). In order to exclude nonspecific cytotoxicity that may be seen with stool filtrates, neutralization of the cytotoxic effect, using anti–*C. difficile* antiserum, must be demonstrated.
  - **Toxigenic culture:** *C. difficile* may be isolated from stool using a spore selection technique (by heat shock or alcohol pretreatment of a stool suspension prior to media inoculation) and selective media. Because not all *C. difficile* isolates produce the toxins associated with disease, culture supernatants must be tested for toxin production to make a diagnosis of *C. difficile*–associated disease.
  - **Toxin detection using immunodiagnostic procedures:** A number of commercially available latex agglutination or EIA kits have been developed for the detection of

C. difficile toxin A and/or toxin B in stool samples. These assays provide a more rapid turn-around time compared with culture or cytotoxicity assays.

- **C. difficile glutamate dehydrogenase antigen detection:** Detection of *C. difficile* glutamate dehydrogenase antigen may be used to screen stool for the presence of *C. difficile*. Because glutamate dehydrogenase is not specific for toxigenic *C. difficile*, positive specimens must be tested for toxin to confirm the diagnosis of *C. difficile*–associated disease.
- **Molecular diagnostic methods:** Molecular diagnostic methods for detection of the toxin or other informative genes of *C. difficile* are being developed and may emerge as the most sensitive methods for detection of disease.
- **Turnaround time:**
  - Molecular diagnostic, immunodiagnostic assays, and the glutamate dehydrogenase assays: 24 hours
  - Cytotoxicity assays: 24–72 hours
  - Culture: 96 hours
- Liquid stool specimens collected in clean containers with tight-fitting lids should be transported to the laboratory at room temperature within 2 hours. If transport will be prolonged, the specimen should be held at refrigerator temperature. Do not freeze.

> ## Interpretation
- **Expected results:** negative

> ## Limitations
- The available assays vary somewhat in sensitivity and specificity for diagnosis of *C. difficile* disease. The choice of diagnostic methods must take cost, assay performance, turnaround time, and other factors into consideration.
- *C. difficile* toxin may be detected in the stool of healthy infants without signs of diarrheal illness or colitis.

CORYNEBACTERIUM DIPHTHERIAE CULTURE (RULE OUT)

> ## Definition and Use
- This culture is used to detect *Corynebacterium diphtheriae* in clinical specimens.
- It should be considered in patients who present with signs and symptoms consistent with diphtheria, which is caused by local infection, most commonly respiratory or cutaneous infection, or systemic disease caused by the action of diphtheria toxin, primarily on the heart, central or peripheral nervous system, liver, and kidney. Diphtheria is now uncommon in countries that have implemented widespread vaccination programs against this pathogen.
- Method:
  - Respiratory or cutaneous specimens are inoculated onto SBA or CNA agar, as well as agar media containing cystine and tellurite, such as cystine-tellurite blood agar or modified Tinsdale agar. The SBA and CNA are used to identify group A *Streptococcus*, *Arcanobacterium hemolyticum*, or other causes of severe pharyngitis. Heavy growth of *C. diphtheriae* may also be seen on SBA plates.
  - On cystine-tellurite agar, *C. diphtheriae*, *Corynebacterium ulcerans*, and *Corynebacterium pseudodiphtheriae* produce black colonies surrounded by a dark halo (modified Tinsdale media). Gram staining is necessary for suspect colonies because organisms such as *Staphylococcus aureus* produce black colonies on these media.

- The identification of suspect colonies must be confirmed. Toxin-producing and non–toxin-producing strains of *C. diphtheriae* may be isolated from clinical specimens. *C. diphtheriae* isolates should be referred for toxin-production testing.
- **Turnaround time:** 48–72 hours for initial isolation. Additional time is required for confirmation of the identity, toxin testing, and further characterization of suspicious isolates.

➤ Special Collection and Transport Instructions

- The laboratory should be alerted before specimen submission to ensure that appropriate media is available for culture inoculation.
- Swab specimens are collected from multiple inflamed sites of the pharynx or other respiratory mucosal surfaces. Collection of specimens from near or under any diphtheritic membrane is recommended.
- Sampling from multiple inflamed sites increases the sensitivity for detection.
- Aspirate, swab, or tissue samples for detection of cutaneous diphtheria are collected following general collection recommendations for skin lesions.
- Routine transport media can be used for transport. Specimens should be delivered to the laboratory as soon as possible—within 24 hours.

➤ Interpretation

- **Expected results:** no growth
- **Positive results:** isolation of toxigenic strains of *C. diphtheriae* from upper respiratory or cutaneous lesions is diagnostic of diphtheria.
- **Negative results:** submission of multiple specimens may be required for *C. diphtheriae* isolation.

➤ Limitation

- Submission of poorly collected or single specimens may limit the sensitivity of cultures to rule out *C. diphtheriae*.

CRYPTOCOCCUS ANTIGEN TEST

➤ Use

- This test may be ordered for the early diagnosis of infections caused by *Cryptococcus neoformans*. It is usually appropriate for immunocompromised patients presenting with clinical signs of meningitis.
- Testing is most informative when CSF is submitted for diagnosis of cryptococcal meningitis. Testing serum has a lower sensitivity for meningitis or infection at other sites. An antigen titer may be determined by testing twofold serial dilutions of the specimen.
- Method
  - There are several formats for commercially available cryptococcal antigen tests, most commonly latex agglutination assays. In these assays, latex particles are coated with polyclonal or monoclonal antibodies directed against antigens of *C. neoformans*.
  - Agglutination at dilutions of 1:8 or greater indicate active disease. Approximately 95% of patients with cryptococcal meningitis are detectable by cryptococcal antigen testing of the CSF.
  - The sensitivity for CSF is 93–100%, and for serum it is 83–97%. Specificity for both specimen types is typically >95%.

- Special collection and transport instructions
  - CSF specimens are collected according to recommendations for spinal fluid culture.
  - There are no special recommendations for collection of serum specimens.
- **Turnaround time:** <24 hours

➤ Interpretation

- **Expected results:** negative
- **Positive results:** cryptococcal infection very likely. Positive results should be confirmed by culture.
- **Negative results:** cryptococcal infection unlikely. Use fungal culture to definitively rule out cryptococcal infection.

➤ Limitations

- False-negative reactions may occur, especially due to a prozone effect in serum sample. (Pronase treatment of serum samples decreases the incidence of the prozone phenomenon.) Some isolates from profoundly immunocompromised patients may produce very little polysaccharide capsular material, resulting in false-negative tests.
- There are several sources of false-positive reactions. Positive reactions caused by rheumatoid factor (RF) may be reduced by pretreatment of the specimen with pronase, EDTA, or reducing agents. The syneresis fluid from agar media can cause false-positive results; an aliquot of the specimen for cryptococcal antigen testing should be removed before media inoculation. Finally, several uncommon pathogens, including *Trichosporon beigelii* and *Capnocytophaga canimorsus*, can cause false-positive cryptococcal agglutination reactions.
- **Common pitfalls:**
  - Positive cryptococcal antigen titers should be confirmed by culture to document active infection and rule out false-positive reactions.
  - Some infected patients may have very low antigen titers. All specimens submitted for cryptococcal antigen testing should be accompanied by cultures of spinal fluid, blood, or other potentially infected material for fungal isolation.

➤ Other Considerations

- Antigen titers are usually higher in patients with AIDS compared with those seen in HIV-negative patients with cryptococcal infection. In patients with AIDS, baseline CSF antigen titers less than 1:2048 are associated with improved prognosis.
- Antigen titers should fall with effective antifungal therapy. (The same test methodology should be used for titer determination.) Steady or increasing cryptococcal antigen titers, even with sterilization of cultures, are an indication of likely treatment failure and recurrence of infection.

CRYPTOSPORIDIUM ANTIGEN DETECTION

➤ Use

- This test is used to evaluate diarrheal disease in patients at risk for cryptosporidiosis, specifically for the identification of *Cryptosporidium parvum* in stool specimens.
- Method
  - EIAs are used. They have very high sensitivity (near 100%) and specificity (near 100%) compared with a series of stool O & P examinations. For information about microscopic *Cryptosporidium* detection, see Ova and Parasite Examination, Stool (p. 466).

- Different EIA assays for fecal parasite detection have different specimen requirements (fresh vs. preserved) and transport conditions. Laboratories should provide assay-specific information for their providers.
- **Turnaround time:** 24–48 hours

➤ Interpretation

- **Expected results:** negative

➤ Limitations

- Several specimens may have to be examined in patients with light infection. Repeat testing improves sensitivity of detection. A series of O & P examinations is recommended in patients with repeatedly negative immunoassays in whom parasitic infection is still suspected.
- Submission of the incorrect type of specimen for the assay is a common pitfall. In order for immunoassays to perform accurately, the correct specimen type (preserved or fresh) and procedures, as specified in kit instructions, must be followed exactly.

➤ Suggested Readings

CLSI. *Procedures for the Recovery and Identification of Parasites from the Intestinal Tract; Approved Guideline.* 2nd ed. CLSI document M47-A. Wayne, PA: Clinical and Laboratory Standards Institute; 2005.

Garcia LS. *Diagnostic Parasitology*, 5th ed. ASM Press (Washington, DC). 2007.

CYTOMEGALOVIRUS (CMV) CULTURE (RULE OUT)

➤ Definition and Use

- CMV is a ubiquitous viral pathogen. Most infections in immunocompetent patients are asymptomatic or mildly symptomatic, including a self-limited mononucleosis syndrome. In immunocompromised patient populations, including neonates, patients with AIDS, and transplant patients, serious localized (e.g., retinitis, colitis, polyradiculopathy, encephalopathy) or systemic infection may occur.
- This test may be ordered to establish a specific diagnosis of CMV infection.
- Method
  - Specimens for CMV culture are usually inoculated onto monolayers of human fibroblasts (e.g., foreskin, fetal lung). The shell vial cultures technique may be used. Shell vial cultures provide a more rapid turnaround time than tube cultures but are somewhat less sensitive for detection. Tube cultures should always be used with shell vial cultures.
  - Presumptive CMV infection may be inferred by typical cytopathic effect, but positive cultures should be confirmed by immunologic techniques, such as DFA staining with CMV-specific reagents.
- **Turnaround time:** Specimens with high viral loads, such as urine, may give positive results within several days, but negative cultures may require incubation for up to 4 weeks before signing out as negative. Shell vial cultures may be positive within 48–72 hours after inoculation.

➤ Special Collection and Transport Instructions

- Specimens should be collected according to general recommendations for virus culture of the specimen type.
- Specimens should be collected early in acute infection.

- Urine is most often recommended for evaluation of neonates with suspected CMV infection. For evaluation of patients with suspected viremia, heparinized whole blood or isolated buffy coat cells are used to inoculate cultures.
- CMV is a fastidious virus and should be delivered to the laboratory as quickly as possible. The virus may not survive freezing if prolonged transport is needed. Most specimens should be placed in viral transport medium and transported on wet ice (4°C).

> ## Interpretation
- **Expected results:** negative. Negative cultures do not rule out CMV infection; they may be due to loss of viability after collection or low viral load in the specimen submitted.
- **Positive results:** Positive cultures usually indicate active CMV infection. Occasionally, positive cultures represent asymptomatic shedding of virus that may be clinically insignificant.

> ## Limitations
- Positive cultures may be due to deregulation of controlled disease or asymptomatic shedding and correlation with histopathology, and other clinical signs and symptoms may be needed to ensure specific diagnosis.

> ## Other Considerations
- Viral culture may be used to provide a patient isolate for antiviral susceptibility testing or further characterization.
- CMV antigenemia studies or CMV viral load determination are more effective than viral culture for identification of the impending emergence of clinical CMV infection in transplant and other immunocompromised patients.

EPSTEIN-BARR VIRUS (EBV) SEROLOGY SCREEN ANTIBODY PROFILE

> ## Definition
- EBV is the etiologic agent of infectious mononucleosis (IM) and is a widely disseminated herpesvirus that is spread by intimate contact between susceptible persons and EBV shedders. EBV spreads primarily via passage of saliva but is not a particularly contagious disease. The virus can persist in the oropharynx of patients with IM for up to 18 months following clinical recovery. EBV has also been isolated in both cervical epithelial cells and in male seminal fluid, suggesting that transmission may also occur sexually.
- This test comprises four serologic markers: EBV-NA (nuclear antigen IgG); EBV-VCA (viral capsid antigen) IgG and IgM; infectious mononucleosis antibody; and EBV-EA IgG (early antigen IgG).
- **Normal range:** negative
- Tests for EBV
  - **IgG-VCA:** Indicates past infection and immunity. May be present early in illness, usually before clinical symptoms are present. Detected at onset in 100% of cases; only 20% show a fourfold increase in titer after visiting a physician. Decreases during convalescence but detectable for many years after illness; therefore, not helpful in establishing diagnosis of IM.
  - **IgM-VCA:** detected at onset in 100% of cases; high titers present in serum 1–6 weeks after onset of illness, starts to fall by third week and usually disappear in 1–6 months. Sera are often taken too late to be detected. It is almost always present in active EBV infection and, thus, most

sensitive and specific to confirm acute IM. May be positive in other herpesvirus infections (especially CMV); therefore, confirmation with IgG and EBV-NA assays is recommended.

- **Early antigen:** IgG antibodies to early antigen are present at the onset of clinical illness. There are two subsets of EA IgG: anti-D and anti-R. The presence of anti-D antibodies is consistent with recent infection, since titers disappear after recovery; however, their absence does not exclude acute illness because the antibodies are not expressed in a significant number of patients. Anti-R antibodies are only occasionally present in IM.
- Early antigen anti-D titers rise later (3–4 weeks after onset; is transient) in course of IM than AB-VCA and disappear with recovery; combined with IgG-VCA suggests recent EBV infection; only found in 70% of patients with IM due to EBV. High titers are found in nasopharyngeal carcinoma due to EBV.
- Early antigen anti-R antibodies occur rarely in primary EBV infection, 2 weeks to months after onset, may persist for a year; more often in atypical or protracted cases. No clinical significance; high titers are found in chronic active EBV infection or Burkitt lymphoma.
- Epstein-Barr nuclear antigen are the last antibodies to appear and are rare in acute phase; develops 4–6 weeks after onset of clinical illness and rises during convalescence (3–12 months) and persists for many years after illness. Absence when IgM-VCA and anti-D are present implies recent infection. Appearance early in illness excludes primary EBV infection. Appearance after previous negative test evidences recent EBV infection.

➤ Use
- Diagnosing IM
- In patients with suspected IM and a negative heterophile test

➤ Interpretation (Table 3-2)

➤ Limitations
- EBV serology testing should not be performed as a screening procedure for the general population. The predictive value of a positive or negative result depends on the prevalence of analyte in a given patient population. Testing should only be done when clinical evidence suggests the diagnosis of EBV-associated infectious mononucleosis.

TABLE 3-2. Interpretation of Epstein-Barr Virus (EBV) Serologic Status

Serologic Status	EBV VCA IgM	EBV VCA IgG	EBV-NA IgG	EBV-EA IgG
Primary acute	Positive	Positive	Negative	Positive
	Positive	Negative	Negative	Positive
	Positive	Negative	Negative	Negative
Acute primary/late	Positive	Positive	Negative	Negative
Late acute	Positive	Positive	Positive	Positive
	Positive	Positive	Positive	Negative
	Negative	Positive	Positive	Positive
Primary acute/ recover	Negative	Positive	Negative	Positive
Previous infection	Negative	Positive	Negative	Negative
	Negative	Positive	Positive	Negative
Susceptible	Negative	Negative	Negative	Negative

- Antibodies to EBV have been demonstrated in all population groups with a worldwide distribution; approximately 90–95% of adults are eventually EBV seropositive. EBV acquired during childhood years is often subclinical; <10% of children develop clinical infection despite the high rates of exposure.
- The false-negative rates are highest during the beginning of clinical symptoms (25% in the first week; 5–10% in the second week, 5% in the third week).
- Approximately 10% of mononucleosis-like cases are not caused by EBV. Other agents that produce a similar clinical syndrome include CMV, HIV, toxoplasmosis, HHV-6, hepatitis B, and possibly HHV-7.
- IgM and IgG antibodies directed against viral capsid antigen have high sensitivity and specificity for the diagnosis of IM (97% and 94%, respectively).

ESCHERICHIA COLI (ENTEROHEMORRHAGIC, SHIGA TOXIN–PRODUCING *E. COLI*, STEC, *E. COLI* O157:H7) CULTURE (RULE OUT)

➤ Definition
- This test is a specialized stool culture for the detection of GI infection caused by *Escherichia coli* strains associated with enterohemorrhagic infection. These strains produce a Shiga toxin and are most commonly, but not exclusively, associated with *E. coli* O157:H7 strains.
- Enterohemorrhagic *E. coli* O157:H7 gastroenteritis commonly presents with abdominal pain with vomiting and diarrhea. Stool may become bloody with signs of colitis. Low grade fever may be present. In most patients, the symptoms resolve within a week after onset of symptoms. Rare patients, usually the elderly or very young patients, develop HUS with onset commonly occurring 7 days or more after onset of diarrheal symptoms.

➤ Use
- This culture is used to diagnose GI infection caused by Shiga-toxin producing *E. coli*. (Stool may be tested directly for the presence of Shiga toxin as an alternative to culture isolation.)
- Special media are used to screen stool. Suspicious isolates are tested further by serotyping and/or Shiga toxin production.
- *E. coli* O157:H7 strains are almost all sorbitol negative. Diarrheal stool may be screened by inoculation onto sorbitol-MacConkey agar (sorbitol used instead of lactose); sorbitol nonfermenting colonies are confirmed with O157:H7 antisera or specific Shiga-toxin testing.
- **Turnaround time:** 48–72 hours. Additional time is needed for positive cultures to confirm final identification.
- **Special collection and transport instructions:** Specimens are collected and transported according to recommendation for routine stool culture.

➤ Interpretation
- **Expected results:** negative. A single negative culture does not rule out infection caused by enterohemorrhagic *E. coli*. Negative results may be due to resolution of the active phase of gastroenteritis, infection caused by sorbitol-positive O157 strains or Shiga toxin-positive non-O157 *E. coli* strains, or other causes.
- A positive test indicates infection by *E. coli* O157:H7 in patients with a compatible clinical presentation.

➤ Limitations

- Cultures are usually positive only in acute, early infection. The use of stool culture for evaluation of patients with HUS is limited.
- The use of sorbitol-MacConkey agar is not sensitive for the detection of non-O157 Shiga toxin producing strains of E. *coli*; alternative testing methods should be used in areas where toxigenic non-O157 strains are prevalent or during outbreaks caused by non-O157 strains.
- Antibiotic therapy of E. *coli* O157:H7 infection may induce Shiga toxin production and disease severity.
- Other E. *coli* serotypes may produce Shiga toxin, but non-O157 toxigenic strains are uncommon in the United States.

ENTEROVIRUS CULTURE (RULE OUT)

➤ Definition

- Poliovirus, coxsackie viruses (A and B) and echoviruses are enteroviruses (EVs). As the name implies, EVs most commonly replicate in the GI tract, and fecal–oral transmission is typical.
- Most clinical manifestations of EV infection are outside the GI tract. EV infection is most commonly considered in children who present with signs and symptoms of aseptic meningitis or meningoencephalitis, usually in summer months. EVs also cause a severe sepsis syndrome in neonates (<2 weeks of age), pleurodynia, myocarditis and cardiomyopathy, and respiratory and oral mucosal diseases.
- Except for neonatal sepsis syndrome and endemic or vaccine related poliomyelitis, EV infection is usually followed by complete recovery.

➤ Use

- This test is used to detect viral infections caused by EVs.
- A number of different cell lines are susceptible to EV infection. Different EVs show differing infectivity for specific cell lines, so a number of different lines are typically inoculated for EV isolation. Monkey kidney cells may be used for poliovirus, coxsackie B virus, and echoviruses. WI-38 and human embryonic lung fibroblast cells may be used for coxsackie A virus.
- **Turnaround time:**
  - Tube cultures may be incubated for up to 4 weeks before signing out as negative.
  - CSF cultures are usually positive within 7 days (when positive).
  - Stool cultures, or other specimen types with higher concentrations of virus, are often positive within several days.
- **Special collection and transport instructions:**
  - Specimens should be collected within the first week after onset of symptoms.
  - Specimens should be collected according to general recommendations for virus culture of the specimen type. For patients with aseptic meningitis, CSF should be transported to the laboratory on wet ice (4°C). Submission of stool for viral culture may improve the detection of EV CNS infection.

➤ Interpretation

- **Expected Results:** Negative

➤ Limitations
- **Common pitfall:** Submission of specimens >7 days after onset of acute infection is associated with decreased sensitivity.
- Cell culture is negative in 25% or more of patients presenting with typical EV infection. EVs may grow slowly in culture. Coxsackie A isolates grow poorly in culture; sensitivity for detection is fairly low.
- RT-PCR techniques have recently emerged as sensitive and specific alternatives for the detection of EV aseptic meningitis.

FECAL LEUKOCYTES EXAMINATION

➤ Definition
- The presence of fecal leukocytes is an indication of an inflammatory process of the colon, including colitis caused by invasive enteric pathogens. A number of GI infections are typically associated with the presence of fecal leukocytes: Infections caused by *Shigella* spp., *Salmonella* spp., *Campylobacter* spp., *Yersinia* spp., enteroinvasive *E. coli*, and *C. difficile*, and amebic dysentery.

➤ Use
- This test is used to detect leukocytes in stool.
- A fecal leukocyte examination may be indicated for patients with a clinical diarrheal syndrome and signs of colitis.
- A fixed smear or wet mount of diarrheal stool is stained with methylene blue and examined for the presence of PMNs using a high-power objective.
- **Turnaround time:** <24 hours.
- Stool is collected according to recommendations for stool culture and transported to the laboratory within 2 hours.

➤ Interpretation
- **Expected results:** Negative
- Negative fecal leukocyte examination does not rule out significant bacterial enteric infection.
- Positive results support a diagnosis of invasive gastrointestinal infection. Enteroinvasive GI infections are usually associated with 3+ to 4+ fecal leukocytes (1-4 PMN/HPF or >5 PMN/HPF) with sensitivity >50% for specimens with results of 3+ or greater. The positive predictive value increases with increasing numbers of PMN/HPF.

➤ Limitations
- Significant infections caused by a number of enteric pathogens, including *Vibrio* spp., enterohemorrhagic *E. coli*, and viral agents, do not show an increase in fecal leukocytes
- An increase in fecal leukocytes is not specific for infection, and may be caused by other conditions, such as inflammatory bowel disease.

FRANCISELLA TULARENSIS CULTURE (RULE OUT)

➤ Definition
- *Francisella tularensis* is a slow-growing, fastidious, gram-negative bacillus capable of producing severe infection, including localized and systemic disease. Infections have typically been

acquired by zoonotic tick-borne transmission or direct contact. The common reservoir for organisms includes rabbits, rodents, deer, squirrels, and other wild mammals. Domestic animals may harbor the organism. This organism is easily transmissible, so it is critical that the laboratory be informed whenever tularemia is suspected. Typical disease syndromes include glandular, oculoglandular, and ulceroglandular tularemia; oropharyngeal tularemia; typhoidal tularemia; and pneumonic tularemia.
- There is great concern regarding the use of this organism for a bioterror-related attack.

➤ Use
- This culture is used to isolate *F. tularensis* from clinical specimens.
- Method
  - Specimens for *F. tularensis* isolation should be inoculated onto enriched agar media. Blood-cysteine-glucose agar is recommended; most clinical isolates will grow on chocolate, Thayer-Martin, and nonselective buffered charcoal-yeast extract (BCYE) agar. Enriched broth media, such as thioglycollate broth, should also be inoculated. Blood and MacConkey agar are typically inoculated for clinical specimens.
  - Because of the risk of laboratory acquired infection and because isolation of *F. tularensis* may represent a sentinel event in a bioterror attack, most clinical microbiology laboratories limit the work-up of suspected isolates to simple tests to rule out suspicious colonies, referring isolates that fail to "rule out" to their local public health laboratory for identification and further characterization. Final results for testing, therefore, may be delayed compared to common bacterial isolates.
- **Turnaround time:** Isolation and a preliminary identification are usually available within 5–7 days. Additional time is required for transfer to the local public health laboratory, confirmation of identification, and further testing.

➤ Special Collection and Transport Instructions
- Lymph node aspirate, ulcerative lesions, sputum, BAL, or other localized specimens, depending on the clinical presentation, are usually submitted for diagnosis.
- Culture of multiple specimens from different infected tissues may improve detection.
- Blood cultures are recommended for evaluation of patients with suspected tularemia.
- Serologic testing is recommended for diagnosis in patients with suspected tularemia.

➤ Interpretation
- **Expected results:** negative. After the acute phase of infection, cultures may become negative. Tularemia cannot be confidently ruled-out by negative cultures.
- **Positive:** Isolation of *F. tularensis* is diagnostic of tularemia. Tularemia is a reportable disease; positive cultures must be reported to the local department of health.

➤ Limitations
- Because *F. tularensis* organisms are tiny and faintly staining, direct detection by Gram stain of clinical specimens is uncommon.
- Cultures late in infection may be negative. Serologic diagnosis may be helpful in patients with disease consistent with tularemia, but negative cultures.
- **Common pitfalls:**
  - The diagnosis of tularemia may not be entertained until after the most acute phase of illnessa, a time when cultures are less likely to be positive.
  - Clinicians may fail to request specific cultures for tularemia or alert the laboratory of their clinical suspicion.

FUNGAL CULTURE (MOLD, YEAST, DIMORPHIC, AND DERMATOPHYTE PATHOGENS)

➤ Definition and Use

- Fungal cultures are indicated when clinically significant fungal infection is suspected. Symptomatic fungal infections commonly can be characterized as follows:
  - Superficial (skin/nail/hair)
  - Subcutaneous (chromoblastomycosis, mycetoma, phaeohyphomycotic cyst, sporotrichosis)
  - Systemic mycosis (e.g., coccidiomycosis)
  - Opportunistic mycosis (e.g., aspergillosis)
- These cultures are used as the most sensitive routine laboratory method for detection of fungal infections.

Method

- The media inoculated vary, depending on the specimen submitted and type of pathogen suspected.
- Direct examination, such as wet mount or calcofluor white staining, should be performed for most specimen types. Specimens for routine fungal culture are inoculated onto nonselective media, such as BHI or Sabouraud dextrose-BHI agar. A blood-containing media, such as BHI blood agar, is inoculated to improve recovery of dimorphic fungal pathogens. For specimens likely to be contaminated, selective media, such as inhibitory mold agar, are inoculated. Antibiotics, such as cycloheximide, aminoglycosides, fluoroquinolones, and chloramphenicol, are commonly used to render media selective. Nonselective media should always be inoculated with selective media because some pathogens may be inhibited by the antibiotics.
- Special media may be inoculated for some types of specimens or suspected pathogen: Bird (niger) seed agar for *Cryptococcus neoformans*; chromogenic agar for differentiation of *Candida* isolates; dermatophyte test medium for dermatophytes. If *Malassezia furfur* is suspected, media supplemented with a source of long-chain fatty acids (like olive oil) is inoculated.
- Inoculated media are typically incubated at 25–30°C in room air for up to 4 weeks. Cultures for isolation of systemic, dimorphic pathogens may be incubated at 35–37°C, but the incremental yield, versus 30°C incubation, is minimal. Cultures for fastidious pathogens are incubated for up to 8 weeks.
- Media inoculated for aerobic bacterial culture will support the growth of the common yeast pathogens, *Candida* species, so specific culture for yeast is not usually required. Cultures for common yeast pathogens are inoculated and incubated like generic fungal cultures, but may be finalized after 7 days of incubation.
- See p. 405, Blood Culture, Fungal for information regarding the detection of fungemia.

Turnaround Time

- Cultures for yeast are incubated for 7 days. Routine fungal cultures are incubated for up to 4 weeks. Cultures for systemic dimorphic pathogens are incubated for up to 8 weeks.
- Additional time is needed for isolation and identification of isolates.

➤ Special Collection and Transport Instructions

- Specimens are collected using sterile technique and transported in a sterile container within 2 hours. Store specimens at 4°C if transport will be delayed.

- Most specimens for fungal culture are collected following standard specimen collection instructions.
  - Collection of specimens using swabs is not recommended, except for samples from mucous membranes for the diagnosis of candidiasis.
  - SPS anticoagulation is recommended for blood and bone marrow specimens.
  - Pluck multiple hairs (10 or more) and scrape scalp from involved areas.
  - Wipe affected nail with 70% alcohol. Submit nail clippings and scrapings from beneath nails in a clean container.
  - Wipe affected skin lesions with 70% alcohol. Scrape the advancing margin to remove superficial cells and keratinized material; submit in a clean container.

➤ Interpretation
- **Expected results:** no growth
- **Positive:** Positive cultures must be carefully interpreted to ensure that endogenous fungal flora and culture contaminants are recognized.

➤ Limitations
- The results of fungal cultures may not be available when decisions regarding therapy of acute infection are required. Empiric therapy may be required.
- **Common pitfalls:** Isolation of endogenous *Candida* species or mold contaminants may be interpreted as clinically significant and result in unneeded treatment.

➤ Other Considerations
- Clinical information, such as travel history, immune status, and animal exposure, should be included on the requisitions for fungal cultures.
- Histopathologic and immunologic testing are important methods for diagnosis of invasive fungal infections. Specific molecular diagnostic testing shows promise for sensitive and specific diagnosis with short turnaround time.
- A diagnosis of vaginal and oral candidiasis (thrush) can be made reliably by direct microscopic examination (Gram stain or wet mount) of scrapings of mucosal surfaces without need for fungal culture.
- Detection of antigen or fungal products, such as cryptococcal antigen, histoplasma antigen, or mannan, may be useful for diagnosis of specific fungal pathogens.
- The India ink wet mount is less sensitive than cryptococcal antigen testing for meningitis caused by *C. neoformans*.

FUNGAL WET MOUNT (KOH, CALCOFLUOR)

➤ Definition
- A direct examination for fungal elements may provide a rapid detection of fungal infection and is recommended for most types of specimens submitted for fungal culture.

➤ Use
- This test is used for the direct detection of fungal forms in patient specimens.
- The specimen is processed to form a liquid suspension of the patient sample.
  - Solid specimens, such as tissues, should be minced to facilitate suspension.
  - The specimen may be suspended in saline or a 10% KOH solution. Use of KOH may improve liquefaction of the specimen and also lyses host cells and keratin, whereas fungal

cells are resistant to KOH digestion. The action of KOH makes fungal elements more easily detected by elimination of some of the background signal caused by host materials.
* A cover slip is added for examination with regular or phase contrast light microscopy.
* Calcofluor white, a fluorogenic dye that binds to specific polysaccharide bonds found in fungal cell walls, may be added to the KOH solution. When viewed by fluorescence microscopy, fungal cell walls fluoresce brightly.
* **Turnaround time:** 24 hours
* Specimens should be collected and transported according to guidelines for fungal culture of the specimen type.

➤ Interpretation

* **Expected result:** negative
  * **Positive:** If present, fungal elements will produce apple green or blue-white fluorescence, depending on the excitation-barrier filter set used on the fluorescent microscope. The pathogen may be characterized preliminarily on the basis of morphology (e.g., budding yeast, aseptate hyphae, and conidia-forming structures consistent with *Aspergillus* species)
  * **Negative:** nonfluorescent, faintly counterstained background material

➤ Limitations

* The morphology of fluorescent objects must be examined carefully to exclude artifacts caused by nonspecific absorption of dye to nonfungal objects, such as capillaries.

GENITAL CULTURE

➤ Definition

* Genital cultures should be collected from patients with signs and symptoms of localized genital tract infection or sexually transmitted disease, including discharge, dysuria, or lower abdominal pain.

➤ Use

* This culture is used to detect common bacterial pathogens from genital specimens. Target pathogens typically include *N. gonorrhoeae*, yeast (*C. albicans*), groups A and B beta-hemolytic streptococci, *Staphylococcus aureus* and *Listeria monocytogenes*. *Gardnerella vaginalis* should be reported if predominant and isolated in moderate to heavy growth. Invasively collected specimens should be cultured for isolation of these, as well as a broad range of invasive pathogens.
* Method
  * A Gram stain should be prepared from specimens submitted for genital culture. In male patients, the presence of many intracellular gram-negative diplococci is consistent with a diagnosis of gonorrhea. In female patients, the Gram stain may be used to identify "clue cells"; the absence of lactobacilli may be a marker of disruption of the normal vaginal flora, as with bacterial vaginosis.
  * Specimens are plated onto selective and nonselective media that supports growth of fastidious pathogens:
    * Blood and chocolate agar
    * CNA and MacConkey agar, or comparable selective agar for gram-positive and gram-negative isolation

- Selective agar for *N. gonorrhoeae*, such as Thayer-Martin, Martin-Lewis, NYC, or comparable media.
- **Turnaround time:** Routine genital cultures are incubated for up to 72 hours. Additional time is required in positive cultures for isolation, final identification, and further testing.

➤ Special Collection and Transport Instructions
- Male: a urethral swab should be collected. It may be possible to collect discharge expressed from the penile urethra. Collection of urethral discharge after prostatic massage may improve detection in patients with symptoms of prostatitis.
- Female:
  - Urethral swabs or swabs from the cervical os are recommended. The cervix is visualized using a speculum lubricated only with water. Prior to collection of cervical specimens, mucus from the exocervix should be removed by use of a cleaning swab.
  - Vaginal specimens are not recommended for routine genital cultures. Vaginal specimens may be useful for diagnosis of vaginal candidiasis, *Trichomonas vaginalis* infection or *S. aureus* superinfection.
  - Other specimens usually require more invasive sampling techniques, such as endometrial curettage, Bartholin's gland aspiration, and culdocentesis.

➤ Interpretation
- **Expected results:** Cultures should yield only endogenous flora for the specimen submitted.
  - **Positive:** The interpretation of positive cultures may depend on the organism isolated and the quantity. *N. gonorrhoeae* is never normal flora and indicates gonorrhea.
  - **Negative:** A single negative culture does not rule out infection with *N. gonorrhoeae*. Sampling several sites, like cervix and urethra, and serial sampling may improve detection.

➤ Limitations
- The symptoms related to genital infections may overlap with those of UTI, so urine cultures are recommended for most patients for whom genital cultures are submitted. Routine genital cultures are most often submitted for diagnosis of an STD caused by *N. gonorrhoeae*. A number of STDs will not be detected by routine bacterial genital culture, including *C. trachomatis*, *Treponema pallidum*, *Haemophilus ducreyi*, *Ureaplasma urealyticum*, *T. vaginalis*, HSV, and HPV. Special cultures or procedures are needed for detection of infections with these pathogens.
- Special cultures of rectal and vaginal swabs are recommended at 35–37 weeks of pregnancy for detection of group B beta-hemolytic *Streptococcus* carriage.
- Additional information
  - If *N. gonorrhoeae* is suspected in infections of nongenital sites, such as the rectum or throat, the clinician should order special cultures to rule out this pathogen from the specimen.
  - Molecular diagnostic techniques provide improved sensitivity for diagnosis of genital infections caused by *N. gonorrhoeae* and *C. trachomatis*.
  - Genital cultures (and culture for sexually transmitted pathogens at other relevant sites) should be collected for the evaluation of sexual abuse or rape.
  - Isolation of a sexually transmitted pathogen from a child must be investigated as a sign of possible abuse.

GIARDIA ANTIGEN DETECTION

➤ Definition and Use
- The *Giardia* antigen detection test is used for the identification of *Giardia lamblia* in stool specimens. It is used to evaluate diarrheal disease in patients at risk for giardiasis.
- Giardia EIA has a very, has a very high sensitivity (near 100%) and specificity (near 100%) compared with a series of stool O & P examinations. For information about microscopic *G. lamblia* detection, see p. 437.
- Different immunoassays have different specimen requirements (fresh versus preserved) and transport conditions. Laboratories should provide assay specific information for their providers.
- **Turnaround time:** 24–48 hours

➤ Interpretation
- **Expected results:** negative

➤ Limitations
- Several specimens may be required in patients with light infection. Repeat testing improves sensitivity of detection.
- A series of O & P examinations is recommended in patients with repeatedly negative immunoassays in whom parasitic infection is still suspected.
- **A common pitfall** is submission of the incorrect type of specimen for the assay. To perform immunoassays accurately, the correct specimen type (preserved or fresh) and procedures, as specified in kit instructions, must be followed exactly.

➤ Suggested Readings
CLSI. *Procedures for the Recovery and Identification of Parasites from the Intestinal Tract; Approved Guideline*—Second Edition. CLSI document M28-A2. Clinical and Laboratory Standards Institute; 2005.
Garcia LS. *Diagnostic Parasitology*, 5th ed. ASM Press (Washington, DC). 2007.

GRAM STAIN

➤ Definition and Use
- Indications
  - This test should be routinely performed for certain specimen types submitted to the laboratory for bacterial culture (e.g., lower respiratory, wound, tissue, abscess and drainage, sterile fluids, CSF, genital samples).
  - Because Gram stain is less sensitive than culture for detection of bacteria, culture of specimens should always be performed with Gram stains with a few possible exceptions. Gram stain without culture may provide accurate detection of vaginal and oropharyngeal thrush (mucosal *Candida albicans* infections).
- The Gram stain is used for the direct detection and initial presumptive identification of bacteria and yeast in patient specimens. It is an effective rapid diagnostic technique for several types of specimens.
- Specimens should be collected and transported according to instructions for specific specimen types.

- Potentially infected patient specimens are used to make smears on glass microscope slides. After fixation, slides are sequentially stained with crystal violet followed by iodine solution. The intracellular crystal violet–iodine complexes formed are too large to escape through the thick peptidoglycan cell wall of gram-positive organisms by alcohol, rendering them dark blue. But the crystal violet–iodine complexes can be rinsed through the thinner, fenestrated cell wall of gram-negative organisms, leaving them colorless. After the rinsing step, the unstained gram-negative organisms are counterstained with safranin, resulting in mild to intense pink staining.
- The Gram stain is, therefore, a differential staining technique, with which staining characteristics (e.g., pink or blue) and morphology (e.g., cocci or bacilli), and other characteristics of the primary pathogens may be ascertained. This information may contribute to informed decisions regarding initial empirical therapy while awaiting definitive culture results.
- The Gram stain can also demonstrate host cells and other evidence of inflammation, or other types of cells, like epithelial cells derived from mucosal or cutaneous surfaces that are not involved in an inflammatory response. The presence of such cells may imply the possibility of contamination of the specimen with the patient's endogenous flora.
- **Turnaround time:** <4 hours

➤ Interpretation
- **Expected results:**
  - Smears prepared from specimens from sterile sites should be negative for microorganisms. Smears from nonsterile sites, such as mucosal surfaces, usually demonstrate organisms of various morphology and concentration typical for the endogenous flora of the site (e.g., respiratory, vaginal, enteric).
  - PMNs and other signs of an inflammatory reaction are not typical for normal tissue specimens and suggest infection (or other inflammatory condition) at the site of collection.
- **Positive results**
  - Microorganisms (usually a single morphotype), in moderate or heavy amounts, with PMNs, and other inflammatory markers are typical of pyogenic infections.
  - Pathogens present in the specimen in concentrations greater than approximately 10^3 to 10^4 organisms per milliliter should be detected by Gram stain and will typically yield at lease moderate growth in culture. Concentration of some specimens, using techniques such as centrifugation, improves detection of microorganisms in sterile fluids.
  - Any type of organisms seen by Gram stain should be isolated by culture if appropriate cultures were inoculated. Monitoring the correlation of Gram stain and bacterial culture results, therefore, may be used as an important quality assurance (QA) tool. For example, demonstration of 4+ faintly staining gram-negative coccobacilli by Gram stain, while routine bacterial culture from the specimen yielded growth of no comparable organism, might suggest that an anaerobe, like *B. fragilis*, is playing an important role in infection, but was not isolated because appropriate media for anaerobic isolation was not inoculated.
- **Negative results:**
  - Infections may be associated with low concentrations of pathogens (<10^3 organisms/mL). For example, in adults with overwhelming bacteremia and sepsis, the concentration of organisms in the bloodstream is typically ~1–10 organism/mL (well below the detection level by Gram stain microscopy).

- PMNs and other signs of inflammation may increase suspicion of infection in smears negative for microorganisms.

➤ Limitations
- Some pathogenic microorganisms fail to stain avidly with the Gram stain technique. Special modifications or stains may improve detection, like the use of fuchsin as a counterstain for the Gram stain, or Acridine orange as a fluorogenic alternative to the Gram stain.
- Poor specimen collection, such as not sampling the site of infection, may give false-negative or misleading results.

➤ Suggested Reading
Winn Jr. WC, SD Allen, WM Janda, et al. *Koneman's Color Atlas and Textbook of Diagnostic Microbiology*. 6th ed. Lippincott Williams & Wilkins (Baltimore, MD and Philadelphia, PA). 2006.

HEPATITIS A VIRUS (HAV) ANTIBODIES (IgM AND TOTAL)

➤ Definition
- The detection of HAV-specific antibodies, both IgG and IgM, occurs early in the acute infection, with IgG persisting for years. Diagnosis of HAV infection requires positivity for IgM. HAV never causes chronic infection, but acute relapses occasionally occur.
- **Normal range:** negative

➤ Use
- Indicated, in conjunction with other serologic and clinical information, as an aid in the clinical laboratory diagnosis of individuals with acute or past hepatitis A virus infection
- Aid in the identification of HAV-susceptible individuals prior to HAV vaccination

➤ Limitations
- The total assay detects the presence of anti-HAV total (both IgG and IgM combined). A positive result indicates that the patient had hepatitis A either recently or in the past.
- IgM antibodies against HAV are detected soon after the onset of symptoms. Persistence of the IgM response is extremely variable, with specific IgM detected for less than one month in some cases to greater than one year in others. In most cases, IgM antibodies against HAV persist for a period of 3–6 months, after which they decline to levels that are below detection.

HEPATITIS B CORE ANTIBODY (HBcAb; TOTAL AND IgM)

➤ Definition
- Hepatitis B core antibodies appear shortly after the onset of symptoms of hepatitis B infection and soon after the appearance of HBsAg. Initially, anti-HBcAb consists almost entirely of the IgM class, followed by appearance of anti-HBc IgG, for which there is no commercial diagnostic assay.

* The anti-HBc total antibodies test, which detects both IgM and IgG antibodies and the test for anti-HBc IgM antibodies, may be the only markers of a recent hepatitis B infection detectable in the "window period." The window period begins with the clearance of HBsAg and ends with the appearance of antibodies to HBsAg. Anti-HBc total antibody may be the only serologic marker remaining years after exposure to hepatitis B.
* **Normal range:** negative

➤ Use

* Differential diagnosis of hepatitis; diagnosis of recent or past resolved hepatitis B infection
* Determination of occult hepatitis B infection in otherwise healthy HBV carriers with negative test results for HBsAg, anti-HBs Ab, anti-HBc IgM Ab, HBeAg, and antibodies to HBeAg.

➤ Interpretation
Increased In

* Acute, chronic, or past resolved hepatitis B infection

Decreased In

* Normal finding

➤ Limitations

* Positive anti-HBc total antibody test results should be correlated with the presence of other HBV serologic markers, elevated liver enzymes, clinical signs and symptoms, and a history of risk factors.
* Low levels of IgM-core antibodies can sometimes be present in chronic hepatitis B, particularly during flares of activity and at times of conversion from positive antigen to positive antibody.
* Neonates (<1 month old) with positive anti-HBc total antibody results from this assay method should be tested for anti-HBc IgM antibody to rule out possible maternal anti-HBc total antibody causing false-positive results. Repeat testing for anti-HBc total antibody within 1 month is also recommended in these neonates.

HEPATITIS B SURFACE ANTIBODY (HBsAb)

➤ Definition

* The presence of HBsAb (>12 mIU/mL) in the serum generally means there is protection against hepatitis B infection. With naturally occurring hepatitis infections, anti-HBs usually appear in serum several weeks after disappearance of HBsAg.
* Also known as HBsAb, anti-HBs, Australia Bs antibody, and HBV antibody
* **Normal range:**
  * <5.00 mIU/mL: negative
  * ≥ 5.00 mIU/mL and <12.0 mIU/mL: indeterminate
  * ≥12.0 mIU/mL: positive

➤ Use

* Identifying current and previous exposure to HBV
* Determining adequate immunity from hepatitis B vaccination

➤ Interpretation

Increased In

- Recovery from acute or chronic HBV infection, or acquired immunity from HBV vaccination.
- Positive results (quantitative anti-HBs levels of ≥ 12 mIU/mL) indicate an adequate immunity to hepatitis B from previous HBV infection or HBV vaccination.
- Screen for individuals at high risk for exposure, such as hemodialysis patients, persons with multiple sex partners, persons with a history of other STDs, IV drug abusers, infants born to infected mothers, individuals residing in long-term residential facilities or correctional facilities, recipients of blood- or plasma-derived products, allied health care workers, and public service employees who come in contact with blood and blood products.

Decreased In

- Inadequate immune response to HBV vaccination

➤ Limitations

- Passively acquired anti-HBs (i.e., transfusion of whole blood or plasma, recent immune globulin treatment) can yield positive results without indicating permanent immunity to HBV infection.
- Anti-HBs levels from previous hepatitis B or HBV vaccination may fall below detectable levels over time.
- Not useful for diagnosis of acute HBV infection
- Coexistence of HBsAg/HBsAb reported in 24% patients. In most cases, the antibodies are unable to neutralize circulating virions. These are regarded as carriers.

HEPATITIS B SURFACE ANTIGEN (HBsAg)

➤ Definition

- Serologic hallmark of HBV infection. First serologic marker to appear (1–10 weeks of acute exposure). Patients who subsequently recover; undetectable after 4–6 months. Persistent for >6 months in chronic infection.
- **Normal range:** negative

➤ Use

- Diagnosis of acute, recent, or chronic hepatitis B infection
- Determination of chronic hepatitis B carriage

➤ Limitations

- Individuals, especially neonates and children, who recently received hepatitis B vaccination may have transient positive HBsAg test results because of the large dose of HBsAg used in the vaccine relative to the individual's body mass.
- Some rare mutations result in false-negative test results. In these suspected cases, the presence of virus can be deduced by testing for HBcAb, surface antigen antibodies, and HBV DNA.
- Specimens with initially reactive test result but negative (not confirmed) by HBsAg confirmation test are likely to contain cross-reactive antibodies from other infectious or immunologic disorders. Repeat testing is recommended at a later date when clinically indicated.

HEPATITIS BE ANTIGEN AND ANTIBODY (Hbeag AND Hbeab)

➤ Definition
* Presence of HBeAg in the serum indicates active replication of virus and is usually associated with HBV DNA. HBeAg to HBeAb seroconversion occurs early in patients with acute infection, prior to HBsAg to HBsAb seroconversion. However, HBeAg seroconversion may be delayed for years to decades in chronic infection. HBeAg to HBeAb seroconversion usually associated with disappearance of HBV DNA in serum.
* Presence of HBeAg in the serum usually indicates that the virus is no longer replicating.
* **Normal range:** negative

➤ Use
* Diagnosis and monitoring of HBV infectivity
* Recognition of resolution of hepatitis B infection with seroconversion of HBeAg to HBeAb

➤ Interpretation
* Increased in hepatitis B

➤ Limitations
* Persistence of HBeAg is associated with chronic liver disease
* Presence of HBeAg implies infective HBV present in the serum, but its absence on conversion to HBeAb does not rule out infectivity, especially in persons infected with genotypes other than A.
* During the HBeAg-positive state, usually 3–6 weeks, hepatitis B patients are at increased risk of transmitting the virus to their contacts, including babies born during this period. Exposure to serum or body fluid positive for HBeAg and HBsAg is associated with 3–5 times greater risk of infectivity than when HBsAg positivity occurs alone.
* HBeAg negative strains respond similarly to antiviral treatment.
* Measurement of HBV-DNA is now recommended, especially in persons with increased ALT but negative HBeAg.

HEPATITIS C VIRUS (HCV) ANTIBODY

➤ Definition
* HCV is now known to be the causative agent for most, if not all, blood-borne non-A, non-B hepatitis. The presence of anti-HCV indicates that an individual may have been infected with HCV and may be capable of transmitting HCV infection.
* Also known as HCV antibody, non-A, non-B hepatitis
* **Normal range:** negative

➤ Use
* Screening for past (resolved) or chronic hepatitis C

➤ Interpretation
Increased In
* Hepatitis C infection: current and past exposure

Decreased In
* Normal finding

➤ Limitations
* Presence of HCV antibodies in serum does not imply protective immunity. False-positive anti-HCV results are rare in certain clinical settings, because the majority of persons being tested have evidence of liver disease and the sensitivity and specificity of the screening assays are high. However, among populations with a low prevalence of HCV infection, false-positive results do occur. This is of concern when testing is performed on asymptomatic persons for whom no clinical information is available, when persons are being tested for HCV infection for the first time, and when testing is being used to determine the need for postexposure follow-up.
* All HCV antibody-positive samples require reflex to confirmatory serologic (RIBA) or nucleic acid supplemental testing according to the testing algorithm recommended by CDC.
* HCV antibodies and RIBA often do not become positive during an acute infection; thus repeat testing several months later is required if HCV RNA is negative.
* HCV serologic testing is not useful for detection of early/acute HCV infection, and it is not useful for differentiating between past (resolved) and chronic hepatitis C.
* Infants born to HCV-infected mothers may have false-reactive HCV antibody test results due to transplacental passage of maternal HCV IgG antibodies. HCV antibody testing is not recommended until at least 18 months of age in these infants.
* May remain negative in immunosuppression and renal failure, although it appears to be a rare finding

HEPATITIS C VIRUS (HCV) ANTIGEN

➤ Definition
* This test, based on detection of a 21 kDa protein made by a stable region of the HCV genome, may be used in research settings to aid in the diagnosis of HCV infection. It is a major component of the viral capsid. It is not clear whether it circulates freely or is only in viral particles. A commercial immunoassay to detect HCV antigen, is available for research use.
* Level strongly correlates with HCV RNA.
* **Normal range:** negative

➤ Use
* To predict a sustained virologic response early during therapy (4 weeks), reaching an optimal performance at month 3.
* The determination of total HCV core antigen levels in serum constitutes an accurate and reliable alternative to HCV-RNA for monitoring and predicting treatment outcome in patients receiving PEG-interferon/ribavirin combination therapy.

➤ Interpretation
* Increased in hepatitis C exposure

➤ Limitations
* Lacks sensitivity in early detection
* HCV antigen has similar sensitivity in infection with all genotypes of HCV.

HEPATITIS C VIRUS (HCV) BY CHIRON RECOMBINANT IMMUNOBLOT ASSAY (RIBA)

➤ Definition
* The Chiron RIBA HCV SIA is a strip immunoblot assay for antibodies to HCV, the etiologic agent of non-A, non-B hepatitis.
* It is a qualitative method of categorizing specific immunoreactivities in serum or plasma to recombinant HCV-encoded antigens and synthetic HCV-encoded peptides that have been immobilized as discrete bands on nitrocellulose test strips.

➤ Use
* Used as a second-tier test to characterize the specificity of an individual's immune response to the component proteins of HCV by identifying the presence, relative level, and pattern of reactivities to the complete set of the viral proteins.
* Routinely used as a confirmatory test for specificity of seroconversion, following a more sensitive but less specific screening test for general reactivity to HCV.

➤ Interpretation
* Reactivity scores: Specimen reactions with the HCV antigen bands are first scored in terms of relative reaction intensity versus the reaction intensity of the IgG low and high control bands incorporated into the strips. A reactivity score of "1+" or greater signifies a specimen reactivity at least equal to that for the IgG low control.
* Test interpretation
  * **Positive:** Reactivity scores of "1+" or greater for at least two of the four clinically significant HCV bands—corresponding to antigens NS5, c33c, and peptides c22(p)p24, c100(p)/5-1-1(p)
  * **Indeterminant:** Reactivity score of "1+" or greater for only one of the four HCV bands, or a score of "1+" or greater for the hSOD (human superoxide dismutase) band in conjunction with a score of "1+" or greater for at least one of the four HCV bands
  * **Negative:** Absence of any reactive bands with a score of "1+" or greater, or a score of "1+" or greater for the hSOD band

➤ Limitations
* Like any second-tier test, the positive predictive value for the Chiron RIBA is a function of the a priori likelihood of the disease by clinical criteria, whereas the negative predictive value is not as well defined because of the variability of the immune response among infected individuals.
* Anti-HCV reactivity may be undetectable in early stages of infection. The presence of anti-HCV is indicative of past or present infection by HCV, but does not necessarily constitute a definitive diagnosis of non-A, non-B hepatitis. It is recommended that individuals for whom results are "Indeterminant" be retested after 6 months using the original specimen *in addition to* a freshly drawn specimen. A specimen that is reactive by a licensed anti-HCV screening test but negative by the Chiron RIBA does not exclude the possibility of infection with HCV.

HEPATITIS C VIRUS (HCV) GENOTYPING ASSAY

➤ Definition
- The HCV genotyping assay identifies HCV genotypes 1–6 in human serum or EDTA plasma samples. Availability of subtype information depends on the method used for testing. The methods may differ in their ability to genotype samples with low viral load or mixed infection.
- **Normal range:** negative

➤ Use
- Methods:
  - Invader (Third Wave)
  - True Gene (Bayer)
  - LiPA (Innogenetics)
  - TaqMan (Abbot Diagnostics)
  - "Home brew" sequencing
- The HCV genotyping assay should be used in the management of HCV-infected individuals undergoing antiviral therapy

➤ Limitations
- Samples with low viral load may be untypable
- Sequencing methods are less effective than hybridization methods in genotyping samples with mixed genotypes.

HEPATITIS C VIRUS (HCV) RNA, QUANTITATIVE VIRAL LOAD: MOLECULAR ASSAY

➤ Definition
- The HCV viral load assay quantifies HCV RNA in the plasma of HCV-infected individuals. The HCV test is standardized against the first WHO international standard for HCV RNA for nucleic acid amplification technology assays (NIBSC code 96/790)
- **Normal range:** not detected when the result is below the level of detection of the assay.

➤ Use
- Methods
  - Branched DNA assay (bDNA; Siemens): a signal amplification technology that detects the presence of specific nucleic acids by measuring the signal generated by branched, labeled DNA probes; a reliable method that provides consistent results in the higher range of the assay
  - Real-time PCR: reverse transcription followed by amplification and quantification of the targeted DNA molecule; generally offers both a wider range of quantification and a lower limit of detection than the bDNA method.
- Used in the management of HCV-infected individuals undergoing antiviral therapy.

➤ Limitations
- PCR inhibitors in the specimen may lead to underestimation of viral quantitation or false-negative results in rare cases.

HEPATITIS D VIRUS (HDV; DELTA HEPATITIS) ANTIBODY

➤ Definition
* HDV is a subviral agent that is dependent on the HBV virus for its life cycle; therefore, HDV infection cannot occur in the absence of HBV infection
* **Normal range:** negative

➤ Use
* Diagnosis of concurrent HDV infection in patients with fulminant acute HBV infection (acute coinfection), chronic HBV infection (chronic coinfection), or acute exacerbation of known chronic HBV infection (HDV superinfection).

➤ Interpretation
* Increased in previous or current hepatitis D infection

➤ Limitations
* The role of HDV antibody testing is controversial because the incidence of infection with HDV has declined markedly in the United States with use of HBV vaccine.
* Interferon treatment may decrease the antibody levels.
* This testing should be ordered only when patient has an acute or chronic hepatitis B infection.

HEPATITIS E VIRUS (HEV) ANTIBODY (IgM AND IgG)

➤ Definition
* HEV is a small nonenveloped virus that causes an acute, usually self-limited, infection that is spread by the fecal–oral route. HEV is endemic in Southeast and Central Asia, with several outbreaks observed in the Middle East, northern and western parts of Africa, and Mexico. In developed countries, HEV infection occurs mainly in persons who have traveled to disease-endemic areas.
* Transmission of HEV may also occur parenterally. Direct person-to-person transmission is rare. Unusually high mortality (approximately 20%) occurs in patients infected in the third trimester of pregnancy. There is no carrier state associated with HEV.
* Viremia and virus shedding occur in the preicteric phase and last up to 10 days into the clinical phase. After an incubation period ranging from 15–60 days, HEV-infected patients develop symptoms of hepatitis with appearance of anti-HEV IgM antibody in serum, followed by detectable anti-HEV IgG antibody within a few days. Anti-HEV IgM remains positive for up to 6 months after onset of symptoms, whereas anti-HEV IgG levels usually persist for years after infection. Anti-HEV IgG is the serologic marker of choice for diagnosis of past HEV infection.
* **Normal range:** negative

➤ Use
* HEV antibody IgM: diagnosing acute or recent (<6 months) hepatitis E infection
* HEV antibody IgG: diagnosis of past hepatitis E

➤ Interpretation
* Increased in previous or current hepatitis E infection

HERPES SIMPLEX VIRUS (HSV) CULTURE (RULE OUT)

➤ Definition and Use

- Clinically detected HSV usually involves vesicular rashes of the oropharyngeal or genital sites, although HSV is capable of causing serious disseminated disease, including infection of multiple organ systems. Vertical transmission may result in neonatal infections, involving disease localized to the skin, eyes and mouth, systemic, disseminated infection, or encephalitis. Other sites of infection in normal or immunocompromised patients include skin, conjunctiva, and the CNS. HSV can cause severe disseminated disease in immunocompromised patients, resulting in multiorgan dysfunction and failure.
- This test may be used to isolate HSV when specific diagnosis is required for patient management.
- Patient specimens are inoculated onto cultured eukaryotic cells, like human foreskin fibroblast or Vero cell cultures. Tube or shell vial cultures may be used for HSV isolation. Cytopathic effect is usually manifested within 24–48 hours in specimens with heavy virus loads, such as vesicular lesions. Cultures showing cytopathic effects should be confirmed using immunologic techniques, such as staining with tagged monoclonal antibodies.
- Specific HSV-1 and HSV-2 antibody reagents may be used to further characterize HSV culture isolates, as needed.
- **Turnaround time:** Most positive cultures are detected within 2 days. Negative tube cultures are typically incubated for up to 7 days. Shell vial cultures are usually finalized within 48–72 hours.

➤ Special Collection and Transport Instructions

- General recommendations for viral culture apply.
- Specimens should be collected early in acute infection.
- Specimens should be collected according to general recommendations for virus culture of the specimen type. Specimens from cutaneous or mucous membranes are most commonly submitted for viral culture to rule out HSV. Samples should be taken from fresh, wet lesions, ideally from intact vesicles after unroofing.
- Most specimens should be placed in a viral transport medium and transported on wet ice (4°C).

➤ Interpretation

- **Expected results:**
  - **Positive:** Cell cultures positive for HSV indicate probable active infection. Occasionally, positive cultures represent asymptomatic shedding of virus that may be clinically insignificant.
  - **Negative:** Negative cell cultures do not rule out HSV infection, especially for CSF and other nonvesicular lesions.

➤ Limitations

- There may be poor sensitivity for certain specimen types, such as CSF. Molecular diagnostic testing may improve detection from these specimens.
- **Common pitfalls:** collection of specimens from dried, overcrusted lesions.
- HSV-specific DFA, performed on cells from the base of vesicles or wet ulcers, provides rapid and specific identification of HSV infection.
- PCR is the most sensitive method for HSV detection and is most useful for diagnosis of CNS infections.

- Culture isolates may be typed, but clinical management decisions can generally be made without typing results. Typing is used mainly for epidemiologic purposes.

HERPES SIMPLEX VIRUS (HSV) DIRECT DETECTION (DIRECT FLUORESCENT ANTIBODY [DFA])

➤ Definition and Use

- This test may be ordered in patients presenting with a vesicular rash in whom specific and rapid diagnosis of HSV infection is important for therapy or management. It is used to diagnose HSV infection by detection of HSV antigens in typical skin lesions.
- Cells scraped from the base of a vesicle or a wet ulcerated lesion are used to make a smear on a glass slide. After fixation, the smear is stained with an HSV-specific antibody reagent tagged with a fluorescent label. After washing away excess reagent, the slide is examined by fluorescence microscopy for the presence of cells showing specific staining.
- Cells are collected from the base of wet skin ulcers or vesicles (after unroofing) with a swab or edge of a scalpel. Slides are prepared by gently rolling the swab or spreading cells collected by scalpel onto the slide surface.
- **Turnaround time:** <24 hours.

➤ Interpretation

- **Expected results:** negative, with no cells showing fluorescent staining.
- **Positive result:** The presence of any cells showing +2 or greater specific fluorescent staining.

➤ Limitations

- The slide must be assessed to ensure cells are present in the smear. If no cells are present, the slide is uninterpretable.
- The number of staining cells drops with evolution of the skin lesion from vesicle to crusted/healing ulcer.
- Faint staining may be an indication of problems with the staining technique or reagents.
- Common pitfalls: poor collection of cells from the lesion base; sampling crusted, healing lesions.

HERPES SIMPLEX VIRUS (HSV) SEROLOGY TESTS, TYPE 1 AND TYPE 2 SPECIFIC ANTIBODIES, IgG AND IgM

➤ Definition

- HSV is a common STD worldwide. Although HSV type 2 (HSV-2) remains the main causative agent for the preponderance of virologically confirmed infections, HSV type 1 (HSV-1) is associated with an increasing proportion of cases of genital herpes.
- HSV-1 generally infects the mucous membrane of the eye, mouth, and mucocutaneous junctions of the face, and it is also one of the most common causes of severe sporadic encephalitis in adults. HSV-2 is usually associated with mucocutaneous genital lesions. Recently, an increasing number of genital herpes infections have been shown to be due to HSV-1. HSV-1 causes primary episodes indistinguishable from HSV-2, but with less frequent recurrence.

- Pregnant women who develop genital herpes near the time of delivery are at high risk for transmission to the neonate. Transmission of HSV infection to neonates is associated with high morbidity and mortality rates if untreated.
- Because HSV-1 and HSV-2 share common antigenic determinants, antibody detected against one viral type may cross-react with the other viral type. Truly type-specific antibody tests are based on glycoprotein G1 (from HSV-1) and glycoprotein G2 (from HSV-2), as these proteins exhibit very limited homology. The CDC recommends the use of type-specific glycoprotein G based assays when serology is performed.
- Other names: herpes simplex serology, HSV antibody titer
- **Normal range:** negative

➤ Use
- To diagnose a patient with a history of genital lesions who did not have a diagnostic work-up
- To diagnose a past or present HSV infection in a patient with an atypical presentation
- To determine susceptibility of a sexual partner of a patient with documented genital HSV infection
- To identify asymptomatic HSV infection in pregnant women who are at risk for shedding at the time of delivery with potential transmission to the infant.
- To help predict the risk of recurrence.

➤ Interpretation
- HSV IgM combined positive result (i.e., the presence of IgM class HSV 1 and/or 2 antibodies) indicates recent infection. The presence of HSV 1 and/or 2 antibodies may indicate a primary or reactivated infection but cannot distinguish between them.
- The IgG antibody assay differentiates between types 1 and 2 HSV antibodies. The presence of IgG antibodies specific for HSV type 1 or 2 indicates previous exposure to the corresponding serotype of the virus.

➤ Limitations
- A clinical diagnosis of genital herpes should be confirmed with laboratory testing. The diagnosis can be made by viral culture, PCR, DFA, Tzanck preparation, and type-specific serologic tests. The choice of test varies with the clinical presentation.
- The prevalence of HSV antibodies can vary depending on a number of factors such as age, gender, geographic location, socioeconomic status, race, sexual behavior, testing method used, specimen collection and handling procedures, and the clinical and epidemiologic history of individual patients.
- A negative result does not necessarily rule out a primary or reactivated infection, since specimens may have been collected too early in the course of disease, when antibodies have not yet reached detectable levels, or too late, after IgM levels have declined below detectable levels.
- False-positive test results may occur in patients infected with EBV, in primary or reactivated varicella virus infection, and in the presence of rheumatoid factor antibodies.

HUMAN IMMUNODEFICIENCY VIRUS 1, 2 ANTIBODY SCREEN

➤ Definition
- HIV is a highly variable virus that mutates readily. Based on genetic similarities, the numerous virus strains may be classified into types, groups, and subtypes. There are two types of

HIV: HIV-1 and HIV-2. Both types are transmitted by sexual contact, through blood, and from mother to child, and they appear to cause clinically indistinguishable AIDS. However, it seems that HIV-2 is less easily transmitted, and the period between initial infection and illness is longer in the case of HIV-2.

* The diagnosis of HIV infection is established by one of the following methods: detecting antibodies to the virus; detecting the viral p24 antigen; detecting viral nucleic acid (NAT); or culturing HIV. By far, the most widely used test is the detection of antibody to HIV. The serologic tests for HIV infection are based on detection of IgG antibody against HIV-1 antigens in serum. These HIV antigens include p24 (a nucleocapsid protein) and gp 120 and gp 41 (envelope proteins). Antibodies to gp41 and p24 antigens are the first detectable serologic markers following HIV infection. IgG antibodies appear 6–12 weeks following HIV infection in the majority of patients and by 6 months in 95 percent of patients. IgG antibodies to HIV generally persist for life. Positive tests should be confirmed with repeat tests or by corroborating laboratory data (e.g., western blot assays). Assays for IgM antibodies are not used because they are relatively insensitive.

* HIV has evolved into several groups: M, N, O, and P. Group M ("main") is considered the pandemic strain and comprises most strains of HIV. Group O ("outlier") represents far fewer strains from Cameroon, Gabon, and Equatorial Guinea. Group N ("non-M/non-O") and group P are represented by very few isolates and have only been documented in Cameroon. Viruses from group M are subsequently divided into 10 distinct subtypes (A–J). HIV testing was originally developed to detect HIV subtype B, the most common subtype in the United States and Europe. The estimated frequency of non-B subtypes in the United States is approximately 2%. The CDC does not recommend routine testing for HIV-2 in settings other than blood centers.

* **Normal range:** negative

➤ Use

* Screening of HIV-1 and/or HIV-2 infection
* Screening organ transplant donors
* Testing individuals who have documented and significant exposure to other infected individuals
* Testing exposed high-risk individuals for detection of antibody (e.g., persons with multiple sex partners, persons with a history of other STDs, IV drug users, infants born to infected mothers, allied health care workers, and public service employees who have contact with blood and blood products)

➤ Interpretation

* Positive in HIV infection; a positive screen test is considered "preliminary" and requires confirmation by a western blot. The patient with a positive test should be told of the result and advised on avoiding risk of transmitting HIV while the western blot test is pending.
* A negative screen test is regarded as a true negative, and requires no confirmation; the patient may be informed that the test is negative.

➤ Limitations

* Common causes of false-negative results can occur due to acute infection and failure to detect certain HIV subtypes.
* Rare causes of false-negative results include immune dysfunction due to defective humoral response or agammaglobulinemia, immunosuppression due to malignancy or medications,

delay in seroconversion following early initiation of antiretroviral therapy, and fulminant HIV infection.
* False-positive test results for HIV infection have been documented after participation in an HIV vaccine trial.
* Indeterminate results may occur due to partial seroconversion during acute HIV infection, advanced HIV infection with decreased titers of p24 antibodies, or infection with HIV-2.
* Other causes for an indeterminate test result in persons who are not infected with HIV include:
  * Cross-reacting alloantibodies from pregnancy
  * Autoantibodies (collagen-vascular diseases, autoimmune diseases, and malignancy)
  * Receipt of an experimental HIV-1 vaccine
  * Influenza vaccination

HUMAN IMMUNODEFICIENCY VIRUS CONFIRMATORY WESTERN BLOT ASSAY

➤ Definition
* A person is considered HIV positive only if preliminary and confirmatory tests are positive. The western blot (WB) assay is a method in which individual proteins of an HIV-1 lysate are separated according to size by polyacrylamide gel electrophoresis. The viral proteins are then transferred onto nitrocellulose paper and reacted with the patient's serum. Any HIV antibody from the patient's serum is detected by an antihuman IgG antibody conjugated with an enzyme that in the presence of substrate will produce a colored band. During the incubation period, HIV-1 antibodies present in the specimen bind to major HIV-1 antigens (p17, p24, p31, gp41, p51, p66, gp120, gp160).
* HIV-2 is a retrovirus and the highest prevalence is the West African nations and Portugal. There have been a small number of reported cases in the United States since 1987. HIV-2 cross-reacts with HIV-1 in serologic tests. A positive screen test for HIV 1 and 2 antibodies with a negative or indeterminate WB suggests positive HIV-2 infection.
* Other names include HIV-1 WB and HIV-2 confirmation test.
* **Normal range:** negative

➤ Use
* Confirmatory detection of HIV-1 and/or HIV-2 antibodies in patients with reactive antibody screen or rapid HIV antibody results.

➤ Interpretation
* **Positive:** As established by CDC the interpretive criteria for HIV-1 is defined by the presence of any two of the following bands; p24, gp41, and gp120/160.
* For HIV-2 WB test, no single standard can currently be applied to all tests. The CDC recommends that each test be interpreted by the criteria suggested by the kit manufacturer.

➤ Limitations
* This test should be ordered only on sera that are reactive by HIV-1 or HIV-2 screening EIA or rapid HIV antibody tests.

- An immunofluorescence assay for HIV-1 antibodies has recently been licensed by the FDA and can be used instead of WB.
- Persons at increased risk for HIV-2 infection include:
  - Persons from or with extensive travel to Africa
  - Sex partners of persons from or with extensive travel to Africa
  - Sex partners of persons known to be infected with HIV-2
  - Persons who received a blood transfusion or a nonsterile injection in Africa
  - Persons who shared needles with a person from or with extensive travel to Africa
  - Children born to women who have risk factors for HIV-2 infection or who are infected with HIV-2

HUMAN IMMUNODEFICIENCY VIRUS TYPE 1 (HIV-1) RNA, QUANTITATIVE VIRAL LOAD (MOLECULAR ASSAY)

➤ Definition

- The HIV-1 viral load assay quantifies HIV-1 RNA in the plasma of HIV-1 infected individuals. One copy of HIV-1 RNA is equivalent to 1.7 ± 0.1 IU based on the WHO first international standard for HIV-1 RNA for nucleic acid–based techniques (NAT) (NIBSC 97/656).
- **Normal range:** not detected when the result is below the level of detection of the assay.

➤ Use

- Methods
  - Branched DNA assay (bDNA; Siemens): a signal amplification technology that detects the presence of specific nucleic acids by measuring the signal generated by branched, labeled DNA probes; a reliable method that provides consistent results in the higher range of the assay.
  - Real-time PCR: reverse transcription is followed by amplification and quantification of the targeted DNA molecule; generally offers both a wider range of quantification and a lower limit of detection than the bDNA method.
- Used in the management of HIV-1–infected individuals undergoing antiviral therapy.

➤ Limitations

- PCR inhibitors in the specimen may lead to underestimation of viral quantitation or false-negative results in rare cases.

INFLUENZA VIRUS DIRECT DETECTION BY ENZYME IMMUNOASSAY (EIA) AND DIRECT FLUORESCENT ANTIBODY (DFA) TESTS

➤ Definition

- Tests for the direct detection of influenza viruses provide results much sooner than results from respiratory virus culture. Therefore, they may serve a critical role in patient management and infection control during winter respiratory virus seasons.

- EIA tests have only moderate sensitivity, but high specificity, for detection of influenza virus infection; they are commonly used for screening.
- DFA tests have high sensitivity and specificity compared to respiratory viral culture and they are a cost-effective definitive diagnostic technique.

➤ Use

- EIA and DFA tests are used to provide early detection for influenza virus infection. Patients may present with febrile respiratory virus infection during winter months. Direct tests may be used sequentially for influenza screening and confirmation.
- Method
  - **EIA:** There are a number of kit formats for EIA tests. Commonly, antibodies directed at specific influenza A, influenza B, or both influenza A and B antigens are immobilized on the surface of a membrane of a test device. The specimen is added to the reaction surface, allowing influenza antigen in the specimen to react with the device antibodies. After washing, a second tagged influenza antibody reagent is added. After washing away excess detection antibody, a label-specific detection reagent is added and the test read as positive or negative.
  - **DFA:** Cells collected by nasopharyngeal swab or wash are fixed onto a microscopic slide. The slide is dried, fixed, and stained with a reagent containing labeled antibodies directed against specific influenza A or influenza B antigens. The label is typically fluorogenic. Stained slides are examined by fluorescence microscopy using excitation and barrier filter appropriate for the specific fluorogenic label.
- **Special collection and transport instructions:** Specimens are collected as recommended for samples for viral culture. Nasopharyngeal specimens, especially nasopharyngeal wash specimens, typically provide specimens with the greatest sensitivity for detection of infected patients.
- **Turnaround time:** 24–48 hours. Some EIA kits allow testing with a turnaround time <4 hours.

➤ Interpretation

- **Expected results:**
  - **Positive:** Specimens showing a significant number of cells with 2+ or greater fluorescence are considered positive. Slides must be examined to ensure that the specimen contains enough respiratory epithelial cells to provide informative testing. Laboratories should establish a lower limit of cells present below which the test is considered uninterpretable. Specimens that demonstrate only few, faintly staining cells should be considered equivocal; repeat testing may provide clear positive or negative results.
  - **Negative:** a cellular specimen without staining by the labeled reagent.

➤ Limitations

- There is variable sensitivity for different commercially available EIA tests. Sensitivities for seasonal influenza may range from 50–80%. The sensitivity depends on the type of specimen and quality of specimen collection. Specimen types acceptable for the kit, collected according to kit instructions, provide maximal sensitivity. The specificity of EIA and DFA kits is typically very high.
- The PPV of antigen detection tests depends on the prevalence of influenza in the region. Testing results should be interpreted with caution, if performed at all, during periods when there is a low prevalence of influenza in the patient's region.

- **Common pitfall:** Poor test performance may be seen when specimens are submitted which have not been validated for the platform/kit used for testing. Anterior nasal swabs, for example, may be submitted instead of nasopharyngeal swabs, resulting in an increased number of false-negative results.

LEGIONELLA ANTIGEN SCREEN

➤ Definition
- Legionellosis refers to two clinical syndromes caused by bacteria of the genus *Legionella*—Legionnaires' disease and Pontiac fever. Legionnaires' disease is considered an atypical pneumonia. *Legionella pneumophila* is responsible for approximately 90% of infections. Most cases are caused by *L. pneumophila*, serogroup 1. Although a number of prominent clinical manifestations are distinctive for *Legionella* infection, none of them are pathognomonic or highly specific. Therefore, laboratory testing using specialized tests for *Legionella* should be considered for all patients hospitalized with community-acquired pneumonia.
- Culturing for *Legionella* species is the single most important laboratory test. Urinary antigen testing is rapid, sensitive, and specific, but it is only useful for the diagnosis of *L. pneumophila* type 1 infection. The combination of culture of an appropriate respiratory specimen and urinary antigen testing are optimal as a diagnostic approach. Serologic tests are generally far less useful for the diagnosis of an individual patient. Although PCR-based tests exist, to date they do not exceed the sensitivity of culturing the organism.
- **Normal range:** negative

➤ Use
- In conjunction to culture for the presumptive diagnosis of past or current Legionnaire's disease (*L. pneumophila* serogroup 1)

➤ Interpretation
- **Positive:** Presumptive positive for *L. pneumophila* serogroup 1 antigen in urine, suggesting current or past infection.
- **Negative:** Presumptive negative for *L. pneumophila* serogroup 1 antigen in urine, suggesting no recent or current infection. Infection due to *Legionella* cannot be ruled out, since other serogroups and species may cause disease, antigen may not be present in urine in early infection, and the level of antigen present in the urine may be below the detection limit of the test

➤ Limitations
- There is no single confirmatory laboratory test for Legionnaire's disease. Culture results, serology, and antigen detection methods may all be useful, in conjunction with clinical findings, for diagnosis.
- The *Legionella* antigen test will not detect infections caused by other *L. pneumophila* serogroups and by other *Legionella* species. Culture is recommended for suspected pneumonia to detect causative agents other than *L. pneumophila* serogroup 1 and to recover *L. pneumophila* serogroup 1 when antigen is not detected.
- Excretion of *Legionella* antigen in urine may vary depending on the individual patient. Antigen excretion may begin as early as 3 days after onset of symptoms and persist for up to a year afterward.

- A positive *Legionella* urinary antigen test result can occur due to current or past infection and, therefore, is not definitive for infection without supporting evidence.

LEGIONELLA SPECIES CULTURE (RULE OUT)

➤ Use
- This test is requested for diagnosis of legionellosis by culture of patient specimens, usually of the lower respiratory tract. This test may be ordered to evaluate patients with atypical pneumonia consistent with legionellosis. Special testing, usually performed outside of clinical microbiology laboratories, is needed for evaluation of environmental cultures for isolation of *Legionella* species.
- Method:
  - All specimens should be inoculated onto nonselective and selective BCYE agar. Antibiotics are used in selective BCYE to inhibit non-*Legionella* flora.
  - For specimens that are likely to be heavily contaminated by endogenous flora, inoculation of additional cultures after a 0.2M KCl acid wash (pH = 2.2) is recommended to improve isolation of *Legionella*. After the acid-wash treatment, aliquots are inoculated onto selective and nonselective BCYE media as for unwashed specimens.
- **Turnaround time:** Cultures are inspected for up to 7 days after inoculation. Additional time is required after isolation for confirmation and further characterization.

➤ Special Collection and Transport Instructions
- Specimens should be submitted early in the acute phase of infection.
- Sputum (expectorated or induced), BAL, bronchial brush, lung biopsy, or tracheal aspirate specimens are usually submitted for culture to rule out *Legionella*.
- Submission of multiple specimens is recommended to improve sensitivity of detection because shedding may be intermittent for this intracellular pathogen.
- Blood, cardiac valve, or other specimen types are occasionally submitted when extrapulmonary legionellosis is suspected. (If *Legionella* endocarditis is suspected, alert the laboratory because special processing and culture techniques are required.)

➤ Interpretation
- **Expected results:** negative. Because *Legionella* may be shed intermittently, a negative culture does not rule out legionellosis.
- **Positive results:** Isolates from *Legionella* cultures must be confirmed as *Legionella* species by further testing and characterization.

➤ Limitations
- *Legionella* are typically present in low concentrations in patient specimens. Extrapulmonary specimens are unreliable for isolation of *Legionella*.
- Because cultures show limited sensitivity for definitive diagnosis of legionellosis, additional diagnostic techniques are recommended for patient evaluation. *Legionella* urine antigen testing may provide sensitive detection for infections caused by *L. pneumophila*, serotype 1. Specific serology may be useful, especially when the diagnosis is considered after the most acute phase of infection. *Legionella* DFA of patient specimens has limited reliability and is not recommended for routine use.

- **Common pitfalls:**
  - The rejection criteria applied to sputum specimens for routine bacterial cultures should not be applied to specimens submitted for *Legionella* culture.
  - *Legionella* may be present in very low concentrations in respiratory secretions. Therefore, BAL and bronchial brush specimens should be directly inoculated onto BCYE media before dilutions are prepared for quantitative bacterial cultures.

MACROSCOPIC EXAMINATION, ARTHROPOD

➤ Use
- This test is used to identify arthropods by visual examination. This test is indicated for identification of ticks, mites, fleas, spiders, lice, maggots and other insects that may be associated with human infection, infestation, disease, or disease transmission.

➤ Method
- These agents are submitted in clean containers with tight fitting lids. Specimens for scabies detection may be collected by skin scraping.
- Plucked hair may be submitted for identification of nits and the eggs of lice. Maggots may be expelled spontaneously, surgically, by vacuum extraction, or other methods.
- The submitted arthropods and insects are inspected by the naked eye or with low-power microscopy, like stereomicroscopy. Identification is based on morphologic features.
- **Turnaround time:** 24–48 hours

➤ Interpretation
- **Expected results:** negative

MACROSCOPIC EXAMINATION, PARASITES

➤ Definition and Use
- Occasionally, large parasitic pathogens may be isolated from patients. Examples include single proglottids or chains of tapeworm segments, pinworms, or ascarid worms.
- This test is used for identification of parasites by visual inspection.
- Submitted specimens are usually parasites that have been expelled spontaneously and collected by patients.
- The submitted parasite is inspected by the naked eye or with low-power microscopy, such as stereomicroscopy. Identification is based on specific morphologic features. Speciation of *Taenia* proglottids may be attempted by injection of India ink through the genital pore, and then counting the lateral uterine branches.
- **Turnaround time:** 24–48 hours.

➤ Interpretation
- **Expected results:**
  - **Positive:** A human parasitic pathogen is identified.
  - **Negative:** A nonhuman pathogen or artifact is identified.

➤ Limitations

*   There may be limited material available for examination. The specimen may have been fragmented or damaged during collection or transport so that specific identification is impossible.
*   **Common pitfall:** Nonhuman pathogens, like earthworms, may be submitted for examination.
*   The eggs of *T. solium* can infect humans. Therefore, great care must be taken in the laboratory when examining *Taenia* proglottids.

MEASLES SEROLOGY SCREEN (MEASLES [RUBEOLA] IgG AND IgM)

➤ Definition

*   Measles is a highly contagious, acute, exanthematous disease caused by the measles (rubeola) virus. It is generally self-limiting and without serious consequences, although complications such as bronchopneumonia and otitis media do occur. The most serious consequence, encephalomyelitis, is fortunately rare (about 1 in 10,000 cases). Natural infection with measles virus confers permanent immunity. Measles infection poses a serious threat to immunosuppressed, or immunocompromised patients. For these reasons, the laboratory diagnosis of measles has become increasingly important, notwithstanding the reduction in the incidence due to the introduction of vaccines.
*   The usual means of laboratory diagnosis of acute measles is serologic, either by the demonstration of a fourfold or greater rise in virus-specific IgG antibody in acute and convalescent serum pairs, or by the detection of virus-specific IgM antibody in a single, early serum specimen.
*   **Normal range:** negative

➤ Use

*   To assist in the diagnosis of acute-phase infection with rubeola (measles) virus
*   To assist in identifying nonimmune individuals

➤ Interpretation

*   Positive IgM results, with or without positive IgG results, indicate a recent infection with measles virus.
*   Positive IgG results coupled with a negative IgM result indicate previous exposure to measles virus and immunity to this viral infection.
*   Negative IgG and IgM results indicate the absence of prior exposure to rubeola and nonimmunity.
*   Equivocal results should be followed up with a new serum specimen within 10–14 days.

➤ Limitations

*   If the assay is used with cord blood as the specimen source, positive results should be interpreted with caution. The presence of IgG antibodies to measles in cord blood may be the result of passive transfer of maternal antibody to the fetus. A negative result, however, may be helpful in ruling out infection.

METHICILLIN-RESISTANT *STAPHYLOCOCCUS AUREUS* CULTURE (RULE OUT)

➤ Definition and Use

- This test is usually ordered to detect methicillin-resistant *S. aureus* (MRSA) carriage in asymptomatic patients for infection control purposes. It is indicated to screen patients at risk for transmitting MRSA to close contacts, such as other hospitalized patients. The test may also be requested to document clearance of MRSA carriage.
- Patient specimens are plated onto selective agar, typically containing 4–6 µg/mL of oxacillin. (Oxacillin in used instead of methicillin because it is more stable and reliable for *in vitro* testing.)
- A base agar selective for gram-positive organisms (like PEA) or staphylococci (mannitol-salt agar) is often used to improve sensitivity of detection of MRSA. Selective chromogenic agar is commercially available for cultures to screen for MRSA carriage. These agars provide increased sensitivity for detection of MRSA with decreased turnaround time to MRSA detection.
- **Special collection and transport instructions:** Swab specimens of anterior nares, throat, axilla, perineum, and/or umbilicus (neonates) are usually submitted for MRSA screening cultures.
- **Turnaround time:** 48 hours

➤ Interpretation

- **Expected results:** negative
- Any growth of *S. aureus* likely represents MRSA; confirmation of oxacillin resistance and identification is recommended for most MRSA-screening protocols.

➤ Limitations

- **Common pitfall:** The MRSA screening culture is usually not indicated for evaluation of potentially infected material. Because only selective media is used, other potential pathogens would be missed if MRSA screening culture only is requested. MRSA isolates grow well in wound and other cultures submitted for evaluation of infected specimens.
- Commercially available molecular diagnostic methods have been developed for detection of MRSA carriage. These assays have been shown to be more sensitive for detection of MRSA carriage, but the clinical implication for detection of very low level MRSA carriage has not been clearly defined.

MICROSPORIDIA EXAMINATION

➤ Definition and Use

- This test should be requested for the evaluation of stool specimens in patients with diarrhea and who are at risk of microsporidial infection. It is used for the direct detection of the intracellular microsporidial parasitic pathogens.
- Permanent smears of diarrheal stool are stained with modified trichrome stains (chromotrope 2R), or similar stains.
- Fresh and preserved specimens are collected and transported to the laboratory according to recommendations for stool submitted for routine O & P examination.
- **Turnaround time:** 24–72 hours

➤ Interpretation
* **Expected results:** negative

➤ Limitations
* Multiple specimens may be required for diagnosis in light infections.

➤ Suggested Readings
CLSI. *Procedures for the Recovery and Identification of Parasites From the Intestinal Tract; Approved Guideline*—2nd ed. Wayne, PA: Clinical and Laboratory Standards Institute; 2005.
Garcia LS, *Diagnostic Parasitology*, 5th ed. ASM Press (Washington, DC) 2007.

MUMPS SEROLOGY SCREEN (MUMPS IgG AND IgM)

➤ Definition
* Mumps is a generalized illness characterized by fever and by inflammation and swelling of the salivary glands, particularly the parotid glands. Mumps is usually not severe in children, but in the adult the inflammation may involve the ovaries or testes (orchitis).
* Inflammation and swelling of the parotid glands (parotitis) in mumps infection is usually sufficiently diagnostic to preclude serologic confirmation. However, inasmuch as one third of mumps infections are subclinical, viral isolation and / or some other serologic procedure may be required.
* **Normal range:** negative

➤ Use
* Virus isolation is cumbersome and time consuming and is usually an impractical procedure for the typical clinical laboratory. Serodiagnosis of mumps infection has been accomplished by neutralization, hemagglutination-inhibition (HI), indirect immunofluorescence, and complement fixation (CF). These methods lack specificity, which limits their usefulness in determining immune status. The HI test also requires pretreatment of test sera to remove nonspecific inhibitors of hemagglutination.
* Enzyme immunoassays (EIA, ELISA) are sensitive and specific and their sensitivity equals that of the neutralization test, and is greater than CF or HI. They are, therefore, reliable tests for the determination of immune status. Serum IgM antibody testing should be obtained no earlier than 3 days following initial onset of symptoms. The test typically remains positive for up to 4 weeks but may be negative in up to 50–60% of specimens from individuals with acute disease who were previously immunized. A negative IgM titer in vaccinated individuals, therefore, does not rule out mumps. Immunity to mumps is established by demonstrating IgG antibodies on ELISA.
* The test is used to assist in the diagnosis of acute-phase infection with mumps virus and to assist in identifying non-immune individuals

➤ Interpretation
* Positive IgM results, with or without positive IgG results, indicate a recent infection with mumps virus.
* Positive IgG results coupled with a negative IgM result indicate previous exposure to mumps virus and immunity to this viral infection.

- Negative IgG and IgM results indicate the absence of prior exposure to mumps and nonimmunity.
- Equivocal results should be followed up with a new serum specimen within 10–14 days.

➤ Limitations
- If the assay is used with cord blood as the specimen source, positive results should be interpreted with caution. The presence of IgG antibodies to mumps in cord blood may be the result of passive transfer of maternal antibody to the fetus. A negative result, however, may be helpful in ruling out infection.

MYCOBACTERIA (AFB, TB) CULTURE

➤ Definition
- Samples of infected patient specimens should be submitted for mycobacterial culture when mycobacteria are specifically suspected or are in the differential diagnosis of serious infections. Mycobacteria may cause acute and chronic infections. Infections may be localized or systemic and there is significant overlap with signs and symptoms of fungal and other bacterial infections.
- Mycobacteria are usually acquired via the respiratory route, and the lower respiratory tract is the site of most serious mycobacterial infections, and *M. tuberculosis* is the most common pathogen associated with these infections. Other mycobacterial species, including other species in the *M. tuberculosis* complex and *M. avium* complex (MAC), may cause chronic pulmonary infections.
- Organisms may disseminate from the site of primary infection to cause localized or systemic infection. Virtually all organ systems may be involved. The CNS, bone, and urinary tract are common sites of extrapulmonary infection. Mycobacteria may be isolated from stool, most commonly in HIV-infected patients, but the role of mycobacteria as a cause of GI infection has been questioned.
- Superficial mycobacterial infections, such as "swimming pool granuloma" caused by *M. marinum* and wound infections caused by rapidly growing mycobacteria, may be caused by direct inoculation of environmental non-*M. tuberculosis* species.

➤ Use
- Mycobacterial culture is used to detect mycobacterial pathogens causing infections and to provide isolates for susceptibility testing and further characterization, such as clonality testing.

Method
- AFB smears should be performed on all specimens submitted for mycobacterial culture. The detection of AFB by smear depends on the concentration of mycobacteria in the specimen, as judged by the number of colonies grown in culture. Approximately 96% of patients with culture-positive, active pulmonary TB will have at least one positive AFB smear when three or more well-collected samples are examined.
- Large-volume liquid specimens should be concentrated, usually by centrifugation, and specimens likely to be contaminated by endogenous flora should be decontaminated and concentrated prior to media inoculation. Because decontamination procedures may also be toxic to

mycobacteria, some laboratories may perform decontamination only on specimens that demonstrate growth on routine bacterial culture.

- Liquid and solid media are inoculated. Most cultures are incubated at 37°C; cultures from skin or superficial lesions should also be incubated at 30–32°C to improve isolation of mycobacteria that are common pathogens at these sites, such as *M. marinum*, *M. ulcerans*, and *M. haemophilum*. Cultures are incubated in 3–10% CO_2. Broth media may be monitored on automated platforms, allowing earlier detection time and providing organisms for identification using molecular genetic tests. Clear, agar-based solid media, like Middlebrook media, provide sensitive isolation of *M. tuberculosis*, early detection of "microcolonies," and preliminary, presumptive identification by microcolony morphology. Selective media, which contain a variety of antibiotic agents, may be inoculated for specimens when heavy contamination is likely. Because pathogenic mycobacteria may be inhibited by selective media, nonselective media must always be included. If *M. haemophilum* skin or superficial infection is suspected (immunocompromised hosts), media supplemented with blood, hemin (X factor strip), or ferric ammonium citrate should be inoculated. Inoculation of parallel cultures, with one culture exposed to light and one incubated in the dark only, can be used to determine characteristics of pigment formation.
- Once mycobacterial growth has been detected and confirmed, further testing for identification and susceptibility, as appropriate, are performed.
  - Growth rate and pigment formation, including photoreactivity, are used to initially characterize nontuberculous mycobacteria and help to determine the panel of tests required for full identification. The rate of growth to mature colonies in subcultures of mycobacterial isolates is used to identify rapidly growing mycobacterial species.
  - Newer technologies for definitive identification of isolates have replaced biochemical and phenotypic testing in many laboratories. The NAP (p-nitro-acetylamino-hydroxypropiophenone) test may be used to rapidly identify *M. tuberculosis*. Nucleic acid probes are available for identification of *M. tuberculosis* complex, *M. avium* complex (MAC), *Mycobacterium kansasii*, and *M. gordonae*. Nucleic acid sequencing technology is emerging as an important tool for identification of mycobacteria in reference laboratories.
  - Using optimal growth, identification and susceptibility testing systems, complete identification and susceptibility testing should be completed for the majority of *M. tuberculosis* isolates within 4 weeks of submission of specimen to the lab.

Special Collection and Transport Instructions

- Specimens should be collected using procedures that minimize the contamination of specimens with the patient's endogenous flora.
- Because routine bacterial, fungal, and other types of infections may be in the differential diagnosis when mycobacterial infection is suspected, ensure that a sufficient volume of infected material is collected to ensure that all testing can be performed.
- For the diagnosis of TB, a minimum of three sputum specimens should be submitted for culture. Patients must be carefully instructed in the proper technique for sputum collection.
- Early morning specimens are preferred because of pooling of secretions at night. A minimum of 5–10 mL of sputum should be submitted for each specimen.
- Collection of sputum induced by inhalation of nebulized hypertonic saline improves detection of pulmonary TB.
- Twenty-four-hour sputum collections should not be submitted.

- First morning gastric aspirates may be collected for patients unable to produce sputum, like small children and the frail elderly.
- Up to five, first-morning urine specimens should be submitted for patients with suspected renal TB.
- Lysis-centrifugation, bi-phasic, and automated mycobacterial culture techniques are optimal for blood and bone marrow specimens submitted for detection of systemic mycobacterial disease.
- Specimens should be transported to the laboratory as soon as possible in sterile containers with tight-fitting lids.
- If same-day AFB stain results are needed, the specimen should arrive in the laboratory early enough in the day to allow enough time for specimen processing (decontamination and concentration) and smear interpretation.
- Specimens for mycobacterial culture should not be collected using swabs.

Turnaround Time
- Cultures may require up to 8 weeks of incubation, although optimal culture techniques yield growth of *M. tuberculosis* within 4 weeks in a majority of positive cultures.
- Several additional weeks may be required for isolation, identification, susceptibility testing, and further characterization, as needed.

➤ Interpretation
- **Expected results:** no growth
- **Positive:** Growth of mycobacteria in culture is usually very specific for mycobacterial infection. *M. gordonae* (tap water bacillus), however, may be isolated in culture but is rarely associated with disease; its growth is most likely caused by contamination of the specimen, or transient contamination of the patient, with organisms from external water sources.
- **Negative:** The post-test probability of mycobacterial infection is significantly diminished if cultures are negative. However, sensitive detection depends on the number of specimens submitted, the quality and quantity of specimen collection, the presence of contaminating flora, and other factors. Correlation of culture results with clinical information is critical and continued isolation may be recommended, pending final culture results, for patients with a high clinical suspicion, even when AFB smears are negative.

➤ Limitations
- Detection of mycobacterial pathogens requires careful specimen collection. Three or more specimens may be required for sensitive detection. The final results of testing may not be available for up to 2 months after collection; decisions regarding empirical therapy and management may be required before culture results are available.
- **Common pitfalls:** Poor quality specimens and insufficient volume of material for culture are commonly submitted, limiting the sensitivity of culture results.

➤ Other Considerations
- The following mycobacterial species are most commonly associated with human disease:
  - *M. tuberculosis* complex: *M. tuberculosis*, *M. africanum* (rare), *M. bovis*, including BCG, and *M. microti* (rare)—pulmonary and other localized infections and systemic disease
  - *M. avium* complex (MAC): systemic infection in immunocompromised patients, like patients with AIDS or chronic pulmonary disease
  - *M. kansasii*—pulmonary disease

- Rapid growers: *M. fortuitum*, *M. chelonae*, *M. abscessus*—wound infections, localized and systemic infection
- *M. scrofulaceum*—cervical lymphadenitis
- *M. marinum*, *M. ulcerans*, *M. haemophilum*—skin and superficial infections
- *M. xenopi*—pulmonary
- *M. szulgai* (uncommon)—pulmonary
- *M. genavense*—disseminated and GI disease in immunocompromised patients
- *M. celatum* (uncommon)—pulmonary
- *M. malmoense*—pulmonary

MYCOBACTERIUM TUBERCULOSIS INFECTION DETECTION, INTERFERON GAMMA RELEASE ASSAY

➤ Definition and Use

- *M. tuberculosis* infection may present with a range of disease syndromes, including acute infection, active infection, latent infection, and reactivation disease. Diagnosis is established by evaluation of clinical presentation, epidemiologic risk assessment, radiographic studies, detection of *M. tuberculosis* by culture or molecular diagnostic methods, and evidence of host response.
- In the past, the tuberculin skin test (TST) was used to detect host response, but the recent development of FDA-approved interferon-gamma release assays (IGRAs) has provided an alternative method for detecting immunologic response to *M. tuberculosis* antigens. IGRAs may be used in the evaluation of patients for latent TB or active (acute or reactivation) TB.

Method

- Three FDA-approved IGRAs are currently available:
  - QuantiFERON-TB Gold assay (QFT-G) (Cellestis Limited, Carnegie, Victoria, Australia)
  - QuantiFERON-TB Gold In-tube assay (QTF-GIT) (Cellestis Limited, Carnegie, Victoria, Australia)
    - T-SPOT TB Test (TSPOT) (Oxford Immunotec Limited, Abingdon, United Kingdom)
- These tests measure immune reactivity of a patient's WBCs when challenged with synthetic antigens present in all strains of *M. tuberculosis* but absent in BCG strains. Immune reactivity is measured by the interferon-gamma concentration, or number of interferon-gamma producing cells, after exposure of viable WBCs to these antigens.
- Advantages of IGRAs include:
  - IGRAs require only a single patient visit to conduct the test.
  - Results are available within 24 hours, which may facilitate patient evaluation and contact investigation.
  - IGRA testing does not boost the immunologic response in subsequent tests.
  - Prior BCG vaccination does not cause false-positive reaction in IGRAs.
- The assessment of IGRA test accuracy depends on the populations studied, the comparator method, and other factors. In general, the sensitivity of the IGRAs is high and comparable to TSTs. Studies suggest that the specificity of IGRAs is slightly higher that the specificity of TSTs. IGRAs may be used and considered acceptable medical and public health practice in all situations in which the CDC recommends TST to aid in the diagnosis

of TB. Nevertheless, there are situations for which an IGRA or a TST may be the preferred method for testing.

- Routine patient testing with TST and IGRA is not recommended. Both tests may be recommended in special circumstances, however.
  - If the initial, primary test is negative, and:
    - The risk for poor patient outcome (severe or progressive disease) is high, as for young children or HIV-infected patients.
    - The clinical suspicion for TB, based on other criteria, is high.
    - A positive result from a second test would be interpreted as increased sensitivity and evidence of infection.
  - If the initial, primary test is positive, and:
    - Additional evidence of infection may encourage a patient's acceptance of the diagnosis and compliance with therapy.
    - To rule out a false-positive result in patients with a low probability, based on other factors, of *M. tuberculosis* infection or progressive disease.
    - To follow-up indeterminate or equivocal test results in patients in whom TB cannot be ruled out by other factors.

Special Collection and Transport Instructions
- Specimens must be collected into tubes specified by the manufacturer.
- Specimens must be collected strictly following the manufacturer's instructions.
- Specimens must be inverted or shaken vigorously according to manufacturer's instructions.
- Transport at room temperature. Specimens should not be refrigerated or frozen during transport.

➤ Interpretation
- **Expected Results:** negative
- **Positive:** Positive results suggest that infection with *M. tuberculosis* is likely, but cannot determine the stage of infection. Reactive specimens support a diagnosis of acute, active infection, latent infection or reactivation TB.
- **Negative:** Infection with *M. tuberculosis* is unlikely.
- **Indeterminate or borderline:** Uncertain likelihood of *M. tuberculosis* infection. Alternative or sequential testing may resolve the diagnosis.

➤ Limitations
- Specimens must be collected, transported, tested, and interpreted using protocols consistent with the FDA-approved methods.
- The performance of IGRAs has not been adequately evaluated in certain patient populations, like pregnant women, children, patients with malignancies and other chronic infections, patients treated with medications that affect immune response and patients with extended therapy with antituberculous agents. Limitations of the specific test used, in the context of the patient history, should be reviewed prior to use.
- Negative test results cannot exclude a diagnosis of TB.
- As with other tests of host immune response, results, especially negative responses, must be interpreted in the context of the patient's state of immunocompetence.

- TSTs are preferred for the evaluation of children, especially those younger than 5 years of age.
- Test results must be interpreted in the context of other patient data.
- Patient samples must be transported to the laboratory and processed within 8–16 hours, depending on the IGRA used.
- For patients with latent TB, IGRAs cannot be used to predict which patients will progress to reactivation disease.
- IGRAs are expensive. The use of IGRAs, versus TSTs, as a first-line diagnostic tool must be determined on the basis of several factors, including patient population served, likely compliance of patients with return visits, prior vaccination with BCG, and access to laboratory processing in a timely manner.
- Although the interpretation of IGRAs does not require the return of a patient after 48–72 hours, patient follow-up is required for positive tests; further patient evaluation may be required to follow-up clinical suspicion of active or latent TB.
- The effect of recent live-virus vaccination on the performance of IGRAs has not been well studied. Therefore, IGRAs may be performed prior to, or on the same day as live-virus vaccination. Otherwise, the IGRA should be delayed for 4–6 weeks after vaccination.
- The effect of lymphopenia on IGRAs is unknown.
- **Common pitfalls:**
  - IGRAs (and TSTs) are not recommended for patients at very low risk for infection with *M. tuberculosis.*
  - The antigens used in IGRAs (ESAT-6 and CFP-10) are present in *Mycobacterium kansasii, M. szulgai, M. marinum* and several other non-*M. tuberculosis* species. Infection with other mycobacterial species should be considered, and ruled out as appropriate, in patients with positive IGRA test results.
  - Delayed transport or improper specimen handling during transport may decrease the viability of lymphocytes and result in false-negative results.

➤ Suggested Reading

Centers for Disease Control and Prevention. Updated guidelines for using interferon gamma release assays to detect mycobacterium tuberculosis infection—United States, 2010. *MMWR Morbid Mortal Wkly Rep.* Vol. 59, No. RR-5, June 25, 2010.

NEISSERIA GONORRHOEAE, AMPLIFIED NUCLEIC ACID DETECTION (URINE, CERVICAL, URETHRAL)

➤ Definition

- Amplified nucleic acid (NA) techniques are the basis for the most sensitive tests for detection of *N. gonorrhoeae* in urine and urogenital specimens. Culture techniques for detection of *N. gonorrhoeae* require optimized culture and transport conditions that are often not realized in clinical practice.

➤ Use

- *N. gonorrhoeae*–amplified NA testing may be submitted for evaluation of sexually active patients with symptoms consistent with STDs. Commercially available amplified NA tests may be used with urine and urogenital specimens. They are not validated for use with other

types of specimens and should not be used for the sole testing technique in the evaluation of rape or child abuse.
- Several amplification techniques have been used in FDA-approved kits for diagnosis of gonococcal (GC) infection, including transcription-mediated amplification (Gen-Probe, San Diego, CA), strand displacement amplification (BD Diagnostics, GeneOhm, San Diego, CA), and PCR (Roche Molecular Diagnostics, Pleasanton, CA). Combination tests for simultaneous detection of *N. gonorrhoeae* and *C. trachomatis* are available.
- Specimens must be collected and transported according to instructions of specific kits and restricted to specimen types for which the kit is validated.
- **Turnaround time:** 24–72 hours

➤ Interpretation
- **Expected results:** negative

➤ Limitations
- **Common pitfalls:** use of incorrect swabs for specimen collection; improper filling of urine transport tubes; submission of inappropriate specimen types.

➤ Other Considerations
- The CDC has recommended confirmation of positive GC tests in patients from low or moderate prevalence (1–7%) populations; however, recent publications have demonstrated limited clinical utility for the results of routine confirmatory testing for positive specimens. If confirmatory testing is needed, it should be performed with a different type of test or target sequence.
- Specimens may yield "equivocal" results on initial testing. For these specimens, confirmation testing should be performed. Such testing may be performed on a new specimen collected from the patient or performed on the original specimen, ideally with a test that uses a comparable, but different technique (e.g., culture, NA test with a different specific target). It is recommended that specimens that yield "equivocal" results on initial testing, but "negative" or "equivocal" results on confirmatory testing be reported as "equivocal," with a request for a follow-up specimen.
- Amplified NA tests should not be used for test of cure evaluations (within 4 weeks of treatment) because DNA may be detectable even after viable organisms have been eliminated.
- Laboratories that use amplified NA tests should evaluate the possibility of laboratory contamination and false-positive tests by performing "wipe tests" of surfaces in the laboratory and by monitoring their rates of GC infection detected by amplified NA techniques. (Significantly increasing rates may be due to laboratory contamination and should be investigated.)

➤ Suggested Readings
Moncada J, Donegan E, Schachter J. Evaluation of CDC-recommended approaches for confirmatory testing of positive *Neisseria gonorrhoeae* nucleic acid amplification test results. *J Clin Microbiol.* 2008;46:1614–1619.

OVA AND PARASITE EXAMINATION, STOOL

➤ Definition
- This test is ordered for diagnosis of common enteric parasitic pathogens in fecal specimens.
- Parasitic infections present with a remarkable diversity of signs and symptoms. Indications for testing for endemic parasitic infections may be fairly straightforward. Clinicians must

have a high index of suspicion for parasitic infection when patients present with symptoms after travel to regions where other parasites are endemic.

➤ Use
* Specimens should be examined visually to identify any macroscopic parasitic forms, like pinworms or tapeworm proglottids.
  * The routine O & P examination of stool includes three components: a direct wet mount (unpreserved liquid stool only), wet mount of stool concentrate (formalin fixed specimen), and preparation of a permanent stained smear (polyvinyl alcohol [PVA]–fixed specimen). The direct wet mount may provide a rapid diagnosis and demonstrate motility of trophozoites in heavily infected patients.
  * The concentrated stool wet mount, prepared from the formalin fixed stool specimen by sedimentation or flotation, provides for detection of protozoal cyst forms, oocyst of coccidian parasites, microsporidia, and helminth eggs and larvae.
  * The permanent smear, made from the PVA-preserved stool specimen, provides the best morphology for identification of parasites and recognition of artifacts as well as providing a permanent slide that can be referred for identification, if necessary. Permanent stains should be used to confirm the identification of any parasite detected by wet mount.
* **Turnaround time:** 48–72 hours

➤ Special Collection and Transport Instructions
* Stool should be submitted in clean containers with tight-fitting lids. It is not necessary to use sterile containers. Stool specimens collected by swab, from the toilet, or on toilet paper are not appropriate. The detection of parasites may be inhibited by intestinal contrast (barium sulfate), mineral oil, bismuth medications, anti-diarrheals, and medications with antiparasitic action. Delay specimen collection for 1–2 weeks after the use of these agents.
* Submit stool during the diarrheal phase of disease. Trophozoite forms may be detected only in diarrheal stool; cyst forms are more common in formed stool.
* At least three stool specimens, collected on separate days, should be submitted within 10 days. A purgative agent, such as magnesium sulfate, improves the detection of intestinal parasites. Six specimens, collected on different days over a 2 week period, should detect more than 90% of amebic infections.
* Stool specimens should be transported to the laboratory as quickly as possible. Stool must be examined within one hour of passage (30 minutes for liquid or semi-liquid stool) if direct wet mount is needed for detection of motile forms. If the transport to the laboratory will be delayed, the stool should be placed into preservative. Stool collection kits generally contain a vial of 10% formalin and a vial of PVA solution. The PVA vial is inoculated to give a 3:1 ratio of fixative to stool. The ratio for formalin should be 3:1 or greater. The stool must mixed be thoroughly with the preservative to ensure that parasitic elements do not degrade with storage. The formalin suspension is used to prepare a direct wet mount from concentrated material. The PVA-fixed material is used to prepare smears for permanent stains.
* Three O & P examinations should be performed after therapy: 3 or 4 weeks after treatment for protozoal infection and 5 or 6 weeks after treatment for *Taenia* infection.
* Special techniques are required for collection of duodenal specimens, or specimens collected by endoscopy or other invasive techniques.

➤ Interpretation
- **Expected results:** negative
- **Positive:** Positive O & P examinations are associated with a high probability of parasitic infection or colonization.
- **Negative:** A single negative test does not effectively rule out enteric parasitic infection.

➤ Limitations
- For some enteric parasitic infections, specimens other than stool, like duodenal contents, may be required for diagnosis. Special techniques, like egg-hatching techniques, may be needed for sensitive detection of certain parasites.
- **Common pitfalls:**
  - The submission of too few specimens limits the performance of stool O & P examination.
  - Special staining techniques are required for effective detection of certain enteric parasitic pathogens, like *Cryptosporidium parvum* or microsporidia.
- Mercury in PVA solutions provides the best morphology in permanent stains, but local restrictions on mercury use have led to the development of zinc- or copper-containing preservatives. Alternative preservatives include MIF (merthiolate-iodine-formalin), which provides some staining of preserved material, and SAF (sodium acetate-acetic acid-formalin) solution, which is best used with iron hematoxylin staining.

PINWORM EXAMINATION

➤ Definition
- This test should be considered in patients, most often children, who present with pruritus ani. Sleep disturbances are common.

➤ Use
- This test is used to diagnose enteric infection with the parasitic pathogen *Enterobius vermicularis* (pinworm).
- Eggs or adult female worms are identified in specimens collected from skin of the perianal area. Specimens are collected with clear cellophane tape or a commercial pinworm collection device. The sticky side of the tape or collection device is pressed onto the perianal skin. Because the female worm emerges from the anus to lay eggs during the night, specimens should be collected in the early morning, before the patient passes a bowel movement, and ideally before arising.
- **Turnaround time:** 24–48 hours

➤ Interpretation
- **Expected results:** negative
- **Positive results:** Typical ova of *E. vermicularis* are usually seen. An adult female *E. vermicularis* is occasionally seen.

➤ Limitations
- The sensitivity of a single examination is fairly low. The examination of multiple specimens is typically required for diagnosis; empirical treatment for enterobiasis may be a cost-effective alternative to therapy based on specific diagnosis.

• **Common pitfall:** The examination of only one or two specimens will often result in a false-negative diagnosis.

PNEUMOCYSTIS JIROVECI (FORMERLY PNEUMOCYSTIS CARINII), MICROSCOPIC DETECTION

➤ Definition

• *Pneumocystis jiroveci*, formerly known as *P. carinii*, was initially characterized as a parasite, but molecular taxonomic studies have shown that it is a fungal pathogen. It is ubiquitous in nature, with low pathogenic potential. In severely immunocompromised patients, especially patients with AIDS, however, it is responsible for serious, potentially fatal respiratory disease.

➤ Use

• This test is used to detect infection with the fungal pathogen *P. jiroveci* in lower respiratory specimens. This test may be used to evaluate immunocompromised patients who present with severe atypical pneumonia.
• Method
  • Direct examination of respiratory specimens for *P. jiroveci* can be performed using several staining methods. Detection is based on the identification of organisms with typical morphology; different reagents may stain the "cyst" form, "trophozoite" form, or both.
  • Giemsa-based stains are convenient but may be difficult to read because of staining of background material. Sensitivity is ~50%. Stains using tagged monoclonal antibody reagents provide the highest sensitivity, ~91%. Calcofluor white staining has sensitivity ~74%. GMS staining provides sensitivity ~79%. Other stains, such as Papanicolaou and modified toluidine blue O, have been described. All staining techniques have excellent specificity when interpreted by experienced microbiologists.
• **Special collection and transport instructions:**
  • Acceptable specimens include material obtained by BAL or sputum induced using nebulized hypertonic saline.
    • Transbronchial or surgical biopsy specimens are acceptable specimens for *Pneumocystis* detection.
    • Expectorated sputum and respiratory secretions obtained by suction through an endotracheal tube or after percussive respiratory therapy are not acceptable for *Pneumocystis* testing.

➤ Limitations

• The performance of tests for direct detection of *P. jiroveci* depends on numerous factors, including the prior probability of infection, type of specimen submitted, specimen processing, and staining method used.
• Submission of expectorated sputum, tracheal aspirates, or specimens other than induced sputum, BAL or biopsy specimens results in poor detection of *P. jiroveci*.

➤ Suggested Readings

Cruciani M, Marcati P, Malena M, et al. Meta-analysis of diagnostic procedures for *Pneumocystis carinii* pneumonia in HIV-1-infected patients. *Eur Respir J.* 2002;20:982–989.

Procop GW, Haddad S, Quinn J, et al. Detection of *Pneumocystis jiroveci* in respiratory specimens by four staining methods. *J Clin Microbiol.* 2004;42(7):3333–3335.

Thomas CF Jr, Limper AH. Pneumocystis pneumonia. *N Engl J Med.* 2004;350:2487–2498.

RESPIRATORY ADENOVIRUS CULTURE (RULE OUT)

➤ Definition

- Adenovirus respiratory infections most commonly occur in young children and typically present with nonspecific findings of febrile viral respiratory tract infection. Adenoviruses may also cause conjunctivitis, enteric infection, hemorrhagic cystitis, and other infections.
- Respiratory adenovirus infections do not show as strong a seasonal variability (winter months) as the other common respiratory viral pathogens.

➤ Use

- This test is used to detect respiratory viral infections caused by adenoviruses.
- Respiratory specimens for adenovirus are inoculated onto human cell lines; A549, HeLa, HEp-2, and MRC-5 cell lines are commonly used. Tube cultures or shell-vial cultures may be used. A presumptive diagnosis may be made on the basis of typical cytopathic effect and then confirmed by immunologic techniques. Testing for adenovirus detection may be included in viral culture panels for respiratory viruses.
- **Turnaround time:** Most cultures are positive within 2 weeks. Tube cultures may be incubated for up to 4 weeks before signing out as negative. Shell vial cultures are stained within 7 days of incubation.

➤ Special Collection and Transport Instructions

- Specimens should be collected in the first week after onset of symptoms.
- Nasopharyngeal swabs or aspirates are recommended; other respiratory tract specimens may be acceptable for culture.
- It is recommended that specimens be inoculated into viral transport medium and transported to the laboratory on wet ice (4°C).

➤ Interpretation

- **Expected results:** negative

➤ Limitations

- Submission of specimens >7 days after onset of acute infection is associated with decreased sensitivity.
- Children with respiratory adenovirus infection frequently demonstrate leukocytosis (>15,000/mm³) and increased ESR and CRP, in contrast to the lack of these signs in other common viral respiratory tract infections.

RESPIRATORY CULTURE, RULE OUT BACTERIAL PATHOGENS

➤ Definition

- Most infections are relatively mild and resolve spontaneously within several days. Cultures may be considered in patients who present with unusually severe signs and symptoms consistent with sinusitis, otitis media, or other para-respiratory infection or symptoms that persist for more than 7 days.
- Viral infections have been implicated as primary agents or contributing infections in a significant number of patients. The common bacterial pathogens include *Moraxella catarrhalis*, *Streptococcus pneumoniae*, *Haemophilus pneumoniae*, and *Staphylococcus aureus*. Anaerobic bacteria

have been implicated, but primarily with chronic infection or acute infection associated with trauma. Opportunistic molds, such as *Mucor* species, may cause severe, invasive upper respiratory tract infections in immunocompromised patients, especially in patients with DM.

➤ Use
- This culture may be used to isolate a specific pathogen in infections adjacent to the respiratory tract. Pathogens are usually derived from the patient's endogenous upper respiratory flora.
- Specimens are typically inoculated onto SBA and MacConkey agar. CNA agar may be inoculated. Anaerobic media is inoculated if requested.
- **Turnaround time:** Cultures are examined for at least 48 hours. Several days are required for isolation and identification, susceptibility testing, and further characterization of isolates.

➤ Special Collection and Transport Instructions
- Swab specimens should be considered unacceptable for culture, except for those collected by direct visualization by an otolaryngologist. Swab specimens are not optimal for isolation of anaerobic pathogens in chronic infections or acute abscesses.
- Pus collected by surgical aspiration or drainage, or by sinus aspiration should be transported to the laboratory under anaerobic transport conditions as quickly as possible.

➤ Interpretation
- **Expected results:** no growth (light growth of endogenous respiratory flora is common)
- **Positive:** Because common causes of para-respiratory infections are usually upper respiratory tract endogenous flora, positive culture must be interpreted cautiously in the context of quantity or bacterial growth, purity of culture, Gram stain findings and clinical signs and symptoms.

➤ Limitations
- **Common pitfall:** Noninvasively collected specimens, which are more likely to represent endogenous rather than pathogenic flora, are often submitted for patient evaluation.

RESPIRATORY CULTURE, RULE OUT VIRAL PATHOGENS

➤ Definition
- Many of the respiratory viral syndromes that occur in winter months are relatively mild and self-limited. Occasionally, however, severe disease may develop for which specific diagnosis is needed to optimize therapeutic and management decisions. Viral culture may be used to provide isolates for antiviral susceptibility testing or further characterization for epidemiologic reasons.
- Adenovirus culture may be included in respiratory viral panels. The adenoviruses are not as typically seasonal as other respiratory viruses.
- Other viruses, such as human metapneumovirus and rhinoviruses, show seasonal variability, but these infections are usually managed symptomatically without the need for specific diagnosis.

➤ Use
- This test may be ordered to make a specific diagnosis for severe seasonal respiratory viral illness. Agents cultured typically include influenza virus A and B, RSV, and parainfluenza virus types 1, 2, and 3.

- Method
  - A number of upper and lower respiratory tract specimens may be submitted for culture. Nasopharyngeal wash specimens, or swabs, are usually associated with the best sensitivity of culture.
  - Specimens are typically inoculated onto several different types of cell lines to help ensure growth of all of the target pathogens. Shell vial cultures may be inoculated in addition to tube cultures. Because influenza and parainfluenza viruses are usually not identified by cytopathic effect, immunologic techniques, like staining with virus-specific tagged monoclonal antibodies, is usually performed at set time intervals after inoculation.
- **Turnaround time**
  - Shell vial cultures may be positive within 48–72 hours.
  - Most respiratory viral pathogens can be detected in tube cultures by blind staining with immunologic reagents at 7 days after inoculation.

➤ Special Collection and Transport Instructions

- Specimens should be collected according to general recommendations for virus culture of the specimen type.
- Specimens should be collected early in acute infection.
- Nasopharyngeal specimens are often optimal for diagnosis.
- RSV is a fastidious virus and should be delivered to the laboratory as quickly as possible. This virus may not survive freezing if prolonged transport is needed. Most specimens should be placed in viral transport medium and transported on wet ice (4°C).
- Specimens for molecular diagnostic, DFA, EIA, or other diagnostic testing for respiratory viruses should be submitted according to laboratory recommendations.

➤ Interpretation

- **Expected results:** negative. Negative cultures do not rule out respiratory virus infection.
- **Positive results:** Positive cultures for specific viruses indicate active infection with that agent.

➤ Limitations

- Negative cultures may be caused by poor specimen collection technique, collection of specimens after acute disease as viral concentrations are dropping, and so on.
- Molecular diagnostic techniques have shown that coinfection with two or more respiratory viral pathogens are relatively common. The impact of coinfection with specific viral pathogens, such as human metapneumovirus, awaits further characterization, as improved diagnostic techniques allow for better clinical–laboratory assessment of patients.
- Coinfection with several respiratory viral pathogens may not be well detected using a general respiratory viral culture.

RESPIRATORY SYNCYTIAL VIRUS (RSV) DIRECT DETECTION (EIA AND DFA)

➤ Definition and Use

- These tests are used to provide early detection of RSV infection. EIAs have only moderate sensitivity for detection of RSV virus infection, so they are commonly used for screening.

DFAs have high sensitivity and specificity compared to respiratory viral culture and represents a cost-effective, definitive diagnostic technique.

- EIA and DFA tests may be used sequentially for RSV screening and confirmation. The tests are used to diagnosis RSV in patients presenting with febrile respiratory virus infection during the winter months.
- **Turnaround time:** 24–48 hours. Some EIA kits allow testing with a turnaround time of <4 hours.
- There are a number of kit formats for EIA tests. Commonly, antibodies directed at specific RSV antigens are immobilized on the surface of a membrane of a test device. The specimen is added to the reaction surface, allowing RSV antigen in the specimen to react with the device antibodies. After washing, a second, tagged RSV antibody reagent is added. After washing away excess detection antibody, a label-specific detection reagent is added and the test read as positive or negative.
- For DFA testing, cells collected by nasopharyngeal swab or wash are fixed onto a microscopic slide. The slide is dried, fixed, and stained with a reagent containing labeled antibodies directed against specific RSV antigen. The label is typically fluorogenic. Stained slides are examined by fluorescence microscopy using excitation and barrier filter appropriate for the specific fluorogenic label.
- **Special collection and transport instructions:** Specimens are collected as recommended for respiratory samples for viral culture. Nasopharyngeal specimens, especially nasopharyngeal wash specimens, typically provide specimens with the greatest sensitivity for detection of infected patients.

➤ Interpretation
- **Expected results:**
  - **Positive:** Specimens showing a significant number of cells with 2+ or greater fluorescence are typically considered positive. Slides must be examined to ensure that the specimen contains enough respiratory epithelial cells to provide informative testing. Laboratories should establish a lower limit of cells present below which the test is considered uninterpretable. Specimens that demonstrate only few, faintly staining cells should be considered equivocal; repeat testing may provide clear positive or negative results.
  - **Negative:** a cellular specimen without staining by the labeled reagent

➤ Limitations
- There is kit to kit variability for sensitivity of commercially available EIA tests. Sensitivities for RSV EIAs may range from 50–80%. The sensitivity depends on the type of specimen and quality of specimen collection. Specimen types acceptable for the kit, collected according to kit instructions, will provide maximal sensitivity. The specificity of EIA and DFA kits is typically very high.
- The positive predictive value of antigen detection tests depends on the prevalence of RSV in the region. Results should be interpreted with caution, if performed at all, during periods when there is a low prevalence of RSV in the patient's region.
- **Common pitfall:** Poor test performance may be seen when specimens not validated for the platform/kit used for testing are submitted. Anterior nasal swabs, for example, may be submitted instead of nasopharyngeal swabs, resulting in an increased number of false-negative results.

RESPIRATORY VIRUS PANEL (RVP) MOLECULAR ASSAY

➤ Definition

* The RVP assay is a comprehensive panel of tests for the detection of multiple viral strains and subtypes. Various molecular assays differ in the specific list of respiratory viruses tested, but most include influenza A (and subtypes), influenza B, parainfluenza, adenovirus, metapneumovirus (HMPV), RSV, and rhinovirus.
* **Normal range:** not detected

➤ Use

* The RVP molecular assay tests for the major respiratory viruses commonly tested for surveillance and patient management.
* In addition, the RVP molecular assay is frequently used for the confirmation of negative results obtained by other methods, such as the rapid antigen assay, direct immunofluorescence, or EIA.

➤ Limitations

* The low limit of detection varies depending on the methods and viruses tested.

ROTAVIRUS FECAL ANTIGEN DETECTION

➤ Definition and Use

* This test is used for the diagnosis of enteric infections caused by Rotavirus.
* This test may be ordered for patients, usually young children, who present with a sudden onset of watery diarrhea, which is often preceded by vomiting.
* Unpreserved stool is submitted for testing.
* Rotavirus antigen in stool is detected by immunologic techniques using Rotavirus-specific antibodies. LA and EIA formats are typically used. Sensitivity and specificity of commercial EIA assays are reported in the high 90% range.
* **Turnaround time:** <24 hours

➤ Interpretation

* **Expected results:** negative

➤ Limitations

* LA tests have reported sensitivities less than the sensitivities of EIA assays.
* Assays may be less reliable in neonates.

RUBELLA SEROLOGY SCREEN (RUBELLA IgG AND IgM)

➤ Definition

* Rubella virus causes German measles, a mild subclinical infection with a characteristic exanthem that affects both children and adults. Rubella is transmitted directly by contact or by droplets from the nasopharynx of infected individuals and can cause significant birth defects if disease occurs early in fetal life. It has an incubation period of 14–21 days. Individuals may

shed virus for up to 2 weeks prior to the outbreak of rash; therefore, patients are typically infectious for some time before the infection becomes clinically obvious. Virus shedding decreases significantly after the appearance of the rash, a period coinciding with the development of neutralizing antibodies.

- Rubella is no longer endemic in the United States as a result of an intensive vaccination campaign. Minor epidemics occurred in the United States every 5–7 years and major epidemics every 10–30 years.
- **Normal range:** negative

➤ Use
- Determination of rubella immune status
- Assist in the diagnosis of rubella infection
- Determine susceptibility to rubella, particularly in pregnant women

➤ Interpretation
- **Positive** ($\geq$10 IU/mL): indicative of past infection or vaccination
- **Equivocal** ($\geq$ 5 $\leq$ 10 IU/mL): considered to be "indeterminate"
- **Negative** ($<$5 IU/mL): does not preclude recent primary infection

➤ Limitations
- In general, 90% of the U.S. population has either been vaccinated or exposed to rubella, with rubella IgG values of $\geq$10 IU/mL.
- The presence of IgG antibodies in a single specimen is not sufficient to distinguish between active infection and past infection. The results of the test must be taken within the context of the patient's clinical history, symptomatology, and other laboratory findings.
- Patients suspected of having primary, active infection should be tested for the presence of IgM antibodies to rubella virus.

SPECIAL SUSCEPTIBILITY TESTING: MINIMUM BACTERICIDAL CONCENTRATION (MBC) AND SERUM BACTERICIDAL TESTS (SBT, SCHLICHTER TEST)

➤ Definition
- The interpretation of routine antimicrobial susceptibility tests (Sensitive, Intermediate, Resistant) is based on inhibition of bacterial growth. The inhibited organisms are ultimately eliminated by the host immune response.
- The endpoints of MBC and SBT tests are based on killing of organisms by an antibiotic.

➤ Use
- Under certain circumstances, tests that measure killing of the infecting organism, rather than just inhibition, may be needed. Examples may include certain immunocompromised patients, patients with altered metabolism or pharmacokinetics for the antimicrobial agent of choice, or for certain deep-seated infections.
- Clinical data do not support the use of "cidal" tests for the vast majority of infectious diseases. These tests should only be ordered in consultation with infectious disease consultants and clinical microbiologists.

- Method: In bactericidal tests, a standard inoculum of a clinical isolate is suspended in a series of dilutions of an antimicrobial "solution." The "solution" may represent an exact concentration of the antimicrobial agent in saline or other diluent in the laboratory (MBC). Alternatively, the antimicrobial "solution" may be prepared from patient serum, typically collected at the time of peak antimicrobial activity (SBT). In the SBT, the exact concentration of the antimicrobial agent may not be known with certainty and depends on the collection time after drug administration, drug pharmacokinetics, drug metabolism, and other factors. Just after addition of the bacterial inoculum, a measured aliquot of the suspension is subcultured to agar media for quantification. Repeat quantification of viable organisms is performed for each dilution at the endpoint, typically after 20–24 hours incubation. For time-kill MBC studies, viable microorganisms are quantified at several time points during incubation at specific informative antibiotic concentrations.
- **Specimen collection:** There are no critical collection issues for MBC testing. For SBT, collection of patient serum should be ordered at the time of peak or trough antibiotic level. The tube and requisition form should clearly indicate the antibiotic phase.
- **Turnaround time:** MBC and SBT assays are not widely available in clinical microbiology laboratories and may require shipment of the clinical isolate (and patient serum for SBT) to a reference laboratory. The turnaround time for these assays is 2–7 days.

➤ Interpretation

- The MBC is commonly defined as the lowest concentration of the antimicrobial agent that results in a 99.9% (3 $\log_{10}$) or greater reduction of the concentration (CFU/mL) of organisms after incubation compared to the starting concentration. The MBC of an organism can be compared to the organism's MIC, or to measured concentration of the antimicrobial agent in patient serum (or at the site of infection), to assess likely success or failure of treatment. Tolerant strains show a MBC-to-MIC ratio of 1:32 or greater, that is, poor killing relative to inhibition.
- Several phenomena may complicate the interpretation of MBC results. A small proportion of organisms (<0.1%) may survive, even in the presence of high antibiotic concentrations. These may represent dormant or slowly replicating cells and are unlikely to be of clinical consequence. In the "paradoxical effect," the proportion of surviving cells increases as the concentration of antimicrobial agent increases above the MBC. This may be due to drug effects, like inhibition of protein synthesis, that occur at high concentration and interfere with the primary effect of the agent.
- For SBT, the end point titer is defined as that dilution of the patient serum that results in a 99.9% (3 $\log_{10}$) or greater reduction of the concentration (CFU/mL) of organisms after incubation compared to the starting concentration. The titer is often reported as the inverse of the dilution. The best predictors for outcome have not been established for SBTs. Some studies have shown that outcome is improved with SBT titers of 16 or 32 when serum is drawn at peak drug concentration. Alternatively, some authors have shown that trough SBT titers (serum drawn just prior to administration of the antimicrobial agent) >2 correlate best with improved outcome.

➤ Limitations

- As discussed, the interpretation of MBC and SBT assays may not be straightforward. Consultation with infectious diseases and microbiology consultants is recommended.

- These tests must be interpreted with consideration of the site of infection. Results may be less useful, and potentially misleading, for infections at sites at which the concentration of antimicrobial agent is not in equilibrium with serum.

➤ Suggested Readings

NCCLS. *Methodology for the Serum Bactericidal Test; Approved Guideline.* NCCLS document M21-A. NCCLS (Wayne, PA). 1999.

NCCLS. *Methods for Determining Bactericidal Activity of Antimicrobial Agents; Approved Guideline.* NCCLS document M26-A. NCCLS (Wayne, PA). 1999.

SPUTUM CULTURE (ROUTINE)

➤ Definition

- Lower respiratory tract (LRT) infections may involve any of the anatomic areas inferior to the larynx. Infections include tracheobronchitis (large airway disease), bronchiolitis (small airway disease), and pneumonia (alveolar disease). The common etiologies depend on the site of infection, age and underlying health of the patient, season, and other factors.
- Patients with LRT infections typically present with a constellation of symptoms of varying severity, including fever, cough, sputum production, difficulty breathing, and shortness of breath. Common bacterial pathogens are less commonly associated with coryza and rhinorrhea than are respiratory viruses and mycoplasmas. Symptoms and clinical examination may help distinguish tracheobronchitis, bronchiolitis, and pneumonia from one another.

➤ Use

- These cultures are used to identify bacterial pathogens responsible for LRT infections, including pneumonia. A wide variety of human pathogens may cause lower respiratory infections, and there is a large overlap in the clinical signs and symptoms.
- Method
  - Noninvasive and minimally invasive techniques for specimen collection may result in contamination of the specimen with the patient's endogenous upper respiratory flora. Because LRT infections are commonly caused by a patient's flora, such contamination may compromise the interpretation of sputum cultures. Therefore, Gram stain examination of sputum should be performed to ensure that poor quality specimens are not processed for routine sputum culture. A number of screening strategies have been proposed. Sputum specimens are scored on the basis of the presence and quantity of PMNs and SECs.
  - Acceptable specimens are inoculated onto nonselective enriched and supportive media, like chocolate agar and SBA, and to selective-differential media, like MacConkey agar.
  - Routine specimens for sputum culture are not acceptable for anaerobic culture because they are commonly contaminated with endogenous anaerobes unrelated to infection. If anaerobic infection is suspected, specialized techniques, like needle aspiration, are required.
- **Turnaround time**
  - Cultures are incubated for 48–72 hours.
  - Additional time is required for isolation, identification, susceptibility, and other testing, as required.

➤ Special Collection and Transport Instructions

* For expectorated sputum samples, patient instruction is critical for collection of a good quality, informative sample.
* Specimens must be collected in sterile transport containers with tight-fitting lids.
* First morning specimens are usually most sensitive because of pooling of secretions during sleep.
* Contamination is reduced for patients who brush their teeth and gargle just before specimen collection.
* The patient must understand that sputum from a deep cough is needed, and saliva should not be expectorated into the collection cup.
* Sputum production may be improved by chest wall percussive techniques.
* Specimens obtained by more invasive procedures, such as sputum induction, BAL, tracheal aspirate, and lung puncture, are collected by physicians or respiratory therapists trained with specific collection protocols.
* Specimens must be transported to the laboratory as quickly as possible at room temperature.

➤ Interpretation

* **Expected results:** Light or rare growth of normal endogenous respiratory tract flora (or no growth).
* **Positive:** Positive cultures must be interpreted carefully in the context of Gram stain results and other laboratory findings, imaging studies, and clinical presentations. Possible endogenous organisms, such as *S. pneumoniae* and *H. influenzae*, are part of the etiology of community-acquired pneumonia and other LRT infections.
* **Negative:** A negative culture does not exclude LRT infection. Poor specimen quality and transport conditions may prevent the isolation of fastidious pathogens. Pathogens may be inhibited by or "lost" among contaminating flora. Other LRT pathogens, such as *Bordetella pertussis*, are not detected reliably by routine sputum culture.

➤ Limitations

* The sensitivity and specificity of routine sputum cultures are relatively low for diagnosis of LRT infections. Diagnoses may be improved by submission of blood cultures, urinary antigen tests (*Legionella, S. pneumoniae*), serology, and molecular diagnostic techniques and tests for other types of LRT pathogens, such as *Mycoplasma* species.
* **Common pitfalls**
  * Poor specimen collection and transport are the major causes for compromised information from sputum cultures.
  * Rejection criteria may be inappropriately applied to special LRT specimens submitted for isolation of fastidious pathogens, such as *Legionella*, mycobacteria, fungi, or viruses.

STOOL CULTURE (ROUTINE)

➤ Definition

* Routine stool culture should be considered for patients with acute diarrheal illness who are producing frequent, loose stools. Nausea, abdominal pain, and vomiting may be present. Fever may be present, but is not a prominent feature in uncomplicated enteric infection.

Fluid loss, especially in infants and small children, may be severe and associated with complications including electrolyte imbalance and cardiovascular instability.

➤ Use

* The routine stool culture is used to detect GI infections caused by enteric bacterial pathogens. The target pathogens identified by routine stool culture may vary somewhat among laboratories, but all should be capable of detecting *Salmonella*, *Shigella*, and *Campylobacter* species. Other pathogens may be included, like shiga-toxin producing *E. coli*, depending on local prevalence. Detection of other enteric pathogens may require special testing.
* Method: Stool specimens are typically inoculated onto several agar media, including a nonselective medium (e.g., SBA), a mildly selective differential medium (e.g., MacConkey agar) and a moderately selective differential medium (e.g., Hektoen enteric agar). Some laboratories have used selective broth enrichment (e.g., Selenite broth) prior to plate inoculation, but the cost-effectiveness of these strategies has been questioned. Selective agar media and incubation at increased temperature (42°C) and microaerophilic conditions are used for isolation of enteric *Campylobacter* species.
* **Turnaround time:** Cultures are examined for growth at 24 and 48 hours. Suspicious colonies are isolated and confirmatory testing performed.

➤ Special Collection and Transport Instructions

* Acceptable specimens: stool (feces), rectal swab
* Sterile collection containers are not required. Specimens may be collected in clean containers. The container should be free of detergent or preservative.
* Specimens should be transported promptly to the laboratory. If transport will be delayed >2 hours, use of a transport media, like Cary-Blair, is recommended.
* Three specimens, collected on consecutive days, are recommended for sensitive detection of enteric pathogens, especially for patients at risk for complication or at increased risk for transmission of enteric pathogens, like food handlers.
* Specimens collected on toilet paper or diapers are not acceptable. Specimens contaminated by urine are not acceptable.

➤ Interpretation

* **Expected results:** Negative
* **Positive:** Any growth of *Salmonella*, *Shigella*, *Campylobacter* or other enteric pathogen.

➤ Limitations

* Effective detection of enteric infection due to enterohemorrhagic *E. coli* (e.g., *E. coli* O157:H7), *Yersinia enterocolitica*, *Vibrio* species, *Aeromonas* species, *C. difficile*, or other bacterial pathogens requires special cultures for sensitive detection.
* Diarrheal illness caused by parasitic or viral pathogens require special test methods.
* *C. difficile* testing should be considered as an alternative to routine enteric pathogen testing for inpatients >6 months of age.
* Stool culture may be negative in invasive enteric infections, like typhoid fever. Blood cultures are recommended for primary gastrointestinal infections that progress to significant fever associated with signs of systemic infection.
* *Shigella* species may not survive broth enrichment techniques.

- **Common pitfalls:**
  - Rectal swabs can collect only a small amount of feces; their use should be restricted to infants.
  - *Shigella* species are fastidious and may not survive changes in stool pH that occur after passage. Rapid transport and/or the use of transport media is important for reliable isolation by culture.

➤ Other Considerations

- Absence of normal fecal flora or the presence of predominant growth of yeast, *S. aureus* or *Pseudomonas aeruginosa* can be recognized by inspection of the SBA plate, providing clinically relevant information about alternative diagnoses.
- Oxidase testing may be performed on SBA isolated with heavy growth to screen for unexpected enteric infection caused by *Vibrio*, *Aeromonas*, or *Plesiomonas* species.

STREPTOCOCCUS, GROUP A, DIRECT DETECTION (ANTIGEN, NUCLEIC ACID)

➤ Definition

- The results of direct tests for group A streptococci may guide early therapy. In antigen tests, the group A cell wall polysaccharide is extracted from a throat swab.

➤ Use

- Direct detection tests for group A beta-hemolytic streptococci (*Streptococcus pyogenes*) are used for early diagnosis of streptococcal pharyngitis. Patients may present with sore throat, fever, headache, and abdominal pain.
- Method
  - Extracted antigen is detected by specific antibodies directed against the antigen, usually using standard immunologic techniques, such as LA or EIA. The sensitivity of antigen tests vary by technique and specific kit used, ranging from 60–95%; the specificity of most tests exceeds 95%. Therefore, throat culture should be performed to confirm negative antigen tests but is not needed to confirm positive tests.
  - The Group A Streptococcus Direct Test (Gen-Probe, San Diego, CA) is an FDA-approved molecular diagnostic assay for the detection of *S. pyogenes* in pharyngeal specimens. Group A streptococci are detected using a specific DNA probe directed against specific *S. pyogenes* rRNA sequences. Sensitivity of the assay is 88–95% with specificity of 98–99.7%. The high sensitivity and specificity for this test allow test results to stand without the need for confirmation of positive or negative tests.
- **Special collection and transport instructions:** Throat swab specimens are collected as recommended for throat cultures.
- **Turnaround time:** <4 hours for antigen tests; <24 hours for molecular tests

➤ Interpretation

- **Expected results:** Negative/not detected. Negative antigen tests decrease the likelihood of group A streptococcal pharyngitis but must be confirmed by a more sensitive technique, such as throat culture or molecular detection.
- **Positive:** Positive results are diagnostic of group A streptococcal pharyngitis in patients with consistent clinical findings.

➤ Limitations

- γ-Irradiated swabs cannot be used for the Gen-Probe assay. Only use swabs specified by the laboratory.

STREPTOCOCCUS, GROUP B, BETA-HEMOLYTIC (*STREPTOCOCCUS AGALACTIAE*) CULTURE (RULE OUT)

➤ Use

- This culture is used to detect rectal or vaginal carriage of group B beta-hemolytic *Streptococcus* (GBS). Specific GBS carriage testing is used in culture-based screening strategies for prevention of neonatal group B *Streptococcus* infection. (*S. agalactiae* grow well in routine bacterial cultures, so requesting GBS screening cultures is not needed when testing samples of potentially infected patient specimens.)
- GBS screening cultures of rectal and vaginal swab specimens are recommended for all pregnant women at 35–37 weeks of gestation.
- Method
  - Broth enrichment: Swabs are inoculated into selective broth medium, such as Todd-Hewitt broth supplemented with antibiotics to suppress growth of endogenous flora (e.g., gentamicin and nalidixic acid, or colistin and nalidixic acid). Enrichment broths that incorporate chromogenic pigments may be used, and these may provide earlier detection of positive specimens.
  - The broth culture is incubated for 18–24 hours at 35–37°C in ambient air or 5% CO_2.
  - GBS isolation: The broth is subcultured to a SBA plate. After incubation for 18–24 hours at 35–37°C in ambient air or 5% CO_2, the plates are inspected for organisms suggestive of GBS. If GBS is not identified after incubation for 18–24 hours, plates are re-incubated and then inspected at 48 hours to identify suspected organisms.
  - GBS identification: Suspect organisms are definitively identified using any of various methods, including specific latex agglutination, nucleic acid probe techniques (direct or amplified) or the CAMP test. Direct latex agglutination or nucleic acid detection techniques may be used on the enriched selective broth.
  - Identification and susceptibility testing: Penicillin is the drug of choice for prophylaxis during labor, so susceptibility testing is needed only for penicillin allergic patients.
- **Turnaround time:** 48–72 hours

➤ Special Collection and Transport Instructions

- Both rectal and vaginal swab specimens should be submitted for GBS carrier culture. A swab of the lower vagina (vaginal introitus) should be collected, followed by collection of a swab from the rectum (i.e., insertion of the swab through the anal sphincter) using the same swab or two different swabs.
- A speculum should not be used for specimen collection.
- The following specimens are *not* acceptable for screening cultures for GBS carriage: cervical, perianal, perirectal, or perineal.
- Swabs should be placed into non-nutritive transport medium, like Amies or Stuart's. Vaginal and rectal swabs, if collected separately, may be placed into the same transport medium.
- Susceptibility testing for clindamycin and erythromycin should be ordered for women at high risk for anaphylaxis due to penicillin allergy. Susceptibility testing and interpretation

should follow CLSI guidelines, including a D-test or comparable method to detect inducible clindamycin resistance.

➤ Interpretation

- Results of culture-based screening for rectovaginal GBS carriage are used in the algorithms for GBS intrapartum prophylaxis recommended by the CDC, American College of Obstetricians and Gynecologists, American College of Nurse-Midwives, American Academy of Pediatrics, American Academy of Family Physicians, Society for Healthcare Epidemiology of America, American Society of Microbiology, and other experts.
- **Expected results:** negative. Intrapartum GBS prophylaxis is not indicated for patients with negative rectovaginal GBS screening cultures obtained within 5 weeks prior to delivery, regardless of intrapartum risk factors.
- **Positive results:** Intrapartum prophylaxis is indicated for patients with positive rectovaginal GBS screening cultures (unless a cesarean delivery is performed before the onset of labor and prior to rupture of membranes).

➤ Other Considerations

- Intrapartum GBS prophylaxis is also recommended for:
  - Women with a history of a previous infant with invasive GBS disease
  - Women with GBS bacteriuria during any trimester of the current pregnancy
  - Women with unknown GBS carrier status at the onset of labor, and onset of labor before 37 weeks of gestation, or amniotic membrane rupture >18 hours, or intrapartum temperature >38.0°C. Results of screening cultures for GBS carriage, collected at the time of presentation for such patients with preterm labor or preterm premature rupture of membranes, may be used in determining subsequent prophylactic therapy.

➤ Limitations

- Swabbing both the lower vagina and rectum (i.e., through the anal sphincter) increases the yield substantially compared with sampling the cervix or sampling the vagina without also swabbing the rectum.
- If direct agar plating is used without prior selective enrichment broth culture, up to 50% of GBS carriers may have false-negative culture results. Therefore, use of enrichment broth is recommended for all specimens for detection of rectovaginal GBS carriage. Direct plating may be performed in addition to enrichment broth culture to improve turn-around-time.
- Collection of only rectal or vaginal swabs significantly reduces the detection of GBS carriage.
- Studies have demonstrated that, with appropriate instruction, patients are able to self-collect good quality rectal and vaginal specimens for GBS carrier testing.
- Chromogenic enrichment broths do not accurately detect non–beta-hemolytic strains of GBS. Therefore, all negative chromogenic enrichment broths must undergo further testing, such as latex agglutination or nucleic acid probe, to rule out nonhemolytic GBS.

➤ Suggested Readings

Centers for Disease Control and Prevention. MMWR. Prevention of Perinatal Group B Streptococcal Disease: Revised Guidelines. August 16, 2002/Vol. 51/No. RR-11. Available at http://www.cdc.gov/mmwr/PDF/rr/rr5111.pdf .

Centers for Disease Control and Prevention. Provisional Recommendations for the Prevention of Perinatal Group B Streptococcal Disease. July 29, 2010. Available at http://www.cdc.gov/groupBstrep/guidelines/downloads/provisional-recommendations-508.pdf

STREPTOZYME, ANTISTREPTOCOCCAL ANTIBODIES, ANTISTREPTOLYSIN O [ASO], ANTI-DNASE-B [ADB])

➤ Definition

* There are several disease-causing strains of streptococci (groups A, B, C, D, and G), which are identified by their behavior, chemistry, and appearance. Each group causes specific types of infections and symptoms. Group A streptococci are the most virulent species for humans and are the cause of "strep" throat, tonsillitis, wound and skin infections, blood infections, scarlet fever, pneumonia, RF, Sydenham chorea (formerly called St. Vitus dance), and GN. Although symptoms may suggest a streptococcal infection, the diagnosis must be confirmed by tests. The best procedure, and one that is used for an acute infection, is to take a sample from the infected area for culture. However, cultures are useless about 2–3 weeks after initial infection, so the ASO, streptozyme, and ADB screen tests are used to determine if a streptococcal infection is present.
* Streptozyme
  * The streptozyme test is often used as a screening test for antibodies to the streptococcal antigens NADase, DNase, streptokinase, streptolysin O, and hyaluronidase. This test is most useful in evaluating suspected poststreptococcal disease following *S. pyogenes* infection, such as rheumatic fever. Streptozyme has certain advantages over ASO and ADB. It can detect several antibodies in a single assay, it is technically quick and easy, and it is unaffected by factors that can produce false positives in the ASO test.
  * The disadvantages are that, although it detects different antibodies, it does not determine which one has been detected, and it is not as sensitive in children as in adults. In fact, borderline antibody elevations, which could be significant in children, may not be detected at all.
* ASO
  * The ASO titer is used to demonstrate the body's reaction to an infection caused by group A beta-hemolytic streptococci. Group A streptococci produce the enzyme streptolysin O, which can destroy (lyse) red blood cells.
  * ASO appears in the blood serum one week to one month after the onset of a strep infection. A high titer is not specific for any type of poststreptococcal disease, but it does indicate if a streptococcal infection is or has been present. Serial ASO testing is often performed to determine the difference between an acute or convalescent blood samples. The diagnosis of a previous strep infection is confirmed when serial titers of ASO rise over a period of weeks, and then fall slowly. ASO titers peak during the third week after the onset of acute symptoms of a streptococcal disease; at 6 months after onset, approximately 30% of patients exhibit abnormal titers.
  * Elevated titers are seen in 80–85% patients with acute RF and 95% in acute GN.
* Anti-DNase B or ADB
  * This test also detects antigens produced by group A streptococcus and is elevated in most patients with RF and poststreptococcal GN.
  * This test is often done concurrently with the ASO titer. When ASO and ADB are performed concurrently, 95% of previous strep infections are detected.
* **Normal values** may vary with season of the year, age, and geographic location of the patient. **Expected values** for normal adults as reported in the literature are typically less than 100 IU/mL. The ULN ASO titer for pediatrics is <100 IU/mL; in school age children or young adults, it is between 166 and 250 IU/ml. A twofold increase in the ASO value,

using serial analysis, within 1–2 weeks of the initial result is supportive of a prior strepto-coccal infection. In the absence of complications or reinfection, the ASO level usually falls to preinfection activity within 6–12 months.

- **Normal range:** ULN, 116 IU/mL

➤ Use

- Direct diagnostic value in scarlet fever, erysipelas, and streptococcal pharyngitis and tonsil-litis
- Indirect diagnostic value in RF, GN, detection of subclinical streptococcal infection, and dif-ferential diagnosis of joint pains of RF and RA

➤ Interpretation

- Increased in pyoderma, postimpetigo nephritis caused by GAS, RF, and pharyngitis

➤ Limitations

- When evaluating patients with acute RF, the American Heart Association recommends the ASO titer rather than ADB. Even though the ADB is more sensitive than ASO, its results are too variable. It also should be noted that, although ASO is the recommended test, when ASO and ADB are done together, the combination is better than either ASO or ADB alone.
- With the ASO test, false-positive results are observed with increased levels of serum beta lipoproteins produced in liver disease and contamination of serum with *Bacillus cereus* or *Pseudomonas* species. In addition, these titers are not formed as a result of streptococcal pyo-derma. Technically, false-positive results occur due to the oxidation of reagents.
- A single ASO analysis may not be meaningful due to the variability of ASO values within the normal population. Both clinical and laboratory findings should be considered in reaching a diagnosis.
- Streptococcal infections already treated with antibiotics may not produce increased results.

SYPHILIS SEROLOGY TESTS

➤ Definition

- Syphilis is an STD caused by the bacterium *Treponema pallidum*. Symptoms of infection are often subtle and easily confused with other STDs such as genital herpes infection. Syphilis is passed from person to person through direct contact with infectious exudates from obvious or concealed, moist, early lesions of skin and mucous membranes of infected people during sexual contacts. Exposure almost always occurs during oral, anal, or vaginal intercourse. A pregnant woman with the disease can pass it to her newborn child.
- The diagnosis of syphilis is most commonly made by serologic testing, and is typically per-formed in two settings: screening of patients at increased risk and evaluation of patients with suspected disease.
- There are two types of serologic tests for syphilis: nontreponemal tests such as the rapid plasma reagin (RPR) test and Venereal Disease Research Laboratory (VDRL) test, and spe-cific treponemal tests such as the *Treponema pallidum* particle agglutination assay (TP-PA), fluorescent treponemal antibody absorption (FTA-ABS) test, and the microhemagglutina-tion test for antibodies to *Treponema pallidum* (MHA-TP).
- **Normal range:** negative

➤ Use

* An aid in the diagnosis of active or past *T. pallidum* infection
* Nontreponemal tests are based upon the reactivity of serum from patients with syphilis to a cardiolipin-cholesterol-lecithin antigen. These tests measure IgG and IgM antibodies and are used as the screening test for syphilis in most settings. Positive tests are usually reported as a titer of antibody, and they can be used to follow the response to treatment in many patients.
* Treponemal tests are more complex and are usually used as confirmatory tests when the nontreponemal tests are reactive. These tests all use *T. pallidum* antigens and are based upon the detection of antibodies directed against treponemal cellular components. These tests are qualitative and are reported as reactive or nonreactive.

➤ Interpretation (Figure 3-1)

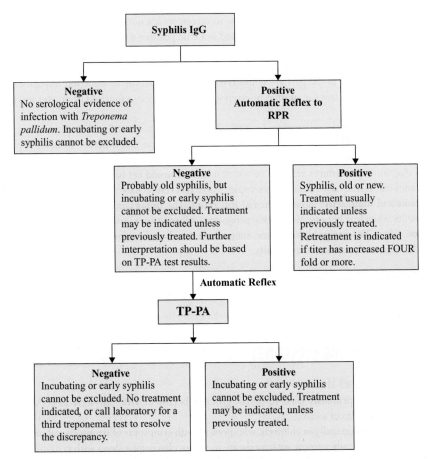

Figure 3-1. Nontraditional algorithm for syphilis testing RPR, rapid plasma reagin (test); TP-PA, *Treponema pallidum* particle agglutination (test).

➤ Limitations

- A nonreactive result does not totally exclude a recent (within the last 2–3 weeks) *T. pallidum* infection. Therefore, results need to be interpreted with caution.
- Detection of treponemal antibodies may indicate recent, past, or successfully treated syphilis infections and, therefore, cannot be used to differentiate between active and cured cases.
- False-positive tests for syphilis can occur with both nontreponemal and treponemal tests. A false-positive test result may be identified by a reactive nontreponemal test followed by a non-reactive treponemal test. It is estimated that 1–2% of the U.S. population has false-positive nontreponemal test results. False-positive tests are particularly common during pregnancy.
- The syphilis serology tests may be reactive with sera from patients with yaws (*T. pallidum* subspecies pertenue) or pinta (*Treponema carateum*).
- With nontreponemal tests, biologic false-positive reactions have been reported in diseases such as infectious mononucleosis, leprosy, malaria, SLE, vaccinia, narcotic addiction, auto-immune diseases, and viral pneumonia.
- Standard (traditional) testing algorithm is to screen with a nontreponemal test such as the RPR; a reactive specimen is then confirmed as a true positive with a treponemal test such as the TP-PA test. When results are reactive to both treponemal and RPR tests, persons should be considered to have untreated syphilis unless this is ruled out by treatment history. Persons who were treated in the past are considered to have a new syphilis infection if quantitative testing on an RPR test (or another nontreponemal test) reveals a fourfold or greater increase in titer.
- Nontraditional testing algorithm: In 2008, the CDC reported that four New York City laboratories had reversed the traditional order of screening and confirmatory tests for syphilis (i.e., specific treponemal testing [EIA] prior to nonspecific treponemal testing). This change in diagnostic procedures resulted in test results that would *not* have been identified by the traditional testing algorithm. For example, 3% of test results have a reactive treponemal test result and nonreactive nontreponemal test result. The importance of these paired testing results is unclear because no specific prognostic information exists to guide patient evaluation. The CDC has published some suggestions for diagnostic management for clinicians who receive these discordant results.

➤ Suggested Reading
Syphilis testing algorithms using treponemal tests for initial screening–four laboratories, New York City, 2005–2006. *MMWR Morb Mortal Wkly Rep.* 2008;57:872.

THROAT CULTURE (ROUTINE)

➤ Definition and Use
- This culture is primarily used to detect group A beta-hemolytic *Streptococcus* (GABHS, *S. pyogenes*) from throat swabs.
- This test is used, usually in children, who present with symptoms of streptococcal pharyngitis. Patients typically present with moderate to severe pharyngitis along with systemic symptoms, including fever, malaise, headache, and abdominal pain. Runny nose, cough, diarrhea, and other symptoms are more suggestive of another cause, usually viral.

- A GABHS throat culture is recommended to confirm negative *S. pyogenes* antigen screening tests in children. Confirmatory cultures are not needed for adults with negative antigen test results if the sensitivity of the specific antigen test used is >80%.
- The importance of diagnosis of GABHS pharyngitis is for the prevention of nonsuppurative sequelae. Antibiotic treatment given during the acute phase of GABHS infection is effective in prevention of RF, glomerulonephritis, and other complications. GABHS pharyngitis may also be complicated by peritonsillar abscess or other suppurative para-respiratory infections.
- A GABHS throat culture is not recommended for test of cure after therapy for documented strep throat; cultures may demonstrate clinically insignificant low-level carriage after successful therapy.
- Throat swabs are inoculated onto SBA; selective agar (by addition of antibiotics) is inoculated by some laboratories to suppress the growth of normal endogenous flora and to facilitate isolation of GABHS. Cultures are commonly incubated for 24 hours; however, incubation of plates for 48 hours may result in significantly increased detection, especially for cultures using selective media.
- *S. pyogenes* isolates remain predictably susceptible to penicillin, the treatment of choice. Antimicrobial susceptibility testing is not performed unless requested because of penicillin allergy.
- **Turnaround time:** Cultures are examined for 24–48 hours. An additional day may be required for isolation and identification of suspected isolates from heavily contaminated specimens.
- **Special collection and transport instructions:**
  - Affected tonsillar and posterior pharyngeal mucosa is rubbed vigorously with a swab, carefully avoiding contamination by the tongue, buccal, or other mucosal surface.
  - The swab is transported to the laboratory in transport media according to routine recommendations for bacterial specimens.

➤ Interpretation
- **Expected results:** No growth of Group A beta-hemolytic *Streptococcus*.
  - **Positive:** Positive cultures, in the setting of a clinical diagnosis, are diagnostic of GABHS pharyngitis. In the absence of symptoms, positive cultures may indicate carriage and not infection.
  - **Negative:** Throat cultures may be negative if there is poor specimen collection or heavy growth of endogenous flora.

➤ Limitations
- Cultures are typically negative in patients presenting with symptoms consistent with non-suppurative complications of GABHS infection. Serologic tests, like ASO and other anti-*S. pyogenes* antigens, may provide support for the diagnosis.
- **Common pitfall:** A throat culture is not optimized for the detection of organisms other than *S. pyogenes*. (Groups C and G beta-streptococci and/or *A. hemolyticum* are identified in throat cultures in some laboratories.)
- Submission of a throat culture is not recommended for detection of carriage or infection by other organisms. To determine the cause of sinusitis or other para-respiratory infections, special procedures for collection and culture (e.g., upper respiratory tract bacterial culture) are required.

➤ Other Considerations

- Other causes of pharyngitis include viruses (most common), mycoplasmas, group C and G beta-hemolytic streptococci, and *Arcanobacterium hemolyticum*. *N. gonorrhoeae* should be considered in patients at risk. *C. diphtheriae*, and related species, are uncommon in the United States but should be considered in patients with typical presentations after possible exposure in endemic areas. Special testing is usually required to detect pathogens other than *S. pyogenes* from throat cultures.
- GABHS may cause infection at other sites, especially cellulitis. Routine bacterial cultures appropriate for these sites should be requested.

THROAT CULTURE, PATIENTS WITH CYSTIC FIBROSIS

➤ Use

- This culture is used to detect the bacterial pathogens that commonly cause lower respiratory tract infections in patients with CF. Pharyngeal specimens are most useful to document carriage/chronic infection, whereas lower respiratory specimens are recommended for the evaluation of clinically evident, acute infection.
- Pneumonia and other lower respiratory tract infections are a cause of significant morbidity and mortality in patients with CF. The etiology of these infections is significantly different than the etiology of pneumonia seen in other patient groups. *P. aeruginosa* (including mucoid variants), *Burkholderia cepacia* complex organisms, *Stenotrophomonas maltophilia*, *H. influenzae*, and other glucose fermenting and nonfermenting gram-negative bacilli, as well as *S. aureus* and *S. pneumoniae*, are commonly isolated from lower and upper respiratory tract specimens submitted from patients with CF.
- Sputum from patients with CF should not be screened by Gram stain, as recommended for routine sputum cultures submitted from patients without CF.
- Method
  - A variety of supportive, selective, and differential agar media are inoculated. Commonly inoculated media include:
    - SBA as a supportive media capable of supporting the growth of many pathogens, including *S. pneumoniae*.
    - CNA agar for gram-positive pathogens; mannitol-salt agar for isolation of *S. aureus*.
    - MacConkey agar for nonfastidious gram-negative bacilli, including *P. aeruginosa* and *S. maltophilia*.
    - *B. cepacia* selective agar
    - Chocolate agar for isolation of *H. influenzae*
  - Cultures for mycobacterial, fungal, viral, or other respiratory pathogens are also recommended in addition to bacterial cultures.
- **Turnaround time:** cultures are examined daily for 96 hours. Several days are required for isolation, susceptibility testing, and identification of suspected isolates.
- **Special collection and transport instructions:**
  - Deep, aggressively collected posterior pharyngeal swabs may be submitted.
  - Expectorated sputum or invasively obtained lower respiratory specimens are recommended for evaluation of chronic carriage/infection and acute exacerbation of pulmonary infection.
  - Specimens are transported as for routine sputum specimens.

➤ Interpretation

- Patients with CF often show respiratory tract colonization that changes little over time, even in response to antimicrobial therapy. The interpretation of cultures demonstrating such "abnormal flora" may be challenging; clinical and therapeutic decisions must be based on a variety of clinical and other factors, in addition to culture results.
- The work-up and interpretation of CF respiratory cultures is typically based on several factors, including type of specimen submitted, organism(s) isolated, and the predominance of a specific pathogen compared to other flora.

➤ Limitations

- Although rapidly growing mycobacteria and mold may be isolated with CF respiratory cultures, special cultures are needed for sensitive detection of nontuberculous mycobacteria, *Aspergillus* species and other molds, and viruses that may cause acute respiratory infections in these patients.
- It is difficult to differentiate isolates that represent chronic colonization versus acute exacerbation on the basis of laboratory criteria.
- **Common pitfalls:**
  - Clinicians must order special throat or lower respiratory cultures for evaluation of patients with CF; routine cultures are not optimized for evaluation of the flora typically isolated from such specimens.
  - Laboratories should not apply sputum rejection criteria based on Gram stain screening recommended for routine sputum cultures submitted from other patients.

TOXOPLASMA SEROLOGY SCREEN (*TOXOPLASMA GONDII*, IgG AND IgM)

➤ Definition

- *Toxoplasma gondii* is an obligate intracellular parasite capable of infecting most mammals, including humans. Toxoplasmosis usually is asymptomatic, but primary infection during pregnancy can result in congenital disease. The domestic cat is the only definitive host for *T. gondii* and is the reservoir of the infective oocysts that are passed in the feces. Human infection may be acquired by consuming cysts in uncooked or undercooked meat of infected animals or by contact with oocysts from the feces of an infected cat.
- Acute toxoplasma infection can pose a serious threat to immunocompromised individuals and newborns who acquire the infection in utero. Immunosuppressed patients may develop encephalitis, myocarditis, or pneumonitis. Congenital infections usually result as a consequence of asymptomatic acute maternal infection. This infection can cause premature delivery, spontaneous abortion, or stillbirth.
- Management of toxoplasmosis requires serologic monitoring of infected individuals, as the organism is not readily available for culture.
- **Normal range:** negative

➤ Use

- Aids in the diagnosis of toxoplasmosis
- First line test in endemic areas for identifying *T. gondii* infection in pregnant women

- Testing for the presence of toxoplasma IgG can be useful to determine prior infection and indicate reactivation of the infection.
- Testing for the presence of toxoplasma IgM is useful to determine acute infection.

➤ Interpretation

- Positive in toxoplasma infection
- Individuals infected with the toxoplasma organism typically exhibit detectable levels of IgM antibody immediately before or soon after the onset of symptoms. IgM titers normally decline within 4–6 months, but may persist at low levels up to a year. Patients with active toxoplasma chorioretinitis usually have undetectable levels of IgM.

➤ Limitations

- IgG is not useful for diagnosing infection in infants <6 months of age, because they are usually the result of passive transfer from the mother.
- Low levels of IgM antibodies may occasionally persist for >12 months post-infection. For the determination of seroconversion from nonreactive to reactive, two serum samples should be drawn 3–4 weeks apart, during the acute and convalescent stages of the infection. The acute phase sample should be stored and tested in parallel with the convalescent sample.
- CDC suggests equivocal or positive results should be retested using a different assay from another reference laboratory specializing in toxoplasmosis testing (IgG dye test, IgM ELISA, reflex to avidity, and/or other tests).

URINE CULTURE (ROUTINE)

➤ Definition

- The range of UTI syndromes is broad, including asymptomatic bacteriuria through pyelonephritis with systemic symptoms. Patients with uncomplicated UTIs often present with dysuria and frequency, whereas pyelonephritis may be associated with signs of sepsis including fever, flank pain, and nausea.
- The risk of UTI, including complicated UTI, is increased in patients with urinary tract prosthetic materials, like stents, GU tract malformations, history of GU surgery, and medical conditions, such as pregnancy, neurologic disorders, and DM.

➤ Use

- Urine culture is used for the detection of UTI caused by common uropathogenic bacteria and yeast.
- Potentially pathogenic isolates are identified and susceptibility testing performed, as appropriate.
- Urine is cultured quantitatively. For most patients, one microliter of urine is inoculated onto SBA and onto a selective, differential agar for isolation of gram-negative bacilli. Therefore, urine specimens with fewer than 10^3 organisms per milliliter of urine will typically yield "no growth" on the media.
  - For patients at risk for clinically significant UTI at lower concentrations of uropathogens, 10 µL of urine may be inoculated, resulting in a lower detection level of 10^2 organisms per milliliter. Uropathogens present in concentrations between 10^2 and 10^3 organisms per

milliliter may be clinically significant in symptomatic patients. Repeat culture has shown that some of these patients may progress rapidly to higher concentrations of bacteria.

- The extent of work-up and susceptibility testing is determined by the type of specimen submitted, concentration and species isolated, and patient risk factors. Limited work-up of mixed cultures, which usually represent specimen contamination with endogenous flora, is recommended.
- **Turnaround time:** Urine cultures from patients at low risk for complicated UTI should be incubated for a minimum of 16 hours. Cultures from patients at risk for complicated UTI should be incubated for a minimum of 48 hours before signing out as negative. Several additional days may be required for final identification and susceptibility testing in positive cultures.

➤ Special Collection and Transport Instructions

- **Acceptable specimens:** Clean-catch midstream urine, straight catheterization ("in and out"), newly placed indwelling catheters and suprapubic aspirates are commonly submitted and should be associated with low contamination rates.
  - Urine collected from an indwelling catheter or from pediatric collection bags are more frequently contaminated. Negative cultures may be helpful in ruling out UTI; positive cultures should be interpreted with caution. Urine for culture should never be taken from a collection bag attached to an indwelling catheter.
  - Collection of urine from ileal conduits or by invasive procedures (like percutaneous nephrostomy or by cystoscopy) is obtained by personnel specifically trained in these techniques.
- The specimen should be transported to the laboratory within 2 hours after collection. If transport is delayed, the specimen may be refrigerated for up to 24 hours.
  - Alternatively, urine may be inoculated into a preservative collection system, allowing transport up to 48 hours. Preservative systems must be inoculated according to the manufacturer's instructions. Preserved specimens are transported at room temperature.
  - There are several commercially available systems that allow culture media to be directly inoculated at the site of collection. These systems may be incubated prior to transport to the laboratory.

➤ Interpretation

- **Expected results:** $<10^3$ colonies/mL for routine urine cultures; $<10^2$ colonies/mL for special cultures taken from patients at high risk for complicated UTI.
- **Positive:** Clinically significant positive cultures are typically positive for a common uropathogen at concentrations $>10^4$ colonies/mL as a sole or predominant isolate. Isolation of *Staphylococcus saprophyticus* may be considered significant in women at levels of 10^3 colonies per milliliter.

➤ Limitations

- Prior antimicrobial therapy can inhibit the growth of uropathogens, resulting in false-negative cultures.
- **Common pitfalls:**
  - Contamination, due to poorly collected or transported urine samples, limits the value of a significant proportion of specimens submitted to the laboratory.
  - Clinically significant polymicrobial UTI is uncommon ($<5\%$). Interpret mixed cultures with caution—they most likely indicate contaminated specimens.

- Urine is frequently transported in collection cups on which the caps are not firmly tightened, resulting in leakage and possible contamination.
- Urethritis and vaginitis may be associated with pyuria and clinically mimic cystitis.

➤ Suggested Reading

McCarter YS, Burd EM, Hall GS, Zervos M. *Cumitech 2C, Laboratory Diagnosis of Urinary Tract Infections.* Washington, DC: ASM Press; 2009.

VANCOMYCIN-RESISTANT ENTEROCOCCUS (VRE) SCREEN CULTURE

➤ Definition and Use

- This test is usually ordered to detect VRE carriage in asymptomatic patients for infection control purposes. It is indicated to screen patients at risk for transmitting VRE to close contacts, like other hospitalized patients. The test may also be requested to document clearance of VRE carriage.
- A patient specimen is plated onto selective agar, typically containing 6 µg/mL vancomycin. Any growth of *Enterococcus* likely represents VRE, but vancomycin resistance and identification should be confirmed by subsequent testing of the isolate.
- Swab specimens of rectum or perianal skin are recommended for VRE screening cultures.
- **Turnaround time:** 48 hours

➤ Interpretation

- **Expected results:** negative

➤ Limitations

- **Common pitfall:** The VRE screening culture is usually not indicated for evaluation of potentially infected material. Because only selective media is used for screening, other potential pathogens would be missed if VRE screening culture only is requested. VRE grow well in wound and other cultures submitted for evaluation of infected specimens.

VARICELLA-ZOSTER VIRUS (VZV) CULTURE (RULE OUT)

➤ Definition

- VZV is most commonly associated with chickenpox and shingles. Clinical diagnosis is usually straightforward for these infections. Occasionally, specific diagnosis may be needed for unusual, serious infections, including disseminated disease, or infections in pregnant, immunocompromised, and other high-risk patients.

➤ Use

- This test may be used to isolate VZV if specific diagnosis is required.
- Patient specimens are usually inoculated onto human lung fibroblast cell cultures, like WI-38. Cell morphology is monitored; cultures showing cytopathic effect typical for VZV should be confirmed using specific immunologic techniques, like staining with tagged monoclonal anti-VZV antibodies.
- **Turnaround time:** Up to 4 weeks. Most positive cultures are detected within 7 days.

➤ Special Collection and Transport Instructions
- General recommendations for viral culture apply.
- Specimens should be collected early in acute infection.
- Specimens should be collected according to general recommendations for virus culture of the specimen type. Specimens from cutaneous or mucous membranes are most commonly submitted for viral culture to rule out VZV. Samples should be taken from fresh, wet lesions, ideally from intact vesicles after unroofing.
- Most specimens should be placed in viral transport medium and transported on wet ice (4°C).

➤ Interpretation
- **Expected results:**
  - **Positive:** Cell cultures positive for VZV indicate active infection.
  - **Negative:** Negative cell cultures do not rule out VZV infection, especially for CSF and mucosal surface samples.

➤ Limitations
- There may be poor sensitivity for certain specimen types.
- **Turnaround time** for VZV culture may be prolonged, limiting their utility for acute management of critically ill patients.
- **Common pitfall:** collection of specimens from dried, over-crusted lesions.

VARICELLA-ZOSTER VIRUS (VZV) DIRECT DETECTION (DFA)

➤ Use
- This test is used to diagnose VZV infection by detection of VZV antigens in typical skin lesions. It may be ordered in patients presenting with a vesicular rash in whom specific and rapid diagnosis of VZV infection is important for therapy or management.
- Cells scraped from the base of a vesicle or wet ulcerated lesions are used to make a smear on a glass slide. After fixation, the smear is stained with a VZV-specific antibody reagent tagged with a fluorescent label. After washing away excess reagent, the slide is examined by fluorescence microscopy for the presence of cells showing fluorescent staining.
- **Turnaround time:** <24 hours.
- **Special collection and transport instructions:** Cells are collected from the base of wet skin ulcers or vesicles (after unroofing) with a swab or edge of a scalpel. Slides are prepared by gently rolling the swab or spreading cells collected by scalpel onto the slide surface.

➤ Interpretation
- **Expected results:** negative
- **Positive:** The presence of any cells showing +2 or greater specific fluorescent staining.
- **Negative:** No cells showing fluorescent staining.

➤ Limitations
- The slide must be assessed to ensure cells are present in the smear. If no cells are present, the slide is uninterpretable.
- The number of staining cells drops with evolution of the skin lesion from vesicle to crusted/healing ulcer.

- Faint staining may be an indication of problems with the staining technique or reagents.
- **Common pitfalls:** poor collection of cells from the lesion base; sampling crusted, healing lesions.

VARICELLA-ZOSTER VIRUS (VZV) SEROLOGY SCREEN (IgG AND IgM)

➤ Definition

- VZV infection causes two clinically distinct forms of disease. Primary infection with VZV results in varicella (chickenpox), characterized by vesicular lesions in different stages of development on the face, trunk, and extremities. Herpes zoster, also known as "shingles," results from reactivation of endogenous latent VZV infection within the sensory ganglia. This clinical form of the disease is characterized by a painful, unilateral vesicular eruption, which usually occurs in a restricted dermatomal distribution.
- The diagnosis of these two diseases is usually made clinically. However, the use of diagnostic assays may be important in specific situations.
- Other names include chickenpox serology testing
- **Normal range:** negative

➤ Use

- To assist in the diagnosis of acute-phase infection with varicella virus
- To assist in identifying non-immune individuals

➤ Interpretation

- A positive IgG result coupled with a positive IgM result indicates recent infection with VZV.
- A positive IgG result coupled with a negative IgM result indicates previous exposure to VZV and immunity.
- A negative IgG result coupled with a negative IgM result indicates the absence of prior exposure to VZV and no immunity. However, a negative result does not rule out a VZV infection. Negative results in suspected early VZV infections should be followed by testing a new serum specimen in 2–3 weeks.
- Equivocal results should be followed up with testing a new serum specimen within 10–14 days.

➤ Limitations

- Test for VZV IgG antibodies is of use when clinical symptoms are present or infection suspected. Screening of the general population leads to no appreciable diagnostic advantage. Results from immunosuppressed patients should be interpreted with caution.
- Many different antibody tests are available with a wide range of performance standards. The fluorescent antibody to membrane antibody (FAMA) is the most extensively validated assay and correlates best with susceptibility to and protection against varicella. However, this test is not widely used because it is labor intensive and requires expert interpretation.
- Many commercially available ELISAs are available that are considered generally less sensitive than FAMA, although specificities are comparable.
- Commercial ELISA assays are suitable for screening for VZV susceptibility among health care workers. The rationale for this is that the risk of vaccinating an adult with a false-negative test

result is much lower than the risk of natural infection in an individual falsely identified as seropositive.
* Routine screening for varicella in individuals born in the United States before 1980, who are not health care workers, is not recommended because of extremely high rates of seropositivity in this population.

VIBRIO CULTURE (RULE OUT)

➤ Definition
* *Vibrio* species are an uncommon cause of bacterial enteric infections in this country, but endemic infections occur in many countries. Epidemic outbreaks are well described, generally associated with inadequately treated sewage or contaminated water. *Vibrio* species are halophilic, and brackish water and shellfish serve as an important reservoir for organisms. Although infection may be relatively mild and self-limited, some patients develop cholera: severe disease with vomiting and profuse watery diarrhea (rice water stools). The severe diarrhea may rapidly lead to life-threatening dehydration and electrolyte imbalance.
* Stool culture to rule out *Vibrio* species should be considered for patients who develop diarrhea, especially severe watery diarrhea, after travel to an endemic area, ingestion of contaminated sea food, or exposure to brackish water of the Gulf Coast.

➤ Use
* This culture is used to detect enteric infection caused by *Vibrio cholerae* or related *Vibrio* species.
* Colonies from routine stool culture may be screened for cytochrome oxidase positive isolates, which should be further tested to rule out *Vibrio* species. Detection is improved by the use of thiosulfate citrate bile sucrose (TCBS) media, differential and selective media for *Vibrio* isolation. Broth enrichment using alkaline peptone water may be used to improve isolation.
* **Turnaround time:** Cultures are incubated for 48 hours. Additional time is required for isolation and identification.

➤ Interpretation
* **Expected results:** no growth

➤ Limitations
* *Vibrio* enteric infection may be missed if specific cultures are not requested.

WOUND CULTURE

➤ Definition and Use
* Wound cultures are used to identify pathogenic bacteria causing infections of wounds.
* Traumatic injury of tissue may be complicated by infection. Infections may be caused by organisms introduced from the external environment, like bite, surgical and traumatic wounds, or by organisms derived from the patient's endogenous flora, like sinusitis, peritonitis associated with ruptured appendix, and dental abscesses. Wound culture should be considered when a wound shows signs and symptoms typical of infection: swelling, redness, exudate or pus formation, sinus tract formation, pain, swelling, or other.

- Most specimens for bacterial wound cultures should be examined by Gram staining. Specimens from superficial wounds showing a significant numbers of epithelial cells are likely to be contaminated by endogenous flora unrelated to the infection. Additional specimens collected with improved superficial decontamination or by more invasive means, like aspiration or biopsy, should be considered.
- Specimens are inoculated onto supportive and enriched nonselective media, like SBA and chocolate agar, and selective media, like MacConkey, PEA, and CNA agar. Some laboratories include a broth media, like thioglycollate broth, to routine cultures. Anaerobic media is inoculated for appropriate specimens collected and submitted under anaerobic conditions.
- **Turnaround time:** Cultures are incubated for 48–72 hours. Additional time is required for isolation, identification, susceptibility testing, and further characterization, as needed.

➤ Special Collection and Transport Instructions
- Wash and decontaminate the collection site using a soap and 70% alcohol.
- Specimens should be collected from the site of active infection. Adjacent areas may show "sympathetic" signs of inflammation, but may not yield relevant pathogens.
- Collection of infected tissue or aspirate, at least one gram, is recommended. Collection using swabs is not recommended.
- Collection and transport under anaerobic conditions is recommended, especially for closed wounds. Specimens should be transported to the laboratory within 2 hours. Specimens may be held at 4°C for a short time if transport is delayed.

➤ Interpretation
- **Expected results:** no growth
- **Positive:** Cultures of infected wounds often show growth of several types of organisms. Cultures must be interpreted carefully. Mixed cultures may be caused by contamination due to poor specimen collection. However, mixed cultures may represent synergistic polymicrobial infections, especially when anaerobes are isolated.

➤ Limitations
- Significant pathogens may not be isolated in mixed cultures due to contamination or polymicrobial infections.
- Multiple cultures may be required to identify the cause of chronic infections. The structure and milieu of abscesses may prevent effective medical treatment. They are avascular spaces and their outer capsule may prevent entry of antimicrobial agents. In addition, antibiotics may be inactivated by the acidic environment and degradative enzymes present. Surgical therapy may be required, especially for large collections of pus.
- **Common pitfall:** Collection of specimens from sites other than the active site of infection, such as sinus tracts, often yield growth of endogenous flora unrelated to the infection.

➤ Other Considerations
- Pyogenic infections are usually associated with heavy growth (10^5 CFU/mL or greater) of the responsible pathogen.
- Gram stain should be performed on specimens submitted for wound culture.
- Polymicrobial infections are often treated successfully with surgical and/or empirical antimicrobial therapy. Extensive culture analysis with identification and susceptibility of multiple isolates is usually not clinically indicated.

• Certain pathogens are associated with specific types of wound infections, such as *P. aeruginosa* with penetrating foot wounds through sneakers and *P. multocida* with cat bites.

YERSINIA ENTEROCOLITICA CULTURE (RULE OUT)

➤ Definition

• *Yersinia enterocolitica* is an infrequent cause of bacterial enteric infection, usually in children and more commonly diagnosed in winter months.
  • Infection has been associated with ingestion of undercooked pork, dairy products, and tainted water. Infection can also be transmitted by the fecal–oral route.
  • Symptoms are fairly nonspecific: fever, abdominal pain, and diarrhea, which may be bloody. Abdominal pain in adults may mimic appendicitis.
• This test is a specialized stool culture for the detection of GI infection caused by *Y. enterocolitica*.

➤ Use

• *Y. enterocolitica* may be isolated using selective media, like MacConkey agar. *Y. enterocolitica* isolation may be improved by incubation at 25°C. Many laboratories use a more selective medium, like CIN agar (cefsulodin-ingrasan-novobiosin), to improve recovery. Cold enrichment, holding stool suspended in buffered saline at 4°C prior to subculture onto enteric media, may improve recovery in heavily contaminated specimens.
• **Turnaround time:** Cultures are examined for 48 hours. Several days are required for isolation and identification of suspected isolates.

➤ Interpretation

• **Expected results:** no growth

➤ Limitations

• The symptoms of yersiniosis are not specific and this enteric pathogen may not be suspected unless specific risk factors or epidemiologic evidence suggests this infection.
• Cold enrichment is rarely required for isolation.
• Isolates are sucrose positive, so isolates may be missed by laboratories using EMB agar for enteric cultures. (EMB medium contains sucrose so isolates will look similar to normal enteric flora.)

Cardiovascular Disorders

Guy Vallaro

This chapter provides the latest information for the diagnosis of cardiac diseases and reviews familial dyslipidemias, atherosclerosis, hypertension, vasculitis, infectious heart diseases, chest pain, and cardiac failure. Each entry is organized with a brief definition of the disorder, and information regarding clinical presentation, laboratory findings, and limitations, if appropriate.

HYPERLIPIDEMIA

➤ Definition

- Hyperlipidemia is an elevation of lipids (cholesterol, cholesterol esters, phospholipids, and triglycerides) in the bloodstream; is a risk factor for coronary heart disease (CHD); and promotes atherosclerosis. Lipids are transported as lipoproteins in the body; there are five major types: chylomicrons, VLDLs, intermediate-density lipoproteins (IDLs), LDLs, and HDLs. The protein portion of the lipoprotein are referred as apolipoprotein, of which there are six major classes (A, B, C, D, E, and H) and numerous subclasses (AI, AII, AIV, AV, B48, B200, CI, CII, CIII, and CIV).
- There are a variety of lipid disorders. The diagnosis of primary hyperlipidemia is made after the secondary causes are evaluated and ruled out or attempt is made to treat or eliminate the underlying cause. Secondary causes of dyslipidemia and associated lipid changes include some underlying disease, organ failure, or some drugs. It is not uncommon to have some overlap, with dyslipidemia being attributed to both primary and secondary causes (Table 4-1).
- Historically, primary dyslipidemias, such as the familial dyslipidemias, have been grouped according to the electrophoretic activity. The primary dyslipidemias are associated with overproduction and/or impaired removal of lipoproteins. A potentially more useful presentation of primary lipidemias is to classify them according to the principal lipid abnormality (Table 4-2).

➤ Who Should be Suspected?

- There are typically no symptoms associated with hyperlipidemia, and it tends to be discovered during routine examination or evaluation for atherosclerotic cardiovascular disease. Detection of cholesterol disorders and other CHD risk factors occurs primarily through clinical case findings. On occasion, symptoms can include xanthomas around the eyes, Achilles tendons, and the extensor tendons of the hands, particularly with familial forms of the disorder.
- Individuals with higher lipid levels may develop lipemia retinalis (white appearance of the retina), arcus senilis (white discoloration of the peripheral cornea), or pancreatitis.

➤ Laboratory Findings

- Core laboratory: Standard lipid profile—total cholesterol (TC), LDL cholesterol, HDL cholesterol, and triglycerides (TGs)—should be obtained at least once every 5 years in adults age 20 and older.
  - Low-risk persons: Further testing is not required if the HDL-cholesterol level is ≥40 mg/dL and TC is <200 mg/dL.
  - High-risk persons: Lipoprotein measurement is recommended as a guide to clinical management. More frequent measurements are required for persons with multiple risk factors or, in those with 0–1 risk factors, if the LDL level is only slightly below the goal level.
- Apolipoprotein (LpA): Elevated in the presence of concomitant hypercholesterolemia or hypoalphalipoproteinemia—may aid in risk assessment for CHD.
- Lipoprotein electrophoresis: Shows a specific abnormal pattern in <2% of Americans; may be indicated if serum TG >300 mg/dL; fasting serum is lipemic; or if significant

TABLE 4-1. Diseases That May Cause Dyslipidemia and Associated Lipid Changes

Cause	Changes
Diabetes mellitus	TG↑, HDL-C↓
Hypothyroidism	LDL-C↑
Acromegaly	TG↑
Anorexia nervosa	LDL-C↑
Lipodystrophy	TG↑, HDL-C↓
Glycogen storage disorders	TG↑
Nephrotic syndrome	Mixed hyperlipidemia (LDL-C↑ predominates)
Chronic renal failure	TG↑
Obstructive liver disease	LDL-C↑, lipoprotein X↑
Alcohol	TG↑
Immunoglobulin excess: paraproteinemia	Mixed hyperlipidemia
Medications	
β-Adrenoceptor antagonists (selective)	HDL-C↓, TG↑
Thiazide diuretics	LDL-C↑, TG↑ or no change
Glucocorticoids	LDL-C↑ or no change, TG↑ or no change, HDL-C↑
Cyclosporine	LDL-C↑, TG↑
Interferons	TG↑
Antiviral medications (HIV protease inhibitors)	TG↑, LDL-C↑, HDL-C↓
Exogenous estrogens	TG↑, HDL-C↑, LDL-C↓
Retinoic acid derivatives	LDL-C↑, TG↑, HDL-C↓

HDL-C, high density lipoprotein-cholesterol; LDL-C, low density lipoprotein-cholesterol; TG, triglyceride; ↑, increased levels; ↓, decreased levels.

hyperglycemia, impaired glucose tolerance, or glycosuria is present. There is increased serum uric acid >8.5 mg/dL and/or strong family history of premature CHD.

- Molecular tests: Pharmacogenomic studies have shown a genetic predisposition for individuals to develop heart disease. Genetic tests are currently being developed that will allow for personalized medicine for the treatment of dyslipidemias.
- Considerations:
  - If lipid screen is normal, further testing should be performed with consideration paid to the measurement of Lp(a) and apolipoproteins B and A-I. A standard serum lipid profile consists of total cholesterol, TG, and HDL-cholesterol.
  - Measure serum TC, HDL cholesterol, and TG after a 12- to 13-hour fast to minimize the influence of postprandial hyperlipidemia (total and HDL cholesterol can be measured in fasting or nonfasting individuals because the difference is clinically insignificant). Average results of two or three tests; if a difference of ≥30 mg/dL appears, repeat tests 1–8 weeks apart and average the results of three tests.
- Use TC for initial case finding and classification and monitoring of diet therapy. Do not use age- or sex-specific cholesterol values as decision levels.
- Consider values in association with clinical risk factors (e.g., age, gender, obesity, smoking, hypertension, and family history).

TABLE 4-2. Classification of Familial Dyslipidemias According to Predominant Lipid Abnormality and Etiology

Increased Cholesterol	Increased Triglyceride	Increased Cholesterol and Triglyceride	Decreased HDL	Increased HDL
Familial hypercholesterolemia	Familial hypertriglyceridemia	Familial combined hyperlipidemia	Familial hypoalphalipoproteinemia of unknown genetic defect	Familial hyperalphalipoproteinemia of unknown etiology
Polygenic hypercholesterolemia	Deficiency of lipoprotein lipase	Familial dysbetalipoproteinemia	Apoprotein A1 deficiency	CETP deficiency
Familial defective apoprotein B100	Deficiency of apoprotein CII		LCAT deficiency	Apoprotein A1 overexpression
Familial combined hyperlipidemia			Fish-eye disease	
			Tangier disease	

CETP, cholesteryl ester transport protein; HDL, high-density lipoprotein; LCAT = lecithin cholesterol acyltransferase; TG = triglyceride.

DISORDERS OF LIPID METABOLISM

ACID LIPASE DEFICIENCIES

➤ **Definition**
* Acid lipase deficiencies are characterized by the inability to hydrolyze lysosomal TG and cholesteryl esters.

➤ **Laboratory Findings**
* Decreased acid lipase in lymphocytes or fibroblasts
* Increased serum TG, LDL-C, and cholesterol esters

METABOLIC SYNDROME (SYNDROME X)

* Metabolic syndrome is a recently recognized constellation of findings, possibly caused by insulin resistance, including hypertension, abdominal obesity, and prothrombotic and proinflammatory states. Glucose intolerance with fasting blood glucose is 110–125 mg/dL.

ATHEROGENIC DYSLIPIDEMIA

* TG >150 mg/dL, HDL-C <40 mg/dL in men and <50 mg/dL in women, with small dense LDL particles.
* Abnormalities in fibrinolysis and coagulation
* Exclusion of other causes of dyslipidemia (e.g., cholestasis, hypothyroidism, chronic renal failure, nephrotic syndrome).

HYPERALPHALIPOPROTEINEMIA (HDL-C EXCESS)

* This condition is inherited as a simple autosomal dominant trait in families with longevity, or it may be caused by alcoholism, extensive exposure to chlorinated hydrocarbon pesticides, or exogenous estrogen supplementation.
* It occurs in 1 in 20 adults with mildly increased TC levels (240–300 mg/dL) secondary to increased HDL-C (>70 mg/dL). LDL-C is not increased, and TG is normal.

SEVERE HYPERTRIGLYCERIDEMIA (TYPE I) (FAMILIAL HYPERCHYLOMICRONEMIA SYNDROME)

➤ **Definition**
* Hypertriglyceridemia is a rare autosomal recessive trait due to deficiency of lipoprotein lipase (LPL) or apo C-II or circulating inhibitor of LPL.
* There is marked heterogeneity in causative molecular defects.

➤ Laboratory Findings
* Core laboratory: changes due to fatty liver (increased serum transaminase)
  * Persistent very high TG (>1000 mg/dL) with marked increase in VLDL and chylomicrons.
  * Deficiency of apo C-II is shown by isoelectric focusing or two-dimensional gel electrophoresis of plasma.

FAMILIAL HYPERCHOLESTEROLEMIA (TYPE II)

➤ Definition
* Familial hypercholesterolemia is inherited as an autosomal dominant disorder. Homozygous patients are very rare (1 per million).
* Clinical manifestations include increased TC (xanthomata, corneal arcus, CAD that causes death usually before age 30 years). Heterozygous patients present with premature CAD; tendinous xanthomas and corneal arcus are often present.

➤ Laboratory Findings
* Homozygous
  * TC is very high (600–1000 mg/dL) with corresponding increase in LDL.
  * Neonatal diagnosis requires finding increased LDL-C in cord blood; serum TC is unreliable. Because of marked variation in serum TC levels during the first year of life, diagnosis should be deferred until 1 year of age. Prenatal diagnosis of homozygous fetus can be made by estimation of binding sites on fibroblasts cultured from amniotic fluids; useful when both parents are heterozygous.
* Heterozygous
  * Increased serum TC (300–500 mg/dL) and LDL (two to three times normal) with similar change in a parent or first-degree relative; serum TG and VLDL are normal in 90% and slightly increased in 10% of these cases.
  * Gene frequency occurs in 1 in 500 in the general population, but 5% in survivors of acute myocardial infarction (AMI) <60 years old. Plasma TG is normal in type II-A but increased in type II-B. This is not the most common cause of phenotype II-A.
  * LDL receptors in fibroblasts or mononuclear blood cells are <25% in homozygous and 50% of normal levels.

POLYGENIC HYPERCHOLESTEROLEMIA (TYPE IIA)

➤ Definition
* Polygenic hypercholesterolemia can be diagnosed only after secondary causes of hypercholesterolemia and autosomal dominant traits have been excluded.
* Premature CAD occurs later in life than with familial combined hyperlipidemia. Xanthomas are rare.

➤ Laboratory Findings
* Persistent TC elevation (>240 mg/dL) and increased LDL without familial hypercholesterolemia or familial combined hypercholesterolemia
* In type IIB disease, both LDL and VLDL are increased.

FAMILIAL COMBINED HYPERLIPIDEMIA (TYPES IIB, IV, V)

➤ Definition
* Familial combined hyperlipidemia occurs in 0.5% of general population and 15% of survivors of AMI <60 years old. Premature CAD occurs later in life (after age 30 years) than with familial hypercholesterolemia.
* Xanthomas are rare. Patients are often overweight.

➤ Laboratory Findings
* There may be any combination of increased LDL-C and VLDL and chylomicrons; HDL-C is often low.
* Different family members may have increased serum TC or TG or both.

FAMILIAL DYSBETALIPOPROTEINEMIA (TYPE III)

➤ Definition
* Familial dysbetalipoproteinemia occurs in 1 per 5,000–10,000 persons.
* Atherosclerosis is more common in peripheral than coronary arteries. Tuberous and tendinous xanthomas and palmar and plantar xanthomatous streaks are present.

➤ Laboratory Findings
* Diagnosis by combination of ultracentrifugation and isoelectric focusing that shows abnormal apoprotein E pattern.
* Abnormality of apoprotein E with excess of abnormal lipoprotein (beta mobility-VLDL); TC >300 mg/dL plus TG >400 mg/dL should suggest this diagnosis.
* VLDL cholesterol-to-TG ratio = 0.3 (normal ratio = 0.2).

➤ Familial Hypertriglyceridemia (Type IV)
* Familial hypertriglyceridemia is an autosomal dominant condition present in 1% of general population and 5% of survivors of AMI <60 years of age. The distinction from familial combined hyperlipidemia is made only by extensive family screening.
* There is elevated TG (usually 200–500 mg/dL) and VLDL with normal LDL-C and decreased HDL-C.

ABETALIPOPROTEINEMIA (BASSEN-KORNZWEIG SYNDROME)

➤ Definition
* Abetalipoproteinemia is a rare autosomal recessive disorder in which the liver and intestine cannot secrete apo B.
* It should be ruled out in children with fat malabsorption, steatorrhea, failure to thrive, neurologic symptoms, pigmented retinopathy, and/or acanthocytosis.

➤ Laboratory Findings
* Hematology
  * Abnormal RBCs (acanthocytes) are present in the PBS; may be 50–90% of RBCs and are characteristic. Decreased RBC life span may vary from severe hemolytic anemia to mild compensated anemia. Abnormal pattern of RBC phospholipids.
  * ESR is markedly decreased (e.g., 1 mm/h).

- Core laboratory
  - Marked decrease in serum TG (<30 mg/dL) with little increase after ingestion of fat, and in TC (20–50 mg/dL). Chylomicrons, LDL-C, VLDL, apo B-48, and apo B-100 are absent; HDL-C may be lower than in normal persons.
  - Low serum carotene levels.
  - A variant is normotriglyceridemic abetalipoproteinemia in which patient can secrete apo B-48 but not apo B-100, resulting in normal postprandial TG values but marked hypocholesterolemia; associated with mental retardation and vitamin E deficiency.
  - There may be decrease of serum β-lipoprotein and cholesterol. Plasma lipids are normal in heterozygotes.
  - Low serum fat-soluble vitamin (A, K, and E) levels.
- Histology: Biopsy of small intestine shows characteristic lipid vacuolization, but this is not pathognomonic (occasionally seen in celiac disease, tropical sprue, juvenile nutritional and megaloblastic anemia).

HYPOBETALIPOPROTEINEMIA

➤ Definition
- Hypobetalipoproteinemia is an autosomal dominant disorder with increased longevity and lower incidence of atherosclerosis.
- At least one parent will show decreased β-lipoprotein.

➤ Laboratory Findings
- There is a marked decrease in LDL-C and LDL-C-to-HDL-C ratio.
- Homozygous patients have decreased serum TC (<50 mg/dL) and TG and undetectable or trace amounts of chylomicrons, VLDL, and LDL.
- Heterozygotes are asymptomatic and have serum TC, LDL-C, and apo B values that are 50% of normal (consistent with codominant disorder); may also be caused by malabsorption of fats, infection, anemia, hepatic necrosis, hyperthyroidism, AMI, acute trauma.

TANGIER DISEASE

➤ Definition
- Tangier disease is a rare autosomal recessive disorder caused by mutations at chromosome 9q31 causing a defect in the metabolism of apo A, in which there is a marked decrease (heterozygous) or absence (homozygous) of HDL.
- Deposits of cholesterol esters in reticuloendothelial cells cause enlarged liver, spleen, and lymph nodes; enlarged orange tonsils; and small orange-brown spots in rectal mucosa. Patients may have premature CAD, mild corneal opacification, and neuropathy in homozygous type.

➤ Laboratory Findings
- Plasma levels of apo A-I and apo A-II are extremely low.
- In homozygotes, HDL-C is usually <10 mg/dL and apo A-I is usually <5 mg/dL.

* In heterozygotes, HDL-C and apo A-I are ~50% of normal. Serum TC (<100 mg/dL), LDL-C, and phospholipids are decreased; TG = 100 to 250 mg/dL. Pre-β-lipoprotein is absent.

LECITHIN-CHOLESTEROL ACYLTRANSFERASE DEFICIENCY (FAMILIAL)

➤ Definition
* Lecithin-cholesterol acyltransferase deficiency is a very rare autosomal recessive disorder of adults.
* It is associated with premature CAD, corneal opacities, and glomerulosclerosis.

➤ Laboratory Findings
* Serum TC is normal but cholesterol esters are virtually absent. Plasma free cholesterol is extremely increased. HDL-C is low.
* Normochromic anemia with large RBCs that are frequently target cells.
* Proteinuria

➤ High HDL-C Lipidemia
* High HDL-C is a rare autosomal recessive disorder causing cholesteryl ester transfer protein gene defects.
* It may be due to active lifestyle, drugs (e.g., estrogens, alcohol, phenytoin, phenobarbital, rifampicin, griseofulvin).

➤ Low HDL-C Lipidemia
* Familial hypoalphalipoproteinemia (autosomal dominant disorder with HDL-C)
* It may be due to deficiency of apo A-I and apo C-III, abetalipoproteinemia, hypobetalipopro-teinemia (<30 mg/dL in women and <40 mg/dL in men), or drugs (isotretinoin, anabolic steroids).

➤ Suggested Reading
Hachem S, Mooradian A. Familial dyslipidaemias: an overview of genetics, pathophysiology and management. *Drugs*. 2006;66(15):1949–1969.

ATHEROSCLEROSIS

➤ Definition
* Atherosclerosis is the condition in which the atheroma (plaque) is the characteristic lesion found in the intima of medium-sized and large arteries as an inflammatory response to injury. The plaques contain lipids, smooth muscle cells, connective tissue, inflammatory cell, and other extracellular constituents.
* The plaque stability is variable and can rupture, triggering thrombosis, which may embolize, leading to potential acute ischemic events.

➤ Who Should be Suspected?
* Atherogenesis occurs over years and is initially asymptomatic until ischemia is clinically manifested. Clinical manifestation is dependent on the particular circulatory bed affected.

Manifestations include myocardial infarction and angina, intermittent claudication and gangrene, stroke, mesenteric ischemia or renal artery stenosis, aneurysms, and arterial dissection.
* Risk factors for atherosclerosis include cigarette smoking, DM, endothelial dysfunction, dyslipidemia, and hypertension.

➤ Laboratory Findings
* Core laboratory: Lp(a) and homocysteine are increased. Elevated CRP (if first result is >3.0 mg/L, repeating the test at least 2 weeks later when patient is in metabolically stable state free of infection or acute illness is recommended).
* Imaging: noninvasive procedure for immunoscintigraphy. Invasive procedures include intravascular ultrasonography, angioscopy, plaque thermography, optical coherence tomography, and elastography.

➤ Suggested Reading
Faxon DP, Fuster V, Libby P, et al. Atherosclerotic Vascular Disease Conference: Writing Group III: Pathophysiology. *Circulation.* 2004;109:2617–2625.

HYPERTENSION

➤ Definition
* Hypertension is present in 18% of adults in the United States, and most (>90%) have essential or primary hypertension, the causes of which are idiopathic. Secondary hypertension is caused by an underlying condition.
* An individual is considered to have hypertension based on the average of two or more or more blood pressure readings, at two or more visits following an initial assessment (Table 4-3).

➤ Who Should be Suspected?
* Mild to moderate essential hypertension is usually asymptomatic. Accelerated or malignant (diastolic >120 mm Hg) hypertension is associated with neurologic symptoms due to intracerebral or subarachnoid bleeding (headache, nausea, vomiting, somnolence, confusion, seizures, coma) and/or visual disturbance (retinal hemorrhages and exudates or papilledema).
* Secondary hypertension symptoms are associated with the underlying pathology including endocrine, renal, CNS, and other diseases (e.g., toxemia of pregnancy, polycythemia, acute porphyria). Drugs and toxic substances may be involved.

TABLE 4-3. Blood Pressure Classification Suggested by the Joint National Committee

Classification	Systolic Pressure (mm Hg)		Diastolic Pressure (mm Hg)
Normal	<120	and	<80
Prehypertension	120–139	or	80–89
Stage 1 hypertension	140–159	or	90–99
Stage 2 hypertension	≥160	or	≥100

Source: The Seventh Report of the Joint National Committee on Prevention, Detection, Evaluation, and Treatment of High Blood Pressure. *Hypertension.* 2003;42:1206.

➤ Laboratory Findings

* Core laboratory: Decreased potassium. Increased calcium. Abnormal renal function tests (microalbuminuria, BUN, creatinine, uric acid). Impaired fasting glucose.
* Laboratory findings due to the underlying disease: TSH and T_4 decreased
* Considerations:
  * It is important to rule out underlying conditions that may be causing hypertension.
  * When hypertension is associated with decreased serum potassium, rule out antihypertensive medication, Cushing syndrome, aldosteronism, and diuretic administration.
  * Laboratory findings due to administration of some antihypertensive drugs, such as:
    * Oral diuretics (e.g., benzothiadiazines): hyperuricemia, hypokalemia, or hyperglycemia or aggravation of preexisting DM; less commonly, bone marrow depression, aggravation of renal or hepatic insufficiency, cholestatic hepatitis, or toxic pancreatitis.
    * Hydralazine: syndrome may not be distinguishable from SLE. ANA may be found in ≤50% of asymptomatic patients.
    * Methyldopa: ≤20% of patients may have positive direct Coombs test, but relatively few have hemolytic anemia. When drug is discontinued, Coombs test may remain positive for months, but anemia usually reverses promptly. Abnormal liver function tests indicate hepatocellular damage without jaundice. Rheumatoid factor (RF) and SLE tests may occasionally be positive.
    * Monoamine oxidase inhibitors (e.g., pargyline hydrochloride): wide range of toxic reactions, most serious of which are blood dyscrasias and hepatocellular necrosis.
* Imaging studies: angiography, magnetic resonance angiography, CT angiography, and Doppler ultrasound (least invasive imaging test for renal artery stenosis).

➤ Suggested Readings

Aram VC, Bakris GL; Black HR, et al., and the National High Blood Pressure Education Program Coordinating Committee. The Seventh Report of the Joint National Committee on Prevention, Detection, Evaluation, and Treatment of High Blood Pressure. *JAMA.* 2003;289:2073–2082.

Papadakis MA, McPhee SJ. *Current Medical Diagnosis and Treatment 2009.* New York: McGraw-Hill Professional; 2008.

VASCULITIS

➤ Definition

* Vasculitis describes a heterogeneous group of disorders that are characterized by leukocyte migration in the vessel wall resulting in damage of blood vessels, which leads to tissue ischemia and necrosis.
* Size and shape of both arteries and veins are affected due to a primary process or secondary to an underlying pathology.

➤ Classification By
Etiology

* Primary: polyarteritis nodosa, Wegener granulomatosis, giant cell arteritis, hypersensitivity vasculitis
* Secondary

- Infections: bacteria (e.g., septicemia caused by gonococcal organisms or *Staphylococcus*), mycobacteria, viruses (e.g., CMV, hepatitis B), rickettsia (e.g., Rocky Mountain spotted fever), spirochetes (e.g., syphilis, Lyme disease)
- Associated with malignancy (e.g., multiple myeloma, lymphomas)
- Connective tissue diseases (e.g., RA, SLE, Sjögren syndrome)
- Diseases that may simulate vasculitis (e.g., ergotamine toxicity, cholesterol embolization, atrial myxoma)

Size of Involved Vessel (Noninfectious Vasculitis)

- Large vessel: dissection of aorta (dissecting aneurysm), Takayasu arteritis, giant cell (temporal) arteritis
- Medium-sized vessel: polyarteritis nodosa (or small), Kawasaki disease, primary granulomatous CNS vasculitis
- Small vessel: ANCA-associated vasculitis (Wegener granulomatosis, Churg-Strauss syndrome, drug-induced, microscopic polyangiitis), immune complex–type vasculitis (Henoch-Schönlein purpura, cryoglobulinemia, rheumatoid vasculitis [or medium], SLE, Sjögren syndrome, Goodpasture syndrome, Behçet syndrome, drug-induced, serum sickness), paraneoplastic vasculitis (lymphoproliferative, myeloproliferative, carcinoma), inflammatory bowel disease
- Any size vessel (pseudovasculitis): antiphospholipid syndrome, emboli (e.g., myxomas, cholesterol emboli, bacterial or nonbacterial endocarditis), drugs (e.g., amphetamines)

► Who Should be Suspected?

- Patients may present with fatigue, weakness, fever, myalgias, arthralgia, headache, abdominal pain, hypertension, nosebleeds, palpable purpura, and/or mononeuritis.

► Laboratory Findings

The gold standard in the diagnosis of most vasculitides is based on pathologic findings in a biopsy of the involved tissue.

- Hematology: ESR is increased in 90% of cases, often to very high levels; CRP correlates with disease activity even better than ESR. Normochromic anemia of chronic disease, thrombocytosis, and mild leukocytosis occur in 30–40% of patients; eosinophilia may occur but is not a feature. Leukopenia or thrombocytopenia occurs only during cytotoxic therapy.
- Urinalysis: hematuria, proteinuria, and azotemia
- Core laboratory: Serum globulins (IgG and IgA) are increased in ≤50% of cases. Serum C3 and C4 complement levels may be increased. RF may be present in low titer. ANA positive in vasculitis secondary to connective tissue disorders. ANCA determination provides valuable information and is highly specific for the diagnosis of small-vessel vasculitides, particularly Wegener's granulomatosis
- Imaging studies: arteriogram, MRI, and ultrasound
- Considerations
  - c-ANCA (anti-proteinase 3; coarse diffuse cytoplasmic pattern) is highly specific (>90%) for active Wegener granulomatosis. Sensitivity is >90% in systemic vasculitic phase, ~65% in predominantly granulomatous disease of respiratory tract, and ~30% during complete remission.
  - ELISA titer does not correlate with disease activity; a high titer may persist during remission for years. c-ANCA is also occasionally found in other vasculitides (polyarteritis

nodosa, microscopic polyangiitis [e.g., lung, idiopathic crescentic and pauci-immune GN], Churg-Strauss vasculitis).

* p-ANCA (against various proteins [e.g., myeloperoxidase, elastase, lysozyme; perinuclear pattern]) occurs only with fixation in alcohol, not formalin. A positive result should be confirmed by ELISA. The test has poor specificity and 20–60% sensitivity in a variety of autoimmune diseases (microscopic polyangiitis, Churg-Strauss vasculitis, SLE, inflammatory bowel disease, Goodpasture syndrome, Sjögren syndrome, idiopathic GN, chronic infection). However, pulmonary small vessel vasculitis is strongly linked to myeloperoxidase antibodies.
* Both p-ANCA and c-ANCA may be found in non–immune-mediated polyarteritis and other vasculitides.
* Atypical pattern (neither c-ANCA nor p-ANCA; unknown target antigens) has poor specificity and unknown sensitivity in various conditions (e.g., HIV infection, endocarditis, CF, Felty syndrome, Kawasaki disease, ulcerative colitis, Crohn disease).

ANTIPHOSPHOLIPID SYNDROME*

➤ Definition
* Antiphospholipid syndrome (APS) is defined by the simultaneous presence of clinical and laboratory criteria.
* It is characterized clinically by the occurrence of either venous or arterial thrombotic events in various vascular beds or obstetrical complications.

➤ Who Should be Suspected?
* Medical patients: APS occurs either as a primary condition, or in the setting of an underlying disease, most commonly SLE, or other connective tissue disorders, infections, or drugs. Patients develop venous thrombosis (DVT), pulmonary embolism (PE), arterial vasoocclusive events (myocardial infarction or stroke), transient ischemic attack, amaurosis fugax, autoimmune thrombocytopenia, hemolytic anemia, and livedo reticularis.
* Obstetric patients: unexplained fetal death, recurrent pregnancy loss, severe preeclampsia diagnosed before 34 weeks of gestation, early onset (second or early third trimester) of severe intrauterine growth restriction, SLE, and biologically false-positive serologic test for syphilis

➤ Diagnosis
* The diagnosis of APS requires the persistence of antibodies for at least 12 weeks. Lupus anticoagulants (LAs) are more commonly associated with thrombotic events than are the anticardiolipin antibodies (ACLAs), which are directed against phospholipid-binding plasma proteins. aPL comprise a heterogeneous family of auto- and alloantibodies (IgG and IgM subclasses) directed against specific plasma proteins with affinity for phospholipid surfaces. The antigenic targets are b (beta)2-glycoprotein I, factor II (prothrombin), and possibly protein C, protein S, kininogens, complement factor H, and annexin V. The most commonly

*This section was contributed by Liberto Pechet, MD, from an original draft written by Daniel Baiyee, MD.

detected subgroups of APLA include ACLA, antiprothrombin antibodies, and anti-b (beta)2-glycoprotein I antibodies (anti-b2 GP I).

➤ Laboratory Findings

- A panel of tests should be ordered. The laboratory criteria are the presence in blood of an LA (see p. 249), b (beta)2 glycoprotein I ELISA, and anticardiolipin ELISA antibodies of the IgG or IgM isotype (see p. 51), possibly associated with thrombocytopenia. The following is the sequence of coagulation-based tests for LA used at the University of Massachusetts Memorial Health Care Laboratory:
  1. PT is used mostly to rule out the effect of oral or other anticoagulants. This is followed by two screening tests:
  2. PTT using an LA-sensitive PTT reagent
  3. PT using a dilute reagent, which confirms the suspicion of an LA if elongated. If either (2.) or (3.) is prolonged
  4. Staclot LA test (confirmatory) involves the inhibition of the antibodies by hexagonal phase phospholipid. If an LA is present, the prolonged clotting time in (2.) or (3.) will be corrected.
  5. In addition, a dilute Russell viper venom time (dRVVT) (see p. 159) is performed; the coagulation cascade is initiated with Russell viper venom and a confirmatory test is included.
- Additional coagulation tests (performed in different laboratories) include the kaolin clotting time, which uses no added phospholipid, and the platelet neutralization test, in which the addition of an increased amount of platelet phospholipid neutralizes the LA activity.
- Factor II level determination is indicated in patients with greatly prolonged PT and/or bleeding manifestations. In these patients, antibodies to factor II may be present.
- Immunoassays
  - ELISA tests are used for the detection of IgG or IgA ACA
  - Anti-b (beta)2 GP I ELISA
  - ANA assay may be positive in low titers (1;40 to 1:160)
- CBC to assess possible anemia, leukopenia, and especially thrombocytopenia
- Renal function tests (e.g., BUN, creatinine)

➤ Limitations

- Abnormal PT or PTT. The PT is commonly prolonged, but it may be only borderline prolonged or even normal. Not all reagents for the PTT assay will demonstrate a prolongation, because many are insensitive to the LA. ACA and anti-b (beta)2 GP I are detected by immunoassays that measure immunoreactivity to phospholipids or phospholipid-bound proteins.
- The detection of LA is more difficult (but not impossible) in the presence of heparin or oral anticoagulant therapy. The laboratory should be notified about anticoagulant therapy when the assays are ordered.

➤ Suggested Readings

Boffa MC, Boinot C, Carolis SD, et al. Laboratory criteria of the obstetrical antiphospholipid syndrome. *Thromb Haemost.* 2009;102:25–28.

Giannakopoulos B, Passam F, Ioannou Y, Krollis SA. How we diagnose the antiphospholipid antibody syndrome. *Blood.* 2009;113:985–994.

CHURG-STRAUSS SYNDROME (ALLERGIC GRANULOMATOSIS AND ANGIITIS)*

➤ Definition
* This multisystem disorder is characterized by asthma, allergic rhinitis, peripheral blood and tissue eosinophilia, extravascular granuloma formation, and vasculitis of multiple organs.
* These manifestations are associated with ANCAs.

➤ Who Should be Suspected?
* Candidates include patients with severe asthma and a necrotizing eosinophilic vasculitis. In addition to pulmonary and sinus involvement, other manifestations are mononeuritis multiplex, skin, and less commonly but possibly fatal, heart disease.

➤ Laboratory Findings
Laboratory diagnosis relies on a combination of tissue biopsy (eosinophilic infiltrates, necrosis, eosinophilic giant cell vasculitis) and blood investigations. There are no pathognomonic laboratory assays.
* Hematology: Leukocytosis with peripheral blood eosinophilia (between 5000 to 9000/μL) is found at some point in >80% of patients. It may be missed because of spontaneous fluctuations or corticosteroid therapy preceding the diagnosis. Normochromic, normocytic anemia. Markedly elevated ESR and CRP.
* Core laboratory: Circulating ANCAs are present in 48–66% of patients, but it is not specific for this syndrome. The majority of ANCA-positive patients have antibodies against myeloperoxidase with a perinuclear staining pattern (P-ANCA). Hypergammaglobulinemia with elevated α2 globulins. Elevated serum IgE during the vasculitic phase. Circulating immune complexes. Positive RF at low titer. Normal or elevated complement components C3, C4, CH50.

➤ Suggested Reading
Noth I, Strek ME, Leff AR. Churg-Strauss syndrome. Lancet. 2003;361:587–594.

DISSECTION OF AORTA (DISSECTING ANEURYSM)

* Dissection of the aorta is caused by cystic medial degeneration or unknown causes. Rapid electroimmunoassay of smooth-muscle myosin heavy-chain protein >2.5 ug/L is reported to have S/S >90%/98% during the first 3 hours and to rapidly decrease thereafter. Higher values for proximal than distal dissection.
* Laboratory changes are due to complications/sequelae (e.g., rupture or infarcts of brain, kidney, gut, limbs) or of predisposing conditions (e.g., Marfan syndrome, hypertension, arterial cannulation, unknown).

---

*This section was contributed by Liberto Pechet, MD.

GIANT CELL (TEMPORAL) ARTERITIS*

➤ Definition
- This disorder is a systemic panarteritis of the large and medium-sized vessels, involving especially the cranial branches of the arteries that originate form the aortic arch.
- Visual loss is a major complication of the disease, and failure to make the diagnosis may lead to irreversible visual loss.

➤ Who Should be Suspected?
- Patients older than 50 years with severe bitemporal headache; visual disturbances including partial, transient monocular visual loss, jaw claudication, polymyalgia rheumatica (40% of cases); or other constitutional symptoms.

➤ Diagnosis
- This involves biopsy of the involved arterial segment, commonly the temporal artery; imaging studies; and pertinent, but not specific, laboratory studies.

➤ Laboratory Findings
- Hematology: Increased ESR ($\geq$50 mm/h, mean 88 mm/h) and CRP. A normal sedimentation rate practically rules out giant cell arteritis. Mild to moderate normocytic, normochromic anemia in 50% of patients. Possible macroangiopathic hemolytic anemia.
- Core laboratory: Mildly abnormal liver function tests, particularly increased ALP levels. Increased levels of IgG and complement. Laboratory findings reflect specific organ involvement.

➤ Suggested Reading
Smetana GW, Shmerling RH. Does this patient have temporal arteritis? *JAMA*. 2002;287:92–101.

POLYARTERITIS NODOSA*

➤ Definition
- This systemic necrotizing arteritis affects medium-sized muscular arteries, and rarely, small muscular arteries.

➤ Who Should be Suspected?
- Candidates are middle aged or elderly individuals, more commonly male, who present with nonspecific symptoms of fatigue, arthralgias, or fever, associated with hypertension, renal insufficiency, neurologic dysfunction, skin lesions, muscle involvement, or abdominal pain, or any combination of systemic symptoms and signs.
- The condition may have been preceded by hepatitis B or C.

---

*This section was contributed by Liberto Pechet, MD.

➤ Laboratory Findings

The diagnosis of polyarteritis nodosa is based on the clinical manifestations, biopsy of involved organs, and supplemented by laboratory studies.

- Hematology: elevated ESR and CRP; abnormal cryoglobulin (only occasionally associated with polyarteritis nodosa).
- Serology: used mostly to rule out other autoimmune disorders.

HENOCH-SCHÖNLEIN PURPURA*

➤ Definition

- Henoch-Schönlein purpura is a self-limited hypersensitivity systemic vasculitis of the small vessels. It involves the skin, and to variable degrees joints, kidneys, and GI tract. The small vessel and renal involvement is caused by IgA deposition.

➤ Who Should be Suspected?

- This condition is seen more commonly in children (90% of cases), but it may affect adults as well.
- In adults, renal disease is common. The renal picture may vary, with minimal urinary abnormalities occurring for years. Patients may present with palpable purpura without thrombocytopenia or a coagulopathy and acute abdominal pain, or with purpura and joint symptoms.

➤ Laboratory Findings

Diagnosis is made clinically; there are no pathognomonic laboratory findings.

- Histology: Renal or skin biopsy supports the diagnosis; it shows focal segmental necrotizing GN that becomes more diffuse and crescentic with IgA and C3 deposition.
- Urinalysis: RBCs, casts, and slight protein in 25–50% of patients. The renal picture varies from minimal urinary abnormalities for years to end-stage renal disease within months. Gross hematuria and proteinuria are uncommon.
- Hematology: Coagulation tests are normal.
- Core laboratory: BUN and creatinine may be increased.

➤ Suggested Reading

Trapani S, Micheli A, Grisolla F, et al. Henoch Schönlein Purpura in childhood: epidemiological and clinical analysis of 150 cases over a 5-year period and review of the literature. *Semin Arthritis Rheum*. 2005;35:143–153.

KAWASAKI SYNDROME (MUCOCUTANEOUS LYMPH NODE SYNDROME)

➤ Definition

- Kawasaki syndrome is a variant of childhood polyarteritis of unknown etiology, with a high incidence of coronary artery complications.

---

*This section was contributed by Liberto Pechet, MD.

➤ Laboratory Findings
- Histology: Diagnosis is confirmed by histologic examination of the coronary artery (same as for polyarteritis nodosa).
- Hematology: Anemia (~50% of patients). Leukocytosis (20,000–30,000/μL) with shift to left occurs during first week; lymphocytosis appears thereafter, peaking at the end of the second week, and is a hallmark of this illness. Increased ESR.
- CSF findings: Increased mononuclear cells with normal protein and sugar.
- Urinalysis: Increased mononuclear cells; dipstick negative.
- Joint fluid findings: Increased white blood cell (WBC) count (predominantly PMNs) in patients with arthritis.
- Core laboratory: Laboratory changes due to AMI. Acute-phase reactants are increased (e.g., CRP, α-1-antitrypsin); these usually return to normal after 6–8 weeks.

TAKAYASU SYNDROME (ARTERITIS)

➤ Definition
- Takayasu syndrome is the term for granulomatous arteritis of the aorta.
- Diagnosis is established by characteristic arteriographic narrowing or occlusion or histologic examination. Laboratory tests are not useful for diagnosis or to guide management.

➤ Laboratory Findings
Findings are due to involvement of coronary or renal vessels.
- Hematology: Increased ESR is found in ~75% of cases during active disease but is normal in only 50% of cases during remission. WBC count is usually normal.
- Core laboratory: Serum proteins are abnormal, with increased γ globulins (mostly composed of IgM). Female patients have a continuous high level of urinary total estrogens (rather than the usual rise during the luteal phase after a low excretion during follicular phase).

THROMBOANGIITIS OBLITERANS (BUERGER DISEASE)

- Thromboangiitis obliterans is the vascular inflammation and occlusion of medium and small arteries and veins of limbs; it is related to smoking. Histology shows characteristic inflammatory and proliferative lesions. Laboratory tests are usually normal.

THROMBOPHLEBITIS, SEPTIC

➤ Definition
- Thrombophlebitis is vascular inflammation due to a blood clot.

➤ Laboratory Findings
Findings are due to associated septicemia, complications (e.g., septic pulmonary infarction), and underlying disease.

- Hematology: Increased WBC count (often >20,000/uL), with marked shift to left and toxic changes in neutrophils. DIC may be present.
- Core laboratory: azotemia.
- Culture: Positive blood culture (*Staphylococcus aureus* is the most frequent organism; others are *Klebsiella, Pseudomonas aeruginosa*, enterococci, *Candida*).

WEGENER GRANULOMATOSIS

See Chapter 12, Immune and Autoimmune Diseases

HEART DISEASE

INFECTIOUS*

ENDOCARDITIS

➤ Definition
- Infective endocarditis (IE) is a noncontagious infection of the heart valves (native or prosthetic) or lining. Prosthetic valve endocarditis may account for up to one-fourth of cases of endocarditis overall.

➤ Who Should be Suspected?
- A number of signs and symptoms are common in patients with IE, but none is invariable. Fever, night sweats, anorexia, malaise, and weight loss are common patient complaints. Physical examination usually reveals a heart murmur, which has often been detected previously; the severity or nature of the murmur may have changed. Stigmata of endocarditis may include petechiae of skin, conjunctivae, and mucosal surfaces. Splinter hemorrhages, Roth spots, Janeway lesions, and Osler nodes may be seen.
- Risk factors: preexisting valve disease, nosocomial infection, bone marrow transplant, DM, and rheumatic heart disease.

➤ Diagnosis
- Diagnosis is based on pathologic or clinical criteria, including microbiologic and imaging studies (usually echocardiography).
- The modified Duke criteria use pathologic and clinical criteria for IE diagnosis. Patient history, pathologic and clinical findings, ECG, imaging studies, and laboratory studies are used to determine definitive IE, possible IE, or rejected IE. For complete details of the modified Duke criteria, see Li et al. Additional information about the Duke criteria is available online.

➤ Laboratory Findings
- Culture: Persistent positive blood cultures. Typical organisms (*Streptococcus viridans* [~50% of cases], *S. bovis, Staphylococcus aureus*, HACEK [*Haemophilus, Actinobacillus, Cardiobacterium, Eikenella, Kingella*], enterococci) in ≥2 blood cultures in absence of primary focus, or

---

*The section "Heart Disease, Infectious" was contributed by Michael Mitchell, MD.

TABLE 4-4. Typical Microorganisms in Infective Endocarditis

Organism	Native Valve (%)*		Prosthetic Valve (%)*	
	Neonate	Older#	Early	Late
Streptococcus species	15–20	45–65	1	30–33
Staphylococcus aureus	40–50	25–35	20–24	15–20
Coagulase-negative staphylococci	8–12	4–7	30–35	10–12
Enterococcus species	<1	5–10	5–10	8–12
Gram-negative bacilli	8–12	4–10	10–15	4–7
Fungi	8–12	1–3	5–10	1
HACEK organisms¶ and culture-negative infectious endocarditis	2–6	3–10	3–7	3–8
Diphtheroids	<1	<1	5–7	2–3
Polymicrobial	3–5	1–2	2–4	3–7

*Percentages are approximate.
#Estimated rates for patients >2 mo of age. Rates do vary somewhat among non-neonates. For example, the rate of enterococcal infective endocarditis is greater in patients >60 years of age.
¶HACEK = Haemophilus parainfluenzae, Aggregatibacter actinomycetemcomitans and A. aphrophilus (formerly of the genus Haemophilus), Cardiobacterium hominis, Eikenella corrodens, Kingella kingae.
Adapted from Mylonakis E, Calderwood SB. Infective endocarditis in adults. N Engl J Med. 2001;345(18):1318–1330.

persistently positive blood cultures drawn >1 hour apart. See Table 4-4 for a list of micro-organisms.

- Hematology
  - ESR and CRP are commonly elevated (CRP >100 mg/L or ESR >30 mm/h if <60 years old or >50 mm/h if >60 years old). Progressive normochromic, normocytic anemia is a characteristic feature.
  - WBC count is normal in ~50% of patients and elevated to ≤15,000/μL in the rest, with 65–86% neutrophils. A higher WBC count indicates presence of a complication (e.g., cerebral, pulmonary). Occasionally there is leukopenia. Monocytosis may be pronounced. Large macrophages may occur in peripheral blood. Platelet count is usually normal, but occasionally it is decreased.
- Urinalysis: Hematuria (usually microscopic) may occur in patients due to glomerulitis or renal infarct or focal embolic or diffuse GN.
- Core laboratory: Albuminuria is almost invariable, even without specific renal complications. Nephrotic syndrome is rare.
- Considerations
  - Findings associated with complications, including neurologic complications, metastatic sites of infection, and CHF may be seen.
  - Laboratory findings are due to underlying or predisposing diseases or complications, such as mitral valve prolapse, rheumatic valve disease, CHD, nosocomial infections (GI or GU systems, long-term indwelling IV catheters, especially those with HIV), and mycotic aneurysms.

➤ Suggested Readings

Brouqui P, Raoult D. Endocarditis due to rare and fastidious bacteria. *Clin Microbiol Rev.* 2001;14:177–207.

CLSI. *Principles and Procedures for Blood Cultures; Approved Guideline.* CLSI document M47-A. Wayne, PA: Clinical and Laboratory Standards Institute; 2007.

Houpikian P, Raoult D. Blood culture-negative endocarditis in a reference center: etiologic diagnosis of 348 cases. *Medicine (Baltimore).* 2005;84:162–173.

Li JS, Sexton DJ, Mick N, Nettles R, Fowler VG Jr, Ryan T, et al. Proposed modifications to the Duke criteria for the diagnosis of infective endocarditis. *Clin Infect Dis.* 2000;30:633–638.

MYOCARDITIS

➤ Definition

- Myocarditis, inflammation of the heart muscle, may present with a broad range of symptoms, reflecting the various causes of disease.
- It can be due to infections (bacterial, fungal, viral), immune mediated (SLE, Kawasaki disease), or as a result of toxic injury (e.g., drugs, metals).

➤ Who Should be Suspected?

- Most cases are asymptomatic. Symptomatic disease may present with subtle, nonspecific symptoms (e.g., dyspnea, chest pain) to fulminant disease with cardiogenic shock and death.

➤ Laboratory Findings

- Core laboratory: Elevated acute-phase reactants (ESR, CRP, mild to moderate leukocytosis). Elevated cardiac markers CK-MB, CK-total, troponin T, and troponin I).
- Histology: Definitive diagnosis is based on the presence of myocytolysis and lymphocytic infiltration in endomyocardial biopsy.
- Serology: Altered IgM antibody. Rheumatologic assessment and testing is recommended.

➤ Suggested Readings

Cooper Jr, LT. Myocarditis. *N Engl J Med.* 2009;360:1526–1538.

Leeper NJ, Wener LS, Dhaliwal G, et al. Clinical problem-solving. One surprise after another. *N Engl J Med.* 2005;352:1474–1479.

PERICARDITIS (ACUTE) AND PERICARDIAL EFFUSION

➤ Definition

- The pericardium is a double-walled sac that surrounds the heart. The inner visceral pericardium is normally separated from the outer, fibrous parietal pericardium by a small volume (15–50 mL) of fluid, a plasma ultrafiltrate. Inflammation of the pericardium results in pericarditis, with or without an associated pericardial effusion.
- The common causes of pericardial inflammation include infection, trauma, malignancy, hypersensitivity, and autoimmune diseases.

➤ Who Should be Suspected?

- Typical signs and symptoms of acute pericarditis include chest pain, pericardial friction rub, ECG changes (e.g., ST elevation, PR depression), and pericardial effusion.

• Not all patients will manifest all of these features; the absence of an effusion does not exclude the diagnosis.

➤ Diagnostic and Laboratory Findings

• Echocardiography: Most useful imaging technique for the evaluation of acute pericarditis and is critical for patients if tamponade is suspected. Small pericardial effusions, undetectable by routine examinations, may be detected, providing support for diagnosis of pericardial disease.
• Electrocardiography: ECG abnormalities, like low QRS voltage, may support a diagnosis or suggest alternative diagnoses, such as myocardial infarction.
• Chest x-ray: May detect specific abnormalities, like increased cardiac silhouette ("water-bottle heart"), pleural effusion, or other informative finding.
• Tuberculin skin test or interferon-gamma release assay: Evaluation to rule out TB is recommended for all patients. Additional diagnostic testing for TB, like AFB cultures, should be performed on patients at increased risk on the basis of epidemiologic and clinical factors.
• Cultures: Cultures of blood and other potentially infected specimens should be submitted for patients with significant fever, signs of sepsis, or systemic or local infection.
• Histology: Pericardiocentesis and pericardial biopsy may be performed for patients with clinically significant tamponade or persistent effusions. Pericardiocentesis and biopsy are also recommended for patients in whom pyogenic, tuberculous, or malignant pericardial disease is suspected.
• Recommended tests for pericardial fluid include:
  • Histopathologic and cytologic examination of tissue and fluid
  • Bacterial and mycobacterial stains and culture
  • Triglyceride concentration for chylous fluid
  • Adenosine deaminase and *M. tuberculosis* PCR, if tuberculous pericarditis is suspected
  • Other specific diagnostic tests, like fungal cultures or PCR are performed based on clinical suspicion.
• Recommended core laboratory tests:
  • Core laboratory: CBC, electrolytes, tests of renal function and thyroid function, and serial plasma troponin concentrations. ANA titers, anti-dsDNA, and serum complement are recommended for patients when an autoimmune cause is suspected. Note: Protein, glucose, LDH, RBC count, and WBC count cannot distinguish exudative from transudative effusions and are usually noncontributory in establishing a diagnosis.
• Serology: HIV should be considered. Pericardial disease is relatively common in HIV-infected patients. Furthermore, HIV infection predisposes patients to mycobacterial infections. Viral diagnostic testing, including serology, has low diagnostic yield and is not routinely recommended.

➤ Suggested Readings

Ben-Horin S, Bank I, Shinfeld A, et al. Diagnostic value of the biochemical composition of pericardial effusions in patients undergoing pericardiocentesis. *Am J Cardiol*. 2007;99:1294–1297.
Hidron A, Vogenthaler N, Santos-Preciado JI, et al. Cardiac involvement with parasitic infections. *Clin Microbiol Rev*. 2010;23:324–349.
Lange RA, Hillis D. Acute pericarditis. *N Engl J Med*. 2004;351:2195–2202.
Levy PY, Cory R, Berger P, et al. Etiologic diagnosis of 204 pericardial effusions. *Medicine (Baltimore)*. 2003;82:385–391.

ACUTE RHEUMATIC FEVER

➤ Definition
* Acute rheumatic fever (ARF) is a nonsuppurative sequela of group A streptococcus (GAS) pharyngitis.
* The acute clinical manifestations, as described below, occur 2–4 weeks after the pharyngitis and resolve spontaneously. Damage to the heart valves, however, may lead to chronic disease and increased risk of endocarditis.

➤ Who Should be Suspected?
* ARF usually occurs in children between the ages of 5 and 10 years.
* Physical examination may demonstrate cardiac damage (murmurs), subcutaneous nodules or rash, or transient arthritis of multiple joints. Some patients may display neurologic complications, including Sydenham chorea (involuntary, nonrhythmic movements), and weakness.

➤ Diagnosis
Diagnosis of ARF is made using a combination of laboratory, evidence of preceding GAS infection, and clinical (Jones) criteria. Additional information about the Jones criteria is available online.
* Culture: Positive throat culture. Throat culture may be negative because the onset of ARF symptoms occurs several weeks after acute pharyngitis.
* Hematology: Elevated ESR. WBC may be normal but usually is increased (10,000–16,000/uL) with shift to the left; increase may persist for weeks after fever subsides. Microcytic anemia, with hemoglobin 8–12 g/dL, is common; anemia gradually improves as activity subsides. Fibrinogen is increased.
* Core laboratory: Elevated CRP. Serum proteins are altered, with decreased serum albumin and increased $\alpha 2$ and γ globulins. (Streptococcus A infections alone do not increase $\alpha 2$ globulin.) Serum AST may be increased, but ALT is normal unless the patient has cardiac failure with liver damage. Increased serum cardiac enzymes or biochemical markers of CHF may be seen with acute myocardial damage in patients with severe carditis.
* Serology: Increased titers to streptococcal antigens. The titer is elevated for one or more antigens in 95% of patients with ARF; if all are normal, a diagnosis of ARF is less likely.
* Urinalysis: Mild abnormality of urine may be seen, including albuminuria, casts, RBCs, and WBCs suggesting mild focal nephritis.

➤ Suggested Reading
Ferrieri P. Jones Criteria Working Group. Proceedings of the Jones Criteria workshop. *Circulation*. 2002;106:2521–2523.

CHEST PAIN

➤ Definition
* Ischemic heart disease is a condition in which there is an insufficient supply of blood and oxygen to a portion of the myocardium, and it often occurs when there is a disparity between oxygen supply and demand.

- The term *acute coronary syndrome* refers to a range of acute myocardial ischemic states that encompasses unstable angina, non-ST segment elevation myocardial infarction (non-STEMI; ST segment elevation generally absent), and ST segment elevation infarction (STEMI; persistent ST segment elevation usually present).
- Infarction describes necrosis or death of myocardial cells. Atherosclerotic heart disease is the most common underlying cause of myocardial infarction. The left ventricle is the principal site of infarction; however, right ventricular infarction occasionally occurs with infarction of the inferior wall of the left ventricle. Other causes include embolization, trauma, arteritis, hypercoagulable state, substance abuse (e.g., cocaine), congenital anomalies (e.g., anomalous origin of left coronary from pulmonary artery or sinus of Valsalva), metabolic diseases (e.g., homocystinuria, Hurler syndrome, Fabry disease), and others (coronary artery spasm, aortic dissection, carbon monoxide poisoning, polycythemia vera, thrombocytosis, amyloidosis, anemia).

➤ Etiology
The clinical assessment of chest pain emphasizes distinguishing among a number of potential causes.
- Cardiac sources: acute coronary syndrome (STEMI), non-STEMI, and unstable angina pectoris), stable angina pectoris, aortic dissection, aortic stenosis, mitral valve prolapse, myocarditis, pericarditis, tamponade.
- Noncardiac sources: GI (GERD, esophageal rupture, medication-induced esophagitis), pulmonary (pneumonia, pulmonary embolism, pulmonary hypertension, sarcoidosis, effusion, esophageal rupture, pneumothorax, pleuritis, serositis), musculoskeletal, and psychosomatic.

➤ Stable Angina Pectoris
- Typical presentations of stable angina pectoris is that of chest discomfort and associated symptoms brought on by exercise with minimal or nonexistent symptoms at rest.
- Symptoms are usually short-lived (less than 15 minutes following cessation of precipitating activities or nitrates) and resume when activity resumes.

➤ Unstable Angina
Unstable angina (UA) is defined as angina pectoris that changes or worsens has a less predictable course than stable angina and, therefore, can lead to an MI. Unstable angina can have a variety of different presentations, which include:
- Angina occurs at rest (or with minimal exertion), usually lasting >10 min.
- New onset angina
- Angina occurs with a crescendo pattern, more severe, prolonged, or frequent than previously.
- When angina is not responsive to nitrates
- When angina is associated with dyspnea, severe nausea, sweating, palpitation, or syncope.
- Considered to be present in patients with ischemic symptoms suggestive of an ACS and no elevation in troponins or CK-MB, with or without ECG changes indicative of ischemia
- Since an elevation in troponins and/or CK-MB may not be detectable for up to 12 hours after presentation, UA and NSTEMI are frequently indistinguishable at initial evaluation.

➤ Who Should be Suspected?
- The presentation of myocardial ischemia is frequently acute chest pain often radiating into the jaw, shoulder, or arm. Symptoms may also include shortness of breath, nausea, vomiting, diaphoresis, rapid pulse, nausea, vomiting, or difficulty in breathing; in some cases, these symptoms may occur without chest pain (particularly in older individuals and in those with

diabetes). These symptoms may also be accompanied by a change in blood pressure. In women, symptoms are often less dramatic and more likely to be misinterpreted as due to another cause than in men.

- The term *myocardial infarction* should be used when there is evidence of myocardial necrosis in a clinical setting consistent with myocardial ischemia. Under these conditions, any one of the following criteria meets the diagnosis for myocardial infarction:
- Detection of rise and/or fall of cardiac biomarkers (preferably troponin) with at least one value above the 99th percentile of the upper reference limit (URL), together with evidence of myocardial ischemia with at least one of the following:
  - Symptoms of ischemia
  - ECG changes indicative of new ischemia (new ST-T changes or new left bundle branch block (LBBB)
  - Development of pathologic Q waves on ECG
  - Imaging evidence of new loss of viable myocardium or new regional wall motion abnormality
- Sudden, unexpected cardiac death, involving cardiac arrest, often with symptoms suggestive of myocardial ischemia, and accompanied by presumably new ST elevation, or new LBBB, and/or evidence of fresh thrombus by coronary angiography and/or at autopsy, but death occurring before blood samples could be obtained, or at a time before the appearance of cardiac biomarkers in the blood.
- For percutaneous coronary interventions (PCIs) in patients with normal baseline troponin values, elevation of cardiac biomarkers above the 99th percentile URL are indicative of peri-procedural myocardial necrosis. By convention, increases of biomarkers greater than 3×99th percentile URL have been designated as defining PCI-related myocardial infarction. A subtype related to a documented stent thrombosis is recognized.
- For coronary artery bypass grafting (CABG) in patients with normal baseline troponin values, elevations of cardiac biomarkers above the 99th percentile URL are indicative of peri-procedural myocardial necrosis. By convention, increase of biomarkers greater than 5×99th percentile URL plus either new pathologic Q waves or new LBBB, or angiographically documented new graft or native coronary artery conclusion or imaging evidence of new loss of viable myocardium, have been designated as defining CABG-related myocardial infarction.
  - Pathologic findings of an acute myocardial infarction

➤ Diagnosis

The diagnosis of acute coronary syndrome depends on the characteristics of the chest pain, and specific associated symptoms, abnormalities on ECG, and levels of serum markers of cardiac injury (Figure 4-1). A patient with a possible acute coronary syndrome (ACS) should be treated rapidly. Therefore, initial management steps must be undertaken before or during the time the diagnosis is being established.

- Electrocardiogram: The 12-lead ECG provides the basis for initial diagnosis and management. The initial ECG may be normal in patients with ACS. The ECG should be repeated at 5–10 minute intervals if the initial ECG is normal but the patient remains symptomatic and there is a high clinical suspicion for MI. There are four major types of acute coronary artery syndromes, in which myocardial ischemia leads to different ECG manifestations.
  - Noninfarction subendocardial ischemia (classic angina), manifested by transient ST segment depressions without QRS changes.

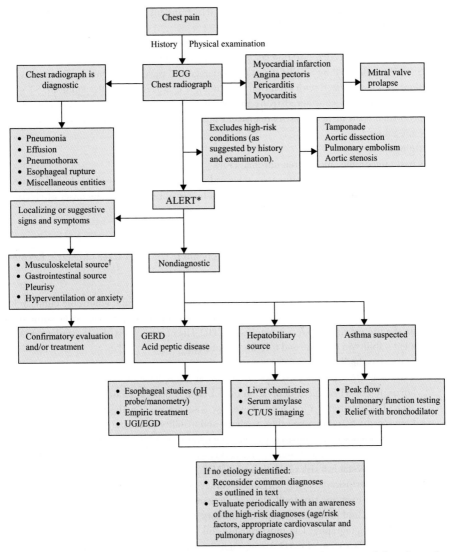

Figure 4-1. Algorithm for the diagnosis of chest pain. *This algorithm is intended to direct the work-up in patients with chest pain of unclear etiology. †Many of these patients will be discovered to have musculoskeletal syndromes that are diagnosed through a detailed history and physical examination. Musculoskeletal diagnoses to specifically consider include overuse syndromes, costochondritis, pectoral girdle syndrome, and xiphodynia. CT, computed tomography; ECG, electrocardiogram; EGD esophagogastroduodenoscopy; GERD gastroesophageal reflux disease; UGI upper gastrointestinal series; US ultrasound.

- Noninfarction transmural ischemia manifested by transient ST segment elevations or paradoxical T wave normalization.
- Non-STEMI (non-Q wave) MI, manifested by ST depressions or T wave inversions without Q waves with corroborating laboratory evidence of infarction.
- STEMI, manifested by ST elevations (or hyperacute T waves), and then by T wave inversions, often associated with evolution of pathologic Q waves. Clinically significant ST segment elevation is considered to be present if it is >1 mm in at least two contiguous precordial leads or in at least two adjacent limb leads and is not attributable to nonischemic causes.
- Imaging studies:
  - Chest radiographs: most often unremarkable
  - Echocardiography: A transthoracic echocardiogram can indicate regional wall motion abnormalities due to severe ischemia that can be visualized prior to the onset of electrocardiographic changes or the development of symptoms.

➤ Laboratory and Other Findings

- Core laboratory: Elevated cardiac enzymes, troponin I/T is the marker of choice. Recommend CBC to rule out severe anemia.
- Stress testing
  - The pretest probability of CHD is based on the clinical history and guides the clinician in choice of test modalities. The sensitivity and specificity of the specific test can be combined with the pretest risk to give a prognosis of CHD. The choice of test also dependent on the patient's ability to exercise and tolerate various drugs.
  - Exercise treadmill test:
    - CAD is likely if patient develops chest pain at a low level of exercise associated with horizontal or ST-segment depression of >1 mm. A drop in blood pressure and significant ST depression at a low level of exercise is suggestive of widespread ischemia.
    - Low sensitivity, predictive value, accuracy and inability to accurately identify and quantify ischemias when compared to stress imaging techniques. Best performed on those patients with at least a moderate probability of CAD. Duke Prognostic Treadmill Score attempts to establish risk of death from CAD.
- Radionuclide perfusion imaging: Greater accuracy and higher positive and negative predictive value than exercise treadmill alone. Can assess myocardial viability, qualitatively left ventricular size, and prognosis for severe coronary artery disease.
- Radionuclide angiography: The most reliable and well-validated procedure for identifying and determine the extent of CAD. Angiography is considered the "gold standard" for diagnosis. May be useful for risk stratification post MI. Invasive and costly, it is appropriate as an initial diagnostic study in only a subset of the population.
- Echocardiography: Is recommended as the initial stress test in patients who can exercise but have baseline ECG abnormalities that interfere with interpretation of exercise ECG testing. With sensitivities and specificity similar to those of angiography, it identifies and quantifies coronary heart disease. False-negative results are more likely with submaximal heart rate during exercise, single vessel disease, and moderate stenoses. Stress test performance is generally lower in women due in part to a lower prevalence of disease.
- Pharmacologic (dobutamine) stress testing: Accurately identifies CAD in patients who are unable to exercise. It is more specific in the identification of CAD in patients with LBBB than

exercise perfusion imaging. It is contraindicated in patients with aortic aneurysm and may lead to ventricular arrhythmias in patients with severe CAD.

➤ Suggested Reading

Fraker TD, Fihn SD. (2007) Chronic Angina Focused update of the ACC/AHA. (2002) Guidelines for the Management of Patient With Chronic Stable Angina. *J Am Coll Cardiol*. 2007;50:2264–2274.

CONGESTIVE HEART FAILURE

➤ Definition

- Heart failure (HF) is a condition representing the end-stage of different cardiac diseases that results in the reduced efficiency of the myocardium due to damage or overload, leading to reduced cardiac output. Therefore, there is insufficient blood flow to meet the body's needs.
- Common causes are heart disease, hypertension, systolic dysfunction, diastolic dysfunction, valve disease, left ventricular hypertrophy inflammation, drugs (e.g., alcohol, cocaine, amphetamines, Herceptin (trastuzumab), anthracycline, chemotherapeutic agents), and toxins (e.g., carbon monoxide, arsenic, lead).

➤ Who Should be Suspected?

- Clinical manifestations include dyspnea, orthopnea, ascites, and peripheral edema foot and ankle swelling.

➤ Laboratory Findings

- Hematology: ESR may be decreased because of decreased serum fibrinogen.
- Urinalysis: Slight albuminuria (<1 g/d) is common. Isolated RBCs and WBCs, hyaline, and (sometimes) granular casts. Urine is concentrated, with specific gravity >1.020. Oliguria is a characteristic feature of right-sided failure.
- Core laboratory: Serum albumin and total protein are decreased. Altered liver function tests. Decreased serum potassium concentration due to diuretic. Elevated brain natriuretic peptide (BNP) or N-terminal pro-BNP. Moderate azotemia (BUN usually <60 mg/dL) is evident with severe oliguria; may increase with vigorous diuresis. (Primary renal disease is indicated by proportionate increase in serum creatinine and low specific gravity of urine, despite oliguria.) Development of hyponatremia or anemia may be a sign of disease progression.
- Electrocardiogram: A 12-lead ECG may demonstrate evidence of ischemic heart disease, right and left ventricular hypertrophy, and presence of conduction delay or abnormalities (e.g., LBBB).
- Imaging studies: Echocardiography is the gold standard used to support a clinical diagnosis of heart failure, with decrease ejection fraction in systolic heart failure. left ventricular hypertrophy. Chest radiography is frequently used to indicate cardiomegaly or pulmonary disorders. Radionuclide ventriculography, MRI, or CT may also provide useful information.

➤ Suggested Readings

Hunt SA, Abraham WT, Chin MH, et al. "ACC/AHA 2005 Guideline Update for the Diagnosis and Management of Chronic Heart Failure in the Adult." *Circulation*. 2005;112 (12):e154–235.
Hunt SA, Abraham WT, Chin MH, et al. *Circulation*. 2009;119(14):e391–479. Epub 2009 Mar 26.

CHAPTER 5

Central Nervous System Disorders

Juliana Szakacs

INTRODUCTION

This chapter updates the individual disease sections with the latest information for the diagnosis of neurologic disease. These have been divided into several categories, including autoimmune disorders; trauma; miscellaneous disorders, with functional abnormalities and degenerative disorders; neoplasia; and vascular disorders, plus a section on infectious disorders. Each entity is presented with a succinct description of the disorder, including signs and symptoms. Evaluation of the nervous system requires a multidisciplinary approach to the patient and where appropriate, pertinent clinical findings, radiologic procedures and laboratory tests have been included to aid in the diagnosis.

AUTOIMMUNE DISORDERS

PRIMARY AUTOIMMUNE AUTONOMIC FAILURE

Primary autoimmune autonomic failure (also known as autoimmune autonomic ganglionopathy, acute panautonomic neuropathy, or acute pandysautonomia) is an autoimmune disorder possibly due to antiganglionic acetylcholine receptor antibodies (AChRs) causing dysfunction of efferent sympathetic and parasympathetic pathways and resulting in orthostatic hypotension, anhydrosis, decreased production of saliva and tears, erectile dysfunction, and impaired bladder emptying. It is responsive to plasma exchange. Antibodies to ganglionic AChR are present in about two thirds of all subacute cases and in one third of chronic cases.

➤ Laboratory Findings

Testing varies according to the presentation and history of autonomic symptoms. Testing should be directed to differentiate between acute inflammatory demyelinating polyneuropathy (Parkinson disease, drug or toxin exposure, and hereditary etiologies) from primary autoimmune autonomic failure.

Detection of antibodies binding to neuronal ganglionic AChRs is performed by radioimmunoprecipitation. There may also be decreased plasma norepinephrine levels.

SECONDARY AUTOIMMUNE AUTONOMIC FAILURE

Secondary causes of autoimmune autonomic failure include DM, amyloidosis, paraneoplastic syndromes, Lambert-Eaton syndrome, botulism, syphilis, HIV infection, collagen vascular disease, and porphyria.

➤ Laboratory Findings

Tests that rule out disorders that may cause autonomic symptoms include:
* Glycosylated hemoglobin to test for diabetes
* Anti-Hu antibody titers, which may be used to test for paraneoplastic syndromes
* Anticalcium channel antibody titers for Lambert-Eaton myasthenic syndrome
* Stool for botulinum by culture and detection of toxin for botulism
* Serum and urine protein electrophoresis to evaluate myeloma due to amyloidosis, or genetic testing to evaluate for familial amyloidosis
* Rapid plasma reagent (RPR) or VDRL to test for syphilis
* HIV serology for AIDS .
* ANA levels, ESR, and other autoimmune tests (e.g., rheumatoid factor [RF] and Sjogren's Syndrome SS-A and SS-B antibodies) to evaluate for collagen vascular disease
* Urinary porphyrins and erythrocyte porphobilinogen deaminase levels for porphyria

➤ Suggested Readings

Klein CM, Vernino S, Lennon VA, et al. The spectrum of autoimmune autonomic neuropathies. *Ann Neurol.* 2003;53:752–758.

Sandroni P, Vernino S, Klein CM, et al. Idiopathic autonomic neuropathy: comparison of cases seropositive and sero-negative for ganglionic acetylcholine receptor antibody. *Arch Neurol.* 2004;61(1):44–48.

Schroeder C, Vernino S, Birkenfeld AL, et al. Plasma exchange for primary autoimmune autonomic failure. *N Engl J Med.* 2005;353:1585.

Vernino S, Freeman R. Peripheral autonomic neuropathies. *Continuum Lifelong Learning Neurol.* 2007;13(6):89–110.

GUILLAIN-BARRÉ SYNDROME

Acute immune-mediated polyneuropathies are classified under the name Guillain-Barré syndrome (GBS), for the authors who described the disease. It is a heterogeneous condition with several variant forms. Most often, GBS presents as an acute monophasic paralyzing illness provoked by a preceding infection. Acute GBS (<2 months' duration) presents with a demyelinating symmetrical polyneuropathy caused by autoantibodies. In 70% of cases it is reversible, but 10% of patients die and 20% have residual defects. Dysautonomia occurs in 70% of patients; severe autonomic dysfunction is occasionally associated with sudden death.

➤ Laboratory Findings

The CSF shows albumin–cytologic dissociation with normal cell count and increased protein (average 50–100 mg/dL). The protein increase parallels increasing clinical severity, and the increase may be prolonged. The CSF may be normal at first.
* A biopsy of the nerve shows evidence of demyelination and remyelination.
* Electrophysiologic changes may be negative for the first 1–2 weeks.

Laboratory findings due to associated disease may be present (e.g., evidence of recent infection with *Campylobacter jejuni* in 15–40% and CMV in 5–20% of cases; EBV and *Mycoplasma pneumoniae* in <2% of cases in developed countries, other viral and rickettsial infections, immune disorders, DM, exposure to toxins [e.g., lead, alcohol], neoplasms). No agent was identified in ≤70% of cases.

➤ Suggested Readings

Köller H, Kieseier BC, Jander S, Hartung HP. Chronic inflammatory demyelinating polyneuropathy. *N Engl J Med.* 2005;352:1343–1356. Review.

Ropper AH. The Guillain-Barré syndrome. *N Engl J Med.* 1992;326:1130–1136.

Sivadon-Tardy V, Orlikowski D, Rozenberg F, et al. Guillain-Barré syndrome, greater Paris area. *Emerg Infect Dis.* 2006;12:990.

Zochodne DW. Autonomic involvement in Guillain-Barré syndrome: a review. *Muscle Nerve.* 1994;17:1145–1155.

MULTIPLE SCLEROSIS

Multiple sclerosis (MS) is the most common autoimmune inflammatory demyelinating disease of the CNS. It presents as distinct episodes of neurologic deficits separated in time and is caused by demyelination of distinct foci of white matter that are separated in space. Women are twice as likely to be affected as men and the disease is rare in children or in patients >50 years of age. Histology of the brain reveals multifocal areas of demyelination with loss of oligodendrocytes and astroglial scarring. Diagnosis should not be made by CSF evaluation alone unless there are *multiple clinical lesions in time* (by clinical history) and *anatomic location* (by MRI, evoked potentials, or physical examination).

➤ Laboratory Findings

CSF changes are found in >90% of patients with MS. The opening pressure, and glucose and albumin levels are normal and leukocyte count is normal in two thirds of patients. Less than 5% of patients have a white blood cell (WBC) count >50 cells/µL. Cells are predominantly T lymphocytes. There are two significant CSF tests that are positive in MS: oligoclonal bands (OCBs) and the IgG index.

Oligoclonal IgG Bands

The qualitative test of IgG on unconcentrated CSF is the single most informative test. It is best performed using Iso-Electric Focusing (IEF) with immunodetection by blotting or fixation run with a simultaneous serum sample on an adjacent track with positive and negative controls. A diagnostic study will show one of five recognized staining patterns of oligoclonal banding.

- Type 1: No OCBs in CSF and serum samples
- Type 2: OCBs in CSF but not serum, indicating intrathecal IgG synthesis
- Type 3: OCBs in CSF with additional identical OCBs in CSF and serum but still indicating intrathecal IgG synthesis
- Type 4: Identical OCBs in CSF and serum, indicating a systemic immune reaction with a normal or abnormal blood–CSF barrier and passive transfer of OCBs to the CSF
- Type 5: Monoclonal bands in CSF and serum, indicating the presence of a monoclonal gammopathy

The lumbar puncture and CSF analysis should be repeated if clinical suspicion for MS is high but results are equivocal, negative, or show only a single band on IEF.

Quantitative IgG analysis is an informative complementary test but not considered a substitute for the qualitative test, which has the highest sensitivity and specificity. Ninety percent of patients with MS have OCBs in their CSF, at least two of which are *not* present in simultaneously examined serum. A few patients with definite MS may have normal CSF immunoglobulins and lack OCBs. OCBs are found in 85–95% of patients with definite MS and 30–40% with possible MS (specificity = 79%); it is the most sensitive marker for MS. Positive results also occur in ≤10% of patients with noninflammatory neurologic disease (e.g., meningeal carcinomatosis, cerebral infarction) and ≤40% of patients with inflammatory CNS disorders (e.g., neurosyphilis, viral encephalitis, progressive rubella encephalitis, subacute sclerosing panencephalitis, bacterial meningitis, toxoplasmosis, cryptococcal meningitis, inflammatory neuropathies, trypanosomiasis).

OCBs are not known to correlate with severity, duration, or course of MS, and they persist during remission. With steroid treatment, the prevalence of OCBs and other gamma globulin abnormalities may be reduced by 30–50%. The evaluation of light chains may help in cases of equivocal oligoclonal IgG patterns.

OCBs in serum may occur in leukemias, lymphomas, some infections, and inflammatory diseases and immune disorders.

IgG Index

The immunoglobulin level, predominantly IgG, is elevated in the CSF relative to other proteins in MS. This finding is expressed as the IgG index (the normal value is less <0.66). It is an indication of IgG synthesis in the CNS. An increase in *production* of IgG is expressed as the ratio of CSF to serum albumin to rule out increased IgG due to disruption of the blood–brain barrier. Ninety percent of MS patients have an index of >0.7. CSF IgM and IgA may also be increased but are not useful for diagnosis.

The CSF IgG does not correlate with duration, activity, or course of MS. It may also be increased in other inflammatory demyelinating diseases (e.g., neurosyphilis, acute GBS), 5–15% of patients with miscellaneous neurologic diseases, and a few normal persons. Recent myelography is said to invalidate the test. The CSF IgG synthesis rate (3.3 mg/day) is increased in 90% of MS patients and 4% of non-MS patients. PCR demonstrates an expansion of B-cell clones.

Other Useful Tests

The presence of **myelin basic protein** indicates recent myelin destruction. It is increased in 70–90% of patients with MS during an acute exacerbation and usually returns to normal within 2 weeks. A weakly reactive result (4–8 ng/mL) indicates an active lesion >1 week old. Normal is <1 ng/mL.

Myelin basic protein is useful for following the course of MS but not for screening; it may be helpful very early in the course of MS before OCBs have appeared or in ~10% of patients who do not develop these bands. It is frequently increased in other causes of demyelination and tissue destruction (e.g., meningoencephalitis, leukodystrophies, metabolic encephalopathies, SLE of CNS, brain tumor, head trauma, amyotrophic lateral sclerosis, cranial irradiation and intrathecal chemotherapy, and 45% of patients with recent stroke) and other disorders (e.g., diabetes mellitus, chronic renal failure, vasculitis, carcinoma of vasculitis, immune complex diseases, and pancreas). It is falsely increased by CSF contamination with blood. It is associated with certain histocompatibility antigens (e.g., Caucasian patients with B7 and Dw2 antigen).

The **albumin index** (ratio of albumin serum to CSF) is a measure of integrity of the blood-to-CSF barrier. Use of this index can prevent false misinterpretation of increased CSF IgG concentrations. An increase indicates CSF contaminated with blood (e.g., traumatic tap) or increased permeability of the blood–brain barrier (e.g., aged persons, obstruction of CSF circulation, diabetes mellitus, SLE of CNS, GBS, polyneuropathy, cervical spondylosis).

CSF total protein is usually normal or may be mildly increased in ~25% of patients and is not a very useful test by itself. Decreased values or values >100 mg/dL should cast doubt on the diagnosis of MS.

CSF gamma globulin is increased in 60–75% of patients regardless of whether the total CSF protein is increased. Gamma globulin ≥12% of CSF total protein is abnormal if there is not a corresponding increase in serum gamma globulin, but may also be increased in other CNS disorders (e.g., syphilis, subacute panencephalitis, meningeal carcinomatosis) and may also be increased when serum electrophoresis is abnormal due to non-CNS diseases (e.g., RA, sarcoidosis, cirrhosis, myxedema, multiple myeloma).

Peripheral blood studies and routine CSF tests yield no changes of diagnostic value. Anti-myelin antibodies initially were thought to be a marker of MS and progression of disease. However, subsequent evidence suggests that these antibodies are not associated with an increased risk of progression or with MS disease activity.

➤ Suggested Readings

Barclay L. New guidelines for standards for CSF analysis in MS. *Arch Neurol.* 2005;62:865–870.

Lampasona V, Franciotta D, Furlan R, et al. Similar low frequency of anti-MOG IgG and IgM in MS patients and healthy subjects. *Neurology.* 2004;62:2092.

McDonald WI, Compston A, Edan G, et al. Recommended diagnostic criteria for multiple sclerosis: guidelines from the International Panel on the diagnosis of multiple sclerosis. *Ann Neurol.* 2001;50:121–127.

TRAUMA

CENTRAL NERVOUS SYSTEM TRAUMA

Laboratory findings vary depending on the type of brain injury (e.g., contusion, laceration, subdural hemorrhage, extradural hemorrhage, subarachnoid hemorrhage). There may also be laboratory findings due to complications of the brain injury (e.g., pneumonia, meningitis).

In possible skull fractures, disruption of the barriers between the sinonasal cavity and the anterior and middle cranial fossae can lead to the leak of CSF into the nasal cavity. This communication with the CNS can lead to infectious complications, resulting in morbidity and mortality.

➤ Laboratory Evaluation for CSF Rhinorrhea

Beta-2-transferrin is produced by neuraminidase activity within the CNS; it is found in the CSF, perilymph, and aqueous humor. Immunofixation electrophoresis with anti-transferrin-precipitating antibody is performed to differentiate CSF desialated transferrin from nasal secretions. The assay has a high sensitivity and specificity. This is currently the recommended laboratory test for identifying the presence of CSF in sinonasal fluid.

Testing for the glucose content in rhinorrhea with the use of glucose oxidase paper is not recommended for the following reasons: Reducing substances in lacrimal-gland secretions and nasal mucus may cause false-positive results; and meningitis may lower the glucose level in the CSF leading to a false-negative result. The test is not specific for the side or site of leak.

Beta-trace protein, also known as prostaglandin D synthase, has been used to diagnose CSF rhinorrhea in multiple studies, with a sensitivity of 92% and specificity of 100%. It is synthesized primarily in arachnoid cells, oligodendrocytes, and the choroid plexus; but it is also present in testes, heart, and serum, and it is nonspecific for CSF. Prostaglandin D synthase may also be altered in renal failure, MS, cerebral infarction, and certain CNS tumors. This test is not specific for side or site of leak and can be difficult to collect if the leak is intermittent.

➤ Suggested Readings

Lindstrom DR, Toohill RJ, Loehrl TA, Smith TL. Management of cerebrospinal fluid rhinorrhea: the Medical College of Wisconsin experience. *Laryngoscope.* 2004;114(6):969–974.

Porter MJ, Brookes GB, Zeman AZ, et al. Use of protein electrophoresis in the diagnosis of cerebrospinal fluid rhinor-rhoea. *J Laryngol.* 1992;106(6):504–506.

Ryall RG, Peacock MK, Simpson DA. Usefulness of beta 2-transferrin assay in the detection of cerebrospinal fluid leaks following head injury. *J Neurosurg.* Nov 1992;77(5):737–739.

Welch KC, Stankiewicz J. CSF Rhinorrhea: Workup http://emedicine.medscape.com/article/861126-diagnosis. Updated: Sep 28, 2009.

ACUTE EPIDURAL HEMORRHAGE

Epidural hemorrhage is a rare but serious complication of head injury. It is found in 1–4% of traumatic head injury cases and in 5–15% of autopsy series. Lumbar puncture is contraindicated in cases where epidural hemorrhage is suspected, due to the risk of herniation.

CSF is usually under increased pressure; it is colorless unless there is associated cerebral contusion, laceration, or subarachnoid hemorrhage.

➤ Suggested Readings
Bullock MR, Chesnut R, Ghajar J, et al. Surgical management of acute epidural hematomas. *Neurosurgery.* 2006;58:S7.

Mayer S, Rowland L. Head injury. In: Rowland L, ed. *Merritt's Neurology.* Philadelphia: Lippincott Williams & Wilkins; 2000:401.

SUBDURAL HEMATOMA

Acute subdural hematoma complicates approximately 11% of mild to severe head injuries that require hospitalization and approximately 20% of severe traumatic brain injuries. Twelve percent to 38% of patients have a transient "lucid interval" after the acute injury, which is followed by a progressive neurologic decline to coma. Lumbar puncture is contraindicated due to the risk of herniation.

CSF findings are variable: clear, bloody, or xanthochromic, depending on recent or old associated injuries (e.g., contusion, laceration).

Chronic subdural hematoma may present with the insidious onset of headaches, light-headedness, cognitive impairment, apathy, somnolence, and occasionally seizures. Symptoms may not become evident until weeks after the initial injury and may be transient or fluctuating. Lumbar puncture is contraindicated due to the risk of herniation.

CSF is usually xanthochromic and the protein content is 300 to 2,000 mg/dL.

Anemia is often present in infants.

➤ Suggested Readings
Bullock MR, Chesnut R, Ghajar J, et al. Surgical management of acute subdural hematomas. *Neurosurgery.* 2006;58:S16.

Kaminski HJ, Hlavin ML, Likavec MJ, Schmidley JW. Transient neurologic deficit caused by chronic subdural hematoma. *Am J Med.* 1992;92:698.

Victor M, Ropper A. Craniocerebral trauma. In: Victor M, Ropper A, eds. *Adams and Victor's Principles of Neurology.* 7th ed. New York: McGraw-Hill; 2001:925.

Wilberger JE Jr, Harris M, Diamond DL. Acute subdural hematoma: morbidity, mortality, and operative timing. *J Neurosurg.* 1991;74:212.

MISCELLANEOUS DISORDERS

ALZHEIMER DISEASE (SENILE DEMENTIA)

Alzheimer disease is the most common cause of dementia in the elderly. It begins insidiously and progresses over 5–10 years to severe cortical dysfunction. The major pathology is cortical atrophy with accumulation of plaques containing abnormal proteins. The dominant abnormal protein is A-beta peptide, a form of amyloid. A-beta 40 and 42 are cleaved from a larger amyloid precursor protein whose gene resides on chromosome 21.

The incidence of Alzheimer disease doubles every 5 years, starting at 1% in the 60- to 64-year-old age group and rising as high as 40% in the 85- to 89-year-old age group. In patients older than 60 with dementia the usual causes are Alzheimer-type, 75%; drugs and alcohol, 13%; endocrine, 4%; low serum iron folate or cobalamin, 8%; and GU tract infection, 2.5%.

➤ Laboratory Findings

There is no definitive laboratory test for the diagnosis of Alzheimer disease. Laboratory tests are useful to rule out other forms of dementia that may resemble Alzheimer disease but are amenable to therapy. The gold standard for the diagnosis of Alzheimer disease is histology of the brain by biopsy or on autopsy.

CSF obtained by lumbar puncture in patients with dementia may show increased Tau proteins and decreased beta amyloid 40 and 42, which suggests a diagnosis of Alzheimer disease.

Recommended tests in all patients with a new onset of dementia should include CBC, urinalysis, electrolyte and blood chemistry panel, screening metabolic panel, serum vitamin B_{12} and folate measurements, thyroid studies, and a serologic test for syphilis.

AD7C-NTP (neural thread protein) is a 41-kD brain protein that is selectively elevated in Alzheimer disease. AD7C-NTP is associated with neurofibrillary tangles, and overexpression of the AD7C-NTP gene is associated with cell death. A newly developed competitive ELISA has been developed to test urine samples and CSF; this test is being investigated as a biochemical marker of Alzheimer disease. (The AD7CTM test, is developed by Nymox Pharmaceutical Corporation.)

➤ Suggested Readings

Galasko D, Clark C, Chang L, et al. Assessment of CSF levels of tau protein in mildly demented patients with Alzheimer's disease. *Neurology*. 1997;48:632.

Kahle PJ, Jakowec M, Teipel SJ, et al. Combined assessment of tau and neuronal thread protein in Alzheimer's disease CSF. *Neurology*. 2000;54:1498.

Sunderland, T, Linker, G, Mirza, N, Putnam, KT. Decreased beta-amyloid1-42 and increased tau levels in cerebrospinal fluid of patients with Alzheimer disease. *JAMA*. 2003;289:2094.

COMA AND STUPOR

Patients with coma or stupor are poorly or nonresponsive to external stimuli. The causes are many and can be divided into several etiologic categories (see subsequent text). The goal of diagnostic testing is to identify treatable conditions including infection, metabolic abnormalities, seizures, intoxications/overdose, and surgical lesions as rapidly as possible.

➤ Causes

- Poisons, drugs, or toxins:
  - Sedatives (especially alcohol, barbiturates)
  - Enzyme inhibitors (especially salicylates, heavy metals, organic phosphates, cyanide)
  - Other (e.g., paraldehyde, methyl alcohol, ethylene glycol)
- Cerebral disorders:
  - Brain contusion, hemorrhage, infarction, seizure, or aneurysm
  - Brain mass (e.g., tumor, hematoma, abscess, parasites)
  - Subdural or epidural hematoma
  - Venous sinus occlusion
  - Hydrocephalus
  - Hypoxia
    - Decreased blood O_2 content and tension (e.g., lung disease, high altitude)
    - Decreased blood O_2 content with normal tension (e.g., anemia, carbon monoxide poisoning, methemoglobinemia)
- Infection (e.g., meningitis, encephalitis)
- Postictal state
- Vascular abnormalities (e.g., subarachnoid hemorrhage, hypertensive encephalopathy, shock, acute myocardial infarction, aortic stenosis, Adams-Stokes Disease, tachycardias)
- Metabolic abnormalities
  - Acid–base imbalance (acidosis, alkalosis)
  - Electrolyte imbalance (increased or decreased sodium, potassium, calcium, magnesium)
  - Porphyrias
  - Aminoacidurias
  - Uremia
  - Hepatic encephalopathy
  - Other disorders (e.g., leukodystrophies, lipid storage diseases, Bassen-Kornzweig syndrome)
- Nutritional deficiencies (e.g., vitamin B_{12}, thiamine, niacin, pyridoxine)
- Endocrine
  - Pancreas (diabetic coma, hypoglycemia)
  - Thyroid (myxedema, thyrotoxicosis)
  - Adrenal (Addison disease, Cushing syndrome, pheochromocytoma)
  - Panhypopituitarism
  - Parathyroid (hypofunction or hyperfunction)
- Psychogenic conditions that may mimic coma
  - Depression, catatonia
  - Malingering
  - Hysteria, conversion disorder

➤ Diagnosis

Testing should be prioritized according to the clinical presentation:

1. Urgent CT scan for possible structural abnormalities such as papilledema, focal neurologic changes, acute stroke, expanding mass lesion, or herniation syndrome.
2. Lumbar puncture for fever to rule out bacterial meningitis or viral encephalitis. Neuroimaging prior to lumbar puncture in a comatose patient is recommended to avoid precipitating transtentorial herniation. CSF may exclude subarachnoid hemorrhage when CT

is normal, and may help in the diagnosis of demyelinating, inflammatory, and neoplastic disease.

➤ Screening Laboratory Tests

* For patients presenting in coma of uncertain cause:
  * CBC
  * Serum electrolytes, calcium, magnesium, phosphate, glucose, urea, creatinine, and liver function tests
  * ABG
  * PT and PTT
  * Drug screen including ethyl alcohol, acetaminophen, opiates, benzodiazepines, barbiturates, salicylates, cocaine, amphetamines, ethylene glycol, and methanol
* If the cause of coma remains obscure, additional testing recommended:
  * Adrenal and thyroid function tests
  * Blood cultures
  * Blood smear: screen for thrombotic thrombocytopenic purpura (fragmented erythrocytes) and DIC with LDH, D-dimer, and fibrinogen.
  * Antiphospholipids if a coagulation problem is suspected
  * Carboxyhemoglobin if carbon monoxide poisoning is suggested
  * Serum drug concentrations for specific drugs

➤ Suggested Reading

Hasbun R, Abrahams J, Jekel J, Quagliarello VJ. Computed tomography of the head before lumbar puncture in adults with suspected meningitis. *N Engl J Med.* 2001;345:1727.

INTELLECTUAL DISABILITY (MENTAL RETARDATION)

Intellectual disability (ID) is an unchanging encephalopathy that may be due to a number of etiologies. Developmental screening with standard screening tools should be performed at every well child visit. A comprehensive history and physical should include measurements of height, weight, and head circumference, including growth velocity, dysmorphic features, neurologic and sensory development, and a detailed observation of behavior.

➤ Causes

Prenatal

Infections (e.g., syphilis, rubella, toxoplasmosis, CMV)

Metabolic abnormalities (e.g., DM, eclampsia, placental dysfunction)

Chromosomal disorders (e.g., Down syndrome, 18 trisomy, cri-du-chat syndrome, Klinefelter syndrome)

Metabolic abnormalities

* Amino-acid metabolism (e.g., phenylketonuria, maple syrup urine disease, hemocystinuria, cystathioninuria, hyperglycemia, argininosuccinicaciduria, citrullinemia, histidinemia, hyperprolinemia, oasthouse urine disease, Hartnup disease, Joseph syndrome, familial iminoglycinuria)
* Lipid metabolism (e.g., Batten disease, Tay-Sachs disease, Niemann-Pick disease, abetalipoproteinemia, Refsum disease, metachromatic leukodystrophy)
* Carbohydrate metabolism (e.g., galactosemia, mucopolysaccharidoses)
* Purine metabolism (e.g., Lesch-Nyhan syndrome, hereditary orotic aciduria)

- Mineral metabolism (e.g., idiopathic hypercalcemia, pseudopseudohypoparathyroidism and pseudohypoparathyroidism)

Other syndromes (e.g., tuberous sclerosis, Louis-Bar syndrome)

Perinatal
- Infections (e.g., syphilis, rubella, toxoplasmosis, CMV, HIV, HSV)
- Kernicterus
- Prematurity
- Anoxia
- Trauma

Postnatal
- Poisoning (e.g., lead, arsenic, carbon monoxide)
- Infections (e.g., meningitis, encephalitis)
- Metabolic abnormalities (e.g., hypoglycemia, malnutrition)
- Postvaccinal encephalitis
- CVA
- Trauma

➤ Laboratory Findings
Genetic Studies
Children with global developmental delay have a 4% incidence of abnormal cytogenetic studies. A karyotype should be routinely performed on all affected patients even if dysmorphic features are not present. Additional factors that should prompt genetic testing include: family history of multiple miscarriages, unexplained infant death, parental consanguinity, or developmental regression or loss of milestones.

Chromosomal microarray analysis identifies subtelomeric chromosomal rearrangements, which may be seen in an additional 5% of children with ID. FISH may be used if microarray diagnosis is not available or if a specific telomeric disorder such as cri-du-chat syndrome is suspected.

Down syndrome (trisomy 21) is the most common form of inherited ID followed by fragile X syndrome, caused by an abnormal expansion mutation of a CGG triplet repeat in the Fragile X Mental retardation 1 gene (FRM1) gene. Testing for fragile X mutations should be considered in male and female patients, especially in those with a family history of ID. Because Down syndrome often presents with nonspecific global developmental delay in young children, there should be a low threshold for this investigation.

Metabolic Studies
ID is a clinical feature of some inborn errors of metabolism these may be identified by newborn screening.

Thyroid Screening
Congenital hypothyroidism may result in ID; thyroid testing is not indicated unless clinical features suggest dysfunction.

Lead Screening
Lead is the most common environmental neurotoxin. At concentrations greater than 10 mcg/dL (0.48 micromol/L) it has been associated with cognitive deficits. Children should be screened at 1–2 years of age. Risk factors for increased levels of lead include living in a community where >12% of children have blood lead levels of >10 mcg/dL and living in a house built before 1950.

➤ Suggested Readings

Hagerman PJ. The fragile X prevalence paradox. *J Med Genet.* 2008;45:498.

Moeschler JB, Shevell M. Clinical genetic evaluation of the child with mental retardation or developmental delays. *Pediatrics.* 2006;117:2304.

Ropers H.H. Genetics of intellectual disability. *Curr Opin Genet Dev.* 2008;18:241–250.

Screening for elevated blood lead levels. American Academy of Pediatrics Committee on Environmental Health. *Pediatrics.* 1998;101:1072.

Shevell M, Ashwal S, Donley D, et al. Practice parameter: evaluation of the child with global developmental delay: report of the Quality Standards Subcommittee of the American Academy of Neurology and The Practice Committee of the Child Neurology Society. *Neurology.* 2003;60:367.

POLYNEUROPATHY (NEURITIS/NEUROPATHY, MULTIPLE)

Polyneuropathy is a generalized, homogeneous process affecting multiple peripheral nerves. It is characterized by symmetric distal sensory loss, burning, or weakness. Etiologies vary and include medication side effects or manifestations of systemic disease. The rate of progression of the polyneuropathy and type (axonal or demyelinating) can help identify its etiology.

Polyneuropathy must be distinguished from mononeuropathy, mononeuropathy multiplex (multifocal neuropathy), and disorders of the CNS. Mononeuropathy is a focal involvement of a single nerve, usually due to a local cause such as trauma, compression, or entrapment. Mononeuropathy multiplex is the involvement of noncontiguous nerve trunks usually due to a systemic vasculitic process that affects the vasa nervorum.

Diseases of the CNS such as a brain tumor, stroke, or spinal cord lesion occasionally present with symptoms that are difficult to distinguish from polyneuropathy.

The etiology of polyneuropathy varies and includes infections, metabolic and immune disorders, neoplasms, and many other diseases, including postvaccinal effect.

➤ Laboratory Findings

For the most specific use of the laboratory, blood tests should be deferred until the results of electromyography and nerve conduction studies are known. Testing may then be performed based on the recommendations of the American Academy of Neurology for axonal or demyelinating diseases.

* Laboratory tests for axonal abnormalities:
  * Serum glucose
  * Serum protein electrophoresis and immunofixation
  * B_{12} level
  * ANA
  * ESR
  * RPR
  * Glycohemoglobin
  * Urine/blood for heavy metals
  * Urine/blood for porphyrins
  * RF
  * Sjögren's syndrome testing (anti-Ro, anti-La antibodies)
  * Lyme testing
  * HIV

- Methylmalonic acid and homocysteine levels (in patients with borderline low serum B_{12} levels)
- Hepatitis screen (for types B and C)
- Laboratory tests for demyelinating disorders
  - Serum protein electrophoresis and IEP
  - Urine protein electrophoresis
  - Hepatitis screen (for types B and C)
  - Lumbar puncture for inflammatory demyelinating polyneuropathies, increase in CSF protein with minimal elevation in CSF white cells (albuminocytologic dissociation)
  - Anti-myelin–associated glycoprotein (MAG) testing (in patients with predominantly sensory symptoms)
  - Anti-GM1 test (in patients with predominantly motor symptoms)
  - HIV
  - Genetic testing for Charcot-Marie-Tooth Disease.
- Additional laboratory tests for infectious disorders
  - Leprosy
  - Diphtheria: CSF protein is 50–200 mg/dL
  - EBV (mononucleosis associated: CSF shows increased protein and up to several hundred mononuclear cells)
  - Lyme disease
- Additional laboratory information that may be contributive
  - Blood
  - Tests to rule out toxic conditions due to drugs and chemicals (especially lead, arsenic, etc.) should be considered.
  - Testing may be performed to rule out underlying metabolic conditions, including pellagra, beriberi, collagen vascular disease, pregnancy, porphyria, and DM.
  - CSF
    - The CSF is usually normal; however, in ~70% of patients with diabetic neuropathy the CSF protein is increased to >200 mg/dL.
    - In some cases of chronic uremia the CSF protein is 50–200 mg/dL.
    - In collagen vascular disease (polyarteritis nodosa has nerve involvement in 10% of patients) the CSF is usually normal.
    - In neoplasms (leukemia, multiple myeloma, carcinoma) the CSF protein is often increased and may be associated with an occult primary neoplastic lesion outside the CNS.
    - In alcoholism the CSF is usually normal.
- Other etiologic agents of polyneuropathy include:
  - Amyloidosis
  - Sarcoidosis
  - Bassen-Kornzweig syndrome
  - Refsum disease
  - Chédiak-Higashi syndrome
  - Immune mediated (e.g., Guillain-Barré syndrome)

➤ Suggested Reading

England JD, Gronseth GS, Franklin G, et al. Practice Parameter: evaluation of distal symmetric polyneuropathy: role of laboratory and genetic testing (an evidence-based review). Report of the American Academy of Neurology, American Association of Neuromuscular and Electrodiagnostic Medicine, and American Academy of Physical Medicine and Rehabilitation. *Neurology.* 2009;72:185.

CRANIAL NERVE, MULTIPLE

Neuropathies of the cranial nerves are most commonly due to local compression by trauma, infection or tumor, vascular and collagen vascular disorders, and some metabolic diseases.

➤ Laboratory Findings

Laboratory findings may be helpful to determine the underlying etiology:

* Peripheral blood for glucose, HgbA1c, BUN, creatinine, AST, and ALT may reveal a metabolic disorder (e.g., DM, renal failure, chronic liver disease, myxedema, porphyria).
* Serology and/or culture may be helpful in identification of infection (e.g., herpes zoster or benign polyneuritis associated with cervical lymph node TB).
* Tissue biopsy of the nerve or adjacent soft tissues may diagnose sarcoidosis and tumors (e.g., meningioma, neurofibroma, carcinoma, cholesteatoma, chordoma) Imaging studies are most useful for the detection of trauma and aneurysms.

MONONEUROPATHY (NEURITIS OF ONE NERVE OR PLEXUS)

Mononeuropathy is a focal involvement of a single nerve, usually due to a local cause such as trauma, compression, or entrapment (e.g. Carpal tunnel syndrome). Mononeuropathy multiplex refers to the involvement of noncontiguous nerve trunks due to multiple nerve infarcts from a systemic vasculitic process that affects the vasa nervorum. Other causes of mononeuropathy include:

* DM
* Infections (e.g., HIV, diphtheria, herpes zoster, leprosy)
* Sarcoidosis
* Polyarteritis nodosa
* Tumor (leukemia, lymphoma, carcinomas)
* Trauma
* Serum sickness
* Bell's palsy
* Idiopathic
* Drugs, toxic substances
* Chronic renal failure
* Thyroid disorders

➤ Laboratory Findings

* Blood tests:
  * Fasting glucose and glycohemoglobin in patients with possible diabetic amyotrophy, idiopathic radiculopathy, or polyneuropathy.
  * Lyme titers in patients with polyradiculopathy, especially in endemic areas.
  * Genetic tests for hereditary neuropathy with predisposition to pressure palsy for patients with multiple mononeuropathies (usually affecting at least two to three extremities), and Chédiak-Higashi syndrome.
  * Lumbar puncture: Evaluation of CSF is warranted in patients with unusual presentations. CSF should be examined for evidence of inflammation, elevated CSF protein, and serologic testing for Lyme disease, syphilis, and CMV. Cytologic evaluation for tumor cells may be warranted.

FACIAL PALSY, PERIPHERAL ACUTE

Patients with Bell's palsy (idiopathic facial palsy) typically present with the sudden onset (usually over hours) of unilateral facial paralysis. Secondary facial nerve palsy may be caused by a variety of disorders that can be confused with Bell's palsy.

➤ Laboratory Findings

Testing should be designed to rule out causes of underlying diseases.

Idiopathic facial palsy or Bell palsy may occasionally present with a slight increase in cells in the CSF.

➤ Causes

* Infection:
  * Lyme disease may produce bilateral palsy. Facial nerve palsy is the most common cranial neuropathy associated with Lyme meningitis. Early negative blood serology does not exclude the diagnosis. A lymphocyte pleocytosis in the CSF is suggestive, and the finding of specific oligoclonal IgG in the CSF is a sensitive indicator.
  * Herpes simplex virus activation has become widely accepted as the likely cause of facial palsy in most cases.
  * Herpes zoster is the second most common viral infection associated with facial palsy.
  * Other infectious causes of facial palsy include CMV, EBV, adenovirus, rubella virus, mumps, influenza B, and coxsackievirus.
  * Bacterial infections such as Lyme disease, syphilis, leprosy, diphtheria, cat scratch disease, *M. pneumoniae,* and otitis media may also be causative.
  * Rickettsial infections have also been reported.
  * Ehrlichiosis can present as facial diplegia.
  * Parasitic (e.g., malaria) infections may cause facial palsy.
  * Local inflammation (otitis media, mastoiditis, osteomyelitis, petrositis) may be causative.
* Structural defects (require imaging) include trauma, tumor (acoustic neuromas, tumors invading the temporal bone), cholesteatoma, and Paget disease of bone. These should be suspected if the onset of facial palsy is gradual.
* Granulomatous disease such as sarcoidosis should be considered, especially in patients with bilateral facial palsy.
* Connective tissue disease, Sjögren's syndrome, is an unusual cause.
* Metabolic disorders, including DM, uremia, and hypothyroidism, may cause neuropathy.
* Drug reaction, particularly to dental injections, may cause local neuropathy.
* Postvaccinal effect and Guillain-Barré syndrome may cause bilateral facial palsy.
* Melkersson-Rosenthal syndrome is characterized by facial paralysis, episodic facial swelling, and a fissured tongue in adolescents. Perivascular granulomas are seen in the edematous tissue, but the cause is unknown.

➤ Suggested Readings

Bitsori M, Galanakis E, Papadakis CE. Facial nerve palsy associated with *Rickettsia conorii* infection. *Arch Dis Child.* 2001;85:54.

Craft JE, Grodzicki RL, Steere AC. Antibody response in Lyme disease: evaluation of diagnostic tests. *J Infect Dis.* 1984;149:789.

Hadithi M, Stam F, Donker AJ, Dijkmans BA. Sjögren's syndrome: an unusual cause of Bell's palsy. *Ann Rheum Dis.* 2001;60:724.

Hansen K, Cruz M, Link H. Oligoclonal *Borrelia burgdorferi*-specific IgG antibodies in cerebrospinal fluid in Lyme neuroborreliosis. *J Infect Dis.* 1990;161:1194.

Jackson CG, von Doersten PG. The facial nerve. Current trends in diagnosis, treatment, and rehabilitation. *Med Clin North Am.* 1999;83:179.

Lee FS, Chu FK, Tackley M, Wu AD. Human granulocytic ehrlichiosis presenting as facial diplegia in a 42-year-old woman. *Clin Infect Dis.* 2000;31:1288.

Levenson MJ, Ingerman M, Grimes C, Anand KV. Melkersson-Rosenthal syndrome. *Arch Otolaryngol.* 1984;110:540.

Morgan M, Nathwani D. Facial palsy and infection: The unfolding story. *Clin Infect Dis.* 1992;14:263.

Mountain RE, Murray JA, Quaba A, Maynard C. The Edinburgh facial palsy clinic: A review of three years' activity. *J R Coll Surgeons Edinb.* 1994;39:275.

Peitersen E. Bell's palsy: the spontaneous course of 2,500 peripheral facial nerve palsies of different etiologies. *Acta Otolaryngol Suppl.* 2002;(549):4–30.

Rosa PA, Schwan TG. A specific and sensitive assay for the Lyme disease spirochete *Borrelia burgdorferi* using the polymerase chain reaction. *J Infect Dis.* 1989;160:1018.

Schirm J, Mulkens PS. Bell's palsy and herpes simplex virus. *APMIS* 1997;105:815.

Teller DC, Murphy TP. Bilateral facial paralysis: a case presentation and literature review. *J Otolaryngol.* 1992;21:44.

HEMIANOPSIA, BITEMPORAL

Visual impairment is caused by suprasellar expansion of a mass, leading to compression of the optic chiasm. The presentation is decreased vision in the temporal fields (bitemporal hemianopsia). The most common cause is pituitary adenoma, but any mass lesion may be causative, including metastatic tumor, sarcoidosis, Hand-Schüller-Christian disease, meningioma of sella, and aneurysm of the circle of Willis.

Diagnosis is predominantly made by neuroimaging. Laboratory findings may help identify the underlying disease particularly of tumor by biopsy.

OPHTHALMOPLEGIA

Internuclear ophthalmoplegia is an impairment of horizontal eye movement with weak adduction of the affected eye and abduction nystagmus of the contralateral eye. It results from a lesion in the medial longitudinal fasciculus of either the pons or the midbrain. Causes of ophthalmoplegia include MS, cerebrovascular disorders (infarction), infection, trauma, and tumor.

▶ Laboratory Findings
Testing is directed at identifying the causative disease and may be helpful in the diagnosis of DM, vasculopathies, and MS. Testing may help exclude myasthenia gravis and hyperthyroid exophthalmos.

▶ Suggested Reading
Frohman EM, Zhang H, Kramer PD, et al. MRI characteristics of the MLF in MS patients with chronic internuclear ophthalmoparesis. *Neurology.* 2001;57:762.

OCULOMOTOR NERVE PALSY

Dysfunction of the third cranial nerve (oculomotor nerve) can result from lesions anywhere along its path. The diagnosis varies according to the age of the patient, characteristics of the palsy, and the presence of symptoms. The most common causes include intracranial aneurysm, ischemia, trauma, and migraine. Ischemic diabetic third nerve palsies, are the most common etiology in adults. Traumatic third nerve palsy arises only from severe blows to the head. Ophthalmoplegic 'migraine' has been reclassified as a cranial neuralgia by the International Headache Society in 2004.

➤ **Laboratory Findings**
Testing can help in the diagnosis of diabetes and vasculopathies. Testing may help exclude myasthenia gravis, which is in the differential diagnosis, and can mimic pupil-sparing ophthalmoplegia.

➤ **Suggested Reading**
Headache Classification Committee of the International Headache Society. The International Classification of Headache Disorders. *Cephalalgia*. 2004;24:1.

TRIGEMINAL NEURALGIA (TIC DOULOUREUX)

Trigeminal neuralgia is one of the most common causes of facial pain. It is a sudden, usually unilateral, severe, brief, stabbing, recurrent pain in the distribution of one or more branches of the fifth cranial (trigeminal) nerve. Eighty percent to 90% of cases are caused by compression of the trigeminal nerve root, by an artery or vein leading to demyelination. Compression may also be caused by vestibular schwannoma (acoustic neuroma), meningioma, epidermoid or other cyst, or, rarely, a saccular aneurysm or arteriovenous malformation. Demyelination of one or more of the trigeminal nerve nuclei may also be caused by MS.

➤ **Laboratory Findings**
Diagnosis is performed predominantly by neuroimaging and electrophysiologic testing. Laboratory findings may assist in identifying MS or herpes zoster. Tissue biopsy may be needed in the diagnosis of schwannoma, meningioma, and cysts.

➤ **Suggested Reading**
Love S, Coakham HB. Trigeminal neuralgia: pathology and pathogenesis. *Brain*. 2001;124:2347.

RETROBULBAR NEUROPATHY (OPTIC NEURITIS)

Retrobulbar neuropathy results in pain behind the affected eye, impaired vision, and rarely blindness. The causes include encephalomyelitis, posterior uveitis, lesions of the retinal artery or vein, tumors, fungal infections, and medications (chloramphenicol, ethambutol, isoniazid, penicillamine, phenothiazines, phenylbutazone, quinine, and streptomycin). Retrobulbar neuropathy may be associated with MS, which ultimately develops in 30–50% of these patients over 15 years.

➤ **Laboratory Findings**
Lumbar puncture is helpful in the diagnosis. CSF may be normal or reveal increased protein and $\leq 200/\mu L$ lymphocytes. Oligoclonal bands may be present.

➤ **Suggested Reading**
Yanoff M, Duker JS. Ophthalmology. St Louis: Mosby; 1999:6.2–6.4.

AUTONOMIC NEUROPATHY

See also Polyneuropathy.

The most common cause of autonomic neuropathy is DM. A wide range of symptoms affecting many different organ systems can occur, including the cardiovascular, GI, GU, pupillary, and neuroendocrine systems.

The etiology of autonomic dysfunction is broad. Disorders that may cause autonomic dysfunction include: amyloidosis, Guillain-Barré syndrome, hereditary neuropathies, infections (e.g., Chagas disease, HIV, botulism, diphtheria, and leprosy), toxicities including drugs (vincristine, cis-platinum, Taxol, thallium, and heavy metals), collagen vascular disease (e.g., Sjögren's disease, systemic lupus, RA), PA, porphyria, uremia, alcoholic neuropathy, hepatic disease, paraneoplastic syndromes, Lambert-Eaton syndrome, and medications (antihypertensives, tricyclics, MAO inhibitors, and dopamine agonists).

➤ Laboratory Findings

Laboratory testing most helpful to determine the causative disease or toxin should be based on the presenting symptoms and history of the patient to rule out the preceding disorders.

➤ Suggested Reading

Freeman R. Autonomic dysfunction. In: Samuels M, Fesky S, eds. *The Office Practice of Neurology*. 2nd ed. Philadelphia: Churchill Livingstone; 2003;14:141–145.

PSEUDOTUMOR CEREBRI

Idiopathic intracranial hypertension, also known as pseudotumor cerebri, results in the neurologic findings of headache and papilledema. The CSF is normal except for increased opening pressure. The primary means of diagnosis is one of exclusion, and consists of neuroimaging to rule out a mass lesion or ventricular obstruction.

➤ Laboratory Findings

Laboratory findings may help in the diagnosis of "secondary pseudotumor cerebri," which is due to an underlying condition. Lumbar puncture should be performed only after neuroimaging to measure the opening pressure and evaluate for cell count, differential, and glucose and protein levels. Culture and cytology may be indicated based on the clinical situation. Obesity has been associated with increased CSF opening pressures.

Testing may be helpful to rule out Addison disease, infection, and metabolic disorders including acute hypocalcemia and other "electrolyte disturbances," empty sella syndrome, and pregnancy. Testing for drugs that may be implicated in secondary pseudotumor cerebri include psychotherapeutic drugs, sex hormones and oral contraceptives, and a reduction in dosage of corticosteroids. Immune diseases may be implicated, including SLE, polyarteritis nodosa, and serum sickness. Other conditions that may be tested for as the symptoms warrant include sarcoidosis, Guillain-Barré syndrome, head trauma, various anemias, and chronic renal failure.

➤ Suggested Reading

Corbett JJ, Mehta MP. Cerebrospinal fluid pressure in normal obese subjects and patients with pseudotumor cerebri. *Neurology*. 1983;33:1386.

REYE SYNDROME

Reye syndrome is an acute noninflammatory encephalopathy with fatty changes of the liver and kidney. Rarely, fatty changes are also seen in the heart and pancreas. The syndrome occurs typically in children recovering from influenza, varicella, or nonspecific viral illness and is associated with use of aspirin. Reye syndrome presents with nausea, vomiting, headache, and delirium with frequent progression to coma. Because aspirin was identified as a major precipitating factor for the development of Reye syndrome, this complication has virtually disappeared.

➤ Laboratory Findings

The diagnostic criteria for Reye syndrome include a markedly increased CSF pressure with no other abnormalities. The serum AST, ALT, or ammonia may be 3 times greater than the upper limit of normal (ULN). On biopsy of the liver, noninflammatory, panlobular fatty changes are seen.

➤ Suggested Reading

Belay ED, Bresee JS, Holman RC, et al. Reye's syndrome in the United States from 1981 through 1997. *N Engl J Med.* 1999;340:1377.

SEIZURES THAT MAY HAVE LABORATORY ABNORMALITIES

A seizure is a sudden change in behavior that is the consequence of brain dysfunction. Seizures are categorized as *epileptic* (resulting from electrical hypersynchronization of neuronal networks in the cerebral cortex), *provoked* (occur in the setting of metabolic derangement, drug or alcohol withdrawal, and acute neurologic disorders such as stroke or encephalitis), and *nonepileptic* seizures (resemble epileptic seizures but are not associated with the typical neurophysiologic changes).

➤ Laboratory Findings

Laboratory diagnosis is directed at determining an underlying cause of a provoked or nonepileptic seizure. Most important are blood tests for electrolytes, glucose, calcium, magnesium, hematology studies, renal function tests, liver function tests, and toxicology screens. Testing for underlying conditions should be performed as indicated by the history and physical examination. A lumbar puncture is helpful if there is an acute infectious process involving the CNS or the patient has a history of cancer. In other circumstances the test may be misleading, since a prolonged seizure can cause CSF pleocytosis.

Conditions associated with seizure activity include brain tumors, abscess, and space-occupying lesions; circulatory disorders such as thrombosis, hemorrhage, embolism, hypertensive encephalopathy, vascular malformations, and angiitis; hematologic disorders such as sickle cell anemia, leukemia, and TTP; and metabolic abnormalities. Carbohydrate metabolism abnormalities may result in seizures with hypoglycemia (<40 mg/dL), or hyperglycemia (>400 mg/dL). Glycogen storage diseases are also known to cause seizures. Disrupted amino acid metabolism as in phenylketonuria and maple syrup urine disease, and lipid metabolism abnormalities such as the leukodystrophies and lipidoses, may result in seizures. Electrolyte imbalance results in neurologic change when sodium is <120 or >145 mEq/L, calcium is <7 mg/dL, or magnesium is low. Hyperosmolality >300 mOsm/L may also result in seizure activity.

Other disorders that may give rise to seizures include porphyria, eclampsia, hyperthyroidism, and renal failure. Drugs that may result in seizures include crack cocaine, amphetamines, ephedrine, and other sympathomimetics. Allergic disorders including drug reactions and postvaccinal reactions may be causative.

Infections, meningitis, encephalitis, and postinfectious encephalitis (measles, mumps) and in the fetus rubella, measles, and mumps may all cause seizures.

Degenerative brain diseases may also be causative.

➤ Suggested Reading

Krumholz A, Wiebe S, Gronseth, G, et al. Practice Parameter: evaluating an apparent unprovoked first seizure in adults (an evidence-based review): report of the Quality Standards Subcommittee of the American Academy of Neurology and the American Epilepsy Society. *Neurology.* 2007;69:1996.

NEOPLASTIC LESIONS

BRAIN TUMOR

Brain tumors are a diverse group of neoplasms with varying growth rates and symptoms. They may produce headache, seizure, nausea and vomiting, syncope, cognitive dysfunction, weakness, loss of sensation, and aphasia. The primary diagnostic modality for brain tumor is neuroimaging including CT, MRI, PET, and SPECT scanning, followed by biopsy for tissue diagnosis.

➤ Laboratory Findings

Evaluation of the CSF may help in the diagnosis. The CSF is usually clear, but it may occasionally reveal xanthochromia or be frankly bloody if there is hemorrhage into the tumor. The WBC count may be increased ≤ 150 cells/μL in up to 75% of patients and normal in others. Protein is usually increased. *Protein is particularly increased with meningioma of the olfactory groove and with acoustic neuroma.*

Tumor cells may be demonstrable in 20–40% of patients with all types of solid tumors, but failure to find malignant cells does not exclude meningeal neoplasm. Atypical WBCs may be seen in leukemia or lymphoma. Tumor antigens/markers may indicate the source of some metastatic tumors. Glucose may be decreased if cells are present.

Brainstem gliomas, which are characteristically found in childhood, are usually associated with normal CSF. The CSF is usually normal in "diencephalic syndrome" of infants due to glioma of the hypothalamus.

GLOMUS JUGULARE TUMOR

This tumor arises from the glomus bodies within the ear, and is the most common tumor of the middle ear. It is a slow-growing, vascular tumor, with blood supply from the external and/or internal carotid artery. It is most common in women and may result in hearing loss with pulsing/ringing in the ear, dizziness, and ear pain.

➤ Laboratory Findings

The diagnosis is made by neurophysiologic testing and CT or MRI. Blood tests for endocrine work-up and urine tests should be performed. Evaluation of the CSF may reveal an increase in protein.

LEUKEMIC INVOLVEMENT OF THE CENTRAL NERVOUS SYSTEM

See Chapter 10, Hematologic Disorders.

➤ Laboratory Findings

Intracranial hemorrhage is the principal cause of death in leukemia (may be intracerebral, subarachnoid, or subdural). It is more frequent when the WBC count is >100,000/μL and with rapid increases in the WBC count, especially in blast crises. The platelet count is frequently decreased. Often there is evidence of bleeding elsewhere.

Evaluation of the CSF may be diagnostic. There may be intracranial hemorrhage and infiltration of leukemic cells into the meninges and fluid. The CNS is involved in 5% of patients with ALL at diagnosis and is the major site of relapse. PCR is used to detect minimal residual cells that are not recognized morphologically. Involvement of the CSF by CLL and plasmacytoid leukemias is very rare.

The CSF may show an increased opening pressure and protein level. The glucose may be decreased to <50% of the blood level. Abnormal cells may be identified by cytochemical, immunohistochemical, immunofluorescent, or flow cytometric techniques to help diagnose leukemia. Malignant cells are found in 60–80% of patients with meningeal involvement.

Evaluation of the CSF may also help in identifying complicating meningeal infection (e.g., various bacteria, opportunistic fungi).

LYMPHOMATOUS INVOLVEMENT OF THE CENTRAL NERVOUS SYSTEM

See Chapter 10, Hematologic Diseases.

➤ Laboratory Findings

Pathologic evaluation of material from the CSF may provide sufficient diagnostic material, thereby avoiding brain biopsy in some patients.

The meninges are involved in <30% of patients with malignant lymphoma. Involvement is most prevalent in diffuse large cell ("histiocytic"), lymphoblastic, and immunoblastic lymphoma, and occurs in 30–50% of patients with Burkitt lymphoma and 15–20% of patients with non-Hodgkin lymphoma.

Hodgkin disease seldom involves the CNS.

Evaluation of the CSF often reveals an elevated protein and a lymphocyte-predominant pleocytosis. The glucose level is usually normal, but may be decreased if there is leptomeningeal disease. Abnormal cells found in the CSF may be differentiated by immunohistochemistry, immunofluorescence, or flow cytometry. PCR may also be used for identification of clonality.

The demonstration of neoplastic lymphocytes in the CSF is sufficient for the diagnosis of CNS lymphoma and may prevent open brain biopsy.

➤ Suggested Readings

Abrey LE, Batchelor TT, Ferreri AJ, et al. Report of an international workshop to standardize baseline evaluation and response criteria for primary CNS lymphoma. *J Clin Oncol.* 2005;23:5034.

Fischer L, Martus P, Weller M, et al. Meningeal dissemination in primary CNS lymphoma: prospective evaluation of 282 patients. *Neurology.* 2008;71:1102.

SPINAL CORD TUMOR

Spinal cord tumors occur within or adjacent to the spinal cord. They may be primary or metastatic. Primary spinal cord tumors account for 2–4% of all primary CNS tumors. Extradural tumors are usually metastatic and can cause spinal cord compression. Tumors arising within the dura, outside of the spinal cord, are termed intradural–extramedullary and comprise the nerve sheath tumors. Tumors arising within the spinal cord itself are called intramedullary tumors, and the majority are gliomas (astrocytomas or ependymomas).

➤ Laboratory Findings

Evaluation of the CSF reveals increased protein. The level may be very high and is associated with xanthochromia when there is a block of the subarachnoid space.

The protein concentration is higher with complete block in cord tumors located at lower levels. Tumor cells may be demonstrable.

➤ Suggested Readings

Kim MS, Chung CK, Choe G, et al. Intramedullary spinal cord astrocytoma in adults: postoperative outcome. *J Neurooncol.* 2001;52:85.

Kleihues P, Burger PC, Collins VP, et al. Glioblastoma. In: Kleihues P, Cavenee WK, eds. *Pathology of the Nervous System: World Health Organization Classification of Tumors.* Lyon, France: IARC (International Agency for Research on Cancer); 2000:29.

Reimer R, Onofrio BM. Astrocytomas of the spinal cord in children and adolescents. J Neurosurg. 1985;63:669.

VASCULAR DISORDERS

CEREBROVASCULAR ACCIDENT, NONTRAUMATIC STROKE

Brain ischemia may be transient or persistent and may be due to thrombosis, embolism, or hypoperfusion. Neurologic symptoms may not accurately represent the underlying pathology. The following characteristics may apply to stroke.

1. It may be intrinsic to a vessel, such as in atherosclerosis, lipohyalinosis, inflammation, amyloidosis, arterial dissection, malformation, aneurysm, and venous thrombosis.
2. It may be remote, such as in embolization.
3. It may involve decreased blood flow, such as is seen with hypotension and increased blood viscosity.
4. It may involve vascular rupture, such as is seen with subarachnoid hemorrhage due to berry aneurysm.

The diagnosis of stroke is made by history and physical examination and neurologic imaging to identify bleeding and rule out brain tumor. If the blood pressure is normal, consider berry aneurysm, hemorrhage into tumor, angioma, or coagulopathy.

Stroke may be hemorrhagic or ischemic.

- Hemorrhagic causes include:
  - Ruptured berry aneurysm (45% of patients)
  - Hypertension (15% of patients)
  - Angiomatous malformations (8% of patients)
  - Miscellaneous causes (e.g., brain tumor, blood dyscrasia)—infrequent
  - Undetermined cause (rest of patients)

- Ischemic causes include:
  - Thrombosis or embolism (80% of patients)

➤ Laboratory Findings

Blood testing at the time of suspected stroke should include CBC, PT and PTT, lipid panel, hypercoagulable panel including LA, anticardiolipin, protein C, protein S, and factor V Leiden. Testing to rule out SLE may be indicated. Additional tests may include a fibrinogen level, ESR, serology for Lyme disease, and HIV, and toxicology to rule out cocaine and other drugs.

➤ Tests Under Development

- The plasma DNA concentration measured by PCR assay for the β-globin gene is reported to correlate with stroke severity and predict mortality and morbidity.
- Preliminary studies indicate that S-100b (marker of astrocytic activation) and B-type neurotrophic growth factor may be a useful adjunct to CT scanning.
- Autoantibodies to brain-specific antigen N-methyl-d-aspartate receptor may assist diagnosis of stroke or assess risk of transient ischemic attack.

➤ Suggested Readings

Dambinova SA, Khounteev GA, Izykenova GA, et al. Blood test detecting autoantibodies to N-methyl-D-aspartate neuroreceptors for evaluation of patients with transient ischemic attack and stroke. *Clin Chem.* 2003;49:1752–1762.

Rainer TH, Wong LK, Lam W, et al. Prognostic use of circulating plasma nucleic acid concentrations in patients with acute stroke. *Clin Chem.* 2003;49:562–569.

Reynolds MA, Kirchick HJ, Dahlen JR, et al. Early biomarkers of stroke. *Clin Chem.* 2003;49:1733–1739.

Rothwell PM, Howard SC, Power DA, et al. Fibrinogen concentration and risk of ischemic stroke and acute coronary events in 5113 patients with transient ischemic attack and minor ischemic stroke. *Stroke.* 2004;35:2300.

BERRY ANEURYSM (SACCULAR ANEURYSM)

Most subarachnoid hemorrhages are due to ruptured saccular aneurysms. The incidence of saccular aneurysms is approximately 5% among the general population. The risk of rupture varies with aneurysm size. The largest number of subarachnoid hemorrhages due to aneurysm rupture occurs in the 40- to 60-year-old age group, with a slight increase in women over men. African Americans have a higher incidence than Caucasians.

Risk factors for saccular aneurysm include smoking, hypertension, genetic diseases (adult dominant polycystic kidney disease, aldosteronism, Ehlers Danlos syndrome), family history, and sympathomimetic drugs such as phenylpropanolamine and cocaine, and decreased estrogen as is seen in postmenopausal women.

➤ Laboratory Findings

The diagnosis of saccular aneurysm rupture is made by identification of symptomatology and laboratory tests. The most common presenting symptom is sudden headache. CT scan will identify subarachnoid clot. Lumbar puncture reveals increased opening pressure and elevated RBC count that does not diminish from tubes 1 through 4. In early subarachnoid hemorrhage (<8 hours after onset of symptoms), the test for occult blood may be positive before xanthochromia develops. After bloody spinal fluid occurs, the white to red cell ratio may be higher in CSF than in the peripheral blood. Bloody CSF clears by the 10th day in 40% of patients. The CSF is persistently abnormal after 21 days in 15% of patients. Approximately 5% of cerebrovascular episodes due to hemorrhage are wholly within the parenchyma, and CSF findings are normal.

➤ **Suggested Readings**

Broderick JP, Brott T, Tomsick T, et al. The risk of subarachnoid and intracerebral hemorrhages in blacks as compared with whites. *N Engl J Med.* 1992;326:733.

de Rooij, NK, Linn, FH, van der, Plas JA, et al. Incidence of subarachnoid haemorrhage: a systematic review with emphasis on region, age, gender, and time trends. *J Neurol Neurosurg Psychiatry.* 2007;78:1365.

HEMORRHAGE, CEREBRAL

Intracerebral hemorrhage is the second most common cause of stroke. It causes 8–15% of all first time strokes, with a higher incidence in Asians, Hispanics, and African Americans. Under-lying conditions are seen in many of the patient's including hypertension, amyloidosis, aneurysms, vascular malformations, alcoholism, and decreased cholesterol, LDL, and triglycerides.

The diagnosis of intracranial hemorrhage is made by neurologic imaging including MRI and CT scans.

➤ **Laboratory Findings**

Lumbar puncture reveals an increased WBC count (15,000–20,000/µL), higher than in cerebral infarct (e.g., embolism, thrombosis).

Tests that may be helpful include an elevated ESR and urinalysis, which may reveal transient glycosuria or concomitant renal disease. Additional tests may be obtained to rule out causes of intracerebral hemorrhage such as leukemia, aplastic anemia, polyarteritis nodosa, SLE, and other coagulopathies.

➤ **Suggested Readings**

Flaherty ML, Woo D, Haverbusch M, et al. Racial variations in location and risk of intracerebral hemorrhage. *Stroke.* 2005;36:934.

Gebel JM, Broderick JP. Intracerebral hemorrhage. *Neurol Clin.* 2000;18:419.

THROMBOSIS, CEREBRAL VEINS AND SINUSES

Cerebral vein and dural sinus thromboses are less common causes of stroke. More occur in neonates than children or adults. The causes of thrombosis include prothrombotic conditions in 85% of cases (oral contraception, pregnancy, malignancy), infection (e.g., otitis, mastoiditis, sinusitis, meningitis), and head injury. Genetic disorders may also be implicated, including antithrombin III deficiency, protein C and protein S deficiency, factor V Leiden mutation, and hyperhomocysteinemia. Collagen vascular and inflammatory diseases (e.g., SLE, sarcoidosis, and Wegener granulomatosis) may also be causative.

Cerebral thrombosis presents as a headache that increases over several days. Motor weakness and paresis or seizures may also occur. Thrombosis of different veins results in diverse clinical findings. Lumbar puncture can rarely precipitate a cerebral vein thrombosis. Thromboses of the cerebral veins and sinuses produce hemorrhagic infarcts in ~40% of cases.

The diagnosis of cerebral vein thrombosis is made predominantly by neurologic imaging. Laboratory tests are nonspecific but may give clues to the etiology.

➤ Laboratory Findings

Lumbar puncture for evaluation of CSF to rule out infection is required. Thirty percent to 50% of patients may have CSF findings. The CSF may reveal protein to be normal or mildly increased to ≤ 100 mg/dL. The cell count may be normal or ≥ 10 WBC/μL during the first 48 hours and rarely $\geq 2,000$ WBC/μL transiently on the third day. Red cells may be increased.

Additional blood tests may be informative. An increased CRP and ESR are risk factors for development of stroke, and an increased CRP is associated with a poorer short-term prognosis. Hematologic disorders (e.g., polycythemia, sickle cell disease, thrombotic thrombopenia, macroglobulinemia) may be identified (see Chapter 10).

Vasculitis (e.g., polyarteritis nodosa, Takayasu syndrome, dissecting aneurysm of aorta, syphilis, meningitis; see Chapter 4, Cardiovascular Disorders) and hypotension (e.g., myocardial infarction, shock) are other potential causes of cerebral vein thrombosis.

➤ Suggested Readings

Biousse V, Ameri A, Bousser MG. Isolated intracranial hypertension as the only sign of cerebral venous thrombosis. *Neurology*. 1999;53:1537.

Bousser MG, Chiras J, Bories J, Castaigne P. Cerebral venous thrombosis—review of 38 cases. *Stroke*. 1985;16:199.

Ferro JM, Canhão P, Stam J, et al (ISCVT Investigators). Prognosis of cerebral vein and dural sinus thrombosis: results of the International Study on Cerebral Vein and Dural Sinus Thrombosis (ISCVT). *Stroke*. 2004;35:664.

Stam J. Thrombosis of the cerebral veins and sinuses [review]. *N Engl J Med*. 2005;352:1791–1798.

EMBOLISM, CEREBRAL

Embolism is the most common cause of stroke in the elderly. Embolism is caused by particles of debris or tissue traveling through the circulation, which originate distally from vessel walls, the heart, or tumors. These fragments may result in the blockage of arterial blood flow to the brain. Unlike thrombosis, which involves the local vessel, local therapy in embolic stroke is only temporizing. The source of the embolic fragment must be identified and treated or additional events may occur.

* There are four categories of embolic strokes:
  * Those with a known cardiac source
  * Those with a possible cardiac or aortic source
  * Those with an arterial source
  * Those with an unknown source

Embolic stroke should be suspected if the change is sudden with maximal deficit at the onset, the infarct is large, there is a known cardiac or large arterial lesion, the infarct is or becomes hemorrhagic on CT, there are multiple lesions, and if clinical findings improve quickly. It is more common in patients with strokes of the posterior circulation. A possible cardiac source should always be considered even in young patients. Small vessel (lacunar) stroke is most commonly seen in patients with hypertension, DM, or polycythemia.

➤ Laboratory Findings

Lumbar puncture evaluation of the CSF reveals findings similar to cerebral thrombosis. Hemorrhagic infarction develops in one third of patients, usually producing slight xanthochromia. Some patients may have grossly bloody CSF (10,000 RBCs/μL). Septic embolism (e.g., bacterial endocarditis) may cause increased WBC (≤ 200/μL with variable lymphocytes and PMNs), increased RBC ($\leq 1,000$/μL), slight xanthochromia, increased protein, normal glucose, and negative culture.

Laboratory tests to diagnose the underlying causative disease should include blood cultures to rule out bacterial endocarditis, hypercoagulable panels to rule out nonbacterial thrombotic vegetations on heart valves, and cardiac enzymes to rule out underlying myocardial infarction with mural thrombus. Additional imaging studies to rule out myxoma of left atrium, fat embolism in fracture of long bones and air embolism in neck, chest, or cardiac surgery may be indicated.

➤ Suggested Readings

Caplan LR. Brain embolism. In: Caplan LR, Chiowitz M, Hurst JW, eds. *Practical Clinical Neurocardiology.* New York: Marcel Dekker; 1999.

DeRook FA, Comess KA, Albers GW, Popp, RL. Transesophageal echocardiography in the evaluation of stroke. *Ann Intern Med.* 1992;117:922.

Glass TA, Hennessey PM, Pazdera L, et al. Outcome at 30 days in the New England Medical Center posterior circulation registry. *Arch Neurol.* 2002;59:369.

HYPERTENSIVE ENCEPHALOPATHY

Hypertensive encephalopathy is usually associated with a blood pressure of $\geq 180/120$ mm Hg and is an acute, life-threatening disorder presenting with signs of cerebral edema.

Clinical symptoms are characterized by the insidious onset of headache, nausea, and vomiting, followed by nonlocalizing neurologic symptoms such as restlessness, confusion, and, if the hypertension is not treated, seizures and coma. Although these symptoms differ from the abrupt onset of stroke, an MRI scan should be obtained. MRI with T2-weighted images may reveal edema of the white matter of the parietooccipital regions.

➤ Laboratory Findings

Findings on laboratory tests are due to changes in other organ systems and to underlying conditions such as cardiac, renal, and endocrine disorders and toxemia of pregnancy. Testing may also reveal changes that may occur due to progressive disorders following hypertensive encephalopathy such as focal intracerebral hemorrhage. The CSF frequently shows increased pressure and protein ≤ 100 mg/dL.

➤ Suggested Readings

Hinchey J, Chaves C, Appignani B, et al. A reversible posterior leukoencephalopathy syndrome. *N Engl J Med.* 1996;334:494.

Phillips SJ, Whisnant JP, on behalf of the National High Blood Pressure Education Program. Hypertension and the brain. *Arch Intern Med.* 1992;152:938.

Vaughan CJ, Delanty N. Hypertensive emergencies. *Lancet.* 2000;356:411.

SPINAL CORD INFARCTION

Spinal cord infarction is a rare and devastating disorder with many etiologies. Patients present with para- or quadriplegia. The diagnosis is made clinically and with neurologic imaging such as MRI and electromyography.

The differential diagnosis of spinal cord infarction includes compression by neoplasm, transverse myelitis, acute polyneuropathy (Guillain Barré Syndrome), epidural hematoma in postoperative patients, aortic dissection or rupture, polyarteritis nodosa, and iatrogenic causes such as aortic arteriography or clamping of the aorta during cardiac surgery.

➤ Laboratory Findings

Laboratory findings may help to diagnose the underlying cause of the infarct. Lumbar puncture may reveal CSF with increased white cells and protein but is usually within normal limits. Evaluation of CSF may help rule out inflammation due to infection (tuberculoma), cytology may rule out malignant processes, flow cytometry may rule out leukemia or lymphoma, and OCBs rule out MS.

Blood testing to rule out syphilis, Lyme disease, HIV, enterovirus, coxsackie A and B virus, adenovirus, and EBV may be suggested.

Blood tests that may assist in the diagnosis include hypercoagulable panel, toxicology, sedimentation rate, ANA, ANCA, and SS-A and SS-B. In patients with neurosarcoid, the ACE level may be elevated. Laboratory tests may also be performed to rule out genetic conditions such as tuberous sclerosis and neurofibromatosis. Parasites, abscess formation, granulomas, cysts, or migrating lesions including *Taenia solium, Echinococcus*, schistosomiasis, toxoplasmosis, amebiasis, trichinosis, and cryptococcosis may also be causative agents.

THROMBOPHLEBITIS OF CAVERNOUS SINUS

Septic dural sinus thrombosis is an uncommon disease since the advent of antibiotics. The diagnosis is primarily made by imaging studies; however, lumbar puncture can be supportive.

➤ Laboratory Findings

The CSF is usually normal unless there is associated subdural empyema or meningitis. The CSF reveals inflammatory cells in 75% of cases. Fifty percent of these cases suggest a parameningeal focus with elevated neutrophils and/or mononuclear cells, normal glucose, normal or elevated protein, and a negative culture. Thirty percent of patients have a CSF finding consistent with bacterial meningitis with elevated neutrophils, low glucose, high protein, and a positive culture.

Mucormycosis may cause this clinical appearance in diabetic patients.

Lumbar puncture is recommended for differentiating periorbital cellulitis from septic cavernous sinus thrombosis. Culture of the CSF may reveal organisms associated with septic cavernous sinus thrombosis and reflect the primary site of infection. *Staphylococcus aureus* is seen in 70% of all infections and is associated with facial infection or sphenoid sinusitis. Streptococci (including *Streptococcus pneumoniae, Streptococcus milleri*, and viridans group streptococci) are less commonly found. Anaerobes are most often found with accompanying sinus, dental, or tonsillar infections. Fungal pathogens have been less commonly reported.

Additional laboratory findings that may be helpful include the CBC where an elevated peripheral WBC count may suggest an acute bacterial infection, or other causes of venous thromboses such as sickle cell disease, polycythemia, or dehydration.

➤ Suggested Readings

Bengel D, Susa M, Schreiber H, et al. Early diagnosis of rhinocerebral mucormycosis by cerebrospinal fluid analysis and determination of 16s rRNA gene sequence. *Eur J Neurol.* 2007;14:1067.

Cannon ML, Antonio BL, McCloskey JJ, et al. Cavernous sinus thrombosis complicating sinusitis. *Pediatr Crit Care Med.* 2004;5:86.

Deveze A, Facon F, Latil G, et al. Cavernous sinus thrombosis secondary to non-invasive sphenoid aspergillosis. *Rhinology.* 2005;43:152.

Ebright JR, Pace MT, Niazi AF. Septic thrombosis of the cavernous sinuses. *Arch Intern Med.* 2001;161:2671.

Southwick FS, Richardson EP Jr, Swartz MN. Septic thrombosis of the dural venous sinuses. *Medicine (Baltimore).* 1986;65:82.

Watkins LM, Pasternack MS, Banks M, et al. Bilateral cavernous sinus thromboses and intraorbital abscesses secondary to *Streptococcus milleri*. *Ophthalmology.* 2003;110:569.

INFECTIONS OF THE CENTRAL NERVOUS SYSTEM*

Infections of the central nervous system (CNS) are associated with significant morbidity and mortality. Infections are caused by all types of pathogens from viruses to parasites. Organisms gain access to CNS most commonly by:

* Hematogenous seeding from a distal site of infection or colonization (e.g., bacterial endocarditis, nasopharyngeal colonization by *Neisseria meningitidis*)
* Direct extension from a contiguous site of infection (e.g., infected sinus)
* Direct invasion (e.g., trauma, basilar skull fracture)

Pathogenesis and signs and symptoms depend on the pathogen and site of infection, as discussed in subsequent text of this chapter, and in other chapters. Primary infection may occur in the parenchyma of the CNS, as seen in encephalitis and brain abscess. Infections may also occur outside the parenchyma in locations bounded by the meninges:

* Epidural abscesses are localized in the space between the dura mater and the vertebrae.
* Meningitis occurs in the subarachnoid space (between the arachnoid and pia mater).
* Subdural abscesses are localized in the space between the dura mater and arachnoid.

Organisms may be directly visualized and isolated from CSF in patients with meningitis, as discussed later. In localized parenchymal, epidural, and subdural abscesses, organisms do not have access to the CSF, so Gram stain and culture of CSF are usually negative, unless the abscess ruptures into the subarachnoid space. On the other hand, the immune response to abscesses may result in inflammatory changes detectable in the CSF, like increased WBC (usually without clear PMN predominance) and mildly elevated protein; CSF glucose is typically normal.

CENTRAL NERVOUS SYSTEM ABSCESSES

As in other tissues, CNS abscesses are localized infections with formation of pus. Disease may be caused by tissue destruction and inflammation caused by the primary infection or by the physical forces of the rigid bony structures acting against the swelling nervous system parenchyma. The infection may occur in the parenchyma of the brain, in the epidural or subdural space, or in other anatomic sites in the CNS. Hematogenous seeding should be suspected in patients with multiple abscesses.

---

*Written by Michael Mitchell, MD.

A very wide variety of pathogens have been implicated in the etiology of brain abscesses. Monomicrobial and polymicrobial infections are well defined. The etiology depends on a number of factors, including:

* Age of the patient
* Anatomic site of infection
* Immune status of the patient
* Site of primary infection or source of organisms
* Virulence of the infecting organism(s)

A broad etiology must be considered, especially in immunocompromised patients, including fungal and parasitic pathogens. *Toxoplasma gondii* reactivation should be considered in patients with defects in cell-mediated immunity, like HIV infection. Other parasitic pathogens, like *Taenia solium* or *Entamoeba histolytica*, must be considered in patients who have emigrated from endemic areas. Patients with arteriovenous malformations or other right-to-left shunts are at significantly increased risk for brain abscess.

Anaerobic organisms are frequently isolated, often as part of a polymicrobial flora. The species reflect, to some extent, the primary source of infection, which is commonly related to oropharyngeal, intraabdominal, or pelvic infections. Pathogens include *Bacteroides*, *Prevotella*, *Fusobacterium*, *Propionibacterium*, and other species.

A wide variety of aerobic species are also implicated, including *Streptococcus* species, enteric gram-negative bacilli, and *S. aureus*. *Citrobacter* species have been implicated in brain abscesses and meningitis in neonates. *Klebsiella pneumoniae* has been implicated in brain abscesses associated with primary liver abscess.

➤ Clinical Presentation

Severe, sometimes localized headache unrelieved by over-the-counter analgesics is the most common symptom of brain abscess. Patients may have neck stiffness. Vomiting, change in mental status, and focal neurologic signs are signs of severe disease.

➤ Diagnosis and Laboratory Findings

Definitive diagnosis in usually made by aerobic and anaerobic culture, with Gram stain, of infected material. Patients with CNS abscesses should be carefully evaluated for increased intracranial pressure, especially prior to collection of CSF by lumbar puncture.

Typical laboratory findings include:

* Aspirate of infected pus should be cultured for aerobic and anaerobic bacteria, fungi, and mycobacteria, with Gram, AFB, and fungal stains.
* Histopathologic examination may provide specific diagnosis.
* CSF shows signs of inflammation, typically:
  * WBC ~25 to 300/μL with increased neutrophils and lymphocytes
  * CSF Protein may be normal, or minimally or markedly increased (75 to >300 mg/dL)
  * CSF Glucose is often normal
  * Bacterial cultures are usually negative, but laboratory signs of acute purulent meningitis may be seen if the abscess ruptures.
* Blood cultures are positive in ~10% of patients
* Toxoplasma serology is recommended in patients with HIV infection. Other specific serologic testing is performed on the basis of epidemiologic risk.
* Laboratory findings due to associated primary disease

ENCEPHALITIS

Encephalitis is a disease characterized by diffuse or localized inflammation of the brain associated with neurologic dysfunction. Historically, viruses have been primary in the infectious etiology of encephalitis. Effective vaccination has reduced the incidence of several of the viruses that have been prominent causes of encephalitis, like mumps and measles viruses. The range of pathogens capable of causing encephalitis is broad. A specific diagnosis cannot be established in a significant number of patients with suspected infectious encephalitis. In patients in whom a diagnosis is established, ~70% are viral, ~20% bacterial, and ~10% other causes (prion, parasitic, fungal). Of note, *M. pneumoniae* has been recognized as the cause of encephalitis in a significant proportion (~30%) of children. Specific anti-*M. pneumoniae* serology was insensitive for detection. In addition, encephalitis and encephalopathy may be caused by a variety of non-infectious medical conditions.

A number of viruses are capable of causing encephalitis, either by direct infection or as an immune-mediated post-infection syndrome. Influenza; measles, mumps, rubella; and varicella-zoster viruses have all been implicated in postinfectious encephalitis.

- **Herpes simplex virus:** HSV, usually type 1, is a common cause of sporadic encephalitis.
- **Arboviruses** (St. Louis, eastern equine, western equine, Venezuelan equine, West Nile): Arboviral encephalitis had been uncommon until the emergence of West Nile virus, which is now the most common cause of arboviral infection in the United States. These viruses show seasonal variability reflecting the distribution and activity of their mosquito vectors.
- **Rabies:** Rabies is uncommon in regions with effective vaccination programs, but low-level endemic infection is seen in host species inaccessible to vaccination, like bats and raccoons. Travel and animal exposure history are critical for timely diagnosis and treatment.
- **Other viruses:** Encephalitis caused by other viruses is uncommon in the United States, but sporadic or epidemic encephalitis is seen in other countries caused by agents such as arenavirus (lymphocytic choriomeningitis virus) and Nipah and Hendra viruses.

➤ Clinical Presentation

Patients present with headache, nausea, and vomiting; fever may be present. Patients usually develop changes in mental status, from subtle behavioral changes to frank obtundation. Seizures are common. Focal neurologic abnormalities may occur. Nuchal rigidity suggests a meningeal component (meningoencephalitis or isolated meningitis).

➤ Diagnosis and Laboratory Findings

A careful physical examination as well as clinical and exposure history may provide important diagnostic clues. Some agents, such as rabies, may have restricted routes of transmission; other agents may show geographic restriction due to the range of the pathogen or intermediate vectors. Temporal lobe involvement suggests HSV infection. Preceding flaccid paralysis is suggestive of West Nile virus infection. Initial diagnostic testing should prioritize agents with the highest pretest probability based on presenting signs, symptoms, and epidemiology.

- CSF usually shows signs of inflammation, but these may be nonspecific. Findings overlap with aseptic meningitis and paraspinal abscesses.

   There is usually mild to moderate CSF pleocytosis (<250 cells/mm^3), with lymphocyte predominance. The presence of significant numbers of RBCs suggests a necrotizing encephalitis, like HSV.

Protein may be mildly elevated (<150 mg/dL). CSF glucose is usually not decreased (>50% of simultaneous serum glucose concentration).

- CSF viral culture has a low diagnostic yield for CNS infections, especially for nonenteroviral and non-HSV CNS infections.
- West Nile virus should be carefully considered because of its frequency of occurrence.
- HSV should be ruled out by PCR in all patients with acute encephalitis of unknown cause because of its prominence in the differential diagnosis and the severity of sequelae in untreated infection.
- PCR is the diagnostic method of choice for most patients with acute encephalitis that is likely to be infectious. The specific target pathogens are prioritized on the basis of pre-test probability.
- Specific PCR for *M. pneumoniae* on CSF and throat specimens is recommended for children with acute encephalitis in whom another cause is not identified.
- Serologic testing is of limited value for patients with acute encephalitis, but may be useful in patients in whom initial testing is not diagnostic. Serologic tests that may support specific diagnoses include detection of intrathecal antibody formation, production of serum or CSF IgM, or rise in antibody titer in acute and convalescent (typically >3 weeks after onset of symptoms) serum specimens.

    Demonstration of specific IgM in CSF provides a diagnosis of West Nile virus encephalitis.
- Brain biopsy, with routine and immunohistologic staining, may provide specific diagnosis for patients in whom initial testing by noninvasive testing is uninformative.
- In patients with postinfectious encephalitis, the virus responsible for the inflammatory response cannot be isolated from affected tissue.

MENINGITIS

Meningitis generally refers to infection in the subarachnoid space, the space between the middle (arachnoid) layer and the layer adjacent to the neural tissue (pia mater). Because the subarachnoid space is the major reservoir of CSF, CSF is usually the specimen of choice for tests to diagnose meningitis. The subarachnoid space is intrinsically "immunocompromised" outside of barrier defenses. There are relatively few phagocytic cells and the concentrations of complement and antibodies are low. Bacteria that gain access to the subarachnoid space are able to proliferate efficiently. There is a high morbidity and mortality associated with acute bacterial meningitis, even when antibiotics are promptly administered. "Aseptic" meningitis refers generically to syndromes associated with signs and symptoms of meningeal irritation, but negative routine bacterial cultures.

Aseptic meningitis is usually caused by viruses, most commonly enterovirus. A number of these viruses are also able to cause parenchymal infection, and distinguishing between meningitis, encephalitis, and meningoencephalitis can be challenging. Encephalitis is primarily characterized by neurologic dysfunction, whereas patients with aseptic meningitis most commonly present with photophobia, stiff neck, headache, and fever. Patients with severe aseptic meningitis, however, may develop seizures and altered mental status and progress to significant neurologic dysfunction.

A wide variety of viruses have been implicated as causing aseptic meningitis; the most common viruses are:

- Enteroviruses. The incidence of enteroviral meningitis peaks in late summer and early fall, but enteroviruses cause low-level, endemic disease year-round.
- HSV-2: A significant percentage of patients with primary genital herpes simplex infection also demonstrate signs and symptoms of aseptic meningitis. HSV-2 may also cause recurrent aseptic meningitis associated with flares of genital infection.
- HIV: A subset of patients with primary HIV infection will develop signs and symptoms of aseptic meningitis or meningoencephalitis, which is usually self-limited.
- Lymphocytic choriomeningitis virus: Virus is transmitted by the urine or feces of mice and other small rodents. There is an increased rate of infection during the winter months, presumably due to increased exposure. Aseptic meningitis caused by lymphocytic choriomeningitis is unusual because CSF may show decreased glucose concentrations and WBC counts greater than $1,000/mm^3$. Diagnosis is usually established serologically.
- Mumps virus: Aseptic meningitis is a fairly frequent complication of mumps infection, but the incidence has significantly decreased due to effective vaccination programs. This diagnosis may be suspected in patients with concurrent or recent parotitis.

A meningitis presentation may be associated with CNS infection by parasitic, mycobacterial, fungal, and bacterial pathogens, as described in other sections. Other infectious agents to consider, based on clinical and laboratory findings, include:

- Spirochetes (e.g., *Treponema pallidum, Borrelia burgdorferi*)
- Tick-borne agents (e.g., *Rickettsia* and *Ehrlichia* species)
- *Mycobacterium tuberculosis*
- Fungal pathogens (*Cryptococcus neoformans, Coccidioides immitis*), especially in immunocompromised patients.
- Parasites: (e.g., *Angiostrongylus*—suspect in patients with increased CSF eosinophils and risk based on epidemiology; amebas)

Aseptic meningitis may also be caused by malignancies, drugs, and other noninfectious causes.

Acute bacterial meningitis (ABM) is a medical emergency. Outcome depends on early administration of effective antibiotics and appropriate medical and neurosurgical interventions. Overall, *N. meningitidis* and *S. pneumoniae* cause a majority of cases of ABM, but the etiology of ABM depends on multiple factors. Age and route of transmission are major determinants:

- Neonates (<1 month): *Streptococcus agalactiae, E. coli, Listeria monocytogenes,* other enteric gram-negative bacteria)
- Infants (1–23 months): *S. pneumoniae, N. meningitidis, S. agalactiae, Haemophilus influenzae, E. coli*
- Older children and adults (2–50 years): *N. meningitidis, S. pneumoniae*
- Elderly (>50 years): *N. meningitidis, S. pneumoniae, L. monocytogenes,* enteric gram-negative bacteria
- Basilar skull fracture: *S. pneumoniae, Streptococcus pyogenes, H. influenzae*
- Penetrating head trauma and postneurosurgical infections: staphylococci (coagulase positive and coagulase negative), aerobic gram-negative bacilli, *Propionibacterium acnes* (CSF shunts)

➤ Clinical Presentation

A significant proportion of adult patients with community-acquired ABM do not present with all of the classic clinical features (headache, fever, stiff neck, and altered mental status), but the majority will show at least two of the four. A significant minority of patients may be comatose on admission or show focal neurologic abnormalities. Seizures are present in ~5% of patients.

Overall, the mortality rate is 20–25%; pneumococcal meningitis has a higher mortality rate than meningococcal (30% versus 7%). Factors associated with increased mortality risk include:
- Age (>60 years)
- Otitis or sinusitis
- Absence of rash
- Low admission score on Glasgow Coma Scale
- Tachycardia (>120 beats/min)
- Labs: Positive blood culture, increased ESR, decreased platelet count, low CSF WBC count (<1000 cells/mm^3)

Nonspecific symptoms are more frequent in infants and the elderly.

ABM may also be caused by invasive medical procedures or by trauma, and associated with a different etiology of infecting organisms. Signs and symptoms depend on the infecting organism as well as the predisposing event; those related to the trauma may overlap with those of the subsequent infection and may delay diagnosis and intervention.

Craniotomy results in bacterial meningitis following fewer than 2% of procedures. Two thirds of these infections occur within the first 2 weeks after the procedure.

Internal intraventricular catheters become infected in ~5–15% of cases, usually within the first month after placement, and usually represent intraoperative transmission. The incidence of infection of external CSF drainage catheters is <10%.

The risk of CNS infection caused by lumbar puncture is very low (~1:50:000).

The risk of meningitis is ~5–10% following compound skull fractures. The risk is increased when the wound is heavily contaminated with external material. Basilar skull fractures, which result in communication of the subarachnoid space with sinus cavities, are associated with a risk of meningitis up to 25%, with onset in the second week after trauma. Persistent CSF leak may be associated with recurrent bacterial meningitis.

➤ Diagnosis and Laboratory Findings

Acute bacterial meningitis should be ruled out by appropriate testing, followed by empirical antibiotic therapy for patients with a high suspicion for ABM. HSV should be ruled out in patients if encephalitis may be present.
- Diagnostic testing performed on CSF represents the primary approach to specific meningitis diagnosis. However, collection of CSF may be hazardous in patients with increased intracranial pressure (ICP). Cranial CT scan should be performed prior to lumbar puncture is clinical presentation suggests increased ICP. (Note: Imaging studies should not delay administration of antibiotics and dexamethasone therapy; blood cultures may be collected prior to imaging studies.) Clinical features significantly associated with increased ICP in adults include:
  - Positive history of CNS disease
  - Immunocompromised state
  - Papilledema
  - Abnormal level of consciousness
  - Focal neurologic abnormalities
- Primary testing usually includes aerobic bacterial culture, Gram stain, and CSF concentration of protein and glucose. The opening pressure should be measured at the time of lumbar puncture.

- Blood cultures, CBC, and other basic metabolic tests should be undertaken for initial evaluation of all patients with suspected ABM.
  - CBC often shows changes related to acute infection (e.g., increased number of band forms, toxic granulations, Döhle bodies, vacuolization of PMNs)
  - ESR, CRP, or other tests may indicate an intense inflammatory response.
  - Infection may result in significant metabolic dysregulation.
- Gram stain is positive for the infecting organism in 25% of patients when organisms were present at 103 cfu/mL; sensitivity increased to 97% when organisms were present at 105 cfu/mL. The sensitivity of detection organisms by culture and Gram stain is improved by concentrating CSF by centrifugation or filtration.
- The sensitivity of Gram stain depends on the infecting organism. Gram stain is positive in 90% of cases caused by staphylococci and pneumococci, 85% of cases caused by *H. influenzae*, 75% of cases caused by *N. meningitidis*, but only 30–50% of cases caused by gram-negative enteric bacilli. If antibiotics have been given before CSF obtained, Gram stain may be negative.
- Acridine orange staining may provide slightly greater sensitivity for detection of faintly staining organisms, but the technique requires use of a fluorescent microscope and technologist experience for smear interpretation.
- Testing for specific bacterial antigens may be used for rapid diagnosis in ABM. CSF is recommended if testing untreated patients; urine may provide increased sensitivity for treated patients. Although tests show acceptable sensitivity and specificity, clinical studies suggest that the results of bacterial antigen testing rarely affect patient management. Kits are commercially available for detection of bacterial cell wall or capsular polysaccharide antigens of:
  - *H. influenzae* type b
  - *N. meningitidis* serogroups A, B, C, Y, and W135
  - *Streptococcus*, group B
  - *S. pneumoniae*
- Other methods for direct detection of organisms in CSF include the limulus lysate assay (gram-negative bacilli), CIE, quelling reaction, and gas-liquid chromatography.
- The most frequent and important differential diagnosis is between ABM and aseptic meningitis. The most useful test results are:
  - CSF identification of organism by stain or culture, specific nucleic acid, or antigen by PCR
  - Decreased CSF glucose, or decreased CSF-to-serum glucose ratio if CSF glucose is normal
  - Increased CSF protein >1.72 mg/dL (1% of aseptic meningitis cases and 50% of ABM cases)
  - CSF WBC >2000/ mm^3 in 38% of ABM cases and PMN >1180/ mm^3 but low counts do not rule out ABM
  - Peripheral WBC count is only useful if WBC (>27,200/ mm^3) and total PMN (>21,000/ mm^3) counts are very high, which occurs in relatively few patients; leukopenia is common in infants and elderly.
- CSF from patients with aseptic meningitis typically shows no organisms by Gram stain. WBC may be mildly elevated (<500 cells/mm^3) with a lymphocyte predominance; protein may be moderately elevated; glucose level is usually normal.
- CSF from patients with ABM typically show markedly increased WBC count (>1000 cells/ mm^3), with a PMN predominance, increased protein (>100 mg/dL), and decreased glucose

($<$50% of serum glucose concentration). Opening pressure is increased (normal 100–200 mm Hg)

- In 50% of cases caused by *L. monocytogenes*, Gram stain may be negative; the cellular response is usually monocytic, which may cause this meningitis to be mistaken for aseptic meningitis.
- Overall, CSF culture has a good sensitivity (70–92%) and high specificity (95%).
- A sufficient amount of CSF must be collected to allow the testing required. Priority must be given to rule out ABM and HSV, when suspected. Repeat sampling may be needed if initial testing is not informative. A minimum of 3–5 mL of CSF should be collected for diagnostic testing for mycobacteria or fungi.
- PCR methods have been developed for detection of some bacterial pathogens causing ABM, though FDA-approved methods are not available.
- Gram stain of scrapings from petechial skin lesions demonstrate pathogen in ~70% of patients with meningococcemia; Gram stain of buffy coat of peripheral blood, and, less often, peripheral blood smear may reveal this organism.
- Laboratory findings due to preceding diseases/conditions:
  - Pneumonia, otitis media, sinusitis, skull fracture prior to pneumococcal meningitis
  - *Neisseria* epidemics prior to this meningitis
  - Bacterial endocarditis, septicemia, and so on
  - *S. pneumoniae* in alcoholism, myeloma, sickle cell anemia, splenectomy, immunocompromised state
  - *Cryptococcus* and *M. tuberculosis* in steroid therapy and immunocompromised state
  - Gram-negative bacilli in immunocompromised state
  - *H. influenzae* in splenectomy
  - Lyme disease
- Primary diagnostic testing may also include other laboratory diagnostic tests for patient in whom clinical presentation, epidemiologic risk factors, or signs and symptoms suggest a high prior probability of a pathogen outside the normal etiology of bacterial meningitis.
- Laboratory findings due to complications (e.g., Waterhouse-Friderichsen syndrome, subdural effusion)

(See discussions of parasitology, virology, mycology, and mycobacteriology for recommendations related to diagnosis of related pathogens.)

▶ Suggested Readings

Al Masalma M, Armougom F, Scheld WM, et al. The expansion of the microbiological spectrum of brain abscesses with use of multiple 16S ribosomal DNA sequencing. *Clin Infect Dis.* 2009;48:1169–1178.

Bitnun A, Ford-Jones EL, Petric M, et al. Acute childhood encephalitis and *Mycoplasma pneumoniae*. *Clin Infect Dis.* 2001;32:1674–1684.

Darouiche RO. Spinal epidural abscess. *N Engl J Med.* 2006;355:2012–2020.

Dumpis U, Crook D, Oksi J. Tick-borne encephalitis. *Clin Infect Dis.* 1999;28:882–890.

Glaser CA, Honarmand S, Anderson LJ, et al. Beyond viruses: clinical profiles and etiologies associated with encephalitis. *Clin Infect Dis.* 2006;43:1565–1577.

Hayden RT, Frenkel LD. More laboratory testing: greater cost but not necessarily better. *Pediatr Infect Dis J.* 2000;19:290–292.

Marciano-Cabral F, Cabral G. *Acanthamoeba* spp. as agents of disease in humans. *Clin Microbiol Rev.* 2003;16:273–307.

Matin A, Siddiqui R, Jayasekera S, Khan NA. Increasing importance of *Balamuthia mandrillaris*. *Clin Microbiol Rev.* 2008;21:435–448.

Maxson S, Lewno MJ, Schutze GE. Clinical usefulness of cerebrospinal fluid bacterial antigen studies. *J Pediatr.* 1994;125:235–238.

Polage CR, Petti CA. Assessment of the utility of viral culture of cerebrospinal fluid. *Clin Infect Dis.* 2006;43:1578–1579.

Pradilla G, Ardila GP, Hsu W, Rigamonti. Epidural abscesses of the CNS. *Lancet Neurol.* 2009;8:292–300.

Tarafdar K, Rao S, Recco RA, Zaman MM. Lack of sensitivity of the latex agglutination test to detect bacterial antigen in the cerebrospinal fluid of patients with culture-negative meningitis. *Clin Infect Dis.* 2001;33:406–408.

Tattevin P, Bruneel F, Clair B, et al. Bacterial brain abscesses: a retrospective study of 94 patients admitted to an intensive care unit (1980 to 1999). *Am J Med.* 2003;115:143–146.

Tunkel AR, Glaser CA, Bloch KC, et al. The management of encephalitis: clinical practice guidelines by the Infectious Diseases Society of America. *Clin Infect Dis.* 2008;47:303–27.

van de Beek D, de Gans J, Tunkel AR, Wijdicks EFM. Community-acquired bacterial meningitis in adults. *N Engl J Med.* 2006;354:44–53.

van de Beek D, de Gans J, Spanjaard L, et al. Clinical features and prognostic factors in adults with bacterial meningitis. *N Engl J Med.* 2004;351:1849–1859.

van de Beek D, Drake JM, Tunkel AR. Nosocomial bacterial meningitis. *N Engl J Med.* 2010;362:146–154.

CHAPTER 6

Digestive Diseases

L. Michael Snyder and Michael J. Mitchell

The current Digestive Diseases chapter combines the sections from the previous eighth edition on pancreatic/hepatobiliary disease and gastroenterologic disease. It lends itself to discussion of the patient's presenting symptoms and/or physical findings. This chapter focuses on several common GI clinical presentations: abdominal pain (acute and chronic); ascites; diarrhea (acute and chronic); GI bleeding upper and lower; hepatomegaly; jaundice and associated diseases, including hepatitis. When appropriate, the discussion includes radiologic and endoscopic procedures as part of the diagnostic evaluation.

DISEASE STATES ASSOCIATED WITH ABDOMINAL PAIN (ACUTE AND CHRONIC)

➤ Definition

Acute abdomen is defined as an episode of severe abdominal pain that lasts several hours or longer and requires medical attention. The acute abdomen usually, but not necessarily, has a surgical cause. However, the term "acute abdomen" should not be equated with a need for emergency surgery. The history and physical examination remain the most important aspects of diagnosis. The key feature in the evaluation of patients with acute abdomen is early diagnosis.

➤ Differential Diagnosis

- The differential diagnosis of an acute abdomen is most appropriately considered by its anatomic location (Table 6-1).
- Common gynecologic causes of lower quadrant pain include mittelschmerz, ovarian cyst, endometriosis, fibroids, ovarian torsion, pelvic inflammatory disease, ovarian tumor, ectopic pregnancy, infection of the uterus, threatened abortion, and round ligament pain secondary to pregnancy.
- Medical conditions that may present as acute abdomen are many. Common examples include lower lobe pneumonias, acute myocardial infarction (MI), DKA, acute hepatitis, porphyria, adrenal hemorrhage, and musculoskeletal problems. Appendicitis is a clinical diagnosis. The triad of right lower quadrant pain, anorexia, and leukocytosis is the most sensitive diagnostic tool. Nausea and vomiting usually follow the onset of pain. The patient may have a low-grade fever and mild leukocytosis. Fevers with higher temperatures or increased WBC counts suggest perforation.

TABLE 6-1. Differential Diagnosis of Acute Abdomen

Right Upper Quadrant Pain	Right Lower Quadrant Pain
Cholecystitis	Appendicitis
Choledocholithiasis	Ruptured ovarian cyst
Cholangitis	Meckel diverticulitis
Hepatitis	Cecal diverticulitis
Liver tumors	Cholecystitis
Hepatic abscess	Perforated colon
Appendicitis	Colon cancer
Peptic ulcer disease (PUD)	Urinary tract infection
Perforated ulcer	Small bowel obstruction
Pancreatitis	Inflammatory bowel disease (IBD)
Gastritis	Nephrolithiasis
Pyelonephritis	Pyelonephritis
Nephrolithiasis	Ectopic pregnancy
Pneumonia	Bowel incarceration
	Pelvic inflammatory disease (PID)

Left Upper Quadrant Pain	Lower Left Quadrant Pain
PUD	Diverticulitis
Perforated ulcer	Sigmoid volvulus
Gastritis	Perforated colon
Splenic disease (e.g., infarct,	Colon cancer
abscess, or rupture)	Urinary tract infection
Gastroesophageal reflux disease	Small bowel obstruction
Dissecting aortic aneurysm	IBD
Pyelonephritis	Nephrolithiasis
Nephrolithiasis	Pyelonephritis
Hiatal hernia	Ectopic pregnancy
Boerhaave syndrome (i.e., rupture of	Incarceration
the esophagus)	PID
Mallory-Weiss tear	
Diverticulitis	
Bowel obstruction	

Midepigastric Pain
PUD
Perforated ulcer
Pancreatitis
Abdominal aortic aneurysm
Esophageal varices
Hiatal hernia
Boerhaave syndrome (i.e., rupture of
the esophagus)
Mallory-Weiss tear

- Thirty percent of patients with appendicitis have an elevated WBC count, whereas 95% have a left shift.
- The intensity of pain is somewhat in proportion to the degree of irritation to the parietal peritoneum. Therefore, a retrocecal appendix (which is the most common location) may cause only a dull ache, given the lack of contact with the parietal peritoneum.

➤ Laboratory Findings
- Laboratory studies are undertaken to support a clinical hypothesis. The evaluation generally includes a CBC, liver chemistries, amylase and lipase, coagulation profile, urinalysis, and urine pregnancy test.
  - Lactic acid level should be obtained for patients with suspected ischemic bowel. An elevated level is associated with tissue hypoperfusion.
  - Beta-hCG levels must be obtained for all women of childbearing age to exclude the possibility of ectopic pregnancy.
- Radiographic studies
  - Chest radiograph should be obtained on all patients with acute abdomen to rule out free air. Pneumonia may present as an acute abdomen.
  - Abdominal radiograph is most effective in detecting either bowel obstruction or pneumoperitoneum. An upright and supine view is necessary.
    - Appendicolith can be seen in 15% of patients with appendicitis, whereas renal stones may also be visualized up to 85% of the time.
    - Other radiographic findings of acute appendicitis include right lower quadrant ileus, loss of psoas shadow, deformity of the cecal outline, free air, and soft tissue density.
- Abdominal ultrasound is the study of choice in patients with possible acute cholecystitis or ovarian cyst. A sonographic Murphy sign is more sensitive than a clinical Murphy sign for acute cholecystitis. An inflamed appendix can be visualized with compression ultrasound (sensitivity ranges from 80–90%).
- CT can also be used to diagnose appendicitis in patients whose clinical symptoms are ambiguous.
  - Air in the appendix or a normal-appearing contrast-filled appendix virtually rules out the diagnosis of appendicitis.
  - CT will provide an alternate diagnosis in 15% of patients when assessing for appendicitis.
- Arteriography is the test of choice for patients with suspected mesenteric ischemia.

DISORDERS OF THE ESOPHAGUS

MALLORY-WEISS SYNDROME

➤ Definition
Mallory-Weiss syndrome is characterized by spontaneous cardioesophageal laceration, usually caused by excessive retching. Laboratory findings are due to hemorrhage from cardioesophageal laceration.

PERFORATION OF ESOPHAGUS, SPONTANEOUS

In spontaneous perforation, gastric contents are found in thoracocentesis fluid.

PLUMMER-VINSON SYNDROME

➤ Definition
Plummer-Vinson syndrome is an iron-deficiency anemia associated with dysphagia, atrophic gastritis, glossitis, and so on. It carries an increased risk of cancer of the esophagus and hypopharynx.

DISORDERS OF THE STOMACH

GASTRITIS, CHRONIC

* A diagnosis of chronic gastritis depends on biopsy of gastric mucosa.

➤ Atrophic (Type A Gastritis, Autoimmune Type)
* Gastric antrum is spared
* Parietal cell antibodies and intrinsic factor antibodies help identify those patients prone to pernicious anemia (PA).
* Characteristics include:
  * Achlorhydria
  * Vitamin B_{12}–deficient megaloblastosis
  * Hypergastrinemia (due to hyperplasia of gastrin-producing cells)
  * Gastric carcinoids
  * Low serum pepsinogen I concentrations
* Laboratory findings may be due to other accompanying autoimmune diseases (e.g., Hashimoto thyroiditis, Addison disease, Graves disease, myasthenia gravis, hypoparathyroidism, type 1 DM)

➤ Nonatrophic (Type B Gastritis)
* Gastric antrum is involved
* Anemia caused by iron deficiency and malabsorption may occur.
* *Helicobacter pylori* infection is detectable in ~80% of patients with peptic ulcer and chronic gastritis. Diagnosis is by biopsy, culture, direct Gram staining, urease test, and serologic tests.
* Hypogastrinemia is caused by destruction of gastrin-producing cells in antrum.
* Chronic antral gastritis is consistently present in patients with benign gastric ulcer.
* Gastric acid studies are of limited value. Severe hypochlorhydria or achlorhydria after maximal stimulation usually denotes mucosal atrophy.

➤ Other Causes
* Infections (other bacteria [syphilis], viral [e.g., CMV], parasitic [e.g., anisakiasis], fungal)
* Chemical (e.g., NSAIDs, bile reflux, other drugs)
* Lymphocytic gastritis
* Eosinophilic gastroenteritis
* Noninfectious granulomatous (e.g., sarcoidosis, Crohn disease)
* Ménétrier disease
* Radiation

CARCINOMA OF THE STOMACH

➤ Laboratory Findings

Carcinoma of the stomach should always be searched for by periodic prophylactic screening in high-risk patients, especially those with PA, gastric atrophy, or gastric polyps.

Cytology: Exfoliative cytology positive in 80% of patients; false-positive result in <2%

Tumor Markers: Increased serum CEA (>5 ng/dL) in 40–50% of patients with metastases and 10–20% of patients with surgically resectable disease. May be useful for postoperative monitoring for recurrence or to estimate metastatic tumor burden. Increased serum AFP and CA 19-9 in 30% of patients, usually incurable. Markers are not useful for early detection.

Gastric Analysis: Normal in 25% of patients. Hypochlorhydria in 25% of patients. Achlorhydria following histamine or betazole in 50% of patients

Core Laboratory: Anemia due to chronic blood loss. Occult blood in stool

DISORDERS OF THE PANCREAS

CARCINOMA OF PANCREAS

Body or Tail

➤ Laboratory Findings

Imaging Studies: Most useful tests are ultrasound or CT scanning followed by ERCP (at which time fluid is also obtained for cytologic and pancreatic function studies). This combination will correctly diagnose or rule out cancer of pancreas in ≥90% of cases. ERCP with brush cytology has S/S = ≤25%/≤100%. Radioisotope scanning of pancreas may be done (75Se) for lesions >2 cm.

Histology: Ultrasound guided needle biopsy has reported sensitivity of 80–90%; false positives are rare.

Tumor Markers: Serum markers for tumor CA 19-9, CEA, and so on) are often normal. In carcinoma of pancreas, CA 19-9 has S/S = 70%/87%, PPV = 59%, and NPV = 92%; there is no difference in sensitivity between local disease and metastatic disease. Often normal in early stages, they are *not useful for screening*. Increased values may help differentiate benign disease from cancer. Declines to normal in 3–6 months if cancer is completely removed so may be useful for prognosis and follow-up. Detects tumor recurrence 2–20 weeks before clinical evidence. Not specific for pancreas because high levels may also occur in other GI cancers, especially those affecting colon and bile duct. CEA level in bile (obtained by percutaneous transhepatic drainage) was reported increased in 76% of a small group of cases.

Testosterone: Dihydrotestosterone ratio <5 (normal ~10) in >70% of men with pancreatic cancer (due to increased conversion by tumor); less sensitive but more specific than CA 19-9 and present in higher proportion of stage I tumors.

Serum Amylase and Lipase: May be slightly increased in early stages (<10% of cases); with later destruction of pancreas, they are normal or decreased. They may increase following secretin-pancreozymin stimulation before destruction is extensive; therefore, the increase is less marked with a diabetic glucose tolerance curve. Serum amylase response is less reliable. See Serum Glycoprotein 2.

Glucose Tolerance: Curve is of the diabetic type, with overt diabetes in 20% of patients with pancreatic cancer. Flat blood sugar curve with IV tolbutamide tolerance test indicates destruction of islet cell tissue. *Unstable, insulin-sensitive diabetes that develops in an older man should arouse suspicion of carcinoma of the pancreas.*

Serum LAP: Increased (>300 units) in 60% of patients with carcinoma of pancreas due to liver metastases or biliary tract obstruction. *It may also be increased in chronic liver disease.*

Other: Triolein ^{131}I test demonstrates pancreatic duct obstruction with absence of lipase in the intestine, causing flat blood curves and increased stool excretion.

Head (see Jaundice)

- The abnormal pancreatic function tests and increased tumor markers that occur with carcinoma of the body of the pancreas may be evident.

➤ Laboratory Findings

Core Laboratory: Serum bilirubin is increased (12–25 mg/dL), mostly conjugated (increase persistent and nonfluctuating). Serum ALP is increased. Urine and stool urobilinogen are absent. Increased serum cholesterol (usually >300 mg/dL) with esters not decreased. Other liver function tests are usually normal. See Serum Glycoprotein 2.

Hematology: Increased PT; normal after IV vitamin K administration

Other: Secretin-cholecystokinin stimulation evidences duct obstruction when duodenal intubation shows decreased volume of duodenal contents (<10 mL/10-minute collection period) with usually normal bicarbonate and enzyme levels in duodenal contents. Acinar destruction (as in pancreatitis) shows normal volume (20–30 mL/10-minute collection period), but bicarbonate and enzyme levels may be decreased. Abnormal volume, bicarbonate, or both is found in 60–80% of patients with pancreatitis or cancer. In carcinoma, the test result depends on the relative extent and combination of acinar destruction and of duct obstruction.

Histology: Cytologic examination of duodenal contents shows malignant cells in 40% of patients. Malignant cells may be found in up to 80% of patients with periampullary cancer.

CYSTIC FIBROSIS OF THE PANCREAS (MUCOVISCIDOSIS)

Core Laboratory: Hypochloremic metabolic alkalosis and hypokalemia. Serum protein electrophoresis shows increasing IgG and IgA with progressive pulmonary disease; IgM and IgD are not appreciably increased. Serum albumin is often decreased (because of hemodilution due to cor pulmonale; may be found before cardiac involvement is clinically apparent). Serum chloride, sodium, potassium, calcium, and phosphorus are normal unless complications occur (e.g., chronic pulmonary disease with accumulation of CO_2; massive salt loss due to sweating may cause hyponatremia). Urine electrolytes are normal. Excessive loss of electrolytes in sweat and stool. Impaired glucose intolerance in ~40% of patients with glycosuria, and hyperglycemia in 8% precedes DM. Protein-calorie malnutrition, hypoproteinemia; fat malabsorption of with vitamin deficiency. Stool and duodenal fluid show lack of trypsin digestion of x-ray film gelatin; useful screening test up to age 4; decreased chymotrypsin production.

Saliva Findings: Submaxillary saliva is more turbid, with increased calcium, total protein, amylase, chloride and sodium but not potassium. These changes are not generally found in parotid saliva.

Other Findings: Overt liver disease, including cirrhosis, fatty liver, bile duct strictures, and cholelithiasis, in ≤5% of cases. Meconium ileus during early infancy. Chronic or acute and recurrent pancreatitis. Pancreatic insufficiency frequency by age 1 year >90%; in adults >95%. Increased incidence of GI tract cancers. GU tract abnormalities with aspermia in 98% due to obstructive changes in vas deferens and epididymis is confirmed by testicular biopsy.

MACROAMYLASEMIA

➤ Definition
Complex of amylase with IgA, IgG, or other high-molecular-weight plasma proteins that cannot filter through glomerulus due to its large size.

➤ Laboratory Findings
Core Laboratory: Serum lipase is normal; normal pancreatic to salivary amylase ratio. Urine amylase normal or low. Serum amylase *persistently* increased (often 1–4X normal) without apparent cause. Amylase-creatinine clearance ratio <1% with normal renal function is very useful for this diagnosis; should make the clinician suspect this diagnosis. Macroamylase is identified in serum by special gel filtration or ultracentrifugation technique.

➤ Limitations
* Macroamylase may be found in ~1% of randomly selected patients and 2.5% of persons with increased serum amylase level. Same findings may also occur in patients with normal molecular-weight hyperamylasemia in which excess amylase is principally salivary gland iso-amylase types 2 and 3.

PANCREATITIS

Pancreatitis, Acute
➤ Laboratory Findings
Lipase: Serum lipase increases within 3–6 hours with peak at 24 hours and usually returns to normal over a period of 8–14 days. Is superior to amylase; increases to a greater extent and may remain elevated for up to 14 days after amylase returns to normal. In patients with signs of acute pancreatitis, pancreatitis is highly likely (clinical specificity = 85%) when lipase ≥5X upper reference limit (URL); if values change significantly with time, and if amylase and lipase changes are concordant. (*Lipase should always be determined whenever amylase is determined*). Urinary lipase is not clinically useful. It has been suggested that a lipase:amylase ratio >3 (and especially >5) indicates alcoholic rather than nonalcoholic pancreatitis). If

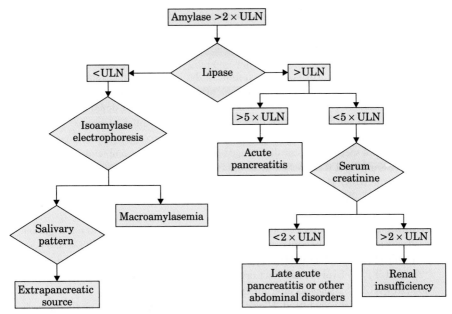

Figure 6-1. Algorithm for increased serum amylase and lipase. (ULN, upper limit of normal.)

lipase ≥5× URL, acute pancreatitis or organ rejection is highly likely but unlikely if <3× URL (Figure 6-1).

Amylase: Increase begins in 3–6 hours, rises rapidly within 8 hours in 75% of patients, reaches maximum in 20–30 hours, and may persist for 48–72 hours. >95% sensitivity during first 12–24 hours. The increase may be ≤40× normal, but the height of the increase and rate of fall do not correlate with the severity of the disease, prognosis, or rate of resolution. In patients with signs of acute pancreatitis, amylase >3× ULN or >600 Somogyi units/dL is very suggestive of acute pancreatitis. An increase >7–10 days suggests an associated cancer of pancreas or pseudocyst, pancreatic ascites, nonpancreatic etiology. Similar high values may occur in obstruction of pancreatic duct; they tend to fall after several days. ≤19% of patients with acute pancreatitis (especially when seen more than 2 days after onset of symptoms) may have normal values, especially with an alcoholic etiology and longer duration of symptoms, even when dying of acute pancreatitis. May also be normal in relapsing chronic pancreatitis and patients with hypertriglyceridemia (technical interference with test). Frequently normal in acute alcoholic pancreatitis. Acute abdomen due to GI infarction or perforation rather than acute pancreatitis is suggested by only moderate increase in serum amylase and lipase (<3× URL), evidence of bacteremia. Of patients with acute alcoholic intoxication, 10–40% have elevated serum amylase (about half are salivary type); they often present with abdominal pain but increased serum amylase is usually <3× URL. Levels >25× URL indicate metastatic tumor rather than pancreatitis. Serum pancreatic isoamylase can distinguish elevations due to salivary amylase that may account for 25% of all elevated values. (In healthy persons, 40% of total serum amylase is pancreatic type and 60% is salivary type). Only slight increase in serum amylase and lipase values suggests a different diagnosis than acute pancreatitis. *Many drugs increase both amylase and lipase in serum.*

Increased urinary amylase tends to reflect serum changes by a time lag of 6–10 hours, but sometimes increased urine levels are higher and of longer duration than serum levels. The 24-hour level may be normal even when some of the 1-hour specimens show increased values. Amylase levels in hourly samples of urine may be useful. Ratio of amylase clearance to creatinine clearance is increased ($>5\%$) and avoids the problem of timed urine specimens; also increased in any condition that decreases tubular reabsorption of amylase (e.g., severe burns, DKA, chronic renal insufficiency, multiple myeloma, acute duodenal perforation). Considered not specific and now discouraged by some but still recommended by others.

Calcium: Serum level is decreased in severe cases 1–9 days after onset (due to binding to soaps in fat necrosis). The decrease usually occurs after amylase and lipase levels have become normal. Tetany may occur. (*Rule out hyperparathyroidism if serum calcium is high or fails to fall in hyperamylasemia of acute pancreatitis.*)

Bilirubin: Serum levels may be increased when pancreatitis is of biliary tract origin but is usually normal in alcoholic pancreatitis. Serum ALP, ALT, and AST may increase and parallel serum bilirubin rather than amylase, lipase, or calcium levels. Marked amylase increase (e.g., $>2,000$ U/L) also favors biliary tract origin. Fluctuation $>50\%$ in 24 hours of serum bilirubin, ALP, ALT, AST suggests intermittent biliary obstruction.

Trypsin: Serum level is increased. High sensitivity makes a normal value useful for excluding acute pancreatitis. But low specificity (increased in large proportion of patients with hepatobiliary, bowel, and other diseases and renal insufficiency; increased in 13% of patients with chronic pancreatitis, 50% with pancreatic carcinoma) and RIA technology limit utility.

CRP: Level peaks 3 days after onset of pain; at 48 hours, sensitivity = 65–100%, PPV = 37–77%. Level of 150 mg/L distinguishes mild from severe disease.

* **Laboratory criteria for severe disease or predictor of mortality:**
* PaO_2 <60 μmol/L
    * Creatinine >2 mg/dL after rehydration
    * Blood glucose >250 mg/dL
    * Hemoconcentration (Hct $>47\%$ or failure to decrease in 24 hours after admission), but Hct may be decreased in severe hemorrhagic pancreatitis
    * GI bleed >500 mL/24 hours
    * Presence, volume, and color of peritoneal fluid
* Methemalbumin may be increased in serum and ascitic fluid (AF) in hemorrhagic (severe) but not edematous (mild) pancreatitis; may distinguish these two conditions but not useful in diagnosis of acute pancreatitis.
* WBC is slightly to moderately increased (10,000–20,000/μL).
* Glycosuria appears in 25% of patients.
* Hypokalemia, metabolic alkalosis, or lactic acidosis may occur.
* **Laboratory findings due to predisposing conditions (may be multiple):**
    * Alcohol abuse accounts for ~36% of cases.
    * Biliary tract disease accounts for 17% of cases.
    * Idiopathic accounts for $>36\%$ of cases.
    * Infections (especially viral such as mumps and coxsackievirus, CMV, and AIDS)
    * Trauma and postoperative factors account for $>8\%$ of cases

* Drugs (e.g., steroids, thiazides, azathioprine, estrogens, sulfonamides; children taking valproic acid) account for >5% of cases.
* Hypertriglyceridemia (hyperlipidemia—types V, I, IV) accounts for 7% of cases
* Hypercalcemia from any cause
* Tumors (pancreas, ampulla)
* Anatomic abnormalities of ampullary region causing obstruction (e.g., annular pancreas, Crohn disease, duodenal diverticulum)
* Hereditary
* Renal failure; renal transplantation
* Miscellaneous (e.g., collagen vascular disease, pregnancy, ischemia, scorpion bites, parasites obstructing pancreatic duct [*Ascaris*, fluke], Reye syndrome, fulminant hepatitis, severe hypotension, cholesterol embolization)
* **Laboratory findings due to complications:**
  * Pseudocysts of pancreas
  * Pancreatic infection or abscess diagnosed by increased WBC count, Gram staining, and culture of aspirate
  * Polyserositis (peritoneal, pleural, pericardial, synovial surfaces). Ascites may develop cloudy or bloody or "prune juice" fluid, 0.5 to 2.0 L in volume, containing increased amylase with a level higher than that of serum amylase. No bile is evident (unlike in perforated ulcer). Gram stain shows no bacteria (unlike infarct of intestine). Protein >3 g/dL and marked increase in amylase.
  * Adult respiratory distress syndrome (with pleural effusion, alveolar exudate, or both) may occur in ~40% of patients; arterial hypoxemia is present.
  * DIC
  * Hypovolemic shock
  * Others

➤ Prognostic Laboratory Findings

* On admission
  WBC >16,000/μL
  Blood glucose >200 mg/dL
  Serum LD >350 U/L
  Serum AST >250 units/L
  Age >55 years
* Within 48 hours
  >10% decrease in Hct
  Serum calcium <8.0 mg/dL
  Increase in BUN >5 mg/dL
  Arterial pO_2 <60 mm Hg
  Metabolic acidosis with base deficit >4 mEq/L
* Mortality
  1%, if 3 signs are positive
  15%, if 3 to 4 signs are positive
  40%, if 5 to 6 signs are positive
  100%, if ≥7 signs are positive
* Degree of amylase elevation has no prognostic significance

• CT scan, MRI, and ultrasound are useful for confirming diagnosis or identifying causes or other conditions.

➤ Suggested Readings

Papachristou GI, Whitcomb DC. Inflammatory markers of disease severity in acute pancreatitis. *Clin Lab Med.* 2005;25:17.
Ranson JHC. Etiological and prognostic factors in human acute pancreatitis: a review. *Am J Gastroenterol.* 1982;77:633.
Whitcomb DC. Acute pancreatitis. *N Engl J Med.* 2006;354:2142.

Pancreatitis, Chronic

• See also Malabsorption.

➤ Laboratory Findings

Laboratory findings are often normal.

Imaging Studies: CT, ultrasound, and ERCP are most accurate for diagnosing and staging chronic pancreatitis. Radioactive scanning of pancreas (selenium) yields variable findings in different clinics.

Cholecystokinin-secretin test: Measures the effect of IV administration of cholecystokinin and secretin on volume, bicarbonate concentration, and amylase output of duodenal contents and increase in serum lipase and amylase. This is the most sensitive and reliable test ("gold standard") for chronic pancreatitis especially in the early stages. However, it is technically difficult and is often not performed accurately; gastric contamination must be avoided. Some abnormality occurs in >85% of patients with chronic pancreatitis. Amylase output is the most frequent abnormality. When all three are abnormal, there is a greater frequency of abnormality in the tests listed below.

• Normal duodenal contents
  • Volume: 95–235 mL/hour
  • Bicarbonate concentration: 74–121 mEq/L
  • Amylase output: 87,000–276,000 mg
• Serum amylase and lipase increase after administration of cholecystokinin and secretin in ~20% of patients with chronic pancreatitis. They are more often abnormal when duodenal contents are normal. Normally serum lipase and amylase do not rise above normal limits.
• Fasting serum amylase and lipase are increased in 10% of patients with chronic pancreatitis.

Serum pancreolauryl test: Fluorescein dilaurate with breakfast is acted on by a pancreas-specific cholesterol ester hydrolase-releasing fluorescein, which is absorbed from gut and measured in serum; preceded by administration of secretin and followed by metoclopramide. Reported S/S = 82%/91%. (Dominguez-Munoz JE, Malfertheiner P. Optimized serum pancreolauryl test for differentiating patients with and without chronic pancreatitis. *Clin Chem* 1998;44:869.)

Glucose tolerance test (GTT): In 65% of patients with chronic pancreatitis and frank diabetes in >10% of patients with chronic relapsing pancreatitis. When GTT is normal in the presence of steatorrhea, the cause should be sought elsewhere than in the pancreas.

Laboratory findings due to malabsorption: Occurs when >90% of exocrine function is lost

• Bentiromide test is usually abnormal with moderate to severe pancreatic insufficiency but often normal in early cases.
• Schilling test may show mild malabsorption of vitamin B_{12} (no longer performed).
• Xylose tolerance test and small bowel biopsy are not usually done but are normal.

- Chemical determination of fecal fat demonstrates steatorrhea. It is more sensitive than tests using triolein [131]I.
- Triolein ^{131}I is abnormal in one third of patients with chronic pancreatitis.
- Starch tolerance test is abnormal in 25% of patients with chronic pancreatitis.

Laboratory findings due to chronic pancreatitis and pancreatic exocrine insufficiency:

- Alcohol in 60–70%
- Idiopathic in 30–40%
- Obstruction of pancreatic duct (e.g., trauma, pseudocyst, pancreas divisum, cancer, or obstruction of duct or ampulla)
- Others occasionally (e.g., CF, primary hyperparathyroidism, heredity, malnutrition, miscellaneous [Z-E syndrome, Shwachman syndrome, alpha$_1$-antitrypsin deficiency, trypsinogen deficiency, enterokinase deficiency, hemochromatosis, parenteral hyperalimentation]).

PSEUDOCYST OF PANCREAS

➤ Laboratory Findings

Imaging Studies: Detected by ultrasound or CT scan.

Core Laboratory: Serum conjugated bilirubin is increased (>2 mg/dL) in 10% of patients. Serum ALP is increased in 10% of patients. Fasting blood sugar is increased in <10% of patients.

Secretin-pancreozymin stimulation: Duodenal contents usually show decreased bicarbonate content (<70 mEq/L) but normal volume and normal content of amylase, lipase, and trypsin.

Pancreatic Cyst Fluid Findings: High fluid viscosity and CEA indicate mucinous differentiation and exclude pseudocyst, serous cystadenoma, other nonmucinous cysts or cystic tumors. Pancreatic enzymes, leukocyte esterase, and NB/70K are increased in pseudocyst fluid. Increased CA 72-4, CA 15-3, and tissue polypeptide antigen are markers of malignancy; if all are low, pseudocyst or serous cystadenoma is most likely. CA 125 is increased in serous cystadenoma.

Other: Laboratory findings due to conditions preceding acute pancreatitis are noted (e.g., alcoholism, trauma, duodenal ulcer, cholelithiasis), infection, perforation, anmd hemorrhage by erosion of blood vessel or into a viscus.

DYSPEPSIA AND PEPTIC ULCER DISEASE

➤ Definition

- Dyspepsia encompasses any or all of a great variety of upper abdominal symptoms, including upper abdominal pain or discomfort, nausea, bloating, heartburn, early satiety, regurgitation, and belching.
- Nonulcerative dyspepsia is defined as persistent or recurrent abdominal pain or discomfort centered in the upper abdomen without definite structural or biochemical explanation. By definition, nonulcerative dyspepsia is a diagnosis of exclusion. Possible mechanisms include dysmotility of the stomach or small intestine, heightened visceral sensitivity, altered intestinal or gastric reflexes, and psychological distress.

* Peptic ulcer disease (PUD)
    * Epigastric abdominal pain is the most common symptom. Pain is nonradiating and is described as a "gnawing" or "hunger pain." Pain occurs 1–2 hours postprandially and is relieved characteristically by food or antacids.
    * Nocturnal pain is more specific for PUD and is due to the physiologic increase in acid secretion, which occurs in the early morning hours.
    * Asymptomatic
        * Patients with PUD induced by NSAIDs are frequently asymptomatic
        * As many as 60% of patients who develop bleeding as a complication of PUD are also asymptomatic.
* Dyspepsia is typically a chronic relapsing condition. Between 65% and 86% of patients with dyspepsia will experience dyspeptic symptoms, at least intermittently, 2 to 3 years after the initial presentation. Long duration of symptoms and intermittent symptoms can also occur in PUD and esophagitis; therefore, these characteristics are not reassuring as to the absence of pathology.
* Gastroesophageal reflux disease (GERD) and dyspepsia have similar symptoms. Gastroesophageal reflux is a normal physiologic process that occurs daily in all individuals. GERD (expressed clinically as heartburn)
* *Helicobacter pylori* infection is clearly implicated in the etiology of recurrent PUD, yet its role in nonulcerative dyspepsia remains unclear. Between 30% and 60% of patients with nonulcerative dyspepsia have *H. pylori*. However, the background prevalence in the general population is also high.

➤ Recommended Tests
* Laboratory investigation may not be necessary in young patients (<45 years of age) who have a normal examination and no indicators for organic disease. The etiology of dyspepsia is presented in Table 6-2.
* In older patients at increased risk, the minimal laboratory work-up should include a CBC, electrolytes, calcium, and liver chemistries.
* Thyroid tests, hCG, amylase, and stool studies should be ordered if specific features of the history or examination are suggestive.
* **Additional studies**
    * **Upper endoscopy** [i.e., esophagogastroduodenoscopy (EGD)]: In the majority of cases, this is the study of first choice when further evaluation of dyspepsia is required, including the ability to obtain biopsies. As many as two thirds of endoscopies are completely normal in younger patients (i.e., <45 years of age). Therefore, it is best applied to older patients and to younger patients with classic symptoms.
    * **Upper GI radiography:** This test is less accurate than upper endoscopy and cannot provide tissue diagnosis. It is best reserved for situations where endoscopy expertise is unavailable, for patients who refuse endoscopy or have low pretest probability of disease, and in situations where endoscopy might be considered unsafe.
* *H. pylori* **testing**
* **Gastric emptying studies:** Gastric scintigraphy and gastroduodenal manometry studies generally do not influence medical management and are reserved for patients with normal laboratory tests and a normal EGD, yet who continue to have frequent or protracted vomiting suggestive of a motility disorder. Even in these cases, empiric treatment with prokinetic agents should probably be tried first. Disorders of the gall bladder (see Biliary Extrahepatic Obstruction, Complete)

TABLE 6-2. Differential Diagnosis of Dyspepsia
Structural Disease Involving the Stomach or Esophagus
Peptic ulcer disease [15–25% of cases] Reflux esophagitis (5–15% of cases) Gastric or esophageal cancer (<2% of cases) Infiltrative disease Eosinophilic gastritis Crohn disease Sarcoidosis
Other Gastrointestinal-related Disease
Gallstones Chronic pancreatitis or pancreatic cancer Celiac disease Lactose intolerance Hepatoma
Medications
Nonsteroidal antiinflammatory drugs Digitalis Theophylline Erythromycin Alcohol Caffeine Nicotine
Other Possible Causes
Hypothyroidism Hypercalcemia Intestinal angina Pregnancy Nonulcerative dyspepsia*
*Nonulcerative dyspepsia occurs in up to 60% of cases, but the diagnosis requires the exclusion of other diagnostic entities.

➤ Suggested Readings

Ferry GD. Causes of acute abdominal pain in children. www.uptodate.com, May, 2009.

Khan F, Sachs H, Pechet, L, Snyder LM. *Guide to Diagnostic Testing*. Philadelphia: Lippincott Williams & Wilkins; 2002.

Penner RM, Majumdar SR. Diagnostic approach to abdominal pain in adults. www.uptodate.com, May, 2009.

ASCITES

➤ Definition
- Ascites is a collection of free fluid in the peritoneal cavity.
- Etiology

- Chronic liver disease (infectious hepatitis and alcoholism) causes 80% of cases of ascites. (see Hepatomegaly, Jaundice)
- Multiple causes, including cirrhosis, peritoneal carcinomatosis, or tuberculous peritonitis, account for 3–5% of cases.
- Carcinomatosis causes <10% of cases of ascites.
- Heart failure is responsible for <3–5% of cases, and nephritic syndrome is a rare cause of ascites.
- Cryptogenic cirrhosis may account for up to 10% of cases.

➤ Classification

- Ascites is currently classified as high gradient or low gradient, depending on the serum ascites albumin gradient (SAAG). Calculation of SAAG involves the difference (not the ratio) between serum values and AF values.
- **High-gradient ascites** results from portal hypertension, whether on the basis of cirrhosis or noncirrhosis. Nephrotic syndrome is an exception and will usually cause low-gradient ascites due to marked hypoalbuminemia.
- **Low-gradient ascites** usually occurs as the result of cardiac failure, malignant carcinomatosis of the peritoneum, infections (such as TB), perforation of the bowel, connective tissues diseases, SLE, and chemical inflammation as in pancreatitis.

➤ Laboratory Findings (Figure 6-2)

- **Culture:** Bedside inoculation of AF in blood culture bottles has increased the positive bacterial yield to interpreted in concert with the cell count. A Gram stain should also be done.

Imaging Studies: Ultrasonography is useful for detecting the presence of ascites as well as for determining the etiology. It may reveal evidence of chronic liver disease, malignancy, hepatomegaly, and pancreatic disorder.

Ascites Fluid Findings: AF examination is the principle diagnostic tool. Using abdominal paracentesis to obtain and study the fluid is crucial to making a diagnosis.

- **Transparent to pale fluid:** is seen in cases of portal hypertension. Neutrophilia in excess of 1,000/mL results in opalescence. A concentration of RBCs in excess of 10,000/mL gives a faint pink tinge, and cell counts >20,000/mL color it red. A traumatic tap is evident by a streak of blood rather than homogeneously red fluid and the tendency to clot. Hepatocellular carcinoma and, rarely metastatic disease, can cause a bloody tap. TB is only a rare cause of hemorrhagic ascites.
- **Chylous or milky ascites:** has a higher triglyceride concentration than serum and >200 mg/dL. It is rarely seen and is usually an indication of cirrhosis rather than lymphoma or TB as was previously thought. The triglycerides are >1,000 mg/dL in truly milky ascites. Dark-brown ascites may be seen in significant hyperbilirubinemia, biliary perforation (when ascitic bilirubin is higher than serum bilirubin), pancreatitis, and, rarely, in malignant melanoma.
- **Bloody ascites fluid:** Once a traumatic tap has been ruled out, 50% of cases are due to hepatocellular carcinoma. TB rarely causes bloody fluid.
- **Staining:** Gram staining has low yield. Even with centrifugation, it has 10% sensitivity in spontaneous bacterial peritonitis. AFB smear for TB have very low sensitivity. In an appropriate clinical setting of low-grade fever, malaise, and weight loss, a high cell count with lymphocytic predominance and low SAAG is suggestive of TB ascites.

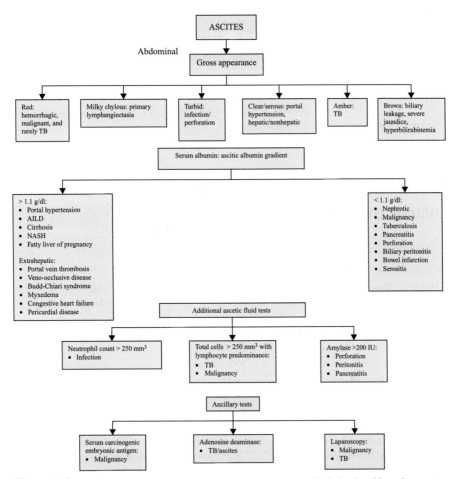

Figure 6-2. Algorithm for the work-up of patients with ascites. *AILD*, alcohol-induced liver disease; *CEA*, carcinoembryonic antigen; *NASH*, nonalcoholic steatohepatitis; *TB*, tuberculosis; *TNC*, total neutrophil count.

- **Protein concentration** of AF categorized ascites into exudative (ascitic protein >2.5 g/dL) or transudative (ascitic protein <2.5 g/dL). The significance of this has never been evaluated adequately and objectively.
- **Cell count and differential.** In uncomplicated cirrhosis, the total WBC count is <500 cells/μL with <250 neutrophils/μL. After diuresis, the total cell count may go up, but the neutrophil count remains below 250 cells/μL. In spontaneous bacterial peritonitis, the total WBC count and neutrophil count are usually but not always raised. In TB and carcinomatosis, the cell count rises but with a predominance of lymphocytes. In traumatic taps, for every 250 RBCs, one neutrophil is subtracted from the total WBC count.

Core Laboratory: The serum and AF glucose concentrations are nearly the same in uncomplicated portal hypertension (large numbers of WBCs, bacteria, or tumor cells consume glucose and may lead to diminished levels). Amylase values may be about 3–5 times higher than the serum values. LD levels rise because of release of LD from the neutrophils. The rise occurs in cases of secondary peritonitis, TB, and pancreatitis.

Cytology: Has limitations in the diagnosis of malignant ascites and has been replaced largely laparoscopic examination of the peritoneum along with biopsy and culture.

➤ Limitations

• Errors may occur if serum albumin is very low or when serum and ascitic samples are not obtained within a short space of time from each other.
• A high globulin level in serum may also give a false result.

DISORDERS OF THE PERITONEUM

CHRONIC LIVER DISEASE (SEE P. 618)

• This disease differs from ascites caused by malignancy.

➤ Laboratory Findings

Albumin: Almost always ≥ 1.1 g/dL in cirrhosis (most common cause), alcoholic hepatitis, massive liver metastases, fulminant hepatic failure, portal vein thrombosis, Budd-Chiari syndrome, cardiac ascites, fatty liver, acute fatty liver of pregnancy, myxedema, mixed (e.g., cirrhosis with peritoneal TB). May be falsely low if serum albumin <1.1 g/dL or patient in shock. May be falsely high with chylous ascites (lipid interferes with albumin assay). Albumin levels <1.1 g/dL in $>90\%$ of cases of peritoneal carcinomatosis (most common cause) TB, pancreatic or biliary ascites, nephrotic syndrome, bowel infarction or obstruction, serositis in patients without cirrhosis.

Ascites Fluid Findings: AF total protein >2.5 mg/dL in cancer is only 56% accurate because of high protein content in 12% to 19% of these ascites as well as changes caused by albumin infusion and diuretic therapies. AF/serum albumin ratio <0.5 in cirrhosis ($>90\%$ accuracy). AF/serum ratio of LD (>0.6) or protein (>0.5) are not more accurate ($\sim56\%$) than only total protein for diagnosis of exudate. AF cholesterol <55 mg/dL in cirrhosis (94% accuracy). Albumin gradient (serum albumin minus AF albumin) reflects portal pressure. Total WBC count is usually $<300/\mu$L (50% of cases) and PMN $<25\%$ (50% of cases).

Core Laboratory: Liver function tests are abnormal.

Other: Cirrhosis findings are similar with or without hepatocellular carcinoma. Cardiac ascites is associated with a blood-AF albumin gradient >1.1 g/dL, but malignant AF shows blood-AF albumin gradient <1.1 g/dL in 93% of cases.

INFECTED ASCITIC FLUID

➤ Laboratory Findings

Culture: AF in blood culture bottles has 85% sensitivity.

Ascites Fliud Findings:

• WBC count $>250/\mu$L: sensitivity = 85%, specificity = 93% and neutrophils $>50\%$ are presumptive of bacterial peritonitis.
• pH <7.35 and arterial-AF pH difference >0.10; both these findings are virtually diagnostic of bacterial peritonitis and absence of the above findings virtually excludes bacterial peritonitis.

- Lactate >25 mg/dL and arterial-AF difference >20 mg/dL are often present. LD is markedly increased. Phosphate, potassium, and gamma-glutamyltransferase may also be increased. Glucose is unreliable for diagnosis. Total protein <1.0 g/dL indicates high risk for SBP.
- Gram stain shows few bacteria in spontaneous bacterial peritonitis (SBP) but many when caused by intestinal perforation. Culture sensitivity = 50% for SBP and ~80% for secondary peritonitis. TB acid-fast stain sensitivity = 20–30% and TB culture sensitivity = 50–70%.

SECONDARY PERITONITIS

- This condition shows polymicrobial infection, total protein >1.0 g/dL, AF/LD greater than serum upper limit of normal, glucose <50 mg/dL compared with spontaneous bacterial peritonitis (SPB).
- Prevalence of SBP 15%; due to *Escherichia coli* ~50%, *Klebsiella*, and other gram-negative bacteria; gram-positive ~25% (especially streptococci).

CONTINUOUS AMBULATORY PERITONEAL DIALYSIS

Monitor dialysate for the following:
- **Infection:** Peritonitis is defined as WBC count >100/μL, usually with >50% PMNs (normal is <50 WBC/μL, usually mononuclear cells), or positive Gram stain or culture (most prevalent: coagulase-negative staphylococci, *Staphylococcus aureus*, *Streptococcus* sp.; multiple organisms, especially mixed aerobes and anaerobes occur with bowel perforation). Successful therapy causes fall in WBC count within first 2 days and a return to <100/μL in 4–5 days; differential returns to predominance of monocytes in 4–7 days with increased eosinophils in 10% of cases. Patients check outflow bags for turbidity. Turbid dialysate can occur occasionally without peritonitis during first few months of placing catheter (due to catheter hypersensitivity) with WBC count 100–8,000/μL, 10–95% eosinophils, sometimes increased PMNs, and negative cultures. Occasional RBCs may be seen during menstruation or with ovulation at midcycle. *Because of low WBC decision level, manual hemocytometer count rather than an automated instrument must be used.*
- **Metabolic change:** assay dialysate for creatinine and glucose; calculate ultrafiltrate volume by weighing dialysate fluid after 4-hour dwell time and subtracting it from preinfusion weight using specific gravity of 1.0.

PANCREATIC DISEASE

- AF amylase level greater than serum amylase level is specific for pancreatic disease, but both levels are normal in 10% of cases.
- Methemalbumin in serum or AF and total protein >4.5 g/dL indicate poor prognosis.

MALIGNANT ASCITES

- Increased fluid cholesterol (>45 mg/dL) and fibronectin (>10 mg/dL) has S/S 90%/82%.
- Positive cytology has S/S 70%/100%.
- Increased AF CEA (>2.5 mg/dL) has S/S 45%/100%.

ASCITES IN FETUS OR NEONATE

➤ Causes

- Nonimmune (occurs in 1 in 3000 pregnancies)
  - Cardiovascular abnormalities causing CHF (e.g., structural, arrhythmias) (40% of cases)
  - Chromosomal (e.g., Turner and Down syndromes are most common; trisomy 13, 15, 16, and 18) (10–15% of cases)
  - Hematologic disorders (any severe anemia) (10% of cases)
  - Inherited (e.g., α-thalassemia, hemoglobinopathies, G6PD deficiency
  - Acquired (e.g., fetal-maternal hemorrhage, twin-to-twin transfusion, congenital infection [parvovirus B19], methemoglobinemia)
  - Congenital defects of chest and abdomen
  - Structural (e.g., diaphragmatic hernia, jejunal atresia, volvulus, intestinal malrotation) Peritonitis caused by GI tract perforation, congenital infection (e.g., syphilis, TORCH [*tox-oplasmosis, other agents, rubella, CMV, herpes* simplex], hepatitis), meconium peritonitis
  - Lymphatic duct obstruction
  - Biliary atresia
  - Nonstructural (e.g., congenital nephrotic syndrome, cirrhosis, cholestasis, hepatic necrosis, GI tract obstruction)
  - Lower GU tract obstruction (e.g., posterior urethral valves, urethral atresia, and ureterocele) is most common cause
  - Inherited skeletal dysplasias (enlarged liver causing extramedullary hematopoiesis)
  - Fetal tumors, most often teratomas and neuroblastomas
  - Vascular placental abnormalities
  - Genetic metabolic disorders (e.g., Hurler syndrome, Gaucher disease, Niemann-Pick disease, G_{M1} gangliosidosis type I, I-cell disease, β-glucuronidase deficiency)
- Immune (maternal antibodies reacting to fetal antigens [e.g., Rh, C, E, Kell])

PERITONITIS, ACUTE

- See Figures 6-3 and 6-4.

Primary Peritonitis

Ascites Fluid Findings: Gram stain of direct smear and culture of peritoneal fluid usually shows streptococci in children. In adults is caused by *E. coli* (40–60%) or *S. pneumoniae* (15%), other Gram-negative bacilli and enterococci; usually one organism. May be caused by *Mycobacterium tuberculosis*. Marked increase in WBC ($\leq$50,000/μL) and PMN (80–90%).

Peritoneal Lavage Fluid Findings: Shows WBC count >200/μL in 99% of cases.

Other: Laboratory findings due to nephrotic syndrome and postnecrotic cirrhosis and occasionally bacteremia in children and cirrhosis with ascites in adults.

Secondary Peritonitis

Occurs and recurs very frequently in continuous ambulatory peritoneal dialysis.
Laboratory findings due perforation of hollow viscus (e.g., appendicitis, perforated ulcer).

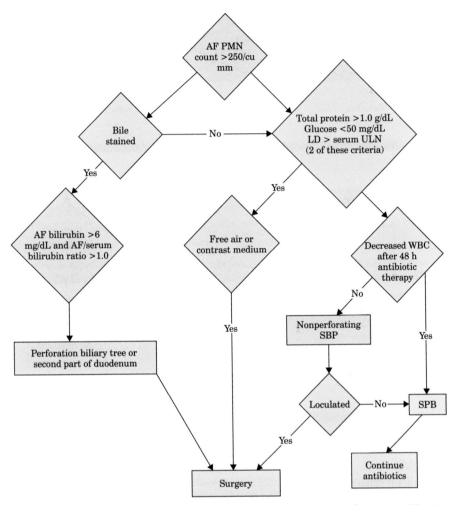

Figure 6-3. Algorithm for differentiating secondary from spontaneous bacterial peritonitis. AF, ascitic fluid; PMN, polymorphonuclear leukocytes; LD, lactate dehydrogenase; ULN, upper limit of normal; WBC, white blood cell; SBP, spontaneous bacterial peritonitis.

Dialysate Findings: Turbid (indicates >300 WBC/μL); Gram stain, culture, and leukocytosis may be absent. Caused by gram-positive bacteria in ~70%, enteric gram-negative bacilli and *P. aeruginosa* in 20% to 30%, others in 10–20%, sterile in 10–20%. *If more than one pathogen is found, rule out perforated viscus.* Usually more than one organism is found.

➤ Suggested Readings

Cárdenas A, Gelrud A, Chopra S. Chylous, bloody, and pancreatic ascites. www.uptodate.com, May, 2009.

Khan F, Sachs H, Pechet, L, Snyder LM. *Guide to Diagnostic Testing.* Philadelphia: Lippincott Williams & Wilkins; 2002.

Runyon B. Diagnosis and evaluation of patients with ascites. www.uptodate.com, May, 2009.

Runyon B. Diagnosis of spontaneous bacterial peritonitis. www.uptodate.com, May, 2009.

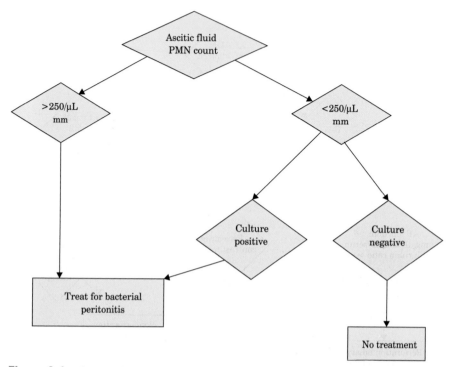

Figure 6-4. Algorithm for spontaneous bacterial peritonitis. PMN, polymorphonuclear leukocytes.

DIARRHEA

➤ Definition
• Diarrhea is defined as >200 g of stool or an increase in the frequency or fluidity of normal stools. It may be acute or chronic, and it is considered chronic when it lasts at least 4 weeks.

➤ Etiology
Diarrhea can result from any of the following mechanisms.
1. Osmosis. Molecules not normally present in the intestinal lumen increase the osmolality of chime, drawing water into the lumen (i.e., lactose)
2. Secretion. Substances can cause intestinal cells to secrete sodium and water (i.e., cholera toxin).
3. Inflammation results in denuding of the intestinal lining, which in turn disrupts normal absorption, thereby allowing compounds from the lining to leak into the lumen resulting in an increased osmosis.
4. Motility. Hypermotility leads to an increased stool volume. Hypomotility can lead to bacterial overgrowth, which causes diarrhea through several different mechanisms.
5. Anal sphincter dysfunction causes fecal incontinence, which can be interpreted by the patient as diarrhea.

➤ Differential Diagnosis

1. Laxative abuse accounts for approximately 15% of all chronic causes. It should be suspected in patients with a mental health disorder.
2. Sorbitol can cause diarrhea. In one study, approximately 17% of people had diarrhea following the ingestion of 4–5 mints containing sorbitol.
3. Both bile salts and fatty acids cause secretion of chloride followed by water into the colon. Excess bile salts also lead to a mild degree of fat malabsorption.
4. Bacterial overgrowth can occur secondary to diabetes, blind loop syndrome, amyloidosis, diverticulitis, and scleroderma, among other causes.
5. Irritable bowel syndrome classically presents with diarrhea alternating with constipation, but it can also occur in a diarrhea-predominant form.
6. Gastric surgery syndrome results in a decreased contact time with the luminal surface and decreased digestive juices mixing with the chyme.
7. Hyperthyroidism usually has increased frequency and amount of diarrhea, but not fluidity. Diarrhea is present in approximately 25% of hyperthyroid cases.
8. Inflammatory bowel disease (IBD)
   * Ulcerative colitis is a relapsing and remitting disease that leads to acute inflammation of the colorectal mucosa. The rectum is involved in 55% of cases. In severe cases, bloody diarrhea often leads to weight loss, anemia, and electrolyte imbalance.
   * Crohn disease is a chronic relapsing disorder characterized by transmural, asymmetric, and segmental inflammation. It typically involves the ilium, colon, or perianal region; right lower quadrant pain associated with bloody diarrhea is present in 80% of patients.
9. Neoplasia
   * Villous adenoma produces prostaglandins, which stimulate chloride and water secretion from the colon.
   * Serotonin from carcinoid cells stimulates gut motility and increases intestinal secretion.
   * Tumor-associated calcitonin stimulates gut motility.
   * Gastrinoma leads to increased gastric acid, which directly causes fluid secretion.
10. Infection
    * Refer to p. 588, Foodborne Infectious Illnesses, and see other sections on specific agents that cause diarrheal disease.

➤ Laboratory Findings

Endoscopy: Lower endoscopy may help. One series has a 20% yield in identifying a pathologic diagnosis. In non–HIV-infected patients, the role of sigmoidoscopy versus colonoscopy is unclear. When clinically suspected, even if no gross abnormalities are noted, consider doing blind biopsies looking for lymphocytic and collagenous colitis. The yield of biopsy with no gross abnormalities ranges from 6–42%. Upper endoscopy is useful for making the diagnosis of sprue, Whipple's disease, and other small bowel infiltrative processes.

Radiology: An upper GI series with small bowel follow-through is most commonly used when evaluating for Crohn's disease. Enteroclysis is superior, with 100% sensitivity and 98% specificity for small bowel involvement with Crohn's disease.

Stool Cultures: Submission of a single specimen is usually sensitive for detection of bacterial causes of diarrhea; repeat cultures may be necessary for detection of *Shigella* or asymptomatic carriage of an enteric pathogen. Routine stool cultures routinely isolate *Salmonella*, *Campylobacter*, and *Shigella*, the three most common causes of bacterial diarrhea in the United States. If another pathogen is suspected on clinical or epidemiologic grounds, pathogen-specific cultures should be ordered (e.g., *E. coli* O157:H7, *Vibrio cholerae*).

Recommended Stool Tests:

* O& P examination
* Fecal leukocytes
* Stool for osmolality gap: The osmolality gap is calculated by the following formula: 2 (stool Na + K). The accuracy is fair in distinguishing between osmotic (if gap is 50) and secretory (if gap is >50) diarrhea.
* Stool for pH: For carbohydrate intolerance (e.g., lactose or sorbitol), one small study found the pH <5.6. For bile acid-induced diarrhea, the pH is usually over 6.8
* Stool for fecal fat: This test is used to detect steatorrhea on the basis of malabsorption.
* Qualitative: Sensitivity is 97–100%, but the specificity varies from 56–86%.
* Quantitative: Based upon a 72-hour collection, the patient should be on a 75–100-g fat diet. A nutritional consult is advised to maximize compliance.

Other Recommended Tests:

* **Nutrition indices.** CBC, albumin , and potassium (sensitivity of hypokalemia is 100% for pancreatic cholera or (VIPoma) are routine studies in the evaluation of chronic diarrhea.
* **Hormonal studies.** TSH, fasting serum gastrin level, calcitonin level, and 24-hour urine collection for 5-Hydroxy Indole Acetic Acid (5-HIAA) are recommended.
* **D-Xylose testing.** This tests for small bowel malabsorption syndromes (e.g., sprue, Crohn disease, amyloidosis). Twenty-five grams of D-xylose are administered. A 5-hour urine collection and a 1-hour serum sample are obtained. A decreased amount of D-xylose in the urine and serum indicates small bowel malabsorption. The sensitivity of the test is decreased in the following situations: creatinine clearance of <30 mg/dL, portal hypertension, ascites, delayed gastric emptying, fiber supplements, glucose load, aspirin, and glipizide.
* **Bentiromide test** (to test for pancreatic exocrine insufficiency). N-Benzoyl-l-tyrosyl para-aminobenzoic acid (NBT PABA) is administered orally. The molecule is cleaved by chymotrypsin; PABA is absorbed, and then measured in a 6-hour urine collection. PABA alone is a somewhat inaccurate measure, so additional markers have been used to increase the accuracy.
* **Serum immune markers.** Several serum immune markers performed by ELISA have been found to be valuable for the diagnosis, stratification, and management of IBD (see Celiac Disease):
  * Deoxyribonuclease (DNAse)–sensitive perinuclear antineutrophilic cytoplasmic antibody (P-ANCA) is positive in 60–80% of adults with ulcerative colitis (UC) and in 83% of children with UC. P-ANCA is positive in 10% of patients with Crohn disease.
  * Anti-*Saccharomyces cerevisiae* antibody (ASCA) is present in 70% of patients with Crohn disease.
  * Pancreatic antibody may be positive in 30–40% of patients with Crohn disease.
  * Outer membrane porin from *E. coli* (OmpC) antibody: An immunoglobulin A (IgA) response to OmpC is seen in 55% of patients with Crohn disease

DIARRHEA, ACUTE

OSMOTIC DIARRHEA

➤ Definition

Defined as diarrhea with a <3-week (upper limit 6–8 week) duration. Increased osmotically active solutes in bowel; diarrhea usually stops during fasting.

Causes

* Exogenous
  * Laxatives (e.g., magnesium sulfate, milk of magnesia, sodium sulfate [Glauber salt], sodium phosphate, polyethylene glycol/saline)
  * Drugs (e.g., lactulose, colchicine, cholestyramine, neomycin, Para-Aminosalicytic Acid (PAS))
  * Foods (e.g., mannitol, sorbitol [in diet candy, chewing gum, soda])
* Endogenous
  * Congenital malabsorption
    * Specific (e.g., lactase deficiency, fructose malabsorption)
    * General (e.g., abetalipoproteinemia and hypobetalipoproteinemia, congenital lymphangiectasia, cystic fibrosis)
  * Acquired malabsorption
    * Specific (e.g., pancreatic disease, celiac sprue, parasitic infestation, rotavirus enteritis, metabolic disorders [thyrotoxicosis, adrenal insufficiency], jejunoileal bypass, bacterial overgrowth, short-bowel syndrome, inflammatory disease [e.g., mastocytosis, eosinophilic enteritis])

SECRETORY (ABNORMAL ELECTROLYTE TRANSPORT) DIARRHEA

➤ Definition

Diarrhea caused by increased water and chloride secretion; normal water and sodium absorption may be inhibited.

Due to:

* Exogenous
  * Drugs
    * Laxatives (e.g., aloe, anthraquinones, bisacodyl, castor oil, dioctyl sodium sulfosuccinate, phenolphthalein, senna)
    * Diuretics (e.g., furosemide, thiazides), asthma (theophylline), thyroid drugs
    * Cholinergic drugs (cholinesterase inhibitors, quinidine, clozapine, ACE inhibitors)
  * Toxins (e.g., arsenic, mushrooms, organophosphates, alcohol)
  * Viral or bacterial toxins (e.g., *S. aureus, E. coli, V. cholerae, Bacillus cereus, Campylobacter jejuni, Yersinia enterocolitica, Clostridium botulinum,* and *Clostridium perfringens*). *C. difficile* is the most common cause of diarrhea in hospitalized patients with onset >3 days after admission. See below (Foodborne Infectious Illnesses), Infectious Diseases, for the discussion of infectious causes of diarrhea.
* Endogenous
  * Hormones (serotonin, calcitonic, VIP)
  * Gastric hypersecretion (Z-E syndrome, Systemic mastocytosis, Short-bowel syndrome)
  * Bile salts (e.g., disease or resection of terminal ileum)

- Fatty acids (e.g., disease of small intestine mucosa, pancreatic insufficiency)
- Congenital (e.g., congenital chloridorrhea, congenital sodium diarrhea)

➤ Laboratory Findings

Stool Fndings: Watery stool, Volume >1 L/day, Blood and pus are absent, stool osmolality close to plasma osmolality with no anion gap.

EXUDATIVE DIARRHEA (INFLAMMATORY CAUSES)

Due to: Infection, injury, ischemia, vasculitis, abscess and/or idiopathic.
Laboratory Findings: Stool contains blood and pus.

MOTILITY DISTURBANCES

Due to:
- Decreased small intestinal motility (e.g., hypothyroidism, DM, amyloidosis, scleroderma)
- Increased small intestinal motility (e.g., hyperthyroidism, carcinoid syndrome)
- Increased colonic motility (e.g., irritable bowel syndrome)

FOODBORNE INFECTIOUS ILLNESSES*

➤ Definition

A foodborne illness is any illness related to food ingestion. Disease is usually manifested by GI tract signs and symptoms but may be manifested by systemic or localized illness without significant GI symptoms (e.g., enteric fever; botulism). A variety of agents may cause foodborne illness, including infectious pathogens and their toxins as well as noninfectious and chemical agents. Most cases are caused by viral agents, but specific diagnosis is often not established because specific tests may not be available or illness may be self-limited. Bacteria are most commonly identified in patients when a definitive diagnosis is established. In the United States, the most common bacterial pathogens associated with gastroenteritis are *Salmonella* spp., *Campylobacter* spp., and *Shigella* spp. A foodborne illness may be restricted to a single individual or a small group, or represent a large outbreak with many patients linked to a common source of infection. Although unlikely, foodborne pathogens have been intentionally introduced into populations as bioterrorist incidents.

➤ Who Should be Suspected?

Patients with foodborne illness usually present with a variety of symptoms including nausea, vomiting, abdominal pain, diarrhea, and anorexia. Certain foodborne illnesses, however, may be associated with minimal GI symptoms, but have prominent systemic or localized symptoms.

Diarrheal illness may be noninflammatory or inflammatory. Non-inflammatory diarrhea is usually caused by disease of the small intestine resulting in hypersecretion or decreased absorption. There is usually abrupt onset and resolution after a brief duration of illness. Systemic symptoms are usually absent or mild. Dehydration may be a complication, especially in the young or elderly.

---

*The section on Foodborne Infectious Illnesses was written by Michael Mitchell, MD.

Inflammatory diarrhea is characterized by mucosal invasion or cytotoxic damage by the pathogen. The large intestine is most commonly affected. The mucosal invasion typically results in bloody stools with many fecal leukocytes. Systemic symptoms are typical, including fever, abdominal pain and tenderness, nausea and vomiting, headache, and malaise.

When evaluating a patient with a likely foodborne illness, a number of issues should be pursued:
- What is the interval between likely exposure and onset of symptoms?
- What is the duration of clinical symptoms in affected patients?
- What are the prominent signs and symptoms of disease?
- Do any of the patient's recent contacts have similar illness?
- Has the patient eaten any unusual food? Eaten at any function with mass-produced meals? Eaten any raw or incompletely cooked or pasteurized food?
- Has there been new contact with animals: domesticated, farm, or wild?
- Has the patient had recent travel to regions where foodborne illness is endemic?
- Does the patient, or does a close contact, attend or reside in a daycare center, long-term care facility, or other facility at which transmission of an agent may be facilitated?
- The following list provides summaries of common agents for foodborne illnesses. In addition to the clinical presentation, epidemiologic risk should be considered when determining diagnostic and therapeutic strategies. Additional information is provided for a number of agents in other sections.
  - Gastroenteritis with vomiting as the prominent symptom. Suspect:
    - Enteric virus (rotavirus in infants; norovirus or other in older patients)
    - Preformed toxin (*S. aureus*, *B. cereus*)
    - Heavy metal poisoning
  - Noninflammatory diarrhea (watery without marked fecal WBCs or RBCs). Suspect:
    - Enterotoxigenic *E. coli*
    - *V. cholerae*
    - Enteric virus (astrovirus, norovirus or other calicivirus, adenovirus, rotavirus)
    - *Cryptosporidium*
    - *Cyclospora cayetanensis*
    - *Giardia lamblia*
  - Inflammatory diarrhea as the prominent symptom (grossly bloody stool, pus or increased fecal WBCs, fever, and systemic signs and symptoms). Suspect:
    - *Shigella*
    - *Campylobacter*
    - *Salmonella*
    - Enteroinvasive or enterohemorrhagic *E. coli*, including serotype O157:H7
    - *Vibrio parahaemolyticus*
    - *Y. enterocolitica*
    - *Entamoeba histolytica*
  - Persistent diarrhea as the prominent symptom (2 weeks or longer). Suspect:
    - *Cryptosporidium*
    - *C. cayetanensis*
    - *E. histolytica*
    - *G. lamblia*
  - Neurologic manifestation as the prominent symptom (paraesthesia, respiratory depression, cranial nerve palsy, respiratory difficulty). Suspect:

- *C. botulinum* toxin
- Guillain-Barré syndrome (after *Campylobacter jejuni* gastroenteritis)
- Intoxication/poisoning (scombroid fish poisoning, ciguatera fish poisoning, *Tetraodon* [fish] poisoning, shellfish poisoning)
- Mushroom poisoning
- Organophosphate/insecticide poisoning
- Thallium poisoning
- Systemic signs and symptoms as the predominant presentation, with minimal GI symptoms. Suspect:
  - *Brucella* spp.
  - *E. histolytica* liver abscess.
  - HAV and HEV
  - *Listeria monocytogenes*
  - *Salmonella* Typhi or Paratyphi
  - *Toxoplasma gondii*
  - *Trichinella spiralis*
  - *Vibrio vulnificus*

➤ Diagnosis and Reporting

- Because of the diverse etiology and variety of tests required to make a specific diagnosis, consultation with infectious diseases experts and clinical microbiologists may improve diagnostic strategies. If the patient appears to be a part of a large outbreak of foodborne illness, reporting to the local department of public health may be required; public health officials may be able to provide important information concerning ongoing outbreaks or diagnostic support.
- Diagnostic techniques for microbial pathogens are discussed in other sections of this book. Specific diagnostic testing is recommended for immunocompromised patients, and patients with severe or prolonged disease, systemic disease, neurologic symptoms, or signs of inflammatory diarrhea. Cultures for bacterial pathogens require use of selective, differential media optimized for isolation of specific pathogens. The pathogens targeted may vary from laboratory to laboratory. *Campylobacter, Salmonella,* and *Shigella* spp. are typically isolated. Special cultures may have to be requested for isolation of other bacterial pathogens from stool (e.g., *E. coli* O157:H7, *Vibrio* spp., *Aeromonas* spp.). Blood cultures are recommended for patients with enteric fever or systemic illness.
- Although there may be slight variability among different jurisdictions, foodborne illnesses are reportable to local, state, and federal agencies. The CDC collects and analyzes data. Reporting may be triggered by clinical suspicion, like a large or unusual outbreak of illness, or identification of a specific pathogen by the laboratory. Reporting is important so that public health officials may identify or effectively manage outbreaks of foodborne illness, identify the source and interrupt further transmission of illness, assess the possibility of intentional introduction of an agent into a population, and assess trends in diseases.

➤ Conclusion

It is important for health care providers to:
- Consider the possibility of foodborne illness in evaluating a patient's illness.
- Realize that many, but not all, foodborne illnesses present with prominent GI tract illness. Patients may present with predominant systemic, neurologic, or other signs and symptoms.

- Understand the testing required for likely pathogens. When specific diagnosis is required, ensure that appropriate specimens and cultures, or other tests, are submitted for testing.
- Obtain a clinical history that may provide clues regarding the source of the illness as well as assessing the possibility of a larger outbreak.
- Report suspect cases to public health officials, as appropriate. Be aware that a patient may be a part of a larger outbreak in the community.
- Instruct patients about how to prevent further transmission of illness to contacts.

➤ Suggested Readings

Centers for Disease Control and Prevention. Diagnosis and management of foodborne illnesses: a primer for physicians and other health care professionals. *MMWR* 2004;53(No. RR-4):1–33.

DuPont HL. Bacterial diarrhea. *N Engl J Med*. 2009;361:1560–1569.

Guerrant RL, T Van Gilder, TS Steiner et al. Practice guidelines for the management of infectious diarrhea. *Clin Infect Dis*. 2001;32:3313–50.

Thielman NM, RL Guerrant. Acute infectious diarrhea. *N Engl J Med*. 2004;350:38–47.

Voetsch AC, FJ Angulo, T Rabatsky-Ehr, et al., for the Emerging Infections Program FoodNet Working Group. Laboratory practices for stool-specimen culture for bacterial pathogens, including Escherichia coli O157:H7, in the FoodNet Sites, 1995–2000. *Clin Infect Dis*. 2004;38(Suppl 3):S190–197.

DIARRHEA, CHRONIC

➤ Definition
Chronic diarrhea is diarrhea that lasts for more than 4 weeks.

➤ Causes
- Infection (e.g., giardiasis, amebiasis, *Cryptosporidium*, *Isospora*, *Strongyloides*, C. *difficile*) See page 570 Foodborne Infectious Illnesses
- IBD (e.g., Crohn disease, UC, collagenous colitis)
- Carbohydrate malabsorption (e.g., lactase or sucrase deficiency)
- Foods (e.g., ethanol, caffeine, sweeteners such as sorbitol, fructose)
- Drugs (e.g., antibiotics, antihypertensive, antiarrhythmic, antineoplastic, colchicine, cholestyramine; see previous section on acute diarrhea)
- Laxative abuse, factitious
- Endocrine (e.g., DM, adrenal insufficiency, hyperthyroidism, hypothyroidism)
- Hormone-producing tumors (e.g., gastrinoma, VIPoma, villous adenoma, medullary thyroid carcinoma, pheochromocytoma, ganglioneuroma, carcinoid tumor, mastocytosis, somatostatinoma, ectopic hormone production by lung or pancreas carcinoma)
- Injury caused by radiation, ischemia, and so on
- Infiltrations (e.g., scleroderma, amyloidosis, lymphoma)
- Colon carcinoma
- Previous surgery (e.g., gastrectomy, vagotomy, intestinal resection)
- Immune system disorders (e.g., systemic mastocytosis, eosinophilic gastroenteritis)
- Intraluminal maldigestion (Bile duct obstruction, Pancreatic exocrine insufficiency)
- Celiac sprue
- Whipple disease
- Abetalipoproteinemia
- Dermatitis herpetiformis

- Intestinal lymphangiectasia
- Allergy
- Idiopathic

OTHER GASTROINTESTINAL CONDITIONS

DIVERTICULOSIS, COLON

➤ **Laboratory Findings**
Core Laboratory: Hypochromic microcytic anemia, increased WBCs. Increased ESR. Positive occult blood.

ENTEROCOLITIS, NECROTIZING, IN INFANCY

➤ **Definition**
Syndrome of acute intestinal necrosis of unknown cause. It is especially associated with prematurity and exchange transfusions.

➤ **Laboratory Findings**
There may be oliguria, neutropenia, and anemia. Persistent metabolic acidosis, severe hyponatremia, and DIC are a common triad in infants. Bloody stools feature no characteristic organisms; significant organisms are often found by frequent repeated cultures of blood, urine, and stool

INFLAMMATORY BOWEL DISEASE

➤ **Definition**
IBD refers to a chronic relapsing spectrum of disorders of unknown cause with destructive mucosal immune reaction in a genetically susceptible host. It is caused by an aberrant immune response and loss of tolerance to normal intestinal flora, leading to chronic inflammation of the gut.

REGIONAL ENTERITIS (CROHN DISEASE)

➤ **Definition.**
Systemic inflammatory disease with predominantly GI tract involvement. There are no pathognomonic findings for Crohn disease or to distinguish it from ulcerative colitis.

➤ **Laboratory Findings**
Histology: Endoscopic biopsy may show granulomas in >60% of cases of Crohn disease but in only 6% of cases of UC.
Serology: Atypical perinuclear-staining antineutrophil cytoplasmic antibodies (P-ANCA) are found in <15% of cases of Crohn disease but in ≤70% of ulcerative colitis patients. Anti-*S.*

cerevisiae (baker's or brewer's yeast) antibodies (ASCA) are found in ~60% of Crohn disease cases but in only ~10% of cases in ulcerative colitis.

Hematology: Increased WBC, ESR, CRP, and other acute-phase reactants correlate with disease activity. Mild increase of WBC indicates activity, but a marked increase suggests suppuration (e.g., abscess). ESR tends to be higher in disease of colon than of ileum. Anemia due to iron deficiency or vitamin B_{12} or folate deficiency or chronic disease.

Core Laboratory: Decreased serum albumin, increased γ globulins. Hyperchloremic metabolic acidosis, dehydration, decreased sodium, potassium, magnesium. Mild liver function test changes due to pericholangitis (especially increased serum ALP). Laboratory changes due to complications or sequelae (e.g., malabsorption, perforation and fistula formation, abscess formation, arthritis, sclerosing cholangitis, iritis, uveitis).

ULCERATIVE COLITIS, CHRONIC NONSPECIFIC

➤ Definition
There are no pathognomonic findings for this disease, nor are there findings that distinguish it from Crohn disease.

➤ Laboratory Findings
Serology: P-ANCA are found in 70% of ulcerative colitis patients but only occasionally in cases of Crohn disease. Stools are negative for usual enteric pathogens and parasites.

Hematology: With diarrhea and fever, Hb <7.5 g/dL, increased neutrophil count, and ESR >30 mm/h indicate severe disease.

Core Laboratory: Serum ALP often increased slightly. Other liver function tests are usually normal. Stools are positive for blood.

➤ Other Considerations
- Laboratory changes due to complications or sequelae (e.g., hemorrhage, carcinoma, electrolyte disorders, toxic megacolon with perforation).
- The lower sensitivity of combined serologic tests only modestly influences pretest and posttest probability in IBD but is very useful in distinguishing Crohn disease from UC. Serial measurements are not useful and do not correlate with disease activity; titers are stable over time.

➤ Suggested Reading
Bossuyt X. Serologic markers in inflammatory bowel disease. *Clin Chem.* 2006;52:171–181.

MALABSORPTION

➤ Definition
Malabsorption is defective nutrient absorption by the small intestine.

➤ Causes
- Inadequate mixing of food with bile salts and lipase (e.g., pyloroplasty, subtotal or total gastrectomy, gastrojejunostomy)
- Inadequate lipolysis due to lack of lipase (e.g., CF of the pancreas, chronic pancreatitis, cancer of the pancreas or ampulla of Vater, pancreatic fistula, vagotomy)

- Inadequate emulsification of fat due to lack of bile salts (e.g., obstructive jaundice, severe liver disease, bacterial overgrowth of small intestine, disorders of terminal ileum)
- Primary absorptive defect in small bowel
- Inadequate absorptive surface due to extensive mucosal disease (e.g., regional enteritis, tumors, amyloid disease, scleroderma, irradiation)
- Biochemical dysfunction of mucosal cells (e.g., celiac sprue syndrome, severe starvation, or administration of drugs such as neomycin sulfate, colchicine, or PAS)
- Obstruction of mesenteric lymphatics (e.g., by lymphoma, carcinoma, intestinal TB)
- Inadequate length of normal absorptive surface (e.g., surgical resection, fistula, shunt)
- Miscellaneous (e.g., "blind loops" of intestine, diverticula, Z-E syndrome, agammaglobulinemia, endocrine and metabolic disorders)
- Infection (e.g., acute enteritis, tropical sprue, Whipple disease [*Tropheryma whippelii*]; in common variable hypogammaglobulinemia, 50–55% of patients have chronic diarrhea and malabsorption caused by a specific pathogen such as *G. lamblia* or overgrowth of bacteria in small bowel)

➤ Laboratory Findings

Core Laboratory: Serum cholesterol may be decreased. Decreased serum carotene, albumin, and iron; increased stool weight (>300 g/24 hours) and stool fat (>7 g/24 hours).

Hematology: PT may be prolonged because of malabsorption of vitamin K. Increased ESR. Anemia is caused by deficiency of iron, folic acid, vitamin B_{12}, or various combinations, depending on their decreased absorption.

Other: Normal D-xylose test, low serum trypsinogen, pancreatic calcification on radiograph of abdomen establish diagnosis of chronic pancreatitis. If calcification is absent (as occurs in 70–80% of cases), abnormal contents of pancreatic secretion after secretin-cholecystokinin stimulation or abnormal bentiromide tests establish diagnosis of chronic pancreatitis.

➤ Recommended Tests

Fat absorption indices (steatorrhea): Direct qualitative stool examination. ≥2 random stool samples are collected on diet of >80 g of fat daily.

Serum trypsinogen: <10 ng/mL in 75–85% of patients with severe chronic pancreatitis (those with steatorrhea) and 15–20% of those with mild to moderate disease; occasionally low in cancer of pancreas; normal (10–75 ng/mL) in nonpancreatic causes of malabsorption.

Bentiromide: Used to differentiate pancreatic exocrine insufficiency (abnormal result) from intestinal mucosal disease (normal result).

Secretin-cholecystokinin is the most sensitive and reliable test of chronic pancreatic disease.

Carotene tolerance test: Measure serum carotene following daily oral loading of carotene for 3–7 days. Low values for serum carotene levels are usually associated with steatorrhea. Increase of serum carotene by >35 μg/dL indicates previously low dietary intake of carotene and/or fat. Patients with sprue in remission with normal fecal fat excretion may still show low carotene absorption.

Vitamin A tolerance test (for screening steatorrhea): Measure plasma vitamin A level 5 hours after ingestion. Normal rise is $9\times$ fasting level. Flat curve in liver disease. Not useful after gastrectomy. With vitamin A as ester of long-chain fatty acid, flat curve occurs in both pancreatic disease and intestinal mucosal abnormalities; when water-soluble forms of vitamin A are used, the curve becomes normal in patients with pancreatic disease but remains flat in intestinal mucosal abnormalities. An abnormal result indicates a defect in small bowel mucosal absorption function (e.g., sprue, Whipple disease, regional enteritis, TB enteritis, collagen diseases involving the small bowel, extensive resection). Abnormal pancreatic function does not affect the test.

CARBOHYDRATE ABSORPTION INDICES

* Disaccharide malabsorption
  * Causes
    * Primary malabsorption (congenital or acquired) because of absence of specific disaccharidase in brush border of small intestine mucosa
    * Isolated lactase deficiency (also called milk allergy, milk intolerance, congenital familial lactose intolerance, lactase deficiency) (is most common of these defects; occurs in ~10% of whites and 60% of blacks; infantile type shows diarrhea, vomiting, failure to thrive, malabsorption, and so on; often appears first in adults; become asymptomatic when lactase is removed from diet).
  * Sucrose-isomaltose malabsorption (inherited recessive defect)
    * Oral sucrose tolerance curve is flat, but glucose plus fructose tolerance test is normal. Occasionally there is an associated malabsorption with increased stool fat and abnormal d-xylose tolerance test, although intestinal biopsy is normal.
    * Hydrogen breath test after sucrose challenge.
    * Intestinal biopsy with measurement of disaccharidase activities.
    * Sucrose-free diet causes cessation of diarrhea.
  * Glucose–galactose malabsorption (inherited autosomal–recessive defect that affects kidney and intestine)
    * Oral glucose or galactose tolerance curve is flat, but IV tolerance curves are normal.
    * Glucosuria is common. Fructose tolerance test is normal.
  * Secondary malabsorption
    * Resection of >50% of disaccharidase activity. Lactose is most marked, but there may also be sucrose. Oral disaccharide tolerance (especially lactose) is abnormal, but intestinal histology and enzyme activity are normal.
  * Diffuse intestinal disease—especially celiac disease in which activity of all disaccharidases may be decreased, with later increase as intestine becomes normal on gluten-free diet; also cystic fibrosis of pancreas, severe malnutrition, UC, severe *Giardia* infestation, blind-loop syndrome, β-lipoprotein deficiency, effect of drugs (e.g., colchicine, neomycin, birth control pills). Oral tolerance tests (especially lactose) are frequently abnormal, with later return to normal with gluten-free diet. Tolerance tests with monosaccharides may also be abnormal because of defect in absorption as well as digestion.
  * Bacterial overgrowth—see Figure 6-4 and Table 6-3.
    * Culture of duodenal aspirate showing >10^5 colony-forming units of anaerobic organisms is considered diagnostic.
    * ^{14}C-D-xylose breath test has good specificity.
    * Hydrogen breath tests (glucose-H_2, lactulose-H_2)—not recommended because of limited sensitivity and specificity.

TABLE 6-3. Infectious Foodborne Diseases

Organism	Identification	Cases of Foodborne Gastroenteritis (%)
Bacterial[a]		88.6
Bacillus cereus gastroenteritis	Isolation of $\geq 10^5$ *B. cereus* per g of suspected food Isolation of same-serotype *B. cereus* from other ill patients but not from control persons Detection of enterotoxin by special tests (e.g., immunogel diffusion)	0.03
Botulism	Isolation of *Clostridium botulinum* from stool of patients Detection of toxin in stool, serum, or food by mouse test	0.4
Brucellosis	Isolation of *Brucella* organism from blood	0.1
Campylobacteriosis	Increase in blood agglutination titer of fourfold or greater at onset and 3–6 weeks later Isolation of same strain of organism from patient's stool Isolation of organism from suspected food Increase in blood agglutination titer of fourfold or greater at onset and 2–4 weeks later	
Cholera	Isolation of organism from vomitus or stool Isolation of organism from suspected food Demonstration that organism is enterotoxigenic by special biologic tests	
Clostridium perfringens enteritis	Isolation of same serotype of *C. perfringens* from food and from patients but not from control persons Isolation of $\geq 10^5$ organisms from suspected food Fecal spore count 10^6/g in most patients within a few days of onset	18.5

TABLE 6-3. (*Continued*)

Organism	Identification	Cases of Foodborne Gastroenteritis (%)
Escherichia coli	Demonstration of toxin in feces (fluorescent antibody test) Isolation of same serotype of *E. coli* from suspected food and from patients but not from control persons Demonstration that organism strain is enteropathogenic	
Listeriosis	Isolation of organism from tissue of fatal case Isolation of same phage type and serogroup from patient and food Demonstration of virulence by biologic tests	
Salmonellosis	Isolation of organism from stool or rectal swab, urine, or blood Isolation of same organism serovar from suspected food	31.9
Shigellosis	Isolation of organism from stool or rectal swab Isolation of same organism serovar from suspected food	18.0
Staphylococcal poisoning or intoxication	Detection of enterotoxin in suspected food (serologic assay) Isolation of same phage type of organism from patient and suspected food Isolation of $\geq 10^5$ organisms/g of suspected food	16.5
Streptococcus, Group A	See Chapter 13	3.2
Vibrio parahaemolyticus	See Chapter 13	0.03
Yersiniosis	Isolation of *Yersinia enterocolitica* or *Y. pseudotuberculosis* from stool or blood or from suspected food	5.5

(Continued)

TABLE 6-3. Infectious Foodborne Diseases (*Continued*)

Organism	Identification	Cases of Foodborne Gastroenteritis (%)
Viral[b]		
Hepatitis A and E	See Table 6.11	
Norwalk and parvo-like	Fourfold or greater increase of blood antibody titer from acute to convalescent phase Immunoelectron microscopy	
Rotavirus		
Chemical (scombroid)	See footnote	
Amebae (e.g., *Entamoeba histolytica, Blastocystis hominis*)	Identification of cysts or trophozoites in feces, biopsy, aspirate; serology	5.1
Parasitic		0.8
Cryptosporidiosis	Demonstration of organisms in stool or suspected food Detection of antigen in stool	
Giardiasis	Recognition of organism in stool, duodenal contents, or small bowel Detection of antigen in stool	
Balantidium coli infestation	Recognition of organism in stool, tissue biopsy Rarely recovered in United States	
Helminthic		
Cestodiasis (e.g., caused by *Diphyllobothrium latum, Taenia saginata, Taenia solium*)	Eggs and proglottids in stool	
Trichinosis	Recognition of cysts in muscle biopsy Demonstration of larvae in suspected food Demonstration of adults and larvae in stool only during first 1–2 weeks Detection of antigen in stool Serologic tests for antibody	

TABLE 6-3. *(Continued)*

Organism	Identification	Cases of Foodborne Gastroenteritis (%)
Trematodiasis (e.g., caused by *Clonorchis sinensis, Fasciola hepatica, Paragonimus westermani*)	Eggs in stool	
Fungal		
Mushroom poisoning	Demonstration of toxin in urine and suspected gathered mushrooms	

[a]Confirm by culture of food, patient's stool, or food handler's stool.

[b]Suspected by exclusion by negative tests for other causes of the symptoms (e.g., failure to find *Entamoeba histolytica, Shigella, Salmonella*). Fecal white blood cells in 20% of rotavirus cases; absent in Norwalk, Norwalk-like, and adenovirus cases.

Antigen detection: Commercial monoclonal-based antibody kits for rotavirus (enzyme immunoassay [EIA], latex agglutination, enzyme-linked immunosorbent assay) are inexpensive, permit rapid diagnosis, and require only small amounts of stool, which may be frozen until testing. Detection of viral antigen in stool may be negative due to brief period of excretion. Sensitivities of 70–100% and specificities of 50–100% are reported. False-positive rates are high in newborns and in breast-feeding children. Less useful in adults and outside of rotavirus season, when confirmatory testing should be performed. Kits also available for adenovirus. Rapid assays for other viruses are under development.

Antibody detection (e.g., to Norwalk virus, especially caused by ingestion of raw oysters) can be diagnosed by presence of serum IgM or by a fourfold rise in specific IgG antibody titers (EIA) drawn at the first week (acute-phase serum) and after the second week (convalescent serum). Patient will have long since recovered from self-limited illness. Chief use is to identify cause of an outbreak. Stool antigen and serum antibody assay for Norwalk virus are available only in research laboratories at present. Monoclonal antibodies for adenovirus 40 and 41.

Direct electron microscopy of stool can detect (≤90% sensitivity) and identify all the morphologic types of enteric viruses (e.g., rotaviruses, adenoviruses, astrovirus, calicivirus, Norwalk virus) by characteristic morphology. Detection requires ≥1 million viruses per milliliter of stool; usually present only during first 48 hours of viral diarrhea. Required for conclusive diagnosis of Norwalk virus. Immune electron microscopy improves sensitivity by 10–100 times, but technology limits this to few laboratories.

Culture: Rotavirus, adenovirus, astrovirus culture available in research centers; not useful for routine diagnosis. Other viruses cannot be cultured.

Electropherotyping: Detection of rotavirus RNA in stool by gel electrophoresis pattern is 100% specific and >90% sensitive in first days of illness; chiefly research tool in United States.

Dot-hybridization probes for rotavirus are more sensitive and specific than antigen detection but are only available in research centers.

Polymerase chain reaction techniques are being developed.

See appropriate sections in Chapter 13.

Source: Steele JCH Jr, ed. Food-borne diseases. *Clin Lab Med.* 1999;19:469–703.

CELIAC DISEASE (GLUTEN-SENSITIVE ENTEROPATHY, NONTROPICAL SPRUE, IDIOPATHIC STEATORRHEA)

➤ Definition

Celiac disease is an autoimmune multisystem disorder (principally manifested in the GI tract) in genetically susceptible persons that may be caused by a mucosal injury by a complex of gliadin (a protein from dietary gluten in wheat, rye, barley, or oats) with tissue transglutaminase (tTG), a cross-linking enzyme. Findings are caused by malabsorption and autoimmunity.

➤ Laboratory Findings

Although there are no universally accepted tests for the diagnosis of celiac disease, specific serologic testing and small bowel biopsy are very sensitive and specific for making the diagnosis. All tests must be performed while patients are on a diet of food that contains gluten (Figure 6-5).

Histology: Biopsy of jejunum is the diagnostic gold standard; shows characteristic although not specific mucosal lesions. Establishing the diagnosis is essential; patients should not be committed to lifelong gluten-free diet without first assessing intestinal mucosal histology. False-negative results may occur because of patchy distribution of pathology.

Stool Findings: Steatorrhea demonstrated by positive Sudan stain on ≥2 stool samples or quantitative determination of fat in 72-hour pooled stool sample.

Anti-IgA tTG antibodies: (by ELISA) has S/S = >90%/>95%. False-negative results may occur in patients with IgA deficiency (present in 2.5% of patients with celiac disease

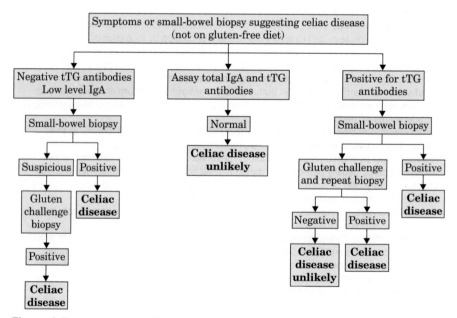

Figure 6-5. Symptoms or small bowel biopsy suggesting celiac disease. tTG, transglutaminase.

for whom corresponding IgG antibody tests may be useful). More reproducible than EMA test.

Anti-IgA deamidated gliadin IgG/IgA antibodies: Deamidated gliadin antibody (DGA) recognizes an antigen related to dietary gluten and is responsible for initiating inflammation in celiac disease. Antigliadin IgA antibodies (by ELISA) have been superseded by these more sensitive tests; has S/S = 80%/80–90%. IgA antigliadin antibodies becomes undetectable 3–6 months after gluten abstinence; may be used to monitor dietary compliance. May be most effective marker for children <3 years of age. Gliadin is a component of gluten. False-negative results may occur in patients on immunosuppressive therapy. If patient is IgA deficient, serology using IgG-tTG or IgG-EMA should be used.

Molecular Tests: HLA variation DQ2 is expressed in ~95% of patients; HLA-DQ8 is expressed in ~5% of patients; absence of these virtually excludes this diagnosis.

Gluten challenge: No longer considered essential to establish the diagnosis. It is done if the diagnosis is uncertain and not documented by biopsy before gluten withdrawal, to determine if symptoms and mucosal changes occur.

Xylose tolerance test: Distinguishes malabsorption caused by impaired transport across diseased mucosa from that caused by impaired digestion in lumen. Normal in many patients with mild to moderate disease not usually performed.

Considerations

* Firm diagnosis requires definite clinical response to gluten-free diet in 3–9 months, preferably with histologic documentation that the mucosa has reverted to normal by repeat biopsy. If patient fails to respond to rigid dietary control, biopsy should be repeated to rule out GI lymphoma, giardiasis, hypogammaglobulinemia, and other causes of villous atrophy, as well as diet should be rechecked.
* Malabsorption may cause folate deficiency with megaloblastic bone marrow and iron deficiency with mild hypochromic macrocytic anemia. Celiac disease should always be considered in cases of iron-deficiency or macrocytic anemia. May also have coagulopathy due to vitamin K deficiency and hypocalcemia and vitamin D deficiency causing osteomalacia. In patients with unexplained diarrhea or malabsorption, celiac sprue should be ruled out by small bowel biopsy.
* Laboratory findings due to frequently associated autoimmune diseases (e.g., thyroid, liver, type 1 DM, dermatitis herpetiformis [≤20% of celiac patients], Addison disease, arthritis) and other diseases (e.g., selective IgA deficiency; hyposplenism, T-cell lymphoma of small intestine; also Down syndrome, IgA nephropathy, IBD). Patients who should be screened include those with steatorrhea, malabsorption, or autoimmune diseases.

➤ **Suggested Readings**

Farrell RJ, Kelly CP. Celiac sprue. *N Engl J Med.* 2002;346:180–188.

Mäki M, Mustalahti K, Kokkonen J, et al. Prevalence of celiac disease among children in Finland. *N Engl J Med.* 2003;348:2517–2524.

ENTEROPATHY, PROTEIN-LOSING

➤ **Definition**

This condition refers to the GI loss of plasma protein in abnormal amounts.

➤ Causes

* Secondary (i.e., disease states in which clinically significant protein-losing enteropathy may occur as a manifestation)
  * Giant hypertrophy of gastric rugae (Ménétrier disease)
  * Eosinophilic gastroenteritis
  * Gastric neoplasms
  * Infections (e.g., Whipple disease, bacterial overgrowth, enterocolitis, shigellosis, parasitic infestation, viral infections, *C. difficile* infection) (see relevant sections in Chapter 13, Infectious Diseases).
  * Nontropical sprue
  * Inflammatory and neoplastic diseases of small and large intestine, including UC, regional enteritis
  * Constrictive pericarditis
  * Immune diseases (e.g., SLE)
  * Lymphatic obstruction (e.g., lymphoma, sarcoidosis, mesenteric TB)
* Primary (i.e., hypoproteinemia is the major clinical feature)
  * Intestinal lymphangiectasia
  * Nonspecific inflammatory or granulomatous disease of small intestine

➤ Laboratory Findings

Core Laboratory: Serum cholesterol usually normal. Serum total protein, albumin, γ globulin, and calcium are decreased. Serum α and β globulins normal. Proteinuria absent.
Hematology: Mild anemia. Eosinophilia (occasionally).
Stool Findings: Steatorrhea with abnormal tests of lipid absorption.
Other: Increased permeability of GI tract to large molecular substances shown by IV iodine-131-polyvinylpyrrolidone (^{131}I-PVP) test (see Malabsorption).

COLITIS, COLLAGENOUS

➤ Definition

Syndrome of chronic nonbloody diarrhea. The incidence is ~3/1,000 in such patients. Diagnosis is established by biopsy of colon in patients thought to have irritable bowel syndrome.

➤ Laboratory Findings

Hematology: ESR is increased, and anemia and hypoalbuminemia occur in some patients. Eosinophil count is increased in some patients.

COLITIS, PSEUDOMEMBRANOUS

* See *Clostridium difficile* discussion in Chapter 13, Infectious Diseases.

GALLSTONE ILEUS

* Laboratory findings caused by preceding chronic cholecystitis and cholelithiasis.

- Laboratory findings caused by acute obstruction of terminal ileum (accounts for 1–2% of patients).

GASTROENTERITIS, EOSINOPHILIC

➤ Definition
Diagnosis requires histologic evidence of predominant eosinophilic (>20 eosinophils/HPF) infiltration of GI tract in absence of parasitic infection or extraintestinal disease.

➤ Laboratory Findings
Hematology: Eosinophilia in 80% of cases.
Other: Eosinophilic ascites with predominant disease of serosal layer. IgE may be increased, especially in children.

➤ Suggested Readings
Bonis PAL, LaMont JT. Approach to the adult with chronic diarrhea in developed countries. www.uptodate.com, May, 2009.
Khan F, Sachs H, Pechet L, Snyder LM. *Guide to Diagnostic Testing.* Philadelphia: Lippincott Williams & Wilkins; 2002.
Wanke C. Approach to the adult with acute diarrhea in developed countries. www.uptodate.com, May, 2009.

GASTROINTESTINAL BLEEDING

UPPER GASTROINTESTINAL BLEEDING (ADULT)

➤ Definition
Upper GI bleeding is defined as emanating from a source above the ligament of Treitz. This is the most common medical emergency for gastroenterologists. The mortality is approximately 8%, and it is not usually due to exsanguination but rather to the adverse effect on comorbid conditions.

➤ Who Should be Suspected?
The patient may present with stigmata of chronic blood loss (anemia and related symptoms) or acute blood loss (weakness or syncope).
Screening. Currently, screening for asymptomatic ulcerated lesions of GI tract is generally recommended, especially for carcinoma of the colon and large adenomas.

➤ Differential Diagnosis of Upper Gastrointestinal Bleeding (Table 6-4)
- PUD (see discussion of acute abdomen under Abdominal Pain) (40–50% of patients) is associated with risk factors including *H. pylori* infection, use of NSAIDs, stress, and increase of gastric acid. It accounts for gastritis 10% of patients, esophagitis 6% associated with gastric reflux (GERD). Risk factors for stress-related bleeding include respiratory failure and coagulopathy. Portal hypertension and varices (18% of patients) indicate the severity of a patient's underlying cirrhosis. These patients have an associated mortality of 50% even after control of the hemorrhage

> **TABLE 6-4. Differential Diagnosis of Upper Gastrointestinal Bleeding**
> - Peptic ulcer disease (40–50%; idiopathic, induced by drug, toxin, or stress, related to an infection, associated with Zollinger-Ellinger syndrome)
> - Erosive esophagitis, gastritis, and duodenitis 25%
> - Portal hypertension and varices (10–15%; esophageal, gastric, duodenal, and portal hypertensive gastropathy)
> - Mallory-Weiss tear (5%)
> - Rare causes: atriovenous malformations, Rendu-Osler-Weber syndrome, watermelon stomach (gastric antral vascular ectasia), Dieulafoy lesion, stomal ulcer, neoplasm (benign, primary, and metastatic malignancy), connective tissue disease (scleroderma, Ehlers-Danlos syndrome), aortic enteric fistula, hemobilia, uremic gastritis, foreign body

- Mallory-Weiss tears (5% of patients) occur in the distal esophagus, at the site of the gastroesophageal junction, usually following a bout of retching. Most tears heal uneventfully within 24–48 hours. The diagnosis is made by endoscopic evaluation, at which time therapeutic interventions may be utilized as well as stratifying the risk of rebleeding.
- Neoplasm of esophagus and stomach accounts for <5% of all cases of severe bleeding. It is generally a late manifestation, and represents a negative prognostic feature. Uncommonly, tumors may metastasize to the gastric mucosa.
- Anticoagulant therapy: GI hemorrhage occurs in 3–4% of patients on anticoagulant therapy; it may be spontaneous or secondary to unsuspected disease (e.g., peptic ulcer, carcinoma, diverticula, hemorrhoids). Occasionally there is hemorrhage into the wall of the intestine with secondary ileus. PT may be in the therapeutic range or, more commonly, is increased. Warfarin (Coumadin) drug action is potentiated by administration of aspirin, antibiotics, phenylbutazone, and thyroxine and by T-tube drainage of the common bile duct, especially if pancreatic disease is present.
- Occult bleeding
- Rendu-Osler-Weber syndrome is associated with telangiectasia of the lips, oral mucosa, and fingertips. Dieulafoy lesion correlates with a dilated aberrant submucosal vessel, which erodes the overlying mucosa in the absence of an ulcer. This should be suspected in the patient with recurrent episodes of undiagnosed upper GI bleeding (GI bleeding in 10–40% of patients).

➤ Causes

- Mass (e.g., carcinoma, adenoma). In addition to the main cause of bleeding, 50% of patients have an additional lesion that could cause hemorrhage (especially duodenal ulcer, esophageal varices, hiatal hernia). With previously known GI tract lesions, 40% of patients bled from an altogether different lesion.
- Inflammation (e.g., IBD, Crohn disease, erosive esophagitis)
- Vascular disorders (e.g., varices, hemangioma)
- Infections (e.g., TB, amebiasis, hookworm, whipworm, strongyloidiasis, ascariasis)
- Other sites (e.g., hemoptysis, epistaxis, oropharynx)
- Others (e.g., factitious, coagulopathies, long distance running)
- Use of fecal occult blood test (see p. 266)

➤ Laboratory Findings
- Initial assessment: assess magnitude of blood loss (CBC, vital signs).
  - Check coagulation (PT, PTT, platelets) and other tests to rule out either an acquired or congenital bleeding disorder.
  - Type and crossmatch number of units appropriate for severity of blood loss.
- Esophagogastroduodenoscopy (EGD) is the diagnostic procedure of choice for patients presenting with acute GI bleeding. Advantages of early EGD include:
  - Confirmation or modification of the working diagnosis, proposed by the history and physical examination
  - Providing therapeutic measures, which lessen transfusion requirements and the need for surgery
  - Potentially averting the need for hospitalization
  - In patients with iron deficiency, recommend upper and lower endoscopy plus work-up for celiac disease

➤ Limitations
- Adenomas <2 cm in greatest diameter are less likely to bleed. Upper GI tract bleeding is less likely than lower GI tract bleeding to cause a positive test.
- Long distance running is associated with positive guaiac test in ≤23% of runners.
- Stools may appear grossly normal with GI bleeding of 100 mL/day.
- Consistent melena requires 150–200 mL blood in the stomach.

GASTROINTESTINAL BLEEDING, SMALL INTESTINE

- The small intestine is an uncommon site of hemorrhage, accounting for only 3–5% of GI bleeding. Patients usually present with occult blood loss and may have evidence of melena or hematochezia.

➤ Differential Diagnosis of Gastrointestinal Bleeding from the Small Intestine (Table 6-5)
- Angiodysplasia accounts for the majority of cases of bleeding from the small intestine (70–80%). Bleeding can be either brisk or occult. An isolated episode of bleeding does not mandate therapy, as the lesions do not usually rebleed (approximately 50%). Angiodysplasia may be an incidental finding and needs to be documented to be considered as a source of blood loss.
- Tumors account for 5–10% of cases of blood from the small intestine. Of these, one third are benign (leiomyoma and adenomas most commonly) and two thirds are malignant (45% adenocarcinoma, usually of the duodenum, 30% carcinoid, 14% lymphoma, and 11% leiomyosarcoma). The three most common malignancies are generally associated with chronic blood loss. Metastatic disease may also occur, most commonly from melanoma and breast cancer.

➤ Laboratory Findings
- Plain abdominal films may show evidence of obstruction suggestive of stricture or tumor, but they are not likely to be diagnostic.
- Contrast radiography

TABLE 6-5. Differential Diagnosis of Gastrointestinal Bleeding from the Small Intestine

- Angiodysplasia
- Small bowel tumors
- Less common causes:
  - Ulcerative diseases (most commonly Crohn disease)
  - Meckel diverticulum (the cause in two thirds of men younger than 30 years of age)
  - Zollinger-Ellison syndrome (causes ulcerations)
  - Infections (e.g., tuberculosis, syphilis, typhoid, histoplasmosis)
  - Medications (e.g., potassium, nonsteroidal anti-inflammatory drugs, 6-mercaptopurine)
  - Vasculitis
  - Radiation enteritis (injury can occur 6–24 months after exposure, secondary to the development of occlusive vasculitis)
  - Jejunal diverticula (<5% actually bleed, but bleeding is usually massive, with mortality as high as 20%)
  - Vascular lesions (varices, venous ectasias, telangiectasias, hemangiomas, atriovenous malformations)

- Small bowel series have a low yield in identifying a bleeding source (i.e., a 5% detection rate). This may be increased to 10% with use of enteroclysis. If the bleeding source is a small intestine malignancy, the yield is considerably better.
- Barium studies cannot diagnose angiodysplasias, but they may be useful in identifying mass lesions and mucosal defects.
- Despite the low diagnostic yield, contrast radiography is the initial study in a patient where small intestinal bleeding is suspected (i.e., when the evaluation of upper and lower GI tracts are nondiagnostic).
- Endoscopic studies
  - Routine EGD reaches the junction of the second and third portions of the duodenum.
  - Conventional push enteroscopy (either a dedicated enteroscope or pediatric colonoscope) can reach the proximal jejunum. Yield with push enteroscopy varies from 24–75% in detecting a bleeding source. Push enteroscopy also has therapeutic value.
  - Sonde enteroscopy is a newer procedure that is being developed to visualize the entire jejunum and ileum. It is a flexible fiberoptic instrument carried through the bowel by peristalsis. It is not a routinely available procedure, and it is best reserved for those patients with comorbid conditions that may preclude intraoperative enteroscopy (video capsule endoscopy).
- Angiography detects a bleeding rate of 0.5 mL/min. It can localize the site of bleeding in 50–72% of cases if bleeding is massive, but in only 25–50% of cases if bleeding has slowed. It has a low yield in diagnosing angiodysplasias and tumors.
- Nuclear imaging
  - Technetium-99 bleeding scan may detect bleeding at a rate as slight as 0.1 mL/min. Like angiography, it is only of value in the setting of active bleeding. It can define a general area of bleeding, but it cannot identify the precise source.

* Technetium-99 Meckel scan, which is taken up by ectopic gastric mucosa in the diverticulum, is not useful if the diverticulum does not contain gastric mucosa.
* Surgical evaluation
  * Intraoperative enteroscopy is a procedure whereby the bowel is manually advanced over an endoscope. It is the most common way to examine the entire small bowel. It is successful in identifying a bleeding source 83–100% of the time.
  * Exploratory surgery is often considered in patients with recurrent GI bleeding of unclear origin. Simple exploration has a low success rate, with a diagnostic yield of only 10% when unaccompanied by other evaluations (i.e., enteroscopy).
* Stepwise approach to evaluation. In a study of 77 patients, the interval from presentation to diagnosis was >20 months, because of the relatively asymptomatic nature of the conditions and the difficulty in evaluating small bowel bleeding sources.
* Determine the source of bleeding
  * In those with a nondiagnostic evaluation of lower and upper GI tracts, small bowel evaluation will be necessary.
  * Once the small bowel is assumed to be the bleeding source (i.e., standard examinations are nondiagnostic), proceed to small bowel series.
* If the source is not identified
  * Proceed to push enteroscopy, before considering repeat EGD or colonoscopy.
  * Sonde enteroscopy may be considered.
  * Withhold bleeding scans and angiography, unless the patient is actively bleeding.
  * Exploratory surgery can be done with intraoperative endoscopy if needed.
  * Video capsule endoscopy

➤ Neoplasms Caused by Primary Diseases of the Small Intestine
* Biopsy of lesions confirms the diagnosis.
* Laboratory findings due to complications (e.g., hemorrhage, obstruction, intussusception, malabsorption).
* Laboratory findings due to underlying conditions (e.g., Peutz-Jeghers syndrome, carcinoid syndrome).

LOWER GASTROINTESTINAL BLEEDING (ADULT), ACUTE

➤ Overview
* Lower GI bleeding is usually defined by bleeding originating from below the ligament of Treitz.
* If the initial assessment does not clearly distinguish between upper and lower sources of GI bleeding, evaluation of the upper tract should be pursued, as this is the more common site of massive GI bleeding.

➤ Differential Diagnosis of Lower Gastrointestinal Bleeding (Table 6-6)
* Angiodysplasia. In elderly patients, angiodysplasia is diagnosed with proportional greater frequency. Angiodysplasia is not visualized by barium enema. The bleeding tends to be self-limited, frequently arising from the right colon.

TABLE 6-6. Differential Diagnosis of Lower Gastrointestinal Bleeding

- Diverticulosis (approximately 33%)
- Angiodysplasia (approximately 28%)
- Neoplasia (benign and malignant approximately 19%)
- Colitis (ulcerative, Crohn, ischemic, pseudomembranous, infectious disease, radiation exposure approximately 18%)
- Hemorrhoid (approximately 3%)
- Less common causes:
  - Solitary ulcers
  - Nonsteroidal antiinflammatory drugs
  - Venous lakes
  - Blue rubber nevus
  - Anastomotic ulcerations and suture lines
  - Mechanical trauma
  - Postbiopsy or polypectomy
  - Coagulopathy and anticoagulation therapy
  - Autoimmune disease (e.g., rheumatoid vasculitis, Henoch-Schönlein purpura)

- Benign anorectal pathology. In younger patients (<35 years of age) benign anorectal pathology (e.g., hemorrhoidal bleeding) is the most common etiology.
- Diverticulosis. Less than 33% of patients with diverticulosis develop significant bleeding. The bleeding is typically painless and occurs in the absence of diverticulitis. Although diverticula are more commonly located on the left side of the colon, right-sided lesions account for a significant portion of diverticular bleeding.
- Colon cancer polyps account for 19% of patients with lower gastrointestinal blood loss in patients older than 50 years of age.
- Coagulopathy usually causes bleeding in patients with a comorbid GI condition. Therefore, a patient with coagulopathy always requires further evaluation.
- Suspect upper GI bleeding in patients presenting with hematochezia.
- Hemorrhoids, bloody diarrhea from inflammation needs to be ruled out.

➤ Diagnostic Evaluation

- Initial assessment
  - Check coagulation studies (PT, PTT, platelets, CBC, BUN, creatinine). Bleeding in uremic patients with angiodysplasia may be a result of acquired coagulopathy.
  - Type and crossmatch number of units appropriate for severity of blood loss.
- Endoscopic studies (assuming an upper GI bleed is excluded by virtue of nonbloody bilious fluid obtained via nasogastric lavage)
  - Anoscopy may be performed to rule out bleeding hemorrhoids in appropriately selected patients.
  - Colonoscopy will identify a bleeding source in approximately 80% of patients and will help control bleeding in up to 40% of patients. Other advantages include assisting in preoperative assessment.
- Neoplasms, Colon: Blood in stool (occult or gross). Annual screening for occult blood detects <50% of cancers and 10% of adenomas.

➤ Suggested Readings

Bonis PAL, Bynum TE. Angiodysplasia of the gastrointestinal tract. www.uptodate.com, May, 2009.

Jutabha R. Etiology of lower gastrointestinal bleeding in adults. www.uptodate.com, May, 2009.

Jutabha R. Approach to the adult patient with lower gastrointestinal bleeding. www.uptodate.com, May, 2009.

Jutabha R, Jensen D. Approach to the adult patient with upper gastrointestinal bleeding. www.uptodate.com, May, 2009.

Khan F, Sachs H, Pechet, L, Snyder LM. *Guide to Diagnostic Testing.* Philadelphia: Lippincott Williams & Wilkins; 2002.

Travis A, Saltzman J. Evaluation of occult gastrointestinal bleeding. www.uptodate.com, May, 2009.

Villa X. Approach to upper gastrointestinal bleeding in children. www.uptodate.com, 1–27, May, 2009.

HEPATOMEGALY

➤ Definition

* Hepatomegaly refers to an enlarged liver with a vertical span >12 cm as percussed in the midclavicular line. Studies have suggested that by ultrasound, a midhepatic (sagittal) diameter >15.5 cm indicates hepatomegaly in 75% of the cases. By radioisotope scanning, a span of >15–17 cm in the midclavicular line indicates hepatomegaly.
* Hepatomegaly may occur in the absence of pathology (i.e., normal variant), or as a result of a depressed right hemidiaphragm, Riedel lobe, or subdiaphragmatic space occupying lesions.

➤ Differential Diagnosis and Work-up (Figure 6-6)

* The causes of hepatomegaly can be subdivided into processes involving
  * Hypertrophy or hyperplasia of cells intrinsic to the normal liver parenchyma
  * Hepatomegaly secondary to infiltration of the liver by cells or organisms not normally present.
  * Vascular causes resulting in congestion of the liver.
* Common causes. Fatty liver (nonalcoholic steatohepatitis) is a common cause of hepatomegaly. The most common cause of fatty liver in the United States is chronic alcoholism. Other causes of fatty liver include diabetes, obesity, hyperlipidemia (metabolic syndrome), protein malnutrition, and prolonged TPN.
  * Other causes. In addition to infectious and drug-related causes, clinically important causes of hepatomegaly include hemochromatosis, α_1-antitrypsin deficiency, Wilson disease, autoimmune hepatitis, SLE, and RA.
  * Cholangiohepatitis is a rare disorder in which intrahepatic and extrahepatic bile ducts become obstructed with bile stones, leading to secondary inflammation of the liver.
  * Congestion from heart failure includes all causes of elevated right heart pressures (e.g., cor pulmonale, tricuspid regurgitation, constrictive pericarditis, ventricular dysfunction).
  * Hepatocellular carcinoma represents approximately 2.5% of all carcinomas in the United States and approximately 30–50% of all carcinomas in Asians living in Asia, where chronic active hepatitis due to hepatitis B virus is common. Other risk factors include chronic hepatitis C or chronic liver disease of any type.
  * Benign tumors include adenomas, focal nodular hyperplasia, and hemangiomas. Adenomas are more commonly seen in women 30–40 years of age, mostly in the right lobe, and can be as large as 10 cm in greatest dimension. There is often a history of oral contraceptive (estrogen) use. Focal nodular hyperplasia often presents as right-sided solid masses.

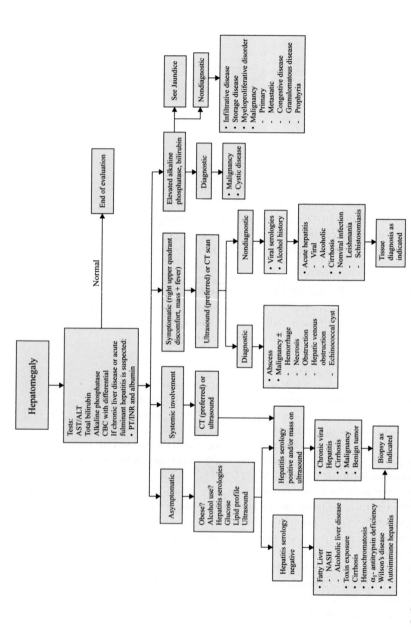

Figure 6-6. Algorithm for the work-up of hepatomegaly, if the vertical span is >12 cm by physical examination or imaging. ALT, alanine aminotransferase; AST, aspartate aminotransferase; CBC, complete blood count; CT, computed tomography; FOBT, fecal occult blood test; GI, gastrointestinal; INR, international normalized ratio; NASH, nonalcoholic steatohepatitis; PT, prothrombin time.

Hemangiomas are most commonly benign, with hemorrhage and malignant transformation occurring rarely.

- Budd-Chiari syndrome (hepatic vein thrombosis) usually presents with hepatomegaly, pain, and severe, intractable ascites. Risk factors included hypercoagulable states, polycythemia vera, myeloproliferative syndromes, paroxysmal nocturnal, hemoglobinuria, and use of oral contraceptive pills.
- Metastatic tumors. After lymph nodes, the liver is the second most common metastatic site, probably due to its high vascularity from a dual arterial/venous blood supply. With the exception of primary brain tumors, any primary tumor can metastasize to the liver. The most common primary tumors derive from the GI tract, lung, breast, and melanoma. The usual presentation is with nonspecific, systemic symptoms such as weight loss, fever, and loss of appetite.
- A tender liver mass in a patient with an elevated WBC count and eosinophilia suggests a liver abscess and possibly parasitic infection.
- Radiologic studies
  - Ultrasound is considered the primary screening examination for hepatic disease. In general, ultrasound is better for focal lesions than for parenchymal disease.
    - The advantages include low cost, portability, and no ionizing radiation. Masses as small as 1 cm can be detected, and cystic masses or abscesses can be distinguished from solid masses. Doppler ultrasonography can assess the patency and direction of blood flow in the hepatic and portal veins (without contrast).
    - The disadvantages include obscured images in the presence of bowel gas and obesity.
  - CT scanning: In general, anatomic definition is more complete than with ultrasound. CT scanning is also better than ultrasound for showing diffuse parenchymal liver disease (fat shows ups as decreased density and hemochromatosis, or secondary iron overload shows up as increased density).
    - The advantages include the ability to image in the setting of obesity and bowel gas.
      - Lesions as small as 1 cm can be distinguished.
      - With IV contrast, abscesses can usually be distinguished from tumors.
      - Dynamic scanning with IV contrast may also show cavernous hemangiomas.
      - Mass lesions can be biopsied under either ultrasound or CT guidance.
    - The disadvantages include cost, radiation, and possible exposure to IV contrast.
  - Magnetic resonance imaging (MRI): Sensitivity is superior to CT scanning for mass lesions.
    - The advantages include lack of ionizing radiation and different planes of imaging.
      - It is the technique of choice to look for hemangiomas
      - It is useful in distinguishing between a regenerating nodule and a tumor in the cirrhotic liver.
      - MRI can be used to monitor the liver for iron and copper deposition and with some modification can identify fatty liver and can produce an estimated quantification of fat content.
      - It can sometimes detect Budd-Chiari syndrome (hepatic vein thrombosis) without the need for IV iodinated contrast media (gadolinium is required).
    - The disadvantages include cost; slow time to acquire images, leading to more artifact; and limitations for patients with metal implants due to the use of a large magnet. MRI cannot distinguish a primary versus metastatic tumor.

- Radioisotope scanning has been largely replaced by ultrasound and CT scanning.
  - Technetium-99m labeled sulfur colloid scanning depends on uptake of phagocytic cells (Küpffer) and can help assess size and shape of the liver. Any disease where Küpffer cells are replaced by tumors, cysts, and abscesses produces a cold spot (adenomas); whereas with focal nodular hyperplasias, the liver will light up. Resolution for mass lesions is approximately 2 cm. Scintigraphy using radioactively labeled antibodies to tumor antigens is being developed as a diagnostic tool.
  - Gallium scanning uses gallium that is preferentially taken up in tissues synthesizing proteins (tumors or abscesses), and such areas show up as hot spots.
- Imaging of the biliary tract
  - ERCP allows for therapy (e.g., stone removal or stenting) as well as diagnosis.
  - Percutaneous transhepatic cholangiography (PTC) allows for imaging of the proximal biliary ducts and some therapy (e.g., stent placement or percutaneous drainage) of the ducts.
  - More recently, magnetic resonance cholangiopancreatography (MRCP) has demonstrated diagnostic accuracy similar to ERCP. The principal disadvantages include spatial resolution, which may not be as good as that achieved with ERCP; lack of therapeutic benefit; and decreased ability to visualize the ampulla.

FATTY LIVER

- Nonalcoholic steatohepatitis in most cases may have a history of metabolic syndrome. Nutritional (e.g., alcoholism, malnutrition, starvation, rapid weight loss)

➤ Causes
- Drugs (e.g., aspirin,[†] glucocorticoids,[*] synthetic estrogens,[*] some antiviral agents,[*†] calcium-channel blockers,[†] cocaine,[†] methotrexate,[*] valproic acid[†])
- Metabolic/genetic (e.g., acute fatty liver of pregnancy,[†] dysbetalipoproteinemia,[*] Weber-Christian disease,[*] cholesterol ester storage,[‡] Wolman disease[‡])
- Other (e.g., HIV infection,[*] B. cereus toxins,[†] liver toxins [e.g., organic solvents, phosphorus[†]], small bowel disease [inflammatory, bacterial overgrowth],[*] fatty liver of pregnancy)

➤ Laboratory Findings
- **Histology:** Biopsy of liver establishes the diagnosis. Fatty liver may be the only postmortem finding in cases of sudden, unexpected death.
- **Core Laboratory:** Most commonly, serum AST and ALT are increased 2–3×; usually ALT > AST in NAFL. Serum ALP is normal or slightly increased in <50% of patients. Other liver function tests are usually normal. Increased serum ferritin (≤5×) and transferrin saturation occur in ~60% of cases.
- **Serology:** Tests for viral hepatitis are negative.
- **Considerations**
- Laboratory findings are due to underlying conditions (most commonly alcoholism; nonalcoholic fatty liver (NAFL) is commonly associated with type 2 DM [≤75%], obesity

---

[*]May principally cause macrovesicular steatosis due to imbalance in hepatic synthesis and export of lipids.
[†]May principally cause microvesicular steatosis due to defective mitochondrial function.
[‡]May principally cause accumulation of phospholipids in lysosomes.

[69–100%], hyperlipidemia [20–81%]; hypertension malnutrition, toxic chemicals). NAFL is distinguished by negligible history of alcohol consumption and negative random blood alcohol assays. Cirrhosis occurs in ≤50% of alcoholic and ≤17% of nonalcoholic cases.

Fatty Liver of Pregnancy, Acute

- The incidence is ≤1 per 15,000 deliveries; usually occurs >35th week of pregnancy.
- This is a medical emergency because of high maternal and fetal mortality that is markedly improved by termination of pregnancy.
- Often associated with preeclampsia (see Chapter 8, Renal and Urinary Tract Diseases)

➤ Laboratory Findings

- **Histology:** Biopsy of liver confirms the diagnosis.
- **Core Laboarotory:** Increased AST and ALT to ~300 U (rarely >500 U) is used for early screening in suspicious cases; ratio is not helpful in differential diagnosis. Serum bilirubin may be normal early but will rise unless pregnancy terminates. Serum uric acid is increased disproportionately to BUN and creatinine, which may also be increased. Blood glucose is often decreased, sometimes markedly. Blood ammonia is usually increased. Neonatal liver function tests are usually normal but hypoglycemia may occur.
- **Hematology:** Increased WBC in >80% of cases (often >15,000/µL). Evidence of DIC in >75% of patients.

NEOPLASMS OF LIVER: HEPATOCELLULAR CARCINOMA (HEPATOMA)

➤ Laboratory Findings

- **Core Laboratory:** Serum AFP may be increased for up to 18 months before symptoms; is sensitive indicator of recurrence in treated patients but a normal postoperative level does not ensure absence of metastases. Levels >500 ng/dL in adults strongly suggest hepatoma. Levels >100× URL have S/S = 60%/100%. In ≤30% of hepatoma cases, AFP <4× URL; such increases are common in chronic HBC and HCV. Serum GGT hepatoma-specific band (HSBs I′, II, II′) by electrophoresis activity >5.5 U/L has S/S = 85%/97%, accuracy = 92%. Does not correlate with AFP or tumor size.
- **Hematology:** ESR and WBC sometimes increased. Anemia is common; polycythemia occurs occasionally. Hemochromatosis (≤20% of patients die of hepatoma).
- **Serology:** Markers of viral hepatitis are frequently present.
- **Tumor Markers:** Serum CEA is usually normal. CEA in bile is increased in patients with cholangiocarcinoma and intrahepatic stones but not in patients with benign stricture, chole-dochal cysts, sclerosing cholangitis. Increases with progression of disease and declines with tumor resection.

Considerations

- Sudden progressive worsening of laboratory findings of underlying disease (e.g., increased serum ALP, LD, AST, bilirubin)
- Relative absence of hepatoma associated with cirrhosis of Wilson disease

- Laboratory findings due to obstruction of hepatic (Budd-Chiari syndrome) or portal veins or inferior vena cava may occur.

➤ **Suggested Readings**

Friedman LS. Congestive hepatopathy. www.uptodate.com, May, 2009.

Khan F, Sachs H, Pechet L, Snyder LM. *Guide to Diagnostic Testing.* Philadelphia: Lippincott Williams & Wilkins; 2002.

Yao DF, Yao DB, Wu XH, et al. Diagnosis of hepatocellular carcinoma by quantitative detection of hepatoma-specific bands of serum γ-glutamyltransferase. *Am J Clin Pathol.* 1998;110:743.

JAUNDICE (SEE HEPATOMEGALY)

➤ **Overview**

- Jaundice is a yellowish staining of the integument, sclerae, and deeper tissues, and is associated with conditions that have increased excretions of bile pigments, which are increased in the plasma.
- Physiology
  - Serum bilirubin accumulates when its production from heme exceeds its metabolism and excretion.
  - An imbalance between the production and clearance of serum bilirubin results either from excess release of bilirubin into the bloodstream, or from physiologic processes that impair the hepatic uptake, metabolism, or excretion of this metabolite.
  - Jaundice is clinically detectable when the serum bilirubin exceeds 2.0–2.5 mg/dL. Because elastin has a high affinity for bilirubin, and scleral tissue is rich in elastin, scleral icterus is usually a more sensitive sign than generalized jaundice.
- Bilirubin metabolism
  - Unconjugated bilirubin. More than 90% of serum bilirubin in normal individuals is in an unconjugated form, circulating as an albumin-bound complex. This is not filtered by the kidneys.
  - Conjugated bilirubin. The remainder is conjugated (primarily as a glucuronide), rendering it water soluble, and thus capable of being filtered and excreted by the kidney.
  - Hepatic phase. Hepatic metabolism has three phases: uptake, conjugation, and excretion.
    - Uptake phase: Unconjugated bilirubin is bound to albumin and is presented to the hepatocyte, where the complex dissociates and bilirubin enters the cell either by diffusion or transport across the membrane.
    - Conjugation phase: bilirubin is then conjugated in a two-step process. This occurs in the endoplasmic reticulum and is catalyzed by glucuronyl transferase. Bilirubin glucuronide is generated.
    - Excretion phase: In an energy-dependent process occurring in the biliary canaliculi, conjugated bilirubin is excreted into the bile. It is important to remember that this is the rate-limiting step. When this phase is impaired, either through obstruction or excretory defects, the conjugated bilirubin is presumed to reflux through the hepatic sinusoids into the bloodstream.
  - Intestinal phase. After excretion into the bile, conjugated bile is transported into the duodenum. It is not reabsorbed by intestinal mucosa. In the intestine, it is either excreted in the feces unchanged or metabolized by intestinal bacteria to urobilinogen. Urobilinogen is

then reabsorbed, where a small portion is metabolized in the liver, and the remainder bypasses the liver and is excreted by the kidney.

➤ Differential Diagnosis of Jaundice (Table 6-7)

* Extrahepatic biliary obstruction
  * The history, physical examination, and initial laboratory assessment have a sensitivity of 90–95%. The specificity, however, is only 76%. When radiologic imaging is factored in, the specificity rises to 98%.

TABLE 6-7. Differential Diagnosis of Jaundice

Conjugated Hyperbilirubinemia

* Hepatocellular jaundice
  * Hepatitis virus
  * Toxin or drugs (alcohol)
  * Cirrhosis
  * Ischemia
* Extrahepatic biliary obstruction
  * Choledocholithiasis
  * Ascending cholangitis
  * Pancreatitis – see Abdominal Pain
  * Sclerosing cholangitis
  * HIV cholangiopathy
  * Biliary stricture or cyst
  * Malignancy
    * Pancreas – see Abdominal Pain
    * Ampullary carcinoma
    * Cholangiocarcinoma
    * Metastatic
* Intrahepatic cholestasis
  * Abscess
  * Tumor
  * Primary biliary cirrhosis
  * Cholestatic jaundice of pregnancy
  * Dubin-Johnson syndrome
  * Rotor syndrome
  * Benign recurrent intrahepatic cholestasis
  * Sepsis
  * Infiltrative disease
    * Sarcoid
    * Amyloid

Unconjugated Hyperbilirubinemia

* Hemolysis
* Gilbert syndrome
* Ineffective erythropoiesis
* Hematoma resorption

- Approximately 40% of patients with this diagnosis present with jaundice.
- In the setting of complete obstruction, alcoholic stools are seen and no urobilinogen is detected in the urine (see cancer head of pancreas acute abdomen).
- In patients with extrahepatic biliary obstruction, ALP would be expected to rise to levels 2–3 times normal. A normal level would be uncommon. Serum transaminases would generally be <300 U/L.
- Intrahepatic cholestasis: Consider intrahepatic etiologies in the differential diagnosis because high levels may be seen in patients with primary biliary cirrhosis and granulomatous hepatitis.
  - This group of disorders is defined by the lack of evidence of mechanical obstruction and cannot be explained on the basis of hepatocellular injury alone. Among these disorders are those characterized by disordered enzyme function (intrinsic/acquired), infiltrative disorders, and drugs.
  - A diagnosis of intrahepatic cholestasis made by clinical assessment and supported by negative findings from ultrasound or CT scan offers 95% specificity. In a patient in whom extrahepatic obstruction is not strongly suspected, no further investigation of the extrahepatic biliary tree is indicated.

HYPERBILIRUBINEMIA

Unconjugated Hyperbilirubinemia
➤ Causes
- Increased destruction of RBCs
  - Isoimmunization (e.g., incompatibility of Rh, ABO, other blood groups)
  - Biochemical defects of RBCs (e.g., G6PD deficiency, pyruvate deficiency, hexokinase deficiency, congenital erythropoietic porphyria, and α- and γ-thalassemias)
  - Structural defects of RBCs (e.g., hereditary spherocytosis, hereditary elliptocytosis, infantile pyknocytosis)
  - Physiologic hemolysis of the newborn
    - Infection (viral, bacterial, and protozoal)
    - Congenital Causes
    - Extravascular blood (e.g., subdural hematoma, ecchymoses, hemangiomas)
    - Erythrocytosis (e.g., maternal-to-fetal or twin-to-twin transfusion, delayed clamping of umbilical cord)

➤ Recommended Laboratory Evaluation
- These studies are of proven benefit in determining the proximate etiologies in the patient presenting with jaundice. With this approach, the clinician can confidently assign probabilities to the major categories that most frequently account for jaundice.
- The first step is to determine the total bilirubin and the bilirubin fractions. This allows the clinician to determine whether the problem is due to an excess production or impaired conjugation (indirect/unconjugated predominant) versus impaired excretion (direct/conjugated predominant).
- ALP elevations out of proportion to the hepatic transaminases would favor extrahepatic or intrahepatic cholestasis.
- Hepatic transaminase elevations out of proportion to the alkaline phosphatase favor hepatocellular etiologies.

- The CBC can be extremely useful. The most important points include the interpretation of or for:
  - Anemia (hemolysis, bleeding). See Chapter 10, Hematologic Disorders
  - Mean corpuscular volume (microcytosis suggests iron deficiency; round macrocytosis suggests chronic liver disease or ineffective erythropoiesis; GI malignancy).
  - Thrombocytopenia (sequestration in portal hypertension, sepsis, autoimmune disease, bone marrow suppression [alcohol])
  - Reticulocytosis (hemolysis). See Chapter 10, Hematologic Disorders
- Urinalysis provides information about bilirubinuria and urobilinogen. In reality, data from urinalysis add little incremental benefit to the decision-making process.
  - The presence of urobilinogen eliminates the possibility of complete biliary tract obstruction. That is, bile has entered the intestine, where it undergoes enterohepatic metabolism.
  - The presence of bilirubinuria, on the other hand, suggests that conjugation is taking place.
- Coagulation studies are useful in two areas.
  - If an invasive intervention is considered, coagulation studies can be used to assess bleeding risk.
  - If the prothrombin time is prolonged and other causes of coagulopathy are unlikely, chronic liver disease or hepatocellular etiologies become increasingly likely.
- Serum amylase would be obtained in cases where extrahepatic obstruction is suspected on the basis of history and physical examination.

➤ Diagnostic Imaging

- It is estimated that 25–40% of common bile duct obstructions are missed by both ultrasound and CT scanning. However, when intrahepatic cholestasis or hepatocellular etiologies are suspected, either of these noninvasive strategies is acceptable.
- Ultrasound: This is the least invasive and most inexpensive of the imaging procedures available to assess obstructive jaundice. Ultrasound determines the presence of obstructive jaundice by detecting dilated bile ducts.
  - The sensitivity is 55–93%, and the specificity is 73–96%.
  - False negatives are generally due to two factors:
    - Inability to visualize the biliary tree (often secondary to interposed bowel gas).
    - Absence of biliary dilation in the presence of obstruction.
  - It may be preferable, given its lower cost and radiation exposure.
- CT scanning is slightly more sensitive (74–96%) and specific (90–94%) than ultrasound in detecting the presence of biliary obstruction.
  - A CT scan is more likely to show the site and cause of obstruction when compared with ultrasound.
  - CT also gives information in instances where staging a suspected neoplasm has clinical significance (see cancer head of pancreas).
  - In patients for whom mass lesions (i.e., malignancy, abscess) are suspected or where technical limitations make ultrasound difficulty to interpret, CT is preferred.
- Percutaneous transhepatic cholangiography (PTC): The technical success rate of this procedure is approximately 90–99%. Its use is limited by a major complication rate of 3–5% and has been largely supplanted by ERCP. ERCP offers a lower complication rate than PTC and provides a greater number of therapeutic options (stone extraction, stent placement).

- This test could reasonably be used in patients with a high likelihood of extrahepatic obstruction (e.g., those who have had recent biliary surgery, symptoms of cholangitis, palpable gallbladder, pain or fever, pancreatitis).
- When palliation is the primary intent, ERCP is an appropriate initial procedure.
- Magnetic resonance cholangiopancreatography (MRCP) is a radiologic technique that produces images of the pancreaticobiliary tree, which are similar in appearance to those obtained by invasive methods. It appears to have diagnostic accuracy similar to that of ERCP.
  - MRCP is indicated for patients with allergies to iodinated contrast media, and patients with altered anatomy (i.e., secondary to surgical procedures or congenital abnormalities).
  - ERCP has advantages over MRCP, which include the ability to perform therapeutic interventions, perform manometry or endoscopic ultrasound, directly visualize the ampulla, and biopsy lesions.

DISEASES ASSOCIATED WITH JAUNDICE

CONJUGATED HYPERBILIRUBINEMIA/HEPATOCELLULAR JAUNDICE

Cirrhosis of Liver

➤ Laboratory Findings

- **Bilirubin:** Serum levels are often increased; may be present for years. Fluctuations may reflect liver status due to insults to the liver (e.g., alcoholic debauches). Most bilirubin is of the unconjugated type unless cirrhosis is of the cholangiolitic type. Higher and more stable levels occur in postnecrotic cirrhosis; lower and more fluctuating levels occur in Laennec cirrhosis. Terminal icterus may be constant and severe. Urine bilirubin is increased; urobilinogen is normal or increased.
- **AST:** Serum levels are increased (<300 units) in 65–75% of patients. Serum ALT is increased (<200 U) in 50% of patients. Transaminases vary widely and reflect activity or progression of the process (i.e., hepatic parenchymal cell necrosis).
- **ALP:** Serum levels are increased in 40–50% of patients.
- **Total protein:** Usually normal or decreased. Serum albumin parallels functional status of parenchymal cells and may be useful for following progress of liver disease, but it may be normal in the presence of considerable liver cell damage. Decreasing serum albumin may reflect development of ascites or hemorrhage. Serum globulin level is usually increased; it reflects inflammation and parallels the severity of the inflammation. Increased serum globulin (is usually gamma) may cause increased total protein, especially in chronic viral hepatitis and posthepatitic cirrhosis.
- **Total Cholesterol:** Normal or decreased. Progressive decrease in cholesterol, HDL, LDL with increasing severity. Decrease is more marked than in chronic active hepatitis. LDL may be useful for prognosis and selecting patients for transplantation. Decreased esters reflect more severe parenchymal cell damage.
- **Other Core Laboratory Findings:** BUN is often decreased (<10 mg/dL); increased with GI hemorrhage. Serum uric acid is often increased. Electrolytes and acid–base balance

are often abnormal and reflect various combinations of circumstances at the time, such as malnutrition, dehydration, hemorrhage, metabolic acidosis, respiratory alkalosis. In cirrhosis with ascites, the kidney retains increased sodium and excessive water, causing dilutional hyponatremia. Increased blood ammonia in liver coma and cirrhosis and with portacaval shunting of blood.

- **Hematology:** WBC is usually normal with active cirrhosis; increased ($<$50,000/µL) with massive necrosis, hemorrhage, and so on; decreased with hypersplenism. Anemia reflects increased plasma volume and some increased destruction of RBCs. If more severe, rule out hemorrhage in GI tract, folic acid deficiency, and excessive hemolysis.

CSF Findings: CSF is normal except for increased glutamine levels, which reflect brain ammonia levels (due to conversion from ammonia). Glutamine $>$35 mg/dL is always associated with hepatic encephalopathy (normal = 20 mg/dL); correlates with depth of coma and is more sensitive than arterial ammonia.

Considerations

- See Tables 6-8 and 6-9.
- Laboratory findings due to complications or sequelae, often in combination
- Abnormalities of coagulation mechanisms (see Chapter 10, Hematologic Disorders) such as prolonged PT (does not respond to parenteral vitamin K as frequently as in patients with obstructive jaundice). Prolonged bleeding time in 40% of cases due to decreased platelets and/or fibrinogen

TABLE 6-8. Causes of Liver Disease with Associated Conditions

Laboratory Findings Due to Causative/Associated Diseases or Conditions	Frequency in United States
Alcoholism	60–70%
Biliary disease (e.g., primary biliary cirrhosis, and sclerosing cholangitis)	5–10%
Cryptogenic	10–15%
Chronic viral hepatitis (HBV with or without HDV; HCV)	10%
Hemochromatosis	5%
Wilson disease	Rare
Alpha$_1$-antitrypsin deficiency	Rare
Autoimmune chronic active hepatitis	
Mucoviscidosis	
Glycogen storage diseases	
Galactosemia	
Porphyria	
Fructose intolerance	
Tyrosinosis	
Infections (e.g., congenital syphilis, schistosomiasis)	
Gaucher disease	
Ulcerative colitis	
Osler-Weber-Rendu disease	
Venous outflow obstruction (e.g., Budd-Chiari syndrome, venoocclusive disease, congestive heart failure)	

TABLE 6-9. Comparison of Different Mechanisms of Jaundice

	Cholestasis	Hepatocellular	Infiltration
Disease Example	Common Duct Stone **Drugs**	Acute viral Hepatitis	Metastatic Tumor, Granulomas, Amyloid
Serum bilirubin	6–20 mg/dL*	4–8 mg/dL	Usually <4 mg/dL, often normal
AST, ALT (U/mL)	May be slightly I, <200	Markedly I, often 500–1000	May be slightly I, <100
Serum ALP	3–5 times N	1–2 times N	2–4 times N
Prothrombin time	I in chronic cases	I in severe disease	N
Response to parenteral vitamin K	Yes	No	

N = normal, I = increase

*Serum bilirubin >10 mg/dL is rarely seen with common duct stone and usually indicates carcinoma.

Increased serum ALP <3× normal in 15% of patients with extrahepatic biliary obstruction, especially if obstruction is incomplete or due to benign conditions. Occasionally AST and LD are markedly increased in biliary obstruction or liver cancer.

- Hepatic encephalopathy (neurologic and mental abnormalities in some patients with liver failure or portosystemic shunt). Diagnosis is clinical; characteristic laboratory findings are supportive but not specific.
- See Table 6-10.
- Markers that may indicate progression to cirrhosis include decreased albumin; increased globulins; AST/ALT ratio >1; increased bilirubin, mainly unconjugated; increased PT; and decreased platelet count.

INFECTIOUS DISEASE: VIRAL HEPATITIS*

➤ Definition

Five hepatitis viruses cause the majority of clinically important viral infections of the liver: HAV, HBV, HCV, HDV, and HEV. They are all RNA viruses except for HBV, which is a DNA virus. All of these viruses can cause acute hepatitis; only HBV, HCV and HDV are able to cause chronic hepatitis infections. Coinfection with two hepatitis viruses or hepatitis virus infection in patients with preexisting liver disease is frequently associated with greater disease severity (Table 6-11). Other viruses or infectious agents may cause liver infection associated with systemic or localized infections. Agents include herpesviruses—like HSV, CMV, and EBV—rubella, *M. tuberculosis*, ameba, and leishmania. See the separate discussions for these infections. A variety of hepatotoxins, autoimmune diseases, and other diseases may also cause hepatitis that is clinically similar to diseases caused by the hepatitis viruses.

---

*The section on hepatitis was written by Michael Mitchell, MD.

TABLE 6-10. Comparison of Three Main Types of Liver Disease Due to Drugs

	Predominantly Cholestatic	Predominantly Hepatocellular	Mixed Biochemical Pattern
Example of drugs	Anabolic steroids,* estrogens*	Cinchophen Isonicotinic acid hydrazide	Phenylbutazone Phenytoin
	Organic arsenicals, antithyroid drugs (e.g., methimazole), chlorpromazine, PAS, erythromycin, sulfonylurea derivatives (including sulfonamides, phenothiazine tranquilizers, oral diuretics, antidiabetic drugs)	Monamine oxidase inhibitors (particularly iproniazid)	PAS and other anti-tuberculosis agents
Serum bilirubin	May be ≥30 mg/dL		
AST, ALT, LD (U/mL)	Mild to moderate increase	More markedly increased	
Serum ALP, LAP	More markedly increased; may remain increased for years after jaundice has disappeared	Less markedly increased	

*ALP, AST, ALT are not increased as much compared with other drugs.

➤ Laboratory Findings

- The earliest laboratory signs of acute viral hepatitis include elevations in ALT and AST, which typically precede elevation of bilirubin levels. In acute illness, the degree of ALT elevation typically exceeds AST elevation. Peak aminotransferase levels >1000 U/L are common. The level of aminotransferase elevation does not reliably predict the severity or prognosis of disease. Total bilirubin may increase to 5–20 mg/dL at peak. ALP is normal or mildly elevated in most cases.
- CBC may show mild neutropenia with a relative lymphocytosis, often with atypical lymphocytes. Serum globulins are normal or mildly elevated. In severe liver disease, synthesis of albumin and coagulation factors may be compromised, resulting in increased PT.

➤ Disease Manifestations

- Viral hepatitis infections show many, but varied, clinical features. One cannot distinguish different types of viral hepatitis by clinical features or routine chemistries; serologic tests are needed. Hepatitis virus infections demonstrate the following clinical phases:
  - Prodrome
  - Acute Liver Damage (Icteric or non-icteric, Cholangiolitic, Acute Hepatic Failure)
  - Post-Acute (Resolution and Chronic Infection—hepatocellular Carcinoma)

TABLE 6-11. Comparison of Different Types of Viral Hepatitis

	A	B	C	D	E
Genome	ssRNA	dsDNA	ssRNA	ssRNA	ssRNA
Classification	Picornaviridae	Hepadnaviridae	Flaviviridae	Unclassified	Caliciviridae?
New cases in the United States, 2007 (www.cdc.gov)	25,000	43,000	17,000	Uncommon. Always associated with HBV; 4% of acute HBV cases have HDV coinfection	Rare; occurs in travelers to endemic areas
Incubation period (days)	15–60	45–160	14–180	42–180	15–64
Transmission					
Enteric	Yes	No	No	No	Yes
Sexual	No	Yes	Possible	Possible	No
Perinatal	No	Yes	Possible	Possible	No
Parenteral	Rare	Yes	Yes	Yes	No
Post-transfusion incidence (%)	None	1 case per 137,000 units transfused	1 case per 2 million units transfused.	Virtually eliminated by HBV screening.	None
Viremia	Transient	Prolonged	Prolonged	Prolonged	Transient?
Fecal excretion of virus	+	–	–	–	+
Onset	Abrupt	Insidious	Insidious	Abrupt	Abrupt
Course	Mild, often subclinical, self-limited	Acute[b] and chronic infection	Acute infection typically mild; high incidence of chronic infection	Increases severity of underlying HBV infection	Usually mild, self-limited[a]

Asymptomatic	Most children	Most children; 50% adults	~75%	Rare	Often
Jaundice	Child: 10% Adult: 70–80%	15–40%[c]	10–25%	Varies	25–50%
Chronic hepatitis after acute infection (%)	0%	1–10% (90% of neonates)	70–85%	Common; high in superinfection	0%
Hepatocellular carcinoma association	No	Yes	Yes	Yes	Unlikely
Acute liver failure	1–2%	0.1–1%	Very rare	5%	1–2%; 20% in pregnancy

[a]Resembles hepatitis A. Case fatality 1%–2% except ≤20% in pregnancy. Usually milder infection and biochemical abnormalities than HBV or HAV infection.

[b]≤20% have serum sickness-like prodroma.

[c]Nonicteric patient is more likely to progress to chronic hepatitis. 1% of icteric cases become fulminant (<8 weeks) and 90% die within 2–4 weeks; associated with encephalopathy; renal, electrolyte, acid–base imbalances; hypoglycemia; coagulation derangements.

➤ Prodromal Period

- After a variable virus-specific incubation period, patients may develop nonspecific symptoms, including low-grade fever, headache, fatigue and malaise, and arthralgias. Anorexia, nausea, and vomiting are common and often associated with abdominal pain (epigastric or right upper quadrant).
- Prodromal symptoms typically last 1–2 weeks before the onset of signs and symptoms of acute liver disease. Dark urine may precede the onset of jaundice. Acholic stools may be seen in HAV and HEV infections.
  - During the prodrome:
    - Specific serologic markers appear in serum (see Figure 6-7)
    - Urinary urobilinogen and total serum bilirubin increase just before clinical jaundice occurs.
    - Serum AST and ALT levels increase during the prodromal phase and show very high peaks (>500 U) by the time jaundice appears.
    - ESR is normal.
    - Leukopenia (lymphopenia and neutropenia) is noted with onset of fever, followed by relative lymphocytosis and monocytosis. Plasma cells and <10% atypical lymphocytes may be seen.

Acute Hepatitis

- Acute hepatitis may be icteric or anicteric. The majority of cases of acute HCV infections and HAV and HBV infections in children are anicteric. Prodromal symptoms usually abate with bilirubin elevation and the appearance of jaundice.
  - Asymptomatic: Many patients infected with hepatitis viruses may remain clinically asymptomatic or show only mild or transient symptoms. The diagnosis of viral hepatitis may be suspected by finding abnormal LFT or other tests collected for other reasons.
  - Symptomatic, icteric
    - Patients develop jaundice; examination of the sclerae may provide the most sensitive site for detection. LFT testing demonstrates parenchymal cell damage in the liver. Fifty percent to 75% of total serum bilirubin is conjugated in the early stage; later, unconjugated bilirubin is proportionately higher. In acute hepatitis, there is usually marked elevation of aminotransferases, with ALT > AST. LD may be mildly elevated. Serum AST and ALT fall rapidly in the several days after jaundice appears and become normal 2–5 weeks later with resolution of infection.
      - Other liver function tests are often abnormal, depending on severity of the disease— bilirubinuria, abnormal serum protein electrophoresis, ALP, and so on Serum cholesterol to ester ratio is usually depressed early; total serum cholesterol is decreased only in severe disease. Serum phospholipids are increased in mild but decreased in severe hepatitis. Plasma vitamin A is decreased in severe hepatitis. Urine urobilinogen is increased in the early icteric period; at peak of the disease it disappears for days or weeks; urobilinogen simultaneously disappears from stool.
  - Symptomatic, anicteric: Laboratory findings are the same as in the icteric type, but abnormalities are usually less marked and there is slight or no increase in serum bilirubin.
- Nonspecific laboratory abnormalities are often associated with the acute phase of viral hepatitis. ESR is increased, but decreasess during convalescence. Serum iron is often increased.

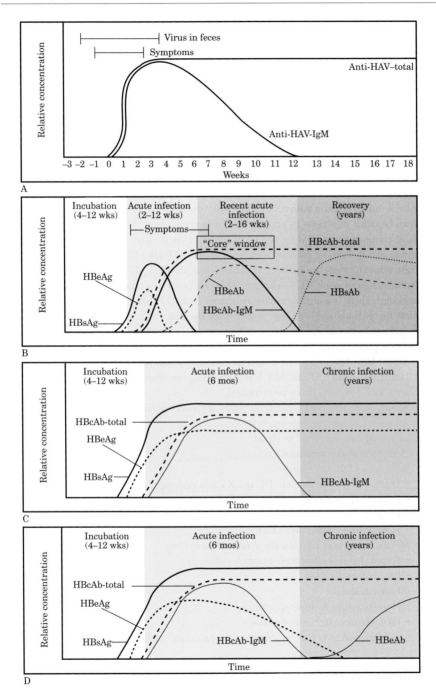

Figure 6-7. Hepatitis serologic profiles. **A.** Antibody response to hepatitis A. **B.** Hepatitis B core window identification. **C, D.** Hepatitis B chronic carrier profiles: no seroconversion **(C)**; late seroconversion **(D).** (Reproduced with permission of Hepatitis Information Center, Abbott Laboratories, Abbott Park, IL.)

Urine examination may show cylindruria, and albuminuria occurs occasionally. The renal concentrating ability is sometimes decreased.

- Cholangiolitic hepatitis: Similar to acute hepatitis, but evidence of obstruction is more prominent (e.g., increased serum ALP and conjugated serum bilirubin), and tests of parenchymal damage are less marked (e.g., AST increase may be 3–6 times normal).
- Acute Fulminant Hepatitis/Acute Liver Failure (ALF)
  - Acute fulminant hepatitis is associated with failure of liver function. Patients present with hepatic encephalopathy and hepatic synthetic dysfunction. The manifestations of encephalopathy may range from drowsiness and confusion to stupor and coma. Synthetic dysfunction is usually manifested by coagulopathy. Multiorgan failure may ensue. Ascites is typical. Bacterial superinfection, especially with streptococci and *S. aureus*, may occur.
  - ALF is more common with coinfection with two hepatitis viruses, like HBV and HDV, or with hepatitis infections in patients with preexisting liver disease. HBV infection is the most common cause of ALF (~1–3% of adults). HAV is associated with ALF only in adults and occurs in 1.8% of patients >60 years of age. ALF after HEV is rare, except for pregnant women, where up to 20% of patients may develop ALF. ALF is an extremely rare complication of acute HCV infection. ALF may occur as a complication of systemic HSV infection. There is a high mortality associated with ALF, but if the patient survives, complete biochemical and histologic recovery are the rule.
- In addition to clinical signs of hepatic failure, significant laboratory abnormalities are common:
  - As the patient's condition deteriorates, titers of HBsAg and HBeAg often fall and disappear.
  - Serum bilirubin progressively increases and may reach very high levels.
  - Increased serum AST and ALT levels are seen, but levels may fall abruptly terminally; serum ALP and GGT may be increased.
  - Serum cholesterol and cholesterol esters are markedly decreased.
  - Albumin and total protein levels are decreased.
  - Increased ammonia level in blood.
  - Hematologic abnormalities
  - Evidence of DIC is common.
    - Decreased factors II, V, VII, IX, and X cause prolonged PT and aPTT.
    - Decreased antithrombin III
    - Platelet count <100,000 in two thirds of patients
    - Hemorrhage, especially in GI tract
  - Metabolic markers are typically abnormal, including:
    - Hypokalemia (early), with metabolic alkalosis
    - Respiratory alkalosis
    - Lactic acidosis
    - Hyponatremia, hypophosphatemia
    - Hypoglycemia in ~5% of patients
  - Renal function tests may be abnormal. Hepatorenal syndrome may develop.

Post Acute Hepatitis

- Resolution: During recovery, systemic symptoms abate. Liver tenderness and biochemical abnormalities may persist. Complete clinical and biochemical recovery occurs 1–2 months after HAV and HEV infections and 3–6 months after uncomplicated HBV. HAV and HEV infections are not associated with progression to chronic infection. HBV, HCV, and HDV may progress to chronic infection. Recovery from acute HBV infection is more likely after clinically apparent, versus unapparent, infection

- Chronic Infection
  - The persistence of clinical and laboratory abnormalities for >6 months after acute hepatitis is characteristic of chronic infection. Chronic liver infection may develop with HCV, HBV, or HBV plus HDV infections. The clinical presentation varies from asymptomatic disease to progression to end-stage liver failure. Signs and symptoms may be fairly constant or marked by flares in severity, increasing the progression of liver injury. Cirrhosis may develop with chronic hepatitis caused by HCV, HBV, or HBV plus HDV. Liver damage is influenced by virus factors, as discussed later, and host factors. Host factors include coexisting diseases, especially liver disease, the host immune response, and alcohol consumption or exposure to other hepatotoxins.
  - The degree of laboratory abnormalities may not accurately reflect the degree of histologic changes. Aminotransferase elevation may be variable. In mild disease, ALT elevation is typically greater than the degree of AST elevation. Marked elevation of bilirubin levels is associated with advanced liver damage and cirrhosis. In advanced cirrhosis, the pattern of aminotransferase elevation is usually reversed, with the degree of AST elevation exceeding that of ALT elevation. The synthetic function of the liver decreases with advanced chronic disease and cirrhosis, with resulting clinical manifestations of coagulopathy, metabolic derangements, and so on.
- Hepatocellular Carcinoma: Hepatocellular carcinoma (HCC) may occur as a complication of chronic viral hepatitis. In HBV infection, HCC may occur in patients with or without cirrhosis. Risk factors for development of HCC in HBV-infected patients include infection early in life, coexisting immunocompromising diseases, and HDV coinfection. HCC may also complicate HCV infection, but occurs only in patients with cirrhosis.

Hepatitis Viruses (Figure 6-8)

- Hepatitis virus infections may be suspected in patients presenting with symptoms suggesting prodromal, acute, or chronic hepatitis or in patients coincidentally identified with abnormal laboratory finding. A limited number of tests may be used to screen patients for acute viral hepatitis:
  - Hepatitis B surface antigen (HBsAg)

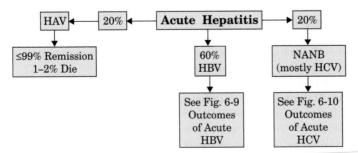

Figure 6-8. Outcomes of acute hepatitis in adults in the United States.

- Total Hepatitis B core antibody (Anti-HBc-Total)
- Hepatitis B core antibody-IgM (Anti-HBc-IgM)
- Hepatitis A antibody-IgM (Anti-HAV-IgM)
- Hepatitis C antibody (Anti-HCV)
- Further testing is determined by results of the initial screening tests. Repeat screening after negative results should be considered for patients with a high clinical suspicion or prior risk to rule out false-negative results due to a window period. Window periods represent intervals prior to immune response or during a transition from phases of antigen predominance to antibody predominance (e.g., HBsAg positive → anti-HBs positive). Specific testing for HDV is not necessary if HBV infection has been ruled out. Testing for HEV is usually unneeded unless a patient has recently traveled to an area where HEV infection is endemic. Specific hepatitis viruses and diagnostic testing are presented in subsequent text of this chapter.
- Hepatitis Viruses Transmitted by Enteric Routes. HAV and HEV infections are transmitted almost exclusively by the enteric route.
  - **HAV**
    - HAV infections, caused by a nonenveloped, single-stranded RNA picornavirus, occur worldwide. Infections usually occur in children. Risk factors include poor sanitation, contaminated water sources, and crowding. The infection may occur by direct fecal–oral exposure or indirectly through contaminated foods.
    - Childhood infections are most commonly asymptomatic, whereas infections in adults are often severe. Most symptomatic infections resolve in 1–2 months. Rare cholestatic variants may remain symptomatic for months, but eventually resolve completely.
    - Fecal excretion of virus begins late in the prodromal phase. IgM appears in the late prodrome; IgM may remain detectable for 6–12 months. After 3 months, IgM levels usually begin to drop, whereas rising IgG levels are detected. IgG levels persist indefinitely. Acute liver failure is uncommon in HAV infection (0.1%). Chronic infection does not occur in HAV infections.
  - **HAV diagnosis**:
    - Anti-HAV-IgM positive: Acute infection
      - Anti-HAV-IgM appears at the same time as symptoms in >99% of cases and peaks within the first month. IgM becomes undetectable within 12 (usually 6) months.
      - The presence of anti-HAV-IgM confirms diagnosis of recent acute infection. Serial testing is usually not needed for diagnosis.
    - Serum bilirubin is usually 5–10 times the normal level. Jaundice lasts a few days to 12 weeks. Patients are usually not infectious after the onset of jaundice.
    - Serum AST and ALT are increased above a hundred for 1–3 weeks.
    - Relative lymphocytosis is frequent.
    - Anti-HAV-IgG positive: Remote infection
      - Anti-HAV-IgG is usually detectable for life after resolution of acute HAV infection and indicates immunity to HAV infection.
    - Anti-HAV-total may be predominantly IgG or IgM, depending on infection status. A negative anti-HAV-total effectively excludes acute HAV, but does not distinguish recent from past infection, for which anti-HAV-IgM test is needed. Tests for anti-HAV-total (minimum detection ~100 mU/mL) may be insensitive for detection of protective antibody after HAV vaccine (minimum protective antibody concentration is <10 mU/mL).
    - Nonspecific elevation of IgM is common in acute HAV infection

- **HEV**
  - HEV infections are caused by an unenveloped, single-stranded RNA virus of the Calci-viridae family and are clinically similar to HAV infections. They are transmitted by the enteric route, and infections are most common in young adults (20–40 years).
  - A cholestatic presentation (duration of infection >3 months), with prolonged jaundice, fatigue, and pruritus occurs more frequently in HEV infections compared to HAV, but infection eventually resolves completely. Acute liver failure may occur in 1–2% of patients overall, but in 10–20% of pregnant women with HEV infection.
- **HEV diagnosis**
  - Anti-HEV-IgM positive: Acute infection
  - Anti-HEV-IgG positive: Remote infection
  - Recent travel to endemic areas should be documented (e.g., Mexico, India, Africa, or Russia)
- Hepatitis Viruses Transmitted by Blood-borne Routes. HBV, HCV, and HDV are all transmitted almost exclusively by blood-borne routes, commonly by percutaneous exposure for all of these viruses. Infection may also be transmitted by perinatal/vertical (especially in HBV in areas with high endemic rate) and sexual routes (now the most common exposure for HBV infection). Transmission by transfusion or transplantation has fallen as a result of screening.
  - **HBV** (see Figures 6-7 and 6-9)

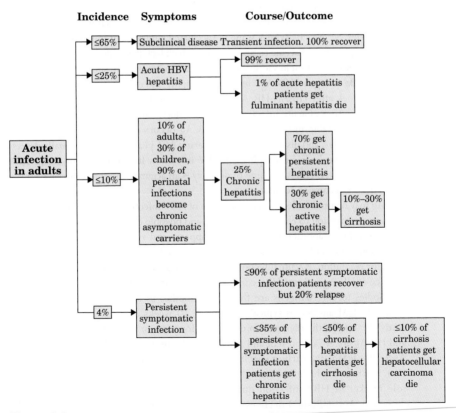

Figure 6-9. Course/outcomes of acute hepatitis B virus infection in adults.

- HBV is a double-stranded DNA hepadnavirus virus and usually infects children and young adults. The disease may have an acute or subclinical onset. HBV infection is associated with acute infection and several types of chronic infections.
- A number of laboratory tests are used to different stages of HBV infection:
  - Hepatitis B surface antigen (HBsAg) is the earliest indicator of active HBV infection. HBsAg is usually detectable within 27–41 days (as early as 14 days) of the onset of infection. HBsAg appears 7–26 days before transaminase abnormalities and peaks as ALT rises. HBsAg detection persists during the acute illness. HBsAg usually disappears 12–20 weeks after onset of symptoms in uncomplicated HBV infection. Detection of HBsAg for >6 months defines chronic infection or a chronic carrier state. Hepatitis B vaccination does not cause a positive HBsAg. Titers are not of clinical value. HBsAg is never detected in some patients; diagnosis of HBV infection is based on presence of HBc-IgM.
  - Antibody to HBsAg (Anti-HBs), without detectable HBsAg, indicates recovery from HBV infection, absence of infectivity, and immunity from future HBV infection. Anti-HBs may be seen after transfusion due to passive transfer. Anti-HBs is found in 80% of patients after clinical cure. The appearance may take several weeks or months after HBsAg has disappeared and ALT has returned to normal, causing a 2–6 week "window" during which sequential or special testing may be needed to identify infectious status. Anti-HBs is the only antibody produced in response to vaccine. Its presence indicates immunity. Antibody develops in ~95% of healthy adults after a three-dose deltoid muscle immunization series. Seroreactivity may wane in vaccinated patients, but immunity to infection is typically preserved. Vaccine escape mutants, which lack the "a" determinant of the vaccine, may cause infection in vaccinated patients who demonstrate anti-HBs.
  - Hepatitis Be Antigen (HBeAg) indicates a highly infectious state. HBeAg appears within 1 week after HBsAg. HBeAg disappears prior to the disappearance of HBsAg during resolution of acute infection. HBeAg is detected only when HBsAg and HBV DNA are detectable in the circulation. HBeAg occurs early in disease, before biochemical changes, and disappears after the serum ALT peaks. Levels are usually detectable for 3–6 weeks in uncomplicated HBV infection. It is a marker of active HBV replication in liver. HBeAg at time of delivery is an accurate predictor of risk (~90%) of vertical transmission to neonates.
  - HBeAg may be used to determine resolution of HBV infection. Persistence >20 weeks suggests progression to chronic carrier state and possible chronic hepatitis. Antibody to HBe (Anti-HBe) appears after HBeAg disappears and remains detectable for years. Detection of anti-HBe is associated with decreasing infectivity and suggests a good prognosis for resolution of acute infection. A positive reaction for anti-HBe and anti-HBc, in absence of HBsAg and anti-HBs, confirms recent acute infection (2–16 weeks).
  - Antibodies to core antigens are the first antibodies to appear after HBV infection. Total and IgM antibodies typically appear 4–10 weeks after appearance of HBsAg. Anti-HBc-total antibodies remain detectable for years or for lifetime. Anti-HBc-total and HBsAg are always present and anti-HBs is absent in chronic HBV infection.
  - Anti-HBc-IgM is the earliest specific antibody to develop in response to HBV infection. It is found in high titer for a short time during the acute disease stage, and is the sole marker of HBV infection during the window between HBsAg and anti-HBs detection. Anti-HBc-IgM declines to low levels during recovery. Because this is the only test unique to recent infection, it may be used to differentiate acute from

chronic HBV. However, because some patients with chronic HB infection become positive for anti-HBc-IgM during flares, it is not an absolutely reliable marker of acute illness. Before anti-HBc-IgM disappears, anti-HBc-IgG appears and lasts indefinitely.

- Detection of HBV DNA by PCR indicates active infection. It is the most sensitive and specific assay for early diagnosis of HBV infection and may be detected when all other markers are negative (e.g., in immunocompromised patients). Detection of HBV DNA indicates active viral replication, even if HBeAg is not detectable. HBV DNA viral load may be used to assess disease status and prognosis, or to monitor the response to therapy. A level of 100,000 copies per milliliter has been proposed for initiation of therapy in HBeAg positive patients. DNA levels decrease in patients who respond to therapy. An increased risk for development of HCC and cirrhosis is seen in chronically infected patients with persistently elevated HBV DNA levels ($>10^5$ copies per milliliter).

- Acute HBV infection usually lasts for 1–6 months with mild or no symptoms. Aminotransferases are increased $>$10-fold. HBsAg gradually arises to high titers and persists; HBeAg also appears. Serum bilirubin is usually normal or only slightly increased in acute disease. Immune complex–mediated diseases may be seen in 10–20% of patients, manifested by serum sickness, arthritis, dermatitis, glomerulonephritis, vasculitis, and so on. Glomerulonephritis or nephrotic syndrome, due to immune complex deposition, may progress to chronic renal failure. Acute HBV usually resolves in 3–6 months in uncomplicated infection. Full recovery is more common after clinically apparent acute HBV infection. Acute liver failure is uncommon, occurring in 0.1 to 1% of patients.

- Continued transaminase elevation for $>$6 months is seen in chronic hepatitis. Chronic HBV infection may last only 1 year or for several decades with mild or severe symptoms. Most cases resolve spontaneously, but some develop progressive liver failure and cirrhosis. AST and ALT fall to 2–10 times normal range. HBsAg usually remains high, and HBeAg remains present. Chronic infection is uncommon, occurring in 1–10% of patients overall, but ~90% perinatal infections.

- A chronic carrier state may develop. Patients are usually, but not always, asymptomatic. AST and ALT fall to normal or $<$2 times normal levels. Anti-HBe is detectable. HBsAg titers fall, although it may still be detectable. The development of anti-HBs marks the end of the carrier stage. Anti-HBc is usually present in high titer ($>$1:512).

- **HBV diagnosis**
  - HBsAg positive, HBeAg, anti-HBc IgM positive: Acute infection. HBV DNA viral load should be elevated.
  - Anti-HBc-IgM positive: Window. Confirm with positive HBV viral load.
  - HBsAg negative, anti-HBs positive, HBeAg negative, anti-HBe positive, anti-HBc IgG positive: Resolving infection. HBV viral load should be negative or rapidly falling.
  - HBsAg positive, anti-HBc-IgG positive, HBeAg positive: Chronic replicative infection. Confirm HBV viral load positive.
  - HBsAg positive, anti-HBs negative, HBeAg negative, anti-HBc-IgG positive, anti-HBc-IgM negative, anti-HBe positive: Non- or minimally replicative phase. HBV viral load may be negative or low-positive.

- Hbsag positive, anti-HBs negative, anti-HBc-IgG positive, anti-HBc-IgM negative, HBeAg negative, anti-HBe positive: Chronic replicative infection with a core or precore HBV mutant. Moderate elevated HBV viral load.
- HBsAg positive, anti-HBc-IgM, anti-HBs negative, anti-HBe negative: Flare of chronic HBV infection. HBV viral load low positive.
- HBsAg negative, anti-HBs positive, anti-HBc IgG negative: Vaccine response pattern.
- Single positive test for HBV infection, like isolated anti-HBc, must be interpreted with caution. Such reactions may represent false positives for the analyte, or false-negative reactions (or levels below the assay detection limit) for other HBV analytes. Repeat testing should be considered.
- Very high serum ALT and bilirubin are not reliable indicators of patient's clinical course.
- Acute fulminant hepatitis may be indicated by triad of prolonged PT, increased PMNs, and nonpalpable liver. A prolonged PT, especially >20 seconds, indicates the likely development of acute hepatic insufficiency; therefore, the PT should be performed with the initial patient evaluation.
- Effective treatment of chronic HBV hepatitis causes ALT, HBeAg, and HBV DNA to become normal.
- **HCV** (see Table 6-11)
- HCV is an enveloped, single-stranded, RNA flavivirus. HCV infections occur worldwide, but with geographic variation in prevalence of infection. In the United States, prevalence rates of 0.5 to 1.8% have been reported. Transmission is almost exclusively by percutaneous exposure. Transmission by sexual and perinatal exposure is rare.
- Major risk factors for HCV infection include:
  - HIV infection
  - History of IV drug abuse, tattoos, body piercing, multiple sexual partners.
  - History of blood product transfusions before 1990.
  - History of long-term hemodialysis.
  - Persistently elevated serum ALT.
- Nonspecific symptoms may follow acute infection as described previously. The acute hepatitis phase is typically mild; >75% of patients remain anicteric. ALF is very rarely seen as a complication of acute HCV infection. Infection persists in 70–85% of patients, with increasing risk for liver disease. Chronic HCV infection, in most patients, is associated with relatively mild clinical disease, but progressive hepatic damage. Risk factors for more severe disease and rapid progression include alcohol (or other hepatotoxins) abuse, coexisting liver disease, immunocompromised status, especially HIV infection, and genetic and other factors. The risk of progression to cirrhosis is markedly increased in patients with hypogammaglobulinemia. Transaminase elevations are typically lower than in HBV infection; episodic fluctuations are common. See Figure 6-10. Occult HBV infection is present in about one third of patients with chronic HCV liver disease.
- Serology: Current EIA assays for HCV antibody are very sensitive; tests are positive at presentation in half of patients and within one month of presentation in ~95% of patients. The specificity is also very high (>99%), but false-positive reactions must be ruled out in asymptomatic patients with a low prior probability of infection, as in blood donor screening. The recombinant immunoblot assay (RIBA) has been used to confirm

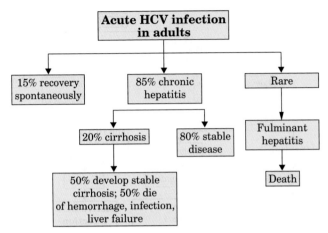

Figure 6-10. Course outcomes of acute hepatitis C virus infection in adults with or without abnormal alanine aminotransferase values. Source: Gupta S, Bent S, Kohlwes J. *Ann Intern Med*. 2003;139:46.

positive EIA tests, but this testing has been largely replaced by qualitative or quantitative testing for HCV RNA or the EIA "cut-off" method. The cut-off method is assay specific. The cut-off point is assigned as the point above which >95% of positive results are true positive results.

- Molecular Diagnostic Testing: HCV RNA detection tests may be qualitative or quantitative. The most sensitive method available should be used to rule out infection in suspect patients. In the past, qualitative HCV RNA assays provided the lowest detectable level of RNA, but real-time (RT)-PCR and other quantitative assays may now able to provide reliable quantification to levels as low as those provided by qualitative assays. An advantage of the use of HCV viral load assays to confirm HCV infection is that they can provide a baseline to predict likely response to antiviral therapy, for determining early virologic response to antiviral therapy and to document sustained viral response after treatment. Patients who do not show a >2 log 10 reduction in HCV viral load after 12 weeks of antiviral therapy are not responsive to therapy.

- There are six different HCV genotypes and many subtypes. The prevalence of different genotypes shows geographic variability. There are genotype-specific differences in response to therapy that are used to determine the duration of antiviral treatment for chronic HCV infection.

- Biochemical Testing: Transaminase levels typically increase within 2–8 weeks after infection. Transaminase levels may show significant variability, and may return to almost-normal levels (formerly called *acute "relapsing" hepatitis*); this pattern is highly suggestive but occurs only in 25% of cases. The degree of ALT elevation is an unreliable predictor of histology in HCV infection; biopsy is needed to define severity.

- HCV infection may be associated with mixed cryoglobulinemia with vasculitis, thyroiditis, Sjögren syndrome, membranoproliferative Glomerular Nephritis (GN), and porphyria cutanea tarda and so on. HCV infection should be ruled out in patients who present with those disorders.

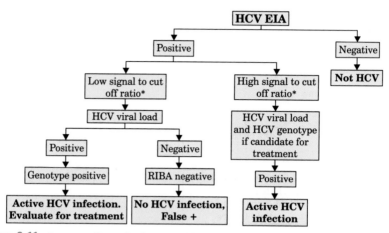

Figure 6-11. Sequence of tests for diagnosis of hepatitis C virus. *The cutoff is a test-specific level above which >95% of results are true positive results.

- **HCV diagnosis** (Figure 6-11)
  - Anti-HCV negative: HCV infection excluded.
  - Positive Anti-HCV EIA results may be confirmed by the "cut-off" method, HCV RNA detection, or RIBA, depending on patient risk factors.
  - Anti-HCV positive (confirmed), HCV RNA positive: Active HCV infection.
  - HCV genotype should be determined for patients with acute or chronic HCV infection.
  - Anti-HCV positive (confirmed), HCV RNA negative: Resolved HCV infection.
  - Anti-HCV positive (not confirmed), HCV RNA negative: May be false-positive EIA or resolved HCV infection. RIBA testing would be positive if resolved infection, but negative if EIA is a false-positive result.
  - An HCV genotype assay should be performed to determine the duration of treatment.
  - Initial HCV viral load concentrations $>10^6$ copies per milliliter and HCV genotype 1 are associated with poor responses to antiviral treatment.
  - HCV viral load should be determined at baseline, at 12 weeks after initiation of antiviral therapy to determine early virologic response, and periodically after completion to document sustained viral response. Viral load assays may provide slightly different quantification results, so serial testing should be performed with a single type of assay.
  - Autoantibodies are frequently seen in chronic HCV infections, including nuclear antibodies, rheumatoid antibodies, and smooth muscle antibodies.
  - Superinfection of HBV with HDV is usually associated with clinical deterioration
- **HDV**
  - HDV, initially called delta antigen when identified in patients with chronic HBV infection, is a small defective single-stranded RNA virus enveloped by hepatitis B surface antigens. HDV requires simultaneous HBV infection but relies on HBV only for envelope proteins, which the HDV particles assemble and release from infected hepatocytes to infect other susceptible cells. The epidemiology of HDV infection is similar to HBV except that sexual and perinatal infection is less efficient. HDV is distributed worldwide, with perhaps 5% of HBV-infected patients coinfected with HDV.

- HDV infection may occur simultaneously with HBV infection. In these patients, clinical manifestations may be similar to patients with HBV infection alone, but coinfection is often more severe in terms of clinical signs and symptoms. In HBV/HDV coinfection, the risk for progression to chronic hepatitis is no greater than is seen in HBV infection alone. In HDV, superinfection of chronic HBV infection, however, usually leads to clinical deterioration, increased chronicity, and may lead to ALF. HDV can also cause superinfection of patients with preexisting chronic HBV infection. These superinfections are usually associated with clinical deterioration.
- HDV infection may be suspected on the basis of exposure in regions of high endemicity, severe HBV disease, or deterioration in chronic HBV infections. Antigen detection is the most reliable laboratory test for diagnosis, but levels may be variable. Serum HDVAg and HDV-RNA appear during the incubation period after the appearance of HBsAg and before a rise in ALT, which often shows a biphasic elevation. HBsAg and HDVAg are transient; HDVAg resolves with clearance of HBsAg. Total anti-HDV supports a diagnosis; anti-HDV-IgM is not reliable for distinguishing between acute and chronic infection but is detectable more often than anti-HDV-IgG. In HBV/HDV coinfections, detectable anti-HDV elevations are not clearly predictable, may be of low titer, and often disappear with resolution of acute infection. In superinfection, however, high anti-HDV levels are seen and these last indefinitely. Determination of the class of anti-HBc, IgG versus IgM, can help distinguish between HDV coinfection and superinfection. Chronic HDV infection is more severe and has higher mortality than other types of viral hepatitis. The risk of HCC is three-fold greater in patients with chronic HBV infection in whom anti-HDV is detected compared to patients who are negative.
- **HDV diagnosis** (see Tables 6-11, 6-12, and 6-13)
  - Anti-HDV positive: HDV infection
    - Anti-HDV positive, HBsAg positive, anti-HBc IgM positive: HBV/HDV coinfection
    - Anti-HDV positive, HBsAg positive, anti-HBc IgG positive: HDV superinfection.

TABLE 6-12. Comparison of Types of Hepatitis D Virus (HDV) Infections			
	Coinfection	Superinfection	Chronic HDV
HBV infection	Acute	Chronic	Chronic
HDV infection	Acute	Acute to chronic	Chronic
Chronicity rate	<5%	>75%	Cirrhosis in >70%
Serology			
HBsAg	+	Usually persistent	Persistent
HBcAb-IgM	+	Negative	Negative
Anti-HDV-total	Negative or low titer	+	+
Anti-HDV-IgM*	Transient +	Transient	High titer
HDV-RNA (HDAg)	Transient +	Usually persistent	Persistent
Liver HDAg	Transient +	Usually persistent	Persistent

+, positive.
*Decrease in anti-HDV-IgM usually predicts resolution of acute HDV. Persistent anti-HDV-IgM typically predicts progression to chronic HDV infection. High titer correlates with active liver inflammation.

TABLE 6-13. Serologic Diagnosis of Hepatitis B Virus (HBV) and Hepatitis D Virus (HDV)

	Test			
HBsAg	**HBcAb-IgM**	**Anti-HDV-IgM**	**Anti-HDV-IgG**	**Interpretation**
Transient+	+High titer	Transient +	Transient low titer	Acute HBV and acute HDV[a]
Transient decrease due to inhibitory effect of HDV on HBV synthesis	Negative or low titers	High titer first, low titer later	Increasing titers	Acute HDV and chronic HBV[b]
May remain + in chronic HBV	Replaced by anti-HBc- IgG in chronic HBV	+correlates with HDAg in hepatocytes	High titers correlate with active infection; may remain+ for years after infection resolves	Chronic HDV and chronic HBV[c]

+, positive.

[a]Clinically resembles acute viral hepatitis; fulminant hepatitis is rare, and progression to chronic hepatitis is unlikely. If HBV does not resolve, HDV can continue to replicate indefinitely.

[b]Clinically resembles exacerbation of chronic liver disease or of fulminant hepatitis with liver failure.

[c]Clinically resembles chronic liver disease progressing to cirrhosis.

• HDV RNA detection is sensitive and specific, but it is not commercially available in the United States.

➤ Suggested Readings

Centers for Disease Control and Prevention. Hepatitis C Information for Health Professionals. Available at http://www.cdc.gov/hepatitis/HCV/Management.htm. Accessed January 31, 2011

Lemon SM, Walker C, Alter MU, Yi MK. Hepatitis C Virus, in Knipe, Dm, PM Howley, DE Griffin, et al. (eds). *Fields Virology*, 5th ed. Philadelphia: Lippincott, Williams & Wilkins; 2007.

Lemon SM. Type A viral hepatitis: epidemiology, diagnosis, and prevention. *Clin Chem.* 1997;43:1494.

Rotman Y, Liang TJ. Hepatitis C Virus, in Richman DD, Whitley RJ, Hayden FG. *Clinical Virology*, 3rd ed. Washington, DC: ASM Press; 2009.

Strader DB, Wright T, Thomas DL, Seeff LB. Diagnosis, management, and treatment of hepatitis C. *Hepatology.* 2004;39:1147–1171.

VASCULAR AND ISCHEMIC DISORDERS OF LIVER

Budd-Chiari Syndrome

➤ Definition

Heterogeneous group of disorders due to obstruction of hepatic venous outflow

➤ Causes

• Thrombosis due to hypercoagulable states (e.g., polycythemia vera [10–40% of cases], essential thrombocythemia, myelofibrosis; antiphospholipid syndrome; and deficiencies of protein C, protein S, and antithrombin III) (See Chapter 10, Hematologic Disorders, Paroxysmal Nocturnal Hemoglobinuria).
• Membranes and webs
• Others (e.g., neoplasms, collagen vascular diseases, cirrhosis, and polycystic liver disease)

➤ Laboratory Findings

• **Core Laboratory:** Due to parenchymal cell necrosis and malfunction (e.g., increased serum AST), ALT may be increased >5 times in acute and fulminant forms. ALP and bilirubin may be increased and serum albumin decreased. Ascitic fluid total protein is usually >2.5 g/dL.
• Radiologic visualization (e.g., ultrasound, CT scan, MRI, hepatic angiography)
• Liver biopsy

➤ Suggested Reading

Menon KVN, Shah N, Kamath PS, et al. The Budd-Chiari syndrome. *N Engl J Med.* 2004;350:578.

Congestive Heart Failure

➤ Laboratory Findings Related to Altered Liver Function

• **Core Laboratory:** Pattern of abnormal liver function tests is variable depending on severity of heart failure; the mildest show only slightly increased ALP and slightly decreased serum albumin; moderately severe also show slightly increased serum bilirubin and GGT; one fourth to three fourths of the most severe will also show increased AST

and ALT ($\leq$200 U/L) and LD ($\leq$400 U/L). All return to normal when heart failure responds to treatment. Serum ALP is usually the last to become normal, and this may be weeks to months later. AST and ALT may be increased 2–3$\times$ normal in less than one third of cases but much higher in severe acute heart failure. Serum albumin is slightly decreased in <50% of patients but is rarely. Serum bilirubin is increased in $\leq$70% of cases (unconjugated more than conjugated); usually <3 mg/dL but may be >20 mg/dL. It usually represents combined right- and left-sided failure with hepatic engorgement and pulmonary infarcts. Serum bilirubin may suddenly rise rapidly if superimposed myocardial infarction occurs. Serum cholesterol and esters may be decreased. Serum ammonia may be increased. Urine urobilinogen is increased. Urine bilirubin is increased in the presence of jaundice.
* **Hematology**: PT may be slightly increased in 80% of cases, with increased sensitivity to anticoagulant drugs. Fails to correct with vitamin K

Portal Hypertension

* This condition may be:
  * Prehepatic (e.g., portal vein thrombosis, splenic arteriovenous fistula)
  * Intrahepatic
    * Presinusoidal (e.g., metastatic tumor, granulomas such as sarcoid, schistosomiasis)
    * Sinusoidal (e.g., cirrhosis)
    * Postsinusoidal (e.g., hepatic vein thrombosis, alcoholic hepatitis)
  * Posthepatic (e.g., pericarditis, tricuspid insufficiency, inferior vena cava web)

BILIARY EXTRAHEPATIC OBSTRUCTION, COMPLETE

DISEASES OF THE GALLBLADDER AND BILIARY TREE (INTRAHEPATIC OR EXTRAHEPATIC) (SEE ABDOMINAL PAIN)

➤ Laboratory Findings

* **Liver Enzymes:** AST is increased ($\leq$300 U), and ALT is increased ($\leq$200 U); they usually return to normal within 1 week after relief of obstruction. In *acute* biliary duct obstruction (e.g., due to common bile duct stones or acute pancreatitis), AST and ALT are increased >300 U (and often >2,000 U) and decline 58–76% in 72 hours without treatment; simultaneous serum total bilirubin shows less marked elevation and decline and ALP changes are inconsistent and unpredictable. Typical pattern of extrahepatic obstruction includes increased serum ALP (>2–3$\times$ normal), AST <300 U/L, conjugated serum bilirubin. In extrahepatic type, the increased ALP is related to the completeness of obstruction. Normal ALP is extremely rare in extrahepatic obstruction. Very high levels may also occur in cases of intrahepatic cholestasis. Serum LAP parallels ALP.
* Conjugated serum bilirubin is increased; unconjugated serum bilirubin is normal or slightly increased. Urine bilirubin is increased; urine urobilinogen decreased. There is decreased stool bilirubin and urobilinogen (clay-colored stools).

* Lipids: Serum phospholipids are increased. Serum cholesterol is increased (acute, 300–400 mg/dL; chronic, $\leq$1,000 mg/dL).
* Hematology: PT is prolonged, with response to parenteral vitamin K more frequent than in hepatic parenchymal cell disease.

Considerations

* Laboratory findings due to underlying causative disease are noted (e.g., stone, carcinoma of duct, metastatic carcinoma to periductal lymph nodes).
* Bile duct obstruction (one): characteristic pattern is serum bilirubin that remains normal in the presence of markedly increased serum ALP.

CANCER OF GALLBLADDER AND BILE DUCTS

➤ Laboratory Findings

* Laboratory findings of duct obstruction are of progressively increasing severity in contrast to the intermittent or fluctuating changes due to duct obstruction caused by stones. A papillary intraluminal duct carcinoma may undergo periods of sloughing, producing the findings of intermittent duct obstruction. These reflect varying location and extent of tumor infiltration that may cause partial intrahepatic duct obstruction or obstruction of hepatic or common bile duct, metastases in liver, or associated cholangitis; 50% of patients have jaundice at the time of hospitalization.
* **Hematology:** Anemia is present.
* **Cytology:** Examination of aspirated duodenal fluid may demonstrate malignant cells.
* **Stool Findings:** Silver-colored stool due to jaundice combined with GI bleeding may be seen in carcinoma of duct or ampulla of Vater.

CHOLANGITIS, ACUTE

➤ Laboratory Findings

* **Culture:** Blood culture positive in ~30% of cases; 25% of these are polymicrobial. Infection of bile ducts usually due to gram-negative (e.g., *E. coli, Klebsiella* sp., gram-positive, and anaerobic [*Streptococcus faecalis*, enterococcus, *Bacteroides fragilis*] organisms usually associated with obstruction
* **Hematology:** Marked increase in WBC ($\leq$30,000/μL) with increase in granulocytes
* **Core Laboroatory:** Increased serum AST and ALT. Increased urine urobilinogen.

Considerations

* Laboratory findings of incomplete duct obstruction due to inflammation or of preceding complete duct obstruction (e.g., stone, tumor, scar). See Choledocholithiasis.
* Laboratory findings of parenchymal cell necrosis and malfunction

CHOLANGITIS, PRIMARY SCLEROSING

* Chronic fibrosing cholestatic inflammation of intra- and extrahepatic bile ducts predominantly in men younger than age 45, rare in pediatric patients; $\leq$75% are associated with IBD, especially UC. Slow, relentless, progressive course of chronic cholestasis to death (usually from liver failure). Twenty-five percent of patients are asymptomatic at time of diagnosis.

➤ Diagnostic Criteria

1. Cholestatic biochemical profile for >6 months
   * Serum ALP may fluctuate but is always increased (usually ≥3 times upper limit of normal).
   * Serum GGT is increased.
   * Serum AST is mildly increased in >90%. ALT > AST in three fourths of cases.
   * Serum bilirubin is increased in 50% of patients; occasionally is very high; may fluctuate markedly; gradually increases as disease progresses. Persistent value >1.5 mg/dL is poor prognostic sign that may indicate irreversible medically untreatable disease.
2. Compatible clinical history (e.g., IBD) and exclusion of other causes of sclerosing cholangitis (e.g., previous bile duct surgery, gallstones, suppurative cholangitis, bile duct tumor or damage due to floxuridine, AIDS, congenital duct anomalies).
3. Characteristic cholangiogram to distinguish from primary biliary cirrhosis.
   * Increased γ-globulin in 30% and increased IgM in 40–50% of cases
     * Anti-neutrophil cytoplasmic (ANCA) is present in ~65% and antinuclear antibodies are noted <35% of cases are present at higher levels than in other liver diseases but diagnostic significance is not yet known.
   * In contrast to primary biliary cirrhosis, antimitochondrial antibody, smooth-muscle antibody, rheumatoid factor, and ANA are negative in >90% of patients.
   * HBsAg is negative.
   * Liver biopsy provides only confirmatory evidence in patients with compatible history, laboratory, and x-ray findings. Liver copper is usually increased but serum ceruloplasmin is also increased.

➤ Other Considerations

* Laboratory findings due to sequelae
* Cholangiocarcinoma in 10–15% of patients may cause increased serum CA 19-9
* Portal hypertension, biliary cirrhosis, secondary bacterial cholangitis, steatorrhea and malabsorption, cholelithiasis, liver failure
* Laboratory findings due to underlying disease (e.g., ≤7.5% of UC patients have this disease; much less often with Crohn disease). Associated with syndrome of retroperitoneal and mediastinal fibrosis

CHOLECYSTITIS, ACUTE

➤ Laboratory Findings

* **Hematology:** Increased ESR, WBC (average 12,000/μL; if >15,000, suspect empyema or perforation), and other evidence of acute inflammatory process.
* **Core Laboratory:** Serum AST is increased in 75% of patients. Increased serum bilirubin in 20% of patients (usually >4 mg/dL; if higher, suspect associated choledocholithiasis). Increased serum ALP (some patients) even if serum bilirubin is normal. Increased serum amylase and lipase in some patients

Considerations
* Laboratory findings of associated biliary obstruction if such obstruction is present
* Laboratory findings of preexisting cholelithiasis (some patients)

* Laboratory findings of complications (e.g., empyema of gallbladder, perforation, cholangitis, liver abscess, pyelophlebitis, pancreatitis, gallstone ileus)

CHOLECYSTITIS, CHRONIC

* May be mild laboratory findings of acute cholecystitis or no abnormal laboratory findings
* May be laboratory findings of associated cholelithiasis
* Laboratory findings of sequelae (e.g., carcinoma of gall bladder)

CHOLEDOCHOLITHIASIS

* Gallstones in bile ducts due to passage from gallbladder or anatomic defects (e.g., cysts, strictures)

➤ Laboratory Findings

* **Core Laboratory:** Increased serum and urine amylase. Increased serum bilirubin in about one third of patients. Increased urine bilirubin in about one third of patients. Increased serum ALP
* **Hematology:** Increased WBC
* **Considerations**
  * Laboratory evidence of fluctuating or transient cholestasis. Persistent increase of WBC, AST, ALT suggests cholangitis.
  * Laboratory findings due to secondary cholangitis, acute pancreatitis, obstructive jaundice, stricture formation, and so on.
  * In duodenal drainage, crystals of both calcium bilirubinate and cholesterol (some patients); 50% accurate (only useful in nonicteric patients)

CHOLELITHIASIS

* Laboratory findings of underlying conditions causing:
  * Hypercholesterolemia (e.g., DM, malabsorption)
  * Chronic hemolytic disease (e.g., hereditary spherocytosis)
* Laboratory findings due to complications (e.g., cholecystitis, choledocholithiasis, gall stone ileus)

ATRESIA, EXTRAHEPATIC BILIARY, CONGENITAL

* Conjugated serum bilirubin increased in early days of life in some infants but not until second week in others. Level is often <12 mg/dL during first months, with subsequent rise later in life.
* Laboratory findings as in complete biliary obstruction
* Liver biopsy to differentiate from neonatal hepatitis
* Laboratory findings due to sequelae (e.g., biliary cirrhosis, portal hypertension, frequent infections, rickets, hepatic failure)
* ^{131}I-Rose bengal excretion test

OTHER CONSIDERATIONS

* Most important to differentiate this condition from neonatal hepatitis, for which surgery may be harmful.
* More than 90% of cases of extrahepatic biliary obstruction in newborns are due to biliary atresia; occasional cases may be due to choledochal cyst (causes intermittent jaundice in infancy), bile plug syndrome, or bile ascites (associated with spontaneous perforation of the common bile duct).

INTRAHEPATIC OBSTRUCTION CHOLESTASIS

* Causes of intrahepatic cholestasis:
  * Intrahepatic obstruction
    * Space-occupying lesions (e.g., amyloidosis, sarcoidosis, metastases; non-Hodgkin lymphoma more often than Hodgkin disease)
    * Drugs (e.g., estrogens, anabolic steroids)—most common cause (Table 6-14)
    * Normal pregnancy
    * Alcoholic hepatitis
    * Infections (e.g. acute viral hepatitis, gram-negative sepsis, toxic shock syndrome, AIDS, parasitic, fungal)
    * Sickle cell crisis
    * Postoperative state following long procedure and multiple transfusions
    * Benign recurrent familial intrahepatic cholestasis—rare condition

INTRAHEPATIC OBSTRUCTIVE (CHOLESTASIS)

* Autosomal recessive condition; attacks begin after age 8, last weeks to months, complete resolution between episodes, may recur after months or years; exacerbated by estrogens

TABLE 6-14. Comparison of Various Types of Cholestatic Disease

Disorder	Bilirubin (mg/dL)	ALP	AST	ALT	Albumin
			Serum Values*		
CBD obstruction					N
Stone	0–10	N–10	N–10	N–10	N
Cancer	5–20	2–10	N	N	N
Intrahepatic					
Drug-induced	5–10	2–10	N–5	10–50	
Acute viral hepatitis	0–20	N–3	10–50	10–50	N
Alcoholic liver disease	0–20	5	<10	<50% of AST	N/sl D

CBD, common bile duct; N, normal; sl D, slightly decreased.
*Serum value, times normal.

➤ Laboratory Findings
- **Core Laboratory:** Increased serum ALP but GGT is usually normal. Serum direct bilirubin may be normal or $\leq$10 mg/dL. Transaminase usually <100 U.
- **Histolohy:** Liver biopsy shows centrolobular cholestasis without inflammation, bile pigment in hepatocytes and canaliculi; little or no fibrosis

CIRRHOSIS, PRIMARY BILIARY (CHOLANGIOLITIC CIRRHOSIS, HANOT HYPERTROPHIC CIRRHOSIS, CHRONIC NONSUPPURATIVE DESTRUCTIVE CHOLANGITIS, ETC.)*

- Slow progressive multisystem autoimmune disease; chronic nonsuppurative inflammation and asymmetric destruction of small intrahepatic bile ducts producing chronic cholestasis, cirrhosis, and ultimately liver failure

➤ Diagnostic Criteria
- Definitive diagnosis requires all three criteria; probable diagnosis requires two criteria
  - Antimitochondrial autoantibodies present
  - Cholestatic pattern (increased ALP) of long duration (>6 months) not due to known cause (e.g., drugs)
  - Compatible histologic findings on liver biopsy
- Serum ALP is markedly increased; is of liver origin. Reaches a plateau early in the course and then fluctuates within 20% thereafter; changes in serum level have no prognostic value. 5'-N and GGT parallel the ALP. *This is one of the few conditions that will elevate both serum ALP and GGT to striking levels.*
- Serum mitochondrial antibody titer is strongly positive in ~95% of patients (1:40 to 1:80) and is hallmark of disease (98% specificity); titer >1:160 is highly predictive of Primary Biliary Cirrhosis (PBC), even in absence of other findings. Does not correlate with severity or rate of progression. Titers differ greatly in patients. Similar titers occur in 5% of patients with chronic hepatitis; low titers occur in 10% of patients with other liver disease; rarely found in normal persons. Titer may decrease after liver transplantation but usually remains detectable.
- Serum bilirubin is normal in early phase but increases in 60% of patients with progression of disease and is a reliable prognostic indicator; an elevated level is a poor prognostic sign. Conjugated serum bilirubin is increased in 80% of patients; levels >5 mg/dL in only 20% of patients; levels >10 mg/dL in only 6% of patients. Unconjugated bilirubin is normal or slightly increased.
- Laboratory findings show relatively little evidence of parenchymal damage.
  - AST and ALT may be normal or slightly increased ($\leq$1–5 times normal), fluctuate within a narrow range, and have no prognostic significance.
  - Serum albumin, globulin, and PT normal early; abnormal values indicate advanced disease and poor prognosis; not corrected by therapy.

---

*Data from: Angulo P. Nonalcoholic fatty liver disease. *N Engl J Med.* 2002;346:1221.

- Marked increase in total cholesterol and phospholipids with normal triglycerides; serum is not lipemic; serum triglycerides become elevated in late stages. Associated with xanthomas and xanthelasmas. In early stages, LDL and VLDL are mildly elevated and HDL is markedly elevated (thus atherosclerosis is rare). In advanced stage, LDL is markedly elevated with decreased HDL and presence of lipoprotein-X (nonspecific abnormal lipoprotein seen in other cholestatic liver disease).
- Serum IgM is increased in ~75% of patients; levels may be very high (4–5 times normal). Other serum immunoglobulins are also increased.
- Hypocomplementemia
- Polyclonal hypergammaglobulinemia. Serum IgM is increased in ~75% of patients with failure to convert to IgG antibodies; levels may be very high (4–5 times normal). Other serum immunoglobulins are also increased.
- Biopsy of liver categorizes the four stages and helps assess prognosis, but needle biopsy is subject to sampling error because the lesions may be spotty; findings consistent with all four stages may be found in one specimen.
- Serum ceruloplasmin is characteristically elevated (in contrast to Wilson disease).
- Liver copper may be increased 10–100 times normal; correlates with serum bilirubin and advancing stages of disease.
- ESR is increased 1–5 times normal in 80% of patients.
- Urine contains urobilinogen and bilirubin.
- Laboratory findings of steatorrhea
  - Serum 25-hydroxyvitamin D and vitamin A are usually low.
  - PT is normal or restored to normal by parenteral vitamin K.
- Laboratory findings due to associated diseases
  - >80% have one, and >40% have at least two, other circulating antibodies to autoimmune disease (e.g., RA, autoimmune thyroiditis [hypothyroidism in 20% of patients], Sjögren syndrome, scleroderma) although not useful diagnostically.

CONGENITAL CONJUGATED HYPERBILIRUBINEMIA

Dubin-Johnson Syndrome (Sprinz-Nelson Disease)

- Autosomal recessive disease (gene located on chromosome 10q24) due to inability to transport bilirubin-glucuronide through hepatocytes into canaliculi but conjugation of bilirubin-glucuronide is normal. Characterized by mild chronic, recurrent jaundice. May have hepatomegaly and right upper quadrant abdominal pain. Usually is compensated except in periods of stress. Jaundice (innocuous and reversible) may be produced by estrogens, birth control pills, or last trimester of pregnancy. May resemble mild viral hepatitis.

➤ Laboratory Findings

- See Table 6-15.
- **Histology:** Liver biopsy shows large amounts of yellow-brown or slate-black pigment in centrolobular hepatic cells (lysosomes) and small amounts in Kupffer cells.
- **Core Laboratory:** Serum total bilirubin is increased (1.5–6.0 mg/dL); rarely ≤25 mg/dL during intercurrent illness; significant amount is conjugated. Normal in heterozygotes.

TABLE 6-15. Differential Diagnosis of Hereditary Jaundice with Normal Liver Chemistries and No Signs or Symptoms of Liver Disease

	Dubin-Johnson Syndrome	Rotor Syndrome	Unconjugated Hyperbilirubinemias			
					Crigler-Najjar Syndrome	
			Gilbert Disease	Type I	Type II	
Incidence	Uncommon	Rare	≤7% of population	Very rare	Uncommon	
Inheritance mode	AR	AR	AD	AR	AD	
Serum bilirubin usual total (mg/dL)	2–7; ≤25	2–7; ≤20	<3; ≤6	>20	<20	
	Direct ~60%	Direct ~60%	Mostly indirect; increases with fasting	All indirect	All indirect	
Defect in bilirubin metabolism	Impaired biliary excretion of conjugated organic anions and bilirubin		Hepatic UDP-glucuronyl transferase activity Decreased		Marked decrease	Marked decrease
Impaired excretion of dyes requiring conjugation (e.g., BSP)	Yes; initial rapid fall, then rise in 45–90 minutes	Yes; slow clearance; no later increase	May be slightly impaired in ≤40% of patients	Absent		
Effect of phenobarbital			Decrease to normal	None	Marked decrease	
Urine coproporphyrin Total	Normal	Increased				

(Continued)

TABLE 6-15. Differential Diagnosis of Hereditary Jaundice with Normal Liver Chemistries and No Signs or Symptoms of Liver Disease (*Continued*)

	Dubin-Johnson Syndrome	Rotor Syndrome	Unconjugated Hyperbilirubinemias			
				Crigler-Najjar Syndrome		
			Gilbert Disease	Type I	Type II	
I/III*	>80%	<80%				
Age at onset of jaundice	Childhood, adolescence	Adolescence, early adulthood	Adolescence	Infancy	Childhood, adolescence	
Usual clinical features	Asymptomatic jaundice in young adults	Asymptomatic jaundice	Appear in early adulthood; often first recognized with fasting; very mild hemolysis in ≤40% of patients	Jaundice, kernicterus in infants, young adults	Asymptomatic jaundice; kernicterus rare	
Oral cholecystogram	GB usually not visualized	Normal	Normal	Normal	Normal	
Liver biopsy	Characteristic pigment	No pigment	Normal	Liver transplant; no response to phenobarbital	Phenobarbital	
Treatment	Not needed	None	Not needed			
Animal model	Corriedale sheep			Gunn rat		

AD, autosomal dominant; AR, autosomal recessive; BSP, sulfobromsulfophthalein; GB, gallbladder; UDP-glucuronyl transferase, uridine-diphosphate glucuronosyl-transferase.
*Normally coproporphyrin III, 75% of total.

Other liver function tests are normal. No evidence of hemolysis. Urine contains bile and urobilinogen.

* **Other:** Urine total coproporphyrin is usually normal but ~80% is coproporphyrin I (normally 25% is coproporphyrin I and 75% is coproporphyrin III); diagnostic of Dubin-Johnson syndrome. Not useful to detect individual heterozygotes. Fecal coproporphyrins are normal. BSP excretion is impaired with late (normal at 45 minutes; increased at 90 and 120 minutes); virtually pathognomonic but is no longer performed.

ROTOR SYNDROME

* Autosomal recessive, familial, asymptomatic, benign defective uptake, and storage of conjugated bilirubin and possibly in transfer of bilirubin from liver to bile or in intrahepatic binding; usually detected in adolescents or adults. Jaundice may be produced or accentuated by pregnancy, birth control pills, alcohol, infection, or surgery.
* See Table 6-15.

CAUSES OF UNCONJUGATED HYPERBILIRUBINEMIA

UNCONJUGATED BILIRUBINEMIA

➤ Causes
* Increased destruction of RBCs
  * Isoimmunization (e.g., incompatibility of Rh, ABO, other blood groups)
  * Biochemical defects of RBCs (e.g., G6PD deficiency, pyruvate deficiency, hexokinase deficiency, congenital erythropoietic porphyria, α- and γ-thalassemias)
  * Structural defects of RBCs (e.g., hereditary spherocytosis, hereditary elliptocytosis, infantile pyknocytosis)
  * Physiologic hemolysis of the newborn
  * Infection

PHYSIOLOGIC JAUNDICE

➤ Definition
Transient unconjugated hyperbilirubinemia ("physiologic jaundice") that occurs in almost all newborns

➤ Laboratory Findings
* In normal full-term neonate, average maximum serum bilirubin is 6 mg/dL ($\leq$12 mg/dL is in physiologic range) that occurs during the second to fourth day and then rapidly falls to ~2.0 mg/dL by fifth day (phase I physiologic jaundice). Declines slowly to <1.0 mg/dL during fifth to tenth day, but may take one month to fall to <2 mg/dL (phase II

physiologic jaundice). Phase I due to deficiency of hepatic bilirubin-glucuronyl transferase activity and six-fold increase in bilirubin load presented to liver. In Asian and Native American newborns, the average maximum serum levels are approximately double (10–14 mg/dL) the levels in non-Asians, and kernicterus is more frequent. Serum bilirubin >5 mg/dL during first 24 hours of life is indication for further work-up because of risk of kernicterus.

* In older children (and adults) icterus is apparent clinically when serum bilirubin is >2 mg/dL, but in newborns clinical icterus is not apparent until serum bilirubin is >5–7 mg/dL; therefore, only half of the full-term newborns show clinical jaundice during first 3 days of life.
* In premature infants—average maximum serum bilirubin is 10–12 mg/dL and occurs during the fifth to seventh day. Serum bilirubin may not fall to normal until thirtieth day. Further work-up is indicated in all premature infants with clinical jaundice because of risk of kernicterus in some low-birth weight infants with serum levels of 10–12 mg/dL.
* In postmature infants and half of small-for-dates infants—serum bilirubin is <2.5 mg/dL and physiologic jaundice is not seen. When mothers have received phenobarbital or used heroin, physiologic jaundice is also less severe.
* When a pregnant woman has unconjugated hyperbilirubinemia, similar levels occur in cord blood but when the mother has conjugated hyperbilirubinemia (e.g., hepatitis), similar levels are *not* present in cord blood.

NONPHYSIOLOGIC JAUNDICE

Cause should be sought for underlying pathologic jaundice if:
* Total serum bilirubin >7 mg/dL during first 24 hours or increases >5 mg/dL/day or visible jaundice
* Peak total serum bilirubin >12.5 mg/dL in white or black full-term or >15 mg/dL in Hispanic or premature infants
* Conjugated serum bilirubin >1.5 mg/dL

HEREDITARY AND/OR CONGENITAL CAUSES OF UNCONJUGATED HYPERBILIRUBINEMIA

CRIGLER-NAJJAR SYNDROME (HEREDITARY GLUCURONYL-TRANSFERASE DEFICIENCY)

* Rare familial autosomal recessive disease due to marked congenital deficiency or absence of glucuronyl-transferase, which conjugates bilirubin to bilirubin glucuronide in hepatic cells (counterpart is the homozygous Gunn rat)

➤ Laboratory Findings
• See Table 6-15.

Type I
Histology: Liver biopsy is normal.
Core Laboratory: Unconjugated serum bilirubin is increased; it appears on first or second day of life, rises in 1 week to peak of 12–45 mg/dL, and persists for life. No conjugated bilirubin in serum or urine. Liver function tests are normal; BSP is normal. Fecal urobilinogen is very low.

➤ Other Considerations
• Untreated patients often die of kernicterus by age 18 months.
• Nonjaundiced parents have diminished capacity to form glucuronide conjugates with menthol, salicylates, and tetrahydrocortisone.
• Type I should always be ruled out when there is persistent unconjugated bilirubin levels of 20 mg/dL after 1 week of age without obvious hemolysis and especially after breast-milk jaundice has been ruled out.

GILBERT DISEASE

• Chronic, benign, intermittent, familial (autosomal dominant with incomplete penetrance), nonhemolytic unconjugated hyperbilirubinemia with evanescent increases of unconjugated serum bilirubin, which is usually discovered on routine laboratory examinations; due to defective transport and conjugation of unconjugated bilirubin.
• Jaundice is usually accentuated by pregnancy, fever, exercise, and various drugs, including alcohol and birth control pills.
• Rarely identified before puberty.
• May be mildly symptomatic; 3–7% prevalence in total population.

NEONATAL JAUNDICE: BREAST-MILK JAUNDICE

• Due to the presence in mother's milk of pregnanediol, which inhibits glucuronyl-transferase activity.

➤ Laboratory Findings
• Severe unconjugated hyperbilirubinemia. Develops in 1% of breast-fed infants by fourth to seventh day. May reach peak of 15–25 mg/dL by second to third week; then gradually disappears in 3–10 weeks in all cases. If nursing is interrupted, serum bilirubin falls rapidly by 2–6 mg/dL in 2–6 days and may rise again if breast feeding is resumed; if interrupted for 6–9 days, serum bilirubin becomes normal.
• No other abnormalities are present.
• Kernicterus does not occur.

LUCEY-DRISCOLL SYNDROME (NEONATAL TRANSIENT FAMILIAL HYPERBILIRUBINEMIA)

* Syndrome is due to some factor in mother's serum only during last trimester of pregnancy that inhibits glucuronyl transferase activity; disappears about 2 weeks postpartum.
* Newborn infants have severe nonhemolytic unconjugated hyperbilirubinemia usually ≤20 mg/dL during first 48 hours and a high risk of kernicterus.

WILSON DISEASE

* Autosomal recessive defect that impairs copper excretion by liver, which may cause copper accumulation in liver and brain resulting in cirrhosis, neuropsychiatric disease, and corneal pigmentation.
* Heterozygous gene for Wilson disease occurs in 1 of 200 in the general population; 10% of these have decreased serum ceruloplasmin; liver copper is not increased (<250 μg/g of dry liver). Serum copper and ceruloplasmin and urine copper are inadequate to detect heterozygous state.
* Homozygous gene (clinical Wilson disease) occurs in 1 of 200,000 in the general population.
  * Liver biopsy may show no abnormalities, moderate to marked fatty changes with or without fibrosis, or active or inactive mixed micronodular–macronodular cirrhosis.

➤ Laboratory Findings
* Findings of liver function tests may not be abnormal, depending on the type and severity of disease. In patients presenting with acute fulminant hepatitis, Wilson disease is suggested if there is a disproportionately low serum ALP and relatively mild increase in AST and ALT. ALP is frequently decreased; ALP/bilirubin ratio <2.0 is said to distinguish Wilson disease as cause of fulminant liver failure with S/S = 100%/100%.
* Radiocopper incorporation into ceruloplasmin is reduced significantly compared with heterozygotes or normal persons. ^{64}Cu is administered IV or PO and serum concentration is plotted against time. Serum ^{64}Cu disappears within 4–6 hours and then reappears in persons without Wilson disease; secondary reappearance is absent in Wilson disease because incorporation of ^{64}Cu into ceruloplasmin is decreased. Useful when liver biopsy is contraindicated but rarely used since advent of transjugular liver biopsy. Can use mass spectroscopy rather than radioactive Cu.
  * Chelating agent (e.g., D-penicillamine) produces urine Cu excretion of 2–4 mg/day.

➤ Other Considerations
* Diagnosis should be ruled out in any patient with hepatitis with negative serology for viral hepatitis, Coombs-negative hemolysis (due to copper released from necrotic liver cells), or neurologic symptoms to allow for early diagnosis and treatment of Wilson disease.

➤ Suggested Reading
Ferenci P. Diagnosis and current therapy of Wilson disease. *Aliment Pharmacol Ther.* 2004;19:157.

TRAUMA

* May be laceration, hematoma, or vascular

➤ Laboratory Findings

* **Core Laboratory:** Serum LD is frequently increased (>1,400 units) 8–12 hours after major injury. Shock due to any injury may also increase LD. Other serum enzymes and liver function tests are not generally helpful.

Endocrine Diseases

Hongbo Yu

➤ Introduction

This chapter focuses on six common groups of endocrine disorders based on organ systems: diabetes mellitus, disorders of the thyroid gland, disorders of the adrenal gland, gonadal disorders, disorders of the pituitary gland, and disorders of the parathyroid gland and mineral metabolism. For each organ system, the diseases are further discussed according to clinical presentations and/or laboratory findings. The differential diagnosis, laboratory work-up, and radiologic studies for each disease are also considered. Of note, male hypogonadism is covered in the Renal and Urinary Tract Diseases chapter 8.

General principles in the diagnosis of endocrine diseases include the following:
- Stimulatory tests should be performed if hypofunction is suspected and suppression tests if hyperfunction is suspected.
- Suppression tests suppress normal glands but not autonomous secretion.
- Patient preparation is particularly important for hormone studies, results of which may be markedly affected by many factors such as stress, position, fasting state, time of day, preceding

diet, drug therapy. These all should be recorded on the laboratory test requisition form and discussed with the laboratory prior to test ordering.
* Appropriate and timely transportation to the laboratory and preparation of specimen are essential.
* No single test adequately reflects the endocrine status in all conditions.
* Multiple gland hypofunction should evaluate the pituitary gland.

DIABETES MELLITUS

➤ Definition
The term "diabetes mellitus" (DM) refers to a group of disorders of abnormal carbohydrate metabolism sharing in common the clinical finding of hyperglycemia. DM is associated with a relative or absolute impairment in insulin secretion, along with varying degrees of peripheral resistance to the action of insulin.

➤ Overview
DM affects approximately 5% of the world population and 8% of the U.S. population. It is the fourth leading cause of death in the United States. Of the estimated 18 million people with primary DM in the United States, 90–95% have type 2 DM.

➤ Types and Classification
The recent classification focuses on the underlying pathophysiologic process, rather than descriptions based upon age at onset or type of treatment.
1. Type 1: immune mediated, results in an absolute insulin deficiency
2. Type 2: relative insulin deficiency due to abnormalities of both insulin secretion and insulin action. Insulin levels are sufficient to prevent lipid mobilization and ketosis.
3. Gestational diabetes: diagnosed during pregnancy. Only 2% of patients with gestational diabetes remain diabetic after delivery. Forty percent of the patients will develop overt diabetes within 15 years, mostly type 2, but occasionally type 1.
4. Specific types of diabetes:
   a. Genetic defects of beta cell function
   b. Genetic defects in insulin action
   c. Diseases of the exocrine pancreas, such as pancreatitis, trauma, pancreatectomy, neoplasia, cystic fibrosis (CF), hemochromatosis, fibrocalculous pancreatopathy
5. Associated with endocrinopathies (i.e., Cushing's syndrome), drugs (i.e., corticosteroids), or chemicals

➤ Who Should be Suspected?
The clinical onset of diabetes can be acute or insidious, depending both on the degree of insulin deficiency as well as on the intercurrent level of physiologic stress. Patients with the following symptoms and signs should be tested:
1. Classic symptoms of hyperglycemia, such as thirst, polyuria, weight loss, visual blurring
2. Serendipitous finding of hyperglycemia or known impaired glucose tolerance
3. Complications of diabetes, such as proteinuria, neuropathy, cardiovascular complications, and retinopathy
4. Evidence of dehydration, orthostatic hypotension, confusion, or coma

➤ Screening for Diabetes Mellitus

A. In the absence of specific symptoms:

Routine screening for type 1 DM is not recommended, since there is no accepted treatment for the asymptomatic phase of type 1 DM.

However, for type 2 DM, the American Diabetes Association (ADA) recommends screening for diabetes or prediabetes in all adults with body mass index (BMI) ≥ 25 kg/m^2 and one or more additional risk factors for diabetes (see subsequent text of this chapter). In individuals without risk factors, testing should begin at age 45 years. Fasting plasma glucose is the recommended screening test, since it is faster, easier to perform, more convenient, acceptable to patients, and less expensive.

B. Risk factors for diabetes

1. Age ≥ 45 years
2. Overweight (body mass index ≥ 25 kg/m^2)
3. Family history diabetes mellitus in a first-degree relative
4. Habitual physical inactivity
5. Belonging to a high-risk ethnic or racial group (e.g., African American, Hispanic, Native American, Asian American, and Pacific Islander)
6. History of delivering a baby weighing >4.1 kg (9 lb) or of gestational DM
7. Hypertension (blood pressure $\geq 140/90$ mm Hg)
8. Dyslipidemia defined as a serum high-density lipoprotein cholesterol concentration ≤ 35 mg/dL (0.9 mM) and/or a serum triglyceride concentration ≥ 250 mg/dL (2.8 mM)
9. Previously identified impaired glucose tolerance (IGT) or impaired fasting glucose (IFG)
10. Polycystic ovary syndrome
11. History of vascular disease

➤ How to Confirm the Diagnosis

ADA Criteria for the diagnosis of diabetes mellitus:

a. Symptoms of diabetes and a casual plasma glucose ≥ 200 mg/dL (11.1 mM). Casual is defined as any time of day without regard to time since the last meal. The classic symptoms of diabetes include polyuria, polydipsia, and unexplained weight loss.
Or

b. Fasting plasma glucose ≥ 126 mg/dL (7.0 mM). Fasting is defined as no caloric intake for at least 8 hours.
Or

c. Two-hour plasma glucose ≥ 200 mg/dL (11.1 mM) during an oral glucose tolerance test (OGTT). The test should be performed using a glucose load containing the equivalent of 75 g anhydrous glucose dissolved water.
Or

d. Glycosylated hemoglobin A1c (HbA1c) $\geq 6.5\%$. In 2010, ADA added this as another criteria for the diagnosis of DM. The diagnostic test should be performed using a method that is certified by the National Glycohemoglobin Standardization Program (NGSP) and standardized or traceable to the Diabetes Control and Complications Trial reference assay. Point-of-care HbA$_{1c}$ assays are not sufficiently accurate at this time to use for diagnostic purposes. HbA1c is an extremely valuable clinical tool useful both in the diagnosis and in management of diabetic patients. HbA1c has a circulating lifespan of about 90 days, and thus measurement of HbA1c provides information about the level of glycemic control

TABLE 7-1. Diagnostic Thresholds for Diabetes and Prediabetic Conditions

Category	Fasting plasma glucose	2-hour plasma glucose	Glycosylated hemoglobin A$_{1C}$
Normal	<100 mg/dL (5.6 mM)	<140 mg/dL (7.8 mM)	<5.7%
Impaired fasting glucose	100–125 mg/dL (5.6–5.9 mM)		
Impaired glucose tolerance		140–199 mg/dL (7.8–11.0 mM)	
Increased risk			5.7–6.4%
Diabetes mellitus	≤126 mg/dL (7.0 mM)	≥200 mg/dL (11.1 mM)	≥6.5%

over a 3-month period. However, if the patient's red blood cells have abnormal survival time, the value of HbA1c may not be reliable. It will be falsely low in patients with hemolytic anemias, and it may be falsely elevated in patients with polycythemia vera or postsplenectomy. It cannot be used as reliable index for glycemic control in patients with chronic liver diseases due to increased erythrocyte turnover.

In the absence of unequivocal hyperglycemia, the diagnosis of DM must be confirmed on a subsequent day by measuring any one of the three criteria (b, c, and d). However, in symptomatic patients with blood glucose ≥200 mg/dL (11.1 mM) or patients with ketonuria and clear manifestations of type 1 DM, the diagnosis is established and further evaluation is not needed.

Patients with prediabetic conditions (Table 7-1) should be counseled on issues related to lowering their risk for macrovascular diseases (smoking cessation, use of aspirin, diet, and exercise), should have measurements of blood pressure and serum lipids, and should also be encouraged to modify their lifestyle and reduce their weight.

➤ Complications

Evaluation for complications of diabetes should be done routinely in diabetic patients.
A. Routine eye examination
B. Routine foot examination
C. Screening for microalbuminuria
D. Screening for coronary heart disease

Acute Complications

Excessive and prolonged hyperglycemia associated with uncontrolled diabetes can cause fluid and electrolyte imbalance, which may be life-threatening.
A. Diabetic ketoacidosis (mostly in type 1 DM, may also be seen in type 2 DM). Absolute insulin deficiency leads to the unopposed action of the counterregulatory hormones, including glucagon on the liver, adipose tissue, and muscle, leading to unchecked gluconeogenesis and lipolysis.
   a. Signs and symptoms
      1. Dehydration, fruity breath smell, orthostatic hypotension, tachypnea, tachycardia, abdominal pain, nausea, vomiting, and confusion
      2. Antecedent history of viral or bacterial illness, trauma, or emotional stress

b. Laboratory findings
1. Hyperglycemia (generally ≥300 mg/dL), glucosuria, ketonemia and ketonuria, low bicarbonate, elevated blood urea nitrogen, elevated creatinine, pH usually less than 7.3
2. Decreased total body potassium and phosphorus. Serum levels may be normal due to acidosis and shifts to the extracellular space

B. Hyperosmolar hyperglycemic nonketotic coma. Hyperglycemia in patients with type 2 DM can lead to hyperosmolar coma. The degree of hyperglycemia and dehydration that develop are often far more severe than in patients with type 1 DM.
a. Signs and symptoms
1. Usually occurs in elderly patients with decreased ability to obtain free water; precipitated by illness or drugs
2. Deceased mentation, coma
3. Dehydration
b. Laboratory findings
1. Hyperglycemia (often ≥600 mg/dL)
2. Serum osmolarity often ≥320 mOsm/kg
3. Bicarbonate remains ≥15 mEq/L
4. pH remains ≥7.3

Chronic Complications

A. Microvasculopathy
a. Diabetic nephropathy
1. Diabetes is now the most common cause of end-stage renal disease in Western countries.
2. Twenty percent to 30% of patients with diabetes will develop evidence of nephropathy.
3. The earliest evidence of nephropathy is the appearance of low levels of albumin (30 mg/day or 20 µg/min) in the urine, termed microalbuminuria.
4. Eighty percent of type 1 DM and 20–40% of type 2 DM patients who develop microalbuminuria will progress to overt nephropathy (≥300 mg/day or 200 µg/min) over a period of 10–15 years if not treated.
5. Of those patients who develop overt nephropathy, end-stage renal disease can be expected to develop in 75% of patients with type 1 DM and 20% of patients with type 2 DM over 20 years.
b. Retinopathy and neuropathy

B. Macrovasculopathy and vascular atherosclerosis are also major complications of DM.

➤ Suggested Readings

McCulloch DK. Diagnosis of diabetes mellitus. UpToDate. Rose B, ed. Waltham, MA: UpToDate, Inc.; 2009.

McCulloch DK. Overview of medical care in adults with diabetes mellitus. UpToDate. Rose B, ed. Waltham, MA: UpToDate, Inc.; 2009.

McCulloch DK. Screening for diabetes mellitus. UpToDate. Rose B, ed. Waltham, MA: UpToDate, Inc.; 2009.

Laffel L, Svoren B. Epidemiology, presentation, and diagnosis of type 2 diabetes mellitus in children and adolescents. UpToDate. Rose B, ed. Waltham, MA: UpToDate, Inc.; 2009.

Levitsky LL, Misra M. Epidemiology, presentation, and diagnosis of type 1 diabetes mellitus in children and adolescents. UpToDate. Rose B, ed. Waltham, MA: UpToDate, Inc.; 2009.

Khan F, Sachs H, Pechet L, Snyder LM. Guide to Diagnostic Testing. Philadelphia, PA; Lippincott Williams & Wilkins; 2002.

Kronenberg HM, Melmed S, Polonsky KS, Larsen PR. Williams Textbook of Endocrinology, 11th ed. Philadelphia, PA: Saunders, Elsevier Inc.; 2008.

DISORDERS OF THE THYROID GLAND

THYROTOXICOSIS/HYPERTHYROIDISM

➤ Definition

Thyrotoxicosis refers to the classic physiologic manifestations of excessive quantities of the circulating thyroid hormones. The term hyperthyroidism is reserved for disorders that result from sustained overproduction of the hormone by the thyroid itself. Thyrotoxicosis can be caused by hyperthyroidism, or by exogenous thyroid hormone, iatrogenic, or self-administered.

➤ Overview

The clinical manifestations of thyrotoxicosis are largely independent of its cause. However, the disorder that causes thyrotoxicosis may have other effects. The most common form is Graves' disease, comprising 70–80% of the cases.

➤ Common causes

1. Graves' disease (diffuse toxic goiter) is the prototypic autoimmune hyperthyroid condition. Prevalence is approximately 1–2% in women; in men, the prevalence is about one tenth of that. Patients commonly have a family history of thyroid dysfunction (hyperthyroidism or hypothyroidism). It may be accompanied by an infiltrative orbitopathy and ophthalmopathy. In patients and their relatives, there is an increased frequency of other autoimmune disorders, such as DM, pernicious anemia, and myasthenia gravis. The radioactive iodine uptake (RAIU) is typically elevated unless the patient has been exposed to excess iodine or acutely to large dose of glucocorticoids. The circulating autoantibodies specific to Graves' disease are directed against the thyroid-stimulating hormone (TSH) receptor and can be measured directly.

2. Toxic multinodular goiter (MNG) is a disorder in which hyperthyroidism arises in a multinodular goiter, usually of long standing. The overproduction of thyroid hormone is usually less than in Graves' disease and is almost never accompanied by infiltrative ophthalmopathy. All patients with MNG should be screened annually with a serum TSH.

3. Toxic adenoma is usually caused by a single adenoma sometimes referred to as hyperfunctioning solitary nodule or toxic nodule. It often shows a suppressed TSH, which appears in a radioiodine thyroid scan as a localized area of increased radioiodine accumulation.

4. Chorionic gonadotropin–induced hyperthyroidism can be physiologic during pregnancy (transient gestational thyrotoxicosis) or associated with trophoblastic tumors.

5. Iodide-induced hyperthyroidism. Administration of supplemental iodine to subjects with endemic iodine-deficiency goiter can result in iodide-induced hyperthyroidism. Amiodarone, an antiarrhythmic medication, is the most common drug that has been reported to be associated with iodine-induced thyrotoxicosis.

6. Autoimmune (Hashimoto's) thyroiditis can associate with transient thyrotoxicosis, which is caused by thyroid cell breakdown, and the hyperthyroid symptoms are of abrupt onset and short duration.

7. Subacute thyroiditis is an acute inflammatory disorder of the thyroid gland, which is caused directly or indirectly by a viral infection. The symptoms of fever, malaise, and neck soreness frequently overshadow the symptoms of hyperthyroidism. Characteristic findings are of a tender thyroid gland, an elevated erythrocyte sedimentation rate, and a low RAIU.

8. Excess thyroid hormone ingestion can be either iatrogenic or factitious. The presence of a low, rather than elevated, serum thyroglobulin level in a patient with thyrotoxic manifestations and a low RAIU is very suspicious for exogenous hormone ingestion rather than thyroid hyperfunction.

9. Thyroid storm (accelerated hyperthyroidism) represents an extreme accentuation of thyrotoxicosis. It is an uncommon but serious complication, with a mortality of 10–75%. Manifestations include severe fever, marked tachycardia, cardiac arrhythmias, tremulousness, and altered mental status.

10. Subclinical (mild) hyperthyroidism refers to the situation that there are no signs or symptoms of thyrotoxicosis but the serum TSH is subnormal despite normal serum free thyroid hormone concentrations. The diagnosis requires several subnormal TSH concentration results spaced months apart.

11. Ectopic thyroid hormone excretion from ovary (struma ovarii)

➤ Who Should be Suspected?

Signs and symptoms of thyrotoxicosis include:

1. Anxiety, emotional lability, nervousness, and irritability
2. Heat intolerance and increased perspiration
3. Weight loss despite a normal or increased appetite
4. Tremor, palpitations, tachycardia, proximal muscle weakness, and exophthalmos
5. Oligomenorrhea in women; gynecomastia and erectile dysfunction in men

➤ Laboratory Findings

The availability of sensitive and reliable assays for serum TSH and free thyroxine (T_4) has made the laboratory diagnosis of hyperthyroidism rather straightforward (Figure 7-1).

- Serum TSH is the most cost-effective screening test. If the value is normal, the patient is very unlikely to have hyperthyroidism. In hyperthyroidism, serum TSH is below normal and frequently <0.1 uIU/mL. TSH may remain decreased for many months in treated formerly hyperthyroid patients; therefore, thyroid hormone levels more accurately reflect the clinical situation.

- Serum free T_4 is important to confirm and determine the degree of hyperthyroidism in a patient with a low TSH.

- Serum T_3 is usually elevated with hyperthyroidism. Assessment of T_3 levels is important to determine the severity of the hyperthyroidism and to monitor the response to treatment.

- RAIU is often elevated in Graves' disease. However, the diagnostic accuracy of RAIU in hyperthyroidism does not approach that of the serum TSH plus free T_4 measurement. Therefore, determining RAIU is not useful in the diagnosis of straightforward Graves' disease but is useful in excluding thyrotoxicosis not caused by hyperthyroidism. Very low values of RAIU in association with thyrotoxicosis signal the presence of factitious thyrotoxicosis, ectopic thyroid tissue, subacute thyroiditis, or the thyrotoxic phase of autoimmune thyroiditis.

- Thyrotropin receptor autoantibodies are present in 70–100% of the patients with Graves' disease, their measurement is not usually necessary for diagnosis, but it may be helpful in prognosis because patients who have high titers that do not decrease with antithyroid drug treatment are unlikely to go into remission. Measurement of thyrotropin receptor autoantibodies is important in pregnancy, because a high titer at the end of pregnancy correlates with an increased risk of neonatal hyperthyroidism.

- Abnormal TSH can also been seen in various nonthyroidal disease. Simultaneous measurement of TSH with free FT_4 is useful in evaluating the differential diagnoses.

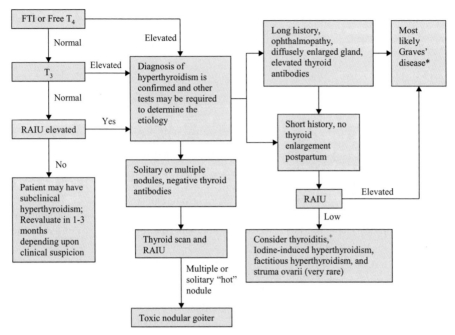

Figure 7-1. Algorithm for the diagnosis of hyperthyroidism. *Graves' disease can be confirmed by measuring thyroid antibodies. + Suspect postpartum thyroiditis if within 6 months of delivery, subacute thyroid if associated with tender gland and constitutional symptoms, and silent thyroiditis if neither. T_4, thyroxine; FTI, free thyroxine index; RAIU, radioactive iodine uptake; T_3, triiodothyronine; TSH, thyroid-stimulating hormone.

➤ Suggested Readings

Khan F, Sachs H, Pechet L, Snyder LM. *Guide to Diagnostic Testing.* Philadelphia, PA: Lippincott Williams & Wilkins; 2002.

Kronenberg HM, Melmed S, Polonsky KS, Larsen PR. *Williams Textbook of Endocrinology,* 11th ed. Philadelphia, PA: Saunders, Elsevier Inc.; 2008.

Ross DS. Diagnosis of hyperthyroidism. UpToDate. Rose B, ed. Waltham, MA: UpToDate, Inc.; 2009.

Ross DS. Overview of the clinical manifestations of hyperthyroidism in adults. UpToDate. Rose B, ed. Waltham, MA: UpToDate, Inc.; 2009.

HYPOTHYROIDISM

➤ Definition
Hypothyroidism refers to a condition in which the amount of thyroid hormones in the body is below normal.

➤ Overview
The diagnosis of hypothyroidism relies heavily upon laboratory tests because of the lack of specificity of the typical clinical manifestations. The prevalence of hypothyroidism is approximately 5% in adults and 15% in women older than 65 years of age. Hypothyroidism is less common in men, with a 5–8 times lower incidence. Hypothyroidism is far more common than hyperthyroidism.

Hypothyroidism is usually easily treated with thyroid hormone replacement. It is now hypothesized that autoimmune hyperthyroidism (Graves' disease) and hypothyroidism (Hashimoto's thyroiditis) represent two extremes of one spectrum of autoimmune thyroid disease.

➤ Common Causes

I. Primary hypothyroidism
   A. Hashimoto's thyroiditis is the most common cause of hypothyroidism in areas of the world in which dietary iodine is sufficient. It usually presents with goiter, hypothyroidism, or both. Goiter usually develops gradually. The diagnosis of Hashimoto's thyroiditis is confirmed by the presence of thyroid autoantibodies, including thyroid peroxidase (TPO) antibody and thyroglobulin antibody.
   B. Iatrogenic: Thyroidectomy and radioiodine therapy or external irradiation for treatment of carcinoma, hyperthyroidism, or goiter can lead to hypothyroidism.
   C. Iodine deficiency (endemic goiter) almost always occurs in areas of environmental iodine deficiency. The incidence of endemic goiter has been greatly reduced by the introduction of iodized salt.
   D. Drugs: thioamides, lithium, amiodarone, interferon, interleukin-2
   E. Infiltrative diseases such as fibrous thyroiditis, hemochromatosis, sarcoidosis
   F. Transient hypothyroidism is defined as a period of reduced free T_4 with suppressed, normal, or elevated TSH levels that are eventually followed by an euthyroid state. This form of hypothyroidism usually occurs in the clinical context of subacute (postviral) thyroiditis, lymphocytic (painless) thyroiditis, or postpartum thyroiditis.
   G. Congenital thyroid agenesis, dysgenesis, or defect in hormone synthesis
   H. Subclinical hypothyroidism is defined as a normal serum free T_4 concentration and a slightly high serum TSH concentration. These patients usually have nonspecific symptoms and a substantial proportion of them eventually develop overt hypothyroidism.
II. Secondary and tertiary (central) hypothyroidism refers to hypothyroidism induced by deficiency of either TSH or thyrotropin-releasing hormone (TRH). This type of hypothyroidism is much less common than primary hypothyroidism, and the symptoms are usually milder than in primary hypothyroidism.
III. Generalized thyroid hormone resistance

➤ Who Should be Suspected?

Signs and symptoms of hypothyroidism include:
1. Fatigue, weight gain, depression, and cold intolerance
2. Dry skin, brittle hair, constipation, and muscle cramps
3. Hypermenorrhea in women
4. Thyroid enlargement (goiter), puffy face and hands (myxedema), and delayed ankle reflex relaxation phase
5. Hypothyroidism in infants and children leads to retardation of mental development and growth. Severe hypothyroidism in infancy is termed cretinism.
6. Myxedema coma refers to severe prolonged hypothyroidism, which is manifested by bradycardia, congestive heart failure, hypothermia, hypoventilation, and paralytic ileus. It is an uncommon but life-threatening condition if not detected and treated promptly.
7. Secondary and tertiary hypothyroidism should be suspected in patients with known hypothalamic or pituitary disease, patients with a pituitary mass, or in patients with other hormonal deficiencies.

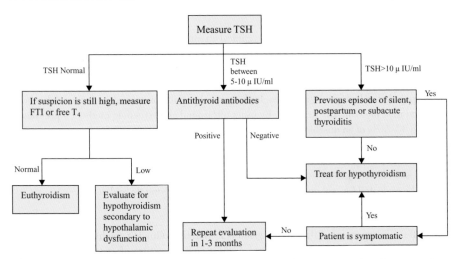

Figure 7-2. Algorithm for the diagnosis of hypothyroidism. T_4, thyroxine; FTI, free thyroxine index; TSH, thyroid-stimulating hormone.

➤ Laboratory Findings (Figure 7-2)

- Laboratory confirmation of the diagnosis of hypothyroidism consists of measuring serum TSH and free T_4. Primary hypothyroidism is characterized by a high serum TSH concentration and a low serum free T_4 concentration. Secondary hypothyroidism is characterized by a low serum TSH concentration as well as a low serum T_4 concentration.
- Total T_4, RAIU, and free T_4 index are usually decreased in hypothyroidism, but they are less sensitive than TSH and free T_4 measurement.
- Antithyroid peroxidase (TPO) antibodies are detected in almost all patients with Hashimoto's disease and its variants, in 70% of patients with Graves' disease, and in a smaller number of patients with various other thyroid disorders such as MNG, nontoxic goiter, and thyroid carcinoma.

➤ Suggested Readings

Khan F, Sachs H, Pechet L, Snyder LM. *Guide to Diagnostic Testing*. Philadelphia, PA: Lippincott Williams & Wilkins; 2002.

Kronenberg HM, Melmed S, Polonsky KS, Larsen PR. *Williams Textbook of Endocrinology*, 11th ed. Philadelphia, PA: Saunders, Elsevier Inc.; 2008.

Ross DS. Diagnosis of and screening for hypothyroidism. UpToDate. Rose B, ed. Waltham, MA: UpToDate, Inc.; 2009.

Ross DS. Subclinical hypothyroidism. UpToDate. Rose B, ed. Waltham, MA: UpToDate, Inc.; 2009.

GOITER AND THYROID NODULES

➤ Definition

Goiter refers to an enlargement of thyroid gland. It can be classified in different ways. Toxic goiter refers to goiter with hyperthyroidism. Nontoxic goiter refers to enlarged thyroid gland with normal or low thyroid hormone levels.

A thyroid nodule is defined as a discrete lesion within the thyroid gland that is due to an abnormal focal growth of thyroid cells.

➤ Overview

Thyroid enlargement or nodules come to clinical attention when noted by the patient, or as an incidental finding during routine physical examination, or during a radiologic procedure, such as carotid ultrasonography or neck computed tomography (CT).

The prevalence of goiter, diffuse or nodular, differs widely depending on the iodine intake by the population living in a given area. In the general population, prevalence of 4.6% has been reported as being clinically detected. By using ultrasound as a screening method, a prevalence of up to 30–50% of an unselected adult population has been described as having goiter.

The clinical importance of thyroid nodules is related primarily to the need to exclude thyroid cancer, which accounts for 4–6.5% of all thyroid nodules in nonsurgical series. The diagnostic goal is to efficiently identify those patients who require surgical intervention. A solitary nodule should be evaluated for malignancy no matter what the underlying thyroid disorder.

➤ Common Causes

I. Diffuse enlargement of the thyroid gland is seen in the following conditions:
- Diffuse toxic goiter—Graves' disease; most common cause of endogenous hyperthyroidism
- Diffuse nontoxic (simple) goiter—relative deficiency of thyroid hormone
- Hashimoto's thyroiditis
- Organification defect (abnormality in the incorporation of iodine into thyroid hormone precursors)

II. Nodular enlargement of the thyroid gland is seen in the following situations:
- A. Benign solid nodule
  - Hyperplastic (or colloid) nodule
  - Follicular adenoma
- B. Malignant tumors
  - Thyroid carcinomas, including papillary, follicular, anaplastic, and medullary carcinomas

    Papillary/follicular/anaplastic carcinomas arise from thyroid follicular epithelial cells. Papillary and follicular cancers are considered differentiated cancers, and patients with these tumors are often treated similarly despite numerous biologic differences. Most anaplastic (undifferentiated) cancers appear to arise from differentiated cancers.

    Medullary carcinoma arises from calcitonin-secreting C cells, and can occur in both sporadic and hereditary forms. The sporadic (noninherited) form accounts for 80% of cases and is usually unilateral. The hereditary form makes up 20% of the cases, is usually multicentric, and can be transmitted as a single entity, part of multiple endocrine neoplasia (MEN) types 2A and 2B, and familial non-MEN.
  - Lymphomas. Most primary thyroid lymphomas arise in patients who have chronic autoimmune thyroiditis.
- C. Multinodular goiter can present with or without thyrotoxicosis. A retrospective study showed that the risk of malignancy was similar in patients with multinodular goiter and one or more dominant nodules to the patients with solitary nodule. Therefore, a dominant nodule in a multinodular goiter should be evaluated as if it were a single nodule.
- D. Simple cyst

➤ Who Should be Suspected?

As mentioned earlier, thyroid nodules can be noted by patient on self-examinations or by physician on routine physical examinations. In addition, the presence of goiter or thyroid nodules should be suspected in patients with the following symptoms or signs.

1. Pain, pressure, or fullness in the neck
2. Hoarseness or change in voice
3. Trouble swallowing

➤ Laboratory Findings (Figure 7-3)

1. Serum TSH should be measured in any patient with a goiter or nodules. It may be used as a first-line screening test. In multinodular goiter, TSH usually is in normal or low-normal range; it is rarely increased.

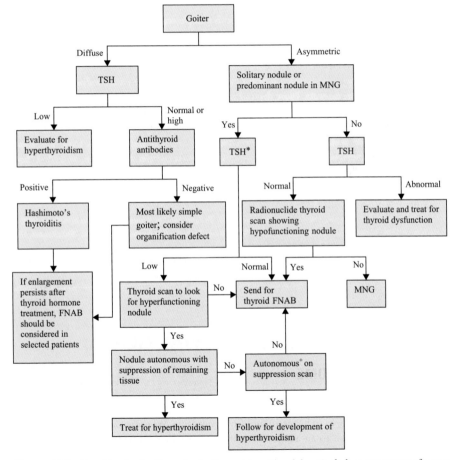

Figure 7-3. Algorithm for the diagnosis of goiter and thyroid nodules. *Include measurement of serum calcitonin if there is a family history of medullary cancer or multiple endocrine neoplasm, type 2 (MEN2). +Autonomy is defined as the ability to concentrate radioactive iodine despite TSH suppression. FNAB, fine–needle aspiration biopsy; MNG, multinodular goiter; TSH, thyroid-stimulating hormone.

2. Calcitonin level is increased in virtually all patients with clinical medullary carcinoma. However, it is not cost-effective or necessary in patients without clinical suspicion due to rarity of the disease and high frequency of false-positive results.
3. Measurement of serum antithyroid peroxidase antibody and antithyroglobulin antibody levels may be helpful in diagnosis of chronic autoimmune thyroiditis, especially if the serum TSH level is elevated.
4. Fine-needle aspiration (FNA) biopsy of the nodule is the most time- and cost-efficient evaluation. The reported overall rates of sensitivity and specificity exceed 90% in iodine-sufficient geographic areas. FNA biopsy should be performed in any patient with a solitary or predominant nodule in a multinodular gland, unless the TSH is suppressed, implying autonomous function and, therefore, a low likelihood of malignancy.

➤ Imaging Studies (see Figure 7-3)

1. Ultrasonography should be used to assess both morphology and size of the goiter and assist in screening and follow-up of thyroid nodules that are difficult to palpate. It may also be useful in directing a FNA biopsy in selected patients. However, this technique cannot distinguish between benign and malignant nodules.
2. Thyroid scintigraphy. Radionuclide scans can be performed with either iodine-123 or technetium-99m pertechnetate. Most thyroid carcinomas are inefficient in trapping and organifying iodine and appear as cold nodules. Unfortunately, most benign nodules also do not concentrate iodine and, therefore, are cold nodules. The only situation in which an iodine scan can exclude malignancy with reasonable certainty is in the case of a toxic adenoma, which is characterized by significantly increased uptake within the nodule, so-called "hot" nodule, and markedly suppressed or absent uptake in the remainder of the gland.

➤ Suggested Readings

Khan F, Sachs H, Pechet L, Snyder LM. *Guide to Diagnostic Testing.* Philadelphia, PA: Lippincott Williams & Wilkins; 2002.

Kronenberg HM, Melmed S, Polonsky KS, Larsen PR. *Williams Textbook of Endocrinology,* 11th ed. Philadelphia, PA: Saunders, Elsevier Inc.; 2008.

Ross DS. Clinical manifestations and evaluation of obstructive or substernal goiter. UpToDate. Rose B, ed. Waltham, MA: UpToDate, Inc.; 2009.

Ross DS. Diagnostic approach to and treatment of thyroid nodules. UpToDate. Rose B, ed. Waltham, MA: UpToDate, Inc.; 2009.

DISORDERS OF THE ADRENAL GLAND

CUSHING'S SYNDROME

➤ Definition

Cushing's syndrome refers to hypercortisolism of any cause. Whereas Cushing's disease refers to hypercortisolism due to an adrenocorticotropic hormone (ACTH)–producing pituitary adenoma.

➤ Overview

The incidence of Cushing's disease is 5–25 cases per 1,000,000 people per year. Other causes of Cushing's syndrome are much less common.

➤ Common Causes

Cushing's syndrome may be either ACTH-dependent or ACTH-independent.

I. ACTH-dependent Cushing's syndrome

   A. Cushing's disease is the most common cause of Cushing's syndrome and comprises 65–70% of the cases. Almost all patients with Cushing's disease have a pituitary adenoma. The adenomas are frequently small, and even a gadolinium-enhanced, high-resolution Magnetic resonance imaging (MRI) of the sella identifies only 50% of them. Pituitary adenoma cells have a higher than normal set point for cortisol feedback inhibition. This feature is clinically important because it permits the use of dexamethasone suppression to distinguish between pituitary and ectopic ACTH secretion; the latter is usually very resistant to glucocorticoid negative feedback.

   B. Ectopic ACTH secretion by nonpituitary tumors accounts for 10–15% of the cases of Cushing's syndrome. A wide variety of tumors, usually carcinomas rather than sarcomas or lymphomas, have been associated with ectopic ACTH secretion. The most common causes are small cell carcinomas of the lung, bronchial or pulmonary carcinoid tumors, and pancreatic islet cell tumors and thymic tumors. Ectopic secretion of ACTH causes bilateral adrenocortical hyperplasia and hyperfunction.

   C. Ectopic corticotropin-releasing hormone (CRH) syndrome constitutes <1% of Cushing's syndrome. CRH secretion by nonhypothalamic tumors causes pituitary hyperplasia, hypersecretion of ACTH, and bilateral adrenal hyperplasia.

II. ACTH-independent Cushing's syndrome

   A. Adrenal tumors account for 18–20% of the cases of Cushing's syndrome. It is important to be sure of the biochemical diagnosis prior to performing any adrenal imaging, since 4% of patients have an adrenal incidentaloma.

   B. Iatrogenic or factitious Cushing's syndrome is usually caused by the use of prednisone; or potent inhaled, injected, and topical glucocorticoids, such as beclomethasone and fluocinolone. Exogenous glucocorticoids inhibit CRH and ACTH secretion, leading to bilateral adrenocortical atrophy. Plasma ACTH, serum cortisol, and urinary cortisol excretion are all low.

➤ Who Should be Suspected?

Symptoms and signs of Cushing's syndrome include hypertension, type 2 DM, and menstrual and psychiatric disorders. Physical examination findings include central obesity, proximal muscle weakness, wide purple striae, spontaneous ecchymoses, and facial plethora (moon face).

➤ Laboratory Findings

I. Diagnosis of Cushing's syndrome involves three steps (Figure 7-4). The first step is to suspect Cushing's syndrome based on the symptoms and signs. The second step is to confirm the presence of excess cortisol production by biochemical testing. The third step is to determine if the hypercortisolism is ACTH dependent, and, if so, the source of the ACTH.

II. Tests used to establish the diagnosis of Cushing's syndrome are listed in Table 7-2. Urinary cortisol, late night salivary cortisol, and low-dose dexamethasone suppression tests are now recommended as first-line tests. At least two first-line tests should be unequivocally abnormal to establish the diagnosis of Cushing's syndrome. Urinary and salivary cortisol measurements should be obtained at least twice.

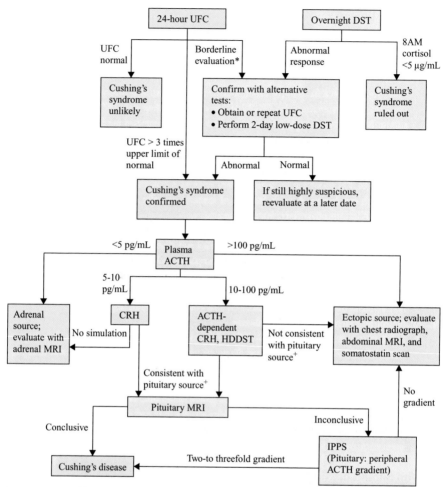

Figure 7-4. Algorithm for the evaluation of Cushing's syndrome. *Patients with alcoholism or depression may have pseudo-Cushing's syndrome and require a CRH test for further evaluation. [+]With a pituitary source, ACTH should increase with CRH, and cortisol production should decrease with HDDST. ACTH, adrenocorticotropic hormone; CRH, corticotropin-releasing hormone; DST, dexamethasone suppression test; HDDST, high-dose dexamethasone suppression test; MRI, magnetic resonance imaging; IPPS, inferior petrosal sinus sampling; UFC, urinary free cortisol.

A. Twenty-four hour urinary cortisol excretion provides a direct and reliable practical index of cortisol secretion. It is an integrated measurement of plasma free cortisol; as cortisol secretion increases, the binding capacity of cortisol-binding globulin is exceeded and results in a disproportionate rise in urinary free cortisol. The two most important factors in obtaining a valid result are collection of a complete 24-hour specimen and a reliable reference laboratory.

TABLE 7-2. Common Tests Used to Establish the Diagnosis of Cushing's Syndrome

Test	Normal Results	Diagnostic
24-hour urinary free cortisol (UFC)	<90 µg cortisol per 24-hour period	>3 times the upper limit of normal
1 mg overnight dexamethasone suppression test (DST) given at 11–12 PM	8 AM plasma cortisol <5 µg/dL	Cushing's syndrome unlikely if cortisol suppresses normally
Low-dose DST (0.5 mg dexamethasone given every 6 hours for 2 days)	UFC <10 µg and 17-OHS <2.5 mg in a 24-hour urine collected on second day	UFC >36 µg/day 17-OHS >4 mg/day
12 midnight cortisol	<5.0 µg/dL	>7.5 µg/dL
12 midnight salivary cortisol	<2.0 ng/mL	>2.0 ng/mL

17-OHS, 17-hydroxycorticosteroid.

B. Late night or midnight salivary cortisol concentration can also be used. Saliva is easily collected and cortisol is stable in saliva for several days even at room temperature. The criteria used to interpret salivary cortisol results vary among different studies. Midnight salivary cortisol is an accurate diagnostic test. A cortisol value >2.0 ng/mL has 100% sensitivity and 96% specificity for diagnosing Cushing's syndrome.

C. Low-dose dexamethasone suppression tests include overnight 1 mg test and standard two-day test. In normal patients, the administration of glucocorticoid results in suppression of ACTH and cortisol secretion. Whereas in Cushing's syndrome of whatever cause, there is a failure of this suppression and the cortisol concentration remains elevated.

D. Midnight serum cortisol is based on the fact that the normal evening or night nadir in serum cortisol is preserved in obese and depressed patients (pseudo-Cushing's syndrome) but not in those with Cushing's syndrome. The test needs to be repeated on at least two nights. Accuracy of midnight cortisol requires an in-dwelling catheter and it is clearly not convenient in an outpatient setting.

III. Tests used to localize the source of the hormone excess. Once the diagnosis of Cushing's syndrome is confirmed, the next step is to distinguish among the three most common causes: a pituitary tumor, ectopic ACTH secretion, and an adrenal tumor. Determining whether elevated cortisol is ACTH-dependent (due to an ACTH-secreting tumor) or whether it is ACTH-independent (due to a primary adrenal disorder) is based primarily on measuring plasma ACTH level.

▶ Imaging Studies (see Figure 7-4)

1. Adrenal imaging is indicated when plasma ACTH levels are <5 pg/mL. Thin section CT or MRI is the next step in evaluating the adrenals. Bilateral adrenal hyperplasia may be present in ACTH-dependent disease.

2. Somatostatin scanning. Ectopic sources of ACTH are notoriously difficult to identify. Because many of these tumors are carcinoids and have somatostatin receptors, scintigraphy with the somatostatin analog indium-111-pentreotide can sometimes localize tumors not found by conventional techniques.

3. Because both incidental pituitary and adrenal tumors are common, biochemical evaluation should be completed before any imaging studies.

➤ Additional Study

Petrosal sinus sampling is used when the anatomic localization fails to identify an unequivocal lesion as suggested by the biochemical testing. This test allows confirmation of the pituitary source of ACTH and identifies the side of the ACTH-secreting lesion. ACTH is measured simultaneously in samples from catheters placed in the left and right inferior petrosal sinuses and compared to peripheral levels. A gradient of two- to threefold is consistent with a pituitary source of ACTH. CRH can also be given during the procedure to enhance its accuracy.

➤ Suggested Readings

Nieman LK. Causes and pathophysiology of Cushing's syndrome. UpToDate. Rose B, ed. Waltham, MA: UpToDate, Inc.; 2009.

Nieman LK. Clinical manifestations of Cushing's syndrome. UpToDate. Rose B, ed. Waltham, MA: UpToDate, Inc.; 2009.

Nieman LK. Establishing the cause of Cushing's syndrome. UpToDate. Rose B, ed. Waltham, MA: UpToDate, Inc.; 2009.

Nieman LK. Establishing the diagnosis of Cushing's syndrome. UpToDate. Rose B, ed. Waltham, MA: UpToDate, Inc.; 2009.

Khan F, Sachs H, Pechet L, Snyder LM. *Guide to Diagnostic Testing*. Philadelphia, PA: Lippincott Williams & Wilkins; 2002.

Kronenberg HM, Melmed S, Polonsky KS, Larsen PR. *Williams Textbook of Endocrinology*, 11th ed. Philadelphia, PA: Saunders, Elsevier Inc.; 2008.

ADRENAL INSUFFICIENCY

➤ Definition

Adrenal insufficiency is defined as a deficiency of hormones synthesized by the adrenal cortex.

➤ Common Causes

I. Primary adrenal insufficiency (Addison's disease): due to intrinsic diseases of adrenal gland
   A. Autoimmune adrenalitis. It is the most common cause of primary adrenal insufficiency and comprises approximately 70–80% of the cases. Some of the patients also have other autoimmune disorders, such as hypoparathyroidism, type 1 DM, Hashimoto's thyroiditis, Graves' disease, or pernicious anemia.
   B. Infections. Common infectious etiologies include tuberculosis, fungi (histoplasmosis, paracoccidioidomycosis), bacteria (meningococcemia, pseudomonas aeruginosa), and viruses (HIV, CMV).
   C. Adrenal hemorrhage or infarction. Adrenal hemorrhage has been associated with meningococcemia (Waterhouse-Friderichsen syndrome) or *pseudomonas aeruginosa*. Anticoagulants are a major risk factor for adrenal hemorrhage.

D. Metastatic disease. Infiltration of the adrenal glands by metastatic cancers is common. The primary site includes lung, breast, stomach, and colon. Similar findings can be seen with melanomas or lymphomas.

E. Drugs. Several drugs may cause adrenal insufficiency by inhibiting cortisol biosynthesis. They include etomidate, ketoconazole, metyrapone, and suramin.

F. Other risk factors include antiphospholipid syndrome, thromboembolic disease, trauma, stress, adrenoleukodystrophy, and abetalipoproteinemia.

II. Secondary adrenal insufficiency: due to inadequate ACTH secretion by the pituitary.

A. Panhypopituitarism. Symptoms are due to a decrease in all pituitary hormones, resulting in hypoadrenalism.

B. Isolated ACTH deficiency

C. Megestrol acetate. Megestrol is used as an appetite stimulant in patients with metastatic breast cancer or AIDS. It suppresses the hypothalamic-pituitary-adrenal axis.

III. Tertiary adrenal insufficiency: due to inadequate CRH secretion by the hypothalamus

A. Following abrupt cessation of high-dose glucocorticoid therapy

B. Following correction of Cushing's syndrome

➤ Who Should be Suspected?

Clinical symptoms and signs of adrenal insufficiency vary depending on the rate and extent of loss of adrenal function, whether mineralocorticoid production is preserved, and the degree of stress.

1. Adrenal crisis: It refers to acute adrenal insufficiency and the predominant manifestation is shock. Other symptoms include anorexia, nausea, vomiting, abdominal pain, weakness, fatigue, lethargy, confusion, or coma. Adrenal crisis may occur in patients with gradual onset who have been stressed either by infection, trauma, or surgery.

2. The most common symptoms of chronic adrenal insufficiency are chronic malaise, anorexia, nausea, vomiting, and generalized weakness.

3. Patients with long-standing primary adrenal insufficiency may present with hyperpigmentation. Other frequent signs are hypotension or orthostatic hypotension. Calcification of the auricular cartilage occurs exclusively in men.

4. Patients with secondary and tertiary adrenal insufficiency usually have intact mineralocorticoid function and do not develop hyponatremia and/or hyperkalemia.

➤ Laboratory Findings (Figure 7-5)

1. Serum cortisol concentration. Cortisol is secreted in a diurnal pattern with highest levels in the morning. Levels measured later in the day are unreliable. Healthy people have early morning serum cortisol concentration of >15 µg/dL. Values <15 µg/dL are suggestive of adrenal insufficiency and require further testing.

2. Basal plasma ACTH concentration. An elevated morning ACTH plasma level in the presence of low cortisol is diagnostic of primary adrenal insufficiency. In contrast, plasma ACTH concentrations are low or low normal in secondary or tertiary adrenal insufficiency.

3. ACTH stimulation tests. If the diagnosis of adrenal insufficiency is being considered and the patients have early morning serum cortisol concentration <15 µg/dL, a short ACTH stimulation test should be performed. A subnormal response confirms the diagnosis of adrenal insufficiency.

4. Corticotropin-releasing hormone test. Differentiation between secondary and tertiary adrenal insufficiency can be done by a corticotropin-releasing hormone test. Patients with

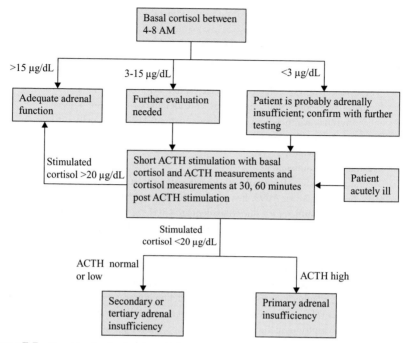

Figure 7-5. Algorithm for the diagnosis of adrenal insufficiency. ACTH, adrenocorticotropic hormone.

secondary adrenal insufficiency show little or no ACTH response, whereas patients with tertiary disease usually have an exaggerated and prolonged ACTH response.

5. Antiadrenal antibodies. Antibodies against 21-hydroxylase (P450c21) are identified in 60–70% patients with autoimmune adrenal insufficiency. They frequently precede the onset of disease. They are also present in 20% of patients with hypoparathyroidism.

6. Patients with suspected adrenal crisis should be treated with dexamethasone, which does not cross-react in the cortisol assay, and confirmatory tests should be performed within 1–2 days.

➤ Imaging Studies

In patients with primary adrenal insufficiency, abdominal CT or MRI with specific attention to adrenals should be obtained to identify the etiology. Enlarged adrenals suggest infectious, hemorrhagic, or metastatic diseases. Pituitary CT or MRI should be performed to look for masses in patients with secondary or tertiary adrenal insufficiency.

➤ Suggested Readings

Nieman LK. Causes of primary adrenal insufficiency (Addison's disease). UpToDate. Rose B, ed. Waltham, MA: UpToDate, Inc.; 2009.

Nieman LK. Causes of secondary and tertiary adrenal insufficiency in adults. UpToDate. Rose B, ed. Waltham, MA: UpToDate, Inc.; 2009.

Nieman LK. Clinical manifestations of adrenal insufficiency in adults. UpToDate. Rose B, ed. Waltham, MA: UpToDate, Inc.; 2009.

Nieman LK. Diagnosis of adrenal insufficiency in adults. UpToDate. Rose B, ed. Waltham, MA: UpToDate, Inc.; 2009.

Nieman LK. Evaluation of the response to ACTH in adrenal insufficiency. UpToDate. Rose B, ed. Waltham, MA: UpToDate, Inc.; 2009.

Khan F, Sachs H, Pechet L, Snyder LM. *Guide to Diagnostic Testing.* Philadelphia, PA: Lippincott Williams & Wilkins; 2002.

Kronenberg HM, Melmed S, Polonsky KS, Larsen PR. *Williams Textbook of Endocrinology,* 11th ed. Philadelphia, PA: Saunders, Elsevier Inc.; 2008.

PRIMARY HYPERALDOSTERONISM

➤ Definition

Primary hyperaldosteronism is a syndrome characterized by hypertension, hypokalemia, and suppressed plasma renin activity associated with increased aldosterone excretion.

➤ Common Causes

1. Aldosterone-producing adenoma accounts for 65% of the cases. Patients tend to have more severe hypertension, lower potassium levels, higher aldosterone secretion, and are of younger age than patients with idiopathic hyperaldosteronism. Unilateral adrenalectomy is curative.
2. Bilateral idiopathic hyperaldosteronism comprises approximately 20–30% of the cases. Bilateral hyperplasia is present.
3. Primary adrenal hyperplasia refers to unilateral aldosterone secretion in patients with physiologic changes similar to those of bilateral idiopathic hyperaldosteronism.
4. Aldosterone-producing adrenocortical carcinoma
5. Ectopic aldosterone-secreting tumors can be of ovarian or renal origin.

➤ Who Should be Suspected?

The classic presenting signs of primary aldosteronism are hypertension, hypokalemia, and edema.

1. Hypertension. The blood pressure in primary aldosteronism is often substantially elevated with mean values of 184/112 and 161/105 mm Hg in patients with adrenal adenoma and adrenal hyperplasia, respectively. However, malignant hypertension rarely occurs.
2. Hypokalemia. Potassium level is low with inappropriate potassium wasting. Plasma potassium tends to be relatively stable at least over the short-term as the potassium-wasting effect of excess aldosterone is counterbalanced by the potassium-retaining effect of hypokalemia itself. Progressive hypokalemia does not occur unless some other factor is added. Hypokalemia may not be the initial presentation, but it is a common finding after administration of diuretics such as furosemide.
3. Metabolic alkalosis
4. Peripheral edema
5. Hypomagnesemia
6. Muscle weakness

➤ Laboratory Findings (Figure 7-6)

1. Plasma aldosterone. High plasma aldosterone concentration (PAC) more than 30 ng/dL is suggestive of hyperaldosteronism. Plasma aldosterone concentrations show diurnal variation with highest concentrations at the time of awakening and lowest in the evening. Aldosterone concentrations are related to extracellular fluid volume, being increased by dietary sodium restriction or diuresis, and decreased by sodium loading. A rise of plasma aldosterone can occur right after assumption of upright position. In practice, most centers draw a morning ambulatory upright sample for assessment of aldosterone and renin levels.

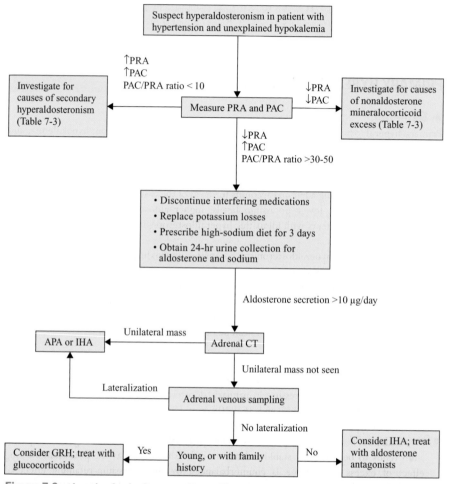

Figure 7-6. Algorithm for the diagnosis of hyperaldosteronism. APA, aldosterone-producing adenoma; CT, computed tomography; GRH, glucocorticoid remediable hyperaldosteronism; IHA, idiopathic hyperaldosteronism; MRI, magnetic resonance imaging; PAC, plasma aldosterone concentration; PRA, plasma renin activity.

2. Urine aldosterone excretion. Elevated 24-hour urinary aldosterone excretion >15 ug/day is suggestive of hyperaldosteronism.
3. Plasma renin activity (PRA). Plasma renin activity relies on endogenous angiotensinogen in the plasma without addition of angiotensinogen. Renin cleaves angiotensinogen to produce angiotensin I, which can be measured by radioimmunoassay. Plasma renin activity is expressed as the amount of angiotensin I generated per unit of time. Plasma renin activity is low in primary hyperaldosteronism. Conversely, high plasma renin activity can be seen with renovascular or malignant hypertension or secondary to diuretic usage.

4. Plasma aldosterone to plasma renin ratio (PAC/PRA ratio). The 2008 Endocrine Society guidelines recommend that the PAC/PRA ratio be used for case detection of primary aldosteronism. Because 30% of the patients with essential hypertension will have low upright renin levels, an elevated plasma aldosterone is required for diagnosis. Hypokalemia must be corrected and the patient must be off diuretics, angiotensin-converting enzyme (ACE) inhibitors, and high-dose beta-blockers. Primary aldosteronism should be suspected when PRA is suppressed and PAC is increased. Secondary hyperaldosteronism (e.g., reno-vascular disease) should be considered when both PRA and PAC are increased and the PAC/PRA ratio is <10. An alternate source of mineralocorticoid receptor stimulation such as hypercortisolism or licorice root ingestion should be considered when both PRA and PAC are suppressed.

5. Aldosterone suppression. Oral sodium loading over 3 days is commonly used in many centers. The patients should receive a high sodium diet for 3 days. The risk of increasing dietary sodium in patients with severe hypertension must be assessed in each case. In addition, because sodium loading typically increases kaliuresis and hypokalemia, serum potassium should be measured daily and vigorous replacement of potassium chloride should be prescribed as indicated. On the third day of the high sodium diet, serum electrolytes are measured and a 24-hour urine specimen is collected for measurement of aldosterone, sodium, and creatinine. The 24-hour urine sodium excretion should exceed 200 meq to document adequate sodium loading. Urine aldosterone excretion 14 ug/day in this setting is consistent with hyperaldosteronism.

6. Other causes of hypertension with associated hypokalemia need to be ruled out. These include secondary hyperaldosteronism and nonaldosterone mineralocorticoid excess. (See Table 7-3.)

7. Patients should be off spirolactone for at least 6 weeks before testing.

8. ACE inhibitors can falsely elevate plasma renin.

9. Patients need to be normokalemic prior to evaluation of aldosterone because hypokalemia suppresses aldosterone secretion.

➤ Imaging Studies

Because of the possibility of "non-functioning" adrenal incidentaloma, adrenal image study is recommended after the biochemical analysis indicates the presence of hyperaldosteronism. Once the diagnosis of primary aldosteronism has been established, a unilateral aldosterone-producing adenoma, or rarely carcinoma, must be distinguished from bilateral hyperplasia, since the treatment is different for the two disorders. Adrenal CT is the recommended initial study to determine subtype. CT is helpful in confirming and locating a unilateral mass, such adenoma or carcinoma. The diagnosis of carcinoma should be suspected when a unilateral adrenal mass is >4 cm in diameter. An abnormality in both glands such as adrenal thickening suggests adrenal hyperplasia. However, patients with hyperplasia may also have normal-appearing adrenal glands on CT.

➤ Additional Study

Adrenal vein sampling can also provide additional information. Measurement of aldosterone in samples of adrenal venous blood, obtained by an experienced radiologist, is the criterion standard test to distinguish between unilateral adenoma and bilateral hyperplasia. Unilateral disease is associated with a marked increase in PAC on the side of the tumor, usually fourfold greater, whereas in patients with bilateral hyperplasia there is little difference between the two sides.

TABLE 7-3. Other Causes of Hypertension Associated with Hypokalemia

Secondary Hyperaldosteronism (high renin and high aldosterone)	Nonaldosterone Mineralocorticoid Excess (low renin and low aldosterone)
Diuretic usage	Congenital adrenal hyperplasia
Renovascular hypertension	Exogenous mineralocorticoids
Renin-secreting tumors	Deoxycorticosterone (DOC)—producing tumor
Coarctation of the aorta	Cushing 's syndrome
Malignant hypertension	Liddle's syndrome
Bartter's syndrome	Chronic licorice ingestion

➤ Suggested Readings

Khan F, Sachs H, Pechet L, Snyder LM. *Guide to Diagnostic Testing.* Philadelphia, PA: Lippincott Williams & Wilkins; 2002.

Kronenberg HM, Melmed S, Polonsky KS, Larsen PR. *Williams Textbook of Endocrinology,* 11th ed. Philadelphia, PA: Saunders, Elsevier Inc.; 2008.

Stowasser M. Assays of the renin-angiotensin-aldosterone system in adrenal disease. UpToDate. Rose B, ed. Waltham, MA: UpToDate, Inc.; 2009.

Young WF, Jr, Kaplan NM, Rose BD. Approach to the patient with hypertension and hypokalemia. UpToDate. Rose B, ed. Waltham, MA: UpToDate, Inc.; 2009.

Young WF, Jr, Kaplan NM, Rose BD. Clinical features of primary aldosteronism. UpToDate. Rose B, ed. Waltham, MA: UpToDate, Inc.; 2009.

ADRENAL MASSES

➤ Definition
Adrenal masses refer to any enlargement of the adrenal glands.

➤ Overview
Adrenal masses can be found in up to 4% of abdominal CT scans done on patients without suspected adrenal problems. The majority of adrenal masses are benign, nonfunctioning adenomas discovered incidentally on abdominal imaging studies (adrenal incidentalomas).

➤ Classification
I. Based on hormonal activity
   A. Hormonally active (functional, hypersecretory)
   - Hypersecreting adrenal adenoma or carcinoma
   - Pheochromocytoma
   - ACTH-dependent Cushing's syndrome with nodular hyperplasia
   - Congenital adrenal hyperplasia
   - Primary aldosteronism
   B. Hormonally inactive (nonfunctional, nonhypersecretory)
II. Based on tumor's biologic behavior
   A. Malignant
   - Adrenal carcinoma
   - Metastatic carcinoma, lymphoma, leukemia

B. Benign
- Adrenal adenoma
- Granulomatous infection
- Hemorrhage or hematoma
- Amyloidosis
- Cysts
- Other benign tumors such as angiomyolipoma, ganglioneuroma, lipoma, hamartoma, teratoma

➤ Who Should be Suspected?

The presence of symptoms or signs suggestive of hormonal activity warrants further evaluation with appropriate biochemical screening tests (Figure 7-7) (Table 7-4).

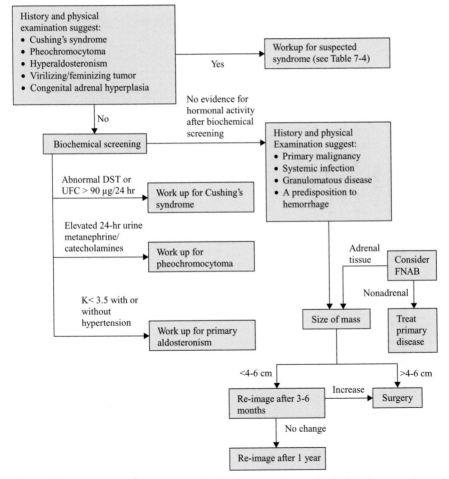

Figure 7-7. Algorithm for the diagnosis of adrenal masses. Consider both clinical presentation and appearance on imaging in deciding cut-off size. DST, dexamethasone suppression test; FNAB, fine needle aspiration biopsy; PE, physical examination; UFC, urinary free cortisol.

TABLE 7-4. Clinical Presentations of Hormonal Hypersecretion and Recommended Screening Tests

Disease	Suggestive Clinical Findings	Screening Recommendations
Pheochromocytoma	Hypertension, paroxysms of headaches, sweating, palpitations, tachycardia, orthostasis, flushing, pallor, glucose intolerance	24-hour urine for fractionated metanephrines, and catecholamines*
Cushing syndrome	Cushingoid habitus, hypertension, thin skin, muscle weakness, facial plethora purplish striae	Overnight 1 mg dexamethasone suppression test, midnight salivary cortisol, or 24-hour urinary free cortisol*
Primary aldosteronism	Hypertension with hypokalemia, metabolic alkalosis	Blood pressure and serum potassium (in salt-replete state)* Upright plasma renin activity and plasma aldosterone concentration 24-hour urine aldosterone
Sex hormone-secreting tumor	Virilization: hirsutism, amenorrhea, frontal balding, acne, clitoromegaly Feminization (very rare): gynecomastia, penile or testicular atrophy	DHEAS, testosterone, urinary 17-ketosteroid for virilizing tumors estradiol for feminizing tumors
Congenital adrenal hyperplasia (especially late-onset 21-hydroxylase deficiency)	In women; acne, hirsutism, amenorrhea, infertility May have suggestive family history	Serum 17α-OHP. If not significantly elevated, perform ACTH stimulation test for 17-OHP (to be considered in patients 21 years of age or younger in the presence of suspicious clinical features).

*Screen in all patients with an incidental adrenal mass.
ACTH, adrenocorticotropic hormone; DHEAS, dehydroepiandrosterone sulfate; 17α-OHP, 17-hydroxyprogesterone.

➤ Laboratory Findings

1. The goal of evaluation is to determine which masses are functional and which ones have the likelihood of being malignant. Benign tumors without hormonal activity need only to be followed, whereas most hormonally active and primary malignant tumors need to be removed. Appropriate biochemical screening tests are listed in the table and algorithm. In patients with no apparent signs or symptoms, a basic biochemical screening is necessary because up to 11% of the cases will have unsuspected abnormal adrenal function.
2. CT and MRI are helpful in determining the likelihood of the adrenal masses being malignant. Size is the most important predictor. Masses >4–6 cm are recommended for surgical removal. Close follow-up is recommended for smaller masses for any change in size.
3. FNA biopsy can differentiate adrenal from nonadrenal masses, but not benign from malignant adrenal tissue. Therefore, it is most useful for evaluation of metastatic disease in patients with a known or suspected cancer outside the adrenal gland.

➤ Suggested Readings

Khan F, Sachs H, Pechet L, Snyder LM. *Guide to Diagnostic Testing.* Philadelphia, PA: Lippincott Williams & Wilkins; 2002.

Kronenberg HM, Melmed S, Polonsky KS, Larsen PR. *Williams Textbook of Endocrinology,* 11th ed. Philadelphia, PA: Saunders, Elsevier Inc.; 2008.

Lacroix A. Clinical presentation and evaluation of adrenocortical tumors. UpToDate. Rose B, ed. Waltham, MA: UpToDate, Inc.; 2009.

Young WF, Jr, Kaplan NM. The adrenal incidentaloma. UpToDate. Rose B, ed. Waltham, MA: UpToDate, Inc.; 2009.

PHEOCHROMOCYTOMA

➤ Definition

Pheochromocytoma refers to catecholamine-secreting tumors arising from the chromaffin cells of the adrenal medulla or the sympathetic ganglia (extra-adrenal).

➤ Overview

Pheochromocytomas are rare neoplasms with an annual incidence of 2–8 cases per 1,000,000 people. This entity constitutes <0.2% of patients with hypertension. These tumors are curable when diagnosed and treated properly, but they are potentially fatal if missed.

➤ Classification

The 10% rules refers to: 10% pheochromocytomas are extra-adrenal, 10% are seen in children, 10% are bilateral, 10% represents recurrence, 10% are malignant, and 10% are familial. Familial syndromes include:

A. Familial pheochromocytomas
B. Multiple endocrine neoplasia (MEN) type 2
   * MEN type 2A: Pheochromocytoma, medullary carcinoma of thyroid, hyperparathyroidism
   * MEN type 2B: Pheochromocytoma, medullary carcinoma of thyroid, mucosal neuromas, marfanoid body habitus
C. Neurofibromatosis 1 (NF1). The main features of NF1 are neurofibromas and dermal café-au-lait spots. NF1 has been associated with a variety of endocrine neoplasms including pheochromocytoma, somatostatin-producing carcinoid tumors of duodenal wall, medullary carcinoma of thyroid, and hypothalamic or optic nerve tumors.
D. Von Hippel-Lindau disease (VHL). It is an autosomal dominant neoplastic syndrome characterized by hemangioblastomas of central nervous system, retinal angiomas, renal cell carcinomas, visceral cysts, pheochromocytoma, and islet cell tumors.

➤ Who Should be Suspected?

The classic triad of symptoms includes episodic headache, sweating, and tachycardia. However, not all patients have the three classic symptoms, and patients with essential hypertension may have the same symptoms. Therefore, pheochromocytoma should be suspected in patients who have one or more of the following:

1. Sustained or paroxysmal hypertension
2. Generalized sweating, palpitations, headache, tremor, panic-attack-type symptoms
3. Familial syndrome of MEN2, NF1, or VHL
4. Family history of pheochromocytoma
5. An adrenal mass incidentally discovered by imaging studies
6. Hypertension and diabetes
7. Onset of hypertension at young age (<20 years)
8. History of gastric stromal tumor or pulmonary chondroma (Carney triad)

➤ Laboratory Findings (Figure 7-8)

Evaluation includes analysis of plasma or urinary catecholamine and their metabolites. The diagnosis is typically confirmed by measurements of urinary and plasma fractionated metanephrines and catecholamines.

1. 24-hour urine catecholamines and metanephrines. It is traditionally relied upon by many institutions for the diagnosis of pheochromocytomas. Sensitivity and specificity of this test is ~98%. Measurement of urinary creatine should also be included to verify an adequate urine collection. A positive test is considered to be twofold elevation above the upper limit of normal in urine catecholamines or metanephrines.

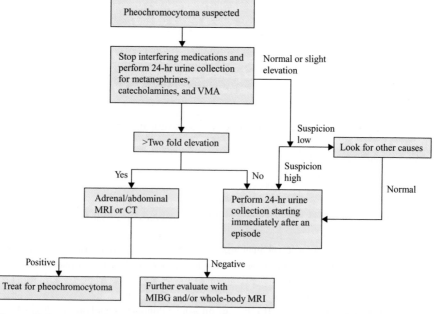

Figure 7-8. Algorithm for the diagnosis of pheochromocytoma. CT, computed tomography; MIBG, [123 I]–metaiodobenzylguanidine; MRI, magnetic resonance imaging; VMA, vanillylmandelic acid.

2. Fractionated plasma free metanephrines. Some groups have advocated fractionated plasma free metanephrines should be a first-line test for pheochromocytoma. The sensitivity of this test is 96–100%, and the specificity is approximately 85–89%. Therefore, the predictive value of a negative test is extremely high.
3. Patients must be off all interfering medications before urine or plasma catecholamines can be measured. Levels can be increased by tricyclic antidepressants, labetalol, levodopa, decongestants, amphetamines, ethanol, and benzodiazepines. Levels can be decreased by metyrosine and methylglucamine, which are present in contrast media. Patients should avoid acetaminophen (Tylenol) during the sample collection.

➤ Imaging Studies

1. CT and MRI will detect most sporadic tumors because they are usually larger than 3 cm in greatest dimension. MRI has some advantage, since pheochromocytomas have a typical hyperintense appearance on T2-weighted images.
2. $[^{123}I]$-metaiodobenzylguanidine (MIBG) scintigraphy is useful in patients with negative CT or MRI.

➤ Suggested Readings

Khan F, Sachs H, Pechet L, Snyder LM. *Guide to Diagnostic Testing.* Philadelphia, PA: Lippincott Williams & Wilkins; 2002.

Kronenberg HM, Melmed S, Polonsky KS, Larsen PR. *Williams Textbook of Endocrinology,* 11th ed. Philadelphia, PA: Saunders, Elsevier Inc.; 2008.

Young WF, Jr, Kaplan NM. Clinical presentation and diagnosis of pheochromocytoma. UpToDate. Rose B, ed. Waltham, MA: UpToDate, Inc.; 2009.

GONADAL DISORDERS

GYNECOMASTIA

➤ Definition

Gynecomastia is defined as excess development of male mammary tissue.

➤ Overview

Gynecomastia is common in infancy, adolescence, and in middle-aged to elderly men. It may be present unilaterally or bilaterally. Gynecomastia develops in response to a variety of causes. The common mechanism of gynecomastia includes an imbalance between the stimulatory effects of estrogens (estradiol, estrone) and the inhibitory effects of androgens (testosterone, androstenedione). Any conditions that alter this balance, including increased production of estrogen, decreased production of androgen, or increased availability of estrogen precursors for peripheral conversion to estrogen, can lead to the proliferation of breast tissue.

➤ Common Causes

Physiologic gynecomastia can occur in neonates and adolescents and usually resolves spontaneously in most cases. The most common causes seen in clinical practice in adult patients includes idiopathic (~25%), persistent postpubertal (~25%), drugs (~10–25%), cirrhosis or malnutrition (~8%), male hypogonadism (10%), testicular tumors (~3%), hyperthyroidism (~1.5%), and chronic renal failure (~1%).

1. Idiopathic. Approximately 25% of the patients have no detectable abnormality. Gynecomastia can occur due to advanced age.

2. Persistent postpubertal gynecomastia. During puberty, serum estradiol concentrations rise to adult levels before the testosterone concentration. Pubertal gynecomastia usually resolves spontaneously within 6 months to 2 years of onset, but in some instances, may persist, leading to postpubertal gynecomastia. It is likely due to estrogen–androgen imbalance.

3. Drugs.
   a. Androgen antagonists and inhibitors. For example, spironolactone, cimetidine, marijuana, flutamide, leuprolide, ketoconazole, finasteride, diazepam, tricyclic antidepressants, phenothiazines, alcohol, chemotherapeutic agents
   b. Estrogenic effects. For example, digitalis, diethylstilbestrol, marijuana, heroin, isoniazid, and alcohol
   c. Increased availability of substrate or activity of aromatase. For example, exogenous administration of gonadotropins, testosterone, or phenytoin
   d. Unknown mechanisms. For example, methyldopa, antihypertensives (ACE inhibitors, calcium channel blockers), narcotics, metronidazole, amiodarone, omeprazole

4. Cirrhosis or malnutrition.
   a. Gynecomastia can occur in up to 67% of cirrhotic patients. There are two mechanisms for this. First, the damaged hepatocytes have an impaired ability to clear androstenedione, which is then available for peripheral aromatase activity and subsequent conversion to estrogens. The second mechanism is through induction of sex hormone–binding globulin (SHBG). Because SHBG binds testosterone with greater affinity than estrogen, any condition that increases SHBG will alter the estrogen–androgen ratio in favor of estrogen.
   b. Malnutrition. During starvation, gynecomastia can occur due to decreased gonadotropin and testosterone levels and normal estrogen production from adrenal precursors. Refeeding is associated with rising gonadotropin, resulting in increased testosterone secretion and marked elevated estrogen production. Therefore, patients during refeeding can develop gynecomastia.

5. Male hypogonadism. Gynecomastia occurs due to androgen deficiency.
   a. Primary hypogonadism. It accounts for approximately 8% of gynecomastia cases. It can be due to a congenital abnormality such as Klinefelter's syndrome, testosterone synthesis defects, or testicular defects (trauma, torsion, or infection)
   b. Secondary hypogonadism. It accounts for approximately 2% gynecomastia cases. It is usually due to a hypothalamic or pituitary abnormality. Pituitary abnormality includes infarction and adenoma. Men with hyperprolactinemia show erectile dysfunction and loss of libido, but can also develop galactorrhea and gynecomastia. Prolactin levels >200 ng/mL are almost always indicative of a pituitary tumor. The principal mechanism is through prolactin's indirect effects on reducing the secretion of gonadotropins, thereby resulting in a shift in the estrogen–testosterone balance favoring estrogen.

6. Testicular neoplasms. The mechanism is related to elevation of the estrogen level either by direct production from the tumor cells or through stimulation of interstitial cells by beta-HCG. Approximately 20% of Leydig cell tumors and 33% of Sertoli cell tumors are associated with gynecomastia. These nongerm cell tumors cause gynecomastia through increased production of estrogen by the tumor cells. Germ cell tumors, on the other hand, under the influence of beta-human chorionic gonadotropin (HCG), cause a disproportionate increase in the production of estrogen over testosterone.

7. Hyperthyroidism. Gynecomastia has been reported in 10–40% of men with Graves' disease.

8. Chronic renal failure. Gynecomastia occurs in approximately 50% of patients treated with maintenance hemodialysis. The mechanism of gynecomastia in renal failure is multifactorial.

a. Renal failure is associated with an increased luteinizing hormone (LH) level, which stimulates the production of estradiol by the Leydig cells.

b. Other etiologies include low testosterone levels related to primary testicular dysfunction, and hyperprolactinemia related to deceased clearance.

c. Increased prolactin levels, linked to secondary hyperthyroidism, may also contribute.

9. Other rare causes include feminizing adrenocortical tumors, ectopic HCG production by tumors of lung, liver, and gastrointestinal tract, true hermaphroditism, androgen insensitivity syndromes, and aromatase excess syndrome.

➤ Who Should be Suspected?

Combination of a careful history and physical examination and a few diagnostic tests can result in the identification of the cause of gynecomastia in the majority of patients.

I. History:
   A. Pain. Gynecomastia tends to present with discomfort, as opposed to breast cancer, which is more typically painless.
   B. Symmetry. Gynecomastia is often bilateral, albeit asymmetrically, whereas breast cancer is often unilateral.
   C. Medication history
   D. Assess for other historical features of family history of cancer, rapid onset, older age, and breast discharge (which suggests breast cancer)
   E. Assess for loss of libido and erectile dysfunction (which suggests hypogonadism).
   F. Check for a history of liver disease, or for risk factors associated with liver disease, chronic renal insufficiency, a pituitary mass, thyroid dysfunction, or Cushing's syndrome.
   G. Check for symptoms of an underlying malignancy, specifically focusing on testicular, lung, and gastrointestinal sources
   H. Assess weight changes and refeeding.

II. Physical examination:
   1. Breast examination.
      a. Breast cancer usually manifests as a hard nodule that is fixed to the underlying soft tissue. Other characteristics include a unilateral presence, nipple discharge, eccentric positioning, skin ulceration, and axillary adenopathy.
      b. Gynecomastia is usually characterized by firm, rubbery, well-defined masses, discoid in shape, mobile, concentric with origination beneath the nipple or areolar region, frequently bilateral, and tender to palpation. Unilateral gynecomastia may be seen as a stage in the development of bilateral gynecomastia. Asymmetry is a frequent finding in patients with gynecomastia.
   2. Testicular examination. Assess for signs of hypogonadism or neoplasm.
   3. Neurologic examination. Assess the visual fields and cranial nerves.
   4. Palpate the thyroid gland for size and nodularity
   5. Assess for stigmata of Cushing's syndrome (strength, striae, fat pad distribution, hirsutism)

➤ Laboratory Findings (Figure 7-9)

1. Initial evaluation should include:
   A. Beta-HCG level, obtained for evaluation of ectopic production.
   B. Serum total and free testosterone, LH, follicle-stimulating hormone (FSH), and estradiol concentrations.
   C. Chest radiograph can be used to rule out pulmonary malignancy.

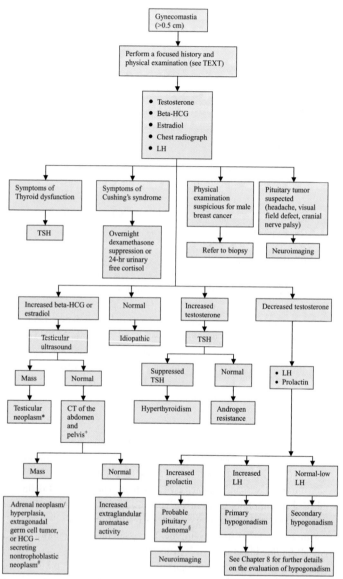

Figure 7-9. Algorithm for the work-up of gynecomastia. CT, computed tomography; HCG, human chorionic gonadotropin; LH, luteinizing hormone; TSH, thyroid-stimulating hormone. *The neoplasm is likely a germ cell tumor if the hCG is elevated, or a nongerm cell tumor if the estradiol is elevated. [+]Abdomen and pelvic images are obtained to identify either an extragonadal germ cell tumor or an HCG–secreting nontrophoblastic neoplasm. An adrenal mass or hyperplasia is sought if the estradiol is elevated. [#]Common nontrophoblastic neoplasms include lung and gastrointestinal sources. [§]An elevated prolactin level may be seen secondary to hypothyroidism, resulting from an elevated TSH. A number of medications can elevate the prolactin level. Before proceeding with neuroimaging, be certain to exclude these possibilities. A prolactin level >200 ng/mL is usually indicative of an adenoma.

2. Supplemental hormonal evaluation is performed as determined by clinical judgement.
   A. Prolactin levels should be obtained in any patients with suspicion of a mass lesion or erectile dysfunction, or when secondary hypogonadism is identified (i.e., low testosterone or low to normal LH).
   B. Dehydroepiandrosterone sulfate (DHEAS) assesses for adrenocortical tumor in the setting of elevated estradiol.
   C. TSH and overnight dexamethasone suppression test (or 24-hour urinary free cortisol)

➤ Imaging Studies (see Figure 7-9)

Neuroimaging should be reserved for those cases in which a mass lesion is suspected (e.g., headache, visual field defect, cranial nerve palsy) or the hormonal evaluation leads one to suspect a pituitary tumor (i.e., elevated prolactin level or Cushing's disease).

➤ Suggested Readings

Braunstein GD. Causes and evaluation of gynecomastia. UpToDate. Rose B, ed. Waltham, MA: UpToDate, Inc.; 2009.

Braunstein GD. Epidemiology and pathogenesis of gynecomastia. UpToDate. Rose B, ed. Waltham, MA: UpToDate, Inc.; 2009.

Khan F, Sachs H, Pechet L, Snyder LM. *Guide to Diagnostic Testing*. Philadelphia, PA: Lippincott Williams & Wilkins; 2002.

HIRSUTISM

➤ Definition

Hirsutism refers to the presence of excess terminal hair in androgen-dependent areas in women, including face, chest, areola, linea alba, lower back, buttock, inner thigh, and external genitalia.

➤ Overview

Hirsutism may affect 5–10% of women of reproductive age. There are two conditions characterized by generalized hair growth that do not represent true hirsutism.

1. Hypertrichosis. It refers to excess terminal hair throughout the body. This is a rare condition that is usually caused by a drug, such as phenytoin, penicillamine, diazoxide, minoxidil, or cyclosporine. It can also occur in patients with systemic diseases such as hypothyroidism, anorexia nervosa, malnutrition, porphyria, and dermatomyositis.
2. Increased vellus hair. It is the soft, unpigmented hair that covers the whole body and it is androgen-independent hair.

➤ Common Causes

Hirsutism is a result of the interaction between circulating serum androgens and the sensitivity of hair follicle to androgens. The most common causes of hirsutism are polycystic ovary syndrome and idiopathic hirsutism (Table 7-5).

➤ Who Should be Suspected?

The clinical approach to a patient with hirsutism includes the degree of androgen excess and its cause. The goal is to identify the small number of women who have potentially serious disorders such as androgen-secreting tumors, or women with polycystic ovary syndrome.

I. History:
   A. Menstrual history. Women with consistently regular menstrual cycles and symptoms of ovulation are unlikely to have severe hyperandrogenemia.

TABLE 7-5. Differential Diagnosis of Conditions Accompanied by Hirsutism and Their Specific Features

Differential Diagnosis	Specific Features
Idiopathic hirsutism	Hirsutism accompanied by no other clinical or biochemical abnormalities
Polycystic ovary syndrome (PCOS)	Onset of hirsutism around the time of puberty, gradual increase in hair growth, menstrual irregularity, obesity, glucose intolerance.
Hyperprolactinemia	Galactorrhea, amenorrhea, or both may be present
Drugs	Danazol, androgenic progestins, phenothiazines, phenytoin, diazoxide, minoxidil; cyclosporine can cause hypertrichosis
Late-onset congenital adrenal hyperplasia	Usually present at birth or in infancy, but the nonclassical form of 21α-hydroxylase deficiency can present prepubertally; 17α-hydroxyprogesterone >1000 ng/dL after administration of adrenocorticotropic hormone; less common from is 11β-hydroxylase deficiency
Hyperthecosis	Increased ovarian testosterone production by luteinized stromal theca cells.
Ovarian tumors	Usually occur later in life, serum testosterone usually >150–200 ng/dL
Adrenal tumors	More often carcinomas, can be with or without evidence of Cushing's syndrome, DHEAS usually 800 µg/dL
Insulin resistant syndromes	Frequently associated with acanthosis nigricans
Menopause	Secondary to altered estrogen–androgen ratios

DHEAS, dehydroepiandrosterone sulfate.

  B. Time course of symptoms. Hirsutism occurring at a later age, with rapid onset, associated with the abrupt cessation of menses, or the presence of other features of virilization, is more often associated with potentially serious disorders, such as adrenal or ovarian tumors.
  C. Weight history
  D. Medication history
  E. Family history
  F. The presence of hirsutism alone is usually a benign condition.
II. Physical examination:
  A. Look for and quantify increased hair in androgen-dependent regions.
  B. Look for evidence of virilization, such as clitoral enlargement, deepening of voice, frontal balding, increased musculature, and loss of female body contour.
  C. Look for evidence of Cushing's syndrome, such as skin striae, thin skin, or bruising.
  D. Body habitus. Height, weight, and a calculation of body mass index (BMI) should be obtained. Many women with polycystic ovary syndrome are obese.
  E. Galactorrhea. The presence of any breast discharge is suggestive of hyperprolactinemia, and a serum prolactin level should be measured.

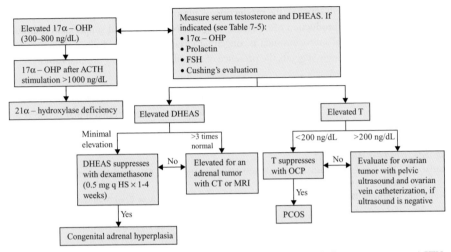

Figure 7-10. Diagnostic algorithm for hirsutism. 17α–OHP = 17α-hydroxyprogesterone; ACTH, adrenocorticotropic hormone; CT, computer tomography; DHEAS, dehydroepiandrosterone sulfate; FSH, follicle-stimulating hormone; MRI, magnetic resonance imaging; OCP, oral contraceptive pill; PCOS, polycystic ovary syndrome; T, testosterone.

F. Abdominal and pelvic examinations. These examinations may reveal mass lesions producing androgen.

➤ Laboratory Findings (Figure 7-10)

1. Serum androgens. Almost all women with hirsutism have an increased production rate of androgens, usually testosterone. Total serum testosterone is adequate to exclude testosterone-secreting tumors, but free testosterone may be necessary to identify smaller increases in testosterone, especially since the carrier protein for testosterone, sex hormone binding globulin, is suppressed by hyperandrogenism and hyperinsulinemia (in patients with polycystic ovary disease). Free testosterone may be elevated, even with a normal total testosterone due to deceased serum binding. Serum DHEAS should be obtained if there is a suspicion of an adrenal androgen-secreting tumor.

2. Serum prolactin. If the patient also has irregular menses, serum prolactin should be measured for evaluation of possibility of hyperprolactinemia.

3. Serum LH. Women with polycystic ovary syndrome tend to have elevated serum LH concentrations and normal or low serum FSH concentrations.

4. 17α–Hydroprogesterone (17α –OHP). Testing for nonclassic 21-hydroxylase deficiency should be considered in women with an early onset of hirsutism, hyperkalemia, or a family history of congenital adrenal hyperplasia. Basal serum 17α–hydroprogesterone concentrations may be only slightly high, especially late in the day. 17α–Hydroprogesterone varies with menstrual cycle and increases with ovulation. A morning value of >300 ng/mL in the early follicular phase strongly suggests the diagnosis of 21-hydroxylase deficiency, which may be confirmed by an ACTH stimulation test. The response to ACTH is usually exaggerated.

5. Dexamethasone suppression testing. Circulating testosterone is derived from both ovarian and adrenal sources and precursors (androstenedione, DHEA, DHEAS). The administration

of dexamethasone will suppress the production of adrenal androgens to a greater extent than it will suppress the production of ovarian androgens. Normal adrenal suppression indicates adrenal production of androgens such as congenital adrenal hyperplasia. Failure of suppression of DHEAS level strongly suggests the presence of an androgen-secreting adrenal tumor.

➤ Imaging Studies (see Figure 7-10)

An adrenal CT scan is recommended to look for an adrenal androgen-secreting tumor when serum DHEAS is markedly elevated. Pelvic ultrasonography with a transvaginal probe is an effective way to look for polycystic ovary or ovarian androgen-secreting tumors.

➤ Suggested Readings

Barbieri RL, Ehrmann DA. Evaluation of women with hirsutism. UpToDate. Rose B, ed. Waltham, MA: UpToDate, Inc.; 2009.

Barbieri RL, Ehrmann DA. Pathogenesis and cause of hirsutism. UpToDate. Rose B, ed. Waltham, MA: UpToDate, Inc.; 2009.

Khan F, Sachs H, Pechet L, Snyder LM. *Guide to Diagnostic Testing.* Philadelphia: Lippincott Williams & Wilkins; 2002.

GALACTORRHEA

➤ Definition

Galactorrhea refers to any persistent discharge of milk or milk-like secretion from the breasts in the absence of a gestational event or beyond 6 months postpartum in a woman who is not nursing.

➤ Overview

Galactorrhea needs to be distinguished from other forms of nipple discharge. Galactorrhea is usually manifested by bilateral milky nipple discharge involving multiple ducts. Green, yellow, bloody, or multicolored fluid should lead the clinicians to look for other causes of nipple discharge. When gross inspection does not permit the identification of the nipple discharge, microscopic examination can be helpful. Milk is rich in lipid content, and thus a fat stain is highly sensitive in confirming the diagnosis of galactorrhea.

➤ Common Causes (Table 7-6)

I. Physiologic causes
   A. Galactorrhea from perpetuation or reactivation of lactation. This accounts for the vast majority of galactorrhea cases. In general, prolactin levels, menses, and fertility are normal. Reactivation of pregnancy-related lactation may occur after a spontaneous first-trimester pregnancy loss, therapeutic abortion, or ectopic pregnancy.
   B. Disorders of the chest wall. Although rare, chest wall injury from surgery such as mastectomy, trauma, infiltrating tumors, and herpes zoster eruptions can produce galactorrhea. Hyperprolactinemia may or may not be present. The mechanism for this milk formation is uncertain, but it may result from chronic neuronal stimulation from the breast to the hypothalamus. Other causes must be ruled out prior to attributing galactorrhea to this cause.
II. Pathologic causes
   A. Pituitary tumors. The most important evaluation in a patient with galactorrhea is the consideration of a pituitary tumor.

TABLE 7-6. Causes of Galactorrhea

Physiologic Causes
- Excessive breast stimulation or tight garments
- Perpetuation or reactivation of postpartum lactation
- Stress, surgery, venipuncture
- Coitus
- Pseudocyesis

Pathologic Causes

Pituitary disorders
- Prolactinomas
- Pituitary angiosarcoma
- Acromegaly
- Cushing's disease
- Empty sella syndrome
- Stalk transsection or compression (postsurgical, head trauma, tumor)

CNS and hypothalamic disorders
- Craniopharyngioma
- Rathke's pouch cyst
- Ectopic pinealomas
- Encephalitis
- Pseudotumor cerebri
- Infiltrative hypothalamic processes (e.g., glioma, histiocytosis, sarcoidosis, tuberculosis)
- Irradiation

Metabolic and endocrinologic disorders
- Adrenal hyperplasia or carcinoma
- Hypothyroidism or hyperthyroidism
- Liver disease
- Chronic renal failure
- Sheehan's syndrome
- Anovulatory disorders (e.g., polycystic ovarian disease, Chiari-Frommel syndrome)
- Idiopathic galactorrhea and amenorrhea

Chest wall lesions

Ectopic prolactin production
- Bronchogenic carcinoma
- Renal cell carcinoma

Pharmacologic Causes
- Antidepressants (e.g., tricyclics, monoamine oxidase inhibitors, selective serotonin reuptake inhibitors)
- Neuroleptics (e.g., phenothiazines and butyrophenones)
- Opiates and narcotics
- H2-blockers (e.g., cimetidine)
- Oral contraceptive pills
- Calcium channel blockers (e.g., verapamil)
- Benzamines (e.g., metoclopramide)
- Alpha-receptor blockers (e.g., reserpine, methyldopa)
- Cocaine
- Amphetamines

Functional/Idiopathic

B. Idiopathic galactorrhea with amenorrhea. Generally the patients in this group have elevated prolactin levels and normal imaging. Possible mechanisms for this disorder include interference of luteinizing hormone-releasing hormone (LHRH), release in the hypothalamus by prolactin, alternation of pituitary sensitivity to LHRH, or interference with steroidogenic action of gonadotropins at the level of the ovary.

C. Anovulatory syndromes

    1. Chiari-Frommel syndrome. It is characterized by galactorrhea and amenorrhea that occurs more than 6 months postpartum in the absence of nursing and in the absence of a pituitary tumor. Approximately 50% of these women will resume normal menses over the next few months. A small minority may have occult microadenomas of pituitary, which may become clinically apparent with time.

    2. Polycystic ovary syndrome (PCOS). It is characterized by obesity, oligomenorrhea, infertility, and hirsutism. Elevated prolactin levels may accompany this syndrome, thereby leading to galactorrhea.

D. Endocrinopathies

    1. Hypothyroidism is a rare cause of galactorrhea. Prolactin levels may be normal or slightly elevated. Galactorrhea is corrected with restoration of euthyroidism.

    2. Galactorrhea is a frequent finding in women with thyrotoxicosis. Serum prolactin is normal, and the mechanism of galactorrhea is unknown.

    3. Cushing syndrome and acromegaly can be associated with galactorrhea. Work-up for these conditions should be undertaken only if specific signs and symptoms are present.

E. Ectopic prolactin production. It is a very rare cause of galactorrhea and other causes should be excluded first. Tumors that have been associated with ectopic prolactin production include renal cell carcinoma and bronchogenic carcinoma.

III. Pharmacologic causes

A. Galactorrhea associated with elevated prolactin levels. Most pharmacologic agents that cause prolactin release either block dopamine receptors (e.g., neuroleptics) or deplete dopamine in the tuberoinfundibular neurons (e.g., centrally acting alpha-blockers). All types of antidepressants can cause galactorrhea, but selective serotonin reuptake inhibitors (SSRIs) do so more commonly than other antidepressants.

B. Galactorrhea associated with oral contraceptive pills (OCPs). Both usage and discontinuation of OCPs can cause galactorrhea. The exact mechanisms are unknown. The abrupt cessation of estrogen and progesterone mimics withdrawal at the time of delivery and can trigger milk production. Estrogen at postmenopausal replacement dose is not associated with galactorrhea.

➤ Who Should be Suspected?

Differential diagnosis of galactorrhea is broad. The goal is to identify the small number of women with pituitary adenoma or other space-occupying lesions as the cause of galactorrhea.

I. History:

A. Menstrual and reproductive history. Galactorrhea can be seen during pregnancy, including ectopic pregnancy, and in the immediate postpartum period. Hyperprolactinemia can lead to hypoestrogenemia, with amenorrhea and infertility. Higher levels of prolactin are associated with more significant menstrual derangements. Galactorrhea in men suggests a pathologic process and should always have an aggressive work-up assessing for a pituitary adenoma and hypogonadism.

B. Medication history

C. History of chest wall surgery, trauma, or herpes zoster eruption

II. Physical examination (Figure 7-11)

A. Eye examination. Check visual acuity and visual fields, and examine the cranial nerves. Assess for symptoms of pituitary diseases such as cranial neuropathies (nerves III, IV, or VI), visual field deficits (bitemporal hemianopsia, optic chiasm, or optic nerve compression), or headache.

B. Breast and chest wall examination. Confirm galactorrhea; palpate for masses, scars, and eruption. Endocrine laboratory testing should be ordered without performing either breast examination or nipple stimulation.

C. Skin examination. Note abnormal skin texture (e.g., myxedema), striae, pigmentation, or hirsutism.

D. Endocrine examination. Assess for thyroid dysfunction, stigmata of Cushing's syndrome (striae, buffalo hump, and central obesity), and acromegaly. Abnormalities of temperature, thirst, and appetite regulation suggest hypothalamic disease.

E. Pelvic examination. Check ovarian and uterine sizes for causes of amenorrhea and anovulation.

➤ Laboratory Findings

1. Serum prolactin. The concentrations may increase slightly during sleep, strenuous exercise, occasionally emotional or physical stress, intense breast stimulation, and high-protein meals. Therefore, a slightly high value should be confirmed before the patient is considered to have hyperprolactinemia. Mildly elevated prolactin levels should prompt investigation for a tumor, even if no other clear cause for the hyperprolactinemia is identified or if symptoms and signs of pituitary and central nervous system (CNS) processes are present. Sample dilutions may be needed in patients with strong suspicion for hyperprolactinemia, but normal or low level of plasma prolactin levels.

2. Beta-HCG level. It should be obtained to exclude pregnancy.

3. Serum TSH. For evaluation of hyper- or hypo-thyroidism.

4. Consider a work-up for less common endocrinopathies such as Cushing's syndrome and acromegaly after excluding more common causes, and only if history and physical findings raise clinical suspicion.

➤ Imaging Studies

High-resolution CT scan or MRI is useful for localization of pituitary tumors.

➤ Suggested Readings

Golshan M, Iglehart D. Nipple discharge. UpToDate. Rose B, ed. Waltham, MA: UpToDate, Inc.; 2009.

Khan F, Sachs H, Pechet L, Snyder LM. *Guide to Diagnostic Testing*. Philadelphia: Lippincott Williams & Wilkins; 2002.

Snyder PJ. Causes of hyperprolactinemia. UpToDate. Rose B, ed. Waltham, MA: UpToDate, Inc.; 2009.

Snyder PJ. Clinical manifestations and diagnosis of hyperprolactinemia. UpToDate. Rose B, ed. Waltham, MA: UpToDate, Inc.; 2009.

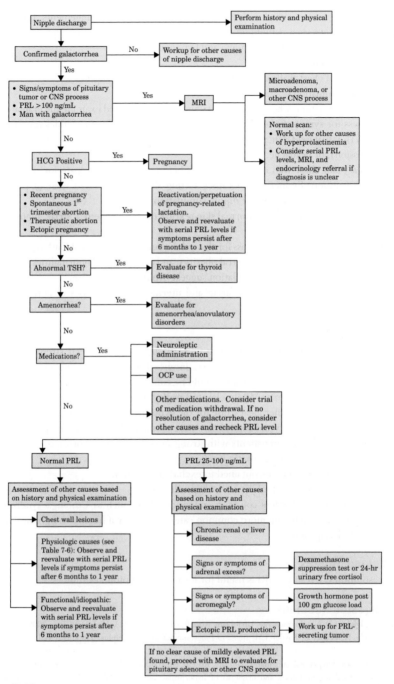

Figure 7-11. Algorithm for the work-up of galactorrhea. CNS, central nervous system; HCG, human chorionic gonadotropin; MRI, magnetic resonance imaging; OCP, oral contraceptive pill; PRL, prolactin; TSH, thyroid-stimulating hormone.

DISORDERS OF THE PITUITARY GLAND

HYPOPITUITARISM

➤ Definition

Hypopituitarism is the deficiency of one or more pituitary hormones resulting from either pituitary or hypothalamic dysfunction. The term panhypopituitarism is used when all the anterior pituitary hormones are absent. When hypothalamic disease is also present, vasopressin deficiency may occur.

➤ Overview

The prevalence of hypopituitarism is 46 cases per 100,000 individuals. The incidence is approximately 4 cases per 100,000 per year.

➤ Causes

Pituitary tumors and other neoplastic processes are the most common causes of acquired hypopituitarism.

I. Pituitary diseases

  1. Mass lesions. They include pituitary adenomas, cysts, lymphocytic hypophysitis, metastatic cancers, and other lesions.

  2. Following surgical or radiation treatment of pituitary

  3. Infiltrative diseases

    a. Hereditary hemochromatosis in the pituitary is characterized by ion deposition in pituitary cells, which leads to hormonal deficiencies.

    b. Lymphocytic hypophysitis often associates with pregnancy and occurs in the postpartum period. It is initially characterized by lymphocytic infiltration and enlargement of the pituitary and then followed by destruction of the pituitary cells. Affected patients typically present with headaches of an intensity out of proportion to the size of the lesion and hypopituitarism.

  4. Pituitary infarction (Sheehan's syndrome). Typically the patients have a history of severe postpartum hemorrhage to cause hypotension and require blood transfusions. Severe hypopituitarism can be recognized during the first days or weeks after delivery by the development of lethargy, anorexia, weight loss, and inability to lactate.

  5. Pituitary apoplexy. Sudden hemorrhage into pituitary gland is called pituitary apoplexy. Hemorrhage often occurs into a pituitary adenoma. It is manifested by sudden onset of headache, cranial nerve defects, visual defects, and hypopituitarism.

  6. Empty sella syndrome. An empty sella refers to an enlarged sella turcica that is not entirely filled with pituitary tissue.

    a. Primary empty sella is due to a congenital defect in the sellar diaphragm.

    b. Secondary empty sella is due to surgery, radiation treatment, or tumor infarction.

  7. Genetic defects. Mutations in genes encoding transcription factors necessary for differentiation of anterior pituitary cells have been identified and they lead to congenital deficiency of one or more pituitary hormones.

II. Hypothalamic diseases

  A. Mass lesions. These include primary benign tumors, such as craniopharyngiomas, and metastatic malignant tumors, such as lung and breast carcinomas.

B. Hypothalamic radiation. It is often associated with radiation treatment for brain tumors and nasopharyngeal carcinomas.

C. Infiltrative diseases. Sarcoidosis and Langerhans cell histiocytosis can cause deficiencies of anterior pituitary hormones.

D. Infections. The most common etiology is tuberculous meningitis.

E. Basal skull fracture or head trauma

➤ Who Should be Suspected?

Hypopituitarism should be suspected in any patient with midline defects or pituitary and/or hypothalamic masses. Symptoms are mainly secondary to target gland dysfunction (i.e., thyroid, adrenal, gonads) due to deficiency of TSH, ACTH, growth hormone, or gonadotropin, but can also be related to local symptoms if a mass is present (i.e., headache, visual disturbances). In pituitary apoplexy, symptoms can be dramatic.

➤ Laboratory Findings

I. ACTH and cortisol

1. Basal ACTH secretion. Serum cortisol should be measured between 8 and 9 AM Serum cortisol value ≤ 3 μg/dL is strongly suggestive of cortisol deficiency, and in a patient with pituitary or hypothalamic disease indicates ACTH deficiency. Cortisol values ≥ 18 μg/dL indicate sufficient basal ACTH secretion. Values between 3 and 18 μg/dL, which persist on repeat determination, are an indication for evaluation of ACTH reserve.

2. ACTH reserve

   a. Metyrapone test. Metyrapone blocks the conversion of 11-deoxycortisol to cortisol by CYP11B1 (11β-hydroxylase, P450c11), the last step in the synthesis of cortisol, and induces a rapid fall of cortisol and an increase of 11-deoxycortisol in serum. The metyrapone test can be performed as an overnight single-dose test or as a 2- or 3-day test. Cortisol and 11-deoxycortisol should be measured at 8 AM A normal response is 8 AM serum 11-deoxycortisol concentration of 7–22 μg/dL. A serum cortisol concentration at 8 AM of <5 μg/dL confirms adequate metyrapone blockade and thereby documents compliance and normal metabolism of metyrapone. Serum 11-deoxycortisol concentrations <7 μg/dL with concomitantly suppressed cortisol values indicate adrenal insufficiency.

   b. Insulin tolerance test (insulin-induced hypoglycemia test). Patients should be administered regular insulin 0.1 U/kg intravenously, and glucose and cortisol should be measured at 15, 30, 60, 90, and 120 minutes after injection. If glucose level falls to 35–40 mg/dL, cortisol should increase to >18 μg/dL. Decreased cortisol levels indicate adrenocortical insufficiency secondary to hypopituitarism. The test requires close observation for hypoglycemia and is risky in patients with cardiac or neurologic dysfunction.

   c. ACTH stimulation test. Cosyntropin is synthetic ACTH, which has the full biologic potency of native ACTH. It is a rapid stimulator of cortisol and aldosterone secretion. The response to ACTH varies with the underlying disorder. If the patient has hypopituitarism with deficient ACTH secretion and secondary adrenal insufficiency, then the intrinsically normal adrenal gland should respond to maximally stimulating concentrations of exogenous ACTH if given for a sufficient length of time. The response may be less than in normal subjects and initially sluggish due to adrenal atrophy resulting from chronically low stimulation by endogenous ACTH. If, on the other hand, the patient has primary adrenal insufficiency, endogenous ACTH secretion is already elevated and there should be little or no adrenal response to exogenous ACTH.

II. TSH
   A. Basal function. Low FTI or free T_4 in the absence of appropriately elevated TSH is suggestive of secondary hypothyroidism. Medications that decrease thyroid hormone binding such as phenytoin, salsalate, or high-dose aspirin should be ruled out. Patient should also be taken off glucocorticoid treatment.
   B. TRH test. TRH is administrated intravenously (200–500 μg). Three blood specimens are collected for serum TSH testing, one immediately prior to TRH injection, and one 15 min and one 30 min after TRH injection. A significant rise in serum TSH from a basal level of 2–3 μU/mL is normal. Secondary (pituitary) hypothyroidism shows no rise in the decreased TSH level. A delayed peak is suggestive of hypothalamic rather than pituitary dysfunction, but is relatively nonspecific.

III. Gonadotropins
   A. Low levels of FSH and LH in postmenopausal women or in men with low testosterone are suggestive of gonadotropin deficiency.
   B. Gonadotropin-releasing hormone (GnRH) test. Patients should be given GnRH (100 μg intravenously), and LH and FSH should be measured at 0, 30, and 60 minutes. LH should increase by 10 IU/L and FSH by 2 IU/L.

IV. Growth hormone (GH)
   A. Basal GH and insulin-like growth factor-I (IGF-I) levels are nonspecific.
   B. Provocative tests with insulin, L-arginine, vasopressin, glucagon, or L-dopa should not be used. Peak GH should be >5–10 ng/mL.

V. Vasopressin
   A. Basal serum sodium, osmolality, and urine osmolality. Hypotonic urine in the presence of increased serum sodium and serum osmolality is suggestive of diabetes insipidus. Twenty-four hour urine should be collected for volume and specific gravity measurement.
   B. Water deprivation test. The inability to concentrate urine with a response to exogenous vasopressin is diagnostic of central diabetes insipidus.

➤ Imaging Studies
A. An MRI scan (T1, T2 +/− gadolinium) is the first choice to evaluate the pituitary gland, hypothalamus, and pituitary stalk.
B. A high-resolution CT with thin sections through the pituitary fossa is a reasonable alternative.

➤ Suggested Readings
Khan F, Sachs H, Pechet L, Snyder LM. *Guide to Diagnostic Testing.* Philadelphia: Lippincott Williams & Wilkins; 2002.

Snyder PJ. Causes of hypopituitarism. UpToDate. Rose B, ed. Waltham, MA: UpToDate, Inc.; 2009.

Snyder PJ. Clinical manifestations of hypopituitarism. UpToDate. Rose B, ed. Waltham, MA: UpToDate, Inc.; 2009.

Snyder PJ. Diagnosis of hypopituitarism. UpToDate. Rose B, ed. Waltham, MA: UpToDate, Inc.; 2009.

PITUITARY TUMORS

➤ Definition
Pituitary tumors are represented by any new growth of the pituitary gland, independent of size or symptoms.

➤ Overview
Pituitary adenomas are the most common cause of sellar masses. Most tumors are considered benign.

➤ Classification
1. Hormonally active tumors
   A. Growth hormone–secreting tumors
   B. Prolactin-secreting tumors
   C. ACTH-secreting tumors
2. Hormonally inactive tumors
   A. Nonsecreting pituitary adenoma
   B. Metastatic tumor (breast and lung are the most common primary sites)
   C. Other brain tumors such as craniopharyngioma, meningioma, and glioma

➤ Who Should be Suspected?
Pituitary masses can present with neurologic symptoms, abnormalities related to undersecretion or oversecretion of pituitary hormones, or as an incidental finding on radiologic examination performed for some other reason.

I. Symptoms
   A. Hormonally active tumors can associate with symptoms of secretion or deficiency.
      a. Growth hormone–secreting tumors present with symptoms of acromegaly.
      b. Prolactin-secreting tumors present with symptoms of galactorrhea.
      c. ACTH-secreting tumors present with symptoms of Cushing's syndrome.
   B. Nonsecreting tumors do not become symptomatic until their size becomes sufficient to cause with pituitary hormone insufficiency (e.g., gonadal dysfunction, secondary hypothyroidism, adrenal insufficiency, growth failure, delayed puberty in children).
   C. Neurologic symptoms
      a. Visual defects. Impaired vision is the most common symptom that leads a patient with a nonfunctioning adenoma to seek medical attention. Visual impairment is caused by suprasellar extension of the adenoma, leading to compression of the optic chiasm. The most common complaint is diminished vision in the temporal fields (bitemporal hemianopsia).
      b. Headaches
      c. Diplopia
II. Signs
   A. Pituitary apoplexy. Sudden hemorrhage into the adenoma can cause excruciating headache and diplopia. It usually occurs spontaneously, but occasionally is precipitated by administration of an anticoagulant.
   B. Pituitary incidentaloma. Pituitary masses discovered incidentally on imaging studies are further evaluated based on their sizes. Incidental microadenomas refer to masses <10 mm in diameter. Patients with microadenomas should be evaluated clinically for hormonal hypersecretion and chemically for any hypersecretion suspected clinically.

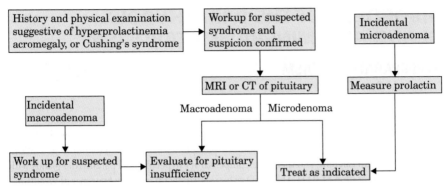

Figure 7-12. Pituitary tumor algorithm. CT, computed tomography; MRI, magnetic resonance imaging.

Serum prolactin level should be measured if there is no clinical suspicion of hormonal hypersecretion. When a macroadenoma ($\geq$10 mm in diameter), evidence for hormonal excess should be sought and assessment of overall pituitary function and formal visual fields is required.

➤ Laboratory Findings (Figure 7-12)

1. A serum prolactin of >200 ng/mL almost always indicates a prolactinoma, although other causes should be considered, such as pregnancy, lactation, stress, dopamine receptor antagonists (e.g., neuroleptics, metoclopramide), primary hypothyroidism, and renal failure. Concentrations between 20 and 200 ng/mL could be due to a lactotroph adenoma or to any other sellar mass. The finding of a large tumor with only minimally elevated prolactin indicates that the tumor is not a prolactinoma but is causing pituitary stalk compression and loss of dopamine inhibition of prolactin secretion.

2. The best test for the diagnosis of acromegaly and growth hormone–secreting tumors is measurement of IGF-I. IGF-I levels need to be corrected for age and sex. Among patients with equivocal values, serum growth hormone secretion after oral glucose administration can be obtained. Random growth hormone measurements are not reliable, since growth hormone is secreted episodically and may be elevated with anxiety, exercise, acute illness, chronic renal failure, and diabetes.

3. Twenty-four hour urine free cortisol quantification, or midnight salivary cortisol test for Cushing's disease.

4. LH, FSH, with testosterone in male patients or estradiol in female patients

5. TSH and free T$_4$ for thyroid function assessment

➤ Suggested Readings

Khan F, Sachs H, Pechet L, Snyder LM. *Guide to Diagnostic Testing.* Philadelphia, PA: Lippincott Williams & Wilkins; 2002.

Kronenberg HM, Melmed S, Polonsky KS, Larsen PR. *Williams Textbook of Endocrinology,* 11th ed. Philadelphia, PA: Saunders, Elsevier Inc.; 2008.

Snyder PJ. Causes, presentation and evaluation of sellar masses. UpToDate. Rose B, ed. Waltham, MA: UpToDate, Inc.; 2009.

Snyder PJ. Clinical manifestations and diagnosis of gonadotroph and other clinically nonfunctioning adenomas. UpToDate. Rose B, ed. Waltham, MA: UpToDate, Inc.; 2009.

Snyder PJ. Pituitary incidentaloma. UpToDate. Rose B, ed. Waltham, MA: UpToDate, Inc.; 2009.

DISORDERS OF THE PARATHYROID GLAND AND MINERAL METABOLISM

HYPERPARATHYROIDISM

➤ Definition

Primary hyperparathyroidism is autonomous hypersecretion of parathyroid hormone (PTH) from the parathyroid glands. Secondary hyperparathyroidism occurs in patients with chronic advanced renal disease that causes retention of phosphate, inadequate vitamin D activation, chronic low serum calcium, and therefore compensatory hyperplasia of parathyroid glands with compensatory secretion of PTH. This chapter focuses solely on primary hyperparathyroidism.

➤ Overview

Primary hyperparathyroidism is frequently identified in asymptomatic patients with an elevated serum calcium concentration. It is estimated to have a prevalence of 1 case per 1,000 people. Primary hyperparathyroidism can occur at any age but the majority of cases occur in patients >45 years of age.

➤ Common Causes

Primary hyperparathyroidism can usually be differentiated from other causes of hypercalcemia by the demonstration of an elevated serum PTH concentration.

1. Parathyroid adenoma is the most common cause of hyperparathyroidism and accounts for approximately 90% of the cases. Most patients have a single enlarged gland with a single adenoma. The remaining glands are usually normal.
2. Parathyroid hyperplasia accounts for approximately 6% of the cases. It involves all four glands and can occur either as isolated or as part of a syndrome such as MEN type 1 or 2, or familial hyperparathyroidism.
3. Parathyroid carcinoma is a rare cause of hyperparathyroidism and constitutes 1–2% of the cases. The diagnosis of carcinoma requires demonstration of either local invasion of contiguous structure, metastases to lymph node, or distant metastases.
4. Familial hypocalciuric hypercalcemia is caused by an inactivating mutation in the calcium-sensing receptor in the parathyroid glands and the kidneys. It is characterized by a family history of hypercalcemia, a young age of onset, lack of symptoms or complications, and specifically by a low urine calcium excretion with Calcium/Creatinine (Ca/Cr) clearance ratio <0.01 in 90% of patients. These patients have normal or only very slightly elevated PTH concentrations.

➤ Who Should be Suspected?

Primary hyperparathyroidism should be suspected in patients with:
1. Elevated serum calcium levels, especially when it persists for years
2. Nephrolithiasis
3. Metabolic acidosis
4. Unexplained osteoporosis, bone pain, and pathologic fractures
5. Osteitis fibrosa cystica, which is characterized by subperiosteal bone resorption on the radial aspect of middle phalanges, tapering of distal clavicles, "salt and pepper" appearance of the skull, bone cysts, and brown tumors of the long bones

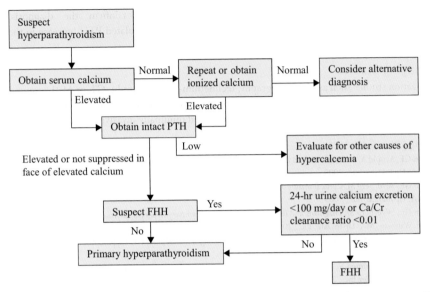

Figure 7-13. Algorithm for the work-up of hyperparathyroidism. Ca/Cr, calcium/creatinine; FHH, familial hypocalciuric calcemia; PTH, parathyroid hormone.

➤ Laboratory Findings

The diagnosis of primary hyperparathyroidism depends on demonstrating elevated serum calcium in the presence of increased PTH (Figure 7-13).

1. Measurement of serum calcium. A single elevated serum calcium concentration should be repeated to confirm the presence of hypercalcemia. Both total and ionized serum calcium concentrations should be obtained. Patient's oral calcium and vitamin D supplements should be withheld before the work-up.

2. Measurement of PTH. Approximately 80–90% of patients with primary hyperparathyroidism have elevated PTH. In the remaining patients, normal or only minimally elevated PTH is detected, but these values are inappropriately high in the setting of an elevated serum calcium level. In patients with nonparathyroid-mediated hypercalcemia, intact PTH is <25 pg/mL. Parathyroid hormone-related protein (PTHrP), which is the humoral cause of cancer-related hypercalcemia, is not detected in the intact PTH assay.

3. Urinary calcium excretion. A 24-hour urine calcium quantitation should be measured if familial hypocalciuric hypercalcemia is suspected. The finding of 24-hour urine calcium excretion <100 mg and Ca/Cr clearance ratio <0.01 confirms the diagnosis.

4. Patients who have a familial history of hyperparathyroidism, or those suspected of having hyperparathyroidism in the context of MEN syndromes should also be evaluated for associated disorders, particularly for pheochromocytoma and thyroid medullary carcinoma.

5. Vitamin D metabolites. Patients with primary hyperparathyroidism convert more calcidiol to calcitrol than normal individuals. Therefore, serum concentrations of calcitrol may be at upper limits of normal or elevated. However, an elevated value is not specific, and thus

measurement of calcitrol is not generally needed to confirm the diagnosis. However, it is helpful to differentiate from the cases with an isolated PTH increase in the absence of hypercalcemia due to vitamin D deficiency.

➤ Imaging Studies

Localization studies such as ultrasonography, technetium-99m sestamibi, CT, or MRI scanning should not be used to establish the diagnosis of primary hyperparathyroidism, but are commonly used to facilitate unilateral neck exploration and minimally invasive surgeries.

➤ Suggested Readings

Fuleihan GE, Arnold A. Pathogenesis and etiology of primary hyperparathyroidism. UpToDate. Rose B, ed. Waltham, MA: UpToDate, Inc.; 2009.

Fuleihan GE, Silverberg SJ. Clinical manifestations of primary hyperparathyroidism. UpToDate. Rose B, ed. Waltham, MA: UpToDate, Inc.; 2009.

Fuleihan GE, Silverberg SJ. Diagnosis and differential diagnosis of primary hyperparathyroidism. UpToDate. Rose B, ed. Waltham, MA: UpToDate, Inc.; 2009.

Khan F, Sachs H, Pechet L, Snyder LM. *Guide to Diagnostic Testing.* Philadelphia, PA: Lippincott Williams & Wilkins; 2002.

Kronenberg HM, Melmed S, Polonsky KS, Larsen PR. *Williams Textbook of Endocrinology,* 11th ed. Philadelphia, PA: Saunders, Elsevier Inc.; 2008.

HYPERCALCEMIA

➤ Definition

Hypercalcemia refers an abnormally high concentration of calcium compounds in the circulating blood.

➤ Overview

Hypercalcemia is a relatively common clinical problem. It results when the entry of calcium into circulation exceeds the excretion of calcium into urine or deposition in bone. Hypercalcemia occurs when there is accelerated bone resorption, excessive gastrointestinal absorption, or deceased renal excretion of calcium. There are many causes of hypercalcemia, but hyperparathyroidism and malignancy are the most common, accounting for >90% of the cases.

➤ Common Causes

Hypercalcemia can be divided into major categories based on the mechanisms of increased bone resorption and increased calcium absorption.
1. Disorders with increased bone resorption
   a. Primary hyperparathyroidism
   b. Secondary and tertiary hyperparathyroidism
   c. Malignancy. The most common etiology with nonmetastatic solid tumor is secretion of PTHrP. Rarely, it is due to a result of ectopic production of PTH.
   d. Thyrotoxicosis
   e. Immobilization
   f. Paget's disease of bone
   g. Tamoxifen used in patients with breast cancer and skeletal metastases
   h. Hypervitaminosis A

2. Disorders with increased calcium absorption
   a. Increased calcium intake. A high calcium intake alone rarely causes hypercalcemia, but it can lead to hypercalcemia when combined with decreased urinary excretion.
   b. Chronic renal failure. It occurs in patients who are treated with calcium carbonate or calcium acetate to bind dietary phosphate.
   c. Milk-alkali syndrome. Excess intake of calcium- and alkali-containing antacids (such as calcium carbonate or sodium bicarbonate) leads to hypercalcemia, metabolic alkalosis, and renal failure. It typically occurs in the situation of taking excess calcium carbonate supplementation to treat osteoporosis or dyspepsia.
3. Hypervitaminosis D can cause hypercalcemia by increasing calcium absorption and bone resorption. High concentration of either 25-hydroxyvitamin D (calcidiol) or 1, 25-dihydroxvitamin D (calcitriol) can lead to hypercalcemia. High serum concentration of 1, 25-dihydroxyvitamin D is usually caused by ingestion of calcitriol as treatment for hypoparathyroidism or for the hypocalcemia and secondary hyperparathyroidism of renal failure, but it also can be due to increased endogenous production in patients with granulomatous disease and lymphoma.
4. Miscellaneous causes
   a. Lithium
   b. Thiazide diuretics
   c. Pheochromocytoma
   d. Adrenal insufficiency
   e. Rhabdomyolysis and acute renal failure
   f. Theophylline toxicity
   g. Familial hypocalciuric hypercalcemia
   h. Metaphyseal chondrodysplasia
   i. Congenital lactase deficiency

➤ Who Should be Suspected?

• Patients with mildly elevated serum calcium (<12 mg/dL) may be asymptomatic, particularly if the elevation is chronic, or they may report nonspecific symptoms, such as constipation, fatigue, and depression.
• Patients with moderately elevated serum calcium (12–14 mg/dL) may have symptoms of polyuria, polydipsia, nausea, anorexia, vomiting, constipation, muscle weakness, and change in sensorium. Acute hypercalcemia leads to a shortened QT interval, which reflects the shortened myocardial action potential.
• Severe hypercalcemia (>14 mg/dL) can lead to progression of above symptoms, and confusion, lethargy, stupor, and even coma and death.

➤ Laboratory Findings (Table 7-7) (Figure 7-14)

The main goal of hypercalcemia work-up is to differentiate PTH-mediated hypercalcemia from non–PTH-mediated hypercalcemia.

• Interpretation of serum calcium. Calcium circulates 40–50% protein bound (predominantly to albumin), and only the ionized or free calcium concentration is physiologically important. Hypercalcemia is caused by an elevation in the ionized or free calcium concentration. In patients with hypo- or hyperalbuminemia, the measured calcium concentration should be corrected for abnormality in albumin. Pseudohypercalcemia should be excluded; it is related to increased protein binding due to either severe dehydration and hyperalbuminemia or

TABLE 7-7. Laboratory Results in Common Causes of Hypercalcemia

Disorder	Serum phosphate	Intact PTH	Urine calcium excretion	Miscellaneous
Primary hyperparathyroidism	↓	↑	NL or ↑	Metabolic acidosis
Familial hypocalciuric hypercalcemia	Variable	NL or SL ↑	↓	
Humoral hypercalcemia of malignancy	↓	↓	NL or ↑	↑ PTHrP
Granulomatous disease	NL or ↑	↓	↑↑	↑ 1,25-OH vitamin D, ↑ angiotensin-converting enzyme
Vitamin D toxicity	NL or ↑	↓	↑↑	↑ 1,25-OH vitamin D
Milk-alkali syndrome	NL or ↑	↓	↓	Metabolic alkalosis and decreased GFR
Metastatic bone disease	NL or ↑	↓	↓	
Thiazide diuretics	NL	↓	↓	
Lithium	NL	↑	↓	

NL, normal level; PTHrP, parathyroid hormone-related protein; SL, slightly.
Normal values: Urine calcium: 100–250 mg/24 hours (females) and 100–300 mg/24 hours (males); serum phosphate: 2.5–4.5 mg/dL; PTH (intact): 12–72 pg/mL; 1,25-OH Vitamin D: 14–78 pg/mL; angiotensin-converting enzyme: 17–70 units; PTHrP: <2.8 pmol/L.

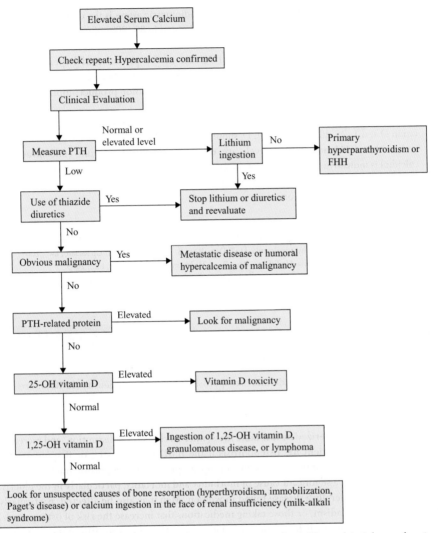

Figure 7-14. Algorithm for the work-up of hypercalcemia. FHH, familial hypocalciuric hypercalcemia; PTH, parathyroid hormone.

production of calcium-binding paraprotein in patients with multiple myeloma. On the contrary, in patients with hypoalbuminemia due to chronic illness or malnutrition, total serum calcium concentration may be normal when serum ionized calcium is elevated.
• Calcium results need to be repeated if abnormal. A single elevated serum calcium concentration should be repeated to confirm the diagnosis.
• Serum calcium should not be measured after a recent high-calcium meal.
• A 24-hour urine calcium quantification is useful in differentiating primary hyperparathyroidism from familial hypocalciuric hypercalcemia (FHH).

- PTH. Measurement of intact PTH via immunoradiometric assays is the current standard for diagnosis of hyperparathyroidism. PTH will be elevated in 80–90% of patients with primary hyperparathyroidism.
- Parathyroid hormone-related protein (PTHrP). In the presence of hypercalcemia, if PTH level is appropriately suppressed, then evaluation for other causes should include measurement of PTHrP. PTHrP is the most common tumor product implicated in the hypercalcemia of malignancy.
- Vitamin D metabolites. Serum concentrations of the vitamin D metabolites, 25-hydroxyvitamin D and 1, 25-dihydroxyvitamin D, should be measured if there is no obvious malignancy and neither PTH nor PTHrP levels are elevated. An elevated serum concentration of calcidiol is indicative of vitamin D intoxication. However, an increased level of calcitriol may be due to direct intake, extrarenal production in granulomatous disease or lymphoma, or increased renal production.

➤ Suggested Readings

Agus ZS. Clinical manifestations of hypercalcemia. UpToDate. Rose B, ed. Waltham, MA: UpToDate, Inc.; 2009.
Agus ZS. Diagnostic approach to hypercalcemia. UpToDate. Rose B, ed. Waltham, MA: UpToDate, Inc.; 2009.
Agus ZS. Etiology of hypercalcemia. UpToDate. Rose B, ed. Waltham, MA: UpToDate, Inc.; 2009.
Khan F, Sachs H, Pechet L, Snyder LM. Guide to Diagnostic Testing. Philadelphia, PA: Lippincott Williams & Wilkins; 2002.

OSTEOPOROSIS

➤ Definition
The World Health Organization defines osteoporosis as bone mineral density (BMD) more than 2.5 standard deviations below the mean of young normal controls (T-score).

➤ Overview
Osteoporosis is characterized by low bone mass, microarchitectural disruption, and increased skeletal fragility. A patient has osteoporosis if the BMD is diagnostic, or if spontaneous, nontraumatic fractures of the wrist, spine, or hip are present. Osteoporotic fractures (especially of the hip) are a significant cause of morbidity and mortality, particularly in the elderly. Osteoporosis is generally a disease found in women. Men may also be affected, particularly those with hypogonadism, or those taking medications that increase the risk of osteoporosis. Patients with osteoporosis have normal bone composition, but too little bone. This is in contrast to patients with osteomalacia, in whom there is failure of normal mineralization of bone matrix.

➤ Who Should be Suspected?
The recommendation is to assess risk factors for fracture in all adults, especially postmenopausal women, men >60 years of age, and in any individual who experiences a fragility or low-trauma fracture.

Risk factors:
1. Caucasian and Asian races
2. Women >55 years of age and men >65 years of age
3. Postmenopausal state or hypogonadism

4. Patients with a history of fragility fractures
5. Long-term glucocorticoid use
6. Acquired osteopenia secondary to disorders such as anorexia nervosa, exercise-associated amenorrhea, delayed puberty, cystic fibrosis
7. Drug use includes anticonvulsants, prolonged administration of heparin, excessive doses of thyroxine, and high doses of methotrexate
8. Sedentary lifestyle
9. Cigarette smoking and alcohol abuse

➤ Laboratory Findings (Figure 7-15) (Table 7-8)

Bone densitometry. Bone density measurements are used in conjunction with fracture risk assessment for osteoporosis screening. Multiple techniques have been developed for the measurement of bone mass, and usage depends mainly on local availability. Dual-energy X-ray

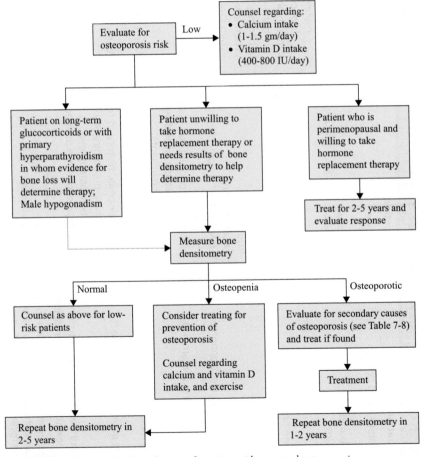

Figure 7-15. Algorithm for the evaluation of a patient with suspected osteoporosis.

TABLE 7-8. Laboratory Evaluation of Patients with Osteoporosis

Evaluation	Indication	Consideration
Complete blood count	Routine	When abnormal, rule out an underlying malignancy
Bicarbonate	Routine	When low, consider metabolic acidosis
Calcium	Routine	When high, consider primary hyperparathyroidism, metastatic cancer, or multiple myeloma. When low, consider osteomalacia or renal failure
Alkaline phosphatase	Routine	When high, consider osteomalacia or another bone disease*
Creatinine	Routine	When high, consider renal failure
TSH	Routine	When low, consider hyperthyroidism
Testosterone	Route in men	When low consider hypogonadism
Serum protein electrophoresis	Low Z-score+, hypercalcemia, or anemia	When abnormal, consider multiple myeloma
Serum 25-hydroxy vitamin D	Elderly with poor intake, history of GI disease, liver disease, or anticonvulsants	When low, consider vitamin D deficiency
Spine radiograph	Significant kyphosis	When the solitary fracture is above T-7, look for an alternative diagnosis
Intact parathyroid hormone	Hypercalcemia, history of renal stones, predominantly cortical osteopenia	When high, consider hyperparathyroidism
Urinary free cortical or overnight dexamethasone suppression test	Cushing's syndrome suspected	When high, consider Cushing's syndrome

GI, gastrointestinal; TSH, thyroid-stimulating hormone.
*Alkaline phosphatase can be transiently elevated with fracture.
+Bone mineral density is >2.5 standard deviations below the mean of age-matched controls.

absorptiometry (DXA) is the most widely used method. Because BMD varies between sites, evaluation at more than one site is recommended.

Laboratory evaluation in a patient with suspected osteoporosis is listed in Table 7-8. It is also important to test for plasma albumin and 25-hydroxycholesterol levels.

➤ Suggested Readings

Raisz LG. Pathogenesis of osteoporosis. UpToDate. Rose B, ed. Waltham, MA: UpToDate, Inc.; 2009.

Raisz LG. Screening for osteoporosis. UpToDate. Rose B, ed. Waltham, MA: UpToDate, Inc.; 2009.

Khan F, Sachs H, Pechet L, Snyder LM. *Guide to Diagnostic Testing*. Philadelphia, PA: Lippincott Williams & Wilkins; 2002.

CHAPTER 8

Renal and Urinary Tract Diseases

Liberto Pechet and Charles Kiefer

This chapter updates the individual disease sections with the latest information for the diagnosis of renal, urinary tract, and prostate diseases. The renal diseases have been divided into noninfectious, congenital, infectious, and tumors. Disorders of the urinary tract, including the prostate gland, are also discussed. Each entry is organized with a brief definition of the disorder, and information regarding clinical presentation, laboratory findings, and limitations, if appropriate.

RENAL DISEASES*

RENAL DISEASES, NONINFECTIOUS

ACUTE TUBULAR NECROSIS

➤ Definition
- The term *acute tubular necrosis* (ATN) is applied to acute disordered renal function that develops in the context of renal ischemia or exposure to nephrotoxins associated with injury to

---

*Submitted by Liberto Pechet MD

the renal tubular epithelial cells. ATN is the most common cause of hospital-acquired acute renal injury.

- Prerenal acute renal failure (see p. 729) and ischemic ATN are part of a spectrum of hypoperfusion renal diseases.

➤ Who Should be Suspected?

- Candidates for investigation include patients (in most cases hospitalized) with exposure to a nephrotoxin (therapy with aminoglycoside or amphotericin B, radiologic contrast materials, heavy metals, cisplatin, or heme pigments) or severe trauma, hemorrhage, surgery, or sepsis, and recent onset oliguria or anuria.

➤ Laboratory Findings

- Typical findings during the acute phases are:
  - Urinalysis (see p. 363)
    - Muddy brown epithelial and granular casts (in prerenal acute renal failure, only hyaline casts are found)
    - Sloughed renal tubular epithelial cells and epithelial casts
    - Urine volume that is typically, but not invariably, low
    - Urinary osmolality that approximates that of plasma (due to impaired urine concentration); in the oliguric phase it is <400 mOsm/kg H_2O
    - Urine sodium usually <40 mEq/L
    - Elevated fractional excretion of sodium (FE_{Na}) ($>2\%$) (see p. 338)
  - Sudden elevation in BUN and creatinine (at a rate >0.3–0.5 mg/dL per day). BUN/creatinine ratio is 10–15:1
- Laboratory findings depend on the phase (initiation, extension, maintenance, or recovery) of ATN when the studies are performed.

AMYLOIDOSIS-ASSOCIATED KIDNEY DISEASE

➤ Definition

- This condition involves amyloid depositions in the kidneys, one of the most frequent complications of amyloid A (AA), amyloid L (AL), and several hereditary amyloidoses.

➤ Who Should be Suspected?

- Candidates with suspected disease include patients with known systemic amyloidosis who develop proteinuria, or, in the absence of this diagnosis, individuals with new-onset proteinuria or the nephrotic syndrome (see p. 727), of unknown etiology.

➤ Laboratory Findings (see also Primary Amyloidosis, p. 865)

- **Urinalysis:** persistent proteinuria that varies from mild, with or without hematuria, to massive, with urinary protein excretion rates as high as 20–30 g per day. The urinary albumin is composed mostly of albumin.
  - Hypoalbuminemia and other findings secondary to the nephrotic syndrome or end-stage renal disease (ESRD), in advanced cases
  - Reduced GFR
  - Nephrogenic diabetes insipidus (DI) may be the result of amyloid deposits in the pericollecting duct tissue

> Suggested Reading

Dember LM. Amyloidosis-associated kidney disease. *J Am Soc Nephrol.* 2006;17:3458–3471.

DIABETIC NEPHROPATHY

> Definition

- Diabetic nephropathy (DN) is persistent proteinuria (present in at least two of three urine collections over a 3- to 6-month period), in the absence of another renal disease. Approximately 40% of patients with type 1 or 2 DM develop DN. The term *Kimmelstiel-Wilson* (or nodular glomerulosclerosis) refers to a subtype of glomerular sclerosis DN characterized by eosinophilic, periodic acid–Schiff–positive glomerular nodules, as demonstrated by kidney biopsy. There is a high correlation between these nodules and the development of diabetic retinopathy.
- DN is recognized after DM has been present for years. Occasionally, DN is associated only with prediabetes. Incidence of ESRD is nearly 30% in type 1 DM and 4–20% in type 2 DM.
- Proteinuria may be the first evidence of DN, and it may be marked, leading in some cases to a frank nephrotic syndrome. Microalbuminuria (see p. 260) is an early sign of the development of DN, and it has very high specificity and PPV for subsequent DN. It appears 5–10 years after the onset of diabetes. It is also highly predictive of cardiovascular events and death in patients with type 1 diabetes.

> Who Should be Suspected?

- Diabetes and DN are more prevalent in African Americans, Native Americans, Polynesians, and Maoris. In addition, risk factors include poorly controlled diabetes, a family history that suggests certain gene polymorphisms, and uncontrolled hypertension.
- Any patient presenting with progressive renal failure should be investigated for the presence of DM. Conversely, all patients with DM should have urinalysis and renal function studies performed periodically.

> Laboratory Findings

- Persistent proteinuria (present in at least two of three urine collections over a 3- to 6-month period) in absence of other renal disease. Proteinuria may be the earliest clinical clue and may be marked (often >5 g/day). Nephrotic syndrome may be associated. Periodic protein testing of urine should be part of routine treatment of all diabetics; dipstick assay detects >200–300 mg/dL. Present in ~25% of type 1 and 36% of type 2 DM patients with negative dipstick test. In type 1 DM, microalbuminuria has S/S of 82%/96% specific and PPV of 75% for subsequent overt nephropathy. In type 2 DM, values are lower.
- Microalbuminuria is associated with a longer duration of diabetes, poorer glycemic control, higher blood pressure, development of more advanced retinopathy and neuropathy, and overt nephropathy and subsequent renal failure, increased vascular damage, and risk for cardiovascular disease.
- Urine shows many hyaline and granular casts and double refractile fat bodies. RBC casts are inconsistent with this diagnosis; if present, HIV, hepatitis, or other disorders should be ruled out by obtaining serology, serum and urine protein electrophoresis, ANA antibodies, or as indicated by associated symptoms. Hematuria is rare.
- Serum protein is decreased.
- BUN and creatinine rise gradually. Azotemia develops gradually after several years of proteinuria.
- See Table 8-1.

TABLE 8-1. Evolution of Renal Disease in Insulin-Dependent Diabetes Mellitus (IDDM)

Stage	Time of Onset	Laboratory Findings*	Morphologic Findings	% of Cases that Progress
Early Renal lesions; no clinical signs	At time of diagnosis 2–3 years after diagnosis	↑ GFR ↑ GFR; albuminuria cannot be detected	Kidney size ↑ ↑ thickness of glomerular and tubular capillary basement membrane; glomerulosclerosis	100 35–40
Incipient nephropathy	7–15 years after diagnosis	Albuminuria 0.03–0.3 g/day. N or sl ↑ GFR; beginning to decline	Glomerulosclerosis progressing	80–100
Clinical diabetic nephropathy	10–30 years after diagnosis	Albuminuria >0.3 g/day. N or sl D GFR; steady fall	Glomerulosclerosis widespread	>75
End-stage renal disease	20–40 years after diagnosis	GFR <10 mL/min; serum creatinine ≥10 mg/dL		

D, decreased; GFR, glomerular filtration rate; I, increased; N, normal; sl, slightly.
*When albuminuria is 0.075–0.1 g/day in IDDM, significant renal disease is present and albuminuria will progress to clinical nephropathy. GFR declines −10 mL/min/year after nephropathy is established.
Source: JV Selby, Fitz-Simmons SC, Newman M, et al. The natural history and epidemiology of diabetic nephropathy. *JAMA.* 1990;263:1954–1960.

TABLE 8-2. Stages of Diabetic Nephropathy	
Stage	Characteristics
I	Asymptomatic Hyperfiltration with increased GFR Reversible microalbuminuria
II	Sustained microalbuminuria that is risk factor for progressive nephropathy and cardiovascular complications
III	GFR approaching normal Overt proteinuria Hypertension
IV	Declining GFR Increasing proteinuria Decreasing renal function
V	Progressive decline in renal function with increasing proteinuria Edema Difficult-to-control hypertension Metabolic disturbances of chronic renal failure (e.g., secondary hyperparathyroidism, metabolic acidosis, anemia) Dialysis or renal transplant
GFR, glomerular filtration rate.	

- Biopsy of kidney is diagnostic.
- DN includes Kimmelstiel-Wilson lesions, UTI (including papillary necrosis), and renal vascular lesions (principally arteriosclerosis).

➤ Course (Table 8-2)
- Type I
  - Onset: hyperfiltration with increased GFR
  - 2–5 years: changes in basement membrane and mesangium
  - 5–10 years: microalbuminuria, often with hypertension
  - >20 years: overt proteinuria, GFR declines, and then increasing creatinine; next 10 years: 50% of patients need dialysis or renal transplant
- Type II
  - At time of diagnosis: microalbuminuria in ≤20%, overt proteinuria in ≤5%, and GFR can decline when microalbuminuria is present
  - 5 years earlier than type I there is overt nephropathy; 10–35% with overt proteinuria develop ESRD

GLOMERULONEPHRITIS

➤ Definition and Classification
- Glomerulonephritis (GN) is a renal disease characterized by inflammation of the glomeruli and/or small blood vessels in the kidneys. It is defined as the abrupt onset of hematuria, often with decreased GFR, proteinuria, edema, hypertension, and sometimes oliguria

* See Tables 8-3 and 8-4 as well as Figure 8-1.
* GN may be considered antibody-mediated or immunologically cell-mediated, infectious or noninfectious, or hypocomplementic or normocomplementic.

Antibody-mediated

* Anti–glomerular basement membrane (GBM) diseases: anti-GBM GN, including Goodpasture syndrome, Alport syndrome, following renal transplantation
* Immune complex–mediated diseases (typically show hypocomplementemia): IgA nephropathy, Henoch-Schönlein purpura, SLE, acute postinfectious GN, membranoproliferative GN (MPGN), membranous GN, fibrillary GN

Cell-mediated

* Wegener granulomatosis, polyarteritis, Churg-Strauss syndrome, ANCA-positive GN, scleroderma

Infectious

* Acute poststreptococcal (group A beta-hemolytic GN)
* Nonpoststreptococcal: bacterial (e.g., infective endocarditis, bacteremias), viral (e.g., HBV, HCV, CMV), parasitic (e.g., trichinosis, toxoplasmosis, falciparum malaria), and fungal

Noninfectious

* Multisystem (e.g., SLE, Henoch-Schönlein purpura, Goodpasture syndrome, Alport syndrome)
* Primary glomerular disease (e.g., IgA nephropathy, MPGN, mesangial proliferative GN)

Hypocomplementic

* Intrinsic renal diseases (especially postinfectious and MPGN)
* Systemic (e.g., SLE, bacterial endocarditis, cryoglobulinemia, serum sickness)

Normocomplementic (Table 8-5)

Glomerulonephritis, Chronic

* Chronic GN syndrome is characterized by proteinuria (may be <3.5 g/1.73 m^2/day), variable abnormalities of urinary sediment, hypertension, and decreased GFR, leading to irreversible end-stage renal failure.
* It develops over years or decades.

➤ Causes

* Poststreptococcal GN: 1–2% progress to chronic GN
* Rapidly progressive GN: 90% progress to chronic GN
* Membranous GN: 50% progress to chronic GN
* Focal glomerulosclerosis: 50–80% progress to chronic GN
* MPGN: 50% progress to chronic GN
* IgA nephropathy: 30–50% progress to chronic GN

➤ Various Clinical Courses

* Early death after marked proteinuria, hematuria, oliguria, progressive increasing uremia, and anemia.
* Intermittent or continuous or incidental proteinuria, hematuria with slight or absent azotemia, and normal renal function tests (may develop into late renal failure or may subside).

TABLE 8-3. Classification of Glomerulonephritis

Glomerular Disorder	Situations in Which May Be Found	Hematuria (% of cases) Micro Present	Hematuria (% of cases) RBC Casts Present	Proteinuria (% of cases) 1–3 g Present	Proteinuria (% of cases) >3 g Present	Renal Function Decreased	Comment
IgA nephropathy (Berger disease)	Focal proliferative GN	100	50	75	25	25% or NS; N in 75%	
IgM mesangial nephropathy		50	Rare	50	50	>75% or NS	
Acute GN secondary to infection (focal GN)	SBE, bacterial pneumonia, viral infections, infection of implanted devices	100	50	75	25	100%	
Crescentic (rapidly progressive) GN Anti-GBM	Goodpasture syndrome in two thirds of patients	100	50	50	50	100%	90% have HLA-DR2 antigen
Immune complex	SLE, mixed cryoglobulinemia, Henoch-Schönlein purpura	100	50	50	50	100%	
Nonimmune complex	Wegener granulomatosis, polyarteritis						See Chapter 15
GN and vasculitis	Wegener granulomatosis, Henoch-Schönlein purpura, mixed cryoglobulinemia; Goodpasture syndrome may occur	100	50	50	50	100%	

(Continued)

TABLE 8-3. Classification of Glomerulonephritis (Continued)

Glomerular Disorder	Situations in Which May Be Found	Hematuria (% of cases) Micro Present	Hematuria (% of cases) RBC Casts Present	Proteinuria (% of cases) 1–3 g Present	Proteinuria (% of cases) >3 g Present	Renal Function Decreased	Comment
SLE							
Mesangial		15		10		N	Most frequent type in SLE
Focal proliferative		50		25		N or D	
Membranous		50			85	N or D	
Diffuse proliferative (<25% of SLE patients)		75			75	Usually D; uremia develops in 50–75%	
Minimal-change disease	Lipid nephrosis, nil disease	20			100	N	85% respond to steroid therapy. Most common cause of NS in children
Focal sclerosis		75		25	75	Usually D	Frequent cause of NS
Membranous nephropathy	Usually idiopathic; occasionally due to heavy-metal toxicity (e.g., gold, mercury), persistent hepatitis B infection, other viruses (e.g., measles, varicella, Coxsackie), other infections (e.g., malaria, syphilis, leprosy,	50		25	75	N early; D late	Frequent cause of NS. Strong association with HLA-DR3. Spontaneous remission in 25%–50%. Persistent proteinuria without progression

	schistosomiasis), neoplasias (e.g., colon carcinoma, lymphoma, leukemia), sarcoidosis, SLE, others					in 25%. Progressive glomerular sclerosis causing renal failure in 50%. Common in adults; uncommon in children
Membranoproliferative GN Type I (idiopathic)	SBE, essential cryo-globulinemia, Henoch-Schönlein purpura, SLE, sickle cell disease, hepatitis and cirrhosis, C2 deficiency, alpha$_1$-antitrypsin deficiency, infected shunts (*Staphylococcus, Corynebacterium*)	75	25	50	50	Usually D; NS at onset in 75%	Renal failure within 5 yrs common in adults but may be delayed 10–20 yrs. Persistent, marked proteinuria is poor prognostic sign. Renal vein thrombosis may occur
Type II (idiopathic)	Infection with streptococci, pneumococci, *Candida*, lipodystrophy					

D, decreased; GBM, glomerular basement membrane; N, normal; NS, nephrotic syndrome; SBE, subacute endocarditis.
Goodpasture syndrome occurs in <5% of cases of GN.
Source: WA Border, RJ Glassock. Progress in treating glomerulonephritis. *Drug Therapy.* 1981;(Apr):97; TR Miller, et al. Urinary diagnostic indices in acute renal failure: a prospective study. *Ann Intern Med.* 1978;89:47; DE Oken. On the differential diagnosis of acute renal failure. *Am J Med.* 1981;71(Dec):916.

TABLE 8-4. Serum Complement in Acute Nephritis

Disorder	Approximate Percentage of Cases
Depressed Serum C3 or Hemolytic Complement Levels	
Systemic disease	
SLE (focal)	75
SLE (diffuse)	90
Subacute bacterial endocarditis	90
"Shunt" nephritis	90
Cryoglobulinemia	85
Renal disease	
Acute poststreptococcal GN	90
Membranoproliferative GN	
Type I	50–80
Type II	80–90
Normal Serum Complement Level	
Systemic disease	
Polyarteritis nodosa	
Wegener granulomatosis	
Hypersensitivity vasculitis	
Henoch-Schönlein purpura	
Goodpasture syndrome	
Visceral abscess	
Renal disease	
IgG–IgA nephropathy	
Idiopathic rapidly progressive GN	
Anti–glomerular basement membrane disease	
Immune complex disease	
Negative immunofluorescence findings	

- Exacerbation of chronic nephritis (with accentuation of proteinuria, hematuria, and decreased renal function) shortly following streptococcal URI.
- Nephrotic syndrome

➤ Laboratory Findings
- Compared with pyelonephritis, chronic GN shows:
  - Lipid droplets and epithelial and RBC casts in urine
  - More marked proteinuria (>2–3 g/day)
  - Poorer prognosis for equivalent amount of azotemia.

Glomerulonephritis, Membranoproliferative

- Types I, II, and III of MPGN are distinguished by morphology and immunofluorescence. The clinical course may be clinically active, or there may be periods of remission; 50% of patients have chronic renal insufficiency in 10 years.

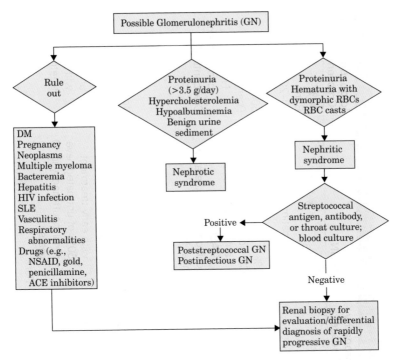

Figure 8-1. Algorithm for evaluation of glomerulonephritis (GN).

➤ Laboratory Findings
- Marked proteinuria and nephrotic syndrome are found in 70% of patients.
- Normal serum C4, but prolonged or permanent depression of C3 is found in 60–80% of patients; clinical course is not related to serum complement levels.
- Renal biopsy and immunofluorescent antibody findings
- GFR <80 mL/min/1.73/m^2 in two thirds of patients
- Associated with systemic diseases, neoplasms, infections (especially HCV with cryoglobulinemia)

Glomerulonephritis, Membranous
- This type of GN is an antibody-mediated disease in which immune complexes localize between outer aspect of basement membrane and epithelial cells. These complexes are in situ or circulating and attach to intrinsic glomerular antigen or exogenous antigen on wall of capillary.
- Usually it occurs in adults, in whom it causes ≤50% of nephrotic syndrome.
- It may be primary (≤75% of cases) or secondary. Secondary membranous GN may be due to connective tissue diseases (e.g., SLE), infections (e.g., HBV, syphilis, malaria, schistosomiasis, leprosy), drugs (e.g., NSAIDs, penicillamine, gold), or neoplasms (non-Hodgkin lymphoma, leukemia, carcinomas, melanoma).

TABLE 8-5. Comparison of Primary Renal Diseases Presenting as Acute GN

	PSGN	IgA Nephropathy (Berger Disease)	MPGN	Idiopathic RPGN (Crescentic)
Acute nephritis	90%	50%	90%	90%
Hematuria	Gross or only microscopic	50%	Rare	Rare
Nephrotic syndrome	10–20%	Rare	70% of patients	10–20%
Acute renal failure	50% (usually transient)	Very rare	50%	60%
Laboratory findings	↑ASOT in 80% Positive streptozyme (95%) ↓C3–C9; normal C1, C4	↑IgA in serum in ≤50% Normal complement	↓C3; normal C4 Positive anti-GBM antibody ↑ASOT 20%	Positive ANCA Normal complement
Renal Pathology	Diffuse proliferation	Focal proliferation Diffuse mesangial	Focal, diffuse proliferation	Crescentic GN
Immuno-fluorescence	Granular IgG, C3 deposits	IgA, IgG, C3; IgA in dermal capillaries	Linear IgG, C3	
Electron microscopy	Subepithelial humps	Mesangial deposits	No deposits	No deposits
Course	95% resolve spontaneously; 5% get RPGN or slowly progress	Slow progression in ≤50% in 5–25 years	75% stabilize or improve with early treatment 50% of untreated have renal insufficiency in 10 years	75% stabilize or improve with early treatment
Hypertension	70%	30–50%	Rare	25%

PSGN, poststreptococcal GN; MPGN, membranoproliferative GN; RPGN, rapidly progressive GN. ↓, decreased; ↑, increased.

➤ Laboratory Findings

- Renal biopsy showing light microscopy, immunofluorescent antibody (IgG and C3), and EM diagnostic findings.
- Marked proteinuria with nephrotic type of syndrome is found in many patients; microscopic hematuria may be present.
- ≤25% of patients progress to ESRD in 20–30 years

Glomerulonephritis, Postinfectious

- Postinfectious GN is due to deposits of immune complexes in the GBM.
- See Table 8-3.

➤ Laboratory Findings

- Evidence of infection, especially group A β-hemolytic *Streptococcus* by throat culture
- Serologic findings indicative of recent infection (e.g., ASOT). Combined use of serologic tests establishes recent streptococcal infection in virtually all cases.
- Urine
  - Hematuria—gross or only microscopic. Microscopic hematuria may occur during the initial febrile URI and then reappear with nephritis in 1–2 weeks. It lasts 2–12 months; usual duration is 2 months.
  - RBC casts and dysmorphic RBCs show glomerular origin of hematuria.
  - WBC casts and WBCs show inflammatory nature of lesion.
  - Granular and epithelial cell casts are present.
  - Fatty casts and lipid droplets occur several weeks later; not related to hyperlipemia.
  - Proteinuria is usually <2 g/day (but may be ≤6–8 g/day); may disappear while RBC casts and RBCs still occur.
  - Decreased urinary aldosterone occurs in the presence of edema.
  - Oliguria is frequent.
- GFR usually shows greater decrease than renal blood flow; therefore, filtration factor is decreased.
- PSP excretion is normal in cases of mild to moderate severity; increases with progression of disease.
- Blood
  - Azotemia is found in ~50% of patients.
  - Leukocytosis with increased PMNs; ESR is increased.
  - There is mild anemia, especially when edema is present (may be caused hemodilution, bone marrow depression, or increased destruction of RBCs).
  - Serum proteins are normal or there is nonspecific decrease of albumin and increase of alpha$_2$ and sometimes of beta and gamma globulins.
  - Serum C3 and total hemolytic complement fall 24 hours before onset of hematuria and return to normal within ~8 weeks when hematuria subsides. If C3 is low >8 weeks, should consider lupus nephritis or MPGN.
  - Antihuman kidney antibodies are present in serum in 50% of patients.
  - Serum cholesterol may be increased.
- Renal biopsy shows characteristic findings with EM and immunofluorescence.
- Chronic renal insufficiency is reported in ≤20% of patients.
- Azotemia with high urine specific gravity and normal PSP excretion usually means acute GN.

Glomerulonephritis, Rapidly Progressive (Crescentic)

➤ Definition

- This type of GN is a glomerular disease of rapid progressive loss of renal function with severe oliguria and renal failure that develops over a period of a few weeks. It may be preceded by a multisystem disease.
- The histopathologic term *crescentic* refers to crescent formation, a nonspecific response to severe injury to the glomerular capillary wall. Patients may have rapidly progressive GN in association with Goodpasture's syndrome, small vessel vasculitis, and ANCA, SLE (see p. 936), or cryoglobulinemia.

➤ Who Should be Suspected?

- Candidates include patients with rapidly developing oliguria or anuria, especially in the presence of an underlying immunologically mediated systemic illness, or following an infection, or administration of certain drugs (allopurinol, hydralazine, rifampin, D-penicillamine).

➤ Laboratory Findings

Laboratory work-up is urgent to initiate therapy, since untreated patients progress rapidly to ESRD. Renal biopsy and immunofluorescent antibodies findings establish the diagnosis and prognosis.

- Urinalysis
  - Oliguria, with urine volume often <400 mL/day
  - Gross hematuria: RBCs, WBCs, and casts
  - Proteinuria beginning about 3 days after injury; it may not be marked because of severe reduction in glomerular filtration
- Rapid, progressive rise in creatinine and BUN
- Laboratory tests to determine underlying etiology (ANCA, anti-GBM antibodies, ANA)
- Serology for infection, including HIV and hepatitis B and C

KIDNEY DISORDERS IN GOUT

- See Pseudogout in Chapter 12. Kidney stones occur in 25% of patients with gout; may occur in absence of arthritis.
- Disorders predispose to GU tract infection
- Characteristics include tubular obstruction and interstitial crystal deposition with tophi formation.
- Arteriolar nephrosclerosis and pyelonephritis are usually associated.
- Early renal damage is indicated by decreased renal-concentrating ability, mild proteinuria, and decreased PSP excretion.
- Later renal damage is shown by slowly progressive azotemia with slight albuminuria and slight or no abnormalities of urine sediment.
- Renal disease causes death in ≤50% of patients with gout.
- It has been suggested that acute uric acid nephropathy may be differentiated from other forms of acute renal failure if ratio of urine urate-to-urine creatinine >1.0 in an adult (many children younger than 10 years of age have ratio >1.0).

TABLE 8-6. Findings in Henoch-Schönlein Purpura

	Hematuria	Proteinuria	Renal Function
Minor urinary abnormality	Microscopic, intermittently gross	<1 g/24 h	Normal
Active renal disease Renal insufficiency		>1 g/24 h	Normal GFR <60 mL/min/1.73 m²

HENOCH-SCHÖNLEIN PURPURA

- See Vasculitis in Chapter 4.
- This condition involves hypersensitivity systemic vasculitis of small vessels with IgA deposition. It is referred to as *Henoch purpura* when abdominal symptoms are predominant and *Schönlein purpura* when joint symptoms are predominant. The renal picture varies from minimal urinary abnormalities for years; ESRD within months is <2%.
- Diagnosis is clinical; there are no pathognomonic laboratory findings.

➤ Laboratory Findings
- Renal biopsy supports the diagnosis; shows focal segmental necrotizing GN that becomes more diffuse and crescentic with IgA and C3 deposition.
- Urine contains RBCs, casts, and slight protein in 25–50% of patients. Gross hematuria and proteinuria are uncommon (Table 8-6).
- In nonthrombocytopenic purpura, hematologic tests are normal. Serum complement is usually normal. BUN and creatinine may be increased.

➤ Suggested Reading
Calviño MC, Llorca J, Garcia-Porrua C, et al. Henoch-Schönlein purpura in children from northwestern Spain. *Medicine*. 2001;80:279–290.

HEPATORENAL SYNDROME

➤ Definition
- This progressive renal failure without demonstrable renal pathology develops in patients with decompensated liver cirrhosis.

➤ Who Should be Suspected?
- Candidates are patients with liver cirrhosis and ascites, especially following fluid loss (e.g. GI hemorrhage, diarrhea, or forced diuresis) or an intercurrent infection.

➤ Laboratory Findings
- Urinalysis
  - Oliguria: concentrated urine with high specific gravity and urine-to-plasma osmolality ratio >1.0
  - Acid pH
  - Small amount of protein

- Bland urine sediment with few hyaline and granular casts, few RBCs
- Decreased to absent urine sodium (<10 mEq/L)
- Stepwise progressive increase in creatinine (>1.5 mg/dL) and BUN (type 1), or stable elevation (type 2), a less ominous situation
- Low GFR (as measured by creatinine clearance) preceding elevations in creatinine/BUN
- Hyponatremia
- Hyperkalemia
- Markedly abnormal liver function tests

➤ Suggested Readings

Arroyo V, Guevara M, Gines P. Hepatorenal syndrome in cirrhosis: pathogenesis and treatment. *Gastroenterology.* 2002;122:1658–1676.

Salerno F, Gerbes A, Gines P, et al. Diagnosis, prevention and treatment of hepatorenal syndrome in cirrhosis. *Gut.* 2007;56:1310–1318.

HYPERCALCEMIC NEPHROPATHY

- This condition is caused by a prolonged increase in serum and urine calcium (due to hyperparathyroidism, sarcoidosis, vitamin D intoxication, multiple myeloma, carcinomatosis, milk-alkali syndrome).

➤ Laboratory Findings

- Early findings are decreased renal concentrating ability manifested by polyuria and polydipsia but no loss of ability to dilute urine; decreased urine osmolality.
- Urine is normal or contains RBCs, WBCs, WBC casts; proteinuria is usually slight or absent.
- Later findings include decreased GFR, decreased renal blood flow, azotemia.
- Renal insufficiency is insidious and slowly progressive; it may sometimes be reversed by correcting hypercalcemia.
- Laboratory findings are due to underlying disorders (e.g., hypercalciuria) and sequelae (e.g., stones).

HYPERCALCIURIA, IDIOPATHIC

➤ Definition

- This condition is generally defined as urine calcium >300 mg per 24 hours in men and >250 mg per 24 hours in women.
- There is increased excretion of urinary calcium >350 mg per 24 hours on a diet containing 600–800 mg/day: >4 mg/kg (either sex). More than 140 mg/g of urinary creatinine is most useful in short or obese patients (either sex).
- Diagnosis requires exclusion of all other causes of hypercalciuria; may be familial. It occurs in ~40% of patients who form calcium renal stones—in 5–10% of the general population.
- Types of hypercalciuria (2-hour urine collection after fasting)
  - Renal: calcium-to-creatinine ratio >0.15. Hypercalciuria persists despite absent dietary calcium in intestine following fasting; due to abnormality of renal tubular reabsorption. It is one-tenth as common as absorptive type.

- Absorptive: <20 mg calcium or calcium-to-creatinine ratio <0.15; 24-hour urine falls to <200 mg per 24 hours following low-calcium diet (400 mg/day) for 3–4 days. It is almost always due to primary increase in intestinal calcium absorption; probably autosomal dominant. This is the most common type.
- Resorptive (nonabsorptive): >30 mg calcium or calcium/creatinine ratio >0.15; due to primary hyperparathyroidism.
- Indeterminate: calcium 20–30 mg per 2-hour urine

➤ Laboratory Findings
- Normal blood calcium levels
- Serum 1,25-dihydroxyvitamin D3 levels are usually high.

IGA NEPHROPATHY

➤ Definition
- This immunologically mediated, focal proliferative GN is the most common form of GN.

➤ Who Should be Suspected?
- Presenting conditions may include persistent or intermittent microscopic hematuria with and variable proteinuria, episodes of painless gross hematuria often associated with (rather than following) 4–10 days infection of any type (usually upper respiratory), nephrotic syndrome, or Henoch-Schönlein purpura.

➤ Laboratory Findings
- Diagnosis is based on renal biopsy with immunofluorescence showing predominant mesangial IgA; IgG and C3 are variably present.
- Plasma IgA increased in ≤50% of patients
- Serum complement is normal.
- Progressive decline in renal function in ≤40% of cases; half of these reach ESRD in 5–25 years. Thirty percent or less have a benign course with persistent microscopic hematuria, proteinuria <1 g/day, and normal serum creatinine.
- IgA deposits may be associated with diseases of the GI tract (e.g., celiac disease), skin (e.g., dermatitis herpetiformis), liver (e.g., cirrhosis); carcinomas (e.g., lung, pancreas), immunologic (SLE, RA), infections (e.g., HIV, leprosy).

➤ Suggested reading
Donadio JV, Grande JP. IgA nephropathy. *New Engl J of Medicine.* 2002;347:738–748.

INFARCTION OF KIDNEY

➤ Causes
- Renal artery embolism (e.g., atrial fibrillation, atheroemboli, after myocardial infarction, myxoma, paradoxical embolism)
- Dissecting aneurysm of aorta or renal artery
- Renal artery vasculitis (e.g., polyarteritis nodosa)

• Renal artery thrombosis (e.g., atherosclerosis, hypercoagulability, angioplasty or catheterization, trauma)

➤ Laboratory Findings
• Microscopic or gross hematuria
• Urine may show no protein or abnormal sediment unless emboli reach glomeruli
• Proteinuria ($\leq 4+$) and pyuria may occur
• Serum LD may be increased markedly (>400 U/dL); it is the most sensitive laboratory abnormality, peaks on the third day, and returns to normal by tenth day. Urine LD may also be markedly increased.
• Increases in serum transaminases, WBC, CRP, and ESR are also increased if the area of infarction is large; the laboratory changes are similar to those developing over time in myocardial infarction.
• Increased serum ALP (from vascular endothelium) occurs in about one third of cases and is the least discriminating enzyme abnormality.
• BUN may increase but creatinine is normal unless other renal disease is present.
• Plasma renin activity (PRA) may rise on second day, peak about at about the 11th day, and remain elevated for more than a month.
• Laboratory findings due to infarction of other organs (e.g., brain, heart, retina, mesentery)
• Atheromatous emboli cause eosinophilia (>350 eosinophils/μL) and eosinophiluria, which are characteristic, occur in 70–80% of cases; increased ESR. Renal biopsy is specific for this diagnosis.
• Confirmed by renal angiography if surgery or fibrinolysis is planned or by CT scan.

➤ Suggested Reading
Hazanov N, et al. Acute renal embolism: forty-four cases of renal infarction in patients with atrial fibrillation. Medicine. 2004;83:292.

INTERSTITIAL NEPHRITIS

Acute

• Typically characterized by the clinical triad of fever, rash, and eosinophilia in patients in acute renal failure.

➤ Causes
• Recent exposure to a causative drug ($\leq 45\%$ of cases), especially antibiotics, diuretics, NSAIDs, anticonvulsants, miscellaneous (e.g., allopurinol, street drugs)
• Following infections, especially group A β-hemolytic streptococcal, diphtheria, brucellosis, leptospirosis, infectious mononucleosis, toxoplasmosis, Rocky Mountain spotted fever, measles
• Metabolic (e.g., calcium, oxalate, uric acid)
• Infiltrative (e.g., sarcoid, lymphoma, leukemia)
• Idiopathic

➤ Laboratory Findings
• Blood
  • Eosinophilia (in 60–100% of patients) with increased blood IgE

- Increased WBCs, neutrophils, and bands
- Anemia with Hb as low as 6.5 g/dL; no evidence of hemolysis or iron deficiency; negative indirect Coombs test; normal bone marrow. Anemia resolves when renal function becomes normal.
  - Increased ESR
  - Serum IgG is usually increased; serum complement is normal.
  - Varying degrees of renal insufficiency with increased BUN and creatinine, hyponatremia, hyperchloremic metabolic acidosis, and decreased serum albumin.
- Urine
  - May be oliguric or nonoliguric
  - Urinary indices similar to those seen in ATN
  - Eosinophiluria reported in ≤100% of patients
  - Microscopic hematuria
  - Proteinuria is usually mild to moderate, <1.0 g/m^2 per 24 hours, unless nephrotic syndrome is present.
  - Sterile pyuria is minimal or absent
  - Casts are uncommon
  - Low osmolality and specific gravity
  - Glycosuria without hyperglycemia may occur.
- Enlarged, poorly functioning kidneys may be demonstrated by IV pyelography, ultrasound, or renal scan.
- Nephrotic syndrome may occur.
- Biopsy of kidney establishes the diagnosis and is usually more severe than indicated by urinalysis and renal studies.

Chronic

- Causes
  - Infections, such as pyelonephritis
  - Not due to infections
    - Analgesic abuse
    - DM (see Diabetic Nephropathy)
    - Drugs: allergic (e.g., antibiotics, diuretics, phenytoin, cimetidine, NSAIDs); toxic (e.g., cyclosporine, lithium, cisplatin, amphotericin B)
  - Toxic substances
    - Exogenous (e.g., lead, mercury, cadmium)
    - Endogenous (uric acid [see Kidney Disorders in Gout], hypercalcemic nephropathy [see above])
    - Oxalate
  - Radiation nephritis
  - Sarcoidosis
  - Others
- Diagnosis is usually by exclusion. Renal biopsy may be helpful in undiagnosed cases.
- May be associated with metabolic acidosis and hyperkalemia out of proportion to degree of renal insufficiency, decreased urine concentrating capacity, and renal salt-wasting.

MINIMAL CHANGE DISEASE

- This condition was formerly called *lipoid nephrosis or nil lesion*.
- It may be associated with Hodgkin disease and non-Hodgkin lymphoma
- It is the most common cause of nephrotic syndrome in children and ≤30% in adults

➤ Laboratory Findings
- Microscopic hematuria occurs in fewer than one third of patients
- Light microscopy is normal.
- Fused epithelial podocytes are visible on EM; no immune deposits on DFA test.

MYELOMA KIDNEY

- See Plasma Cell Myeloma (see p. 859)

➤ Laboratory Findings
- Renal function is impaired in ≤50% of patients; usually there is loss of renal-concentrating ability and azotemia.
- Proteinuria is very frequent due to albumin and globulins in urine; BJ proteinuria may be intermittent. BJ protein occurs in <50% of myeloma patients but in almost all patients with renal failure due to myeloma kidney.
- Severe anemia out of proportion to azotemia occurs.
- Occasional changes due to altered renal tubular function are present.
  - Renal glycosuria, aminoaciduria, decreased serum uric acid, and renal potassium wasting
  - Renal loss of phosphate with decreased serum phosphorus and increased ALP
  - Nephrogenic DI
  - Oliguria or anuria with acute renal failure precipitated by dehydration
- Hyperchloremia or hyperbicarbonatemia with normal or low serum sodium values reduces the AG and should suggest myeloma in an appropriate clinical setting.
- Changes due to associated amyloidosis or hypercalcemia occur.

NEPHRITIC SYNDROME

- This immune disorder with acute onset of hematuria is characterized by urinary dysmorphic RBCs and RBC casts, hypertension, oliguria, and declining renal function (azotemia).

➤ Causes
- Renal (e.g., postinfectious [certain nephritogenic strains of streptococcal, staphylococcal, or pneumococcal infections; mumps, measles, chickenpox, hepatitis B and C]) or MPGN, anti-glomerular membrane disease
- Systemic (e.g., SLE, vasculitides, IgA nephropathy, Henoch-Schönlein purpura)

➤ Laboratory Findings
- Renal biopsy establishes the diagnosis.
- Decreased C3 complement

TABLE 8-7. Relative Frequency of Primary Glomerular Diseases Underlying Nephrotic Syndrome

Primary Glomerular Disease	Children Affected (%)	Adults Affected (%)	
		<60 years	<60 years
Minimal change disease	76	20	20
Membranous glomerulonephritis	7	40	39
Membranoproliferative glomerulonephritis	4	7	0
Focal segmental glomerulosclerosis	8	15	2
Other diseases	5	18	39

- Immunologic tests (e.g., antiglomerular basement, ASOT)
- Some proteinuria, but much less than in nephrotic syndrome

NEPHROTIC SYNDROME

- This syndrome presents as proteinuria >3.5 g/1.73 m^2 per 24 hours, hypoalbuminemia, hyperlipidemia, lipiduria, and edema.

➤ Causes
- Renal (causes 95% of cases in children, 60% in adults)
- Primary glomerular disease ($>$50% of patients) (Table 8-7)
  - Membranous GN: ~65% have spontaneous complete or partial remission of proteinuria, and ~15% develop ESRD
  - MPGN
  - Other proliferative GN (e.g., focal, IgA nephropathy, pure mesangial): 10% in children, 23% in adults
  - Rapidly progressive GN
  - Minimal change disease
  - Focal segmental glomerulosclerosis
- Systemic (most common)
  - Diabetic glomerulosclerosis (15% of adult patients): most common cause of nephrotic proteinuria
  - SLE (20% of adult patients)
  - Amyloidosis (primary and secondary)
- Systemic (less common)
  - Henoch-Schönlein purpura
  - Multiple myeloma
  - Goodpasture syndrome (rare)
  - Berger disease
  - Polyarteritis (rare)
  - Takayasu syndrome
  - Sarcoidosis
  - Sjögren syndrome

- Wegener granulomatosis (rare)
- Dermatitis herpetiformis
- Cryoglobulinemia
- Myxedema
- Venous obstruction
  - Obstruction of inferior vena cava (thrombosis, tumor)
  - Constrictive pericarditis
  - Tricuspid stenosis
  - CHF
- Infections
  - Bacterial (e.g., poststreptococcal GN, bacterial endocarditis, syphilis, leprosy)
  - Viral (HBV, HCV; also HIV, CMV, infectious mononucleosis, varicella)
  - Protozoal (quartan malaria)
  - Parasitic (schistosomiasis, filariasis, toxoplasmosis)
- Allergic (e.g., pollens, poison ivy and oak, bee sting, vaccines, antitoxins)
- Neoplasm-associated in 10% of adults and 15% older than age 60 years (e.g., Hodgkin disease; carcinomas of colon, lung, stomach and others; lymphomas and leukemia); paraproteinemia (multiple myeloma, light chain nephropathy). In adults with minimal change nephrotic syndrome without evident cause, first rule out Hodgkin disease. With membranous lesion, carcinoma may be more likely.
- Drugs, toxins (e.g., heavy metals, heroin, captopril, probenecid, NSAIDs, penicillamine, mephenytoin, ampicillin, anticonvulsants, chlorpropamide, lithium, rifampin, interferon alfa). Heroin may cause focal segmental glomerulosclerosis and progressive renal insufficiency.
- Hereditary/familial (e.g., Alport syndrome, Fabry disease, sickle cell disease). In atypical familial nephrotic syndrome, course is benign; more than one sibling is involved.
- Miscellaneous: toxemia of pregnancy, chronic allograft rejection, renal artery stenosis, malignant nephrosclerosis, ulcerative colitis

➤ Laboratory Findings
- Marked proteinuria: >3.5 g/1.73 m^2 body surface/day—usually >4.5 g/day
- Hyperlipidemia: increased serum cholesterol (free and esters)—usually >350 mg/dL (low or normal serum cholesterol occurs with poor nutrition and suggests poor prognosis); increased serum triglycerides, phospholipids, neutral fats, low-density beta-lipoproteins, and total lipids
- Decreased serum albumin (usually <2.5 g/dL) and total protein
- Serum α_2 and β-globulins are markedly increased, γ-globulin is decreased, and α_1 is normal or decreased. If γ-globulin is increased, rule out systemic disease (e.g., SLE).
- Urine containing doubly refractive fat bodies is seen by polarizing microscopy; many granular and epithelial cell casts
- Hematuria: present in 50% of patients but is usually minimal and not part of syndrome
- Azotemia: may be present but not part of syndrome
- Changes secondary to proteinuria and hypoalbuminemia (e.g., decreased serum calcium, decreased serum ceruloplasmin, increased fibrinogen)
- Serum C3 complement is normal in idiopathic lipoid nephrosis but decreased when there is underlying GN.

- Laboratory findings due to:
  - Primary disease
  - Increased susceptibility to infection (especially pneumococcal peritonitis) during periods of edema
  - Hypercoagulability with thromboembolism; abnormalities in coagulation factors, clotting inhibitors, fibrinolytic system, and platelet function have been described. Associated renal vein thrombosis has been reported in ~35% of patients (≤40% of these will have pulmonary emboli), especially when due to membranous nephropathy, MPGN, or rapidly progressive GN.
- Renal biopsy establishes the diagnosis.
- Urine immunoelectrophoresis should always be performed to rule out myeloma and renal primary (AL) amyloidosis.

NEPHROSCLEROSIS

- Atherosclerotic plaques of the small arteries and arterioles of the kidney secondary to hypertension.
- "Benign" nephrosclerosis ("essential hypertension")
  - Urine contains few or no protein or microscopic abnormalities.
  - 10% of patients develop marked renal insufficiency.
- "Accelerated" nephrosclerosis ("malignant hypertension")
  - Syndrome may occur in the course of "benign" nephrosclerosis, GN, unilateral renal artery occlusion, or any cause of hypertension.
  - Increasing uremia is associated with minimal or marked proteinuria and hematuria.

POLYARTERITIS NODOSA

➤ Definition
- This necrotizing vasculitis of medium-sized or small arteries without GN or vasculitis in arterioles, capillaries, or venules causes renal involvement in 75% of patients.
- See Chapter 4, Cardiovascular Disorders.

➤ Laboratory Findings
- Azotemia is often absent or only mild and slowly progressive.
- Albuminuria is always present.
- Hematuria (gross or microscopic) is very common. Fat bodies are frequently present in urine sediment.
- There may be findings of acute GN with remission or early death from renal failure.
- Always rule out polyarteritis in any case of GN, renal failure, or hypertension that shows unexplained eosinophilia, increased WBCs, or laboratory evidence of involvement of other organ systems.

PRERENAL AZOTEMIA

- This condition is characterized by abnormally high levels of nitrogen-type wastes in the blood.

TABLE 8-8. Sensitivity, Specificity, and Predictive Values of Tests in Predicting Bacteriuria (10^5 colonies/mL)

Test	Sensitivity (%)	Specificity (%)	Predictive Value (%) of Positive Test	Negative Test
>5 WBC/HPF	80	83	46	96
>10 WBC/HPF	63	90	53	93
Nitrite	69	90	57	94
Leukocyte esterase	71	85	47	94
Nitrite + leukocyte esterase (either positive)	86	86	54	97

* It occurs commonly in CHF and may occur in other functional forms of decreased renal perfusion (e.g., hepatorenal syndrome).

➤ **Laboratory Findings**

* Serum creatinine is rarely >4 mg/dL, even when BUN >100 mg/dL in pure prerenal azotemia. BUN/creatinine ratio is >20.
* Urine is hypertonic (increased osmolality) with low sodium concentration (<10 mEq/L).
* Protein excretion is frequently increased but rarely exceeds 2 g per 24 hours.
* Urine sediment may contain granular or hyaline casts, but cellular or pigmented casts are conspicuously absent.

PYELONEPHRITIS, ACUTE

* Involves diagnosis of UTI and determination of antibiotic sensitivity

➤ **Causes**

* Urinary outflow obstruction with ascending infection. See Table 8-8.
* Hematogenous (much less common)
* Vesicoureteric reflux
* Pyuria and bacteriuria

➤ **Limitations**

* When urine is allowed to remain at room temperature, the number of bacteria doubles every 30–45 minutes.
* False-low colony counts may occur with a high rate of urinary flow, low urine specific gravity, low urine pH, presence of antibacterial drugs, or inappropriate cultural techniques (e.g., tubercle bacilli, *Mycoplasma*, *Chlamydia trachomatis*, anaerobes).
* High doses of vitamin C may cause false-negative test for nitrite on dipstick.
* *Trichomonas* may cause a positive leukocyte esterase reaction.

➤ **Interpretation**

* Dipstick test for pyuria for detection of WBC, sensitivity is 100% for >50 WBCs per HPF, 90% for 21–50 WBCs, 60% for 12–20 WBCs, 44% for 6–12 WBCs. For detection of bacteria, sensitivity is 73% for "large" numbers and 46% for "moderate" numbers.

- Combined positive esterase and nitrate strips are sufficient indication for colony count to identify bacteriuria.
- Dipstick of first-catch urine is a cost-effective way to detect asymptomatic urethritis (*Chlamydia, Neisseria*) in males.
- Leukocyte esterase of neutrophil granules (intact or degenerated) does not detect lymphocytes. It has an NPV >90% and a PPV of 50% for bacterial infection. False-negative reaction may be caused by glycosuria, large doses of vitamin C, and some drugs. False-positive reaction may be caused by contaminated collection, indwelling catheters, foreign bodies, neoplasms, appendicitis, among others.
- Dye tests (bacterial reduction of dietary nitrate to nitrite; tetrazolium reduction) do not detect 10–50% of infections. False-negative reaction may be caused by some important bacteria that do not reduce dye (gram-positive) (e.g., coliforms are more likely to be detected than enterococci; bacteria show great variability in rate of dye reduction), urine has not incubated in patient's bladder for ≥4 hours, large doses of vitamin C. False-positive reaction may be due to contaminated collection and artifacts (e.g., amorphous urates and phosphates).
- Direct microscopic examination of uncentrifuged urine, either unstained or gram-stained that shows 1 PMN or 1 organism per HPF has sensitivity of 85% and specificity of 60% for bacteriuria. It may show >10% false-positive results.
  - Uncentrifuged urine showing 1 organism per oil-immersion field (threshold of detection for microscopy) correlates with count ≥10,000 colonies/mL.
  - Gram stain of cytospin specimen has >90% sensitivity and >80% specificity for ≥10^5/mL. With pyuria and bacteriuria, a Gram stain to differentiate gram-positive cocci (e.g., enterococci or *Staphylococcus aureus*) from gram-negative bacilli will indicate appropriate immediate initial therapy.
  - Less than 50% of patients with chronic UTI and asymptomatic bacteriuria may not show significant numbers of WBCs on urine microscopic examination; however, pyuria is associated with bacteriuria in ~90% of cases.
  - Presence of both bacteria and WBCs has a higher predictive value than either alone.
  - Large numbers of squamous epithelial cells may indicate a specimen that contains greater numbers of bacteria from the vagina or perineum rather than the urinary tract.
  - High ratio of WBCs to epithelial cells suggests infection.
- Bacteriuria and pyuria are often intermittent; in the chronic atrophic stage of pyelonephritis, they are often absent. In acute pyelonephritis, marked pyuria and bacteriuria are almost always present; hematuria and proteinuria may also be present during first few days.
- WBC casts are very suggestive of pyelonephritis. Glitter cells may be seen. A colony count should be performed under the following conditions: a midstream, clean-catch, first morning specimen is submitted in a sterilized container; the specimen is refrigerated until the colony count is performed; the periurethral area has first been thoroughly cleaned with soap. Transport tubes have an inhibitory effect and should be used. Suprapubic sterile needle aspiration is the most reliable sampling technique, and the presence of any organisms on culture is virtually diagnostic of UTI (97% sensitivity); it is the only acceptable method in infants, as urine collection bags have a very high false-positive rate; compared to urethral catheterization of adults, it is more accurate, simpler, and less traumatic.
  - Count of >100,000 bacteria/mL indicates active infection (>85% sensitivity).
  - Count of <10,000/mL in the absence of therapy largely rules out bacteriuria but pathogenic organisms may be clinically relevant.
  - Count of 10,000 to 100,000/mL should be repeated and cultured.

* Count of <100,000/mL with clinical findings of acute pyelonephritis with no obvious explanation such as recent use of antibiotics, suggests urinary tract obstruction or perinephric abscess.
* A culture should be performed for identification of the organism and determination of antibiotic sensitivity when these screening tests are positive. This antibiogram is useful to subsequently identify the same organism in relapsing infections.
* If culture shows a common gram-positive saprophyte, it should be repeated because the second culture is often negative.
* Causative bacteria are usually gram-negative rods (especially *Escherichia coli*); 5–20% are gram-positive cocci.
* Positive significant single culture or predominant organism should be considered positive in symptomatic patients (95% reliable), and repeat is unnecessary.
* Three or more species with none being predominant (i.e., >80% of the growth) almost always represents specimen contamination and culture should be repeated, but true mixed infections may occur after instrumentation or with chronic infection.
* *Pseudomonas* or *Proteus* may indicate an anatomic abnormality in the patient. If organism other than *E. coli* is found, the patient probably has chronic pyelonephritis, even if this is the first clinical episode of infection.
* In women, >80% of UTIs are caused by *E. coli*; a smaller percent are caused by *Staphylococcus saprophyticus*, and less often are caused by other aerobic gram-negative bacilli. In men, gram-negative bacilli cause ~75% of UTIs but *E. coli* causes only ~25% of infections in men and <50% of infections in boys.
* Other common gram-negative bacilli are *Proteus* and *Providencia* species. Gram-positive organisms (especially enterococci and coagulase-negative staphylococci) cause about 20% of infections in men and boys, but *S. saprophyticus* is rare. *Gardnerella vaginalis* is found in <3% of bacteriuric men.
* If *Candida* are isolated, should rule out contaminated specimen, diabetes mellitus, papillary necrosis, indwelling catheter, broad-spectrum antibiotic exposure, immunosuppressive chemotherapy, malignancy, and malnutrition.
* "Sterile" (i.e., pyogenic infection is absent) pyuria (≥10 WBC/HPF in centrifuged urine) and absence of bacilli (<1 bacillus in multiple oil immersion fields or 20–40 bacteria/HPF in centrifuged sediments) should cast doubt on diagnosis of untreated bacterial UTI and may occur in renal TB, chemical inflammation, mechanical inflammation (e.g., calculi, instrumentation), early acute GN prior to appearance of hematuria or proteinuria, polycystic kidney disease, papillary necrosis, chronic prostatitis, interstitial cystitis, transplant rejection, sarcoidosis, GU tract neoplasm, uric acid and hypercalcemic nephropathy, lithium and heavy metal toxicity, extreme dehydration, hyperchloremic renal acidosis, genital herpes, nonbacterial gastroenteritis, and respiratory tract infections, as well as after administration of oral polio vaccine. It may persist for several months after transurethral prostatectomy.
* When urine cultures are persistently negative in the presence of other evidence of pyelonephritis, a specific search should be made for tubercle bacilli.
* With pyuria and bacteriuria, persistent alkaline pH may indicate infection with urea-splitting organism (e.g., *Proteus*; less often *Pseudomonas* or *Klebsiella*), suggesting a calculus.
* Bacteria should be cleared from urine within 48 hours of antibiotic therapy; persistence indicates need to change antibiotic treatment or search for another explanation.

- Asymptomatic bacteriuria occurs in ≤15% of pregnant women. Routine urinalysis is done on first prenatal visit because 20–40% of untreated patients with positive culture develop acute pyelonephritis during pregnancy (occurs in only 1% of women with negative cultures).
- Persistent or recurrent infection may be caused by stones or obstruction. Greater than 10^5/mL colonies of a single organism found on culture of midstream specimen indicates significant bacteriuria.
- Bacteriuria may be found in
  - ≤15% of patients who are pregnant
  - 15% of patients with DM
  - 20% of patients with cystocele
  - ~50% of patients with dysuria
  - 70% of patients with prostatic obstruction
  - ≤5% of patients during catheterization
  - 95% of patients (untreated) with an indwelling catheter for >4 days
  - Should be searched for in elderly patients with altered mental status and infants with failure to thrive, persistent fever, or lethargy
  - Bacteriuria plus a positive dipstick test identified in specimens obtained by suprapubic aspiration, cystoscopy, nephrostomy, and renal transplant, suggests infection but with a negative dipstick test suggests colonization.
- Acute pyelonephritis shows two consecutive colony counts ≥100,000 organisms/mL with or without upper GU tract symptoms (flank pain, fever, costovertebral angle tenderness, fever, chills, nausea, vomiting, leukocytosis).
- Acute urethral syndrome and acute cystitis have a colony count ≥100 organisms/mL and lower GU tract symptoms (dysuria, frequency, urgency, suprapubic pain). Urine dipstick for WBC (leukocyte esterase) detects 8–WBCs per HPF. Pyuria is rarely present unless bacterial count >10,000/mL.
- Catheterization for <30 days or intermittent catheterization—criterion for bacteriuria is ≥100 organisms/mL; >95% of patients progress to >100,000 organisms/mL within days; multiple organisms are common.
- Catheterization for >30 days—mixed infections >100,000 organisms/mL in >75% of cases; organisms constantly change with new ones appearing every ~2 weeks
- Decreased glucose in urine (<2 mg/dL) in properly collected first-morning urine (no food or fluid intake after 10 PM, no urination during night) correlates well with colony count.
- Positive test for antibody-coated bacteria (using fluorescein-conjugated antihuman globulin) is said to indicate bacteria of renal origin and be 81% predictive of upper GU tract infection but negative in bacteria from lower tract infection. False-positives may occur with heavy proteinuria, prostatitis, or contamination with vaginal or rectal bacteria. False-negatives may occur in early infection. The test is less reliable in children and adults with neurogenic bladder. Test is not recommended for routine use.
- Albuminuria is usually <2 g per 24 hours (≤2+ qualitative) and, therefore, helps differentiate pyelonephritis from glomerular disease, in which albuminuria is usually >2 g per 24 hours; may be undetectable in a very dilute urine associated with fixed specific gravity.
- Beta$_2$ microglobulin is increased in 24-hour urine in pyelonephritis (due to tubular damage) but not in cystitis.

- LD-4 and LD-5 are increased in urine in renal medullary damage (pyelonephritis); less useful than beta$_2$ microglobulin to distinguish upper from lower urinary tract damage.
- Hyperchloremic acidosis (due to impaired renal acid excretion and bicarbonate reabsorption) occurs more often in chronic pyelonephritis than in GN.
- Decreased concentrating ability occurs relatively early in chronic renal infection but not bladder infections. Persistent dilute urine (low specific gravity or osmolarity) suggests renal rather than bladder infection if patient is not forcing fluid. Not a sensitive or specific test because of overlapping values, even though it is more marked in bilateral than unilateral infection and concentrating ability increases with cure.
- Renal blood flow and glomerular filtration show parallel decrease proportional to progress of renal disease. Comparison of function in right and left kidneys shows more disparity in pyelonephritis than in diffuse renal disease (e.g., nephrosclerosis, GN).
- Fluctuation in renal insufficiency (e.g., due to recurrent infection, dehydration) with considerable recovery is more marked and frequent in pyelonephritis than in other renal diseases.
- There is a decrease in 24-hour creatinine clearance before a rise in BUN and blood creatinine occurs.
- Laboratory findings of associated diseases (e.g., DM, urinary tract obstruction [e.g., stone, tumor]), neurogenic bladder dysfunction, are present. UTI in infant <1 year of age is associated with an underlying GU tract anomaly in 55% of male and 35% of female infants.
- Laboratory findings due to sequelae (e.g., papillary necrosis, bacteremia) are present.
- "Cured" patients should be followed with routine periodic urinalysis and colony count for at least 2 years because asymptomatic recurrence of bacteriuria is common

RADIATION NEPHRITIS

- This type of nephritis involves exposure (one or both kidneys) to >2,000 rads for 2–5 weeks. Injury related to total dose and duration.
- The latent period is >6–12 months.

➤ Acute
- Laboratory findings: abrupt onset hematuria; proteinuria; severe hypertension; severe normochromic, normocytic anemia (may be disproportionate)
- After >10 years, most affected individuals progress to chronic nephritis with diminishing renal function and severe hypertension

➤ Chronic
- Stable isolated proteinuria, mild-to-moderate hypertension, slow progression to renal failure
- Laboratory findings due to other complications of radiation (e.g., retroperitoneal fibrosis obstructing ureters, radiation neuropathy causing neurogenic bladder)

RENAL ARTERY STENOSIS

➤ Definition
- Narrowing of the renal artery secondary to atherosclerosis often leads to chronic renal insufficiency and ESRD. See Figure 8-2.

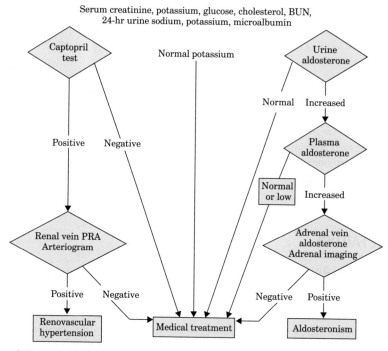

Figure 8-2. Algorithm for diagnosis of suspected renovascular hypertension (PRA, plasma renin activity.)

➤ Laboratory Findings
- Mild proteinuria occurs often.
- BUN and creatinine may show recent increase.
- PRA in peripheral vein is increased and may cause hypokalemic metabolic alkalosis.
- Urine sodium concentration may be low.
- There may be asymmetrical renal function or size (e.g., scan, ultrasound, pyelogram). IV pyelogram, arteriography, MRI, or Doppler sonography of renal arteries may support diagnosis.
- Late (>age 55) or early (<age 20) onset hypertension is often severe; stenosis is the cause in >70%.
- Ischemic nephropathy with irreversible parenchymal damage may occur.

RENAL ARTERY THROMBOSIS

➤ Definition
- This condition involves narrowing of one or both renal arteries or their branches. Bilateral involvement is present in half the cases.
- It is caused by atherosclerosis and less frequently by fibromuscular dysplasia. The common cause in the middle-aged and elderly is an atheromatous plaque at the origin of the renal artery.
- If not treated, it may lead to end-stage kidney failure.

➤ Who Should be Suspected?

• Candidates include patients with new-onset hypertension, rapid blood pressure swings, or increase in severity of known hypertension, especially if it becomes refractory to antihypertensive therapy.
• Old age, the existence of other atherosclerotic lesions, and the presence of chronic kidney disease are risk factors.

➤ Laboratory Findings

Laboratory tests are generally nonspecific. The diagnosis is made by imaging studies.

• Urinalysis: mild proteinuria; low urine sodium concentration
• BUN and creatinine may show recent increase

➤ Suggested Reading

Dworkin LD, Cooper CJ. Clinical practice: renal-artery stenosis. *N Engl J Med.* 2009;2009;361:1972–1978.

RENAL FAILURE

Renal Failure, Acute

➤ Definition

• Acute renal failure (ARF) is a rapid decline in function that limits the kidney's ability to maintain homeostasis and eliminate nitrogenous waste. The distinction between acute and chronic renal failure is not always clear. It is reflected by a rise in plasma creatinine (see p. 136), an abnormality in urinalysis (see p. 372), or electrolyte and acid–base abnormalities that have developed over a few hours to a few days.
• The causes resulting in ARF can be divided into three categories: those resulting from impaired kidney perfusion (prerenal azotemia), those resulting from injury to the nephrons themselves (intrinsic), and those resulting from obstruction of the urinary flow (postrenal).

➤ Who Should be Suspected?

Patients with ARF present in a variety of ways:

• Patients with symptoms suggestive of uremia. (The term *uremia* describes the clinical syndrome associated with the retention of the end products of nitrogen metabolism that occurs with severe reduction in renal function. It can be a consequence of either acute or chronic renal failure.)
• Patients with *oliguria* (urine outflow of <500 mL/day) or *anuria* (<100 mL/day urine output).
• Patients with an elevated serum creatinine.
• Hospitalized patients with severe losses of extracellular fluid, the use of nephrotoxic drugs, sepsis, or following the use of radiographic contrast agents and above described symptoms or findings.

➤ Laboratory Findings

Laboratory findings are essential. Patients with postrenal disease are diagnosed by clinical presentation and imaging studies.

• Urinalysis is the most important noninvasive test in the diagnosis of ARF and its etiology. Microscopic examination is normal in most instances of prerenal disease (for abnormalities in intrinsic renal disease, see p. 736). The presence of RBC casts indicates glomerular disease. Finding cellular debris or granular casts suggests ischemic or nephrotoxic ARF.

- Urine sodium is low in prerenal disease and high in acute kidney injury. Calculation of FE_{Na} (see p. 338), which refers to urine and plasma sodium, as well as urine and plasma creatinine, is an accurate method to differentiate between prerenal and renal ARF. It distinguishes ATN (elevated) from prerenal azotemia (decreased to $<1\%$).
- Urine osmolality. If high, it suggests prerenal disease; if low, it may be a marker of ATN. Urine osmolality and urine specific gravity are of limited value in establishing the etiology of ARF.
- Urine volume is low in prerenal disease; it may be low or normal in patients with ATN.
- Plasma or serum creatinine is elevated at diagnosis and continues to rise. The rate of rise may be helpful in diagnosing different etiologies of ARF.
- GFR (see p. 139) gives an approximate estimation of the number of functioning nephrons. Estimation of GFR has a prognostic rather than diagnostic utility with respect of type of ARF.
- BUN/plasma creatinine ratio is normal in intrinsic renal disease (10–15:1), but elevated ($>20:1$) in prerenal disease.
- Urine to plasma creatinine concentration. The ratio is high in patients with prerenal disease but low in renal causes of ARF.
- New biomarkers to diagnose parenchymal renal disease are under investigation.
- Ancillary laboratory assays may point to specific etiologies.
  - Anemia is more often present in chronic renal failure. When it is severe and of recent onset it suggests hemolysis, plasma cell dyscrasia, or TTP/HUS.
  - Acid–base balance abnormalities reflect the severity of electrolyte imbalance.
  - Hyperphosphatemia eventually develops in ARF.
  - A combination of hyperkalemia, hyperphosphatemia, hypocalcemia, and elevations in uric acid and CK (MM isoenzyme) suggest rhabdomyolysis.
  - Hyperuricemia in association with hyperkalemia, hyperphosphatemia, and increased levels of LDH may indicate acute urate nephropathy and tumor lysis syndrome.
  - A wide anion and osmolal gap indicates the ingestion of methanol or ethylene glycol

➤ Limitations
- In patients with preexisting renal disease, none of the laboratory criteria for the diagnosis of prerenal disease is present
- FE_{Na} may give misleading information in certain clinical conditions: urinary tract obstruction, acute glomerular disease where urinary excretion of sodium may be low, prior administration of diuretics, and in preexisting renal disease.

➤ Suggested Reading
Post TW, Rose BD. Diagnostic approach to the patient with acute or chronic kidney disease. UptoDate. Rose B, ed. Waltham, MA: UptoDate, Inc.; 2009.

Renal Failure, Chronic
➤ Definition
- Chronic renal failure (CRF) occurs when there is a progressive, irreversible reduction in the number of nephrons, as reflected by a gradual increase in BUN and creatinine, and/or albuminuria. CRF is said to be present when the renal disease exists for >3 months. CRF

becomes more prevalent with increasing age. The distinction between acute, subacute, and chronic kidney disease is not always clearcut but it is important, since ARF (see p. 736) may be reversible, whereas CRF is not. A reduced size of the kidney (demonstrated by ultrasound) indicates the chronic phase. Renal disease is divided into five stages on the basis of severity. Stage 5, the most advanced, is also called *end-stage renal disease* (ESRD).

* The majority of cases of CRF are due to:
  * Glomerular disease (e.g. nephritic syndrome, renal vascular disease, benign nephrosclerosis, DN, renal artery stenosis, and cholesterol atherothrombotic disease), or following GN or pyelonephritis
  * Tubular and interstitial disease
  * Long-standing obstructive uropathy

➤ Who Should be Suspected?

* Patients who have had acute renal injury or GN, or those who have diabetes or uncontrolled hypertension.
* Those in whom symptoms develop insidiously, suggesting uremia (easy fatigability [result of chronic, progressive anemia], anorexia, vomiting, mental status changes, seizures), or generalized edema.
* Those in whom renal function or urinalysis abnormalities are discovered incidentally; the changes may be slowly progressive.
* Those with a family history of CRF, who may have a congenital renal abnormality.

➤ Laboratory Findings

Laboratory studies are indicated once renal disease is suspected. Note that until renal insufficiency is severe, adaptation of tubular function allows the excretion of relatively normal amounts of water and sodium.

* Serum (or plasma) creatinine and BUN increase in parallel.
* Creatinine clearance (see p. 136), established via well-accepted formulas, is used to estimate the GFR. This parameter is useful in stable patients to evaluate the degree of impaired renal function; it has no etiologic diagnostic value. Repeated determinations, in conjunction with creatinine values, establish whether the patient has stable or progressive disease.
* Urinalysis (see p. 363)
  * Microscopic examination is the most important tool in determining the etiology of CRF. WBC, RBC, and casts are usually found.
  * Dipstick examination for albumin, glucose, pH, and blood contribute to determining the etiology of CRF (bacterial cultures and free pigments [Hb, myoglobin]).
* Blood pH: acidosis is a frequent complication of advanced CRF.
* Serum phosphate (hyperphosphatemia)
* Serum potassium (hypokalemia, uncommon), superseded by hyperkalemia
* Serum sodium (hyponatremia)
* Serum calcium (hypocalcemia)
* Serum magnesium (hypermagnesemia)
* Serum uric acid is increased
* Serum amylase is frequently increased
* Serum protein (hypoalbuminemia is common in the nephrotic syndrome [see p. 727]). Hypergammaglobulinemia with monoclonal gammopathy suggests myeloma kidney as the etiology of CRF.

TABLE 8-9. Chief Causes of Chronic Insufficiency in Patients Presenting for Dialysis

Glomerulonephritis	44%
Diabetic nephropathy	15%
Nephrosclerosis and renal vascular disease	12%
Congenital or hereditary disease (including polycystic kidney)	10%
Chronic pyelonephritis	6%
Others and unknown	15%

- Serum lipids: increased triglycerides, cholesterol, and VLDL lipoprotein levels are common; severe hyperlipidemia accompanies the nephrotic syndrome (see p. 727)
- Metabolic acidosis
- Anemia develops with reductions of renal function to 30–50% of normal; it is caused by reduction in the synthesis of erythropoietin
- Coagulation studies may be affected by uremic by-products such as guanidinosuccinic acid and exuberant production of nitrous oxide by uremic vessels, resulting in abnormal platelet function

▶ **Suggested Reading**

Levey ASW, Coresh J, Balk E, et al. National Kidney Foundation practice guidelines for chronic kidney disease: evaluation, classification, and stratification. *Ann Intern Med.* 2003;139:137–147.

DIALYSIS FOR END-STAGE RENAL DISEASE, LABORATORY TESTS FOR MANAGEMENT

- See Table 8-9 and further details in appropriate sections.

▶ **Conditions to Evaluate Routinely**

- Azotemia (creatinine and BUN; tests for residual renal functions, including 24-hour urine volume)
- Electrolyte and mineral balance (e.g., serum calcium, potassium, chloride, bicarbonate, phosphorus)
- Liver function tests (serum total protein, albumin, LD, ALP, AST); HBsAg (if seronegative or if antibodies are present after HBV vaccination)
- Renal osteodystrophy (osteomalacia) (serum calcium and phosphorus and quarterly serum PTH for secondary hyperparathyroidism)
- Anemia (CBC)
- Coagulation disorders (clotting time with each dialysis; weekly PT if on warfarin)

▶ **Conditions to Evaluate Nonroutinely**

- Tests for bleeding or clotting disorders
- Heart disease (e.g., uremic pericarditis, hypertension, hyperlipidemia)
- Bone disease (hyperparathyroid bone disease due to hyperphosphatemia and low $1,25(OH)_2$ vitamin D_3 levels)
- Hepatitis
- Symptomatic endocrine problems

* Uremic neuropathies
* Acute complications associated with dialysis (e.g., catheter infection, infective endocarditis, peritonitis if peritoneal dialysis)
* Tests for aluminum toxicity as cause of encephalopathy, vitamin D-resistant osteodystrophy, and iron-resistant anemia. Histochemical staining of bone biopsy (if serum level >100 µg/L) or atomic absorption of serum (>200 µg/L = toxic; >100 µg/L "view with concern"; 60–100 µg/L appears to cause no problem). Serum assay every 6–12 months or every 3 months especially in pediatric patients; serum level may not reflect tissue content.
* Iron overload (due to frequent transfusions; now replaced by erythropoietin therapy)
* Special tests for specific conditions (e.g., acquired renal cystic disease causing renal cell carcinoma, control of DM)

RENAL TRANSPLANTATION

➤ Laboratory Criteria for Kidney Donation
* Living donor
  * Three successive urinalyses and cultures must be negative
  * There must be no evidence of HBV, HCV, HIV, CMV, malignancy, history of renal disease, or severe hypertension.
* Cadaveric donor
  * Likewise, there must be no evidence of HBV, HCV, HIV, CMV, malignancy, history of renal disease, or severe hypertension.
* Donor and recipient must show
  * ABO and Rh blood group compatibility
  * Leukoagglutinin, mixed lymphocyte culture compatibility
  * Platelet agglutinin compatibility

➤ Indications of Rejection
* Total urine output is decreased.
* Proteinuria is increased.
* Cellular or granular casts appear.
* Urine osmolality is decreased.
* BUN and creatinine increase.
* Hyperchloremic renal tubular acidosis may be an early sign of rejection or indicate smoldering rejection activity.
* Renal clearance values decrease.
* Sodium iodohippurate ^{131}I renogram is altered.
* Biopsy of kidney shows a characteristic microscopic appearance allowing definitive diagnosis.
* Sequential measuring of subsets of activated T cells by flow cytometry is useful for diagnosis of rejection and monitoring reversibility of rejection.
* Messenger RNA recovered from cells in urine encoding cytotoxic proteins perforin and granzyme B are reported to be increased by PCR in acute rejection
* Recurrent diseases following rejection

* GN, especially dense deposit disease, anti-GBM disease, focal glomerulosclerosis, membranous nephropathy
* Diabetic intercapillary glomerulosclerosis (Kimmelstiel-Wilson syndrome)
* Amyloidosis

➤ Suggested Reading

Li B, Hartono C, Ding R, et al. Noninvasive diagnosis of renal-allograft rejection by measurement of messenger RNA for perforin and granzyme B in urine. *N Engl J Med.* 2001;344:947.

RENAL TUBULAR ACIDOSIS

* Renal tubular acidosis (RTA) involves the nonuremic defects of urine acidification due to renal bicarbonate loss. It results in hyperchloremic metabolic acidosis

➤ Distal (Type 1)

* Collecting ducts do not secrete sufficient H^+ to form ammonium or backleak of secreted H^+ out of collecting tubule lumen; occurs predominantly in females (70%).
* Hyperchloremic acidosis, low plasma bicarbonate concentration; should be suspected in any patient with metabolic acidosis with normal AG and inappropriately high urine pH (>5.3 in adults, >5.6 in children).
* Incomplete type 1 RTA should be suspected with normal plasma bicarbonate concentration, urine pH persistently >5.3, and calcium stone disease, or positive family history.
* Alkaline urine (pH 6.5–7.0) that persists at any level of plasma bicarbonate
* Ammonium loading test (NH_4Cl 0.1 g/kg) shows inability to acidify urine below pH 6.5 and depressed rates of excretion of titratable acid and ammonium.
* No other tubular defects
* Often presents with complications (e.g., nephrocalcinosis, interstitial nephritis renal calculi, rickets, and osteomalacia) as well as growth retardation
* Most commonly caused by autoimmune disorders (e.g., Sjögren syndrome) or hypercalciuria in adults and hereditary form in children

Hypokalemic or Normokalemic Type

* Primary (inability of tubular cell to secrete enough H^+)
* Secondary
  * Increased serum globulins (especially gamma) (e.g., SLE, Sjögren syndrome, Hodgkin disease, sarcoidosis, chronic active hepatitis, cryoglobulinemia)
  * Pyelonephritis
  * Medullary sponge kidney
  * Ureterosigmoidostomy
  * Hereditary insensitivity to ADH (vasopressin)
  * Various renal diseases (e.g., hypercalcemia, potassium-losing disorders, medullary cystic disease, polyarteritis nodosa, amyloidosis, Sjögren syndrome)
  * Various genetically transmitted disorders (e.g., Ehlers-Danlos syndrome, Fabry disease, hereditary elliptocytosis)
  * Starvation, malnutrition
  * Hyperthyroidism, hyperparathyroidism
  * Vitamin D intoxication

Hyperkalemic Type (Due to Impaired Sodium Reabsorption in Cortical Collecting Tubules)

- Hypoaldosteronism
- Obstructive nephropathy
- SLE
- Sickle cell nephropathy
- Cyclosporine toxicity

➤ Proximal (Type 2)

- Results from defective bicarbonate reabsorption in the proximal tubule
  - Low plasma bicarbonate concentration with hyperchloremic acidosis
  - Alkaline urine that becomes acid if extracellular bicarbonate level is decreased below the patient's maximum reabsorptive limit
- Normal urine pH in the absence of bicarbonate in the urine
- IV NaHCO$_3$ ($\leq$1.0 mEq/kg/hour) causes rapid increase in urine pH even though plasma HCO$_3^-$ has increased but is still less than normal (24–26 mEq/L).
- Proximal RTA is diagnosed by fractional excretion of bicarbonate >15% when plasma bicarbonate is >20 mEq/L.
- Most commonly due to increased excretion of monoclonal Ig light chains in multiple myeloma or carbonic anhydrase inhibitor (e.g., acetazolamide for glaucoma) in adults and cystinosis or idiopathic cause in children

Primary (defect in bicarbonate reabsorption)

- Usually occurs in males
- Only clinical manifestation is retarded growth; renal and metabolic complications are absent
- Good prognosis with clinical response to alkali therapy, which is usually not permanently required

Secondary

- Idiopathic or secondary Fanconi syndrome (cystinosis, Lowe syndrome [X-linked recessive disorder with congenital cataracts, neurologic involvement], tyrosinemia, glycogen storage disease, Wilson disease, hereditary fructose intolerance, heavy metal intoxication, toxic effect of drugs such as outdated tetracycline)
- Vitamin D–deficient rickets
- Medullary cystic disease
- Following renal transplantation
- Nephrotic syndrome, multiple myeloma, renal amyloidosis

➤ Incomplete or Mixed (Type 3)

- May be seen in obstructive uropathy and in hereditary fructose intolerance.

➤ Hypera Aldosteronism (Type 4)

- Consists of a variety of conditions characterized by:
  - Mild to moderate renal impairment
  - Hyperchloremic acidosis
  - Hyperkalemia
  - Acid urine pH

- Reduced ammonium secretion
- Frequently, tendency to lose sodium in urine
- Decreased mineralocorticoid secretion in some patients due to isolated hypoaldosteronism; others have decreased tubular response to aldosterone.

RENAL VEIN THROMBOSIS

➤ Definition

- This vascular disorder involves occlusion of one or both main renal veins by a thrombus.
- It occurs as a secondary event in a variety of settings: nephritic or nephrotic syndromes; compression by tumors, especially lymphatic ones; trauma; invasion by carcinomas; severe dehydration in infants; DIC; pregnancy; and use of oral contraceptives in the presence of underlying thrombophilia (see p. 887). The nephrotic syndrome itself (see above) is considered a hypercoagulable state.

➤ Who Should be Suspected?

- Infants with acute loss of renal function
- Patients with subacute or chronic deterioration of renal function with hematuria and proteinuria in the appropriate setting, including those with thrombophilia or an underlying renal disease
- Frequently associated with deep venous thrombosis or pulmonary embolism.

➤ Laboratory Findings

- Urinalysis: hematuria, proteinuria (variable from day to day). microscopic pyuria
- Elevated creatinine and decreased creatinine clearance
- Leukocytosis and anemia
- Elevated fibrin degradation products and D-dimers
- Evidence of RTA
- Hypercholesterolemia
- Hyperosmolality
- Various laboratory findings according to the underlying disease. The definitive diagnosis is made by imaging studies.

➤ Suggested Reading

Wysokinski WE, Gosk-Bierska I, Green EL, et al. Clinical characteristics and long-term follow-up of patients with renal vein thrombosis. *Am J Kidney Dis.* 2008;51:224–232.

SCLERODERMA (PROGRESSIVE SYSTEMIC SCLEROSIS), RENAL DISEASE

- Renal involvement occurs in two thirds of patients; one third die of renal failure.
- See Chapter 12, Immune and Autoimmune Diseases.
- Clinical cause of slowly progressive renal insufficiency with moderate proteinuria often <2 g/day and hypertension, or less commonly, ARF, which may be associated with malignant hypertension, CHF, microangiographic hemolytic anemia, and marked increase in PRA.

SICKLE CELL NEPHROPATHY

- Renal functional abnormalities are very common.
- Albuminuria (macro- and micro-) occurs in ≤68% of patients; usually 1–2 g/day
- Gross hematuria is relatively common.
- Early decrease of renal concentrating ability is evident in heterozygotes as well as homozygotes; more pronounced in HbSS and HbSC. Progressively decreases with age. The decrease is temporarily reversed in children by transfusion but not in adults.
- Even with normal BUN, GFR, and renal plasma flow sickle cell nephropathy may occur in sickle cell trait
- Chronic renal failure occurs only with HbSS (4.2%) or HbSC (2.4%) diseases.
- Papillary necrosis occurs in 39% of Hb SS patients.
- RTA may produce severe hypokalemia.

SYSTEMIC LUPUS ERYTHEMATOSUS NEPHRITIS

- See Table 8-10 [cross refer to SLE in the Autoimmune section].

➤ Who Should be Suspected?
- Renal involvement occurs in two thirds of patients with SLE.

TABLE 8-10. Comparison of Clinical and Morphologic Types of Systemic Lupus Erythematosus Nephritis

	Mesangial Changes (% of patients)	Focal Proliferative GN (% of patients)	Diffuse Proliferative GN (% of patients)	Membranous GN (% of patients)
% of total patients	39	27	16	18
Hematuria, pyuria	13	53	78	50
Proteinuria	36	67	89	100
Nephrotic syndrome	0	27	56	90
Azotemia	13	20	22	10
Decreased complement	54	77	100	75
Increased anti-DNA	45	75	80	33
Decreased complement and increased anti-DNA	36	63	80	33
Hypertension	22	40	56	50
Prognosis	Better	Worse	Worse	Better

Source: Appel GB. The course of management of lupus nephritis. *Intern Med.* 1981;2:82.

* Nephritis of SLE may occur as acute, latent, or chronic GN, nephrosis, or asymptomatic albuminuria or hematuria.

➤ Laboratory Findings
* Urine findings are as in chronic active GN. Azotemia or marked proteinuria usually indicates death in 1–3 years.
* Laboratory findings of SLE may disappear during active nephritis, nephrosis, or uremia. Examination of needle biopsy should always include immunofluorescent and electron as well as light microscopy. May show normal or minimal disease, mesangial lesions, focal or diffuse proliferative GN, or membranous GN.
* Laboratory findings due to drug therapy:
  * Prednisone
  * Cytotoxic drugs (e.g., azathioprine, cyclophosphamide): leukopenia—nadir WBC kept at 1,500–4,000/μL, infection (e.g., herpes zoster, opportunistic organisms), gonadal toxicity, hemorrhagic cystitis, neoplasia

THIN BASEMENT MEMBRANE NEPHROPATHY (BENIGN FAMILIAL HEMATURIA)

* This relatively common familial disorder is manifested by asymptomatic hematuria (see p. 761) without proteinuria. The genetic defect is similar to that of hereditary nephritis (Alport syndrome), but the patients do not present with hearing loss, ocular abnormalities, or renal failure. Patients with the basement membrane nephropathy can be considered as being carriers of autosomal recessive Alport syndrome.
* The hematuria clears spontaneously with time.
* Possible candidates are patients with a familial history of hematuria (present in 30–50% of patients) and macroscopic hematuria associated with flank pain but without evidence of renal disease.
* Laboratory diagnosis is directed to exclude other glomerular disorders that may cause isolated hematuria, such as IgA nephropathy and Alport syndrome.
* Renal biopsy is unnecessary in most cases, especially in the absence of proteinuria.

➤ Suggested Reading
Tryggvason K, Patrakka J. Thin basement nephropathy. *J Am Soc Nephrol.* 2006;17:813–822.

URIC ACID NEPHROPATHY

➤ Definition
* Hyperuricemia causes several renal problems resulting from kidney deposition of uric acid, all of which may be defined under the umbrella of uric acid nephropathies. Laboratory findings depend on the type of uric acid nephropathy.
* Chronic urate nephropathy, sometimes referred to as urate nephrosis, is a rare form of renal insufficiency caused by deposition of urate crystals in the kidney's medullary interstitium and pyramids.

- Acute uric acid nephropathy is a reversible cause of renal insufficiency resulting from deposition of large amounts of uric acid crystals in the renal collecting ducts, renal pelvis, and ureters. It is characterized by severe oliguria or anuria.
- Uric acid nephrolithiasis may develop as the consequence of hyperuricemia.

➤ Who Should be Suspected?

- Patients with chronic renal insufficiency and severe hyperuricemia
- Patients with acute onset oliguria or anuria, especially following chemotherapy or radiation therapy (tumor lysis syndrome) for a hematologic malignancy or, less commonly, intensive chemotherapy for a nonhematologic tumor; those with Lesch-Nyhan syndrome; and those with Fanconi-like syndrome with decreased uric acid reabsorption in the proximal tubules.
- Patients with gout and attack of renal colic. These are subjects exposed to dehydration in high temperature climate or with chronic diarrhea, diabetic patients with metabolic syndrome; and patients with aggressive myeloproliferative neoplasms and hyperuricemia.

➤ Laboratory Findings

- In uric acid nephrolithiasis, chemical examination of a passed stone reveals uric acid or a nidus of uric acid surrounded by calcium oxalate or calcium phosphate.
- Twenty-four–hour collection (if urine is available) may reveal hyperuricemia. In the acute uric acid nephropathy, the uric acid to creatinine ratio is >1.0, whereas in most forms of ARF with decreased urinary output, the ratio is <1. Uric acid crystals may be visualized in the urine sediment. Otherwise the sediment is relatively bland in uric acid nephropathies.
- Serum uric acid may be elevated (see discussion of pseudogout, p. 932) out of proportion to the degree of renal failure; it is greatly elevated in the tumor lysis syndrome.
- Hyperkalemia, hyperphosphatemia, and hypocalcemia may accompany the acute uric acid nephropathy, especially when it is the result of severe tissue destruction, such as in the tumor lysis syndrome.

➤ Suggested Readings

Rose BD, Becker MA. Uric acid renal disease. UptoDate. Rose B, ed. Waltham, MA: UptoDate Inc.; 2009.
Rose BD, Becker MA. Uric acid nephrolithiasis. UptoDate. Rose B, ed. Waltham, MA: UptoDate Inc.; 2009.

CONGENITAL DISORDERS OF THE KIDNEY

HEREDITARY NEPHRITIS

- This disorder is classified into two types:
  - Fabry disease
  - Alport syndrome: familial X-linked disease of type IV collagen associated with nerve deafness and lens defects is rare, with gene located at Xq13. It is characterized by glomerular hematuria with normal complement, and nephrotic syndrome occurs in 40% of cases. Renal disease is progressive to ESRD.
- Renal biopsy showing EM changes in GBMs and immunohistochemistry of skin biopsy
- Prenatal and presymptomatic diagnosis is by linkage analysis or by direct gene studies in previously tested families.

HORSESHOE KIDNEYS

- This condition involves fusion of two kidneys across midline, usually at lower pole; usually associated with malrotation and other developmental abnormalities (e.g., Turner syndrome).
- Laboratory findings due to complications of ureteral obstruction (e.g., pyelonephritis, renal stones) occur.

POLYCYSTIC KIDNEY DISEASES

- Polycystic kidney disease (PKD) is a genetic disorder characterized by the growth of numerous cysts in the kidney.

➤ Autosomal Dominant Form (ADPKD)

- Usually slowly progressive and asymptomatic until patient is >50 years of age; accounts for ~10% of transplant or dialysis cases. Renal failure is inevitable.
- Type I accounts for ≤90% of cases. Type II accounts for ≤15% of cases, with later onset symptoms, slower progression to renal failure, and longer life expectancy.
- Laboratory findings in ADPKD due to
  - Cysts that may occur in liver, ovary, pancreas, spleen, and CNS
  - Associated intracranial aneurysms that cause cerebral hemorrhage and death in >10% of patients

➤ Familial Nephronophthisis (Autosomal Recessive)

- This form is usually more severe and becomes manifest earlier, and there are few survivors as adults.
- Cysts occur in the medulla at the border of the cortex with bilateral shrunken kidneys.

➤ Medullary Cystic Kidney

- Autosomal dominant traits with bilateral shrunken kidneys occur.
- This condition first appears in adulthood and is clinically milder than nephronophthisis.
- Renal failure is inevitable.

➤ Medullary Sponge Kidney

- Findings are due to complications (e.g., calculi in ≤50% of cases; infection; hematuria).
- Disease is asymptomatic, not progressive, and renal failure is rare.

➤ Other Inherited Conditions (Associated with Renal Cysts)

- Von Hippel-Lindau disease, tuberous sclerosis
- Acquired form: Simple cysts due to aging; multicystic may be seen due to drugs, hormones, chronic renal failure of any etiology, and ≤90% of dialysis (for >10 years) patients
- May show polyuria, salt wasting, progressive renal insufficiency, hypertension, growth retardation. Anemia of renal failure is less severe than in other forms of kidney disease. Polycythemia may occur due to production of erythropoietin that may be increased.
- Polyuria is common.
- Hematuria may be gross and episodic or an incidental microscopical finding.
- Proteinuria occurs in about one third of patients and is mild (<1 g per 24 hours).
- Renal calculi may be associated (≤30% of ADPKD patients).
- Superimposed UTI is frequent (33% of patients).

- Death occurs within 5 years after BUN rises to 50 mg/dL (33% of patients).
- Death usually occurs in early infancy or in middle age, when superimposed nephrosclerosis of aging or pyelonephritis has exhausted renal reserve.
- Increased incidence of gout occurs in patients with polycystic kidneys.
- Prenatal diagnosis is possible using DNA obtained by amniocentesis or chorionic villus sampling.
- Diagnosis is usually made by ultrasound; MRI and CT are more sensitive.

➤ Suggested Reading

Wilson PD. Polycystic kidney disease. *N Engl J Med*. 2004;350:151.

RENAL DISEASE, INFECTIOUS*

BACTERIAL ABSCESS

➤ Definition

- Renal and perinephric abscesses are usually a complication of UTI but may also be caused by hematogenous seeding of necrotic renal tissue or perinephric fat.
- Structural abnormalities (e.g., cysts), functional abnormalities (resulting in reflux), trauma (including surgery), foreign bodies (including stones), and DM predispose to these infections. Perirenal abscess may result from infection, due to various organisms, of a perirenal hematoma (e.g., due to trauma, tumor, polyarteritis nodosa).

➤ Who Should be Suspected?

- Patients usually present with fever, rigors, flank pain, abdominal pain, nausea, and other symptoms similar to pyelonephritis. Renal abscess may be suspected because of delayed response to treatment for pyelonephritis. Onset may be subtle in the elderly and in patients with chronic neurologic disorders.
- The etiology is similar to UTI, with *E. coli* and other uropathogens the most common causes. There is an increased frequency of polymicrobial abscesses, especially those associated with stones and neurologic conditions.

➤ Laboratory Studies

- Urine: For abscesses caused by complicated pyelonephritis, urinalysis generally shows abnormalities consistent with UTI. Urine culture should be positive if effective antimicrobial therapy has not been given. Renal abscesses due to hematogenous spread are usually located in the renal cortex and may be associated with normal urinalysis and sterile urine culture. Renal abscess (often multiple) due to hematogenous seeding should be suspected in patients with urine cultures positive for *S. aureus*.
- Blood culture: A primary or secondary bloodstream infection should be ruled out by collection of two or three sets of blood cultures. Blood culture may be the only source for isolation, with subsequent infectious diseases and susceptibility testing of the causative pathogen.
- Core laboratory: Signs consistent with systemic infection are frequently seen, with elevation and shift of WBCs, elevated ESR and CRP, and other nonspecific signs of inflammation. Laboratory findings due to underlying disease (e.g., obstruction, calculi, diabetes) may be apparent.

---

* Submitted by Michael Mitchell MD

TUBERCULOSIS, RENAL*

* The clinical manifestations of renal TB are variable; many patients show minimal symptoms and may be identified after work-up for pyuria or microhematuria, which are almost universally seen. The disease is caused by hematogenous seeding of the kidney during mycobacteremia that may occur during primary infection or miliary dissemination.
* Diagnosis should be suspected in a patient with a history or increased risk of mycobacterial disease, especially TB, and signs (e.g., microhematuria or pyuria) or symptoms (e.g., dysuria) of UTI. Routine urine culture is negative, although contaminated urine or coincidental UTI may confound the diagnosis.
* Mycobacteria are shed intermittently, so four to six first-morning samples should be submitted for mycobacterial culture. Mycobacterial culture of samples from other potentially infected sites is also recommended, as well as skin (or comparable) testing for TB.
* See discussion of TB for general findings.

TUMORS OF THE KIDNEY

RENAL CELL CARCINOMA

➤ Definition
* This cancer originates from the proximal tubule; ≤80% are the clear cell type.
* Even in the absence of the classic loin pain, flank mass, and hematuria, renal cell carcinoma should be ruled out in the presence of these unexplained (paraneoplastic) laboratory findings, which are associated with a poorer prognosis.

➤ Laboratory Findings
* Abnormal liver function tests (in absence of metastases to liver) are found in 40% of these patients (e.g., increased serum ALP or AST, prolonged PT, altered serum protein values)
* Hypercalcemia
* Polycythemia in 5–10% of patients due to production of erythropoietin
* Thrombocytosis
* Leukemoid reaction
* Refractory anemia and increased ESR
* Amyloidosis
* Cushing syndrome
* Salt-losing syndrome
* Increased serum ferritin (due to hemorrhage within tumor)
* Von Hippel-Lindau disease
* Exfoliative cytology of urine for suspicious tumor cells
* Increased urine enzyme concentration
* Incidental finding of imaging of kidney

---

* Submitted by Michael Mitchell MD

➤ Limitations
- Needle biopsy is not recommended due to possible spread along needle tract as well as false-positive rate of 5% and false-negative rate of ≤25%.

RENIN-PRODUCING TUMORS

- These extremely rare small hemangiopericytomas of juxtaglomerular apparatus are usually benign. Also Wilms tumor; ectopic renin production by lung, pancreas, and ovary cancers.
- PRA is increased, with levels significantly higher in renal vein from affected side.
- PRA maintains circadian rhythm despite marked elevation; responds to changes in posture but not to changes in sodium intake.
- Secondary aldosteronism is evident, with conditions such as hypokalemia.
- Prorenin level may be >50 times higher than active renin (normal = 3–5 times higher), especially in ectopic renin production and Wilms' tumor.
- Laboratory changes (and hypertension) are reversed by removal of tumor.

WILMS TUMOR

➤ Definition
- This tumor is the most common tumor of the kidney in childhood.
- Wilms tumors are associated with a wide range of constitutional and chromosomal abnormalities in 9–17% of cases. The lesion is bilateral in 7% of cases.
- The neoplasm has been associated with loss of function mutation of a number of tumor suppressor genes.
- Wilms tumors are diagnosed by histologic examination of biopsy or of the tumor removed surgically.

➤ Who Should be Suspected?
- Candidates are children between the ages of 3 and 5 years, with an abdominal mass, hematuria, abdominal pain, or hypertension.

➤ Laboratory Findings
- Serum creatinine may be elevated.
- Urinalysis may show proteinuria if the tumor is associated with other syndromes.
- Liver function tests, if abnormal, may indicate the presence of hepatic metastasis.
- Hypercalcemia may accompany other associated syndromes.
- Studies for von Willebrand disease (see p. 879) are indicated since 8% of affected children have acquired von Willebrand disease and may bleed at surgery.
- Genetic studies for tumor suppressor genes (WT1, p53, FWT1, and FWT2 genes) and mutations at the 11.15.5 loci may be of interest.

➤ Suggested Readings
Chintagumpala M, Muscal JA. Presentation, diagnosis, and staging of Wilms tumor. UptoDate. Rose B, ed. UptoDate Inc.; 2009.

Scott RH, Stiller CA, Walker L, Rahman N. Syndromes and constitutional chromosomal abnormalities associated with Wilms tumour. *J Med Genet.* 2006;43:705–715.

DISORDERS OF THE URINARY TRACT AND PROSTATE

BLADDER DISORDERS

CANCER OF THE BLADDER

➤ **Definition**
- This transitional cell epithelium cancer occurs in the urinary bladder. Less frequently, it may develop in the renal pelvis, ureter, or urethra.

➤ **Who Should be Suspected?**
- Candidates are patients older than 40 years of age, more commonly males with a history of cigarette smoking, who present with painless hematuria (see p. 761) or irritative (frequency, urgency, dysuria) bladder symptoms.
- The definitive diagnosis is made by endoscopic evaluation, which includes visualization with biopsy of suspected lesions, and cytologic examination.

➤ **Laboratory Findings**
- Urinalysis sediment: hematuria (>3 red cells per HPF) present throughout micturition. No other abnormalities are present in the urinary sediment. The urine should be kept at room temperature and examined within 30 minutes of collection.
- Cytology: Urine-based markers: numerous such tests have been developed, used mainly for surveillance purpose. Their mortality benefit and cost-effectiveness have not been determined. A 3-year study to determine the value of urinary genetic marker screening has recently been undertaken.

➤ **Suggested Reading**
Getzenberg RH. Urine-based assays for bladder cancer. *Laboratory Medicine*. 2003;34:613–617.

PROSTATE DISORDERS*

BENIGN PROSTATIC HYPERPLASIA (BPH)

➤ **Definition**
- BPH is enlargement of the prostate resulting from hyperplasia of prostatic stromal and epithelial cells. This results in the formation of large, discrete nodules in the periurethral region of the prostate.

➤ **Who Should be Suspected?**
- Candidates are men, generally older than 30, with symptoms of moderate to severe lower urinary tract symptoms (LUTS), decreased peak urinary flow rates, and prostate volume.
- A history, physical examination (including a digital rectal examination of the prostate) and urinalysis (for urinary infection and hematuria) are advised to rule out other or more serious

---

*Submitted by Charles Kiefer PhD

disorders that could cause symptoms similar to those of BPH (bladder calculi, prostate or bladder cancer).

- Serum prostate specific antigen (PSA), maximum urinary flow rate, and post-void residual urine volume are useful measures in most men with suspected BPH, although they are considered optional by the American Urologic Association.

➤ Laboratory Findings

- Serum prostate specific antigen (PSA): In 20% of BPH patients, serum PSA may be increased from the widely used cut-off value of 4.0 ng/mL to 10 ng/mL. In fact, BPH is a more common cause of elevated PSA levels than is prostate cancer. Serum PSA and prostate volume exhibit a log-linear relationship, although the long-term predictive value of baseline PSA levels for the development of LUTS is uncertain.

➤ Suggested Readings

Carter HB, Landis P, Wright EJ, Parsons JK, Metter EJ. Can a baseline prostate specific antigen level identify men who will have lower urinary tract symptoms later in life? *J Urol*. 2005; 173:2040–2043.

Hochberg DA, Armenakas NA, Fracchia JA. Relationship of prostate-specific antigen and prostate volume in patients with biopsy proven benign prostatic hyperplasia. *Prostate*. 2000; 45:315–319.

Jacobsen SJ, Girman CJ, Lieber MM. Natural history of benign prostatic hyperplasia. *Urology*. 2001; 58:5–16.

Roehrborn CG, Boyle P, Gould AL, Waldstreicher J. Serum prostate-specific antigen as a predictor of prostate volume in men with benign prostatic hyperplasia. *Urology*. 1999; 53:581–589.

PROSTATE CANCER

➤ Definition

- Prostate cancer is a form of cancer that develops in the prostate. Most prostate cancers are slow growing, but some cases may be more aggressive.
- The incidence rate for prostate cancer in the US (2001–2005) is 0.158%. Prostate cancer is so indolent that most men die of other causes before the disease becomes clinically advanced.
- Although as an annual screening tool, PSA testing with DRE (digital rectal examination) has little or no proven benefit in reducing mortality from the disease, detection of the disease is higher than by usual care without screening. (less than one in three men with an elevated PSA will have prostate cancer detected on biopsy).

➤ Who Should Be Suspected?

- Symptoms of prostate cancer can include pain, difficulty in urinating, problems during sexual intercourse, or erectile dysfunction. Other symptoms can potentially develop during later stages of the disease.
- For symptomatic males, a test for serum prostate specific antigen (PSA) is warranted. An elevated level of PSA warrants further testing for prostate cancer (Figure 8-3).

➤ Laboratory Findings

- PSA testing has relatively low sensitivity (70–80%) and specificity (60–70%), at the traditional cutoff of 4.0 ng/mL Moreover, the overall positive predictive value for a PSA level >4.0 ng/mL is only 30% (the gold standard method for diagnosis is prostate biopsy).
- For PSA levels between 4.0 and 10.0 ng/mL, the positive predictive value is 25%, and for PSA levels >10.0 ng/mL, the positive predictive value is 42–64%.

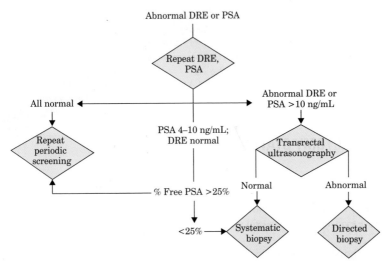

Figure 8-3. Algorithm for prostate cancer screening (DRE, direct rectal examination; PSA, prostate-specific antigen.)

- Within the PSA "gray zone" (4.0 to 10.0 ng/mL), 75% of prostate cancers have been found to be organ-confined and potentially curable.
  - PSA levels in the gray zone are frequently found to be normal on subsequent testing, so it is advisable to confirm an elevated PSA result before proceeding to prostate biopsy.
  - Within the gray zone, free-to-total PSA ratio tends to be lower in men with disease.
- Transient increases in PSA levels may occur through:
  - Physiologic fluctuations (e.g., post-ejaculation)
  - Prostate manipulations (e.g., needle biopsy, transurethral resection, cytoscopy, vigorous bicycling, digital rectal examination, radiation therapy, indwelling catheter, certain drugs – e.g., testosterone)
  - Non-cancerous prostate conditions (e.g., prostatitis, acute urinary retention, BPH, prostatic ischemia)

➤ **Monitoring diagnosed disease:**
For diagnosed prostate cancer, disease stage can be monitored by tracking the PSA level (given below in ng/mL).
- < 4: organ-confined
- 4–10: bone metastases rare
- >10: >50% have extracapsular disease
- >50: most have positive lymph nodes
- >100: predicts bone metastases (accuracy >90%, sensitivity 66%, specificity 96%; PPV 73%)

➤ **Suggested Readings**
Andriole GL, Crawford ED, Grubb RL, 3rd, et al. Mortality results from a randomized prostate-cancer screening trial. *N Engl J Med.* 2009; 360:1310–1319.
Catalona WJ, Partin AW, Slawin KM, et al. Use of the percentage of free prostate-specific antigen to enhance differentiation of prostate cancer from benign prostatic disease: a prospective multicenter clinical trial. *JAMA* 1998; 279:1542–1547.

Crawford ED, DeAntoni EP, Etzioni R, et al. Serum prostate-specific antigen and digital rectal examination for early detection of prostate cancer in a national community-based program. The Prostate Cancer Education Council. *Urology*. 1996;47:863–869.

Eastham JA, Riedel E, Scardino PT, et al. Variation of serum prostate-specific antigen levels: an evaluation of year-to-year fluctuations. *JAMA* 2003;289:2695–2700.

Jemal A, Siegel R, Ward E, et al. Cancer statistics, 2009. CA Cancer *J Clin*. 2009; 59:225–249.

Schröder FH, Hugosson J, Roobol MJ, et al. Screening and prostate-cancer mortality in a randomized European study. *N Engl J Med*. 2009; 360:1320–1328.

POSTVASECTOMY STATUS

➤ Definition

* Following a vasectomy, a series of semen analyses are performed for a defined period to determine the success or failure of the procedure. Azoospermia in a semen specimen is definitive evidence of a successful vasectomy.

➤ Who Should be Evaluated?

* Postvasectomy patients. About four of five patients will be azoospermic after three months and 20 ejaculations. However, this period of time will be shorter if ejaculations are more frequent or if the patient is older.
* In a low percentage of cases, post-vasectomy patients will consistently evidence non-motile sperm, possibly reflecting an undue delay between ejaculation and laboratory analysis. Repeat testing after one and two months may confirm azoospermia, but the continued presence of rare, nonmotile sperm at this point is probably clinically insignificant.

➤ Laboratory Findings

* A fresh specimen should be examined using direct phase-contrast microscopy (25 to 50 high-power fields). If sperm are not seen on the initial slide, a centrifuged specimen should be evaluated.
* If motile sperm are present at the three month checkup, further testing should be performed one to two months later, and again if necessary. If motile sperm are still present three months after the procedure and there have been more than 20 ejaculates, then the vasectomy is considered a failure.

➤ Suggested Readings

Barone MA, Nazerali H, Cortes M, et al. A prospective study of time and number of ejaculations to azoospermia after vasectomy by ligation and excision. *J Urol*. 2003;170:892–896.

Griffin T, Tooher R, Nowakowski K, Lloyd M, Madden G. How little is enough? The evidence for post-vasectomy testing. *J Urol*. 2005;174:29–36.

PRIAPISM

➤ Definition

Priapism is a painful and prolonged erection of the penis (more than four hours) in the absence of sexual arousal. It is a medical emergency requiring urologic treatment to aspirate occluded blood from the corpora cavernosae. Potential complications – ischemia, thrombosis, or vascular damage – may result in impaired erectile function or impotence.

➤ Who Should be Suspected?

Although the neurological and vascular mechanisms underlying priapism are poorly understood, the causes can be classified into six main categories:

- Thromboembolic disease (sickle cell disease or trait, polycythemia, pelvic thrombophlebitis)
- Infiltrative diseases (e.g., leukemia, bladder or prostate carcinoma)
- Penile trauma
- CNS infection (e.g., syphilis, TB) or spinal cord injury or anesthesia
- Intra-cavernous injectables for treatment of erectile dysfunction (papaverine, alprostadil, phentolamine)
- Other medications: antihypertensives, antipsychotics (e.g., chlorpromazine, clozapine), antidepressants (especially trazodone), anticoagulants, testosterone, heparin, recreational drugs (alcohol, cocaine, marijuana, cantharides)

Other causes include prostatitis and retroperitoneal bleeding. Phosphodiesterase type-5 (PDE5) inhibitors (sildenafil, tadalafil, vardenafil) have only rarely been implicated.

➤ Laboratory Findings

- Measurement of intracorporeal pO_2 can be used to differentiate the more dangerous low-flow priapism from high-flow priapism (which is less of a medical emergency).

➤ Suggested Readings

Akinola NO, Stevens SM, Franklin IM, Nash GB, Stuart J. Rheological changes in the prodromal and established phases of sickle cell vaso-occlusive crisis. *Br J Haematol.* 1992; 81:598–602.

Ballas SK, Smith ED. Red blood cell changes during the evolution of the sickle cell painful crisis. *Blood.* 1992; 79:2154–2163.

PROSTATITIS

➤ Definition

- Prostatitis refers, sensu stricto, to histological inflammation of the prostate gland, although the term is used loosely to describe several different conditions. The 1999 classification system of the NIDDK comprises four categories of prostatitis:
  - (I) Acute prostatitis. Route of entry of microorganisms is nearly always via the urethra or bladder through the prostatic duct, with intraprostatic reflux of urine and sometimes concomitant infection of the bladder or epididymis.
  - (II) Chronic bacterial prostatitis. This form occurs in less than 5% of patients with non-BPH lower urinary tract symptoms. Although bacteria are present, symptoms are usually absent until there is a bladder infection.
  - (III) Chronic prostatitis/chronic pelvic pain syndrome. This is the most common form of chronic prostatitis, with an annual prevalence in the general population of 0.5%.
  - (IV) Asymptomatic inflammatory prostatitis. Although patients have no history of genitourinary pain, leukocytosis is discovered during the workup for other conditions. The prevalence ranges from 6–19% (asymptomatic men with dead WBCs in semen).

➤ Who Should be Suspected?

- Symptoms suggesting prostatitis are pain, urination problems, sexual dysfunction, and general health problems (fatigue or depression).

- The key symptom of chronic prostatitis/chronic pelvic pain syndrome is pelvic or perineal pain without evidence of urinary tract infection, lasting longer than 3 months. Post-ejaculatory neurogenic-myofascial pain is a hallmark of this syndrome.

➤ Laboratory Findings

- Acute prostatitis
  - A complete blood count will reveal an increased WBC count.
  - A urine culture usually exhibits a positive colony count. Bacteria causing prostatitis are easily recoverable from urine (prostate massage is contraindicated in suspected acute prostatitis, because it may induce sepsis). Recovered organisms are generally those that induce UTI and urethritis: *Escherichia coli, Klebsiella, Proteus, Pseudomonas, Enterobacter, Enterococcus, Serratia,* and *Staphylococcus aureus.*
  - WBCs are found in the centrifuged urine sediment of the last portion of a voided urine specimen.
- Chronic bacterial prostatitis
  - Using the Stamey four-glass test with an established bacteriuria baseline ($<10^3$/mL), chronic prostatitis is suspected if the leukocyte count in the prostatic secretion is >12 per high power field.
  - Chronic prostatitis is likely if the leukocyte count is >20 per high power field.
  - Although cultures of urine or prostatic secretions are nearly always positive, negative cultures do not necessarily exclude the possibility of chronic bacterial prostatitis.
- Chronic prostatitis/chronic pelvic pain syndrome
  - Although there is no definitive diagnostic test for this syndrome, prostatic fluid usually shows >10 dead WBCs per high power field in the inflammatory form of the syndrome (Category IIIA). In the non-inflammatory form (Category IIIB), no WBCs are present.
  - Cultures of urine, semen, and prostatic fluid are negative. The presence of many lipid-laden macrophages is suggestive.

➤ Suggested Readings

Korrovits P, Ausmees K, Mändar R, Punjab M. Prevalence of asymptomatic inflammatory (National Institutes of Health Category IV) prostatitis in young men according to semen analysis. *Urology.* 2008; 71:1010–1015.

Luzzi GA. Chronic prostatitis and chronic pelvic pain in men: aetiology, diagnosis and management. *J Eur Acad Dermatol Venereol.* 2002; 16:253–256.

Schaeffer AJ. Clinical practice. Chronic prostatitis and the chronic pelvic pain syndrome. *N Engl J Med.* 2006; 355:1690–1698.

Schaeffer AJ. Epidemiology and evaluation of chronic pelvic pain syndrome in men. *Int J Antimicrob Agents.* 2008; 31:S108–111.

URINARY TRACT DISORDERS

CALCULI

➤ Definition

- Hard crystalline particles in the urine are commonly referred to as kidney stones.
- Calcium oxalate alone (acid urine) or with phosphate is the constituent of kidney stones in 85% of male and 70% of female patients. Calcium phosphate stones form with hypercalciuria, hypocitraturia, and alkaline urine (Figure 8-4).

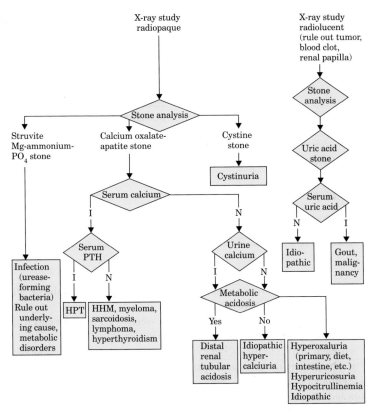

Figure 8-4. Algorithm for diagnosis of renal calculi, as revealed by flank pain, renal colic, hematuria, fever, and urinalysis findings. (I, increased; N, normal; PTH, parathyroid hormone; HPT, hyperparathyroidism; HHM, humeral hypercalcemia of malignancy.)

- Idiopathic hypercalciuria: ~50% of patients (Table 8-11)
- Struvite stones (staghorn calculi): 10–15% of stones. Only occur in UTI urea-splitting bacteria Proteus species (>50% of cases; but should rule out *Klebsiella, Pseudomonas, Serratia, Enterobacter*), and in patients with persistently alkaline urine (Mg, NH_3, Ca, PO_4). Staghorn calculi should be cultured.

➤ Who Should be Suspected?
- 20–30% of patients have:
  - Bone diseases—destructive (e.g., metastatic tumor) or osteoporosis (e.g., immobilization, Paget disease, Cushing syndrome)
  - Milk-alkali (Burnett) syndrome
  - Hypervitaminosis D
  - Sarcoidosis
  - RTA—type I (hypercalciuria, highly alkaline urine, serum calcium usually normal)
  - Hyperthyroidism
  - Gout: 25% of patients with primary gout and 40% of patients with marrow-proliferative disorders have calculi. Stones precede joint symptoms in 40% of cases.

TABLE 8-11. Comparison of Types of Idiopathic Hypercalciuria

	Resorptive	Absorptive	Renal
Due to	Primary hyperpara-thyroidism	Primary increase in intestinal absorption; reabsorption autosomal	Abnormal renal tubular dominant
Frequency	Least common	Most common	1/10 as common as absorptive type
2-hour urine after fasting			
Calcium	30 mg	<20 mg	Increased
Calcium/creatinine ratio	>0.15	<0.15	>0.15

- Primary hyperparathyroidism occurs in ~5% of patients with nephrolithiasis; 50–75% of hyperparathyroidism patients have renal calculi.
- Patients with urine that is more acidic than normal, often <5.5 (e.g., patients with chronic diarrhea, ileostomy); only form in persistently acidic urine.
- Oxalate is present in 65% of stones, but hyperoxaluria is a relatively rare cause of these calculi and may be primary or secondary hyperoxaluria.
- Uric acid is present in 5% of stones. Fifty percent of patients with urinary calculi have normal serum and urine uric acid levels.
- Cystine stones (present in 1–2% of stones) form when urine contains >300 mg/day of cystine in congenital familial cystinuria. Cystine-only stones form only in homozygotes. Tend to have bilateral obstructive staghorn calculi with associated renal failure.
- Hereditary glycinuria is a rare familial disorder associated with renal calculi.
- Patients with anatomic abnormalities such as urinary tract obstruction

➤ Children with Calculi
- Infections account for 13–40% of stones.
- Hypercalciuria is most common noninfectious cause (especially idiopathic but also caused by distal RTA and therapy with furosemide, prednisone, or ACTH).
- Oxaluria accounts for 3–13% of stones.
- Uric acid stones account for 4% of stones.
- Cystinuria is found in 5–7% of children with stones.
- Hypocitraturia is found in 10% of children with stones.
- Xanthine is present in children with inborn error of metabolism.
- Deficiency of adenine phosphoribosyltransferase

➤ Laboratory Findings
- Collect two, 24-hour urine specimens and routine blood chemistries to rule out underlying disorders. Helical CT is preferred imaging modality with S/S 96%/100%; ultrasound S/S 61%/96%.

- Crystalluria is diagnostically useful when there are cystine crystals (occurs only in homozygous or heterozygous cystinuria) or struvite crystals. Cyanide-nitroprusside test is positive (false-positive may occur with sulfur-containing drugs). Calcium oxalate, phosphate, and uric acid should arouse suspicion about possible cause of stones but they may occur in normal urine.
- Microscopic hematuria is found in 80% of patients.
- Leukocytosis may be present if there is infection or stress.
- In renal colic, hematuria and proteinuria are present, and there is an increased WBC due to associated infection.

➤ Suggested Reading
Curhan GC. A 44-year-old woman with kidney stones. *JAMA*. 2005;293:1107.

CARCINOMA OF RENAL PELVIS AND URETER, LEUKOPLAKIA

- Hematuria is present.
- Renal calculi are associated.
- UTI is associated.
- Cytologic examination of urinary sediment for malignant cells may be falsely negative in 20% of patients.

LEUKOPLAKIA OF RENAL PELVIS

- Metastases to kidneys occur in ~12% of cancer patients, most commonly with cancers of lung, breast, ovary, bowel, and other solid cancers. Greater than thirty percent of patients with lymphomas have renal involvement.
- Cell block or Pap smear of urine may show keratin or keratinized squamous cells.
- High-grade (aneuploid) tumors can be detected by flow cytometry of DNA on >90% of cases.

EPIDIDYMITIS*

➤ Definition
- Epididymitis is inflammation of the epididymis.
- Epididymitis can be classified as acute or chronic. The acute form is caused by sexually transmitted diseases or by GU tract infections. The chronic form ensues for more than six weeks, and is characterized by inflammation even in the absence of infection. A differential diagnosis must consider a range of other sources of scrotal pain, such as testicular cancer, varicocele, or a cyst within the epididymis.

➤ Who Should be Suspected?
- Candidates are males with unilateral testicular pain, usually of gradual onset. The scrotum may become red, warm and swollen.
- Asymptomatic urethritis often accompanies sexually transmitted epididymitis.
- Epididymitis from non-sexual causes is more likely to arise in men over 35 years of age, and be associated with recent urinary tract instrumentation or surgery, or anatomic abnormalities.

---

*Submitted by Charles Kiefer PhD

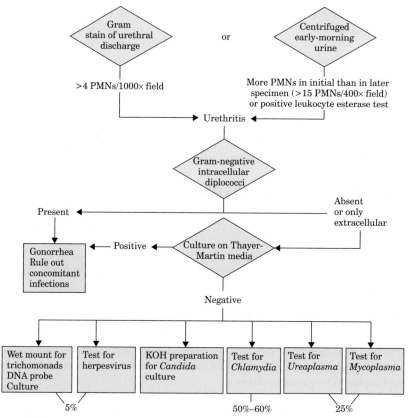

Figure 8-5. Algorithm for diagnosis of urethritis in males.

- In children, epididymitis may be a response following infection by enterovirus, adenovirus or *Mycoplasma pneumoniae*.

➤ Laboratory Findings

- In sexually active men, *Chlamydia trachomatis* and *Neisseria gonorrhoeae* are the most frequent causative agents in patients under 35 years of age. Combined infections by both agents are more frequently found than infections by *N. gonorrhoeae* alone.
- In men over 35 years of age, gram-negative enteric organisms are likely to be found. Less common pathogens include *Ureaplasma*, *Mycobacterium tuberculosis* (although with only 35% having a history of previous TB), cytomegalovirus, or *Cryptococcus* (patients with HIV infection).
- In boys before puberty, *E. coli* is a common cause.
- (Figure 8-5) presents an algorithm for the diagnosis of urethritis in males by causitive agent.

➤ Suggested Readings

Doble A, Taylor-Robinson D, Thomas BJ, et al. Acute epididymitis: a microbiological and ultrasonographic study. *Br J Urol.* 1989; 63:90–94.

Hawkins DA, Taylor-Robinson D, Thomas BJ, Harris JR. Microbiological survey of acute epididymitis. *Genitourin Med.* 1986; 62:342–344.

Workowski KA, Berman SM. Sexually transmitted diseases treatment guidelines, 2006. *MMWR Recomm Rep.* 2006; 55:1–94.

HEMATURIA

➤ Definition

- The term *hematuria* refers to the presence of >2 RBCs per HPF in urine. It should not to be confused with hemoglobinuria, a term reserved for the presence of free Hb in urine (see p. 762).
- Hematuria may be macroscopic—grossly visible as red urine—or it may be microscopic—discovered by dipstick (see p. 372). It can be classified as glomerular or nonglomerular in origin. Centrifugation separates true hematuria (RBC in sediment), from discoloration due to pigment, such as Hb (normal sediment, colored supernatant).

➤ Who Should be Suspected?

- In addition to patients with gross hematuria or accidental finding of RBCs during a routine urinalysis, hematuria should be specifically looked for when screening for possible diagnosis of diseases of the GU tract. It may also be useful in patients on oral anticoagulants and with high INR (see p. 315) (even in these patients, it is necessary to investigate for another source of hematuria). Microscopic hematuria has a broad differential diagnosis, from entirely benign causes, to a potentially life-threatening disease, such as a malignancy of the GU tract.
- Additional causes of isolated hematuria include stones, trauma, prostatitis, sickle cell trait or disease, TB, or *Schistosoma haematobium* infection. Acute cystitis or urethritis in women can cause gross hematuria. Hypercalciuria and hyperuricosuria are also risk factors for unexplained isolated hematuria.
- The term *benign familial* or *recurrent hematuria* refers to asymptomatic, recurrent hematuria without proteinuria or other laboratory abnormalities. Persistent or recurrent hematuria, even if only microscopic, should be investigated, especially in patients >50 years of age. Other family members may be affected. The condition may clear spontaneously.

➤ Laboratory Findings

- The most important test in the evaluation of hematuria is the microscopical analysis of urine. It often distinguishes glomerular from nonglomerular bleeding. In cases of persistent hematuria and no obvious etiology, imaging studies, urinary cytology, cystoscopy, or occasionally renal biopsy may be indicated.
- Urinalysis (see also p. 372):
  - Dipstick is positive for RBCs, hemoglobin, or myoglobin. Proteinuria is also detected by dipstick. A 2+ proteinuria in the presence of microscopic hematuria indicates glomerular disease. The presence of WBCs suggests inflammation or infection.
  - Microscopy of centrifuged urinary sediment should be examined under high dry magnification. Note that <3% of normal persons have ≥3 RBC per HPFs. RBCs or Hb casts indicate that the blood is of glomerular origin. The most common cause of isolated glomerular hematuria are IgA nephropathy, hereditary nephritis (Alport syndrome), and thin basement membrane disease. Presence of clots rules out glomerular origin. Large thick clots suggest bladder origin; small stringy clots indicate upper urinary tract disease.
  - Immunocytochemical staining against human Tamm-Horsfall protein is positive with >80% of RBC of renal origin and <13.1% of RBC of nonrenal origin.

Limitations

* Causes of false-positive results (especially on dipstick)
  * Vaginal bleeding (menstruation)
  * Viral illness
  * Bacteriuria
  * Red diaper syndrome
  * Drugs (rifampin, phenolphthalein, iodides, bromides, copper, oxidizing agents, permanganate)
  * Foods (beets, blackberries, rhubarb)
  * Pigmenturia (myoglobin, porphyrin, hemoglobin)
  * Semen in urine
  * Trauma
  * Vigorous exercise before urine collection
  * Factitious
  * pH >9
* Causes of false-negative results
  * Reducing agents (high doses of vitamin C)
  * pH <5.1

➤ Suggested Reading

Cohen RA, Brown RS. Clinical practice. Microscopic hematuria. *N Engl J Med.* 2003;348:2330–2338.

HEMOGLOBINURIA

➤ Definition

* Hemoglobinuria refers to the presence of free Hb in urine. The renal threshold for hemoglobinuria is 100–140 mg Hg/dL plasma.
* Free Hb directly passing the glomeruli in the ultrafiltrate is relatively uncommon. Most often, RBCs enter the urinary tract and undergo various amounts of lysis. Nevertheless, conditions resulting in intravascular hemolysis have the potential of producing hemoglobinuria once all available plasma haptoglobin is bound by Hb. Hb is readily absorbed by proximal tubules as dissociated dimers, and it catabolizes to ferritin. In turn, ferritin is denatured to hemosiderin that can be found in urine in cases of severe, prolonged hemoglobinuria.

➤ Causes

* Parasites (malaria, Oroya fever)
* Certain infections (*Clostridium perfringens* [previously known as *Clostridium welchii*], *E. coli* bacteremia from transfused blood, *Bartonella*)
* Incompatible transfusion reactions (see p. 894)
* Hemolytic anemias with intravascular hemolysis
  * Paroxysmal nocturnal hemoglobinuria (see p. 810)
  * Paroxysmal cold hemoglobinuria
  * Microangiopathic hemolytic anemias: Thrombotic thrombocytopenic purpura/hemolytic uremic syndrome (see p. 889), prosthetic heart valves, or severely damaged natural valves, especially aortic
  * Severe autoimmune hemolytic anemias (see p. 804)

- Fava bean sensitivity, G6PD deficiency, and other hemoglobinopathies (see p. 796)
- Severe hereditary spherocytosis
- DIC (see p. 883)
- Infusion or bladder irrigation with hypotonic solutions
- Thermal burns
- Diabetic acidosis
- Chemicals (naphthalene, sulfa drugs)
- Strenuous exercise, including march hemoglobinuria
- Infarction of kidney

➤ Who Should be Suspected?
- Candidates include patients with red urine but no red cells in urinary sediment, especially if there is a history suggesting intravascular hemolysis.

➤ Laboratory Tests
- Positive urine dipstick for RBCs but normal sediment
- Hb measured both in urine and plasma by spectrophotometric methods
- Work-up for underlying cause, especially intravascular hemolysis
- Elevated serum conjugated bilirubin
- Decreased serum haptoglobin
- Elevated urine urobilinogen
- Urine hemosiderin in severe, prolonged cases

➤ Limitations
- False-positive results may occur with:
  - Hematuria with hemolysis of RBCs in urine, if the urine was not promptly processed
  - Other pigments (myoglobin, porphyrin) that may give the visual appearance of hemoglobinuria
  - False-positive dipstick in the presence of pus, iodides, or bromides

OXALOSIS

- Rare metabolic disorder resulting in excessive oxalate.
- It may be inherited (autosomal recessive) or acquired.

➤ Secondary
- Causes
  - Increased oxalate in diet (e.g., green leafy vegetables, chocolate, tea)
  - Ingestion of oxalate precursors (e.g., ascorbic acid, ethylene glycol)
  - Methoxyflurane anesthesia
  - Primary diseases of ileum with malabsorption (e.g., bypass surgery, Crohn disease, pancreatitis), causing increased absorption of dietary oxalate
- Urinary oxalate is usually 50–100 mg per 24 hours

➤ Primary (Types 1 and 2)
- Rare, autosomal recessive inherited disorders of glyoxylate metabolism causing recurrent calcium oxalate renal lithiasis, nephrocalcinosis, and uremia.
- Urinary oxalate is usually >100 mg per 24 hours unless renal function is diminished.

RETROPERITONEAL FIBROSIS

* Rare disease characterized by proliferation of fibrous tissue in the retroperitoneum resulting in the blockage of the ureters.

➤ Causes
* Primary (70% of cases)
  * Angiomatous lymphoid hamartoma
* Secondary (30% of cases)
  * Infection
  * Trauma
  * Connective tissue disease
  * Aortic aneurysm
  * Irradiation
  * Drugs (e.g., methysergide; also methyldopa, ergotamine, phenacetin, hydralazine, propranolol)

➤ Laboratory Findings
* ESR is increased.
* Anemia, leukocytosis, and increased ESR may be present.
* Occasionally eosinophilia occurs.
* Serum protein and A/G ratio are normal; if the person is chronically ill, total protein may be decreased and γ-globulins may be increased.
* Laboratory findings due to ureteral obstruction.

CHAPTER 9

Gynecologic and Obstetric Disorders

Liberto Pechet and Mary Williamson

T his chapter refers to disorders of the female genital tract: vulva, vagina, and uterus, including abnormalities related to menstruation. It also refers to the diagnosis and abnormalities of pregnancy.

GYNECOLOGIC DISORDERS

UTERINE CANCER

CANCER OF CERVIX

➤ **Definition**
• This form of cancer is one of the most frequent neoplasms that affect a woman's reproductive system. In the United States, this cancer has a higher prevalence in African American and Hispanic populations than in Caucasians, probably related to less frequent

screening with Pap smears. Cervical cancer is the result of STDs with various strains of the Human Papilloma Virus (HPV), especially (but not exclusively) the oncogenic types 16 and 18.

➤ Who Should be Suspected?

* This cancer may be suspected in women in their 40s with a history of early sexual activity and multiple partners, who present with abnormal or postintercourse bleeding, or vaginal discharge that may be watery, mucoid, or purulent and malodorous. The presence of pelvic or lower back pain suggests advanced disease. The suspicion is high in the presence of abnormal Pap smears.

➤ Laboratory Findings
Diagnosis

The diagnosis is made by punch biopsy, colposcopy with directed biopsy, or conization, if the two other procedures are inadequate.

* Imaging studies: Recommended to evaluate possible involvement of adjacent organs, such as the kidneys.
* Hematology: CBC abnormalities correlate with stage of disease.
* Molecular testing: DNA testing for highly oncogenic strains of HPV types is used mostly for epidemiologic studies. Its role in screening for cervical cancer is still evolving. See p. 766.

CANCER OF UTERINE BODY

➤ Definition

Uterine cancer is the most common gynecologic cancer in North America
Type 1 is estrogen- or tamoxifen related, usually low-grade.
Type 2 is unrelated to estrogen or tamoxifen, usually higher grade

➤ Who Should be Suspected?

A patient with a history of abnormal vaginal bleeding, especially if post menopausal
Diagnosis:

* Pap smear of vagina/cervix is positive in ≤70% of patients with endometrial adenocarcinoma; a false-negative result occurs in 30% of patients. Therefore, a negative Pap smear does not rule out carcinoma.
* Pap smear from aspiration of endometrial cavity is positive in 95% of patients.
* Endometrial biopsy may be helpful, but a negative result does not rule out carcinoma.
* Diagnostic curettage is the only way to rule out carcinoma of the endometrium.

Pap Smear*

* Use
  * Routine screening of asymptomatic women to detect carcinoma of cervix or various atypias. Combined with HPV, DNA testing is being evaluated as primary screening test for uterine cervical abnormalities.
  * Also used to monitor response to therapy for carcinoma, infections, and so on

---

*Submitted by Mary Williamson, PhD.

- Occasionally detects carcinoma from other sites (e.g., endometrium, ovary, fallopian tube)
- Often detects presence of various previously undiagnosed infectious agents (e.g., *Trichomonas vaginalis*, HSV, *Candida*)
- Occasionally useful in chromosome studies
- May be used to estimate ovarian functional hormonal status
- Interpretation
  - Routine screening in the general population may be positive for ~6 of every 1000 women (prevalence); only 7% of these lesions are invasive. The prevalence rate is greatest in certain groups:
    - Women in their 20's should have a pap smear every two years; women in their 30's who have had three consecutive normal Pap smears should undergo screening every three years
    - Women infected with oncogenic types of HPV
    - Women who use birth control pills rather than diaphragm for contraception
    - Women with early onset or long duration of sexual activity
  - Vaginal pool Pap smear has an accuracy rate of ~80% in detecting carcinoma of the cervix. Smears from a combination of vaginal pool, exocervical, and endocervical scrapings have an accuracy rate of 95%.
  - The presence of endocervical cells indicates that the sample was taken from the transformation zone, where cancer is more likely to develop.
  - Biopsy shows important lesions of the cervix in some of these patients. Therefore, an abnormal initial smear requires further investigation of the cervix regardless of subsequent cytologic reports.
  - Women who have undergone noncancerous hysterectomy and/or women aged 65–70, who have three consecutive normal pap smear results with no abnormal findings in the past 10 years can discontinue pap smear screening.
- Limitations
  - False-negative results in ~5–10% of cases
  - Sparse cells—100 abnormal cells is threshold for reliable screening; usual Pap smear contains 50,000 to 300,000 cells.
  - Sampling problems up to 10% samples collected have integrity issues and are considered unsatisfactory due to the presence of blood or mucous, inflammation, insufficient cells or problems with the slide preparation. Malignant cells may not be present if smear is repeated too soon after previous abnormal smear.
  - Certain tumor types are less readily diagnosed (e.g., adenocarcinoma, lymphoma, sarcoma, verrucous carcinoma).
  - Human error in interpreting difficult cells; <3% of preventable cervical cancer is due to misread smears.

Note: The SurePath™ Liquid-Based Pap Test and ThinPrep® Pap Test™ have replaced the conventional pap smear for screening cervical cancer, precancerous lesions and atypical cells due to the ability of laboratories to automate the imaging process. Both liquid based techniques have a lower incidence of sample integrity issues compared to the conventional pap smear.

➤ Suggested Reading

Saraiya M, Ahmed F, Krishnan S, et al. Cervical cancer incidence in a prevaccine era in the United States, 1998–2002. *Obstet Gynecol.* 2007;109:360–370.

PELVIC INFLAMMATORY DISEASE*

➤ Definition

* Pelvic inflammatory disease (PID) is the most common and most important complication of STDs (85%); 15% of cases arise postoperatively. PID involves infection of upper genital tract. It may include the endometrium, myometrium, parametrium, uterine tubes, ovaries, and peritoneum.

➤ Causes

* *Chlamydia trachomatis* (see Chapter 13). PID due to *C. trachomatis* causes less severe symptoms than that due to *Neisseria gonorrhoeae*.
* *N. gonorrhoeae* infection is found in 8% of acute cases (see Chapter 13).
* *Mycoplasma hominis* (see Chapter 13)
* Anaerobic bacteria (e.g., *Clostridium* sp., *Actinomyces* sp.)
* Coliform bacilli
* Polymicrobial in many cases.
* See causes of vulvovaginitis.
* Other organisms that cause STDs
  * *N. gonorrhoeae*
  * *Chlamydia*
  * Streptococcal group A vaginitis
  * *Staphylococcus aureus* with toxic shock syndrome

➤ Conditions Included

* Urethritis
* Cervicitis
  * Cervical Gram stain >10 PMNs/HPF (1000×) in nonmenstruating women
  * Tests for appropriate organism
    * Culture may not correlate with intra-abdominal culture.
    * Direct antigen test (e.g., *Chlamydia*)
* Vulvovaginitis (see below)
* Pelvic abscess—usually polymicrobic (≥3 organisms), aerobic (e.g., *Streptococcus*, *Escherichia coli*) and anaerobic (e.g., *Peptococcus*, *Bacteroides*). *Chlamydia* and *N. gonorrhoeae* are recovered from cervix in approximately one third of cases.
* Perihepatitis (Fitz-Hugh-Curtis syndrome)

➤ Laboratory Findings

* Imaging studies: Pelvic ultrasound, CT scan, x-ray studies abnormal.
* Hematology: Elevated white blood cell (WBC) count; increased neutrophils; elevated ESR.
* Core laboratory: Increased amylase and serum globulin.
* Tumor markers: Elevated CA-125 antigen titer.
* Laboratory findings due to complications (e.g., infertility, ectopic pregnancy, premature birth, neonatal conjunctivitis, infant pneumonia, septicemia, septic shock, peritonitis, pelvic thrombophlebitis).

---

*Contributed by Mary Williamson.

VAGINOSIS AND VAGINITIS (BACTERIAL VAGINOSIS, TRICHOMONIASIS, VULVOVAGINAL CANDIDIASIS)*

➤ Definition

- Vaginitis is used to describe conditions associated with significant inflammation, whereas vaginosis is used when vaginal secretions do not show a marked increase in inflammatory cells. Symptoms attributed to vaginitis may also be due to primary cervicitis, urethritis, or inflammation to other related tissues.
- Changes in the amount or character of vaginal discharge are common presenting complaints of women seeking medical attention. Although there is normal variability in vaginal secretions, infectious and other pathologic causes are common and should be carefully evaluated.

➤ Causes

- Complaints associated with noninfectious causes may be indistinguishable from those caused by genital tract infections. Common noninfectious causes include:
  - Allergy and irritants. Many products, such as detergents, soaps, bubble bath, latex (e.g., condoms), and topical medications, may cause inflammation of the vaginal mucosa and changes in the character and volume of secretions. Clinical management requires elimination of the allergen or irritant.
  - Atrophic vaginitis. This type of vaginitis is caused by estrogen deficiency and is usually associated with menopause, but may be seen in the postpartum period or as a result of medication. Symptoms of estrogen deficiency lead to vaginal dryness and itching rather than an increase in vaginal secretions. Here there are mixed nonspecific gram-negative rods with decreased lactobacilli; vaginal cytology shows an atrophic pattern.
  - Physiologic leukorrhea. Vaginal secretions may vary significantly in normal women, especially related to the menstrual cycle. The volume of vaginal secretion is typically greatest in mid-cycle. Significant symptoms and inflammation are not seen with physiologic leukorrhea; the odor, color, and viscosity of secretions are similar to the characteristics in the absence of leukorrhea.
- Bacterial vaginosis, trichomoniasis, and vulvovaginal candidiasis are the most common causes of clinically significant vaginosis/vaginitis and are described in detail below. Other infectious causes of vaginitis include:
  - Condyloma acuminata. Increased vaginal discharge, pruritus, and pain are common symptoms caused by anogenital warts.
  - Foreign body or traumatic vaginitis. Foreign bodies, like a retained tampon, may cause a change in the normal vaginal flora and mild signs and symptoms of infection. Removal of the foreign body is usually all that is required for clinical management.
  - Group A *Streptococcus* (GAS). *Streptococcus pyogenes* (GAS) may cause acute vaginal infection with pain, edema, erythema, and purulent vaginal discharge. Gram staining shows an increased number of gram-positive cocci in chains; isolation of GAS by bacterial culture confirms the diagnosis. Although group B *Streptococcus* (GBS) is a common component of the vaginal flora of reproductive-aged women and presents a significant risk

---

*This section contributed by Michael J. Mitchell, MD.

of neonatal infection, amnionitis, and endometritis, GBS is not a significant cause of vaginitis.

➤ Clinical Presentation

* In premenopausal women, the volume of vaginal secretions is <5 mL/day. Secretions are typically odorless, transparent, and viscous, and white to yellowish. Normal vaginal pH is 4.0–4.5. Microscopic examination demonstrates a predominance of normal squamous epithelial cells (SECs) and few PMNs; there is a predominance of gram-positive bacilli consistent with lactobacilli (long, slender, may form chains).

Bacterial Vaginosis

* Bacterial vaginosis (BV) is the most common infectious cause of infectious vaginosis, accounting for ~50% of cases. BV is caused by a disruption of the normal microbial flora of the vagina. There is a loss of the predominant *Lactobacillus* species, which produce peroxide and acidify the vaginal secretions. Loss of the lactobacilli allows overgrowth of anaerobes and other microorganisms, including *Gardnerella* and *Mobiluncus, Atopobium vaginae,* and other species. BV is associated with sexual transmission.
* Patients with BV are often asymptomatic, or present with minimal symptoms. Typical symptoms include an increase in the volume of thin, homogeneous vaginal secretions, often with a "fishy" odor. Signs of inflammation are minimal.
* Diagnosis of BV is based on ≥3 of the following (Amsel criteria):
  * Homogeneous, thin, whitish adherent vaginal secretions
  * Positive "whiff" test
  * Presence of clue cells on wet mount
  * Vaginal pH >4.5
* Direct detection: Wet mount of vaginal discharge shows an increased proportion of "clue cells" (>20% of vaginal squamous cells coated with small coccobacilli) in 90% of cases.
* Gram stain: BV is characterized by a loss of gram-positive rods, with overgrowth of mixed flora, including small, curved gram-negative bacilli and gram-variable coccobacilli. Vaginal secretions have been demonstrated to have high positive and negative predictive values (90% and 94%, respectively) compared to diagnosis using the Amsel and Nugent criteria. Interpretation is based on the number of clue cells (≥2 clue cells per 20 fields) and the proportion of bacterial morphotypes (non-*Lactobacillus* > *Lactobacillus*). Specific diagnosis of BV requires laboratory testing (see Table 9-1).

Trichomoniasis

* This sexually transmitted protozoal infection is caused by *Trichomonas vaginalis.*
* Although affected women may be asymptomatic, they typically present with acute, inflammatory vaginitis. Most patients (~70%) present with vaginal and urethral inflammation resulting in burning, itching, dysuria, and other symptoms associated with increased vaginal secretions. Secretions are described as greenish, frothy, and foul-smelling in a minority of patients.
* Specific diagnosis requires laboratory testing (see Table 9-1). *Douching within 24 hours decreases the sensitivity of tests. Do not test during first few days of menstrual cycle.*
  * Culture: Considered the gold standard for diagnosis, but cultures must be incubated for 3-7 days before final results are available.

- Direct detection: Rapid diagnosis may be possible by microscopic examination. Vaginal secretions typically show increased pH (>4.5) and increased numbers of PMNs. Motile trichomonads, with typical falling leaf morphology, are diagnostic, but seen in only 50–70% of cases. Organisms may lose motility as early as 10 minutes after collection.
- Urinalysis: Frequently an incidental finding in routine urinalysis.
- Serology: Qualitative immunochromatographic kit has reported S/S = 99%/98%.
- Molecular tests: Playing an increasing role in diagnosis, providing high sensitivity and specificity with decreased turn-around-time compared to culture.

Vulvovaginal Candidiasis

- *Candida albicans* is responsible for 80–90% of cases of vulvovaginal candidiasis, but *Candida glabrata* and other *Candida* species are capable of causing clinically significant candidiasis. Vulvar inflammation, edema, pain, and pruritus are common symptoms. Thick, adherent, curd-like vaginal secretions are well described, but thin secretions may be seen and are indistinguishable from other causes of vaginal infection. Vulvovaginal candidiasis is not significantly associated with sexual transmission.
- Factors associated with an increased risk of vulvovaginal candidiasis include:
  - Contraceptive use (especially vaginal sponges and intrauterine devices)
  - Current or recent antimicrobial therapy
  - DM, especially when poorly controlled
  - Increased estrogen levels caused by pregnancy or therapeutic estrogen administration
  - Intrinsic or acquired immunodeficiency or immunosuppressive therapy

➤ Diagnosis: General Aspects of Vaginosis

The initial diagnostic evaluation should include a detailed history and laboratory testing. (Note that symptoms may be caused by more than one infectious condition.) A detailed clinical history may provide information that is useful in distinguishing infectious vaginitis from other conditions that may cause changes in the character of vaginal discharge (e.g., urethritis, cervicitis, noninfectious inflammatory conditions). Important factors include:

- Menstrual history: Vaginal secretions may vary with pregnancy and menstrual cycle. Vulvovaginal candidiasis often occurs in the premenstrual period; trichomoniasis often occurs in the postmenstrual period.
- Sexual history: Factors associated with an increased risk of STDs, including BV and trichomoniasis, include: new sexual partner, exposure to multiple sexual partners, and history of STD.
- Recent and current medications: Antibiotics, estrogen and progestin drugs, and other medications may predispose to vaginitis through changes in the vaginal environment or flora.
- Personal hygiene and potential irritants: Hygienic products and practices, frequent or recent douching, soaps and detergents, topical medications, and panty liners and other products may cause vaginal irritation, resulting in symptoms indistinguishable from infectious causes.

➤ Diagnosis: Laboratory Findings

Specific diagnosis requires laboratory testing (see Table 9-1).
- Vaginal pH: Secretions are collected, using a dry swab, from the vaginal sidewall half-way between the cervix and introitus. A narrow-range paper (pH 4.0–5.5) should be used.

TABLE 9-1. Comparison of Various Causes of Vaginitis

Condition	pH	Gram Stain/Saline Mount	10% KOH Mount	Culture	Amine Test
Normal	4.0–4.5	PMN/EC <1; Gram positive rods dominant; 3+ SECs	—		—
Bacterial vaginosis	>4.5	Clue cells; PMN/EC <1; ↓ Gram-positive rods, ↑ gram-negative coccobacilli	—	No value	>70% positive
Vulvovaginal candidiasis	<4.5	PMN/EC <1; hyphae in ~40%; Gram positive rods dominant; 3+ SECs	Hyphae in 70%	If wet mount is negative	—
Trichomoniasis	>4.5	Motile trichomonads in ~60%; 4+ PMNs; mixed flora	—	Use if wet mount is negative.	Often positive

↓, decreased; ↑, increased; PMN/EC, ratio of polymorphonuclear cells to epithelial cells.

- Examination: Saline wet mount preparations are used for direct detection of yeast-like cells and pseudohyphae, trichomonads, and host cells. Vaginal secretions collected by swab are suspended in a drop of normal saline on a microscopic slide. Normal vaginal secretions show a predominance of SECs with a minimal number of PMNs. Note that although *Candida* species are common components of the normal vaginal microflora, visualization of many yeast-like cells or pseudohyphae is abnormal and characteristic of candidiasis. "Clue" cells are squamous epithelial cells covered by coccobacillary organisms, resulting in fuzzy or indistinct cell borders.
- Gram stain: Gram stains are used for direct detection of bacteria, yeast and host cells. Normal vaginal secretions show a predominance of SECs with a minimal number of PMNs. There is a pre-dominance of gram-positive bacilli consistent with *Lactobacillus* species.
- Amine "whiff" test: A drop of 10% KOH may be added to vaginal secretions on a microscopic slide. The immediate release of a "fishy" (volatile amine) odor is typical of BV.
- Culture: Culture of vaginal secretions may improve the sensitivity of detection for candidiasis and trichomoniasis. Special techniques are required for isolation of *T. vaginalis*. Positive cultures for yeast must be interpreted with caution because *C. albicans* and other yeast may represent normal endogenous flora. Bacterial culture, including culture for *G. vaginalis*, is not reliable for diagnosis of BV because no single organism can be specifically implicated in the pathogenesis of BV.
- Serology: Serologic testing does not play a significant role in the diagnosis of vaginitis.
- Molecular tests: Molecular diagnostic tests are increasingly available for diagnosis of infectious vaginitis. For example, nucleic acid hybridization (*Affirm*™ *VPIII* Microbial Identification Test, BD Diagnostic Systems) provided greater sensitivity for detection of agents associated with BV, trichomoniasis, and vulvovaginal candidiasis compared with standard methods.

➤ Suggested Readings

Anderson MR, Klink K, Cohrssen A. Evaluation of vaginal complaints. *JAMA* 2004;291:1368–1379.

Eckert LO. Acute vulvovaginitis. *N Engl J Med.* 2006;355:1244–1252.

Goonan K. Chapter 34: Vaginitis, in Khan F, HJ Sachs, L Pechet, LM Snyder. *Guide to Diagnostic Testing.* Lippincott Williams & Wilkins; 2002.

Hilmarsdóttir I, Hauksdóttir GS, Jóhannesdóttir JD, Daníelsdóttir T, Thorsteinsdóttir H, Ólafsson JH. Evaluation of a rapid gram stain interpretation method for diagnosis of bacterial vaginosis. *J Clin Microbiol.* 2006;44: 1139–1140.

Lowe NK, Neal JL, Ryan-Wenger NA. Accuracy of the clinical diagnosis of vaginitis compared with a DNA probe laboratory standard. *Obstet Gynecol.* 2009;113:89–95.

Mazzulli T, Simor AE, Low DE. Reproducibility of interpretation of gram-stained vaginal smears for the diagnosis of bacterial vaginosis. *J Clin Microbiol.* 1990;28:1506–1508.

Nugent RP, Krohn MA, Hillier SL. Reliability of diagnosing bacterial vaginosis is improved by a standardized method of gram stain interpretation. *J Clin Microbiol.* 1991;29:297–301.

Nygren P, Fr R, Freemzan M, Bougatsos C, Klebanoff M, Guise J-M. Evidence on the benefits and harms of screening and treating pregnant women who are asymptomatic for bacterial vaginosis: An update review for the U.S. preventive services task force. *Ann Intern Med.* 2008;148:220–233.

U.S. Preventive Services Task Force. Screening for bacterial vaginosis in pregnancy to prevent preterm delivery: U.S. preventive services task force recommendation statement. *Ann Intern Med.* 2008;148:214–219.

PREGNANCY & OBSTETRIC MONITORING OF THE FETUS AND PLACENTA*

OBSTETRIC MONITORING OF THE FETUS AND PLACENTA

PREGNANCY

➤ Altered Laboratory Tests

- Hematology: RBC mass increases 20%, but plasma volume increases ~40% causing RBC, Hb, and Hct to decrease ~15%. WBC increases 66%. Platelet count decreased by average 20%. ESR increases markedly during pregnancy, making this a useless diagnostic test during pregnancy. Occasionally cold agglutinins may be positive and osmotic fragility increased.
- Renal function tests: Respiratory alkalosis with renal compensation. Normal pCO_2 = ~30 mEq/L, normal HCO_3^- = 19–20 mEq/L. Serum osmolality decreases 10 mOsm/kg during first trimester. Increased GFR 30–50% early until ~20 weeks postpartum. Renal plasma flow increases 25–50% by mid-pregnancy. BUN and creatinine decrease 25%, especially during first half of pregnancy. BUN of 18 mg/dL and creatinine of 1.2 mg/dL are definitely increased (abnormal) in pregnancy, although normal in nonpregnant women. *Beware of BUN >13 mg/dL and creatinine >0.8 mg/dL.* Serum uric acid decreases 35% in first trimester (normal = 2.8–3.0 mg/dL); returns to normal by term. Serum aldosterone, angiotensins I and II, renin are increased although secondary hyperaldosteronism may also be seen with toxemia of pregnancy.
- Urinalysis: Urine volume is not increased. Glycosuria occurs in >50% of patients due to impaired tubular resorption. Lactosuria should not be confused with glucose in urine. Proteinuria (200–300 mg/24 hour) is common (~20% of patients); worsens with underlying glomerular disease. Urine porphyrins may be increased. Urinary gonadotropins (human chorionic gonadotropin, hCG) are increased. Urine estrogens increase from 6 months to term (≤100 µg/24 hours). Urine 17-ketosteroids rise to upper limit of normal at term.
- Serum protein findings: Serum total protein decreases 1 g/dL during first trimester; remains at that level. Serum albumin decreases 0.5 g/dL during first trimester and 0.75 g/dL by term.
- Serum α-1 globulin increases 0.1 g/dL. Serum α-2 globulin increases 0.1 g/dL. Serum β-globulin increases 0.3 g/dL.
- Core laboratory: Fasting blood glucose decreases 5–10 mg/dL by end of first trimester. Serum calcium decreases 10%. Serum magnesium decreases 10%. No changes are found in serum levels of sodium (normal = ~135 mEq/L), potassium, chloride, or phosphorus. Serum T_3 uptake is decreased and T_4 is increased. T_7 ($T_3 \times T_4$) is normal. TBG is increased. (Check tests for thyroid function.) Serum progesterone is increased.
- Enzyme studies: No changes are found in serum levels of amylase, AST, ALT, LD, ICDH, acid phosphatase, α-hydroxybutyrate dehydrogenase. Serum CK decreases 15% by 20 weeks of gestation; increases at beginning of labor to peak 24 hours postpartum, and then gradually returns to normal. CK-MB is detected at onset of labor in ~75% of patients with peak 24 hours postpartum, and then returns to normal. Serum LD and AST levels remain low. Serum

---

*Contributed by Mary Williamson.

ALP increases (200–300%) progressively during the last trimester of normal pregnancy caused by an increase of heat-stable isoenzyme from the placenta. Serum LAP may be increased moderately throughout pregnancy. Serum lipase decreases 50%. Serum pseudo-cholinesterase decreases 30%.

* Lipid studies: Serum phospholipid increases 40–60%. Serum triglycerides increase 100–200%. Serum cholesterol increases 30–50%.
* Iron studies: Serum iron decreases 40% in women not on iron therapy. Serum vitamin B_{12} level decreases 20%. Serum folate decreases ≥50%. Overlap of decreased and normal range of values often makes this test useless in diagnosis of megaloblastic anemia of pregnancy. Serum transferrin increases 40% and percent saturation decreases ≤70%. Serum ceruloplasmin increases 70%.

➤ Monitoring Assays
Recommended Testing for Prenatal Screening
At first prenatal visit, all pregnant women should have:
* Histology: Pap smear if not done in preceding year
* Hematology: CBC
* Blood bank: Blood type, Rh type, and antibody screen
* Serology/infectious disease: Rubella screen, Rapid plasma reagin (RPR) test for syphilis, HBsAg for HBV infection and HIV test should be offered. High-risk women—test for *N. gonorrhoeae, C. trachomatis*, HBsAg; repeat at 28 weeks.
  * First Trimester (10w3d and 13w6d): Maternal Triple Screen (Pregnancy-Associated Placental Protein A, total hCG and Nuchal Translucency and sonogram for genetic diseases (see Chapter 11)
  * Second Trimester (15w0d and 22w6d): Maternal Quad Screen (Pregnancy-Associated Placental Protein A, total hCG, Nuchal Translucency and Inhibin A) and sonogram for genetic diseases (see Chapter 11)
  * At 36 weeks: Optional screen for group B streptococcus

➤ Recommended Well-Baby Routine Laboratory Tests for Newborns
* Hematology: Hb, Hct, WBC, and differential
* Blood bank: blood type and hold and Coombs' tests if mother is Rh-negative or if jaundice develops by 24 hours
* Microbiology/infectious diseases: syphilis, HBV, and/or toxoplasma
* Core laboratory: urinalysis. Serum bilirubin, glucose, sodium, potassium, chloride, and calcium at appropriate intervals.
* Newborn screening: On day of discharge or follow-up at age 4 days as mandated by state law (e.g., PKU, thyroid function tests, others).

INFANTS AT INCREASED RISK

➤ Risks During Pregnancy
* Infants born before 38th week of gestation. Low birth weight ≤ 2500 g; very low birth weight = 1500 g; extremely low birth weight = 1000 g. Gestational age may not parallel birth weight, although most low–birth weight infants are preterm.

- Other infants at increased risk include high–birth weight infants (>4,000 g), postmaturity infants, infants of high-risk mothers (toxemia, diabetes, drug addiction, cardiac or pulmonary disease), polyhydramnios, oligohydramnios, cesarean delivery, infection, other major illnesses such as hepatitis and thyrotoxicosis.

Risks During Labor and Delivery
- Fetal pH <7.2
- Pulmonary immaturity
- Amnionitis, meconium staining of AF
- Others

Risks During Neonatal Period
- Tests for Respiratory Distress Syndrome (RDS), chronic lung disease (e.g., blood gases [pO_2, pCO_2, and pH] indicated by baby's color, condition, and respiratory symptoms; pneumothorax/pneumomediastinum occurs in ≤3% of full-term newborns).
- Metabolic function: hypoglycemia and hypocalcemia
- Anemia of prematurity due to
  - Insufficient erythropoietin production (most)
  - Shorter RBC life span = ~35 to 50 days (term infant = 60–70 days)
  - Physiologic anemia at 10–12 weeks occurs earlier; more marked than in term newborns; on phlebotomy: >10 nucleated RBCs is highly suggestive of fetal ischemic encephalopathy
  - Rh/ABO immunization
- Nonimmune hydrops fetalis due to various causes (e.g., cardiovascular, respiratory, hematologic, GI, GU, others)
- Infections are more common than in term newborns (e.g., late-onset nosocomial infection by coagulase-negative staphylococci and fungi with central venous catheters; sepsis or pneumonia due to amnionitis)
- GI (e.g., necrotizing enterocolitis, cholestasis with prolonged parenteral feeding)
- Neonatal hyperbilirubinemia (see Chapter 6)

➤ Suggested Reading
Phelan JP. Nucleated red blood cells: a marker for fetal asphyxia? *Am J Obstet Gynecol.* 1995;173:1380.

OBSTETRIC DISORDERS

AMNIOTIC FLUID (AF) EMBOLISM

- Hematology: Consumptive coagulopathy
- Laboratory findings due to pulmonary embolism (see Chapter 14)
- Identification in maternal lung tissue postmortem:
  - Morphologic identification of fetal products (e.g., fat from vernix caseosa, mucin derived from meconium)
  - Immunohistochemical identification of fetal isoantigen A and mucin-type glycoprotein derived from meconium and AF

AMNIOTIC FLUID INFECTIONS*

➤ Definition and Etiology
- Intra-amniotic infection (IAI) represents a significant cause of fetal demise, premature delivery, neonatal sepsis and pneumonia, and maternal bacteremia and sepsis. Such infection most commonly affects preterm deliveries and is increased with premature rupture of membranes. Amniotic fluid infections may manifest with amnionitis, chorioamnionitis, and intrapartum fever.
- Most amniotic fluid infections are caused by vaginal microorganisms that gain access to the uterine cavity. These ascending infections are most common as a result of premature rupture of the fetal membranes. Amnionitis and chorioamnionitis are an important cause of premature delivery and fetal death. Amniotic and fetal bacterial infections may cause bacteremia in the mother with disseminated or localized infection. Fetal infection may also be caused by hematogenous transmission from the maternal circulation. This route is most common for viral pathogens.
- The etiology is broad. Mixed infections are common. IAI pathogens include:
  - Anaerobes, including *Bacteroides* spp., *Fusobacterium* spp., and anaerobic gram-positive cocci.
  - *E. coli, Proteus mirabilis,* and other enteric gram-negative rods
  - *Enterococcus* spp.
  - *G. vaginalis*
  - *Listeria monocytogenes*
  - Streptococci, including group B *Streptococcus* and group A *Streptococcus*
  - *Toxoplasma gondii*
  - *Ureaplasma urealyticum* and *Mycoplasma hominis*
  - Viruses: CMV, HSV, rubella

➤ Who Should be Suspected?
- The mother commonly presents with fever, abdominal pain and uterine tenderness, and leukocytosis. Other laboratory signs and clinical symptoms typical of infectious complications, such as maternal and fetal tachycardia, are common. Foul odor of amniotic fluid is strongly suggestive of IAI.

➤ Laboratory Findings
- Histology: Fetal membranes and tissue and placenta should be submitted for histologic examination, as appropriate.
- Culture: Amniotic fluid specimens are transported to the laboratory as quickly as possible. If transport will be delayed, hold at 4°C to prevent overgrowth of contaminants. Two or three sets of blood cultures should be collected from the mother to evaluate the possibility of bacteremia or fungemia.
- Amniotic fluid findings: Analysis of fluid glucose concentration and WBC count is recommended. Leukocyte esterase (LE), IL-6 concentration, and other markers of inflammation may support the diagnosis of IAI.
- Molecular testing: Molecular diagnostic testing are recommended for viral pathogens and *T. gondii.*

---

*This section contributed by Michael J. Mitchell, MD.

➤ Interpretation

* In women presenting with clinical symptoms of IAI, increased CRP and increased WBC with a left shift support the diagnosis of IAI.
* Isolation of a typical pathogen from amniotic fluid by culture, or detection by PCR, is considered the "gold standard" for diagnosis of IAI.
* Other individual tests have lower sensitivity and specificity, but specificity is increased when several tests are positive. For example, for patients with premature labor, the finding of positive Gram stain, positive LE, increased WBC, and decreased glucose have a sensitivity of 90% and specificity of 80% for predicting positive cultures.

➤ Suggested Readings

Broekhuizen FF, Gilman M, Hamilton PR. Amniocentesis for gram stain and culture in preterm premature rupture of the membranes. *Obst Gynecol.* 1985;66:316–321.

Gauthier DW, Meyer WJ. Comparison of gram stain, leukocyte esterase activity, and amniotic fluid glucose concentration in predicting amniotic fluid culture results in preterm premature rupture of membranes. *Am J Obstet Gynecol.* 1992;1092–1095.

Goldenberg RL, Hauth JC, Andrews WW. Intrauterine infection and preterm delivery. *NEJM* 2000;342:1500–1507.

Hussey M, Levy E, Pombar X, Meyer P, Strassner H. Evaluating rapid diagnostic tests of intra-amniotic infection: Gram stain, amniotic fluid glucose level, and amniotic fluid to serum glucose level ratio. *Am J Obst Gynecol.* 1998;179:650–656.

Romero R, Gomez R, Chaiworapongsa T, et al. The role of infection in preterm labour and delivery. *Paediat Perinat Epidemiol.* 2001;15:41–56.

Sperling RS, Newton E, Gibbs RS. Intraamniotic infection in low-birth-weight infants. *J Infect Dis.* 1988;157:113–117.

ECTOPIC (TUBAL) PREGNANCY

➤ Definition

* Ectopic pregnancy is implantation of blastocyst elsewhere than endometrium.

➤ Laboratory Findings

* Human chorionic gonadotropin (hCG): Tests for hCG should recognize the following three important forms. Intact hCG, H-hCG (hyperglycosylated hCG produced by invasive cytotrophoblasts; key component in early pregnancy), and free β-hCG that many kits and point-of-care (POC) tests do not recognize.
    * hCG titer doubles about every 2–3.5 days during first 40 days of normal pregnancy (at least two measurements 48–72 hours apart are needed to calculate this); an abnormally slow increase in hCG (<66% in 48 hours during first 40 days of pregnancy) indicates ectopic pregnancy (S/S = 80%/91%) or abnormal intrauterine pregnancy in ~75% of cases.
    * 6500 mIU/mL (equivalent to ~6 weeks of gestation) without an intrauterine gestational sac by transabdominal sonography favors ectopic pregnancy, since at this titer an intrauterine pregnancy should be visualized. May also occur with spontaneous abortion.
    * Intrauterine gestational sac by sonography may not be identified conclusively until 28 days after conception.
    * <6000 mIU/mL without a sac = unknown diagnosis; absent gestational sac at this hCG concentration is associated with ectopic pregnancy in >85% of cases.
    * <6000 mIU with a sac suggests either ectopic or an early normal/abnormal pregnancy.

- ~2000 mIU/mL, transvaginal sonography should identify viable intrauterine pregnancy.
- Decrease of hCG of ≥15% 12 hours after curettage is diagnostic of completed abortion, but hCG that rises or remains the same indicates ectopic pregnancy.
- hCG level >50,000 mIU/mL in ectopic pregnancy is rare. Normally rise to 100,000 mIU/mL and then plateaus.
- Serum hCG is used to monitor methotrexate treatment of ectopic pregnancy (performed weekly until undetectable).
- Urine pregnancy test is more variable.
- Progesterone: Serum progesterone should be used to screen all patients at risk for ectopic pregnancy at time of first positive pregnancy test. Level of ≥25 ng/mL is said to indicate normal intrauterine pregnancy (sensitivity = 98%) and ≤5 ng/mL confirms nonviable fetus (100% sensitivity) permitting diagnostic uterine curettage to distinguish ectopic pregnancy from spontaneous intrauterine abortion.
- Hematology: WBC may be increased; usually returns to normal in 24 hours. Persistent increase may indicate recurrent bleeding. Fifty percent of patients have normal WBC; 75% of the patients have WBC <15,000/µL. Persistent WBC >20,000/µL may indicate PID. Anemia depends on degree of blood loss; often precedes the tubal pregnancy in impoverished populations. Progressive anemia may indicate continuing bleeding into hematoma. Absorption of blood from hematoma may cause increased serum bilirubin.

FETAL DEATH IN UTERO

➤ Causes
- Antepartum (86% of deaths)
  - Chronic hypoxia of different etiologies (30%)
    - Congenital malformations/chromosomal anomalies (20%)
    - Complications of pregnancy, for example, abruptio placentae, Rh immunization (25%)
    - Fetal infections (5%)
    - Idiopathic (25%)
- Intrapartum deaths
  - AF may be brown with markedly increased CK level. Intrauterine fetal death has been said to be reliably indicated by increased CK.
  - DIC may occur, especially if >16 weeks of gestation and retained dead fetus ≥4 weeks.

PROLONGED PREGNANCY

➤ Definition
- Prolonged pregnancy is defined as one lasting >294 days or 42 weeks of gestation.

➤ Laboratory Findings
- Core laboratory: Progressively falling rather than a rising estriol (E3) is usually found.
- Amniotic fluid findings: Lecithin-to-sphingomyelin (L/S) ratio <2 occurs in 6% of cases. A high ratio (~4) can occur before 42 weeks of gestation. Therefore, the L/S ratio is not useful

for this diagnosis. Squalene (derived from fetal sebaceous glands) is markedly increased after 39 weeks. Squalene-to-cholesterol ratio in AF:
<0.40 before 40 weeks
>0.40 after 40 weeks
>1.0 after 42 weeks

MULTIPLE PREGNANCY

* This condition may be caused by fertility drug therapy (e.g., clomiphene, gonadotropins). One third of cases are monozygotic. The hCG may be increased, with increased maternal serum AFP.
* Laboratory findings due to associated conditions (e.g., polyhydramnios)
* Sequelae
  * Preeclampsia
  * Twin-to-twin transfusion
  * Others, such as intrauterine growth retardation

PLACENTAE ABRUPTIO AND PREVIA

➤ Placenta Abruptio
* Placenta abruptio is premature separation of normally implanted placenta after the 20th week of gestation. It causes hemorrhage and 15% of third-trimester stillbirths.
* There are no diagnostic laboratory findings. Laboratory findings are due to hypovolemic shock, acute renal failure, and DIC (is most common cause of DIC in pregnancy).

➤ Placenta Previa
* Placenta previa is abnormal implantation of placenta into the lower uterine segment; covers part (partial) or all (complete) of the internal os. It may cause painless vaginal bleeding.
* Laboratory findings are due to blood loss. Maternal Hct should be maintained at ≥35%.
* Beware of DIC, which occurs in >15% of cases.
* Determine lung maturity by amniocentesis for preterm delivery.
* This condition may be complicated by placenta accrete (placenta attached to myometrium).

PRETERM DELIVERY

➤ Definition
* Preterm delivery occurs when gestational age <37 weeks or 259 days; premature infant weighs <2500 g. A term infant is defined as born between 38 and 42 weeks after onset of mother's last period.

➤ Laboratory Findings
* Fetal fibronectin in cervical secretions >50 ng/mL (immunoassay) or rapid test identifies women who deliver before term with S/S = 60–93%/52%–85%, PPV = 25%. With high-risk patients, S/S = 70%/75%. NPV = 96% rules out labor within 7 days. Normally present

in early pregnancy and within 1–2 weeks of onset of labor at term but normally absent from cervicovaginal fluid after 20 weeks. If present between 24 and 36 weeks, precedes preterm labor/birth by ≥3 weeks.
* Laboratory findings are due to associated conditions (e.g., hyaline membrane disease, intraventricular hemorrhage)

➤ **Suggested Reading**

Foxman EF, Jarolim P. Use of the fetal fibronectin test in decisions to admit to hospital for preterm labor. *Clin Chem.* 2003;50:663.

RUPTURED MEMBRANES

* Direct observation of fluid leaking from cervical os is best proof.
* Laboratory diagnosis of fluid from posterior fornix as AF rather than urine
  * Detection of fetal isoform of fibronectin (immunoassay) in vaginal secretions indicates presence of AF; sensitivity >98% but low specificity. Is 5–10× greater in AF than in maternal plasma; not present in normal vaginal secretions or urine.
  * Other laboratory methods for detecting AF in the vagina
    * "Fern" test is the most reliable test (>96% accuracy). AF air-dried on a glass slide shows a characteristic fernlike pattern microscopically. Results are false positive in the presence of cervical mucus or semen and false negative in the presence of blood, dry swab, or insufficient drying time; they are not affected by meconium or pH.
    * Nitrazine paper changes from blue to yellow if pH >6.5, with accuracy ~93%. Results are false positive due to blood, semen, alkaline urine, trichomoniasis, bacterial vaginosis. Normal vaginal pH in pregnancy = 4.5–4.7; AF pH = 7.1–7.3. Reagent strip test pH ≥7 and protein ≥100 mg/dL indicate AF (Table 9-2).
* To detect premature rupture of membranes in any trimester, saline washings of vaginal fornix reportedly show hCG >50 mIU/mL with high S/S and PPV.
* Measurement of AFP in vaginal secretions is unreliable; same concentration in AF and maternal plasma in third trimester.

➤ **Suggested Reading**

Anai T, Tanaka Y, Hirota Y, et al. Vaginal fluid hCG levels for detecting premature rupture of membranes. *Obstet Gynecol.* 1997;89:261–264.

TABLE 9-2. Predictive Value of Amniotic Fluid Analysis		
	Sensitivity	Specificity
pH alone	85%	83%
Protein alone	90%	87%
Either or both	95%	91%
*Blood, meconium, renal disease, and infection interfere with accuracy. There is microscopic evidence of fat-laden fetal squamous epithelial cells (Nile blue sulfate stain).		

TOXEMIA OF PREGNANCY

➤ Definition

• Preeclampsia is characterized by hypertension and proteinuria and edema (of face, hands, legs) after 20th week of pregnancy on ≥2 occasions 6 hours but <1 week apart.
• Etiology is unknown; there are many theories. One is that renin (produced in kidney) acts on angiotensins I and II. Healthy pregnant women are resistant to vasoconstriction and increase in BP, but in toxemia this is not the case.

➤ Laboratory Findings

• Core laboratory: Serum uric acid is increased in virtually all cases of preeclampsia; correlates with disease severity. Serum creatinine >1.2 mg/dL. BUN may be normal unless the disease is severe or there is a prior renal lesion. (BUN usually decreases during normal pregnancy because of increase in the GFR.) Creatinine clearance is decreased, causing increased BUN and creatinine.
• Urinalysis: RBCs and RBC casts are not abundant; hyaline and granular casts are present.

Mild Preeclampsia

• Diagnostic criteria
  • Hypertension >140/90 but diastolic <110 mm Hg *and*
  • Proteinuria (collected by catheter if membranes have ruptured or in presence of vaginitis) >300 mg/24 hours or >1+ on dipstick on 2 occasions >6 hours but <1 week apart *or* 2 specimens ≥1+ by dipstick 6 hours but <1 week apart *or*
  Single specimen ≤2+ by dipstick *or*
  Single specimen with protein/creatinine ratio ≤0.35
• Proteinuria is variable and usually late sign (1+ dipstick correlates with 30 mg/dL).
• Increased serum inhibin A (at 15–20 weeks) and activin A (at ~30 weeks) may indicate preeclampsia and preterm labor.

Severe Preeclampsia

➤ Definition

• Diagnostic criteria
  • Hypertension >160/110 mm Hg or diastolic ≥110 mm Hg on 2 occasions >6 hours apart on bed rest
  • Persistent severe visual or cerebral disturbances
• Pulmonary edema

➤ Laboratory Findings

• Histology: Biopsy of kidney is pathognomic (swelling of glomerular and mesangial endothelial cells) and also rules out primary renal disease or hypertensive vascular disease.
• Urinalysis: Proteinuria (collected by catheter if membranes have ruptured or in presence of vaginitis) *or* >500 mg/24 hours or >3+ on dipstick on two occasions >6 hours apart *or* Significant new onset proteinuria ≥3.0 to 5.0 g/24 hours *or* >3+ by dipstick on two occasions. Oliguria—urine output ≤500 mL/24 hours

- Hematology: Platelet count $<100,000/\mu L$
- Core laboratory: Abnormal liver function tests with persistent right upper quadrant or epigastric pain.

Eclampsia

➤ Definition
- Indicated by new onset of grand mal seizures without other identifiable cause occurring in woman who meets criteria for preeclampsia. Approximately 20% of women who develop eclampsia have only mild hypertension and often without proteinuria or edema.

➤ Laboratory Findings
- Laboratory findings due to complications (e.g., cerebral hemorrhage, pulmonary edema, renal cortical necrosis)v
- $MgSO_4$ treatment requires urine output ≥ 100 mL/4 hours.
- Beware of associated or underlying conditions (e.g., hydatidiform mole, twin pregnancy, prior renal disease, DM, or nonimmune hydrops fetalis).

➤ Suggested Reading
Cukle H, Sehmi I, Jones R. Maternal serum Inhibin A can predict preeclampsia. *Br J Obstet Gynaecol.* 1998;105:1101.

TROPHOBLASTIC NEOPLASMS

➤ Definition
- Hydatidiform mole—10% become invasive moles; 2.5% progress to choriocarcinoma
- Complete mole—normal amount of DNA that is all of paternal origin (due to fertilization of an anucleate ovum). Seventy-five percent to 85% are homozygous 46 XX; the rest are heterozygous, mostly 46 XY with few 46 XX.
- Partial mole—paternal and maternal DNA present but overabundance of paternal DNA. Fertilization of oocyte by 2 haploid sperm causes triploid 69 XYY, 68 XXY, 69 XXY karyotypes in two thirds of cases; the rest have diploid karyotype (46 XX or 46 XY). β-hCG is not usually very increased and spontaneously regresses in >95% of cases requiring chemotherapy.

➤ Laboratory Findings
- Serum hCG: used for diagnosis and management of both benign and malignant types. Persistently elevated or slowly declining level by end of first trimester indicates persistent trophoblastic disease and the need for systemic therapy for invasive mole or choriocarcinoma. hCG level >500,000 mIU/L is virtually diagnostic. After evacuation of the uterus, hCG is negative by 40 days in 75% of cases. If test is positive at 56 days, 50% have trophoblastic disease. Repeat test every 1–2 weeks with clinical examination for 6 months. Disease remits in 80% without further treatment. Plateau or rise of titer indicates persistent disease. Chemotherapy is indicated if disease persists or metastasizes. Repeat negative titer should be rechecked every 3 months for 1–2 years. High-risk patients are indicated by initial serum titer >40,000

mIU/L. Frequent follow-up titers are indicated after radiation therapy with lifelong titers every 6 months.

- hCG (secreted by placenta syncytiotrophoblasts) is important to identify 15–20% of hydatidiform moles that persist after curettage.
- CSF hCG: Measurement of hCG in CSF (ratio of serum-to-CSF <60:1) is used in diagnosis of brain metastases.
- Histology: Diagnosis is by histologic examination of tissue removed by curettage.

➤ Limitations

Beware of false lows due to artifactual "hook effect" of immunoassays due to large antigen excess (>1 $\times$ 10^6 mIU/L); eliminated by 2-stage immunoassay. Clinical and biochemical evidence of hyperthyroxemia may occur because α subunits of TSH and hCG are identical.

Hematologic Disorders

Liberto Pechet

T his chapter covers blood diseases encompassing pathology of the formed elements of blood (red cells, white cells, and platelets), monoclonal plasmatic dyscrasias, hemorrhagic and thrombotic diseases, and lastly metabolic disorders that have a major impact on hematologic parameters. Principles of transfusion medicine are also included.

RED CELL DISORDERS

ANEMIAS

➤ Definition

- Anemia is a reduction in Hb leading to decrease in oxygen supply to peripheral tissues. Normal Hb range (see p. 202) is established by population studies, but range should be adjusted for different age groups, especially for children, and levels are lower in women and in African Americans. There is some debate whether people of older ages have *physiologically* lower Hg levels. Most likely lower values reflect underlying pathology.
- Hb values are more accurate than Hct values, because Hb is measured directly by automated analyzers, whereas the Hct is a calculated value (see p. 202).

➤ Diagnosis

- There are many ways to classify anemias, but the differential diagnosis of anemia can be narrowed by using the RBC size, as reflected in the MCV (see p. 254) and the reticulocyte count. See Figure 10-1.
- In addition, insight into mechanism and etiology complements the differential diagnosis.
- Onset of anemia has a great impact on diagnosis.

Onset

- Acute
  - Bleeding
  - Hemolysis
  - Acute bone marrow disease (e.g., leukemias)
- Chronic
  - Deficiencies: iron (most common), folic acid, vitamin B_{12}, nutritional
  - Congenital (hemoglobinopathies, hereditary spherocytosis)
  - Neoplasia, especially metastatic or hematologic malignancies
  - Renal disease
  - Chronic inflammatory disorders
  - Many others

When to Suspect Anemia

- Children
  - Young child who fails to thrive and is not as active as expected for age
  - Anemia detected at ages 3–6 months suggests a congenital disorder of Hb synthesis or structure.
- Adults
  - Nonspecific symptoms and signs such as weakness, dizziness, progressive lack of energy, pallor, and shortness of breath in the absence of serious heart or lung disease (overt CHF may develop as a consequence of severe anemia)
  - Protracted GI or vaginal bleeding
  - Family history of anemia
  - Jaundice or red urine

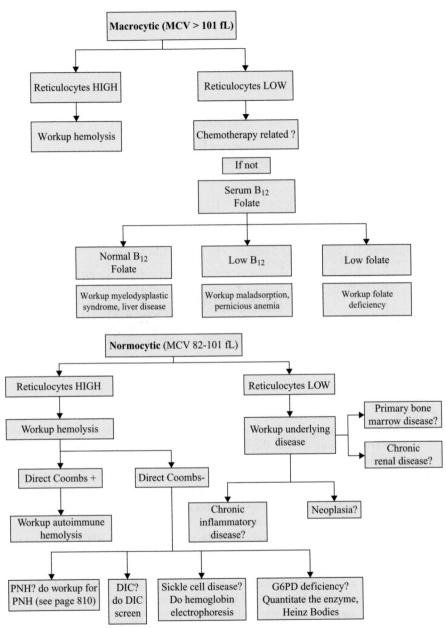

Figure 10-1. Work-up of anemias based on the mean corpuscular volume (MCV) of red cells (hematocrit [Hct] in males <42 vol%; Hct in females <37 vol%).

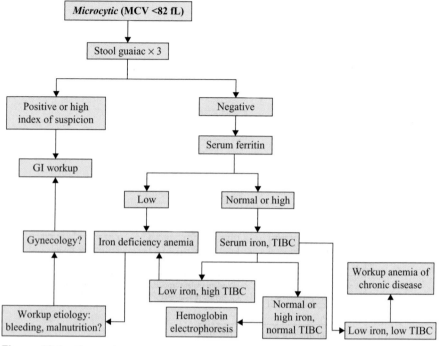

Figure 10-1. (*Continued*)

➤ Tests

- Initial laboratory investigation should include a complete CBC with a reticulocyte count (see p. 323) and examination of the PBS. The reticulocyte count reflects bone marrow response to anemia.
- Once the suspicion of anemia is confirmed by finding a reduction in Hb and Hct (the RBC count may be normal or even higher in certain conditions, such a thalassemia trait), the type of anemia must be determined by subsequent laboratory investigations, based mostly on the MCV, and subdivided by pathophysiology.
- The RDW provides a useful measurement of the variation in size of RBCs, indicating the presence of anisocytosis when elevated (see p. 319)
- Once anemia is documented, subsequent investigations depend on the type of anemia suspected based on indices and the reticulocyte count (see Figure 10-1). More complex laboratory tests or bone marrow biopsy may be indicated to ascertain its precise etiology.
- Various types of anemias are described subsequently.
    - Microcytic (see p. 792)
    - Macrocytic (see p. 791)
    - Normocytic (see p. 793)
    - Aplastic (see p. 794)
    - Hemoglobinopathies (see p. 796)
        - Sickle cell (see p. 796)
        - HbC, HbD, HbE diseases (see p. 800)

- Thalassemias (see p. 801)
- Hemolytic (see p. 804)

➤ Suggested Readings

Beutler E, Waalen J. The definition of anemia: what is the lower limit of normal of the blood hemoglobin concentration? *Blood*. 2006;107:1747–1750.

Tefferi A. Anemia in adults: a contemporary approach to diagnosis. *Mayo Clin Proc*. 2003;78:1274–1280.

MACROCYTIC ANEMIAS

➤ Definition

Anemias in which the RBCs are oval macrocytes, with an MCV larger than normal (>101 fL)

➤ Who Should be Suspected?

- A patient with macrocytic anemia, hypersegmented neutrophils on PBS, and symptoms of malabsorption, poor diet, chronic hemolysis without folate supplementation, chemotherapy, or hypothyroidism. Folate deficiency is seen with alcoholism; in third world countries it is associated with sprue-like syndromes. Vitamin B_{12} (cobalamin) deficiency increases in incidence with aging, and should be searched for, even in the absence of anemia in the elderly with neurologic deficits. Cobalamine and folic acid deficiencies often coexist.
- Other causes of macrocytic anemias are liver cirrhosis, myelodysplastic syndrome (MDS), azidothymidine (AZT) therapy for AIDS, Down syndrome, and normal newborns.

➤ Tests

- Laboratory investigation of macrocytic anemias must differentiate between macrocytic anemias without megaloblastosis and true megaloblastic anemias resulting from vitamin B_{12} and/or folate deficiency. Megaloblastic anemia is a morphologic definition based on bone marrow examination. B_{12} deficiency may be the result of PA (lack of intrinsic factor), or may have other etiologies.
  - CBC
    - Anemia with oval macrocytes, poikilocytosis and anisocytosis, small teardrop cells
    - High RDW (see tests)
    - Thrombocytopenia and leukopenia in severe cases
    - Hypersegmented polymorphonuclears and giant metamyelocytes in megaloblastic anemias
    - Reticulocyte count: inadequate for the degree of anemia
  - Serum or RBC folate and serum cobalamin are obtained if another etiology is not obvious. The specific metabolites methylmalonic acid and homocysteine accumulate in these deficiencies; they are additional assays and may help discriminate between cobalamin and folate deficiencies, and other etiologies for macrocytic anemias. These assays, as well as RBC folate, are more expensive and should be reserved for patients with borderline folate or cobalamin values but strong suspicion of one or the other.
  - Serum cobalamin if <200 pg/mL (see p. 381) is consistent with vitamin B_{12} deficiency.
  - Serum folate if <2 ng/mL (see p. 180) is consistent with folate deficiency.
  - Serum or urine methylmalonic acid (see p. 257 for normal range) if increased confirms vitamin B_{12} deficiency. It may be normal in folate deficiency.
  - Homocysteine (total) (see p. 208) if elevated is compatible with either cobalamin or folate deficiency. If normal, both are excluded.

- Documentation of cobalamin deficiency does not establish the diagnosis of PA, an autoimmune disease characterized by deficiency of intrinsic factor (IF) and lack of HCl gastric secretion. PA was traditionally diagnosed by the absorption of orally administered radiolabeled cobalamin, the Schilling test (no longer available in the United States). In its absence, the assays mentioned above are helpful, but not specific for PA. Fifty percent to 70% of PA patients will have positive serum anti-IF antibodies, thus documenting PA (100% specificity). The patients who are negative for IF antibodies cannot be distinguished from non-PA cases of cobalamin malabsorption, but will respond to oral vitamin B_{12} if not PA. Antiparietal antibodies are less sensitive or specific. Recently, chronic *Helicobacter pylori* infection has been implicated in the etiology of PA and the lack of IF.
- Bone marrow aspirate (indicated in only selected cases) may reveal marked red cell hyperplasia and megaloblastic maturation in both vitamin B_{12} or folate deficiency. Otherwise, it may uncover other reasons for macrocytosis, such as MDS.
- Serum LDH and indirect bilirubin are elevated in folate and vitamin B_{12} deficiency.

➤ Limitations
- In the presence of coexisting iron deficiency, MCV may not be elevated, even in cases of overt folate or cobalamin deficiency.
- Low cobalamin levels develop during pregnancy.
- One hospital meal may normalize serum (but not RBC) folate level. Methylmalonic acid increases in renal insufficiency.

➤ Suggested Reading
Schrier SL. Diagnosis and treatment of vitamin B_{12} and folic acid deficiency. UptoDate. Rose B, ed. Waltham, MA: UptoDate Inc.; 2008.

MICROCYTIC ANEMIAS

➤ Definition
- Anemias characterized by low MCV ($<$82 fL) and hypochromia
- Most common: iron deficiency anemia; to be differentiated from the thalassemias (see p. 801) and occasionally from anemia of chronic diseases (see p. 793). Despite the high frequency of iron-deficiency anemia, patients should not be treated automatically with iron without determining the cause of the deficiency.

➤ Who Should be Suspected?
- Suspect iron deficiency if the following are present:
  - Microcytosis, hypochromia
  - History of GI, vaginal, or massive, repeated urinary bleeding
  - Poor diet

➤ Tests
- First line of investigation: serum ferritin (see p. 174) has a specificity of 98%, but a sensitivity of only 25% for a 12 µg/L threshold. Because ferritin is an acute phase reactant, it may be normal or even increased despite iron deficiency when the patients have serious medical problems, such as chronic inflammatory conditions and active liver disease. As a consequence, a normal ferritin value does not exclude iron deficiency. Very low values

are definitely diagnostic, iron deficiency is confirmed, and there is no need to obtain serum iron and total iron binding capacity (TIBC). Investigation of etiology (history, stool examination for occult blood, GI investigation, pelvic and rectal examinations) are mandatory.

- If serum ferritin is normal or borderline, serum iron and transferrin (usually reported as TIBC) are the next assay to be ordered (see p. 234).
- If the serum iron is very low and TIBC elevated (with ratio serum iron divided by TIBC <16%), diagnosis is confirmed.
- Normal serum iron and TIBC: iron deficiency is excluded in most cases.
- Low serum iron, low TIBC: most likely anemia of chronic disease; work-up underlying etiology
- High serum iron, normal TIBC: the most likely diagnosis is thalassemia (see p. 801).
- Two additional blood tests: the soluble transferrin receptor and the reticulocyte Hb content are optional. When used in conjunction with ferritin, theses tests improve further our ability to accurately diagnose iron deficiency. Not widely used.
- As a last resort, if the diagnosis is still in doubt: bone marrow aspirate/biopsy for Prussian blue stain. If it is negative, iron deficiency is definitely present.

NORMOCYTIC ANEMIAS

➤ Definition
- Anemias with normal MCV

➤ Who Should be Suspected?
- Patients with anemias secondary to an underlying nonhematologic disease (also known as "anemias of chronic disease" [ACD]). The term "anemia of chronic inflammation" may be used too, but it does not cover all situations (see below).
- The most common conditions leading to ACD:
  - Anemia of chronic inflammation (infections, rheumatologic diseases) is the prototype of normocytic anemias; the red cell may occasionally be borderline microcytic.
  - Anemia of chronic renal failure's etiology is in part the reduced production of erythropoietin; additional factors are a shortened red cell survival and frequent bleeding.
  - Anemia in cancer patients is a common, multifactorial finding. Microangiopathic hemolytic anemia and myelophthisic anemia may be an additional feature resulting from disseminated carcinoma.
  - Aplastic anemias (AAs) (see p. 794) can be congenital or acquired. In AA, hematopoiesis fails. All blood lineages are decreased (pancytopenia), with the possible exception of lymphocytes. Pure red cell anemia is a variant of AA in which only, or mostly, the red cell line is affected.

➤ Tests
- CBC: moderate anemia, normal to slightly reduced MCV in inflammatory conditions; normal red cell morphology, with only mild variation in RDW. In anemia of chronic renal failure burr cells can be seen on the PBS.
- Inadequate reticulocyte response.
- Increased serum ferritin; reduced serum iron and TIBC
- Serum erythropoietin is inadequate for the level of anemia, especially in renal failure

APLASTIC ANEMIA (AA)

➤ Definition

* Although the name refers only to anemia, AA is characterized by peripheral blood pancy-topenia. It is the paradigm of bone marrow failure. There is variable bone marrow hypocel-lularity due to diminished or absent hematopoietic precursors, the result of injury to the pluripotent stem cell.
* The absence of a myeloproliferative neoplasm or an MDS is a prerequisite for the diagnosis.

➤ Etiology

* AA may be acquired or congenital (Fanconi anemia; see below). More than 50% of the acquired cases are idiopathic, most likely due to an autoimmune mechanism that destroys or suppresses the hematopoietic stem cell via cytotoxic T lymphocytes and the cytokines they produce.
* Other cases may result from drugs, such as chemotherapy, anticonvulsants, chlorampheni-col, phenylbutazone, quinacrine, sulfa drugs, antihistamines, antidiabetic drugs, gold, sulfa drugs, antithyroid drugs, penicillamine, benzene exposure, and many more.
    * Immunologic disorders such as graft-versus-host disease
    * Thymomas
    * Exposure to ionizing radiation
    * Viral infections: EBV and the putative agent of seronegative hepatitis
    * Severe malnutrition: kwashiorkor, anorexia nervosa
    * Leukemia may be the underlying disease in 1–5% of patients who present with AA
    * PNH (see p. 810) develops in 5–10% of patients with AA; conversely, AA develops in 25% of patients with PNH.

➤ Who Should be Suspected?

* An individual who presents with a clinical picture of increasing symptoms of anemia, or mucosal bleeding, rarely infections, and in whom an initial CBC demonstrates pancytopenia
* Pancytopenia from other causes, such as chemotherapy, should be ruled out (see below).
* The disease is frequent in East Asia.

➤ Tests

* RBC: anemia is normocytic, normochromic, but may be slightly microcytic. Hg may be <7 g/L. RDW is normal.
* PBS: normocytic, occasionally microcytic RBC. There are decreased granulocytes and plate-lets. Abnormal WBC are not seen.
* Reticulocytes are invariably decreased to absent.
* WBC: neutropenia (absolute neutrophil count <1,500/µL) is always present, often accom-panied by monocytosis. Lymphocyte count is normal (false lymphocytosis if one observes the percent of WBC rather than the absolute count).
* Platelets are decreased, but severity varies.
* Bone marrow is hypocellular, with <30% of residual cells being hematopoietic. Hematopoiesis is not megaloblastic. Aspiration and biopsy are both necessary to rule out MDS, leukemias, granulomatous disease, or tumors. The bone marrow also must exclude the viral hemophagocytic syndrome, where macrophages with ingested hematopoietic cells are observed.

- Cytogenetics: normal karyotype
- Flow cytometry phenotyping shows virtual absence of CD34 cells blasts in blood and marrow. In >50% of cases, PNH clones (see p. 810) can be detected by positivity for CD59.
- Serum iron studies are normal.

FANCONI'S ANEMIA (FA)

➤ Definition
- Autosomal recessive syndrome of aplastic anemia in childhood and congenital anomalies of rudimentary thumbs, hypoplastic radii, short stature, renal anomalies, and skin hyperpigmentation. FA is a rare disorder of chromosomal instability. There are 13 genes involved.
- There is an increased incidence of leukemia in patients and relatives.
- The diagnosis is usually made between the ages of 4 and 10 years, but in rare cases it may not been made until the 20s.

➤ Tests
- RBC: The anemia is usually normochromic, but may be macrocytic
- WBC: leukopenia due to granulocytopenia
- Cytogenetics: normal chromosome numbers but structural instability causing breaks, gaps, constrictions, and rearrangements. Exposure to DNA cross-linking agents increases chromosome breakage and specific assays are now used to diagnose FA.
- Genetics: Multiple genes appear to be responsible for the clinical picture. Genetic methodology to subtype FA based on the genes involved is now recommended to finalize the diagnosis and to determine optimal care.
- Fetal Hb is increased (>28%).
- i antigen may be observed.

PURE RED CELL APLASIA (PRCA)

➤ Definition
- PRCA presents with anemia, absent reticulocytes, and absent bone marrow erythroid precursors. (The congenital pure red cell aplasia is described below). It is considered an immune-mediated disease. It may be associated with thymomas, collagen vascular syndromes, CLL, or follow parvovirus B19 infection. It may also be part of the 5q− myelodysplastic syndrome.
- Rarely, PRCA follows administration of certain preparations of erythropoietin due to development of anti-erythropoietin antibodies.

➤ Tests
- CBC: severe reduction in RBCs, but normal WBC and platelet counts
- Reticulocytes are severely depressed or absent.
- Bone marrow: erythroid precursors cells are absent, except for occasional normoblasts (giant normoblasts indicate parvovirus infection). White cell precursors and megakaryocytes (except in the 5q− syndrome) are normal.

DIAMOND-BLACKFAN ANEMIA (DBA)

➤ Definition
* DBA is a congenital pure red cell aplasia.
* It is usually sporadic but may be inherited in an autosomal dominant manner. Onset is before 12 months.
* DBA is associated with congenital anomalies of the kidneys, eyes, skeleton, and heart.
* Spontaneous remissions have been observed in 20% of cases after months or years.

➤ Tests
* RBC: severe normochromic, or slightly macrocytic, anemia that is refractory to all treatments.
* Reticulocytes are <1%
* WBC, differential white cell count, and platelet count are normal.
* Bone marrow shows marked decrease in erythroid precursors. All other cell lines are normal.
* Fetal Hb is increased.
* Adenosine deaminase is increased in RBCs.
* Serum iron and all other hematologic parameters are normal.
* Serum erythropoietin is elevated.

HEMOGLOBINOPATHIES

More than 1000 mutations involving the globin genes have been described; they result from amino acid substitution or from abnormalities of synthesis. Diagnosis is confirmed by Hb variant analysis in most cases. Table 10-1 describes the three most common hemoglobinopathies encountered in North America: sickle cell syndromes, HbC disease, and β and α thalassemias.

Sickle Cell Anemia
➤ Definition
* Sickle cell diseases encompass a group of conditions with autosomal inheritance of abnormal Hb β chain resulting from a substitution of a valine for glutamic acid. They are encountered mostly in persons of African or Arab ancestry, as well as in some Indian groups.
* Sickle cell anemia is the homozygous disease where the majority of Hb is S. This results in the precipitation and polymerization of Hb, causing rigid crystals that deform red cells (sickling), leading to microvascular occlusions and hemolysis.
* Sickle cell trait is the heterozygous form, an asymptomatic condition in which the CBC is normal. Its diagnosis is important for genetic counseling.
* Sickle cell syndromes (diseases) represent combinations of sickle cell trait with other hemoglobinopathies, most commonly with β thalassemia or Hb C.

➤ Who Should be Suspected?
* A young child with a family history of sickle cell disease, failure to thrive, or progressive anemia.
* Vasoocclusive phenomena eventually become common. Clinical manifestations are not present at birth, but become apparent after 3–6 months of life, as the concentration of Hb F declines, and that of Hb S increases.

TABLE 10-1. Hemoglobinopathies

Condition	HbA (%)	HbA$_2$ (%)	HbF (%)	HbS (%)	HbC (%)	Other (%)
Normal	≥94	2–3.5	0.5–1	0	0	
Sickle cell trait	50–70	2–4.5	0.5–1	30–45	0	
Sickle cell anemia	0	2–4	1–25	75–95	0	
HbC trait	50–60	sl ↑	0.5–1	0	30–40	
HbCC (homozygous)	0	<3.5	sl ↑	0	95	
HbS/HbC disease	Trace	0	<1	50–55	45–50	
β Thalassemia minor	90–95	3.5–7	1–5	0	0	
β Thalassemia major	β+: Trace β−: 0	2–sl ↑	60–95 95–98	0	0	
α Thalassemia with 1–2 abnormal genes	Varies with genetic type	2–3.5	0.5–1	0	0	
α Thalassemia: 3-gene defect (HbH disease)	<60	<2	<1–1	0	0	HbH: 5–40
α Thalassemia: 4-gene defect (hydrops fetalis)	0 or trace	<2	0 or trace	0	0	Hb Bart's 70–80
HbS-β Thalassemia	Heterozygous: 70–85 Homozygous: 0	4–6 1–2.1	<1–10 15–30	70–90 0	0 0	
Hereditary persistence of fetal Hb (HPFH)	0	0	100	0	0	

- Aplastic crises are self-limited episodes of erythroid aplasia lasting 5–10 days. They are due to infections (most commonly parvovirus B19) and may require emergency transfusions.
- Bilirubin gallstones are present in 30% of patients by age 18, and 70% by age 30.

➤ Tests

- Gene analysis of fetal DNA may be performed on chorionic villi (7–10 weeks of gestation) or amniocytes (15–20 weeks of gestation). DNA testing may be also useful in newborns or children in cases with high levels of HbF.
- In older children or in adults, a "sickle cell screen" (see p. 337) can be obtained for a rapid preliminary diagnosis. It is positive in sickle cell anemia, sickle cell trait, in some non-S sickling hemoglobinopathies, and in combined sickle cell disease with other hemoglobinopathies.
- Hb variant analysis (HPLC or electrophoresis, [see p. 203]) are used to separate different hemoglobins. Newborns have predominantly HbF with a small amount of HbS and no HbA1. Because other sickle cell syndromes may have similar patterns, it is recommended to study the parents, or repeat the test after one year of age, when the adult pattern is established, with very high HbS and occasionally elevated HbF, especially in patients treated successfully with hydroxyurea.
- The newborn with sickle cell trait will have HbA, HbF, and HbS. Adults have >50% Hb A1 and 35–45% HbS.
- Patients with HbSC disease have equal amount of HbS and C.
- Patients with sickle cell trait–β thalassemia (+) have HbA1, elevated HbA2, and HbS.
- CBC in patients with sickle cell anemia
  - RBC: anemia (Hct 15–30%, Hb 5–10 g/dL)
  - Reticulocytes 3–15% (they account for elevated MCV)
  - MCV is normal (except as noted above); MCHC is elevated.
  - PBS: visible sickle cells, polychromasia, and Howell-Jolly bodies (see p. 322) in older children, reflecting autosplenectomy. Nucleated red cells, basophilic stippling, and Pappenheimer bodies (see p. 322) are usually found.
  - WBCs may be higher than normal.
  - Platelets may be elevated.
  - Bone marrow aspirate (not necessary for diagnosis) is hyperplastic.
  - Serum LDH is elevated.
  - Serum bilirubin is commonly elevated.
  - Serum haptoglobin is elevated.
  - Serum aminotransferase is often elevated.
  - Ferritin becomes very elevated in multiply transfused patients.
  - Urine hemosiderin and urobilinogen are present (not necessary for diagnosis).

Hemoglobin S–Hemoglobin C Disease
➤ Definition

- A moderately severe sickling disease, intermediate between sickle cell anemia and sickle cell trait
- Occurs in 1 of 833 people of African ancestry

➤ Tests

- Hb electrophoresis: HbA is absent; HbS and HbC are present in approximately equal amounts. HbF is ≤76%.

* CBC
  * Anemia: mild to moderate normochromic, normocytic
  * PBS: tetragonal crystals within the RBC in 70% of patients. Target cells (≤85%) and plump/angulated sickle cells, rather than typical sickle cells are identified.
  * MCV is low, or low normal, MCHC is high.

Sickle Cell–α-Thalassemia Disease

* α-Thalassemia modifies the severity of sickle cell anemia. Otherwise it is usually clinically insignificant.

Sickle Cell–β-Thalassemia Disease

➤ Definition
* Condition of mild to moderate severity found in 1 of every 1667 people of African ancestry.

➤ Tests
* Hb electrophoresis: HbS varies between 20% and 90%; HbF is between 2% and 20%. If the HbS is very high and HbA1 is suppressed, the disease is severe. In milder cases HbA1 is 25–50%. HbA2 is increased (due to the presence of β-thalassemia) but it has to be differentiated from HbC, which has a similar migration pattern.
* CBC
  * RBC: hypochromic, microcytic anemia with decreased MCV (iron deficiency must be ruled out).
  * PBS: target cells are prominent; other findings resemble those of sickle cell anemia.

Sickle Cell–Persistent High Fetal Hemoglobin

➤ Definition
* Condition seen in 1 in 25,000 African Americans but also frequent in Arab populations
* May be mimicked in patients with sickle cell anemia responding to hydroxyurea therapy
* Clinical picture and findings intermediate between sickle cell anemia and trait.

➤ Tests
* Hb electrophoresis: HbF is 20–40%; HbA1 and A2 are absent; HgS is ~65%.
* RBC. HbF is unevenly distributed among RBC.

Sickle Cell–Hemoglobin D Disease

➤ Definition
* Condition resembling HbS/HbC disease; less severe than sickle cell anemia.
* Found in 1 in 20,000 individuals of African ancestry
* Clinically a mild syndrome

➤ Tests

* Intermediate between those of sickle cell anemia and sickle cell trait
* Hb electrophoresis cannot distinguish HbS from HbD at alkaline pH but can be separated at pH 6.2

➤ Suggested Readings

Vichinsky EP, Mahoney Jr DH. Diagnosis of sickle cell syndromes. UpToDate. Rose B, ed. Waltham, MA: UpToDate, Inc.; 2008.

Ware RE. How I use hydroxyurea to treat young patients with sickle cell anemia. *Blood.* 2010;115:5300–5311.

Hemoglobin C Disease

➤ Definition

* Hemoglobinopathy is prevalent in West Africa.
* Autosomal transmission.
  * HbC trait: found in 2% of African Americans, less frequently in other groups; asymptomatic, no anemia.
  * Homozygous HbC disease: mild hemolytic anemia.

➤ Tests

* HbC trait: Hb variant analysis shows 50% HbA1 and 30–40% HbC
* Homozygous condition: there is no HbA1, and HbC forms the majority variant Hb; HgF is slightly increased. PBS shows a variable number of target cells ($\leq$40%), a variable number of microspherocytes, occasionally nucleated RBCs, and a few tetragonal crystals within RBCs.

Hemoglobin C–β Thalassemia

* This combination resembles homozygous HbC disease, but with elevated HbA2. It is asymptomatic, although moderate hemolysis is present if HbA1 is absent.

Hemoglobin D Disease

➤ Definition

* Autosomal inherited hemoglobinopathy prevalent in Southeast Asia and in parts of India (HbD Punjab).
* The heterozygous form is asymptomatic with no anemia

➤ Tests

* Hb variant analysis demonstrates the abnormal Hb at acid pH (it has the same mobility as HbS at alkaline pH). There are no other laboratory abnormalities in the heterozygous individual.
* RBC: mild hemolytic, microcytic anemia in homozygous individuals.
* PBS: target cells and spherocytes in the homozygous.

Hemoglobin E Disease
➤ Definition
* Autosomal inherited hemoglobinopathy, prevalent in Southeast Asia (15–30% of the population in Cambodia, Thailand, parts of China, Burma, and Vietnam). Heterozygous individuals have similar findings as patients with mild β-thalassemia trait (see p. 803). Homozygotes exhibit more microcytosis but are asymptomatic.
* The most common structural hemoglobinopathy in the United States after HbS and HbC.

➤ Tests
* Hb variant analysis shows 95–97% HbE in the homozygous (the rest is HbF); 30–35% in HbE trait. Electrophoretic mobility is the same as for HbA2, but it is present in much higher concentrations. It separates from HbC and O on citrate agar electrophoresis at acid pH (see p. 203)
* CBC
  * Mild hemolytic, microcytic (MCV 55–70 fL) anemia or no anemia in the homozygous.
  * Erythrocytosis may be present ($\sim$5,500.000/µL) in both the trait and in the homozygous.
  * PBS shows 25–60% target cells and microcytes in the homozygous individuals.

Hemoglobin E–β-Thalassemia
➤ Definition
* The most common symptomatic thalassemia in Southeast Asia.
* A severe condition that resembles β-thalassemia intermedia or β-thalassemia major (see p. 803).

➤ Tests
* Hemolytic anemia varies from moderate to severe β-thalassemia
* PBS shows severe hypochromia and macrocytosis, and marked anisopoikilocytosis with many teardrop and target red cells. Nucleated RBC and basophilic stippling may be present.

Hemoglobin E–α-Thalassemia
* A mild hemolytic anemia encountered in Southeast Asia. It causes microcytosis. The severity depends on the number of α genes deleted (see p. 803 below)

THALASSEMIAS

This group of chronic inherited microcytic, hemolytic anemias results from reduced or absent production of either β or α chains. The thalassemias are among the most common genetic disorders worldwide. They have an autosomal recessive inheritance resulting in either homozygous (thalassemia major) or subtle (thalassemia minor) clinical abnormalities. The β-thalassemia syndromes are extremely heterogenous. In addition to β-thalassemia trait and major described below, there are combinations with other hemoglobinopathies and variants as described above.

β-Thalassemia intermedia refers to patients who have two β-globin genes carrying a thalassemia mutation, but at least one of the two genes carries a mild mutation. These patients may be symptomatic but require infrequent RBC transfusions. It is a condition with marked disparity between genotypes and phenotypes.

β-Thalassemia Major
➤ Definition
* A severe condition resulting from impaired production of the β globin chains of Hb. The patients have 2 α and 2 γ globin chains. The resulting excess α chains lead to precipitates inside the red cells with dire consequences (severe hemolysis, skeletal changes, liver abnormalities, premature gallbladder bilirubin stones, splenomegaly, aplastic crises, impaired growth, endocrine and cardiopulmonary complications, and hemosiderosis resulting from RBC transfusions). Patients with β (−) mutations produce no β globin and are the most severely affected; patients with β (+) mutations produce a small amount of β chains and are less severely affected.
* The diagnosis is usually established at 6–12 months of age due to increasing symptoms.
* β-Thalassemia is most common in individuals of Mediterranean ancestry but is also found in African Americans and in some groups in India.

➤ Tests
* CBC
    * RBC: profound anemia, microcytosis, reduced MCV and MCHC, very elevated RDW. Heinz bodies (see p. 322). The anemia may become extremely severe, even life-threatening, during aplastic crises, mostly provoked by parvovirus B19.
    * WBC is elevated (in part falsely so, due to enumeration of nucleated RBCs as WBCs by some automated counters)
    * Platelets may be reduced due to hypersplenism
    * PBS: marked poikilocytosis with many target cells, tear drop cells, nucleated RBCs, and basophilic stippling of RBCs
    * Reticulocyte count is inappropriately low
* Bone marrow aspirate shows marked red cell hyperplasia with marked shift to early red cell progenitors due to intramedullary hemolysis, in turn the result of accelerated apoptosis. Extramedullary hematopoiesis develops in skeletal bones, liver, and spleen.
* Hb variant analysis shows absence of HbA1; only HbA2 and HbF are present. HbA2 may increase to 3–6% (unless iron deficiency is also present, in which case this elevation is not seen). HbA1 may be present after RBC transfusions.
* Serum iron and ferritin increase progressively throughout life due to RBC transfusions
* Serum bilirubin is elevated.
* Liver function tests are abnormal, consistent with viral hepatitis as the result of multiple transfusions.
* LDH is elevated.
* Haptoglobin is decreased.
* Endocrine abnormalities are related to the extensive iron deposits, with laboratory evidence of hypogonadism and diabetes.
* Hypercoagulability: abnormalities in the level of clotting factors and their inhibitors have been reported in some cases.

β-Thalassemia Minor
➤ Definition
- Heterozygotes who carry one normal β globin allele, and one β-thalassemic allele. The individuals who carry this genotype are clinically normal but may have a hematologic picture that may mislead for a diagnosis of iron deficiency, if not investigated.

➤ Tests
- CBC shows microcytic anemia. The anemia is milder (Hg 10–13 g/dL), but the microcytosis is more profound (MCV 60–70 fL) than seen in iron deficiency. RBC count may be higher than normal (another contrast to iron-deficiency anemia). RDW is normal, since the RBCs are uniformly microcytic and hypochromic. On PBS, basophilic stippling of RBCs and target cells may be observed.
- Hb variant analysis: HbA2 is elevated, sometimes as high as 7–8% with the ratio HbA2/HbA1 being 1:20 instead of the normal 1:40; HgF is slightly elevated in 50% of cases. A normal concentration of HbA2 does not rule out β-thalassemia trait. Definitive diagnosis can only made by molecular genetic techniques.

Hemoglobin E/Thalassemia
➤ Definition
- One β-globin gene carries a thalassemia mutation (mild or severe), the other β-globin gene carries a point mutation encoding for HgE.

➤ Tests
- CBC: microcytic anemia of variable severity
- Hb variant analysis: reduced HbA1, elevated HbA2, and in some cases HbF; HbE present.

α-Thalassemia Syndromes
➤ Definition
- Normal subjects have 4 α-globin genes, two on each chromosome. The α-thalassemias are caused by mutations or deletions affecting one or more of the 4 α globin genes, resulting in their impaired synthesis. This defect results in excess of β globin chains, which may lead to hemolysis.
- The condition is prevalent in populations of African or Southeast Asian ancestry.

➤ Diagnosis
- The severity of the syndrome depends on the number of α genes affected.
  - Loss of all four α globin loci results in hydrops fetalis with Hb Bart, condition incompatible with extrauterine life. Hb Bart is fast moving on Hb electrophoresis.
  - Loss of three loci results in HbH disease. These patients have a moderate microcytic, hypochromic anemia with inclusion bodies present on the PBS. HbH disease can be acquired in hematologic malignancies, especially in myelodysplastic syndromes. Hb electrophoresis or chromatographic techniques show 5–30% HbH, which is the result of tetrameric β chains.

- Loss of two loci results in α thalassemia-1 trait (α thalassemia minor). Adult patients may have mild microcytic, hypochromic anemia. Hb electrophoresis is normal. Definitive diagnosis can only made by molecular genetic techniques.
- Loss of only one locus results in α thalassemia-2 trait (α thalassemia minima or silent carrier of α thalassemia). There are no hematologic abnormalities, and Hb electrophoresis is normal.

➤ Suggested Readings

Benz EJ. Clinical manifestations and diagnosis of the thalassemias. UpToDate. Rose B, ed. UpToDate Inc.; 2008.
Benz EJ. Newborn screening for α-thalassemia-keeping up with globalization. *New Engl J Med*. 2011;364:770–771.
Forget BG. Thalassemia. *Hematologic Clinics of North America*. 2010;24:1–140.

Hemolytic Anemias

➤ Definition

- Hemolytic anemias result from increase in the rate of RBC destruction, thereby decreasing RBC survival.
- The most common causes of hemolysis in North America are:
  - Acute: immune mechanisms due to autoantibodies or drugs
  - Chronic: sickle cell and thalassemia syndromes, hereditary spherocytosis, mechanical hemolytic anemias

➤ When to Suspect Hemolysis

- Acute onset of anemia with jaundice and spherocytes or schistocytes on the PBS, or family history of anemia, anemia since early childhood, early gallstones
- Mild, fluctuating jaundice, dark urine but normal-colored stools
- Splenomegaly
- Fragmented RBC (schistocytes) or spherocytes on the PBS

➤ Etiology
Classification: Intrinsic Versus Extrinsic

- Intrinsic red cell defects (usually congenital)
  - Hereditary spherocytosis: due to red cell membrane skeletal defect
  - Hereditary elliptocytosis and hereditary ovalocytosis: generally benign red cell membrane defects
  - Enzymopathies: anemias caused by abnormalities in red cell metabolism resulting from deficiencies in RBC enzymes. The most common are G6PD deficiency and PK deficiency.
  - Hereditary pyropoikilocytosis
  - Hereditary stomatocytosis
- Extrinsic red cell membrane injuries (most are acquired)
  - Autoimmune hemolysis: warm-reactive or cold-reactive antibodies
  - Alloimmune hemolysis: transfusional or hemolytic anemia of the newborn
  - Mechanical injuries to red cells (microangiopathic and macroangiopathic), DIC, TTP, HUS; disseminated malignancies, burns; membrane lysins (clostridial sepsis, leptospirosis, snake bites)
  - Water infusion or drowning
  - Drug use

Classification: Site of Destruction

- Intravascular: mechanical injuries by diseased arterial walls or abnormal heart valves, PNH, infusion of hypotonic solutions
- Extravascular: red cell destruction in macrophages (spleen, liver, other): congenital or auto-immune anemias; hypersplenism
- Intramedullary (ineffective erythropoiesis): thalassemias, myelodysplastic, and megaloblastic syndromes (partially), dyserythropoietic anemias (very rare, congenital)

➤ Tests

- CBC: anemia, usually normocytic, normochromic (microcytic in HS, macrocytic when reticulocytes are very elevated)
- PBS: polychromasia (reflects high reticulocyte count); macrocytosis if associated folate deficiency is present; nucleated RBCs
- RBC count (severe cases): deformed red cells (sickle cell anemia, microangiopathic hemolysis); target cells (thalassemia major); spherocytes (microcytic hyperchromic in HS), agglutinated red cells (suspect cold agglutinins)
- RBCs: direct Coombs test if autoimmune anemia is suspected; flow cytometry if PNH is suspected; G6PD quantitation if an enzyme defect is suspected
- Reticulocyte count (mandatory): increased (unless iron deficiency or bone marrow suppression coexist), and except during periods of intercurrent inflammatory disorders
- WBCs and platelets: increased in acute hemolysis
- Serum bilirubin: total and indirect (unconjugated) increased
- Haptoglobin: decreased (lowest levels are present in intravascular hemolysis)
- Plasma Hb: increased in intravascular hemolysis (red plasma)
- LDH isomers 1 or 2: increased
- Hb variant analysis: if a hemoglobinopathy is suspected
- Cold agglutinin titer: positive in cold agglutinin-induced hemolysis
- Urine: hemoglobinuria, hemosiderinuria (especially with intravascular hemolysis)
- Bone marrow aspirate (rarely indicated): red cell hyperplasia

HEMOLYTIC INTRINSIC RED BLOOD CELL DEFECTS

- The most common enzymopathies are G6PD and pyruvate kinase (PK) deficiency. Other rare deficiencies of RBC enzymes occur

Enzymopathy: Glucose-6-Phosphaste Dehydrogenase (G6PD) Deficiency

➤ Definition

- This enzymopathy is an hereditary RBC enzyme deficiency.
- Inheritance of G6PD deficiency is X-linked.
- Incidence is high in regions were malaria is or was prevalent. More than 300 variants have been described.
- G6PD deficiency can be divided into three categories; the normal is designated G6PD type B

- Class 1 (Mediterranean variant, G6PD type B–): <5% of normal RBC enzyme activity. It results in a chronic hemolytic anemia exacerbated by oxidant drugs or febrile illnesses. Very severe hemolytic attacks develop after the ingestion of fava beans (favism).
- Class 2 (African variant, G6PD type A–): <10% of normal RBC enzyme activity; patients have episodic hemolytic attacks produced by certain oxidant drugs or acidosis. It is not triggered by ingestion of fava beans.
- Class 3: 10–60% of the normal enzyme activity. There is no hemolysis except for limited episodes (2–3 days) after ingestion of oxidant drugs or infections.

➤ **Tests**
- Basis of diagnosis
  - Generation of NADPH from NADP as detected by either quantitative spectrophotometric analysis or, more rapidly, by a fluorescent screening test.
  - G6PD levels may be normal during and shortly following a hemolytic episode in type A–, because very young RBCs contain sufficient enzyme. Assays for G6PD should be postponed for at least 6 weeks after the acute episode.
- Female carriers: possible mild hemolytic episodes that are difficult to diagnose with conventional methodology; they can be diagnosed with genetic methods.
- Hemolytic anemia: chronic in class 1 and intermittent in classes 2 and 3. It is seen 2–4 days after ingestion of an oxidant drug (primaquine and sulfa drugs are the most common offending agents), or of fava beans.
- Neonatal jaundice; develops in 5% of affected newborns of African or Mediterranean ancestry after the first 24 hours of life. Serum indirect bilirubin reaches a peak (often >20 mg/dL) at third to fifth day with resulting kernicterus.
- PBS: Heinz bodies in RBCs (require special stain) (see p. 322), nucleated RBCs, spherocytes, poikilocytes, fragmented RBCs
- Reticulocytosis

Enzymopathy: Pyruvate Kinase (PK) Deficiency
➤ **Definition**
- This enzymopathy is a congenital, recessive, nonspherocytic chronic hemolytic anemia with splenomegaly.
- There is a wide range of clinical and laboratory findings. Anemia varies from severe neonatal anemia requiring transfusions to a fully compensated hemolytic process in adults who have 10–20% of the normal enzyme in their RBCs.

➤ **Tests**
- Diagnosis may be difficult. The mild to severe chronic hemolysis may be exacerbated by pregnancy or viral infections.
- PBS shows no characteristic changes.
- A screening test using crude hemolysate detects heterozygous carriers in persons who are hematologically normal. This assay may miss some variants. Quantitation of the enzyme can be performed in specialized laboratories.

Hereditary Spherocytosis (HS)

➤ Definition

* This congenital red cell membrane abnormality results from defects in genes encoding any of the protein components involved in vertical linkages between the skeletal network of the RBCs and the membrane.
* HS is inherited as autosomal dominant transmission in 75% of affected individuals. The condition is recessive or presents as a new mutation in the remaining 25%.
* HS is seen mostly in patients of northern European origin.
  * Patients present with anemia, jaundice, splenomegaly, and cholelithiasis early in life.

➤ Tests

* CBC: anemia of varying severity
  * Moderately severe hemolysis occurs in approximately 70% of cases, and approximately 20% have a mild, compensated hemolysis.
  * Approximately 10% of people have severe, debilitating anemia and are transfusion-dependent, unless splenectomized (splenectomy ameliorates the anemia, but spherocytosis persists).
  * Autohemolysis is always increased.
* Indices: normal MCV (except elevated when the reticulocyte count is very high), elevated MCHC and RDW.
* Reticulocytosis (5–20%).
* PBS: spherocytosis of various degrees is invariably present. Howell-Jolly bodies indicate previous splenectomy. The presence of spherocytes on PBS may be due to acquired hemolytic anemias rather than HS.
* Osmotic fragility (rarely performed today) reveals increased RBC fragility, but it may be abnormal (increased) also in patients with acquired hemolytic anemias
* Haptoglobin: decreased
* Coombs test: negative
* Hb: usually normal at birth but decreases sharply during the subsequent 20 days of life
* Genetic tests: offered in some research laboratories

➤ Other Considerations

* Laboratory findings may reflect cholelithiasis or aplastic crises.
* Falsely elevated potassium (hyperkalemia) is due to potassium leaking from RBCs.

Hereditary Elliptocytosis (HE)

➤ Definition

* This congenital heterogeneous disorder of the membrane skeleton of RBCs, most commonly spectrin, is transmitted by autosomal dominant inheritance. Occasionally, the transmission is recessive.
  * Individuals who are heterozygous for HE are asymptomatic
  * Individuals who are homozygous or compound heterozygous (10% of patients) exhibit mild to severe anemia.

- The disorder is more frequent in African Americans and in patients of Mediterranean origin (previous areas of endemic malaria).
- Affected neonates may have transient overt hemolytic anemia until adult Hb supervenes.

➤ Tests
- PBS: more than 50% of RBCs are ellipsoidal or rod-shaped.
  - Other markers of hemolysis are uncommon, except in the approximately 10% of severely affected patients.
  - In severe cases of HE, severe poikilocytosis is common
- Indices: decreased MCV, MCH, MCHC; increased RDW
- Variant Hb studies and osmotic fragility are normal.

➤ Other Considerations
- Some degree of elliptocytosis may be seen in PBS of other types of anemia.

Hereditary Pyropoikilocytosis
➤ Definition
- Hereditary pyropoikilocytosis is considered a subtype of HE.
- In homozygous individuals, it results in a severe congenital hemolytic anemia.
- It occurs primarily in people of African ancestry.

➤ Tests
- PBS
  - RBCs are markedly misshapen (fragments, microspherocytes, elliptocytes, pyknotic forms). The RBC fragments when heated at 45–46° (normal RBCs show budding and fragmentation only when heated at 49°C).
  - Severe microcytosis and micropoikilocytosis are present.

Hereditary Ovalocytosis
➤ Definition
- Hereditary ovalocytosis is a condition of altered membrane deformability.
- It is very common in Southeast Asia where its prevalence is 5–25% in malaria endemic areas.
- Transmission is autosomal dominant, but so far only heterozygous individuals have been identified.
- Most affected people express minimal hemolysis.

➤ Tests
- PBS: oval-shaped RBCs with 1 or 2 transverse ridges or a longitudinal slit.

➤ Other Considerations
- Hereditary ovalocytosis can be confused with hereditary elliptocytosis.

Hereditary Stomatocytosis (HS)
➤ Definition
* Hereditary stomatocytosis is an uncommon autosomal dominant disease resulting from defective RBC permeability to sodium and potassium ions.

➤ Tests
* PBS
  * Homozygous individuals: >35% of RBCs show slit-like areas of central pallor, producing a mouth-like appearance.
  * Heterozygous individuals: 1–25% stomatocytes.
* Anemia: similar to that of hereditary ovalocytosis
* Homozygous individuals: varying degrees of hemolysis
* Heterozygous individuals: no anemia

➤ Other Considerations
* Stomatocytes may be seen on the PBS of many acquired disorders, such as alcoholism, liver disease, and drug-induced hemolytic anemias

HEMOLYTIC EXTRINSIC RED BLOOD CELL DEFECTS

Autoimmune Hemolytic Anemias (AIHAs)
* AIHAS anemias may be classified on the basis of the type of antibody present: warm (binding optimally at 37°C), cold (binding optimally at 4°C), or occasionally combined warm and cold antibodies.
* Each of these AIHAs may be idiopathic or secondary to other diseases.

➤ Definition
Warm-Reactive AIHAs
* Warm-reactive AIHAs are due to the presence of IgG antibodies that react with RBC antigens at body temperature.
* About 60% are idiopathic, and the remaining 40% are the result of lymphomas, leukemias, other neoplasms, or autoimmune disorders such as SLE. They may also accompany HIV or other viral infections.

Cold-Reactive AIHAs and Cold Agglutinin Disease
* These AIHAs result from the presence of IgM antibodies that react to polysaccharide antigens on the RBC surface at temperatures below that of the body's. The antibodies fix complement.
* Most of the chronic cases, for which the term *cold agglutinin disease* is commonly used, have an underlying B-cell neoplasm (CLL/small lymphocytic lymphoma [SLL], lymphomas, macroglobulinemia) as their etiology. Some cases are idiopathic.
* Acute cases are the result of either viral infections such as mycoplasma pneumonia and infectious mononucleosis or belong to a group known as paroxysmal cold hemoglobinuria (see p. 812).
* There are variable degrees of hemolysis; the disease can be intravascular or extravascular.

- The disease is worse in cold weather; Raynaud's phenomenon are common, with vascular obstruction due to RBC clumps, cyanosis of exposed parts, and pallor.
- Splenomegaly is uncommon; the liver is the site for sequestering the coated RBCs.

➤ Tests
Warm-Reactive AIHA
- Hb moderate to severe decrease, in the range of 7–10 g/dL
- Reticulocytes: elevated in most cases
- Indices: increased MCV due to reticulocytosis; increased MCHC reflects the presence of spherocytes
- PBS: microspherocytes, polychromasia, and occasionally nucleated RBCs
- Coombs test: direct IgG and C3d are positive. The warm antibodies are in most cases directed against IgG1 and less frequently against IgG3.
- Unconjugated bilirubin, LDH, urine and fecal urobilinogen: elevated
- Haptoglobin: decreased

Cold-Reactive AIHA and Cold Agglutinin Disease
- Anemia (severity depends on cold agglutinin titer) with anomalous high MCV and MCHC (artifacts due to RBC clumping at room temperature)
- PBS: RBC clumping
- Reticulocyte count: high
- Anticomplement (C3) Coombs test (positive). Anti-I antibodies are best detected using cord blood red cells.
- Cold agglutinin titers: elevated

Paroxysmal Nocturnal Hemoglobinuria (PNH)
➤ Definition
- PNH is an acquired disorder of hematopoietic stem cells, characterized by attacks of intravascular hemolysis and hemoglobinuria in the absence of another bone marrow disorder. Only 25% of cases present with nocturnal and paroxysmal hemolysis.
- The clinical triad of intravascular hemolysis, venous thrombosis (the leading cause of death), and bone marrow failure is typical. The chronic intravascular hemolysis results in iron deficiency. There is a high risk of evolution into aplastic anemia (see p. 794), myelodysplastic syndrome (see p. 843), or AML (see p. 823).
- Clinically, the polymorphism of PNH can be roughly divided into two presentations:
  - Classic PNH: hemolysis without bone marrow failure
  - Aplastic anemia PNH syndrome (AA-PNH): hemolysis with bone marrow failure

➤ When To Suspect Paroxysmal Nocturnal Hemoglobinuria
- Patients with Coombs-negative intravascular hemolysis, especially if concurrently iron deficient
- Patients with hemoglobinuria
- Patients with venous thrombosis involving unusual sites (mesenteric, hepatic, portal, cerebral or dermal veins, and especially patients with otherwise unexplained Budd-Chiari

syndrome). Such patients should also be investigated for the JAK2 V617F (see p. 236) mutation if the etiology remains unclear.
* Patients with unexplained refractory anemia

➤ Tests
Highly Recommended
* Flow cytometry (high sensitivity and specificity)
  * At least two different monoclonal antibodies, directed against two different glycosylphosphatidylinositol (GPI)–anchored proteins, on at least two different cell lineages, should be used to diagnose a patient with PNH.
  * CD59 and CD55 are the most commonly assessed. The presence of any CD55/CD59-double negative hematologic cells is considered positive for PNH.
* Fluorescently labeled aerolysin (FLAER): PNH white cells are resistant to FLAER because they lack GPI anchor on their surface.

Recommended
* CBC
  * RBC indices: macrocytic anemia evolving into a microcytic picture. Reticulocytes are increased, but not commensurate with the degree of anemia.
  * WBC: leukopenia may be marked.
  * Platelets: thrombocytopenia may be moderate to severe.
* Bone marrow: normoblastic hyperplasia; indicated if an additional underlying hematologic disease is suspected.
* Direct Coombs test: negative
* Haptoglobin: reduced
* Serum iron and ferritin: decreased
* Karyotype: normal
* LDH: increased
* Leukocyte alkaline phosphatase: absent or reduced
* Liver function studies:
  * Unconjugated bilirubin: increased
  * AST/ALT: normal
  * ALP: normal
* Methemalbumin: reduced
* Hb, plasma: increased (hemoglobinemia)
* Urinalysis
  * Hemoglobinuria
  * Hemosiderinuria
  * No intact RBCs in urine sediment

Previously Used Tests No Longer Recommended (Low Specificity)
* Ham's test (acidified serum test)
* Sucrose lysis test
* Complement lysis sensitivity test

➤ Suggested Reading
Brodsky RA. How I treat paroxysmal nocturnal hemoglobinuria. *Blood.* 2009;113:6522–6527.

Paroxysmal Cold Hemoglobinuria (PCH)

➤ Definition

• PCH is an acute hemolytic anemia that results from characteristic antibodies (Donath-Landsteiner) that cross react with P blood group on RBC membrane causing osmotic lysis. This transient, nonrecurring hemolysis occurs following exposure to a cold environment, with sudden hemoglobinuria.

• PCH may be associated with the convalescence phase of an acute viral illness (mumps, measles, infectious mononucleosis), or seen in patients with syphilis.

• PCH may also be idiopathic.

➤ Tests

• Plasma: scarlet-appearing and becoming maroon or brown after a few hours (free Hb is oxidized to metHb, as well as due to formation of methemalbumin)

• PBS: spherocytes, nucleated RBCs, anisocytosis, poikilocytosis

• Donath-Landsteiner test: cold autohemolysins when the blood is cooled, then brought to 37°C, under well-standardized conditions.

• Complement-directed Coombs test: may be positive but the IgG Coombs is negative

Drug-Induced Hemolytic Anemias

• This hemolytic anemia is due to anti-RBC antibodies that develop as the result of drug effects. The drugs most commonly implicated and the mechanisms involved are described in Table 10-2.

Hemolytic Disease of the Newborn

➤ Definition

• Hemolysis occurs when fetal RBCs cross the placenta and the mother is immunized with a fetal RBC antigen that is not present on her RBCs.

• Some women may be immunized with more than one type of RBC antigen. The resulting immune response triggers the production of IgG antibodies that are then transferred to the fetus and cause hemolysis of the fetal RBCs.

TABLE 10-2. Drugs Most Commonly Implicated in Hemolytic Anemias	
Mechanisms	Offending Drugs
Acute intravascular: positive direct Coombs test in the presence of the drug	Sulfonamides, quinidine, quinine, stibophen
Chronic extravascular: positive direct and indirect Coombs test without the drug present	α-Methyldopa, mefenamic acid, levodopa
Unknown mechanism	Ribavirin
Intravascular and extravascular: positive Coombs test in the presence of the drug	High-dose penicillin and analogs, cephalothin, streptomycin

* The most frequent cases are due to immunization against the D antigen of the Rh blood group. Next most common are due to immunization against the Kell antigen.

➤ **Tests**
* Laboratory findings are those of hemolysis in the newborn.
* After birth: the by-products of RBC destruction occur, especially increased unconjugated bilirubin, with attended complications (bilirubin encephalopathy and kernicterus).

Mechanical Hemolysis

➤ **Definition**
* Physical trauma to RBCs damages them, resulting in RBC fragmentation and intravascular hemolysis.
* Mechanical hemolytic anemias can be divided into two groups:
  * Microangiopathic: endothelial cell injury in small blood vessels due to fibrin strands in vessel lumens, as seen in DIC (see p. 883), TTP (see p. 889), HUS (see p. 889), disseminated malignancy; malignant hypertension; vasculitis; HELLP syndrome; scleroderma renal crises; insertion of foreign bodies into the circulation; Kasabach-Merritt syndrome (giant hemangioma); chemotherapy; and the "catastrophic" antiphospholipid antibody syndrome
  * Macroangiopathic: RBC injury from malfunctioning valvular prosthesis, severe cardiac valve deformities, or aortic atheromata (Waring blender syndrome)
* Mechanical hemolysis may also occur in hypersplenism, March hemoglobinuria (runner's hemoglobinuria), and freshwater drowning or inadvertent infusion of water

➤ **Tests**
* Laboratory diagnosis: directed to the causative disease
* Anemia: commensurate with severity of underlying process
* PBS: >5 of 500 RBCs are deformed (schistocytes) or helmet cells (a subtype of schistocytes), or are microspherocytes
* Platelets: varying degrees of thrombocytopenia, occasionally without anemia
* Latex-dimer (see p. 152) and fibrin(ogen) degradation products (FDPs) (see p. 178): elevated if DIC present
* Plasma Hb and urine hemosiderin: elevated
* Plasma haptoglobin: decreased

➤ **Suggested Readings**
Beutler E. Glucose-6-phosphate dehydrogenase deficiency: a historical perspective. *Blood.* 2008;111:16–24.
Brodsky RA. How I treat paroxysmal nocturnal hemoglobinuria. *Blood.* 2009;113:6522–6527.
Mohandas N, Gallagher PG. Red cell membrane: past, present, and future. *Blood.* 2008;112:3939–3948.

Evans Syndrome

➤ **Definition**
* Evans syndrome is characterized by the simultaneous (or sequential) development of autoimmune hemolytic anemia and immune thrombocytopenia (ITP) and/or immune neutropenia, without a demonstrable underlying etiology.

- Evans syndrome may be associated occasionally with SLE (see p. 936), lymphoproliferative neoplasms, or primary immune deficiencies.

➤ Tests
- As described for autoimmune hemolytic anemias (see p. 804 under Anemia, hemolytic) and immune thrombocytopenias (see p. 868 under Platelets, thrombocytopenias).
- When neutropenia is present studies for antileukocyte antibodies should be undertaken.

➤ Suggested Reading
Michel M, Chanet V, Dechartres A, et al. The spectrum of Evans syndrome in adults: new insight into the disease based on the analysis of 68 cases. *Blood.* 2009;114:3167–3172.

WHITE BLOOD CELL DISORDERS

LEUKOCYTOSIS AND LEUKOPENIAS

- Leukocytosis refers to a total white cell count >10,300/µL (in our laboratory). Counts up to 11,000 may be considered physiologic by allowing two standard deviations above the upper limit.
- Leukocytosis may reflect an absolute increase of neutrophils, lymphocytes, eosinophils, monocytes, basophils, or combinations.
- Leukopenia is defined as a total white cell count <4300/µL

➤ Causes of Neutrophilia (Neutrophilic Leukocytosis)
- In adults neutrophilia is defined as an increase in the absolute neutrophil count >7500/µL (or >72%). A relative neutrophilia is seen when the other cellular elements (mostly the lymphocytes) are decreased. The absolute neutrophil count, as reported by automated counters, is a more reliable parameter than the percent count.
- Spurious neutrophilia may be reported by automated counters in the presence of clumped platelets or cryoglobulins. The counters will flag such results as not acceptable.
- Causes of neutrophilia can be divided into primary (clonal) and secondary.

Primary Neutrophilia
- Myeloproliferative neoplasms (see p. 836)
- Neutrophilic leukemia (see p. 836)
- Hereditary, giant neutrophilia (occasional large neutrophils with multiple nuclear lobes)
- Hereditary neutrophilia, a rare autosomal dominant condition without medical problems
- Chronic idiopathic neutrophilia, condition not associated with medical problems

Secondary Neutrophilia
- Acute infections
  - Localized (e.g., pneumonia, meningitis, tonsillitis, abscess, acute otitis media in children)
  - Systemic (e.g., septicemia). Certain bacteria, such as pneumococcal, *staphylococcal*, and clostridial species, may cause very elevated neutrophil and bands counts.
- Inflammation, especially during chronic diseases flare-ups
- Vasculitis (see p. 508)
- Acute rheumatic fever (see p. 520)
- Crohn's disease (see p. 592)

* RA (see p. 935)
* Ulcerative colitis (see p. 593)
* Chronic hepatitis (see p. 620)
* Intoxications
* Metabolic (uremia, acidosis, eclampsia, acute gout)
* Poisoning by chemicals (mercury), venoms (e.g., black widow spider)
* Parenteral (foreign proteins, vaccines)
* Drugs: epinephrine, steroids, lithium, retinoic acid therapy for acute promyelocytic leukemia, therapeutic cytokines, especially granulocyte (or granulocyte–monocyte) colony stimulating factors
* Acute hemorrhage
* Acute hemolysis
* Tissue or tumor necrosis
* Acute myocardial infarction
* Tumor necrosis
* Burns
* Gangrene
* Bacterial necrosis
* Physiologic conditions
  * Strenuous exercise
  * Emotional stress
* Labor
* Smoking
* Leukoerythroblastic reaction (myelophthisis): neutrophilia associated with immature granu- locytes, nucleated red cells, and teardrop red cells; it is associated with tumor invasion of the bone marrow, TB, and other granulomatous diseases.

NEUTROPENIA

* <43% of leukocytes, or an absolute neutrophil and band count <1600/μL (or <1000/μL in people of African ancestry).
* Absence of granulocytes: agranulocytosis (see p. 817)
* A greatly reduced number of neutrophils: granulocytopenia

➤ Causes of Neutropenia
* Decreased bone marrow production
  * Myelodysplastic syndromes (see p. 843)
  * Aplastic anemia (see p. 794)
  * Chemotherapy
  * Acute leukemia (see p. 823)
  * Radiation therapy or accident
  * Folic acid or vitamin B_{12} deficiency
* Increased bone marrow production, but decreased survival of neutrophils
  * Autoimmune and isoimmune neutropenia
  * SLE and RA (see p. 935 and p. 936)

- Felty syndrome (see p. 930)
- Hypersplenism
- T-gamma lymphocytosis
- Viral infections (various mechanisms)
  - Infectious mononucleosis (see p. 1002)
  - HIV infection (see p. 1008)
  - Hepatitis (see p. 620)
  - Influenza
  - Measles (see p. 1017)
  - Rubella (see p. 1016)
  - Psittacosis (see p. 968)
- Bacterial infections
  - Overwhelming sepsis (see p. 958)
  - Miliary TB (see p. 749)
  - Typhoid and paratyphoid
  - Brucellosis (see p. 951)
  - Tularemia (see p. 951)
- Rickettsial infections
  - Scrub typhus (Tsutsugamushi disease)
  - Sandfly fever (caused by Sicilian or Naples virus)
- Other infections
  - Malaria (see p. 1030)
  - Kala-azar (see p. 1030)
- Drugs
  - Sulfa drugs (TMP/SMX)
  - Antibiotics (chloramphenicol, vancomycin, cephalosporin, macrolides)
  - Antimalarials (chloroquine, quinine, amodiaquine)
  - Antifungal agents (amphotericin B, flucytosine)
  - Antidiabetics (chlorpropamide, tolbutamide)
  - Antiinflammatory (sulfasalazine, gold salts, phenacetin, phenylbutazone)
  - Anticonvulsants (carbamazepine, phenytoin, valproate, ethosuximide)
  - Psychotropic drugs (clozapine, phenothiazines, tricyclic and tetracyclic antidepressants, meprobamate)
  - Cardiovascular (procainamide, ticlopidine, ACE inhibitors, propranolol, dipyridamole, digoxin)
  - Diuretics (thiazides, furosemide, spironolactone, acetazolamide)
  - Antithyroid drugs (thioamides)
  - Dermatologic drugs (dapsone, isotretinoin)
- Chronic idiopathic neutropenia
- Neonatal and infantile
  - Maternal immune neutropenia
  - Maternal ingestion of drugs causing neutropenia
  - Maternal isoimmunization to fetal leukocytes
- Congenital neutropenia as seen with certain inborn errors of metabolism and other congenital syndromes

AGRANULOCYTOSIS

➤ Definition
- The term literally means total absence of granulocytes in the peripheral blood. Severe granulocytopenia (neutrophils and bands <500/μL) is casually also referred as agranulocytosis.
- A count <500/μL confers a high risk for sepsis; a count of <200 is certain to lead to overwhelming bacterial infection (for causes of neutropenia, see p. 815).
- Due to:
  - Peripheral destruction of PMNs (often drug related)
  - More generalized bone marrow failure

➤ Who Should be Suspected?
- Most acquired cases of acute agranulocytosis are drug-related. It should be suspected in anyone recently started or restarted on any drug, who suddenly develops fever, chills, and signs of infection.
- Sore throat is a common presenting symptom. Patients may develop overwhelming sepsis.

➤ Tests
- CBC: normal Hb and platelets (except under special circumstances, such as postchemotherapy); absent, or extremely decreased neutrophils and bands. The granulocytes may show pyknosis or vacuolization. Normal lymphocytes and monocytes (but relative lymphocytosis and monocytosis).
- Bone marrow shows an absence of cells in the granulocytic series but normal erythroid and megakaryocytic series.
- ESR is increased
- Other laboratory findings are due to infection
- Hb, RBC count and morphology, platelet count, and coagulation tests are normal.

LYMPHOCYTOSIS

➤ Definition
- Lymphocytosis is defined as an absolute lymphocyte count >3400/μL (or >43%) in adults, >7200 in adolescents, and >9000 in young children and infants.
- Spurious lymphocytosis: neutropenia with relative lymphocytosis, but normal absolute lymphocyte count (e.g. thyrotoxicosis, agranulocytosis)

➤ Primary (Clonal) Lymphocytosis
- Chronic lymphocytic leukemia (CLL) (see p. 829)
- Monoclonal B-cell lymphocytosis (>4000 but <5000 clonal lymphocytes) (see p. 829)
- Acute lymphocytic leukemia (ALL) (see p. 821)
- Prolymphocytic leukemia (see p. 832)
- Hairy cell leukemia (see p. 834)
- Follicular, mantle cell and splenic marginal zone lymphomas in leukemic phase (see p. 847)
- Large granular lymphocytic leukemia (see p. 835)

➤ Secondary (Reactive) Lymphocytosis
* Infections (e.g., pertussis, infectious mononucleosis [EBV], infectious lymphocytosis [especially in children], infectious hepatitis, CMV, mumps, German measles, chickenpox, toxoplasmosis, babesiosis, chronic TB, cat scratch disease)
* Noninfectious causes (e.g. hypersensitivity reactions, stress)
* Drugs: efalizumab (Raptiva)

LYMPHOCYTOPENIA

➤ Definition
* <1600/μL (or <18%) in adults, and <3000/μL in children

➤ Causes
* Corticosteroid therapy or Cushing syndrome; epinephrine injection
* Certain infections (e.g., acute and chronic retroviral infections, TB)
* Sarcoidosis
* Congenital immunoglobulin disorders
* Chemotherapy and radiation therapy
* Neoplastic diseases, especially Hodgkin lymphoma (see p. 857)
* ARDS
* Autoimmune disorders
* Idiopathic CD4+ lymphocytopenia
* CHF (see p. 525)
* Increase loss via the GI tract (e.g., intestinal lymphectasia, thoracic duct drainage, obstruction to intestinal lymphatic drainage)

MONOCYTOSIS

➤ Definition
* Absolute count of >1200/μL, or >12% of a differential count

➤ Causes
* Acute monocytic or myelomonocytic leukemia, chronic myelomonocytic leukemia (as part of myelodysplastic syndromes (see p. 843), or myeloproliferative neoplasms (see p. 836)
* Hodgkin lymphoma, non-Hodgkin lymphomas, multiple myelomas (see p. 859)
* Carcinomas of ovary, stomach, and breast
* Lipid storage diseases (e.g., Gaucher disease) (see p. 906)
* Postsplenectomy
* Recovery from agranulocytosis, chemotherapy, or subsidence of acute infection
* Protozoan infections (e.g., malaria, kala-azar, trypanosomiasis)
* Some rickettsial infections (e.g., Rocky Mountain spotted fever, typhus)
* Certain bacterial infections (e.g., bacterial endocarditis, TB, syphilis, brucellosis)
* Ulcerative colitis, regional enteritis, sprue

- Sarcoidosis
- Connective tissue diseases (e.g., SLE, RA)
- Tetrachloroethane poisoning
- Chronic corticosteroid therapy
- Acute minor viral infections (counts should be rechecked in 1 month)
- Diurnal variations

EOSINOPHILIA

➤ Definition
- Count of >600/μL eosinophils or >8% of the differential count.
- Eosinophilia may be either primary (clonal or idiopathic), reactive, or idiopathic.

➤ Associated Conditions
- Primary
  - Hematologic: hypereosinophilic syndrome (see p. 827)
  - Neoplastic disorders: chronic eosinophilic leukemia (see p. 827), myelomonocytic leukemia with inversion 16 (see p. 833), mastocytosis, and T-cell lymphomas that secrete interleukin-5
- Secondary
  - Allergic diseases: atopic and related diseases, medication-related
  - Infectious diseases: parasitic infections, mostly helminths, some fungal infections, infrequently other infections
  - Collagen vascular disorders
  - Autoimmune disorders such as the vasculitis of the Churg-Strauss syndrome (see p. 512)
  - Tumors with secondary eosinophilia: T-cell lymphomas (e.g., mycosis fungoides, Sézary syndrome), Hodgkin lymphoma
  - Pulmonary diseases: (hypersensitivity pneumonia, Loeffler's pneumonia
  - Endocrine: adrenal insufficiency (see p. 668)
  - Immunologic reactions, transplant rejection
  - Cholesterol embolism syndrome

PERSISTENT EOSINOPENIA

➤ Definition
- No lower limit can be determined because the eosinophil count may be 0% in some normal patients.

➤ Associated Conditions
- Drugs: corticosteroids or epinephrine administration
- Cushing syndrome (see p. 664)
- Infections in conjunction with neutrophilia
- Inflammation: acute

BASOPHILIA

➤ Definition
- Basophilia is defined as >300/μL or >2% of leukocytes. (The basophil is the rarest of leukocytes.)

➤ Associated Conditions
- Basophilia frequently accompanies myeloproliferative neoplasms, and its progression may herald a blast crisis in chronic myelogenous leukemia (see p. 837). The existence of basophilic leukemia is controversial. It was recently described by our group
- Other causes of basophilia are:
  - Hypersensitivity states (drugs, foods, foreign protein injection)
  - Myxedema
  - Anemias, chronic hemolytic, iron deficiency (in some patients)
  - Ulcerative colitis (see p. 593)
  - Postsplenectomy
  - Hodgkin lymphoma (see p. 857)
  - Chronic sinusitis
  - Chickenpox (see p. 1006)
  - Smallpox (see p. 1018)
  - Nephrotic syndrome (see p. 727) (in some patients)

➤ Basophilopenia (no lower limit can be determined because some normal subjects may have 0% basophils)
- Hyperthyroidism
- Irradiation or chemotherapy
- Drugs: corticosteroids
- Ovulation and pregnancy
- Stress

LEUKEMOID REACTIONS

➤ Definition
- A count >50,000/μL in non-leukemic conditions defines a leukemoid reaction. The PBS shows increase in and shift to the left of myeloid cells (bands, metamyelocytes, myelocytes, some promyelocytes, and rare myeloblasts); increased primary granules in the myeloid cells (toxic granulation) and Döhle bodies, cytoplasmic vacuolization.
- If the left shift consists in an elevation of bands only (>700/μL), the term bandemia is applied. Frequently it signals the onset of a septic episode such as acute appendicitis.

➤ Causes of Leukemoid Reactions
- Severe sepsis (osteomyelitis, empyema, disseminated TB)
- Burns
- Tissue necrosis (gangrene, mesenteric vein thrombosis)
- Therapy with granulocyte colony stimulating factor (G-CSF) or granulocyte monocyte colony stimulating factor (GM-CSF)
- Metastatic infiltration of the marrow

ACUTE LEUKEMIAS

LEUKEMIA, ACUTE B LYMPHOBLASTIC (B-ALL)

➤ Definition
- B-ALL is commonly seen in childhood, comprising >85% of leukemias in children, but can occur at any age.
- It is a clonal disease affecting the lymphocytic B line, with heavy infiltration of bone marrow and peripheral blood. If the neoplasm is confined to a mass with no or minimal evidence of peripheral blood or bone marrow involvement, the term B lymphoblastic lymphoma is appropriate.

➤ Who Should be Suspected?
- Children (peak incidence at age 2–3 years) or adults older than 65, presenting with acute onset of fever, infection, bleeding, fatigue, musculoskeletal pain (particularly in adolescents), and characteristic findings on the CBC. Lymphadenopathy and hepatosplenomegaly are present in the majority of patients, but are not massive.
- Predisposing factors: children with certain genetic disorders such as Down syndrome. With modern therapy B-ALL has a good prognosis in children, but not in adults. To what this difference is attributable is not clear.
- Poor prognostic signs at presentation: WBC count >100,000/μL, platelet count <50,000/μL, CD10 negativity, certain karyotypic abnormalities, occurrence of the disease before age 1 (probably having occurred before birth) or after age 10, and induction failure. Mature B leukemic phenotype rather than precursor B-cell is associated with poorer prognosis.

➤ Tests
- Laboratory diagnosis is based on morphology, immunophenotype, and cytogenetic/genetic analysis.

Morphology
- Blood: CBC
  - Anemia, moderate to severe
  - Thrombocytopenia
  - WBC is usually elevated, with lymphocytosis and neutropenia, but approximately 50% of children have WBC counts <10,000 at presentation
  - Lymphoblasts are usually identified on the PBS
  - The French-American-British (FAB) classification is based on appearance of lymphoblasts but has been superseded by the more accurate and detailed WHO classification.
- Bone marrow generally shows >50% lymphoblasts. It should be obtained before starting therapy to determine immunophenotype, cytogenetics, and overall cellularity. Peripheral blood may be sufficient for these studies in cases with high peripheral blood blast count. Once the diagnosis of leukemia is confirmed, definitive assignment of the subtype of B-ALL, as provided by immunophenotyping and cytogenetic studies, is mandatory before deciding on therapeutic protocol.

Immunophenotype
- Seventy percent to 80% of childhood ALL are of B-precursor lineage. The expression of markers on the leukemic lymphoblasts does not correlate strictly with normal lymphoid maturation. B-ALL lymphoblasts are positive for CD19; cytoplasmic CD79a; cytoplasmic

and surface CD 22, 24; PAX5, and TDT. The expression of CD 34 and 20 is variable. Positivity for CD 10 (CALLA antigen) reflects a good prognosis. Myeloid markers CD13 and 33 may also be present. The aberrant immunophenotype serves to identify minimum residual disease in the bone marrow following therapy.

- A simple classification is offered below.
- Mature B-cell phenotype (1–2% of cases in children and 5% in adults). Surface monoclonal immunoglobulins. Indistinguishable from Burkitt lymphoma/leukemia.
- B-progenitor ALL present in 80–85% of childhood B-ALL. Eighty to 90% express CD10. The majority have an immunoglobulin gene rearrangement, predominantly involving the IgH gene. Different subsets are based on various cell markers: (pro-B ALL[CD10−, no cytoplasmic Ig (cIg)], early pre-B ALL [CD10+ but no cIg] and pre-B ALL [CD10+, cIg positive]. The prognosis among these various forms of immature B-ALL depends mostly on their genetic etiology as reflected in karyotypes (see below)

Cytogenetic/Genetic Analysis

- Recurrent abnormalities are used to subclassify B-ALL. Both numerical and structural abnormalities of the chromosomes in B-ALL are associated with prognosis and influence treatment.
  - t(9:22)(q34;q11.2); BCR-ABL (the Ph chromosome) is present in ≤25% of adults and 3% of children. Its presence denotes the poorest prognosis in B-ALL patients, both adults and children, but seems to respond to tyrosine kinase inhibitors;
  - t(v:11q23); MLL gene on chromosome 11 rearranged and fused with other genes, determining the translocation pattern: poor prognosis;
  - t(12:21)(p13;q22); translocation between genes TEL-AML1. Very favorable prognosis
  - t(5:14)(q31;q32); translocation between the IL3 gene and the IGHα gene. Rare. Uncertain prognosis.
  - t(1;19)(q23;p13.3); translocation between E2A and PBX1 genes. Responds readily to therapy
  - Hyperdiploidy (the blasts contain >50, but <66 chromosomes). Very favorable prognosis.
  - Hypodiploidy (the blasts contain <46 or even <44 chromosomes). Poor prognosis
- In addition to the genetic abnormalities demonstrated by chromosome and FISH studies (see above), high-density single nucleotide polymorphism (SNP) arrays and gene expression profiles are being developed, which may further stratify B-ALL patients and determine prognosis and therapeutic protocols.

Additional Information

- CSF may show increased protein and cells, some recognizable as lymphoblasts. Because of high incidence of meningeal involvement, examination of CSF is part of all protocols.
- Serum LDH and sedimentation rate are elevated.
- Hypercalcemia, hyperpotassemia, hyperphosphatemia, and hyperuricemia may be present at diagnosis or develop as the result of therapy.
- Acute lysis syndrome may develop as the result of therapy.

➤ Suggested Readings

Borowitz MJ, Chan JKC. B lymphoblastic leukaemia/lymphoma not otherwise specified. In: *WHO Classification of Tumours of Haematopoietic and Lymphoid Tissues*. 4th ed. Lyon, France: International Agency for Research on Cancer; 2008:168–170.

Borowitz MJ, Chan JKC. B lymphoblastic leukaemia/lymphoma with recurrent genetic abnormalities. In: *WHO Classification of Tumours of Haematopoietic and Lymphoid Tissues.* 4th ed. Lyon, France: International Agency for Research on Cancer; 2008:171–175.

LEUKEMIA, ACUTE MYELOID (AML)

➤ Definition
- AML (formerly known as acute nonlymphocytic leukemia) is a clonal proliferation of the myeloid/erythroid/megakaryocytic hematopoietic stem cells characterized by acquisition of somatic mutations that confer a proliferative or survival advantage and impair normal hematopoiesis.
- AML is a markedly heterogeneous disease with numerous genetic aberrations.

➤ Classification
- AML was classified until recently by the French-American-British (FAB) group in well-defined categories. Despite wide clinical use, it became evident that mutation analysis and cytogenetic studies offer more prognostic significance than the morphologic FAB classification, which will not be used here.
- Instead, the recent (2008) WHO classification will guide the description of AML variants in this section. The WHO divides myeloid neoplasms into six major groups:
  1. AML with recurrent genetic abnormalities: these abnormalities impact prognosis. The most common ones are balanced abnormalities that create a fusion gene encoding a chimeric protein. Best examples: acute promyelocytic leukemia (APL), formerly known as M_3; AML with inv(16)(p13.1q22); AML with t(8;21)(q22;q22)
  2. AML with myelodysplasia-related changes comprises three categories: AML arising from previous MDS or MDS/MPN; AML with an MDS-related cytogenetic abnormality; AML with multilineage dysplasia. This group has a worse survival compared with AML–not otherwise specified (see below) independent of age or cytogenetic risk group.
  3. Therapy-related myeloid neoplasm: the leukemia occurs as a late complication of cytotoxic chemotherapy or radiation therapy
  4. AML not otherwise specified: cases that do not fulfill criteria for the other groups. These cases of AML are classified basically by morphology, and follow closely the FAB classification, except for having eliminated acute promyelocytic leukemia (formerly M3).
  5. Myeloid sarcoma: extramedullary myeloid tumor. It may precede or coincide with overt AML.
  6. Myeloid proliferations related to Down syndrome (DS): DS individuals have a 50–150-fold increase in the incidence of AML in the first 5 years of life. In some AML is acute megakaryocytic. Ten percent of DS newborns have a transient episode of abnormal myelopoiesis expressed mainly as thrombocytopenia and marked leukocytosis.

➤ Who Should be Suspected?
- AML should be suspected during the first months of life (initiating events are in utero), in middle age or in the elderly, in a patient who is acutely ill, and with nonspecific presenting signs and symptoms that reflect profound disturbances in hematopoiesis: fatigue, malaise, infections, ulcerations of mucous membranes, bleeding, diffuse bone tenderness, joint pain, and swelling.

* Other findings:
  * Modest splenic enlargement is present in 50% of cases.
  * Lymphadenopathy is not present. Isolated masses (myeloid sarcoma [chloroma]), which are collection of blasts in extramedullary sites, may precede systemic AML (see above).

➤ Tests

* CBC
  * Anemia, normochromic, normocytic is universally present. Nucleated red cells may be identified on the PBS.
  * Thrombocytopenia is severe in most cases
  * WBC: Leukocytosis with neutropenia is present in more than half the cases; some patients may present with leukopenia, especially if AML follows MDS. Greater than 20% of white cells are blasts. There are few or no intermediate granulocytic cells (myelocytes, metamyelocytes, bands). Auer rods (see p. 392) are present in certain subtypes with granulocytic differentiation, and help to establish the diagnosis, especially by determining myelogenous rather than lymphoid etiology at the first inspection of the patient's PBS.
* Bone marrow aspirate and biopsy are mandatory for cytochemical, immunophenotypic, cytogenetic, and genetic studies. WHO classification defines AML as with either >20% blasts in bone marrow or PBS, or with specific cytogenetic findings. The bone marrow is hypercellular in most cases, with a predominance of early progenitor cells (myeloblasts and promyelocytes, or monoblasts and promonocytes) depending on the leukemic subtype. Initial assessment is based on counting 500 cells on the aspirate. AML-erythroleukemia is established when >50% of precursor cells are erythroid, and myeloblasts comprise >20% of nonerythroid cells. Careful assessment of megakaryocytes and the degree of marrow fibrosis are also part of the initial studies.
* Coagulation studies. Bleeding, a severe complication of AML, is usually due to the severe thrombocytopenia, compounded by platelet functional defects. In addition, patients with the t(15;17) and hypergranular promyelocytes frequently develop a proteolytic state akin to DIC (see p. 883) either spontaneously, or following the initial chemotherapy. The mechanism is thought to be release of tissue factor from the promyelocytes' granules. PT and PTT are elongated, FDP and latex D-dimers (see p. 152) are elevated, and fibrinogen (see p. 177), initially elevated, decreases dramatically.
* Metabolic and electrolyte abnormalities are common; the patients must be monitored carefully, especially during induction chemotherapy. Renal failure from multifactorial causes is common.
  * Hyperuricemia is the most frequent biochemical abnormality.
  * Hyperuricuria may also be present
  * Tumor lysis syndrome may develop during induction chemotherapy. It is characterized by rapid development of hyperuricemia, hyperkalemia, hyperphosphatemia, and hypocalcemia.
  * Acute promyelocytic leukemia (APL) differentiation syndrome (previously the retinoic acid syndrome) develops in 2–27% of patients in the first to third week after initiating all-transretinoic acid (ATRA) therapy. Patients with hyperleukocytosis and abnormal serum creatinine are most susceptible. It is characterized by various clinical and radiographic findings.
  * Lactic acidosis has been described in patients with AML
  * Hypokalemia is common and may be profound
  * Lysozyme is released from blasts and may induce renal tubular damage
  * Hypercalcemia and hypocalcemia have been reported

- CNS involvement is infrequent in AML (5–7% of patients). Examination of CSF for the presence of blasts is indicated when neurologic signs develop.
- Cytochemistry although extremely useful in the past, is taking a secondary role in the era of cytogenetic/genetic and immunophenotyping diagnosis and classification. It plays a role when more sophisticated diagnostic tools are not available, or a rapid result is beneficial, such as rapidly differentiating AML from ALL. The most commonly used stains are:
  - Myeloperoxidase or Sudan Black B: positive in AML with maturation, in myelomonocytic leukemia and in erythroleukemia; strongly positive in APL; negative in ALL, minimally differentiated AML, monoblastic leukemia without differentiation and in megakaryocytic leukemia.
  - Chloracetate esterase: positive in AML with differentiation and in acute myelomonocytic leukemia; negative in ALL, AML without differentiation, in acute monoblastic and erythroleukemia.
  - Nonspecific esterase: positive (and inhibited by sodium fluoride) in acute myelomonocytic or monoblastic leukemia with or without differentiation; negative in ALL, AML with granulocytic line as the main component.
  - Periodic acid–Schiff (PAS): the pattern of granules staining with PAS may differentiate lymphoid from myeloid precursors (e.g., very coarse granules in ALL lymphoblasts).
  - Lysozyme is positive in AML with monocytic differentiation.
    - Immunophenotype. Most cases of AML are characterized by their complex immunophenotypes. There is great variation in immunophenotype depending on the leukemic subtype. Blasts are positive for CD34 (except for APL and some with monocytic differentiation, where CD34 may be weakly expressed or absent) and in some cases HLA-DR (except for APL) and CD117. The AML variants with differentiation toward the granulocytic phenotype express CD13, 33, 15, and 65. Those with monocytic characteristics are positive for CD14, 4, 11b, 11c, 64, and 36. The megakaryoblastic leukemias express platelet antigens, such as CD41 and/or CD61.
    - Cytogenetic/molecular genetic investigations determine to a great extent prognosis and therapeutic protocols, and have become the major criteria WHO uses for subclassification of AML. Complex karyotype has consistently been associated with poor outcome. Although cytogenetic studies are essential for diagnosis and classification, many of the variant translocations can also be detected by real time polymerase chain reaction (RT-PCR) that has higher sensitivity and as such is useful for residual disease monitoring. In the future, gene-expression profiling may lead to further subclassifications of AML, with prognostic and therapeutic implications. Ultimately, it is expected that a proteomic-based classification will emerge.
      - AML with t(8;21)(q22;q22) with RUNX1-RUNX1T1 fusion is found in ~5% of AML cases. Generally shows maturation in the neutrophilic lineage, occurs in a younger population, and may present as myeloid sarcomas. Good response to chemotherapy
      - AML with inv(16)(p13.1q22) or t(16;16)(p13.1;q22) with fusion of the CBFB and MYH11 genes shows monocytic and granulocytic differentiation and abnormal eosinophils in the bone marrow. This rearrangement may be difficult to detect without FISH or PCR. It is important to alert the cytogenetics laboratory if this variant is suspected. Myeloid sarcomas may be present at diagnosis or at relapse. This variant constitutes 5–8% of AML cases. Patients respond well to chemotherapy.

* Acute promyelocytic leukemia (APL) with t(15;17)(q22;q12), with the PML-RARA retinoic acid receptor-α translocation. Five percent to 8% of acute leukemias. Use of FISH analysis for rapid diagnosis may be useful for early initiation of ATRA therapy.
* There are two varieties of APL: the majority (considered typical APL) have hypergranular promyelocytes, many containing large Auer rods (see p. 392) and high incidence of acute DIC; the microgranular (variant) PML, presents with bilobed nuclei and very high WBC. APL provided the first paradigm of molecularly targeted therapy, ATRA. Variant RARA translocations can be detected by classical cytogenetics and by FISH, and are important to distinguish, as not all variants respond to ATRA.
* Prognosis is most favorable among all AML subtypes when treated with ATRA and an anthracycline.
* AML with t(9;11)(p22;q23); the MLLT3 gene on chromosome 11q23 is involved in numerous translocations with different partner genes, most commonly in association with 9p22. Most frequently the morphology is monocytic or myelomonocytic. Detected in 9–12% of pediatric and 2% of adult AML. Intermediate prognosis. Other MLL rearrangements tend to have poorer prognosis.
* AML with t(6;9)(p23;q34) fuses DEK on chromosome 6, with NUP214 on chromosome 9. May have monocytic, basophilic and multilineage dysplastic features. May belong to any of the FAB classifications, except APL. Incidence: 0.7–1.8% of AML. Presents with lower WBC than other AML, and pancytopenia. Poor prognosis.
* AML with inv(3)(q21;q26.2) or t(3;3)(q21;q26.2) with rearrangement of EVII and RPN1 genes may present de novo or evolve from MDS with normal or increased platelet counts and atypical megakaryocytes in the bone marrow. Comprises 1–2% of all AML. Trilineage dysplastic morphology is common; aggressive disease with short survival.
* AML (megakaryoblastic) with t(1;22)(p13;q13). Fusion of RBM15-MKL1 genes. Very rare leukemia that occurs in infants and young children. Marked hepatosplenomegaly.
* AML with MDS-related changes may have complex karyotypes, unbalanced abnormalities, such as −7del (7q−) or −5del (5q−), or balanced abnormalities.
* Therapy-related myeloid neoplasms have abnormal karyotypes in >90% of cases. Approximately 70% of patients have unbalanced chromosomal aberrations, mainly whole or partial loss of chromosomes 5 and/or 7, frequently associated with other chromosomal abnormalities.
* Molecular genetics. In addition to the genetic mutations with cytogenetic abnormalities described above specific gene mutations are also common and may be present in cases with or without detectable cytogenetic abnormalities. Mutations in FLT3 (fms-related tyrosine kinase 3) and NPM1 (nucleophosmin) are of particular prognostic import. In normal karyotype cases, FLT3-ITD (internal tandem duplication) carries an unfavorable prognosis, whereas NPM1 mutation is considered favorable. Similarly, CEBPA (CCAAT/enhancer-binding protein α) mutation in a normal karyotype background is considered favorable
* Monitoring of minimal residual disease (MRD) remains an active field of investigation. Immunophenotypic detection of MRD after induction and consolidation therapy provides negative prognostic information.

► Suggested Readings

Arber DA, Brunning RD, LeBeau MM, et al. Acute myeloid leukaemia with recurrent genetic abnormalities. *WHO Classification of Tumours of Haematopoietic and Lymphoid tissues.* 4th ed. Lyon, France: International Agency for Research on Cancer; 2008:110–123. (See also 124–144.)

Dohner H, Estey RH, Amadori S, et al. Diagnosis and management of acute myeloid leukemia in adults: recommendations from an international expert panel, on behalf of the European Leukemia Net. *Blood.* 2010;115: 453–474.

Rowe JM, Tallman MS. How I treat acute myeloid leukemia. *Blood.* 2010;116:3147–3156.

Weinberg OK, Seetharam M, Ren L, et al. Clinical characterization of acute myeloid leukemia with myelodysplastic-related changes as defined by the 2008 WHO classification system. *Blood.* 2009;113:1906–1908.

Wouters BJ, Lowenberg B, Delvel R. A decade of genome-wide gene expression profiling in acute myeloid leukemia: flashback and prospects. *Blood.* 2009;113:291–298.

LEUKEMIA/LYMPHOMA, ACUTE T LYMPHOBLASTIC (T-ALL)

➤ Definition
- T-ALL is a neoplasm of lymphocytes committed to the T-cell lineage. The term lymphoma is preferred to leukemia when the presenting manifestation is a tumor, rather than peripheral blood involvement.
- The incidence of T-ALL in children with ALL ranges between 10% and 15% and in adults between 20% and 25%.

➤ Who Should be Suspected?
- Presentation is similar as for B-ALL (see p. 821), but there is more predominant extramedullary involvement, including frequent CNS and anterior mediastinal thymic masses.

➤ Tests
- CBC: (see B-ALL at p. 821, but note higher leukocytosis at presentation)
- Immunophenotype. CD3 is T-lineage specific. The lymphoblasts are TdT positive and express CD1a, CD2, CD4, CD5, CD7, and CD8 to variable degrees. CD10 may also be positive.
- Genetics. Clonal rearrangement of the T-cell receptor gene (TCR) is almost always present.
- Cytogenetics. Abnormal karyotypes are present in 50–70% of cases. The most common recurrent abnormality involves the α and Δ TCR loci at 14q11.2

➤ Suggested Reading
Borowitz MJ, Chan JKC. T lymphoblastic leukaemia/lymphoma. In: *WHO Classification of Tumours of Haematopoietic and Lymphoid Tissues.* 4th ed. Lyon, France: International Agency for Research on Cancer; 2008:176–178.

CHRONIC LEUKEMIAS

CHRONIC MYELOGENOUS LEUKEMIAS

(See Myeloproliferative Neoplasms [p. 836])

LEUKEMIA, CHRONIC EOSINOPHILIC (CEL) AND HYPEREOSINOPHILIC (HES) SYNDROMES

➤ Definition
- CEL syndrome is a rare clonal myeloproliferative disease characterized by the overproduction of eosinophils. It must be distinguished from the idiopathic hypereosinophilic syndrome (see below), reactive eosinophilia, or other leukemias with predominant eosinophilia. It may undergo blastic transformation.

- HES is defined as persistent (>6 months duration) eosinophilia of >1500 eosinophils/mL with no demonstrable disease that could cause eosinophilia, no abnormal T-cell population, and no evidence of another clonal myeloid disorder. It leads to end-organ damage because of the proinflammatory role of eosinophils; any organ may be involved. If untreated, HES may be fatal.

➤ 2001 WHO Criteria for CEL and HES

- Persistent peripheral blood eosinophilia ($\geq$1500/μL) for >6 months
- Increased numbers of bone marrow eosinophils
- Myeloblasts <20% in peripheral blood or bone marrow
- Exclude all causes of reactive (secondary) eosinophilia
- Exclude all neoplastic disorders with secondary, reactive eosinophilia
- Exclude other neoplastic disorders in which eosinophils are part of the neoplastic clone
- Exclude T-cell population with an aberrant phenotype and abnormal cytokine production

➤ Who Should be Suspected?

Patients fulfilling WHO criteria (see above) with eosinophilia for longer than 6 months. Presumptives signs and symptoms of organ involvement, especially cardiac or neurologic

➤ Tests

- CBC:
  - Eosinophilia with mostly mature eosinophils; the WBC count is usually <25,000/μL, but may be >90,000, with rare immature forms
  - Mild anemia in half the patients; thrombocytopenia in one third of cases; thrombocytosis may also be present
  - Increase in dysplastic-appearing or immature eosinophils
- Bone marrow:
  - Hypercellular marrow with 25–75% eosinophils, and increase in eosinophil precursors; <2% blasts; no reticulin fibrosis
  - For CEL only: hyperplasia with increase in abnormal eosinophils and eosinophilic precursors
- Cytogenetic or FISH studies are generally normal (see above WHO criteria). The following cytogenetic abnormalities must be excluded by chromosome analysis and/or FISH: BCR-ABL fusion (Ph[1] chromosome), FGFR1 rearrangement, PDGFRB rearrangement, and PDGFRA rearrangement.
- The most common mutation associated with the myeloproliferative variant of the HES is that presenting with the fusion tyrosine kinase FIPIL1/PDGFRA (F/P)
  - F/P is cytogenetically cryptic and requires FISH analysis for detection. Patients with these genetic markers respond to tyrosine kinase inhibitors such as imatinib mesylate and are considered and classified as separate entities.
  - CEL: no specific clonal abnormalities. Certain clonal abnormalities may be demonstrated, most frequently involving chromosomes 5, 7, 8 (the 8p11 syndrome), 10, 15, or 17. The best defined entity in CEL is t(5:12)(q33;p13). The Ph chromosome or inv(16) are absent. In the absence of clonal abnormalities the diagnosis is more difficult and the hypereosinophilic syndrome may be considered.
- Interleukin 5: overproduction in some patients.
- Elevated troponin levels suggest cardiac involvement by HES.

➤ Suggested Readings

Klion AD. How I treat hypereosinophilic syndrome. *Blood.* 2009;114:3736–3741.

Oliver JW, Deol I, Morgan DL, Tonk VS. Chronic eosinophilic leukemia and hypereosinophilic syndromes. *Cancer Genet Cytogenet.* 1998;107:111–117.

Tefferi A. Blood eosinophilia: a new paradigm in disease classification, diagnosis, and treatment. *Mayo Clinic Proc.* 2005;80:75–83.

CHRONIC LYMPHOCYTIC LEUKEMIA (CLL)/ SMALL LYMPHOCYTIC LYMPHOMA (SLL)

➤ Definition

- CLL/SLL is an indolent clonal proliferation of functionally incompetent B-lymphocytes, leading to an accumulation of these cells in the peripheral blood, bone marrow, and extramedullary lymphoid tissues. In the World Health Organization (WHO) classification, CLL is always a disease of neoplastic B-cells, whereas the entity formerly described as T-CLL is now called T-cell prolymphocytic leukemia.
- In addition, in the WHO classification, B-cell CLL is considered identical (one disease at different stages) with the mature B-cell neoplasm small lymphocytic lymphoma (SLL), an indolent non-Hodgkin lymphoma. SLL by itself refers to the nonleukemic cases. This section will present CLL/SLL as one entity.

➤ Who Should be Suspected?

- Individuals who present with persistent (at least 3 months) absolute lymphocytosis of >5000 μL, often discovered accidentally, frequently with lymphadenopathy and splenomegaly.
- Rarely, patients may present with typical "B symptoms" of lymphoma. CLL/SLL is more common in patients >55 years of age, but it may be encountered in young individuals.

➤ Diagnosis

- The simplest way to diagnose CLL is by flow cytometry, where the presence of a clone of CD5 and CD20 positive cells confirms the diagnosis (see below for details).
- Patients with persistent lymphocytosis of >5000 μL should be tested by flow cytometry for prompt diagnosis.

➤ Tests

- CBC
  - Anemia, when present, is normochromic, normocytic when present; it connotes advanced disease. In some cases it is autoimmune, with a positive direct Coombs test (see p. 119). If the etiology of anemia is autoimmune, the anemia by itself does not categorize the disease as being in an advanced stage. Autoimmune hemolytic anemia may also develop as a complication of purine analog therapy.
  - Platelet count is decreased in advanced disease. Occasionally there is an autoimmune component to thrombocytopenia (ITP). In these cases the bone marrow reveals a normal number of megakaryocytes. If thrombocytopenia is solely immune in etiology, it does not indicate advanced disease.
  - WBC count is increased, usually 50,000 to 250,000/μL, with >90% lymphocytes. Recently clonal B-lymphocytes have been identified in patients with counts between 4000

and 5000 lymphocytes: monoclonal B-cell lymphocytosis (MBL). MBL is best defined as the flow cytometry detection of peripheral blood monoclonal B-cell population in the absence of a history of B-cell leukemia or another related lymphoproliferative disease. Some of these patients may eventually evolve into typical CLL and need to be followed closely.

* In stable CLL/SLL the lymphocytes are small, with nonactivated-appearing morphology, clumped chromatin and scanty cytoplasm. Basically, they are normal-appearing lymphocytes. Smudge cells (an artifact of preparation of fragile lymphocytes) are numerous; their presence suggests CLL/SLL, even if the WBC count is not greatly elevated. Survival was shown to be better in patients with a high percentage of smudge cells. Increasing numbers of lymphocytes (lymphocyte doubling time in <1 year), or the development of abnormal-appearing lymphocytes, indicate progressive disease. Granulocytopenia similarly indicates progressive disease, unless it is the result of therapy.
* Bone marrow
  * Bone marrow aspiration and biopsy are seldom required for diagnosis
  * There is typically involvement with >30% monoclonal B-lymphocytes. Progressive replacement of erythroid, myeloid, and megakaryocytic series by lymphocytes takes place over time. In many fields of the aspirate, the normal hematopoietic cells are replaced by the clonal (but normal appearing) lymphocytes. Bone marrow biopsy may show a pattern of nodular, interstitial, combined nodular and interstitial, or diffuse infiltration by lymphocytes. The latter pattern correlates with an adverse prognosis. Remaining lymphocytic nodules may be identified during hematologic remissions.
* Lymph node biopsy: the histopathologic findings in CLL and SLL are identical. They show a pattern of diffuse lymphoma (diffusely effaced nodal architecture) with occasional residual naked germinal centers. The cells in the infiltrate are mostly mature-appearing, small, non-cleaved lymphocytes with condensed chromatin, round nuclei, and occasionally single small nucleoli. There is an admixture of prolymphocytes and paraimmunoblasts usually clustered in pseudofollicles. There is a low mitotic activity.
* Flow cytometry reveals expression of HLA-DR and of B-cell associated antigens CD19, CD20 (weak), CD21, CD22, CD23, CD43, CD79a, and CD11c (weak). CD10, FMC7, CD79b, CD25, and CD103 are negative; CD5, a T-cell associated antigen, is uniformly present on CLL/SLL cells. Although the diagnosis cannot be established in the absence of CD5 positivity, mantle-cell lymphoma cells (see p. 851; Table 10-3) are similarly positive for CD5. Staining for surface IgM/κ or IgM/λ (whichever represents the abnormal clone) is dim. Some cases may have an atypical phenotype. Minimal residual disease assessment in posttherapy hematologic remission is determined by multicolor flow cytometry and compared with the initial pattern.
* Cytogenetics. About half the patients have deletion 13q14.3 by FISH analysis. Other abnormalities include: trisomy 12, 11q22-23 (ATM) deletion, 17p13 (p53) deletion, 6q21 deletion, and IgH rearrangement (see below the prognostic role of the karyotypes under Prognostic markers). Interphase FISH can detect these abnormalities in a peripheral blood sample.
* Prognostic markers
  * The expression on leukemic cells of ZAP-70, CD38, and unmutated immunoglobulin heavy chain variable region are associated with aggressive disease. Of the three assays, positivity for ZAP-70 has emerged as the strongest risk factor. Because of lack of availability and of methodologic standardization, immunoglobulin mutation status assays are not recommended at this time.

TABLE 10-3. Differential Immunophenotypic Markers for Four Chronic Lymphoproliferative Diseases

Marker	CLL/SLL	B-PLL	HCL	Mantle Cell Lymphoma
Surface Immunoglobulin	Dim	Bright	Positive	Bright
CD5	+	+/−	−	+
CD11c	Weakly +	−	+	−
CD22	+	−	+	+
CD103	−	−	+	−
CD23	+	−	−	−
CD25	−	−	+	+
TRAP	−	−	+	−

B-PLL, prolymphocytic leukemia; CLL, chronic lymphocytic leukemia; HCL, hairy cell leukemia; SLL, small lymphocytic lymphoma; TRAP, tartrate-resistant acid phosphatase.

- Cytogenetic studies segregate prognosis as follows (in order of decreasing survival): isolated deletion 13q14.3 (best survival), normal karyotypes, trisomy 12 (intermediate prognosis), 11q/ATM deletion, 17p/p53 deletion (shortest survival). The combination of B-cell count and FISH were shown to be the best predictors of overall survival.
- Genomic studies may emerge in the future as the best tools for determining the clinical course of CLL/SLL. Genetic complexity is associated with aggressive disease. Recently downregulation of miR-29c and miR-223 were associated with adverse prognosis and may help refine stratification. MiR-34a indicates resistance to chemotherapy. This is an area that develops rapidly.
- Serum immunoglobulins: Hypogammaglobulinemia develops and progresses as the disease becomes more advanced. A monoclonal protein, usually of the same class as the surface membrane immunoglobulin is found in 5% of patients.
- LDH and β-2 microglobulin are elevated in more than half the patients. Their increase parallels a worsening prognosis.

➤ Transformation

- CLL/SLL rarely evolves into acute lymphocytic leukemia. The more common transformation is reflected by a progressive increase in prolymphocytes. A transition phase, with prolymphocytes >20% but <55% is called CLL/prolymphocytic leukemia. When ≥55% of the leukemic lymphocytes acquire characteristics of prolymphocytes the disease becomes known as prolymphocytic leukemia (see below). It connotes a grave prognosis.
- Diffuse large cell lymphoma (Richter syndrome), a transformation from CLL/SLL into diffuse large cell lymphoma, occurs in 2–8% of patients. It has an adverse outcome

➤ Suggested Readings

Gribben JG. How I treat chronic lymphocytic leukemia. *Blood*. 2010;115:187–197.

Halle M, Cheson BD, Catovsky D, et al. Guidelines for the diagnosis and treatment of chronic lymphocytic leukemia: a report from the International Workshop on Chronic Lymphocytic Leukemia updating the National Cancer Institute-Working Group 1996 guidelines. *Blood*. 2008;111:5446–5456.

Muller-Hermelink HK, Montserrat E, Catovsky D, et al. Chronic lymphocytic leukaemia/small lymphocytic lymphoma. WHO *Classification of Tumours of Haematopoietic and Lymphoid Tissues.* 4th ed. Lyon, France: International Agency for Research on Cancer; 2008:180–182.

Rassenti LZ, Jain S, Keating MJ, et al. Relative value of ZAP-70, CD 38, and immunoglobulin mutation status in predicting aggressive disease in chronic lymphocytic leukemia. *Blood.* 2008;112:1923–1930.

Rawstron AC, Bennett FL, O'Connor SJM, et al. Monoclonal B-cell lymphocytosis and chronic lymphocytic leukemia. *N Engl J Med.* 2008;359:575–583.

PROLYMPHOCYTIC (PLL) LEUKEMIA OF B- AND T-CELL SUBTYPE

➤ Definition

- B-cell PLL is a rare, aggressive, clonal lymphoproliferative disease composed mainly of B-cell prolymphocytes. It involves peripheral blood, bone marrow, and spleen.
- T-cell PLL is still rarer and will not be discussed further.

➤ Who Should be Suspected?

Patients who present with prominent splenomegaly but no lymphadenopathy, B symptoms, WBC counts of >100,000 comprised nearly exclusively of abnormal appearing lymphocytes, and frequently with anemia and thrombocytopenia. Some have a history of CLL/PLL, which occasionally transforms into B-cell PLL (see p. 832)

➤ Tests

- CBC
  - 50% of patients present with anemia and thrombocytopenia.
  - PBS is heavily populated by medium/large-sized "prolymphocytes," with moderately condensed chromatin and a single, prominent, vesicular nucleolus. The prolymphocytes must exceed 55% of lymphocytes, but are frequently >90%.
- Bone marrow is infiltrated in an interstitial pattern by prolymphocytes.
- Lymph nodes may show vague nodularity, but proliferation centers are absent.
- Immunophenotype
  - The prolymphocytes express bright surface IgM and IgD, and bright CD20 (see Table 10-3) as well as CD19, CD20, CD21, CD22, CD24, CD 79a and b, and FMC7.
  - Expression of CD5 and CD23 is weak or absent. CD25, CD11c, and CD103 are negative.
  - ZAP 70 and CD38 are expressed in half the cases.
- Cytogenetics. There are few studies available. Reported abnormalities include 6q-, t(6;12) (q15;p13), and structural aberrations of chromosomes. FISH detects deletion at 13q14 in half the cases and deletion of ATM. Isochromosome 17q leading to deletion of 17p and TP53 has also been noted. Molecular studies of p53 detect mutations in more than half the cases. The t(11;14) (13;q32), typical of mantle cell lymphoma, should be excluded, as these cases are considered the leukemic variants of mantle cell lymphoma.

➤ Suggested Reading

Campo E, Catovsky D, Montserrat E, et al. B-cell prolymphocytic leukaemia. WHO *Classification of Tumours of Haematopoietic and Lymphoid Tissues.* 4th ed. Lyon, France. International Agency for Research on Cancer; 2008: 183–184.

LEUKEMIA, CHRONIC MYELOMONOCYTIC (CMML)

➤ Definition

- CMML belongs to the group of myelodysplastic-myeloproliferative neoplasms (also called MDS/MPD overlap syndromes) that, according to the 2008 WHO classification, also include: atypical BCR-negative CML, juvenile myelomonocytic leukemia, and myelodysplastic/myeloproliferative neoplasm, unclassifiable.
- CMML is subdivided into two subcategories:
  - CMML-1: blasts (including promonocytes) <5% in the peripheral blood and <10% in the bone marrow;
  - CMML-2: blasts (including promonocytes) 5–19% in the peripheral blood or 10–19% in the bone marrow, or the presence of Auer rods

➤ Who Should be Suspected?

- An elderly patient, more commonly a male, with persistent monocytosis of >3 months duration and splenomegaly.
- Hepatomegaly, lymphadenopathy, tissue infiltrations, or serous effusions may also be presenting findings.

➤ Tests

- CBC: One, two, or all three lineages present dysplastic features.
  - RBC: normocytic, sometimes macrocytic anemia is common
  - WBC: persistent absolute monocyte count of >1000/µL (>10% of leukocytes) in the peripheral blood. The monocytes may be morphologically normal, or may have dysplastic features. In cases without dysplasia, other causes of monocytosis must be excluded. Neutropenia or neutrophilia may also be present, but neutrophil precursors account for <10% of the leukocytes. They may have dysplastic features (see p. 393). In some cases eosinophilia is present (CMML with eosinophilia).
- Platelets: moderate thrombocytopenia with atypical, large platelets may be present.
- Bone marrow is hypercellular with striking granulocytic, and to a less extent monocytic proliferation; an increase in erythroid precursors with dyserythropoietic features may also be present. Abnormal megakaryocytes complete the morphologic picture. Cytochemical and immunohistochemical studies of the peripheral blood or bone marrow are helpful in identifying the immature, dysplastic cells as of monocytic lineage.
- Immunophenotype. Myelomonocytic antigens CD33 and CD13 are positive; CD14, 68, and 64 are variably expressed. Aberrant features are frequently present. An increasing CD34 population forecasts transformation into acute leukemia.
- Immunostain for lysozyme on tissue sections can also help to identify the monocytic cells.
- Genetic studies. PDGFRA or PDGFRB are not rearranged. Rearrangements must be excluded in cases with eosinophilia.
- Cytogenetics. Nonspecific clonal cytogenetic abnormalities are found in 20–40% of patients. The most frequent abnormalities are +8, −7/del(7q), and structural abnormalities of 12p. Some patients with t(5:12)(q33;p13) may have eosinophilia and may respond to therapy with tyrosine kinase inhibitors. This group of patients should probably not be included in the CMML category, since they result from fusions of PDGFRB with other genes (see above).

➤ Suggested Reading

Orazi A, Bennett JM, Germing U, et al. Chronic myelomonocytic leukaemia. *WHO Classification of Tumours of Haematopoietic and Lymphoid tissues.* 4th ed. Lyon, France: International Agency for Research on Cancer; 2008:76–79.

LEUKEMIA, HAIRY CELL

➤ Definition

* Hairy cell leukemia (HCL) is a rare indolent B-cell lymphoproliferative neoplasm, characterized by hairy projections of affected lymphocytes.
* The disease has a 4:1 to 3:1 male to female ratio
* A variant (vHCL) may present with intermediate features between hairy cells and prolymphocytes, and has an aggressive course.

➤ Who Should be Suspected?

* Individuals who present with splenomegaly and cytopenias but no lymphadenopathy.

➤ Tests

* CBC.
    * Anemia and thrombocytopenia are common, in part due to bone marrow infiltration, and in part to hypersplenism.
    * WBC is usually decreased at presentation, but it may also be increased if the abnormal lymphocytes are elevated. Neutropenia and monocytopenia may be present.
    * Usually from 10–90% of lymphocytes in the peripheral blood smear reveal lymphocytes with cytoplasmic projections (hairy). Nucleoli are not visible. In aggressive cases these lymphocytes may be increased to leukemic levels.
* Bone marrow.
    * Aspirate is difficult to obtain because of reticulin fibrosis.
    * Biopsy shows a hyperplastic marrow, with diffuse infiltration by hairy cells in a characteristic loose, widely spaced, fashion, with a well-defined rim of cytoplasm leaving a clear zone around the cells, producing a "fried-egg" appearance. The hairy projections are not seen on the biopsy specimen. No nucleoli are seen. There is no paratrabecular involvement. In some patients there may be a hypocellular marrow that may resemble aplastic anemia (see p. 794).
* Spleen and lymph nodes
    * The leukemic cells are found in the red pulp with infiltration of the cords and sinuses, whereas the white pulp is atrophic. Angiomatous lakes are formed.
* Cytochemistry
    * Tartrate-resistant acid phosphatase (TRAP) is invariably positive (see Table 10-3). It requires peripheral blood smear or bone marrow aspirate. Positivity appears as cytoplasmic granularity.
* Flow cytometry
    * Flow cytometry (see Table 10-3) is positive for CD19, CD20 (bright), CD22, CD25, CD11c, CD52, CD103, and CD123. Cyclin D1 is also positive Most cases lack both CD10 and CD5. Surface immunoglobulin is positive.
    * The hairy cell variant is negative for CD25 and CD123. This distinction is important therapeutically.

* Genetics
  * The presence of unmutated Ig heavy chain variable genes defines a subset of HCL with aggressive behavior. The study of Ig genes has become an integral part of the diagnostic work-up of HCL to determine optimal therapy upfront.
  * Karyotype. No consistent karyotypic abnormalities are found. Abnormalities of 5q may be detected.

➤ Suggested Readings

Foucar K, Falini B, Catovsky D, Stein H. Hairy cell leukemia. *WHO Classification of Tumours of Haematopoietic and Lymphoid Tissues.* 4th ed. Lyon, France: International Agency for Research on Cancer; 2000:188–190.
Grever MR. How I treat hairy cell leukemia. Blood. 2010;115:21–28.

LEUKEMIA, T-CELL LARGE GRANULAR LYMPHOCYTIC (T-LGL)

➤ Definition
* T- LGL belongs to chronic lymphoproliferative disorders of natural killer (NK) cells.
* It is characterized by a persistent (>6 months) increase in the number of clonal peripheral blood large granular lymphocytes (LGLs), usually between 2000 and 20,000/µL (the absolute number of LGLs in normal subjects is 2–400), without a clearly identified cause. T-LGLs may be occasionally associated with other diseases, such as RA or other hematologic disorders.

➤ Who Should be Suspected?
* A middle age or elderly patient with neutropenia and/or anemia, together with peripheral blood lymphocytosis, and moderate splenomegaly. The patient may be asymptomatic for long periods of time or may suffer from repeated bacterial infections.
* If the total lymphocyte count is not elevated, the disease may be suspected if an increased number of LGLs are present on examination of the peripheral blood.

➤ Tests
* CBC may reveal neutropenia, lymphocytosis but rarely thrombocytopenia.
  * RBC: anemia is present in half the patients, occasionally with oval macrocytosis.
  * WBC: neutropenia is present in the majority of patients. LGLs are increased; they have a large size with abundant cytoplasm containing fine or coarse azurophilic granules, and a reniform or round nucleus.
* Bone marrow may show diffuse infiltration with LGL, but the extent of bone marrow involvement is variable. Bone marrow core biopsy immunohistochemistry may be helpful to confirm diagnosis.
* Immunophenotype: Most T-LGL leukemias show a profile of cytotoxic T cells, with CD3+, T-cell receptor (TCR) antibody-positive, CD4– and CD8+. Expression of CD57 and CD16 is seen in more than 80% of the cases. T-LGL cells can also express cytotoxic effector proteins TIA1 and granzyme.
* Genetic studies help define the disease by finding TCR gene rearrangement. Developing technology found a number of genes whose expression was active in LGL T cells, but silent in normal T cells.
* Cytogenetics reveals no consistent karyotypic abnormalities, but abnormalities involving chromosomes 7, 8, and 14 have been described in some patients.

- Serum protein electrophoresis shows hypergammaglobulinemia in half the patients, rarely a monoclonal IgG gammopathy.
- Serologic findings: RF is common, and antinuclear antibodies and circulating immune complexes are present in half the cases.

➤ **Suggested Readings**

Chan WC, Foucar K, Morice WG, Catovsky D. T-cell large granular lymphocytic leukaemia. *WHO Classification of Tumours of Haematopoietic and Lymphoid tissues.* 4th ed. Lyon, France: International Agency for Research on Cancer; 2008:272–273.

Lamy T, Loughran Jr TP. T cell large granular lymphocyte leukemia. UpToDate. Rose B, ed. Waltham, MA: UpToDate, Inc.; 2008.

LEUKEMIA, NEUTROPHILIC

➤ **Definition**

A rare myeloproliferative disease in which the predominant blood peripheral cells are mature PMNs.

➤ **Who Should be Suspected?**

- Patients with persistent neutrophilia in whom a chronic infection, neoplasm, or inflammatory process is excluded.
- Clinical picture of splenomegaly and hepatomegaly of unknown etiology. Twenty-five to 30% of patients present with mucocutaneous bleeding.
- Polycythemia vera, primary myelofibrosis, and essential thrombocythemia should be excluded.

➤ **Tests**

- CBC: characterized by persistent leukocytosis (WBC $\geq 2500 \times 10^9$/mu (micro)/L) due to neutrophilia (segmented neutrophils and bands are >80% of WBC). Immature granulocytes are <10% on the PBS. Hb and platelets are normal early in the disease, but anemia and thrombocytopenia develop as the disease progresses.
- Bone marrow: hypercellular with increase in mature neutrophils, but <5% myeloblasts.
- Cytogenetics and genetic studies: no rearrangement of BCR-ABL1, PDGFRA, PDGRFB, or FGFR1.

➤ **Suggested Reading**

Bain BJ, Brunning RD, Vardiman JW, Thiele J. Chronic neutrophilic leukaemia. *WHO Classification of Tumours of Haematopoietic and Lymphoid tissues.* 4th ed. Lyon, France: International Agency for Research on Cancer; 2008.

MULTILINEAGE DISEASES

MYELOPROLIFERATIVE NEOPLASMS (Mpns)

➤ **Definition**

- Chronic MPNs are a heterogeneous group of clonal malignant disorders that arise from the transformation of hematopoietic stem cells/progenitors and are characterized by their expansion. Clonal overexpansion leads to deranged overproduction of blood cells by one or more subordinate cell lines and a predisposition of the progenitor cells to undergo terminal transformation into leukemic blast cells.

* The three most common nonleukemic MPNs are polycythemia vera, essential thrombocythemia, and primary myelofibrosis. They are characterized by clonal dominance and unregulated increase in the circulation of erythrocytes, leukocytes, or platelets, each lineage alone, or in combination. Diagnostic challenges ensue because of the overlap of clinical and laboratory manifestations among these three disorders (phenotypic mimicry). This mimicry has been enhanced by the discovery of a common mutation *(V617F)* in *JAK2*, which belongs to the Janus family tyrosine kinases.
* Bone marrow biopsies are valuable for distinguishing among the various MPNs and for monitoring disease progression or effect of therapy. Following the discovery of mutations in crucial genes, the diagnosis of MPNs had become both morphologic and molecular.

➤ Classification
* Below is the revised (2008) WHO classification of MPNs
  * Chronic myelogenous leukemia, BCABL+ (see p. 833)
  * Chronic neutrophilic leukemia (see p. 836)
  * Polycythemia vera (see p. 839)
  * Primary myelofibrosis (see p. 841)
  * Essential thrombocythemia (see p. 841)
  * Chronic eosinophilic leukemia, not otherwise classified (see p. 827)
  * Mastocytosis
  * Myeloproliferative neoplasm, unclassifiable (see p. 836)
* The diagnostic approach of these entities will be presented under separate headings.

➤ Suggested Reading
Spivak JL. Narrative review: thrombocytosis, polycythemia vera, and JAK2 mutations: the phenotypic mimicry of chronic myeloproliferation. *Ann Intern Med.* 2010;152:300–306.

LEUKEMIA, CHRONIC MYELOGENOUS (CML)

➤ Definition
* CML is a myeloproliferative neoplasm that results primarily in increase of myeloid cells, and, to a lesser extent, erythroid and platelets in the peripheral blood, and marked hyperplasia in the bone marrow. It is induced by a chimeric gene that results from the fusion of the ABL gene on chromosome 9 with the BCR gene on chromosome 22, leading to the formation of a new leukemia-specific fusion gene that codes for constitutionally activated protein tyrosine kinases of different molecular weight. The Philadelphia chromosome is the abnormal chromosome 22, reflecting the 95% of cases where the translocation between chromosomes 9 and 22 is balanced.
* If untreated, CML progresses from the chronic phase to acute leukemia (blastic transformation) within 3–5 years, frequently with an intermediate "accelerated" phase. It may also present in the accelerated or blastic phase when first diagnosed.

➤ Who Should be Suspected?
* Patients found to have persistent, and not otherwise explained, leukocytosis with increase in the myeloid line.
* Patients with fatigue, anorexia, weight loss, excessive sweating, and an abdominal mass (splenomegaly).

➤ Tests
Chronic Phase
- CBC:
  - WBC count is markedly elevated, usually 50,000–300,000/µL, predominantly neutrophils, bands, metamyelocytes, and myelocytes, with a few blasts and promyelocytes. Basophilia is nearly always present. Eosinophilia may also be present. Absolute monocytosis and normal absolute lymphocytes.
  - Hct/Hb may be normal or slightly decreased or increased; if anemia is present, it is normochromic, normocytic. Normoblasts are usually seen on the PBS. Reticulocyte count is <3%.
  - Platelets may be normal, but in ~50% of cases they are elevated. Occasionally the platelets may be decreased, especially as the disease progresses. Large platelets (megathrombocytes) may be conspicuous.
- Bone marrow
  - Hyperplastic, with increase mainly in the myelocytic line, increased myeloid-to-erythroid ratio
  - Myeloblasts are <5%. Increase in basophiles and eosinophils, including immature forms. Megakaryocytes may be increased. Focal or diffuse reticulin fibrosis in approximately one third of cases.
  - Increased vascularity
- Cytogenetics or FISH
  - Demonstration of the Philadelphia chromosome, t(9,22) involving BCR-ABL1 genes is the gold standard for diagnosis. Approximately 5% of CML patients do not demonstrate the Philadelphia chromosome by karyotyping, but demonstrate the BCR-ABL1 gene fusion by FISH or real-time PCR techniques*. Interphase nuclei FISH appears to be more sensitive for the detection of BCR−ABL+ than chromosome banding analysis.
  - The V617F JAK2 mutation is absent.
- Leukocyte alkaline phosphatase (LAP): Low or absent LAP is not necessary for diagnosis in Philadelphia chromosome–positive patients.
- Uric acid: elevated

Accelerated Phase
- 10–19% blasts in peripheral blood and/or of nucleated bone marrow cells
- ≥20% peripheral blood basophiles
- Persistent thrombocytopenia (<100,000/µL) unrelated to therapy
- Increasing spleen size and increasing WBC count unresponsive to therapy
- Cytogenetic evidence of clonal evolution

Blast Crisis
- ≥20% blasts of peripheral blood cells or of nucleated bone marrow cells
- Extramedullary blast proliferation
- Large foci or clusters of blasts in the bone marrow biopsy

---

*Atypical CML is referred by some hematologists to cases mimicking CML, but without evidence of BCR-ABL gene fusion. These cases are classified by WHO in the group of myeloproliferative/myelodysplastic disorders. Another variant is the rare chronic neutrophilic leukemia (see p. 836), characterized by mature granulocytic hyperplasia and elevated LAP, but absent Philadelphia chromosome.

➤ Laboratory Criteria for Response in Treated Patients

- Disease monitoring is one of the key management strategies of CML to assess the response to therapy and to detect early relapse. The most sensitive approach to detect CML is the quantitative real-time PCR (RT-PCR) of the BCR-ABL messenger RNA. By this methodology, one CML cell can be detected in 100,000 to 1 million cells. Another advantage of this methodology is the use of peripheral blood rather than bone marrow tissue. In cases of complete cytogenetic response, present guidelines suggest molecular testing every 3 months.
- In patients treated with tyrosine kinase inhibitors, monitoring for new mutation in ABL is recommended, because such mutations predict the development of resistance to therapy.

Complete Hematologic Response
- Complete normalization of peripheral blood counts with leukocytes <10,000/µL
- Platelet count <450,000/µL
- No immature cells in peripheral blood

Cytogenetic Response
- Complete: no Ph chromosome positive detected in a minimum of 20 metaphases
- Major: 0–30% Ph-positive metaphases
- Minor: 35–90% Ph-positive metaphases

Molecular Response
- Defined by the magnitude of reduction in BCR-ABL transcripts from a standard value.
- *Complete* molecular response: *BCR-ABL1* mRNA undetectable by RT-PCR
- *Major* molecular response: >3-log reduction of *BCR-ABL1* mRNA; it correlates well with survival. No patient who achieved complete cytogenetic response and a major molecular response at 18 months progressed to accelerated or blast phase at 60 months.

➤ Suggested Readings

Calabretta B, Perrotti D. The biology of CML blast crisis. *Blood.* 2004;103:4010–4022.
Druker BJ. Translation of the Philadelphia chromosome into therapy for CML. *Blood.* 2008;112:4808–4817.
Radich JP. How I monitor residual disease in chronic myeloid leukemia. *Blood.* 2009;114:3376–3381.

POLYCYTHEMIA VERA (PV)

➤ Definition
- PV is the most common clonal chronic myeloproliferative neoplasm (MPN). It is characterized by overproduction of morphologically normal erythroid cells, leading to an elevated red cell mass (RCM).
- An increased RCM alone is insufficient to establish the diagnosis, because the RCM may be increased in conditions associated with hypoxia or with tumors secreting erythropoietin.

➤ Classification
- Proposed revised WHO criteria for the diagnosis of PV (the diagnosis requires the presence of both major criteria and one minor criterion, or the presence of the first major criterion with two minor criteria).

- Major criteria
  - Hb >18.5 in men, >16.5 in women, or other evidence of increased red cell mass.
  - Presence of V617F JAK2 mutation in exon 14, or other functionally similar mutation such as JAK2 exon 12 mutation.
- Minor criteria
  - Bone marrow biopsy showing hypercellularity for age with trilineage growth (panmyelosis) and with prominent erythroid, granulocytic, and megakaryocytic proliferation.
  - Serum erythropoietin level below the reference range of normal.
  - Endogenous erythroid colony formation in vitro (not generally available in clinical laboratories).
  - Some investigators consider the presence of V617F JAK2 mutation in association with low erythropoietin levels as sufficient for the diagnosis of PV.

➤ Who Should be Suspected?

- Patients found to have an elevated Hb and Hct (the disease may be asymptomatic for long time) that cannot be explained otherwise.
- Patients with a history of familial polycythemic disorders and elevated Hb/Hct
- Patients with unexplained thrombotic or bleeding events
- Patients with splenomegaly otherwise unexplained
- Patients with pruritus, erythromelalgia, and transient visual disturbances

➤ Tests

- CBC: elevated Hb, Hct, and red cell count; platelets and granulocytes/monocytes modestly elevated at the time of diagnosis; mildly elevated reticulocyte count.
- Red cell mass (RCM): elevated (requires isotope study availability); plasma volume is normal or elevated. Caveat: iron deficiency should be corrected before performing RCM studies. RCM may be omitted in patients with extreme elevations of Hb/Hct.
- Blood gases: O_2 >92%
- Bone marrow: Hyperplasia of erythroid, granulocytic, and megakaryocytic lines, without increase in immature cells; decreased iron stores; increased reticulin, especially as the disease progresses.
- Molecular genetics: V617F JACK2 mutation is present in 95–97% of PV patients, but it is not specific for PV as it may also be present in essential thrombocythemia and primary myelofibrosis. Increasing amounts of V617F allele correspond to a more pronounced myeloproliferative phenotype, favoring higher Hb levels and leukocyte counts. Other mutations seen in a minority of patients include mutations, insertions, or deletions in exon 12.
- Cytogenetics or FISH: Absence of BCR-ABL1; abnormalities that may be found include 20q−, +8, +9, and 9p−
- Serum erythropoietin: low or immeasurable
- Leukocyte alkaline phosphatase and serum vitamin B_{12} are elevated, but unnecessary for diagnosis.

➤ Suggested Readings

Spivak JL, Silver RT. The revised World Health organization diagnostic criteria for polycythemia vera, essential thrombocytosis, and primary myelofibrosis: an alternative proposal. *Blood*. 2008;112:231–239.

Tefferi A, Thiele J, Orazi A, et al. Proposal and rationale for revision of the World Health Organization diagnostic criteria for polycythemia vera, essential thrombocythemia, and primary myelofibrosis: recommendations from an ad hoc international expert panel. *Blood*. 2007;110:1092–1097.

ESSENTIAL THROMBOCYTHEMIA (ET)

➤ Definition
ET is a chronic myeloproliferative neoplasm (MPN) involving mainly the megakaryocytic lineage, characterized by persistent thrombocytosis.

It is the only MPN without a specific phenotype, making it a diagnosis of exclusion.

➤ Who Should be Suspected?
* Patients with persistent thrombocytosis without underlying cause
* Patients with unexplained splenomegaly
* Patients with unexplained vascular occlusion

➤ Tests
* CBC: sustained platelet count >450,000 (some recommend persistent elevated counts for ≥8 months).
* No evidence of reactive thrombocytosis
  * Bone marrow biopsy showing proliferation of the megakaryocytic lineage with increased numbers of enlarged, mature megakaryocytes; no increase and no left-shift of granulopoiesis or erythropoiesis.
  * Not meeting criteria for polycythemia vera, primary myelofibrosis, chronic myelogenous leukemia, myelodysplastic syndromes, or other myeloid neoplasms.
  * Genetic test: V617F JAK2 mutation can be demonstrated in about half the cases of ET; in its absence, reactive thrombocytosis should be ruled out, especially by demonstrating normal serum ferritin to exclude iron deficiency.
  * Cytogenetics or FISH: absence of Bcr-Abl should be documented to exclude CML; no specific abnormalities have yet been described.

➤ Suggested Reading
Teffery A, Thiele J, Orazi A, et al. Proposal and rationale for revision of the World Health Organization criteria for polycythemia vera, essential thrombocythemia, and primary myelofibrosis: recommendations from an ad hoc international expert panel. *Blood.* 2007;110:1092–1097.

PRIMARY MYELOFIBROSIS (PMF)

➤ Definition
* PMF is a chronic myeloproliferative neoplasm (MPN) characterized by clonal proliferation of myeloid cells and stimulation of marrow fibroblasts.
* PMF is also called chronic idiopathic myelofibrosis in the WHO classification and was formerly known as agnogenic or primary myeloid metaplasia It is the rarest and the most severe Philadelphia-negative chronic MPN.
* PMF is characterized by a leukoerythroblastic blood picture, teardrop poikilocytosis of red cells, and extramedullary hematopoiesis, with progressive hepatosplenomegaly. Other causes of marrow fibrosis must be excluded.

➤ Classification
* The WHO proposal for revision has been recently criticized. The main criticism resides in the difficulty of diagnosing the prefibrotic stage of PMF. The proposed revision:
  * Major criteria

- Presence of megakaryocytic proliferation and atypia, usually accompanied by either reticulin and/or collagen fibrosis; in the absence of significant reticulin fibrosis, the megakaryocytes changes must be accompanied by an increased bone marrow cellularity characterized by granulocytic proliferation and often decreased erythropoiesis (the prefibrotic cellular-phase disease).
- Not meeting WHO criteria for PV, CML, MDS, or other myeloid neoplasms.
- Demonstration of V617F JAK2 or other clonal markers, or in the absence of a clonal marker, no evidence that the bone marrow fibrosis is due to an underlying inflammatory or other neoplastic diseases.
- Minor criteria
  1. Leukoerythroblastosis
  2. Increased serum LDH
  3. Anemia
  4. Palpable splenomegaly

➤ Who Should be Screened for PMF?

- Patients with progressive splenomegaly reaching enormous size and resulting in hypersplenism as manifested by pancytopenia
- Patients age >65 with constitutional symptoms, progressive unexplained anemia with bizarre PBS morphology and leukocytosis
- Patients with thrombosis of splanchnic veins (portal vein and hepatic veins)

➤ Tests

- CBC
  - RBCs. Normochromic, normocytic progressive anemia caused by hemolysis and decreased/ineffective marrow production. Bleeding may also play a role in the etiology of anemia. PBS shows marked anisocytosis and poikilocytosis with teardrop RBCs (dacrocytes) (see p. 318), polychromasia, and nucleated red cells (part of an leukoerythroblastic picture). Reticulocyte count is increased.
  - WBCs may be decreased, normal, or increased; abnormal or immature forms may be present and increase with time. As the disease progresses, the WBCs and blasts may increase (blasts are initially <5%). Basophils and eosinophils may be increased.
  - Platelets may be decreased, normal, or increased. Thrombocytopenia becomes more profound with disease progression. Abnormal or large forms are present. Deficient aggregation with collagen or epinephrine is common.
- Bone marrow shows progressive fibrosis that can be visualized with silver stain for reticulin, and a trichrome stain for mature collagen. Bone marrow sinusoids are expanded and there is intravascular hematopoiesis. Early on the bone marrow may be hypercellular with minimal fibrosis (cellular phase of PMF, difficult to diagnose). Frequently the bone marrow aspirate results in a dry tape. The biopsy shows a progressively hypocellular marrow replaced by fibrosis. Megakaryocytes are the last remaining hematopoietic elements, most of which have abnormal morphology.
- Lymph node biopsy (usually not necessary) shows extramedullary hematopoiesis involving all three cell lines. Foci of extramedullary hematopoiesis may occur in almost any organ.
- Genetics and flow cytometry
  - The V617F JAK2 mutation (done on peripheral blood) is present in approximately 50–60% of cases

- MPL (W515K/L): activating mutations affecting MPL thrombopoietin receptors are present in 5–7% of cases.
- Elevated CD34+ hematopoietic precursors can be detected in peripheral blood and distinguishes PMF from PV and ET in which they are absent in the chronic phases.
- Karyotypic abnormalities occur in 32–48% of patients at diagnosis. Favorable abnormalities include sole deletions in 13q or 20q, or trisomy 9. Rearrangement of chromosome 5 or 7 or ≥ 3 aberrations, trisomy 8 or 12p- predict a poor survival. Patients with abnormalities of chromosome 17 have the poorest survival, with a median survival of only 5 months. Additional karyotypic abnormalities that may develop during the course of the disease may further affect prognosis.
- Cytogenetic studies are recommended not only to determine prognosis, but most importantly to rule out CML through the absence of BCR-ABL translocation (Ph chromosome).
- PT or PTT may be prolonged and laboratory evidence of DIC is occasionally found.
- Leukocyte alkaline phosphatase (LAP) is increased (not routinely recommended).
- LDH, serum uric acid and vitamin B12 are often increased.

➤ Suggested Readings

Levine RL, Gilliland DG. Myeloproliferative disorders. *Blood.* 2008;112:2190–2198.

Spivak JL, Silver RT. The revised World Health Organization diagnostic criteria for polycythemia vera, essential thrombocytosis, and primary myelofibrosis: an alternative proposal. *Blood.* 2008;112:231–239.

Tam CS, Abruzzo LV, Lin KI, et al. The role of cytogenetic abnormalities as a prognostic marker in primary myelofibrosis: applicability at time of diagnosis and later during disease course. *Blood.* 2009;113:4171–4178.

Tefferi A, Thiele J, Orazi A, et al. Proposal and rationale for revision of the World Health Organization diagnostic criteria for polycythemia vera, essential thrombocythemia, and primary myelofibrosis: recommendations from an ad hoc international expert panel. *Blood.* 2007;110:1092–1097.

Tefferi A, Vardiman JW. Classification and diagnosis of myeloproliferative neoplasms: the 2008 World Health Organization criteria and point-of-care diagnostic algorithms. *Leukemia.* 2008;22:1422.

MYELODYSPLASTIC SYNDROME (MDS)

➤ Definition

- MDS is a group of clonal disorders of the bone marrow, characterized by ineffective hematopoiesis. (bone marrow is hypercellular, with dysplasia (abnormal morphology) involving at least 10% of a specific myeloid lineage, peripheral blood cytopenias, and dysplasia within single or multiple lineages.
- Approximately two thirds of patients present initially with low risk disease. Higher grades disease categories tend to progress to acute myeloid leukemia. Refractory cytopenias are the principal cause of mortality and morbidity.
- The differential diagnosis of MDS includes other causes of macrocytic or refractory anemias, alcohol consumption, and thyroid disease.

➤ Who Should be Suspected?

- An elderly patient, more often a male, presenting with cytopenia(s) discovered by routine CBC, or with symptoms resulting from anemia (fatigue, weakness, exercise intolerance, new angina), less frequently infections, bruising, or bleeding. Splenomegaly and lymphadenopathy are absent. The presence of monocytosis is suggestive of chronic myelomonocytic leukemia (CMML) (see p. 833).

- Previous exposure to environmental toxins such as benzene, radiation therapy, or treatment with alkylating agents or topoisomerase II inhibitors may result in secondary MDS.
- Alternatively, young patients with an inherited hematologic disorder are predisposed to develop MDS.

➤ Classification

- The original FAB classification has been succeeded by the WHO classification and will not be described. The WHO classification has proved helpful for prognosis and in selection of therapy and is updated periodically. The 2008 WHO classification of MDS contains eight entities:
  1. Refractory cytopenias with unilineage dysplasia (RCUD)
  2. Refractory anemia (RA): <5% bone marrow blasts, ≤1% blasts in the peripheral blood; <15% of erythroid precursors are ringed sideroblasts (characterized by at least five granules of iron that encircle the nucleus of erythroid precursors). Variants: refractory neutropenia (RN) and refractory thrombocytopenia (RT).
  3. Refractory anemia with ringed sideroblasts (RARS): similar to RA, but with >15% ringed sideroblasts in the bone marrow. Erythroid dysplasia only.
  4. Refractory cytopenias with multilineage dysplasia (RCMD): dysplasia in ≥10% of cells in two or more lineages and <5% bone marrow blasts. ±15% ringed sideroblasts.
  5. Refractory anemia with excess blasts-1 (RAEB-1): 5–9% blasts in the bone marrow but no Auer rods. Cytopenia(s) but <5% blasts in peripheral blood.
  6. Refractory anemia with excess blasts-2 (RAEB-2): 10–19% blasts in bone marrow, Auer rods ±; 5–19% blasts in peripheral blood, cytopenia(s), ≤1000/μL monocytes.
  7. Myelodysplastic syndrome-unclassified (MDS-U): <5% blasts in bone marrow; dysplasia in <10% of cells when accompanied by a cytogenetic abnormality is considered presumptive evidence for a diagnosis of MDS; cytopenias and ≤1% blasts in peripheral blood.
  8. MDS associated with isolated del (5q) (the 5q− syndrome). Bone marrow: normal or increased megakaryocytes with hypolobated nuclei; <5% blasts; no Auer rods; del(5q) as the only cytogenetic abnormality. Peripheral blood: anemia; normal or increased platelet count, no or rare blasts (<1%).
- Syndromes with mixed features of myelodysplastic-myeloproliferative disorders are classified separately as MDS/MPS (see p. 843). The prototype is CMML.

➤ Tests

- Findings vary with subtype of MDS (see above). Common findings will be described, as well as those distinguishing ones for various subtypes.
  - CBC. Monolineage, bilineage, or trilineage cytopenias are common, but in the absence of dysplastic features they are insufficient for the diagnosis of MDS.
    - Red cells: commonly macrocytic anemia (high MCV); hypochromic, microcytic cells in RARS; ovalomacrocytosis; basophilic stippling, Howell-Jolly bodies, and megaloblastoid nucleated red cells may be present on PBS.
    - WBC: leukopenia resulting from neutropenia is present at diagnosis in half the patients. Granulocytes have reduced or absent granulation, reduced segmentation of nuclei (pseudo-Pelger-Huet nuclei), clumped chromatin pattern, ringed-shaped nuclei and nuclear sticks. The granulocytes may be dysfunctional, leading to infections. Lymphopenia due to a reduction of T4 lymphocytes is seen in hyper transfused patients. Mild

monocytosis is common, but if the monocytes are markedly elevated, CMML (p. 833) should be considered.

- Platelets: varying degrees of thrombocytopenia are present at the time of diagnosis in about 25% of patients. Giant or agranular platelets can be seen on PBS. Platelets may be functionally defective, and platelet aggregation is often abnormal. Thrombocytosis may be present in some patients with RARS; thrombocytosis is also part of the 5q⁻ syndrome or in patients with translocations involving chromosome 3.
- Bone marrow examination is routinely done for diagnosis and classification of MDS subtype. Marrow fibrosis is rare; when present it suggests therapy-related MDS or CMML. In most cases the bone marrow is hyperplastic, and red cell hyperplasia, in association with ineffective erythropoiesis, tends to be prominent. The red cell precursors show alterations in their nuclei. Approximately 10–15% of patients have a hypocellular marrow that is difficult to distinguish from aplastic anemia (see p. 794).
- Defective maturation in the myeloid series is common, and counting the number of blasts is essential to determine subtype and prognosis.
- Megakaryocytes numbers are normal or increased; they sometimes occur in clusters.
- Abnormal morphology of megakaryocytes is common.
- Cytochemistry of the bone marrow (especially iron and PAS stains of erythroblasts) is helpful in the diagnosis of the various subtypes of MDS.
- Immunophenotyping of the bone marrow is useful in determining percentage of CD34+ cells, which parallels the number of blasts. An emerging population of CD34 or CD117 positive cells in low-grade MDS suggests the development of more aggressive disease.
- Cytogenetic studies are helpful for diagnosis, may provide prognostic information, and are useful for monitoring response to therapy. Patients with the 5q⁻ anomaly (isolated or in combination with other abnormalities) may be treated differently, as they often respond to lenalidomide. Clonal cytogenetic abnormalities are seen in approximately 50–75% of cases and are not specific to subtypes, although certain cytogenetic abnormalities may be associated with characteristic morphology, for instance the association of *EVI1* rearrangements at 3q26 with abnormal megakaryocytes. Recurrent abnormalities include −5/5q−, −7/7q−, trisomy 8, and 20q−. In the International Prognostic Scoring System (IPSS) for MDS, normal chromosomes, −Y, 5q−, and 20q− are considered good prognosis; −7/7q− or complex karyotype (≥three abnormalities) are considered poor prognosis, and other findings are considered intermediate. Del(17p) is associated with the presence of pseudo-Huët granulocytes containing small vacuoles, a deletion of TP53, and a relatively high risk of leukemic transformation. Abnormalities of *MLL* at 11q23 often represent therapy-related MDS and are associated with poor prognosis. Certain clonal cytogenetic abnormalities, for example, −Y, +8, and 20q−, are not diagnostic of MDS in the absence of positive morphologic findings.
- Serum B₁₂ and folate should be obtained to exclude deficiencies that may mimic MDS morphologically. The karyotype is normal in these deficiencies.
- Hb electrophoresis may reveal acquired Hb H disease, or rarely acquired thalassemic syndrome, but it is not necessary for the diagnosis of MDS.
- Serum immunoglobulins are variably abnormal, with hypogammaglobulinemia, polyclonal hypergammaglobulinemia, and even monoclonal gammopathies reported.
- Studies for PNH (see p. 810) help differentiate the two diseases, or reveal various combinations of PNH with aplastic anemia or refractory anemias as part of a MDS picture.

- Serology for HIV infection may be indicated in some cases, since AIDS may be associated with dysplastic hematopoiesis and cytopenias.

➤ Prognosis

- The International Prognosis Scoring System (IPSS) classifies MDS patients into four prognostic categories based on the number of cytopenias, cytogenetics, and percent of blasts in the bone marrow.

➤ Suggested Readings

Brunning RD, Orazi A, Germing U, et al. Myelodysplastic syndromes/neoplasms, overview. *WHO Classification of Tumours of Haematopoietic and Lymphoid tissues.* 4th ed. Lyon, France: International Agency for Research on Cancer; 2008:88–93.

Doll DC, Landaw SA. Clinical manifestations and diagnosis of the myelodysplastic syndromes. UpToDate. Rose B, ed. Waltham, MA: UpToDate Inc.; 2008.

Nimer SD. Myelodysplastic syndromes. *Blood.* 2008;111:4841–4851.

Stone RM. How I treat patients with myelodysplastic syndromes. *Blood.* 2009;113:6296–6303.

Tefferi A, Vardiman JW. Mechanisms of disease: myelodysplastic syndromes. *N Engl J Med.* 2009;361:1872–1885.

SPLENOMEGALY

➤ Definition

- Enlargement of the spleen that can be demonstrated either by physical examination or by imaging studies.
- Splenomegaly reflects an underlying disease. Finding splenomegaly should trigger systemic investigation of its etiology.

➤ Who Should be Suspected?

- Patients with abdominal fullness, early satiety, or chronic or acute left upper abdominal pain.
- Common causes of splenomegaly are:
  - Infections
    - Infectious endocarditis (see p. 516)
    - Infectious mononucleosis (see p. 1002)
    - Brucellosis (see p. 951)
    - Miliary TB (see p. 978)
    - Parasitic infections: malaria, schistosomiasis, kala-azar)
    - Fungi
  - Vascular (systemic or portal) congestion (congestive splenomegaly)
  - Immune disorders
    - RA (Felty syndrome)
    - SLE (see p. 936)
    - Sarcoidosis
  - Hematologic conditions
    - Hemolytic anemias (see p. 804)
    - Thalassemia major (see p. 802)
    - Hereditary spherocytosis (see p. 807), ovalocytosis (see p. 808)
    - Polycythemia vera (see p. 839)
    - Essential thrombocythemia (see p. 841)
    - Chronic lymphocytic leukemia (see p. 829)

- Non-Hodgkin lymphomas (see p. 847)
- Hodgkin lymphoma (see p. 857)
- Chronic myeloid leukemia (massive) (see p. 837)
- Primary myelofibrosis (massive) (see p. 841)
- Systemic mastocytosis
- Infiltrative splenomegaly
  - Lipid storage diseases—Gaucher disease, (see p. 906), Niemann-Pick disease (see p. 917), and many more
  - Amyloidosis (see p. 865)
  - Sarcoidosis
  - Metastatic disease
- Developmental anomalies
- Multitransfused patients
- In many cases of splenomegaly, the spleen's ability to engulf blood cells is increased (hypersplenism), resulting in mono-, bi-, or pancytopenias.

NON-HODGKIN LYMPHOMAS

➤ Definition

- Non-Hodgkin lymphomas are neoplasms of lymphoid tissues comprising numerous variants. They are a heterogeneous group of distinct disorders, mostly unrelated to one another, with a spectrum of histologic grades and clinical behavior. The present classification, as updated by the WHO in 2008, recognizes three categories of lymphoid neoplasms: B-cell, T-cell and NK-cell lymphomas, and separately Hodgkin lymphoma and plasma cell disorders. Among the non-Hodgkin lymphomas, most are derived from B cells. The present classification is based on currently available morphologic, immunophenotypic, and genetic techniques, with an attempt to correlate the various types with their clinical behavior. The latter is utilized as a guide for predicting prognosis and therapy in the International Prognostic Index.
- Many issues remain unresolved, and the 2008 WHO classification represents evolving concepts. Rapidly evolving genomic technologies, which include gene rearrangement and microarray techniques, reveal multiple subtypes of different molecular etiologies, clinical evolution and response to therapy, all within the presently accepted types of lymphomas.
- In addition, studies of microRNA (miRNA) (small noncoding RNAs that orchestrate many aspects of cell physiology and their deregulation is often linked to distinct neoplasms) have demonstrated clusters, such as 17–92 overexpressed in a variety of B-cell lymphomas.
- Because of the extreme rarity of some lymphomas (B- or T-cell lymphoblastic leukemia/lymphoma, primary cutaneous follicle center lymphoma, aggressive NK-cell leukemia, angioimmunoblastic T-cell lymphoma, peripheral T-cell lymphoma [unspecified], hepatosplenic T-cell lymphoma, T-cell lymphoma, nasal type, adult T-cell leukemia/lymphoma, anaplastic large cell lymphoma, ALK positive or negative, enteropathy-associated intestinal T-cell lymphoma, subcutaneous panniculitis-like T-cell lymphoma, primary cutaneous gamma-delta T-cell lymphoma, primary cutaneous CD30+ T-cell lymphoproliferative disease, lymphomatoid papulosis, and primary cutaneous anaplastic large cell lymphoma) and space constraints, these entities will not be included. The reader is referred to the WHO classification manual, or specialty hematopathology textbooks.

- The following types of non-Hodgkin lymphoma and diagnostic approaches are described in subsequent sections:
  - Diffuse large cell (see p. 850)
  - Follicular (see p. 851)
  - Mantle zone (see p. 851)
  - Marginal zone (see p. 853)
  - Burkitt (see p. 848)
  - Cutaneous (see p. 849)
  - Lymphoplasmacytic (see p. 855)
  - Posttransplantation (see p. 854)

➤ Common Laboratory Findings (type-specific findings will be presented with each lymphoma chapter)

- Abnormalities of humoral immunity: hypogammaglobulinemia and occasionally monoclonal gammopathies
- Autoimmune hemolytic anemia and/or thrombocytopenia
- Laboratory findings due to involvement of other organs (CNS, liver, kidneys, GI tract, testes)
- Laboratory and clinical findings related to therapy:
  - Cytopenias
  - Peripheral neuropathies
  - As the result of infections
  - Gonadal dysfunction
- History of AIDS

➤ Suggested Readings

Jaffe ES, Harris LN, Stein H, Isaacson PG. Classification of lymphoid neoplasms: the microscope as a tool for disease discovery. *Blood.* 2008;112:4384–4399.

Swedlow SH, Campo E, Harris NL, et al. *WHO Classification of Tumours of Haematopoietic and Lymphoid Tissues* 4th ed. Lyon, France: International Agency for Research on Cancer; 2008:158–166.

BURKITT LYMPHOMA (BL)

➤ Definition

- BL is a highly aggressive, extranodal non-Hodgkin lymphoma with distinctive morphologic, genetic, and cytogenetic alterations related to c-myc proto-oncogene overexpression. BL may include a leukemic, ALL-like phase.
- There are three distinctive forms of BL: endemic (in Equatorial Africa), sporadic (in Western countries), and associated with immunodeficiency.

➤ Who Should be Suspected?

1. For the endemic form: children with jaw or facial bones tumors. Nearly all endemic cases are associated with EBV infection.
2. In nonendemic areas tumors of nonhematopoietic organs prevail. The peak incidence is in the second and third decades. BL has a propensity to invade bone marrow and CNS.
3. BL may develop in patients infected by the HIV. In addition to BL, other AIDS-associated lymphomas (see AIDS p. 1008) are diffuse large B-cell lymphoma (see p. 850) with immuno-

blastic-plasmacytoid differentiation, primary effusion lymphoma, and its solid variants that occur specifically in HIV-positive patients.

➤ Tests
- For diagnosis, a biopsy with studies of morphologic, genetic, and cytogenetic analysis, and immunophenotyping is necessary.
  - Immunohistochemistry. CD 10, 19, 20, 22, 38, 43, and 79a, are positive; monotypic sIgM+; CD5 and TDT are negative. Bcl-2 is usually negative. Proliferation fraction by Ki-67 is nearly 100%.
  - Cytogenetics. Translocation *(8:14) (q24;q32)* is found in 80% of cases; in the rest, *t(8:22) (q24;q11)* or *t(2;8)(p11;q24)*. Because these translocations involve the MYC gene at 8q24 they can be rapidly detected by FISH.
  - Genetic studies. C-MYC dysregulation with Bcl-6+ is the key element in BL pathogenesis. Gene profile studies help differentiate atypical BL from diffuse large cell lymphoma, but no uniform criteria have yet been established.

➤ Suggested Readings
Carbone A, Cesarman E, Spina M, et al. HIV-associated lymphomas and gamma-herpesviruses. *Blood.* 2009;113:1213–1224.
Leoncini L, Raphael M, Stein H, et al. Burkitt lymphoma. *WHO Classification of Tumours of Haematopoietic and Lymphoid Tissues.* 4th ed. Lyon, France: International Agency for Research on Cancer; 2008:262–264.

LYMPHOMA, CUTANEOUS T-CELL (CTCL): MYCOSIS FUNGOIDES (MF) AND SÉZARY SYNDROME (SS)

➤ Definition
- CTCL are tumors of the CD4+ helper T cells. MF is the most common; it is an indolent, extranodal non-Hodgkin lymphoma.
- SS is a leukemic variant of CTCL in which typical malignant cells and Sézary cells circulate in the peripheral blood, but can be found also in skin and lymph nodes.

➤ Who Should be Suspected?
- An elderly patient with pruritic patches, plaques, or subcutaneous tumors (MF).
- An elderly patient with a high number of atypical (cerebriform) blood lymphocytes; cutaneous (erythroderma) and extracutaneous infiltrates, with marked lymphadenopathy (SS).

➤ Tests
- Diagnosis is established by the typical morphology of skin biopsy for MF and SS, as well as by the study of peripheral blood for SS. Bone marrow and liver biopsies are usually normal.
  - CBC is normal in MF. Total WBC count is often increased in SS. More than 1000/μL are atypical lymphocytes, easily identifiable, are usually present.
  - ESR, Hb, and platelet counts are usually normal in both conditions.
  - Immunophenotyping may be technically difficult. In MF the cells are positive for CD2, CD3, CD5, and CD4, but, in most cases, negative for CD8. Alterations in the expression of T-cell antigens are commonly seen, with loss of expression of CD7 being the most common. Immunophenotyping helps to distinguish CTCL from reactive or inflammatory lymphoid infiltrates in the skin, which usually express all mature T-cell antigens. An epidermal/

dermal discordance for CD2, CD3, CD5, and CD7 suggests the diagnosis of CTCL. In SS, the neoplastic lymphocytes are markedly expanded in the peripheral blood with a CD4/CD8 ratio of >10.
* Genetic studies. T-cell receptor gene rearrangement may help establish the diagnosis of MF when the skin biopsy and immunophenotyping results are ambiguous.
* Cytogenetics. The tumor cells have complex karyotypes in many patients.

➤ Suggested Reading

Hoppe RT, Kim YH. Clinical features, diagnosis, and staging of mycosis fungoides and Sézary syndrome. UpTodate. Rose B, ed. Waltham, MA: UpTodate, Inc.; 2008.

LYMPHOMA, DIFFUSE, LARGE B-CELL

➤ Definition

* Diffuse large B-cell lymphoma (DLBCL) is an aggressive neoplasm of large B cells, with nuclear size more than twice the size of a normal lymphocyte. It constitutes 20–40% of adult non-Hodgkin lymphomas in Western countries.
* DLBCL is characterized by clinical, morphological, cytogenetic, and molecular heterogeneity. Gene expression profiling has identified three distinct molecular subgroups: germinal center B-cell like, activated B-cell like, and primary mediastinal B-cell lymphoma. They have different survivals and respond differently to therapy.

➤ Who Should be Suspected?

* Patients in their 60s who present with rapidly enlarging lymphadenopathy and/or with tumors at extranodal sites, the most common being the GI tract.
* The bone marrow may also be involved, and in many of these cases lymphoma cells may be detected in the peripheral blood.

➤ Tests

* Diagnosis is best established by biopsy of an enlarged lymph node or another affected organ. The morphologic pattern and immunophenotype establish the diagnosis and its variants. Increasingly, genomic studies offer better differentiation and prognostication.
  * Immunophenotype can be determined by flow cytometry or immunochemistry of the biopsied tissue. In most cases the tumor cells are positive for the B-cell markers CD19, CD20, CD22, CD79a, as well as CD45. Monoclonal cell surface membrane IgM is usually positive. Occasionally, DLBCL cells may be CD5 or CD10 positive.
  * Cytogenetics. There are no karyotypic abnormalities specific for DLBCL. Up to 30% of cases show rearrangement of 3q27, involving the BCL6 gene; 30% carry a t(14;18) (q32;q21) causing a *BCL2-IGH* rearrangement, more typically found in follicular lymphomas and ~10% carry a *cMYC* rearrangement.
  * Elevated serum LDH indicates aggressive disease.

➤ Suggested Readings

Freedman AS. Clinical manifestations, pathologic features, and diagnosis of diffuse large B cell lymphoma. UpToDate. Rose B, ed. Waltham, MA: UpTodate, Inc.; 2008.

Stein H, Warnke, RA, Chan WC, et al. Diffuse large B-cell lymphoma, not otherwise specified. *WHO Classification of Tumours of Hematopoietic and Lymphomatous tissues.* 4th ed. Lyon, France: International Agency for Research on Cancer; 2008:233–237.

LYMPHOMA, FOLLICULAR (FL)

➤ Definition
- FL is defined primarily by its morphologic pattern, and by the translocation t(14;18), that leads to deregulated expression of the antiapoptotic BCL-2 protooncogene.
- FL is the second most common lymphoma in the United States and Western Europe after DLBCL.
- It is considered an indolent lymphoma, but most cases eventually transform into aggressive lymphoma, usually DLBCL (see p. 850). Its clinical course is variable. The prognosis can be determined by the criteria known as The Follicular Lymphoma International Prognostic Index (FLIPI).

➤ Who Should be Suspected?
Patients in their 50s or 60s, complaining of generalized, progressive lymphadenopathy and splenomegaly, but otherwise asymptomatic, despite the high incidence of bone marrow involvement and generalized disease.

➤ Tests
- The primary diagnosis is established by biopsy of an involved lymph node. According to the number of centroblasts present in the neoplastic infiltrate, FL is subdivided into grades 1 to 3A that constitute a biologic continuum. Grade 3B is composed of blasts exclusively and is usually negative for t(14;18).
- Bone marrow biopsy and peripheral blood. Whenever the bone marrow is involved paratrabecular lymphoid aggregates are seen. With leukemic involvement of the peripheral blood, notched or clefted lymphocytes are identified.
- Immunophenotype. FL cells (obtained from lymph node, bone marrow biopsy, or peripheral blood), are positive for CD 19, CD20, CD22, and CD79a. In most cases, the cells are also CD10 positive. Some cases especially in grade 3 (advanced) disease may lack CD10 expression. The cells also express BCL-2 and BCL-6, and lack expression of CD5 and CD43. Immunoglobulins heavy and light chains are rearranged. About half of the affected express IgM and 40% IgG.
- Cytogenetics. The t(14;18) (q32;q21) is present in 90% of cases. This is not a specific finding, since 30% of DLBCL are also positive for these alterations. Moreover, it was found that a majority of healthy persons have this translocation among their circulating lymphocytes, without any evidence of FL. FISH analysis detects deletions at 3q.14 in 27% of patients.
- Hb below 12 g/dL is associated with advanced disease.
- Serum LDH is usually normal, but a high LDH connotes a poor prognosis.

➤ Suggested Readings
Harris NL, Swerdlow SH, Jaffe ES, et al. Follicular lymphoma. *WHO Classification of Tumours of Haematopoietic and Lymphoid Tissues.* 4th ed. Lyon, France: International Agency for Research on Cancer; 2008:220–226.
Solai-Celigny P, Roy P, Colombat P, et al. Follicular lymphoma international prognostic index. *Blood.* 2004;104:1258–1265.

LYMPHOMA, MANTLE CELL (MCL)

➤ Definition
- MCL is a moderately aggressive lymphoma, composed of small to medium-sized lymphoid cells with irregular nuclear contours.

- It accounts for 3–6% of non-Hodgkin lymphomas.
- The t(11;14)(q13;q32) is universally present. The translocation determines the ectopic and deregulated expression of Cyclin D1, which is considered the primary molecular event in the pathogenesis of MCL. The MCL affected cells are usually positive for CD5, creating difficulties in the differentiation from CLL/SLL (see p. 829).

➤ Who Should be Suspected?

- Elderly male patients with generalized nonbulky lymphadenopathy, possibly hepatosplenomegaly, lymphocytosis, bone marrow invasion, multiple lymphomatous polyposis of the intestine, and constitutional symptoms.

➤ Tests

- Laboratory diagnosis of MCL is based mainly on lymph node morphology, flow cytometry, and cytogenetics.
- CBC: anemia and thrombocytopenia are commensurate with the clinical stage, the degree of bone marrow infiltration, or may reflect chemotherapy. Increasing lymphocyte count denotes a poor prognosis.
- Lymph node biopsy shows lymphoid proliferation with vaguely nodular, diffuse, or mantle zone pattern. Lymphocytes are homogenous, small to medium in size with irregular or "cleaved" nuclei, and inconspicuous nucleoli.
- Immunophenotype. Cells express intense surface IgM/IgD and light chain (lambda more frequently than kappa). The cells are positive for CD5, CD19, bright CD20, CD22, CD79a, FMC-7, and CD43. They are negative for CD10, BCL6, and in contrast to CLL/SLL, CD23 is negative or weakly positive. All cases are BCL2 positive, and expression of cyclin D1 (as detected by immunohistochemistry) is almost universal. Some variability exists in antigen expression. Presence of a high proportion of cells positive for Ki-67 denotes a poor prognosis. The Ki-67 proliferation index seems the most powerful predictor of survival in MCL.
- Genetics. Gene expression analysis profiles identified a cohort of 20 "proliferation signature" genes that predict length of patient survival. The technology is not yet applicable in daily practice.
- Cytogenetics. The t(11q;14)(q13;q32) is present in almost all cases of MCL.
- LDH elevation is associated with poor prognosis.

➤ Transformation

- Transformation is characterized morphologically by increase in cell size (blastic variant), frequent mitoses, and an aggressive clinical course.
- Morphologic differentiation from acute lymphocytic leukemia may be difficult.

➤ Suggested Readings

Ghielmini M, Zucca E. How I treat mantle cell lymphoma. *Blood*. 2009;114:1469–1476.

Hoster E, Dreyling M, Klapper W, et al. A new prognostic index (MIPI) for patients with advanced-stage mantle cell lymphoma. *Blood*. 2008;111:558–565.

Perez-Galan P, Dreyling M, Wiestner A. Mantle cell lymphoma: biology, pathogenesis, and the molecular basis of treatment in the genomic era. *Blood*. 2011;117:26–38.

Swerdlow SH, Campo E, Seto M, Muller-Hermelink HK. Mantle cell lymphoma. *WHO Classification of Tumours of Haematopoietic and Lymphoid Tissues*. 4th ed. Lyon, France: International Agency for Research on Cancer; 2008:230–232.

LYMPHOMAS, MARGINAL ZONE (MZL)

➤ Definition

- According to the WHO 2008 classification of lymphomas, MZL includes three distinct B-cell lymphomas: splenic MZL ($\pm$ villous lymphocytes); extranodal MZL of mucosa associated lymphoid tissue (MALT); and nodal MZL. These three lymphoma subtypes are clinically distinct.
- The first two types will be presented in this section.
  A. Splenic marginal B-cell lymphoma is an indolent lymphoma composed of small lymphocytes that surround and replace the splenic white pulp germinal centers. The condition may be associated with villous lymphocytes in the peripheral blood. Splenic hilar lymph nodes and the bone marrow are often involved.
  B. MZL originating at mucosal sites (MALT lymphoma) is a low-grade lymphoma originating in sites normally devoid of lymphoid tissues, such as glandular epithelium, and it is often preceded by chronic inflammation of the affected site or is associated with autoimmune diseases such as Sjögren syndrome and Hashimoto thyroiditis. Whereas most cases present with gastric involvement, other GI tract organs of bronchial epithelium may be involved. Bacterial infection with *Helicobacter pylori* is associated with 92% of gastric MALT lymphomas. The GI tract (salivary glands, small bowel, and stomach) are the most common site of presentation. Usually MALT presents as a localized disease.

➤ Who Should be Suspected?

- Splenic marginal B-cell lymphoma: Elderly patients with abdominal discomfort due to splenomegaly, lymphocytosis, and cytopenias. Peripheral lymphadenopathy and involvement of extralymphatic organs—except bone marrow—are uncommon.
- MZL originating at mucosal sites (MALT lymphoma): a patient with GI symptoms not otherwise diagnosed, or with demonstrated *H. pylori* infection of the stomach and a gastric lesion. The majority of patients present with stage I or II disease.

➤ Tests
Splenic Marginal B-cell Lymphoma

- CBC. Anemia, thrombocytopenia (both may have an autoimmune etiology) and neutropenia are commonly present; lymphocytosis is frequently present, but not essential for diagnosis. The lymphocytes have a round nucleus, condensed chromatin, and abundant basophilic cytoplasm with small surface "villous" projections.
- PTT may be prolonged due to an acquired inhibitor, such as the lupus anticoagulant.
- Bone marrow or lymph node biopsy is indicated in the absence of diagnostic peripheral blood findings or available spleen histology.
- Immunophenotype. The neoplastic lymphocytes express surface immunoglobulins (IgM or IgD +), B-cell antigens (CD19, CD20, CD22, CD79a) and bcl-2. Unlike CLL/SLL they are CD5 negative. They are CD10, CD43, CD23, CD25, and CD103 negative. In contrast with mantle cell lymphoma, cyclin D1 is negative. Negative CD10 and BCL6 help exclude follicular lymphoma.
- Cytogenetics and genetics. No characteristic genetic abnormalities have been identified, but in the majority of the patients an abnormal karyotypes is found with complex chromosomal changes. The most common aberrations are gains of 3q and deletion of 7q22-36. The presence

of 7q31 deletion connotes an aggressive clinical course. A gene expression profile, different from other B-cell lymphomas, has been described.

MZL Originating at Mucosal Sites (MALT Lymphoma)

* For patients presenting with gastric MALT lymphoma the diagnosis is established by endoscopic biopsy
* Microbiology. Studies for *H. pylori* are positive for gastric MALT lymphoma, but other microbes have been implicated in the pathogenesis of other MZL.
* Cytogenetics. Detection of t(11;18) (q21;q21) by FISH suggests widely disseminated disease.

➤ Unfavorable Prognostic Laboratory Findings

* Splenic marginal B-cell lymphoma: Hb <12 g/dL; elevated serum LDH; serum albumin <3.5 g/dL; unmutated immunoglobulin heavy genes

➤ Transformation

* Splenic MZL has the potential to transform into a high-grade lymphoma.

➤ Suggested Readings

Arcaini L, Lazzarino M, Colombo N, et al. Splenic marginal zone lymphoma: a prognostic model for clinical use. *Blood.* 2006;107:4643–4649.

Isaacson PG, Piris MA, Berger F, et al. Splenic marginal zone lymphoma. *WHO Classification of Tumours of Haematopoietic and Lymphoid tissues.* 4th ed. Lyon, France: International Agency for Research on Cancer; 2008:185–187.

LYMPHOPROLIFERATIVE DISORDER, POST TRANSPLANT (PTLD)

➤ Definition

* Lymphoma is the most common malignancy after stem cell or solid organ transplantation. PTLD comprises a spectrum of lymphomas classified by the WHO as early lesions, polymorphic PTLD, monomorphic PTLD (classified according to B/T cell lymphomas they resemble), and classic Hodgkin lymphoma-like PTLD.
* >90% of early cases (<1 year after transplantation) are EBV positive. Later cases (>2 years post transplantation) are less often associated with EBV positivity, and their etiology is uncertain.

➤ Who Should be Suspected?

* Post-transplant patients who present with fever, generalized lymphadenopathy, hepatosplenomegaly, and no documented infection. The GI tract, lungs, and liver may also be involved, occasionally as single organs.
* The incidence of PTLD correlates with the intensity of immunosuppression. It is seen sometimes following unrelated allogeneic stem cell transplantation or umbilical cord blood transplants after intensive immunosuppression.

➤ Tests

* Peripheral blood may show very atypical plasmacytic lymphocytes.
* Lymph node biopsy or fine needle aspiration is essential for diagnosis and classification. It reveals atypical plasmacytoid lymphoid cells.
* Bone marrow biopsy should be done if no other tissue source is easily obtained.

- Flow cytometry of lymph nodes or bone marrow biopsy reveals κ/λ ratio of 5:1.
- EBV clonality and load helps define the etiology.

➤ Suggested Reading

Swerdlow SH, Webber SA, Chadburn A, Ferry JA. Post-transplant lymphoproliferative disorders. *WHO Classification of Tumours of Haematopoietic and Lymphoid Tissues.* 4th ed. Lyon, France: International Agency for Research on Cancer; 2008:343–349.

LYMPHOPLASMACYTIC LYMPHOMA (LPL)/ WALDENSTROM MACROGLOBULINEMIA (WM)

➤ Definition

- A B-cell lymphoma resulting from the accumulation, predominantly in the bone marrow, of clonally related lymphoplasmacytic cells that secrete a monoclonal IgM protein, resulting in elevated serum IgM paraprotein. Most cases of LPL are IgM associated, hence bona fide WM. Less than 5% of cases of LPL are made up of IgA, IgG, and nonsecreting LPL cells, hence falling outside the classical denomination of WM.
- Clinically, WM can be distinguished from lymphoplasmacytic lymphoma (LPL) on the basis of symptoms of hyperviscosity. Moreover, based on clinical definitions, WM can be observed in other types of lymphomas. However, there seems no rationale for separating these entities. We will use the terms interchangeably, as LPL/WM.
- The term LPL/WM should be reserved for a distinct neoplasm of small lymphoid cells that are CD5−, CD10−, CD23−, and have a pan-B-cell marker positive phenotype. There is variable involvement of bone marrow, lymph nodes, and spleen. Monoclonal gammopathy of undetermined significance (MGUS) of IgM class (defined as <10% marrow infiltration and <30g/L of serum monoclonal IgM) has been associated with an increased risk of developing LPL/WM.

➤ Who Should be Suspected?

- Patients with lymphadenopathy, hepatosplenomegaly, nose and gum bleeding, and constitutional symptoms (weakness, fatigue, weight loss, fever, night sweats, recurrent infections—especially pneumonias with pleural effusion), and symptoms characteristic of the hyperviscosity syndrome (blurring or loss of vision, headache, vertigo, nystagmus, dizziness, diplopia, ataxia) and peripheral neuropathy.
- Patients with type I or II cryoglobulinemia (see p. 866) and cold agglutinin hemolytic anemia (see p. 809) should also be investigated for LPL/WM.

➤ Tests

- **CBC**
  - Red cells: moderate to severe normochromic, normocytic anemia with rouleaux formation on the PBS. The anemia is multifactorial, to a large extent being the result of red cell dilution by increased plasma volume. Autoimmune hemolytic anemia may develop on the basis of cold or warm antibodies.
  - WBC: lymphocytosis or monocytosis are common. Occasionally leukopenia is present.
  - Platelets: thrombocytopenia may be present, occasionally immune in etiology. Platelet function is impaired secondary to coating of the platelets surface receptors by IgM

paraproteins, resulting in impaired platelet adhesiveness (no specific assay for platelet adhesiveness is available). Platelet aggregation may show a thrombocytopathy.

- **Immunoglobulins**
- Serum protein electrophoresis, a key assay in the diagnosis of LPL/WM, reveals a homogenous spike (M component), almost always of γ mobility.
- Total serum protein and globulin are markedly increased.
- Quantitation of immunoglobulins reveals increased IgM (>30 g/L in most cases, but no specific cut-off is required for the diagnosis). There can be great heterogeneity among patients between their respective serum IgM levels and bone marrow involvement. There is reciprocal decrease of IgG and of IgA. Serial quantitation of serum IgM is used to monitor effect of therapy or disease progression.
- Immunofixation is a more definitive diagnostic assay because it identifies the M spike as a monoclonal IgM protein.
- Serum light chains: a preponderance of κ or λ light chains, with a reported 4.5:1 incidence ratio. Serum free light chain determination could be used as a surrogate tumor marker.
- A serum monoclonal IgM is not pathognomonic for WM. It may be seen in rare cases of multiple myeloma (WM can be excluded if such patients have osteolytic lesions) and splenic marginal zone lymphoma (see p. 853). In asymptomatic patients, a diagnosis of smoldering LPL/WM may be entertained. If the bone marrow is infiltrated with <10% clonal cells and the patient is asymptomatic, the diagnosis of IgM-MGUS should be considered.
- Serum viscosity: Clinical symptoms of hyperviscosity begin when serum viscosity is >4 centipoise. At a viscosity of >6 centipoise the symptoms become more severe. The frequency of hyperviscosity ranges from 6–20% of cases. There may be great variability in the serum viscosity level at which patients become symptomatic.
- Bone marrow biopsy: it has been proposed that the diagnosis of LPL/WM should be based on bone marrow involvement by the disease. Bone marrow aspirate appears often to be hypocellular. The biopsy specimen, however, demonstrates hypercellularity with ≥10% infiltration by small lymphocytic and plasmacytoid or plasma cells. The pattern of infiltration is usually nodular, (interstitial or paratrabecular), mixed, or diffuse. The abnormal cells have a nuclear spoke-wheel pattern of plasma cells, but have high nuclear/cytoplasmic ratio more typical of small lymphocytes. Nevertheless, typical plasma cells with Russell and Dutcher bodies may be seen. Mast cells are frequently increased.
- Lymph node biopsy shows lymphoplasmacytic infiltration, but the normal architecture is preserved. Distinguishing LPL/WM from other B-cell lymphomas, especially marginal zone B-cell lymphoma, may be difficult.
- Histologic transformation: LPL can transform in a more aggressive form of lymphoma, similar to Richter's transformation in CLL (see p. 829). Transformation can be demonstrated by lymph node or bone marrow biopsy. It connotes an aggressive clinical picture resistant to therapy. Occasionally the disease may evolve into AL amyloidosis (see p. 865).
- CNS infiltration with plasma cells and lymphocytes (the Bing-Neel syndrome) has been described. Peripheral neuropathy is seen in up to 20–25% of patients. The evaluation of anti-myelin-associated glycoprotein antiganglioside MI, and anti-sulfatide IgM antibodies may be appropriate.
- Flow cytometry demonstrates earlier stage of B-cell differentiation than the plasma cells of multiple myeloma. The clonal cells are surface IgM+, CD19+, CD20+, CD22+, CD25+, CD27+, CD38+, CD79a+, FMC7+, BCL2+, PAX5+; CD3−, CD103−,

CD138−. There may be some variability in immunophenotypic findings. Up to 20% of patients may express CD5, CD10, or CD23.
- Cytogenetics. Chromosome abnormalities are common, but not specific for the condition. The most common reported recurrent abnormalities is 6q deletion (encompassing 6q21-25). Also reported are trisomy 4, 5, and monosomy 8. Translocation (9;14) is rare according to some investigators, but it may be present in near 50% of patients, according to others. Cytogenetic examination may be useful in differentiating LPL/WM from IgM myeloma.
- Blood coagulation: thrombin time is prolonged due to inhibition of fibrin polymerization by the paraprotein (impaired coagulation may play a role in the bleeding diathesis).
- Serum β-2 microglobulin is elevated in half the patients.
- Sedimentation rate and C-reactive protein may be very elevated.
- LDH and alkaline phosphatase when elevated correlate with an unfavorable course.
- Hyperuricemia and hypercalcemia have been reported.
- Azotemia may be present on the basis of light chain or amyloid depositions, as well as parenchymal renal involvement by lymphoplasmacytic cells.
- Tests no longer recommended
  - Immunoelectrophoresis (replaced by immunofixation).
  - BJ protein may be replaced in the future by measuring serum light chains (its role remains to be validated) because the amount of IgM excreted in urine may be below detection level and does not correlate well with tumor burden. In addition, obtaining serum light chain analysis obviates the need to collect 24-hour urine.

➤ Limitations
- Spurious results: the high-level IgM may interfere with automated analyzer results, especially producing an artificially low HDL cholesterol or falsely elevated Hb.
- Serum IgM may occasionally be artifactually low because of polymerization of IgM. A warm bath collection should be obtained for blood specimens in patients suspected of having cryoglobulinemia to avoid underestimation of serum IgM.
- Difficulty in cross-matching blood may be encountered.

➤ Suggested Readings
Lin P, Medeiros LJ. Lymphoplasmacytic lymphoma/Waldenstrom macroglobulinemia. *Adv Anat Pathol.* 2005;12: 246–255.
Vijay A, Gertz MA. Waldenstrom macroglobulinemia. *Blood.* 2007;109:5096–5103.
Vitolo U, Ferreri AJM, Montoto S. Lymphoplasmacytic lymphoma-Waldenstrom's macroglobulinemia. *Clinical Rev Oncol Hematol.* 2008;67:172–185.

HODGKIN LYMPHOMA (HL)

➤ Definition
- HL, formerly called Hodgkin's disease, is a neoplasm of transformed B-lymphocytes, characterized morphologically by the presence of Hodgkin cells or Reed-Sternberg cells in biopsies.
- HL is comprised of two disease entities: nodular lymphocyte predominant HL (NLPHL) and classical HL (cHL). Within cHL, four subtypes have been distinguished with distinct morphology and prognosis: nodular sclerosis (NSHL), mixed cellularity (MCHL), lymphocyte-rich (LRHL), and lymphocyte-depleted (LDHL).
- The Ann Arbor modified staging classification is used to determine prognosis and therapy.

➤ Who Should be Suspected?

* Commonly, but not exclusively, a young adult with indolent lymphadenopathy in the cervical or other areas. Occasionally the patient may present with B symptoms (fever, night sweats, weight loss, and pruritus).

➤ Tests

* The diagnosis of HL is based on tissue biopsy of an involved lymph node, primarily on its morphology.
* Bone marrow biopsy is positive for malignant cells in up to 6.5% of advanced cases. It affects therapy only marginally, and in most cases it is not needed.
* CBC
  * Normochromic, normocytic anemia in advanced cases. Anemia or leukopenia at presentation denote a poor prognosis. Eosinophilia occurs in ≈20% of patients. Lymphopenia or monocytosis may also occur.
  * Platelets may be decreased (in some cases immune thrombocytopenia is present) or increased.
* Elevated ESR, elevated LDH, and low serum albumin are associated with advanced disease.
* Liver function tests may be abnormal.
* Serum calcium may be elevated due to bony involvement or overproduction of calcitriol.
* Genomic analysis detects EBV positivity in 40% of LRHL, 70% of MCHL, and nearly 100% of LDHL, but not in NSHL or NLPHL. Activation of NF-κB pathway is a central event in HL pathogenesis.
* Immunophenotype. The neoplastic cells in *cHL* express CD15 and CD30, but lack pan B- and pan T-antigens. The expression of CD20 and epithelial membrane antigen (EMA) is mostly negative. By contrast, in NLPHL the neoplastic cells stain positively for CD 19, 20, 22, 79a, 45, and EMA. They lack CD15 and 30.
* Cytogenetics. There are no typical cytogenetic abnormalities. The majority of cases of classical HL do have clonal cytogenetic abnormalities, but they differ from case to case. Many show 14q abnormalities. It has recently been shown that gains involving the chromosome 16p11.2-13.3 have been associated with a poor prognosis and treatment failure.
* Microbiology. HIV infection may accompany LDHL.

➤ Suggested Readings

Armitage JO. Early-stage Hodgkin's Lymphoma. *New Engl J Medicine.* 2010;363:653–662.

Mauch PM. Initial evaluation and diagnosis of Hodgkin lymphoma in adults. UpToDate. Rose B, ed. Waltham, MA: UpToDate Inc.; 2008.

MONOCLONAL GAMMOPATHIES

* This section describes disorders of plasma cells and of plasma proteins. These neoplasms result from the expansion of a clone of Ig-secreting, terminally differentiated B lymphocytes. These neoplasms are known as monoclonal gammopathies because they express monoclonal products of homogenous immunoglobulins (or fragments) produced by the neoplastic abnormal B cells. The monoclonal proteins may be present in serum, urine, and CSF.
* The section will follow the 4th edition of the *WHO Classification of Tumours of Haematopoietic and Lymphoid Tissues.* It includes plasma cell myeloma, plasmacytoma, the benign precursor

monoclonal gammopathy of undetermined significance (MGUS), and the syndromes defined by the consequence of tissue immunoglobulin deposition, primary amyloidosis (AL) and light and heavy chain deposition disease. Lymphoplasmacytic lymphoma (see p. 85) and the heavy chain diseases (see p. 863) are described separately.

➤ Suggested Reading

Swerdlow SH, Campo E, Harris NL, et al. *WHO Classification of Tumours of Haematopoietic and Lymphoid Tissues.* 4th ed. Lyon, France: International Agency for Research on Cancer; 2008:200–213.

PLASMA CELL MYELOMA*

➤ Definition

- Plasma cell myeloma (formerly multiple myeloma) is a B-cell neoplasm consisting of neoplastic proliferation of plasma cells primarily occurring in the bone marrow. The current WHO classification stratifies this disorder into two distinct categories based on specific criteria: (1) symptomatic plasma cell myeloma and (2) asymptomatic (smoldering) myeloma (see below).
- Clinically, plasma cell myeloma is manifested by osteolytic lesions, renal failure, hypercalcemia, anemia, hyperviscosity, and serum/urine M (monoclonal) protein.

➤ Who Should be Suspected?

- Middle-aged patients in their 60s who present with anemia, bone pain, unexplained fractures, frequent infections, bleeding, symptoms of hypercalcemia (excessive thirst and urination, constipation, nausea, loss of appetite and mental confusion), and neurologic symptoms arising from compression fractures of vertebrae.
- There is a wide clinical spectrum ranging from an asymptomatic state to aggressive forms and disorders due to deposition of immunoglobulin chains in tissues.

➤ Tests

- The diagnosis is based on established criteria (WHO) for plasma cell myeloma:
  - Symptomatic plasma cell myeloma
    - M protein in serum or urine: >30 g/L IgG, or >20 g/L IgA, or >1 g/24 hour urine light chain; some patients with symptomatic myeloma may have lower levels.
    - Bone marrow clonal plasma cells (usually >10% of nucleated cells) or plasmacytoma(s).
    - Related organ or tissue impairment (hypercalcemia, renal insufficiency, anemia, bone lesions, amyloidosis, hyperviscosity or recurrent infections).
  - Asymptomatic (smoldering) myeloma: patients progress into symptomatic myeloma or amyloidosis at a rate of 10% per year in the first 5 years.
    - M protein in serum or urine (>30 g/L IgG, >20 g/L IgA, or >1g/24 hour or urine light chain)
    and/or
    - 10% or more clonal plasma cells in bone marrow
    - No related organ or tissue impairment

---

*Written with Madhu Mennon, M.D., Ph.D.

- Laboratory diagnosis is essential for diagnosis and prognosis upfront, and for determining the presence of a complete remission (CR) following therapy. The current definition of CR is based on serologic and cytologic results, rather than molecular studies.
- Bone marrow biopsy and aspirate. Aspirate and biopsy are recommended for identification and quantitation of plasma cells morphologically and by immunophenotype ($CD138^+$). Plasma cells are seen in sheets or abnormal clusters. Plasmablastic morphology with characteristic cells is present.
- CBC. Normochromic, normocytic anemia with or without leukopenia, thrombocytopenia, and presence of normoblasts in cases with extensive marrow replacement. Rouleaux formation (due to paraproteinemia) is present on PBS.
- Serum protein is markedly elevated with increased globulins (decreased A/G ratio) (50–75% of patients) and hypoalbuminemia. Decrease in polyclonal gamma globulins
- Hypogammaglobulinemia in light chain myelomas that produce only light chains.
- Serum protein electrophoresis (see p. 332) and immunofixation (see p. 332) reveal a monoclonal protein (κ or λ) and identify a specific heavy chain (IgG 50%, IgA 20%, light chain 20%, IgD, IgE, IgM, and biclonal in <10% of cases).
- Urine protein electrophoresis and immunofixation reveal M protein (BJ protein) reflecting urine light chain. With extensive renal damage, albumin and whole immunoglobulin molecules can be found in urine.
- Serum free light chain immunoassay (see p. 219). Normal $\kappa:/\lambda$ is 0.26 to 1.65. The ratio is altered in nonsecretory myeloma, oligosecretory myeloma, and light chain myeloma. This assay is useful for diagnosis, monitoring during and after treatment, and perhaps prognosis of patients with multiple myeloma and an intact immunoglobulin.
- Cold agglutinins or cryoglobulins (see p. 142) may be present.
- Serum calcium (see p. 82) may be elevated due to osteolytic lesions.
- Hypercalciuria results from dehydration and renal tubular dysfunction.
- Serum uric acid (see p. 369) is elevated in 50% of cases.
- ESR (see p. 162) is usually (90% cases) greatly elevated.
- Serum β2 microglobulin (see p. 69) can be elevated. A level >6 µg/mL portends poor prognosis.
- Renal function tests may be abnormal in the presence of monoclonal light chain proteinuria.
- Immunophenotype. The neoplastic plasma cells classically are $CD138^+$, $CD38^{high}$, $CD19^-$, $CD56^+$ (60–80%), $CD79a^{+,}$ and express monotypic cytoplasmic κ or λ. In addition, plasma cells may also aberrantly express CD117, CD20, CD52, CD10, and occasionally myeloid and monocytic antigens. Cyclin D1 expression may be seen in cases with t(11,14) translocation.
- Cytogenetics. Genetic abnormalities can be detected by conventional cytogenetics in 30% of cases and by FISH in >90% cases. Structural abnormalities include t(11,14) (15–18%), t(14,16) (5%), t(4,14) (15%), t(6,14) (3%), and t(14,20) (2%), all of which involve the IG heavy chain locus on chromosome 14q32. Numerical abnormalities involve hyperdiploidy of odd chromosomes 3, 5, 7, 9, 11, 15, 19, and 21. Monosomy or partial 13 deletion, K or NRAS mutations (30–40%), FGFR3 mutation, TP53 (17p13) deletion, MYC translocation, and inactivation of RB1 or $p18^{INK4c}$ represent progression of disease.
- Microbiology: Repeated bacterial infections caused by *Diplococcus pneumoniae, Staphylococcus aureus,* and *Escherichia coli.*
- Test no longer recommended: serum immunoelectrophoresis

➤ Suggested Readings

Harousseau JL, Attal M, Avet-Louiseau H. The role of complete response in multiple myeloma. *Blood* . 2009;114:3139–3146.

Kyle RA, Rajkumar SV. Multiple myeloma. *Blood*. 2008;111:2962–2972.

McPherson RA, Pincus MR. *Henry's Clinical Diagnosis and Management by Laboratory Methods.* 21st ed. Saunders Elsevier; 2007:576.

Swerdlow SH, Campo E, Harris NL, et al. *WHO Classification of Tumours of Haematopoietic and Lymphoid Tissues.* 4th ed. Lyon, France: International Agency for Research on Cancer; 2008:202–208.

MONOCLONAL GAMMOPATHY OF UNDETERMINED SIGNIFICANCE (MGUS)*

➤ Definition

- MGUS is a pre-neoplastic condition characterized by the presence in serum of:
  - M-protein <30 g/L
  - Bone marrow clonal plasma cells <10%
  - No end-organ damage
  - No clinical manifestations or evidence of another B-cell proliferative disorder
- The few neoplastic plasma cells are usually present in the bone marrow; however, IgM-producing cells may be seen originating in spleen and lymph nodes. The risk of progression to an overt plasma cell myeloma, amyloidosis (see p. 865), lymphoplasmacytic lymphoma (see p. 855), or other lymphoproliferative disorder is 1% per year.

➤ Who Should be Suspected?

- MGUS is more common in men (1.5:1) and African American subjects; its incidence is 3% in those older than 50 years and 5% in those older than 70.
- There are no distinctive symptoms or physical findings associated with this disorder.
- 79–82% of patients with the systemic capillary leak syndrome have MGUS.

➤ Tests

- Bone marrow biopsy and aspirate. Plasma cells are increased, but <10; interstitial and in small cluster distribution.
- CBC is usually normal. Rouleaux formation (due to paraproteinemia) may be seen.
- Serum proteins may be elevated with increased globulins (decreased A/G ratio) and hypoalbuminemia.
- Hypogammaglobulinemia may be present in light chain MGUS where only light chains are produced.
- Serum protein electrophoresis and immunofixation reveal a monoclonal protein (κ or λ) and identify preponderance of a specific immunoglobulin chain (IgG 70% of cases, IgA 12%, light chain 20%, IgM 15%, and biclonal 3%).
- Urine protein electrophoresis and immunofixation reveal M protein (BJ protein) in one third of cases, reflecting urine light chain.
- Serum free light chain immunoassay. Normal κ-to-λ is 0.26:1.65. Abnormal ratio in MGUS is a significant risk factor for progression to myeloma.

---

*Written with Madhu Mennon, M.D., Ph.D.

- Renal function tests may be abnormal in MGUS. Light chains and proteinuria may be present.
- Immunophenotype. Flow cytometry analysis frequently shows two populations of plasma cells: one with normal immunophenotype (CD38 bright, CD19+, and CD56−) with polytypic cytoplasmic light chain expression and another with an aberrant phenotype (CD38+, CD19-, CD56+) with monotypic cytoplasmic light chain expression.
- Cytogenetics. Genetic abnormalities are similar to those described for plasma cell myeloma (see p. 859), but demonstrated infrequently.

➤ Suggested Readings

Kyle RA, Rajkumar SV. Multiple myeloma. Blood. 2008;111:2962–2972.

Mehta J, Cavo M, Singhai S. How I treat elderly patients with myeloma. Blood. 2010;116:2215–2223.

Swerdlow SH, Campo E, Harris NL, et al. WHO Classification of Tumours of Haematopoietic and Lymphoid Tissues. 4th ed. Lyon, France: International Agency for Research on Cancer; 2008:200–202.

PLASMA CELL LEUKEMIA (PCL)*

➤ Definition

- PCL is an aggressive form of plasma cell myeloma consisting of clonal plasma cells circulating in the peripheral blood. PCL can occur de novo (primary PCL) or evolve as a late feature in the course of plasma cell myeloma (secondary PCL).
- It has a poor prognosis with a median survival of 7–11 months in treated cases.

➤ Who Should be Suspected?

- PCL is more common in men and in African Americans. The incidence is 0.02–0.03 cases/100,000 population. Secondary PCL occurs in 1–4% of plasma cell myeloma cases.
- Patients with PCL present with clinical features similar to those of plasma cell myeloma (PCM) (see p. 859). Primary cases have smaller M-protein peak in serum, higher platelet count, younger age (55 versus 65 for secondary PCL), and longer survival.
- In addition to peripheral blood and bone marrow, clonal plasma cells are found frequently in spleen, liver, pleural effusions, ascites, and CNS.

➤ Tests

- CBC. Leukocytosis with clonal plasma cells exceeding 2000/micro/L or 20% of differential count. Mild anemia and/or thrombocytopenia can also be observed. The plasma cells have relatively scant cytoplasm and may resemble plasmacytoid lymphocytes. They may also have the morphology of plasmablasts.
- Bone marrow biopsy and aspirate are similar to that for PCM (see p. 859)
- Serum protein electrophoresis and immunofixation (see p. 332) reveal a monoclonal protein (κ or λ) and identify a specific heavy chain. The relative distribution of Ig type is IgG 30%, IgA 20%, light chain 35%, IgD 3%, and IgE 1%.
- Urine protein electrophoresis and immunofixation reveal M protein (BJ protein).
- Serum free light chain immunoassay (see p. 219). Abnormal κ-to-λ ratio may be seen.
- Renal function tests may be abnormal in cases with monoclonal light chain proteinuria.

---

*Written with Madhu Mennon, M.D., Ph.D.

- Immunophenotype. Bright CD38 and/or CD138 with monoclonal cytoplasmic κ or λ are usually observed. Contrary to PCM, CD56 staining is rarely observed. CD19 and/or CD20 are frequently absent.
- Cytogenetics. Abnormal karyotypes (similar to PCM) are frequently found and there is a higher incidence of unfavorable cytogenetics—del 13q14, t(4,14), t(14,16) and del 17q113.

➤ Suggested Readings

Rajkumar SV, Kyle RA, Connor RF. Plasma cell leukemia. UpToDate. Rose B, ed. Waltham, MA: UpToDate Inc.; 2008.

Swerdlow SH, Campo E, Harris NL, et al. *WHO Classification of Tumours of Haematopoietic and Lymphoid Tissues.* 4th ed. Lyon, France: International Agency for Research on Cancer; 2008:203.

MONOCLONAL LIGHT AND HEAVY CHAIN DEPOSITION DISEASES*

➤ Definition
- These disorders include light chain deposition disease (LCDD), heavy chain deposition disease (HCDD), and light and heavy chain deposition disease (LHCDD). They are seen in the context of plasma cell disorders or of lymphomas with plasmacytic differentiation.
- There is abnormal deposition of light chain, heavy chain, or both light and heavy chains in tissues, but in contrast to amyloidosis, they do not form β sheets and do not stain with Congo red. Median survival is 4 years.

➤ Who Should be Suspected?
- Middle-aged (median age 56 years) male patients with symptoms of Ig deposition in various organs: kidney (nephrotic syndrome and renal failure), heart, liver, peripheral nerves, lungs, blood vessels, joints.

➤ Tests
- Bone marrow biopsy and aspirate. Evidence of plasmacytosis, overt myeloma, lymphoplasmacytic lymphoma, or marginal zone lymphoma may be present.
- Tissue biopsy of involved organs (e.g., heart, kidneys, liver) shows evidence of nonamyloid, nonfibrillary, amorphous eosinophilic material. LCCD demonstrates positive anti-light κ or λ chain antibody staining.
- Immunofluorescence with antibodies against κ or λ demonstrates linear deposits of light chains along the outer edge of renal tubular basement membrane.
- CBC is usually normal. Rouleaux formation (due to paraproteinemia) may be seen.
- Serum protein may be elevated and hypogammaglobulinemia may be present.
- Serum complement levels may be decreased in HCDD.
- Serum protein electrophoresis and immunofixation (see p. 332) reveal a monoclonal light chain (κ in 80% cases), heavy chain protein or both.
- Urine protein electrophoresis and immunofixation demonstrate M protein (BJ protein), which is composed of urine light chain.

---

*Written with Madhu Mennon, M.D., Ph.D.

- Serum free light chain immunoassay (see p. 219): altered κ : λ ratio
- Renal function tests may be abnormal in cases with monoclonal light chain proteinuria. Increased serum creatinine is associated with poor prognosis.
- Immunophenotype. Plasma cells have immunophenotype similar to that described for plasma cell myeloma and MGUS (see p. 859 and p. 861).

➤ Suggested Reading

Swerdlow SH, Campo E, Harris NL, et al. *WHO Classification of Tumours of Haematopoietic and Lymphoid Tissues.* 4th ed. Lyon, France: International Agency for Research on Cancer; 2008:209.

PLASMACYTOMA

➤ Definition

- Plasmacytoma(s) refers to single (or multiple) monoclonal plasma cell tumors with no involvement of bone marrow or blood. There are no typical clinical features associated with plasmacytoma.
- Plasmacytomas are classified as either
  1. Solitary plasmacytoma of bone (SPB), a localized bone lesion
  2. Extraosseous plasmacytoma (EP), localized plasma cell neoplasm that arise in tissues other than bone (upper respiratory tract, sinuses, larynx, GI system, lymph nodes, bladder, breast, thyroid, testis, parotid, CNS, and skin)
- SPB and EP constitute 3–5% of all plasma cell neoplasms. Approximately 75% of SPB patients progress to PCM or additional bone lesions develop with a median survival of 10 years. Conversely, EP cases have better prognosis with only 15% progressing to plasma cell myeloma.

➤ Who Should be Suspected?

- Middle-aged patients with bone pain, fractures, or neurologic symptoms related to nerve compression should be suspected for SPB.
- Patients with EP usually present with epistaxis, rhinorrhea, and nasal obstruction related to the tumor mass. Other manifestations depend on the location of EP.

➤ Tests

- Bone marrow biopsy and aspirate are usually normal. They are necessary to rule out PCM.
- Biopsy of SPB or EP. Monoclonal plasma cells are seen. Some plasma cells can have plasmablastic or anaplastic morphology. EP cases might pose a diagnostic challenge, as they might be difficult to distinguish from lymphoplasmacytic lymphomas (see p. 855).
- CBC is usually normal
- Serum protein electrophoresis and immunofixation (see p. 332) may reveal a monoclonal protein (κ or λ) and identify a specific heavy chain (EP patients commonly have IgA).
- Urine protein electrophoresis and immunofixation (see p. 375) may reveal M protein (BJ protein).
- Serum free light chain ratio is useful for predicting prognosis.
- Renal function tests may be abnormal in the presence of monoclonal light chain proteinuria.
- Immunophenotype is similar to that of PCM (see p. 859)

- Cytogenetics. Genetic abnormalities are similar to those described for PCM but are demonstrated infrequently.

➤ Suggested Reading

Swerdlow SH, Campo E, Harris NL, et al. *WHO Classification of Tumours of Haematopoietic and Lymphoid Tissues.* 4th ed. Lyon, France: International Agency for Research on Cancer; 2008:208–209.

PRIMARY AMYLOIDOSIS (PA)*

➤ Definition

- PA is caused by extracellular deposition of either intact or fragments of Ig light chains or rarely heavy chains in the form of insoluble β sheets.
- PA occurs in the setting of plasma cell dyscrasias—MGUS (see p. 855) and PCM (see p. 859) or lymphoplasmacytic lymphoma (see p. 855). Currently, it is also classified as amyloidosis-AL (associated with light chain) type, which should be differentiated from secondary amyloidosis or amyloidosis-AA type. Light chain deposition disease (LCDD; see p. 863) is a different entity characterized by deposition of light chains without formation of amyloid β sheets.

➤ Who Should be Suspected?

- Middle-aged (median age 64) male patients with clinical or laboratory findings of MGUS or PCM.
- Common clinical manifestations include edema due to cardiac failure and nephrotic syndrome, malabsorption, macroglossia, hepatomegaly, purpura, bone pain, peripheral neuropathy, and carpal tunnel syndrome. Bleeding diathesis may be seen due to increased fragility of blood vessels resulting from amyloid deposition, in combination with factor X deficiency (due to renal excretion of factor X).

➤ Tests

- Bone marrow biopsy and aspirate. Evidence of overt myeloma or lymphoplasmacytic lymphoma along with replacement by amyloid is seen. β Sheets stain pink with Congo red. New technologies (e.g., tandem mass spectrometry-based proteomic analysis) for the typing of amyloidosis in biopsy specimens are being developed.
  - Tissue biopsy of involved organs, for example, heart, kidneys, and liver, show evidence of amyloid deposition that demonstrates positive Congo red staining is positive in AL. (LCCD is negative for Congo red staining but positive for anti-κ or λ antibody staining). Secondary amyloidosis (AA) is negative for both.
  - CBC. Usually Rouleaux formation (due to paraproteinemia) may be seen.
  - Serum protein may be elevated and hypogammaglobulinemia may be present.
  - Serum protein electrophoresis and immunofixation (see p. 332) reveal a monoclonal light chain (λ in 70% cases) and rarely monoclonal heavy chain protein.
  - Urine protein electrophoresis and immunofixation (see p. 375) demonstrate M protein (BJ protein), which is composed of urine light chains. Secretion of λ light chain is associated with poor prognosis.

---

*Written with Madhu Mennon, M.D., Ph.D.

* Serum free light chain immunoassay (see p. 219). Altered κ : λ ratio is present in PA.
* Renal function tests may be abnormal in cases of monoclonal light chain proteinuria. Increased serum creatinine is associated with poor prognosis.
* Immunophenotype. Plasma cell immunophenotype is similar to that of PCM and MGUS (see p. 861).
* Cytogenetics. Genetic abnormalities are similar to those described for PCM. Interestingly, t(11;14) is found in higher percentage of amyloidosis cases (>40%) as compared to plasma cell dyscrasias without amyloidosis.

➤ Prognosis
* In PA, the median survival is approximately 2 years from diagnosis, with cardiac failure the major cause of death.

➤ Suggested Reading
Swerdlow SH, Campo E, Harris NL, et al. *WHO Classification of Tumours of Haematopoietic and Lymphoid Tissues.* 4th ed. Lyon, France: International Agency for Research on Cancer; 2008:209–212.

CRYOGLOBULINEMIA

➤ Definition
* Cryoglobulins (CG) are proteins that precipitate in the body at low temperature or on storage of serum at refrigerated temperature. They are insoluble at 4°C and may aggregate at up to 30°C. CG are either immunoglobulins or a mixture of immunoglobulins and complement components. CG can fix complement and initiate inflammatory reactions.
* The term cryoglobulinemia is often used to refer to a systemic inflammatory syndrome or to vasculitis with serum CG, but the majority of people with CG are asymptomatic. CG can also be detected in patients with chronic infection and/or inflammation.

➤ Who Should be Tested for CG?
* Patients with cutaneous manifestations, the hyperviscosity syndrome, vasculitis, sensitivity to cold including Raynaud phenomenon, and the Meltzer triad: arthralgia, purpura, and weakness.

➤ Tests
* CG are tested on serum (to distinguish from cryofibrinogen, which is tested on plasma [see p. 141]). The blood is obtained in test tubes without anticoagulant, prewarmed at 37°C, and let to clot at the same temperature. Serum is incubated at 4°C to detect turbidity or precipitate after 24–72 hours. That is compared with an aliquot of the same patient's serum kept at 37°C, which should have no precipitate.
* The normal value is <80 μg/dL CG in serum. The pathologic values found in cryoglobulinemia range from 500 to 5000 mg/dL. To determine the nature of the CG, they must be redissolved by warming and the sample analyzed. This helps to classify the various cryoglobulinemia types.
* *Other pertinent laboratory findings*
  * Serologic evidence of hepatitis and liver disease
  * Decreased serum components
  * Serologic evidence of HIV infection
  * Renal disease (e.g., membranoproliferative glomerulonephritis) with proteinuria or hematuria

* Skin biopsy may show cutaneous vasculitis.
* ESR and C-reactive protein are generally elevated.

➤ Classification

* *Type I:* monoclonal immunoglobulin, especially IgG or IgM κ type
  * May cause hyperviscosity syndrome in 5–25% of cases.
  * Most commonly associated with PCM and Waldenstrom macroglobulinemia (lymphoplas-macytic lymphoma); other lymphoproliferative neoplasms with M components; it may be idiopathic.
  * The CGs are often present in great amounts (5–10 mg/dL) with cryocrits >70%. The blood may gel when drawn.
  * Severe symptoms (Raynaud syndrome, gangrene without other causes)
  * Skin, kidney, and bone marrow are predominantly involved.
* *Type II (essential mixed cryoglobulinemia):* monoclonal immunoglobulin mixed with at least one other type of polyclonal immunoglobulin, typically IgM or IgA and polyclonal IgG; always associated with RF.
  * Causes 40–60% of cases
  * Associated most often with chronic HCV or HIV infection; less often with HBV, EBV, bacterial and parasitic infections, autoimmune diseases, Sjögren syndrome, and syndrome of essential mixed cryoglobulinemia, immune-complex nephritis.
  * High titer RF without definite rheumatic disease
  * C4 levels are decreased
* *Type III:* mixed polyclonal immunoglobulin, most commonly IgM–IgG, occasionally IgA–IgG combinations, usually with RF. Types II and III generally produce 1–5 mg/dL CG
  * Causes 40–50% of cases
  * Most commonly associated with connective tissue disorders (SLE, Sjögren's syndrome), persistent infections (HIV, HCV), and rarely with lymphoproliferative disorders
  * In types II and III, the skin, peripheral nervous system, and kidneys are predominantly involved.

➤ Limitations

* False-negative results may occur if the blood was cooled below 37°C during collection; if the blood clotted right away centrifugation may remove the CG with the clot. The centrifugation too must be performed in a temperature-controlled centrifuge.
* The presence of CG may cause erroneous WBC counts on electronic counters.

➤ Suggested Reading

Peng SL, Schur PH. Overview of cryoglobulins and cryoglobulinemia. UpToDate. Rose P, ed. Waltham,, MA: UpTo-Date, Inc.; 2009.

CRYOFIBRINOGENEMIA

➤ Definition

* Cryofibrinogen (CF) is generated by a mixture of fibrinogen, fibrin, fibronectin, and fibrin split products that precipitate reversibly at cold temperatures in anticoagulated blood.
* An individual whose plasma, but not serum, forms a cryoprecipitate has cryofibrino-genemia.

➤ Who Should be Suspected?

- Patients with cold-induced thrombotic events, or patients with hematologic and solid neoplasms, transiently in some infections, autoimmune syndromes, including connective tissue disorders, and patients with painful ulcers, purpura, livido reticularis, and painful or pruritic erythema of the extremities.
- The disease is common in patients with HCV.
- Some individuals may be asymptomatic, and CF may be discovered accidentally in the laboratory.

➤ Tests

- Blood must be collected at 37°C on anticoagulant. The plasma is placed in a Wintrobe tube and refrigerated at 4°C for 72 hours. At that time the cryocrit is quantitated by centrifugation while it remains cooled at 4°C. The result is reported as percent of cryocrit. Individual components of the precipitate can be studied if indicated.
- CF may be present in healthy people, but it is usually <50 mg/L.

➤ Limitations

- If collection is not performed at 37°C, the formation of a cryoprecipitate may be missed, which can lead to a falsely negative result. Collection of blood on heparin, or even administration of heparin, may lead to false-positive results.
- CF may cause erroneous WBC counts with electronic counters.

➤ Suggested Reading

Peng SL. Cryofibrinogenemia. UpToDate. Rose B, ed. Waltham, MA: UpToDate, Inc.: 2009.

DISORDERS OF HEMOSTASIS AND THROMBOSIS

DISORDERS OF PLATELETS: THROMBOCYTOPENIAS

Thrombocytopenias represent a reduction in the number of circulating platelets below the lower limit of normal set by the laboratory (see p. 294). They may be classified in various ways. First one must determine if the condition is congenital or acquired. Acquired thrombocytopenias may be acute or chronic. The causes of thrombocytopenias can be classified by etiology (Figure 10-2): increased destruction, decreased production, artifactual, and miscellaneous. TTP/HUS is discussed separately (see p. 889).

IMMUNE THROMBOCYTOPENIC PURPURA (ITP)

➤ Definition

- ITP (formerly known as idiopathic thrombocytopenic purpura) is an immune-mediated acquired disease characterized by transient or persistent decrease of the platelet count due to accelerated destruction by autoantibodies and impaired platelet production.
- Typically, ITP is an isolated thrombocytopenia (unaffected white or red cells), with a platelet count <100,000/micro mL. Depending on the severity of thrombocytopenia and other contributing factors, patients with ITP are at increased risk for bleeding.

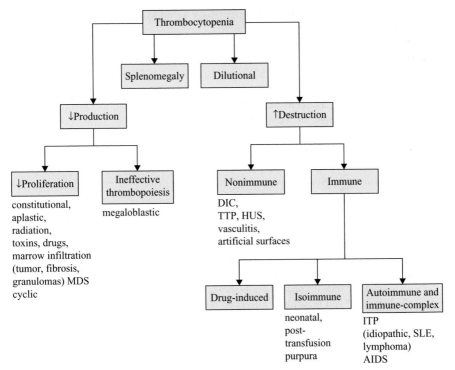

Figure 10-2. The etiology of thrombocytopenia. DIC, disseminated intravascular coagulation; HUS, hemolytic uremic syndrome; TTP, thrombotic thrombocytopenic purpura; MDS, myelodysplastic syndromes.

- ITP is a heterogeneous group of disorders. Most cases are considered primary, whereas others are secondary to other autoimmune conditions that have to be ruled out, such as SLE, as well as HIV and HCV infections.

➤ Who Should be Suspected?

- Individuals with no previous history of bleeding and no hematologic disease who complain of mucosal (especially epistaxis, gum or excessive menstrual bleeding) and subcutaneous bleeding in the form of petechiae or ecchymoses.
- Individuals with absence of splenomegaly (except for young patients where mild splenomegaly may be found) or lymphadenopathy.
- Individuals with no ingestion of drugs that may cause drug-induced thrombocytopenia.
- In children, ITP is often preceded by a viral infection, and most cases remit spontaneously.

➤ Tests

- Laboratory findings are not specific; there is no "gold standard" test that can reliably establish the diagnosis.
- CBC
  - RBC: normal count, unless the bleeding had been excessive and of long duration in which cases anemia may be present and the reticulocyte count elevated

- WBC is normal; in cases with severe hemorrhage a shift to the left (immature cells) may be observed.
- Platelets are markedly decreased in most acute cases with counts of <20,000/μL at presentation. In chronic or in cases that present insidiously, the decrease in platelet counts may be moderate to marginal.
- PBS is normal, except for the decreased number of platelets; the remaining ones are frequently large (early, accelerated bone marrow release) and MPV is elevated (see p. 255). Platelet clumping must be excluded (pseudothrombocytopenia). Schistocytes are not present.
- Bone marrow (not indicated unless an underlying hematologic disease is suspected or in patients >60 years of age) is normal. In some patients there are an increased number of younger appearing megakaryocytes that do not seem to release platelets.
- All coagulation tests are normal.
- Serology to rule out SLE (see p. 936) is mandatory in adult ITP. ANA (see p. 59) may also be helpful.
- Platelet antibody detection and identification assays are available through reference laboratories. ELISA and flow cytometry methods are offered. However, because of the high frequency of false-positive and false-negative tests (antibodies are detected in only 60% of patients), serologic tests for platelet antibodies are not recommended.
- Microbiology: HIV and hepatitis C infections need to be ruled out in populations at risk. *H. pylori* testing may have pertinence since the elimination of certain strains may eradicate ITP.
- Blood group Rh (D) typing is necessary if anti-D Ig is being considered for therapy.
- Baseline Ig levels should be measured.

DRUG-INDUCED THROMBOCYTOPENIA, IMMUNE

➤ Definition
- Acute platelet destruction caused by drug-dependent antibodies. The antibodies react with various epitopes on the platelet surface.

➤ Who Should be Suspected?
- A patient with isolated thrombocytopenia, and a history of medication known to result in drug-induced thrombocytopenia. The most common offenders are: quinine, quinidine, heparin (discussed separately as HIT, see below), sulfa drugs, digoxin, GPIIb/IIIa antagonists, vancomycin, gold compounds, β-lactam antibiotics, valproic acid, levodopa, procainamide, and vaccines against measles-mumps-rubella.

➤ Tests
- Thrombocytopenia (may be severe) without abnormalities in RBC or WBC.
- Laboratory tests to demonstrate the presence of specific antibodies are used in research laboratories, but have not been validated for general use.
- The gold standard for diagnosis is recovery from thrombocytopenia following discontinuation of the drug, which is usually prompt, except for gold-induced thrombocytopenia that may develop long after the therapy had been discontinued and may persist for several months.

HEPARIN-INDUCED THROMBOCYTOPENIA (HIT)

➤ Definition
* HIT is a complication of heparin therapy resulting in a reduction in platelet count.
  * Type 1 HIT refers to a modest drop in platelets, not of immune etiology, seen during the first 2 days of heparin administration; the counts normalize without the need to discontinue heparin.
  * Type 2 HIT is an immune-mediated HIT, with antibodies developing against the complex of heparin and platelet factor 4 (PF4).
* HIT develops in about 3% of patients treated with unfractionated heparin, but rarely (0.2%) in those receiving low–molecular-weight heparin (but there is cross-reactivity of the antibodies between the two) or the pentasaccharide fondaparinux. It develops more frequently in surgical rather than medical patients, particularly after bypass surgery.
* Its seriousness is underlined by the frequent complication of venous and arterial thromboses that result in up to 20% mortality and limb loss rates of 2–3%.
* The term HITT is used for HIT associated with thrombosis.

➤ Diagnosis
* The clinical diagnosis of HIT is based on the "4Ts" criteria:
  1. >50% fall in platelet count, or platelet nadir 20–100,000/μL;
  2. Onset between days 5 and 10 following initiation of heparin, or <1day in patients with exposure to heparin within the previous 100 days;
  3. New thrombosis, skin necrosis, or acute systemic reaction post-heparin bolus;
  4. No other obvious cause for fall in platelet count.
     There are exceptions to these rules. One such situation is seen in patients who develop HIT after discontinuation of heparin. In patients with typical HIT, the platelet count generally recovers within one week after discontinuing heparin administration.

➤ Tests
* There are two types of assays: immunologic and functional. Some patients may develop specific antibodies without clinical manifestations of HIT. In these cases the immunoassays are positive, but the functional ones are not. The immunoassays are sensitive in detecting HIT antibodies, but none is completely specific. To increase the specificity of immunoassays, manufacturers have developed IgG specific assays. The resulting assays have a very high negative predictive value.
* Immunoassays presently available to coagulation laboratories:
  * PIFA Heparin/PF4 is a qualitative particle immunofiltration screening test that detects antibodies to PF4. It has good negative predictive value (NPV), but because of relatively low specificity, a positive result must be followed by a more specific immunologic or functional assay.
  * PF4 IgG^M is an ELISA assay designed to detect antibodies reactive with PF4. It is directed solely against IgG rather than all classes of immunoglobulins. This assay has both excellent NPV (with a cutoff <0.4 Optical Density [OD]) and high positive predictive value (PPV). A good relationship with the serotonin release assay (see below) has been found at OD readings >1.4. Successful performance of the assay requires high technical skills.
  * Flow cytometry for detecting PF4 antibodies is available in research laboratories.

- ^{C}14- platelet serotonin release (PSR) is considered the gold standard for the diagnosis of HIT. It has excellent sensitivity and specificity. Because it uses radioactive serotonin as its principal reagent, this assay is performed only in a few reference laboratories with a turnaround time of at least one week. As a consequence, the assay can be used only for final confirmation of the diagnosis.
- Heparin-induced platelet aggregation is an alternative to the PSR. The assay can be performed in laboratories that offer platelet aggregometry (see p. 291) but it is not well standardized, and although it has excellent specificity, it has low sensitivity. It is hoped that with more sophisticated equipment for platelet aggregation the methodology will be improved.

NEONATAL THROMBOCYTOPENIA

➤ Classification
- Thrombocytopenias in the newborn can classified as due to increased destruction or decreased production.

Increased Destruction
- Neonatal alloimmune thrombocytopenia (NAIT) occurs when fetal platelets contain an antigen inherited from the father that the mother lacks. Fetal and neonate thrombocytopenia is the platelet equivalent of Rh disease; the most commonly involved platelet antigen is HPA-1a or PI^{A1}. When the mother is exposed to fetal platelets during pregnancy, anti-HPA-1a antibodies are generated; they traverse the placenta and the result is fetal thrombocytopenia. Intracranial hemorrhage is a potentially serious complication.
- Laboratory studies:
  - Platelet counts in the neonate are often $<50,000/\mu L$.
  - Platelet antigens are tested in mother and father to establish the incompatibility. HPA 1, 3, and 5 should be screened in all potential cases, as well as HPA 4 if the patient is of Asian descent. Testing must prove both a platelet antigen incompatibility between the parents, and a maternal antibody directed against the antigen. The assays must be performed in very experienced laboratories. It is unclear if antenatal screening should be instituted.
- Autoimmune thrombocytopenia in the newborn is the result of the mother having ITP (see p. 868) with antibodies that cross the placenta and react with the platelets of the fetus.
- Most neonates whose mothers have ITP have mild thrombocytopenia (counts $>50,000/ \mu L$), but occasionally they may be severely affected.
- Other causes of thrombocytopenia due to increased platelet destruction in the neonate:
  - Disseminated intravascular coagulation (DIC) as a complication of an acute underlying illness, or as the result of consumption in DIC with capillary hemangiomas (Kasabach-Merritt syndrome)
  - Severe infection
  - Hypersplenism
  - Drug-related thrombocytopenia in the mother
  - Hypersplenism in neonates with an enlarged spleen
  - Necrotizing enterocolitis
- Laboratory studies are directed to the underlying condition and monitoring the platelet counts.

Decreased Production

- Genetic disorders: thrombocytopenia-absent radius syndrome (see p. 874); congenital megakaryocytic thrombocytopenia; Fanconi anemia (see p. 795); certain chromosome abnormalities; congenital platelet disorders (see p. 874); lipid storage diseases
- Acquired causes: bone marrow diseases (neonatal leukemia, neuroblastoma); toxic injury to megakaryocytes due to drugs or infections; neonates whose mothers have preeclampsia; birth asphyxia; following exchange transfusion

➤ Tests

- Serial platelet counts
- Maternal studies for thrombocytopenia
- DIC screening (see p. 883) in infants at risk for DIC

PSEUDO (SPURIOUS) THROMBOCYTOPENIA

➤ Definition

- A false decrease in reported platelet counts. It may be due to:
  - Platelet clumping induced by collection of blood in EDTA (the routine anticoagulant used for CBC); it is the most common cause for spurious thrombocytopenia (see p. 873).
  - Platelet satellitosis (platelets form rosettes around white cells)
  - Platelet cold agglutinins
  - Giant platelets missed by automated counters
  - Very elevated RBC count
  - Artifacts due to inappropriate technique in blood collection (clots, overfilling vacuum tubes)
- In a good laboratory, the technicians observe all CBC tubes flagged for low platelets for clots and review stained PBS for clumps.

➤ Suggested Readings

Bussel J. Diagnosis and management of the fetus and neonate with alloimmune thrombocytopenia. *J Thromb Haemost.* 2009;7(Suppl 1):253–257.

Cines DB, Bussel JB, Liebman HA, Luning Park ET. The ITP syndrome: pathogenetic and clinical diversity. *Blood.* 2009;113:6511–6521.

Fernandes CJ. Neonatal thrombocytopenia. UpToDate. Rose B, ed. Waltham, MA: UpToDate, Inc.; 2009.

Pouplar C, Gueret P, Fouassier M, et al. Prospective evaluation of the "4Ts" score and particle gel immunoassay specific to heparin/PF4 for the diagnosis of heparin-induced thrombocytopenia. *J Thromb Haemost.* 2007;5:1373–1379.

Provan D, Stasi R, Newland AC, et al. International consensus report on the investigation and management of primary immune thrombocytopenia. *Blood.* 2010;115:168–186.

Rodeghiero F, Stasi R, Gernsheimer T, et al. Standardization of terminology, definitions and outcome criteria in immune thrombocytopenic purpura of adults and children: report from an international working group. *Blood.* 2009;113:2386–2393.

Warkentin TE, Sheppard JI, Moore JC, et al. Quantitative interpretation of optical density measurements using PF4-dependent enzyme-immunoassay. *J Thromb Haemost.* 2008;6:1304–1312.

DISORDERS OF PLATELET FUNCTION

- Disorders of platelet function are also referred as thrombocytopathies. The platelets' major physiologic role is in hemostasis, where they arrest bleeding in small blood vessels. To perform this function optimally, the platelets' number as well as function must be normal.

- Thrombocytopathies can be congenital, but more commonly they are acquired. In most acquired thrombocytopathies, the platelet counts are normal. In some of the congenital disorders, the platelet count is reduced as well.
- Individuals who present with recent or life-long mucocutaneous bleeding should be suspected. Because thrombocytopathies and most von Willebrand's disease cases have similar presentations, work-up for the two conditions should be initiated simultaneously.

INHERITED THROMBOCYTOPATHIES

- Defects in platelet–platelet interaction (aggregation defects)
  - Glanzmann thrombasthenia: severe autosomal recessive bleeding disorder. It is due to absence (type 1) or reduction (type 2) of the platelet integrin receptor GPIIb-IIIa ($\alpha_{2bb}\beta_3$). The platelet count is normal. Bleeding results from the platelets' inability to bind fibrinogen. There is absence, or reduction in aggregation with all agonists, but platelets agglutinate normally with ristocetin) (Table 10-4). There is normal release with strong agonists, such as thrombin. Complete absence of clot retraction was described in type 1 disease.
  - Afibrinogenemia: in the absence of fibrinogen platelet cannot adhere resulting in lack of aggregation.
- Disorders of secretion and signal transduction include storage-pool deficiencies of platelet granules or granule contents as well as primary transduction defects. The bleeding is usually mild.
  - In the gray platelet syndrome, platelets are deficient in α granules. Platelet aggregation studies have produced variable results. Aggregation induced by ADP, epinephrine, arachidonic acid, and agglutination with ristocetin is normal (or nearly normal), but aggregation with collagen has been reported to be decreased or absent. Platelet count varies from 20,000–150,000/µL. On the PBS, platelets are large and appear gray or gray-blue, are vacuolated, or look ghost-like. These patients have a tendency to develop myelofibrosis
  - Δ-storage pool diseases are characterized by the absence of dense bodies. In most cases the second wave aggregation with ADP and epinephrine is absent. There are several subtypes:
    - Δ-storage pool disease without other associations: autosomal dominant.
    - Hermansky-Pudlak syndrome: autosomal recessive inheritance due to deficiency of dense bodies. It is associated with oculocutaneous albinism. Hermansky-Pudlak syndrome has a high prevalence in northwest Puerto Rico and is the most common cause of oculocutaneous albinism in Japan.
    - Chediak-Higashi syndrome: autosomal recessive deficiency of dense bodies; associated with oculocutaneous albinism. Giant cytoplasmic granules are present in neutrophils, monocytes, and lymphocytes.
    - Thrombocytopenia-absent radius syndrome: autosomal recessive. It is associated with hypomegakaryocytic thrombocytopenia.
    - Wiskott-Aldrich syndrome: X-linked recessive condition due to deficiencies of dense bodies and cytoskeletal regulation. It is associated with thrombocytopenia, eczema, and T-cell immune deficiency.
    - May-Hegglin anomaly is an autosomal dominant abnormality of granulocytes and platelets, associated with thrombocytopenia, giant platelets, Dohle-like bodies in neutrophils, and chronic renal disease.

TABLE 10-4. Abnormalities of Platelet Function

Disorder	Features	Collagen	ADP and Epinephrine	Arachidonic Acid	Ristocetin
Glanzmann thrombasthenia	Absent clot retraction	↓	↓↓	↓	N
Storage pool disorders	Absence of α or δ platelet granules	↓	N ↓	N	N
Aspirin ingestion and aspirin-like storage pool disorder	Decreased thromboxane 2 generation	↓	N ↓	↓↓	N
Bernard-Soulier Syndrome	Thrombocytopenia and giant platelets	N	N	N	↓
Von Willebrand Disease, except type 2B	Plasmatic defect that affects platelet function. Normal platelet count	N	N	N	↓ or N
Von Willebrand Disease Type 2B	Thrombocytopenia	N	N	N	↑↑
Platelet-type von Willebrand Disease	Thrombocytopenia	N	N	N	↑

- Signal transduction defects due to abnormal platelets receptors. It is uncertain to what extent single receptor defects result in clinical bleeding.
  - Integrin α2β1 and GPVI (collagen receptor defects)
  - P2Y12 (ADP receptor defect)
  - Epinephrine receptor defect
  - Thromboxane A$_2$ receptor deficiency
- Signal transduction defects due to abnormalities in arachidonic acid pathways and thromboxane A$_2$ synthesis.
  - Patients with abnormal thromboxane A$_2$ synthesis have an aspirin-like defect.
  - Impaired liberation of arachidonic acid
  - Cyclooxygenase deficiency
  - Thromboxane synthase deficiency
- Disorders of platelet–vessel wall interaction (platelet adhesion defects)
  - Bernard-Soulier syndrome: autosomal recessive. Caused by absence or abnormalities in the platelet receptor complex GPIb-IX-V. Presents with moderate to severe thrombocytopenia and giant platelets. Platelets aggregate normally with ADP, epinephrine, collagen, arachidonic acid, but show delayed aggregation with thrombin and no response to ristocetin (see Table 10-4).
  - Platelet-type von Willebrand disease (see p. 879): autosomal dominant condition associated with intermittent thrombocytopenia, normal platelet morphology, and decreased levels of high–molecular-weight vWF multimers. It must be distinguished from von Willebrand disease type 2B.
- Disorders of platelet function related to other defects.
  - Quebec platelet disorder: excessive fibrinolysis resulting from increased expression and storage of the fibrinolytic enzyme urokinase plasminogen activator in platelets, resulting in delayed-onset bleeding after trauma or surgery.
  - Scott syndrome: autosomal recessive disorder due to a defect in platelets' membrane resulting in inability to assemble prothrombinase and intrinsic tenase complexes.
  - The Montreal platelet syndrome was recently documented to be a variant of type 2B von Willebrand disease.

ACQUIRED THROMBOCYTOPATHIES

➤ Drug-Induced

- The majority of acquired thrombocytopathies are drug-induced. The following drugs are associated with reduced platelet function:
  - Strong effect
    - Aspirin and nonsteroidal anti-inflammatory drugs (NSAIDs). Aspirin affects platelets by irreversible acetylation of cyclooxygenase (COX)1. This inhibition impairs formation of thromboxane A2 required for full activation with weak agonists. NSAIDs affect the same pathways, but without permanent acetylation. The effect of aspirin on platelets lasts for approximately 10 days, whereas the effect of an NSAID is of short duration, 24–48 hours.
    - Sulfinpyrazone
    - The thienopyridine derivatives ticlopidine (rarely used now because of the high incidence of TTP), clopidogrel, and other similar drugs being developed are antithrombotic

drugs that inhibit platelet response to ADP by blocking its receptor $P2Y_{12}$. The full effect of clopidogrel requires 4–7 days, and persists for up to 7 days after it is discontinued.
- Anti IIb-IIIa agents are used mainly in acute coronary syndromes: Abciximab, Eptifibatide, Tirofiban
- Dipyridamole
- Antibiotics, especially when administered in large doses: penicillin, carbenicillin, ampicillin, ticarcillin, nafcillin, azlocillin, mezlocillin, cephalosporins, nitrofurantoin
- Plasma volume expanders: dextran, hydroxyethyl starch
- Weak effect
  - Chemotherapeutic drugs: bis-chloronitrosourea (BCNU), anthracyclines, mithramycin
  - Cardiovascular drugs: β blockers, calcium-channel blockers, nitroglycerin
  - Alcohol
  - Anticonvulsants: valproic acid
  - Tricyclic antidepressants: imipramine, amitriptyline
  - Phenothiazines: chlorpromazine, trifluoperazine
  - Anesthetics: halothane
  - Epsilon aminocaproic acid administered in large doses
  - Radiographic contrast agents
  - Certain foods (onions, garlic, ginger, black tree fungus) and food supplements

➤ Disease-Induced or Iatrogenic
- Myeloproliferative neoplasms (see p. 836): moderately severe defect.
- Myelodysplastic syndromes (see p. 843): usually mild defect.
- Uremia: defect due to accumulation of guanidinosuccinic acid. It is partially corrected by dialysis. Platelet counts are normal.
- Liver cirrhosis: normal platelet counts, except in cases with hypersplenism.
- Paraproteinemias: normal platelet counts, except in advanced cases, or as the result of chemotherapy.
- DIC (see p. 883) affects platelet function mostly due to the effect of fibrin degradation products (FDP) on platelets.
- Cardiopulmonary bypass surgery causes marked platelet dysfunction, as well as temporary thrombocytopenia.

➤ Tests
- CBC
- Platelet count may be normal, decreased, or increased, depending on the etiology (see above).
- The PBS may show normal platelets, or giant platelets and thrombocytopenia, depending on etiology.
- Bleeding time may be prolonged, but it is unreliable (see p. 73), hence not recommended.
- Clot retraction, rarely used, is absent in severe Glanzmann thrombasthenia.

➤ Other Considerations
- Platelet aggregation and chemoluminescence studies (see p. 291) with various agonists (ADP, epinephrine, collagen, thrombin, and arachidonic acid), and agglutination studies with ristocetin are presently the best assays to evaluate platelet function. Mixing studies in the presence of ristocetin (patient's platelets with normal plasma and normal platelets with

patient's plasma) are used to differentiate von Willebrand disease type IIb from platelet-type von Willebrand disease (see Table 10-4).
- PFA-100 is a device used for rapid diagnosis of platelet functional defects (see p. 293). If positive, the diagnosis should be refined by studies of platelet aggregation.
- Flow cytometry is a sensitive tool to examine platelet function, but it may not be readily available
- Electron microscopy may determine the status of platelet granules, but its utility is mostly for research purposes.

➤ Suggested Reading
Kottke-Marchant K, Corocoran G. The laboratory diagnosis of platelet disorders. An algorithmic approach. *Arch Path Lab Med.* 2002;126:133–146.

DISORDERS DUE TO COAGULATION FACTOR DEFICIENCIES: CONGENITAL CLOTTING DEFECTS

HEMOPHILIA

➤ Definition
- Hemophilia A (factor VIII [F VIII] deficiency) and hemophilia B (factor IX [F IX] deficiency) formerly also known as Christmas disease, are life-long bleeding disorders, both inherited as X chromosome–linked recessive conditions, hence limited almost exclusively to males.
- Hemophilia B is about one-tenth as prevalent as hemophilia A.
- Factor XI deficiency was classified in the past as hemophilia C; it will be presented separately (see p. 882).
- Acquired hemophilia is a severe bleeding diathesis, resulting from the development of autoantibodies against factor VIII or rarely IX, in a patient with no previous bleeding history. It affects both males and females.

➤ Who Should be Suspected?
- A male with a bleeding family history in other males on the maternal side (one third of cases have a negative family history), and a personal history of spontaneous major bleeding episodes (mostly in joints, but also intracranial, in skeletal muscles, and in other organs), some resulting in chronic disability, or fatalities if not treated appropriately. In infants bleeding at circumcision, on teeth eruption, or when first standing (in knee joints) should raise the suspicion of hemophilia.
- The severity of bleeding is similar for the same levels of factor deficiency in hemophilia A and B.
  Acquired hemophilia should be suspected in postpartum females, patients with lymphoproliferative neoplasms, or in the elderly without other predisposing factors except age.
- The development of alloantibodies (either against F VIII or IX) is suspected in hemophiliacs multiply infused with the respective factor who become refractory to replacement therapy. They develop in 15–30% of hemophilia A and 3–5% of hemophilia B patients. The majority develop before age 20.

➤ Tests

- Screening tests. Platelet counts, PT and PTT are recommended as the initial work-up of patients presenting with a bleeding diathesis. Of those, the platelet count and PT are normal in hemophiliacs, whereas the PTT is variably prolonged.
- Definitive tests. Factor VIII and IX levels are established by quantitation of factors VIII or IX, respectively (see p. 171). Severe hemophiliacs have factors VIII or IX levels between 0 and <2%; moderate hemophiliacs between 2 and 5%, and mild cases from >5% to below the lower limit of the assay. Patients in the latter group do not bleed spontaneously, but may have severe bleeding on traumatic events, sometimes surprisingly, since they present with no previous bleeding history. Mild hemophilia A patients have an unexpected tendency to develop inhibitors.
- Obligate female carriers (mothers to more than one hemophiliac son or daughters of a hemophiliac) do not need to be investigated. Carriers may have coagulant and immunologic factor VIII levels around 50%, but there is a wide scatter in these levels, and when skewed to low levels, may result in clinical bleeding (a "female hemophiliac"). A more definitive diagnosis in suspected carriers or as prenatal diagnosis is through genetic analysis using DNA-based techniques. The most common abnormality found in carriers of severe hemophilia A is intron 22 inversion in the factor VIII gene. The genetic diagnosis is easier in factor IX carriers than in factor VIII ones because of a large deletion in the factor IX gene.
- The diagnosis of inhibitors to factor VIII or IX is established by specific assays, and inhibitor titers are reported in Bethesda units (see p. 171).

➤ Limitations

- Type III and 2N von Willebrand's disease have the same clinical presentation as hemophilia, and both may have very low FVIII values (see p. 881). Detailed laboratory assays are necessary to distinguish these two conditions from hemophilia. Moreover, they are also present in females.

➤ Suggested Readings

Mannucci PM, Tuddenham GD. The hemophiliac—from royal genes to gene therapy. *N Engl J Med.* 2001;344:1773–1779.

Preston FE, Kitchen S, Jennings TA, et al. SSC/ISTH classification of hemophilia A: can hemophilia center laboratories achieve the new criteria? *J Thromb Haemost.* 2004;2:271–274.

VON WILLEBRAND DISEASE (VWD)*

➤ Definition

- VWD is a heterogeneous group of qualitative and quantitative disorders of vWF resulting in a hemostatic defect. In severe cases, coagulation type defect is present. It is the most common inherited bleeding diathesis, seen in up to 1% of the Caucasian population.
- vWF is synthesized in endothelial cells and megakaryocytes and released as large multimers. It is acted on by a metalloprotease, ADAMTS 13, to form variably sized multimers. It mediates

---

*Written with Reema Jaffar, M.D.

platelet adhesion through a platelet receptor, GP1b. It also functions as a carrier for factor VIII. Inheritance is autosomal recessive in most cases.

➤ Who Should be Suspected?

* Patients with a personal history of mucosal bleeding (except for VWD type III, where the bleeding is severe, and type IIN which mimics hemophilia; see below)
* Females with severe menorrhagia presenting at menarche.
* A positive family history of mucosal bleeding is helpful (very low vWF levels are highly heritable, whereas vWF levels at the low end of the population distribution [35–50 IU] show low heritability and cannot be diagnosed definitely as vWD).
* Although VWD is relatively common, not all patients are diagnosed because not all have a bleeding history that is different from what would be considered normal bleeding in a population at large.

➤ Tests

* Because the clinical manifestations of VWD and platelet defects are similar, the laboratory work-up for platelet function and for VWD should be initiated simultaneously, except for cases with a definite family history.
* One should keep in mind that there is a continuum of vWF levels between the normal population and patients with genuine VWD. Better-defined criteria to establish separation cut-off levels, as well as genetic assays, are being developed.
* First-tier tests:
  1. vWF Ag (vWF:Ag)
  2. Factor VIII coagulant
  3. Ristocetin cofactor (vWF:RCo) assay measures vWF activity. A ratio vWF:RCo/vWF:Ag <0.7 is indicative of a qualitative vWF defect.
  4. Some authors have suggested the use of the platelet function analyzer PFA-100 as a screening test for VWD. It has better reproducibility than the bleeding time.
* Second tier tests:
  1. VWF multimers once the diagnosis has been established. Useful to determine various subtypes of the disease.
  2. Ristocetin-induced platelet aggregation (RIPA). In this assay, patient's platelets and plasma are used as a source of vWF (see p. 291).
* Seven clinical variants have been described based on laboratory results and clinical history:
  1. VWD type 1 (70–80% of cases) is a quantitative defect with mild bleeding. The diagnosis can be challenging and might require repeated testing. RIPA is insensitive to mild quantitative defects (see p. 291).
  2. VWD type 2A (10–15% of cases) is a qualitative defect with moderate to severe bleeding. There is absence of high–molecular-weight VWF multimers.
  3. VWD type 2B is a rare qualitative defect with a "gain of function" point mutation in the GP1b binding domain of VWF. Patients have spontaneous platelet agglutination resulting in thrombocytopenia. There is absence of high–molecular-weight VWF multimers. DDAVP administration is contraindicated.
  4. VWD type 2M is a rare, mostly autosomal dominant, qualitative defect with moderate to severe bleeding. There is a defect in the GP1b binding domain of VWF preventing binding to platelets.

TABLE 10-5. Subtypes of von Willebrand Disease

Type	vWF Ag	FVIII	Ristocetin Cofactor	Ristocetin-induced Platelet Aggregation	Multimers
1	↓	↓	↓	N/↓	N (globally ↓)
2A	↓/N	↓/N	↓	↓	HMW absent
2B	↓/N	↓/N	↓/N	↑	HMW absent
2M	N	N	↓	↓	N
2N	N	↓	N	N	N
3	↓	↓	↓	↓	↓ (globally low)
Platelet type	↓/N	↓/N	↓	↑	N

N, normal; ↓, decreased; ↑, increased with low-dose ristocetin; HMW, high molecular weight multimers.

In types 2A, 2B, and 2M there is a low ratio (<0.7) of vWF activity to antigen.

5. VWD type 2N is a rare qualitative defect with moderate to severe bleeding. There is a defect in the FVIII binding domain of vWF. It simulates hemophilia.

6. VWD type 3 is a rare quantitative defect with severe bleeding. These patients may develop alloantibodies to VWF after receiving multiple transfusions.

7. Platelet-type VWD is not a genuine VWD variant (see p. 876), but a qualitative defect in platelets caused by a gain of function in the GP1b receptor on platelets. That leads to increased avidity for VWF resulting in spontaneous platelet agglutination and thrombocytopenia. Platelet type VWD can be differentiated from VWD type IIB by mixing or cryoprecipitate studies. Platelets from Bernard-Soulier syndrome (see p. 876) do not aggregate in the presence of ristocetin. The condition must be differentiated from VWD.

• Acquired VWD is seen in lymphoproliferative neoplasms, multiple myeloma, MGUS, autoimmune diseases, hypothyroidism, aortic stenosis due to sheer stress-enhanced proteolysis, ventricular septal defects, and GI telangiectasia

• The major patterns to differentiate various types of VWD are described in Table 10-5.

➤ Limitations
• vWF Ag and activity levels run 20–30% lower in group O than in individuals with other blood groups.
• VWF levels fluctuate. Both the VWF and factor VIII are acute-phase reactants. Levels may increase 2–5 times from baseline in the third trimester of pregnancy, with strenuous exercise and severe stress. Repeated testing may be required.

➤ Suggested Reading
Nichols WL, Hultin MB, James AH, et al. von Willebrand disease (VWD): evidence-based diagnosis and management guidelines, the National Heart, Lung, and Blood Institute (NHLBI) expert panel report (USA). *Hemophilia.* 2008;14:171–232.

Sadler JE, Budde U, Eikenboom, JC, et al. Update of the pathophysiology and classification of von Willebrand disease: a report of the Subcommittee on von Willebrand Factor. *J Thromb Haemost.* 2006;4:2103–2114.

FACTOR XII (F XII) DEFICIENCY

➤ Definition

- F XII deficiency was first described preoperatively in a Mr. Hageman (hence the synonym Hageman factor) who was found to have a prolonged PTT, no bleeding history, and no deficiency of any known clotting protein. He succumbed to a thrombotic event. Affected patients have no bleeding diathesis. The fact that patients with severe deficiency of F XII, prekallikrein, and low–molecular-weight kininogen do not bleed, even when exposed to severe trauma or surgery, suggest that these proteins play no, or a minimal, role in hemostasis.
- The controversy about an increase incidence of thrombosis and myocardial infarction in patients with severe F XII deficiency has not been resolved.

➤ Decreased Levels

- Congenital: Autosomal recessive inheritance: Levels of F XII are 40–60% in heterozygous state, and are undetectable in homozygotes.
- Acquired
  - Septic shock
  - Severe liver disease
  - Nephrotic syndrome
  - Type II hyperlipoproteinemia
  - Patients with anticardiolipins may have circulating antibodies to F XII in addition to falsely decreased F XII levels in patients with lupus anticoagulant (see p. 249).

FACTOR XI (F XI) DEFICIENCY

- F XI deficiency is in most cases an inherited autosomal recessive disorder. More than 100 mutations have been described in the F XI gene. Although F XI deficiency is rare in the population at large, it is common in Ashkenazi Jews and in some Arab groups.
- Bleeding is highly variable. Patients with mild F XI deficiency can experience bleeding complications, and those with severe deficiencies may not bleed excessively. In general the homozygous patients display a severe deficiency of measurable F XI, from <1% to 20%. It is not usually associated with spontaneous hemorrhage, but these individuals may bleed excessively after injury or surgery, particularly of body areas with high fibrinolytic activity, such as dental surgery. Spontaneous abortions have been seen in one patient with severe F XI deficiency by the author.

➤ Suggested Reading

Lorand L. Factor XIII and the clotting of fibrinogen: from basic research to medicine. *J Thromb Haemost.* 2005;3:1337–1348.

FACTOR XIII (F XIII) DEFICIENCY

➤ Definition

- F XIII deficiency is a rare condition that leads to a bleeding diathesis of varying intensity. It is inherited as an autosomal disorder.

- Congenital
  - A variety of mutations lead to F XIII deficiency. Most patients deficient in F XIII lack the factor in plasma and in platelets.
  - In the homozygous deficiency patients have a severe bleeding diathesis. Bleeding a few days after birth at the umbilical cord site occurs in most severely affected cases. Heterozygous deficient subject may be subjected to delayed bleeding and impaired wound healing.
- Acquired
  - Liver disease, prematurity, plasmacytoma, surgery, DIC
  - Acute promyelocytic and some chronic leukemias
  - Alloantibodies may develop in severely deficient patients after therapeutic exposure to the antigen. Antibody inhibitors may develop after exposure to certain drugs such as phenytoin, isoniazid, penicillin, or valproic acid.
  - Antibodies against F XIII may result in severe bleeding.

➤ **Tests**

- A qualitative assay investigates the clot solubility in 5 molar urea (a plasma clot from a patient deficient in F XIII is easily dissolved in urea, acids, and bases). In the absence of F XIII, the clots remain soluble. If the test is positive, mixing studies are recommended to rule out a factor XIII inhibitor. If no inhibitor is detected, the deficiency should be confirmed by a quantitative test.
- Deficiency of F XIII does not affect PT (INR), PTT, thrombin time, or fibrinogen levels.
- F XIII is unaffected by vitamin K deficiency or oral anticoagulants.

ACQUIRED HEMORRHAGIC DISORDERS OF MULTIFACTORIAL ETIOLOGY

DISSEMINATED INTRAVASCULAR COAGULATION (DIC)

➤ **Definition**

- DIC is an acquired systemic complex syndrome producing both hemorrhages and thrombosis. It is a secondary condition that develops as a complication to a variety of disorders (Table 10-6).
- DIC consists of the systemic activation of coagulation, resulting in multiple thrombi in the microcirculation, consumption of clotting proteins and platelets (in the past, the syndrome has also been called consumption coagulopathy), in turn leading to a hemorrhagic diathesis. The fibrinolytic mechanism becomes activated in parallel, exacerbating the hemorrhagic tendency.
- Most cases of DIC are overt (acute), with the majority of patients being cared for and diagnosed in intensive care units. In cases of nonovert (chronic and low-grade DIC), blood coagulation is continuously or intermittently activated by small amounts of tissue factor, such as may be released from disseminated malignancies.

➤ **Tests**

- The laboratory findings of DIC are variable. They depend on the underlying etiology and stage of the syndrome. Some assays such as fibrinogen, an acute-phase reactant, may be elevated early on, but decrease progressively due to their consumption as the condition progresses. Pathologic fibrinolysis may diminish or disappear in very severe cases when the fibrinolytic proteins are completely consumed.

TABLE 10-6. Common Underlying Etiologies of Disseminated Intravascular Coagulation (DIC)

Infections	Bacterial septicemias, gram positive and negative. High prevalence in meningococcemia Viremia
Shock	Septic Hemorrhagic
Metabolic abnormalities	Acidosis
Obstetrical accidents	Eclampsia, amniotic fluid embolism, retained dead fetus, abruptio placentae
Neoplasms	Metastatic neoplasms, especially pancreas, prostate; adenocarcinomas
Hematologic conditions	Acute leukemias, especially promyelocytic Intravascular hemolysis due to mismatched transfusions Myeloproliferative disorders
Physical injuries	Massive or blunt trauma with extensive tissue injury; extensive surgery Burns
Vascular malformation (chronic disseminated intravascular coagulation)	Capillary hemangiomas (Kasabach-Merritt syndrome); giant hemangiomas; large aortic aneurysm
Toxins	Snake bites, brown recluse spider bites

- Conversely, excessive fibrinolysis may develop without DIC, as with direct infusion of thrombolytic agents and in patient with prostate cancer.
- Because DIC is primarily a bedside diagnosis, the diagnosis is established when, in addition to bleeding and thrombotic events, end-organ injury is documented.
- Repeated laboratory studies are more useful than a single determination. The findings described below are categorized in three groups.
  1. Procoagulant activation and consumption
     - PT, PTT, and thrombin time may be variably prolonged, but are nonspecific, and hence of little diagnostic value.
     - Fibrinogen is useful in serial studies, since it can demonstrate a dynamic process of consumption coagulopathy. As a single determination it is less useful, especially during the initial phase when it may be greatly elevated.
     - Platelet counts may be decreased, but thrombocytopenia is nonspecific. In cases of thrombocytopenia and thrombosis, HIT may have to be excluded (see p. 207).
     - Best markers of hypercoagulability are elevated D-dimer (see p. 152). To avoid false-positive results, a less sensitive assay, such as semi-quantitative latex is recommended

rather than the ELISA-type supersensitive D-dimer tests used to rule out DVT and PE (see p. 152).
- The following assays are reproducible and have a high PPV but are not available in most hospital laboratories: increased prothrombin fragments (F1 and F2), fibrinopeptides A and B, thrombin-antithrombin complexes, and soluble fibrin.
- Many clotting factors or inhibitory proteins (protein C and S) are decreased because of their consumption. The most sensitive and undergoing highest decrease are factors V and VIII. Their determination is generally not necessary for the diagnosis of DIC.
- Because DIC is a microangiopathic syndrome (see p. 813), hemolytic anemia with schistocytes on the peripheral blood smear develops in severe cases.
2. Fibrinolytic activation: Increased levels of fibrin (ogen) degradation products (FDP), latex D-dimer (see above), and soluble fibrin (not widely available). In primary fibrinolysis FDP are greatly elevated, whereas D-dimers are not. Platelet counts are normal.
3. Inhibitor consumption
- Progressive decrease in antithrombin (ATIII) (see p. 64)
- Increased levels of thrombin-antithrombin and plasmin-antiplasmin
- Decrease in α2 antiplasmin (not necessary for diagnosis)

➤ Recommendations
- We have suggested a simple, selective "DIC profile" based on the three categories mentioned above: titration of latex D-dimer, FDP, and ATIII. The ATIII assay is helpful for observing the evolution of the syndrome, since its marked decrease connotes a poor prognosis. FDP and D-dimers are elevated in chronic DIC as well. In addition to the above panel, chemistry panels to assess end-organ injury are mandatory.
- Other recommendations have been published by the International Society on Thrombosis and Haemostasis in 2003 and reviewed in 2007 and by the Japanese Ministry of Health and Welfare in 1987.

➤ Suggested Readings
Toh CH, Hoots WK on behalf of the SSC on Disseminated Intravascular coagulation of the ISTH. The scoring system of the Scientific and Standardization Committee on Disseminated Intravascular coagulation of the International Society on Thrombosis and Haemostasis: a 5-year overview. *J Thromb Haemost.* 2007;5:604–606.

Yu M, Nardella A, Pechet L. Screening tests of disseminated intravascular coagulation: guidelines for rapid and specific laboratory diagnosis. *Crit Care Med.* 2000;28:1777–1780.

HEMOSTATIC FAILURE IN CARDIOPULMONARY BYPASS SURGERY

➤ Definition
- Bleeding is a common complication in patients undergoing open heart surgery. Its etiology is multifactorial, as reflected in multiple laboratory abnormalities. Platelets, the fibrinolytic system, both the extrinsic and intrinsic coagulation pathways, and the complement system are activated.
- The principal causes of bleeding in bypass surgery are: excess heparin, fibrinolysis, and decrease in platelet number and function.

➤ Tests

- Hemostasis, platelet function, and fibrinolysis can be monitored by conventional techniques, or at the surgical room site, by a thromboelastogram.
  - Thrombocytopathy (functional platelet defect): frequent occurrence due to platelet activation during bypass; exacerbated by the use of drugs that interfere with platelet function
  - Thrombocytopenia: platelets decline temporarily. By the end of surgery their number is typically reduced by 40–60% due to hemodilution, activation, and consumption during bypass procedure. Occasionally the decline may be more profound and compromise hemostasis.
  - Hyperfibrinolysis: elevated fibrin(ogen) degradation products (FDP) (see p. 178).
  - The effect of heparin and its neutralization by protamine. Heparin-related causes of bleeding are caused primarily by incomplete inactivation by protamine. "Heparin rebound" is a term that refers to delayed release of heparin from the lymphatic system after protamine has already been cleared from plasma. It may result in bleeding after completion of surgery. "Heparin resistance" may be secondary to antithrombin III deficiency. Excessive infusion of protamine may itself result in bleeding.
  - DIC. The concentrations of D-dimer (see p. 152) and of fibrinopeptides A and B are increased.

COAGULOPATHY OF LIVER DISEASE

➤ Definition

- A syndrome of excessive bleeding, occasionally thrombosis, resulting from severe liver disease. The coagulopathy is multifactorial, due to liver's many functions in hemostasis and thrombosis.
  - Decreased synthesis in clotting factors → bleeding. Prekallikrein and factor VII are ones of the earliest clotting proteins to be decreased in liver disease. Fibrinogen is one of the last ones.
  - Decreased clearing of activated clotting factors (especially factor Xa) → tendency to DIC.
  - Decreased synthesis of plasminogen and antithrombin → tendency to thrombosis.
  - Decreased synthesis of fibrinolytic inhibitors → excessive fibrinolysis with increased bleeding.
  - Synthesis of abnormal clotting factors → bleeding; occasionally risk of thrombosis.
  - Hypersplenism → thrombocytopenia that exacerbates bleeding.
  - The coagulopathy of liver transplantation is extremely complex, with DIC and pathologic fibrinolysis predominating.

➤ Tests

- PT is prolonged (INR is not recommended to evaluate liver function or bleeding diathesis). If PT is >4 seconds longer than the upper limit of the normal range, it is an indicator of poor prognosis.
- PTT is prolonged, but less consistently than PT.
- Factors V, VII, II, IX, X, fibrinogen, but not factor VIII, are decreased.
- Antithrombin III is decreased.
- Fibrinolytic inhibitors: thrombin activatable fibrinolytic inhibitor (TAFI), plasminogen activator inhibitor-1 (PAI-1), and α2-antiplasmin are decreased.

- DIC screen (see p. 883) may be positive. The differentiation between DIC and excessive fibrinolysis may be difficult. The two conditions may coexist.

ANTICOAGULANTS, CIRCULATING

➤ Definition
- Circulating anticoagulants are antibodies that inhibit the function of specific coagulation factors, most commonly factors VIII or IX. They may be acquired following multiple transfusions in hemophiliacs (alloantibodies), or spontaneous (autoantibodies), again, most commonly against factor VIII (see p. 878).
- LA (see p. 249).

➤ Who Should be Suspected?
- A circulating anticoagulant is suspected under two conditions:
  - A patient with hemophilia A or B who has had multiple transfusions whose bleeding does not stop on infusion of the missing factor.
  - A middle-aged person, especially if suffering from lymphoma, or a postpartum patient who develops unprovoked hemorrhages.

➤ Interpretation
- In a patient with hemophilia, serial determinations of the missing factor show no elevations following infusions.
- In a patient with no previous bleeding history, the finding of a prolonged PTT should raise the suspicion of an acquired circulating anticoagulant. If incubation at 37°C of half the normal plasma mixed with half the patient's plasma for 1–2 hours does not correct the prolonged PTT, a circulating anticoagulant is present.
- Specific titration of the inhibitor's potency is performed either for factor VIII or IX inhibitors, and the results reported in Bethesda Inhibitor units.

THROMBOTIC DISORDERS

THROMBOPHILIA*

➤ Definition
- The term thrombophilia refers to the propensity to develop thrombosis due to an abnormality in the coagulation system (i.e., a hypercoagulable state). The abnormality may be congenital or acquired. The thrombosis may have a predilection for arteries or veins. There is no urgency in obtaining thrombophilia tests for patients who present with an acute venous thromboembolism (VTE), because this information does not alter acute therapy decisions.
- Consider obtaining a thrombophilia work-up, if indicated, when the patient has recovered from the acute event and ideally when warfarin and/or heparin administration have been discontinued for at least 2–4 weeks.

---

*Prepared with Reema Jaffar, M.D.

➤ Who Should be Suspected?

I. Suspected inherited thrombophilia
  A. Venous thrombophilia
  - Family history of VTE
  - VTE at a young age (< 45 years)
  - Recurrent VTE without obvious risk factors
  - VTE following minimal or no provocation
  - VTE at an unusual site (upper extremity, mesenteric vein, cerebral vein)
  - Pulmonary embolism (PE) without known etiology
  - Neonatal purpura fulminans
  - Warfarin-induced skin necrosis
  B. Arterial thrombophilia
  - Patients with unexpected/unexplained arterial thrombotic events.
II. Suspected acquired hypercoagulability
  - Patients with unprovoked venous or arterial thromboembolism in the absence of a known family history. Some patients may have both venous *and* arterial thrombotic events.

➤ Tests

I. Suspected inherited thrombophilia
  A. Venous thrombophilia
  - First-tier tests*
    - Activated Protein C Resistance (APCR): functional assay
    - Prothrombin G20210A: genetic assay
    - Protein C activity**: functional assay
    - Protein S activity**: functional assay
    - Antithrombin (AT) activity: functional assay
  - Second-tier tests
    - Factor V Leiden mutation (if APCR is abnormal): Genetic assay
    - Protein C antigen (if functional test is low): Immunologic assay
    - Protein S antigen (total and free) (if functional test is low): Immunologic assay
    - AT antigen (if functional test is low), except in DIC, heparin therapy or liver disease: Immunologic assays are rarely necessary
  - Third-tier tests
    - Thrombin time and fibrinogen for dysfibrinogenemia
    - Selected clotting factors (fibrinogen, factors VII, VIII, IX, vWF) to assess marked elevations–their usefulness is not definitely documented
    - Homocysteine (may be of value for congenital arterial thrombophilia as well)
  B. Arterial thrombophilia***
  - Lipid profile
  - Lipoprotein a
  - Homocysteine

---

*All five first-tier tests should be ordered together, because inherited venous thrombophilia cases are often due to a polygenic effect.

**Warfarin therapy reduces vitamin K–dependent factors including proteins C, S, and Z. Testing for protein Z is not recommended at this time.

***There is no documented indication to order the tests suggested for venous thrombophilia in cases of arterial thrombophilia (except for APCR in pediatric thrombophilia with idiopathic ischemic stroke)

II. Suspected acquired hypercoagulability

- First-tier tests:
  - Lupus anticoagulant
  - Anticardiolipin and anti-β2 glycoprotein 1 antibodies (IgG, and IgM)
  - Antinuclear antibodies (ANA)
  - DIC (recommended DIC panel: FDP, Latex D-dimer, antithrombin) (see p. 883)
  - DVT/PE: a sensitive, quantitative assay for D-dimers (see p. 152) to be used in relation with a probability algorithm
  - Lipid profile
  - Homocysteine
- Second-tier tests:
  - Comprehensive investigation of possible underlying neoplasm or a myeloproliferative disorder, including JAK-2 mutation
  - To be ruled out
    - Pregnancy
    - Paroxysmal nocturnal hemoglobinuria (PNH)–flow cytometry (see p. 810)
    - Chemotherapy, Thalidomide and Tamoxifen
  - If TTP is strongly suspected (see p. 889) start therapy and order ADAMTS 13 assay
  - If promyelocytic leukemia (M3 in FAB classification) is suspected, order diagnostic tests (FISH, karyotype, flow cytometry) on bone marrow aspirate, and start therapy promptly

➤ Suggested Readings

Dahlback B. Advances in understanding pathogenic mechanisms of thrombophilic disorders. *Blood.* 2008;112: 19–27.
Tripodi A, Mannucci PM. Laboratory Investigation of Thrombophilia. *Clin Chem.* 2001;47:1597–1606.

THROMBOTIC THROMBOCYTOPENIC PURPURA/ HEMOLYTIC UREMIC SYNDROME (TTP/HUS)

➤ Definition

- TTP and HUS are severe thrombotic microangiopathies characterized by systemic platelet aggregates causing organ ischemia that involves multiple organ systems, thrombocytopenia, and fragmentation of red cells. These conditions are expressed by microangiopathic hemolytic anemia (see p. 813), thrombocytopenia, neurologic, and renal involvement.
- TTP and HUS are disorders with many similarities. There are, however, sufficient differences between these conditions to be considered separately.

➤ Who Should be Suspected?
TTP

- Classically, patients with TTP present with the following pentad: fever, microangiopathic hemolytic anemia, thrombocytopenia, and impaired renal and neurologic function. In reality, most patients have some, but not all, of the components of the pentad.
- TTP may be congenital, resulting from a deficiency in the protease ADAMTS 13, or acquired, resulting from antibodies against ADAMTS 13, or following certain infections or drugs (Figure 10-3).
- ADAMTS 13 is a metalloprotease, that cleaves very large molecular weight components of the pro-vWF, thereby reducing the propensity of the pro-vWF to agglutinate platelets in

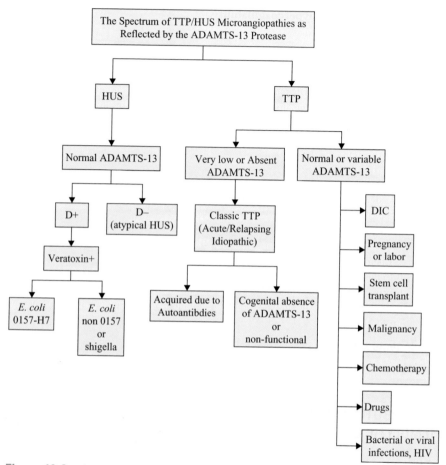

Figure 10-3. The spectrum of thrombotic thrombocytopenic purpura (TTP)/hemolytic uremic syndrome (HUS) microangiopathies as reflected by the ADAMTS 13 protease. *E. coli, Escherichia coli.*

vivo. Its absence results in release into the circulation of very high–molecular-weight vWF multimers.

- Because of wide variation in presentation of TTP, in clinical practice the combination of otherwise unexplained thrombocytopenia (see p. 868) and microangiopathic hemolytic anemia (see p. 804) are sufficient to suspect the diagnosis of TTP.

- TTP can be broadly divided into two categories: the acute idiopathic (classic) TTP seen in about one third of cases, and secondary TTP (in two thirds of cases), those in which a causative condition or agent can be identified: bacterial or viral (including AIDS) infections, pregnancy (especially during the third trimester and postpartum period), certain drugs: ADP inhibitors of platelet function (ticlopidine [rarely used now], and infrequently clopidogrel), quinine, mitomycin C, cisplatinum, bleomycin, α-interferon, cyclosporine, tacrolimus, other immunosuppressive or chemotherapeutic agents, disseminated malignancy, and allogeneic stem cell transplantation. Classic TTP occurs primarily in adults and has a higher incidence in women. The rare congenital type has been described as the Upshaw-Schulman syndrome.

HUS

* HUS is predominantly a pediatric disease. It presents commonly in a child who recently had abdominal pain and bloody diarrhea, and develops acute microangiopathic hemolytic anemia, thrombocytopenia, and acute renal failure. It is a complication of an infection caused by a verotoxin-producing strain of *E. coli* 0157:H7 (most common cause in the United States) or *Shigella* (see Figure 10-3). In different countries other bacteria have been found to be the etiologic agent in HUS. HUS is a self-limited disease.
* Because the preceding diarrhea is not universal, HUS had been divided into two categories: diarrhea-associated (D+) (the common form) and non-diarrhea associated (D−) or atypical HUS, which comprises approximately 10% of cases. Approximately half of the patients with the atypical form have mutations in genes that regulate the complement system with deficiency of complement factor H. In these patients a low serum C3 level may be detected.

➤ Tests
TTP

* CBC
    * Microangiopathic hemolytic anemia with Hb <8g/L
    * WBC may be increased (with neutrophilia) or normal counts
    * Platelets: severe thrombocytopenia (usually <20,000/μL) rapidly responsive to effective therapy.
    * PBS: Fragmented red cells (schistocytes) (see p. 321) represent >1% of RBC (or two or more per HPF); they decrease with response to therapy (schistocytes are absent in rare cases). Characteristics: nucleated red cells; basophilic stippling; polychromasia resulting from reticulocytosis.
* LDH is very elevated (>1,000 U/L at presentation is not unusual); LDH levels decrease with therapy and are useful in assessing response.
* Haptoglobin is decreased
* Indirect bilirubin is elevated
* Direct Coombs test is negative
* Coagulation studies are normal and help in ruling out DIC (see p. 883)
* Increased creatinine may occur, but marked increase favors HUS
* Serology for HIV is necessary to rule out HIV as a causative agent
* ADAMTS 13 (see Figure 10-3)
    * The value of measurements of this protease and its inhibitors at the time of diagnosis remain uncertain. Moreover, because it is performed in only a few reference laboratories, its turnaround time (TAT) may be long (although the technology is improving and shortening of TAT is expected); as a consequence, ADAMTS 13 measurements are helpful retroactively to confirm the diagnosis of TTP, and for follow-up because the assay provides useful prognostic information.
    * *Under no circumstances should the clinician wait for results of ADAMTS 13 levels or antibodies against the enzyme before starting therapy when other criteria for TTP are present.* Undetectable plasma levels of ADAMTS 13 (<5%) are specific for TTP. They have been found in

idiopathic TTP, and in TTP associated with pregnancy, autoimmune diseases, and ADP inhibitors of platelet function. The absence of ADAMTS 13 at the time of diagnosis is predictive of relapsing episodes in about 20–30% of cases. Absence of measurable enzyme during remission predicts relapse in 60% of patients.

* In TTP secondary to allogeneic stem cell transplantation, chemotherapy and other drugs, as well as in HUS (see below) the levels of the protease are normal. ADAMTS 13 testing is not helpful in most patients with secondary TTP. Because >90% of idiopathic TTP cases are acquired and due to anti-ADAMTS 13 antibodies, the antibodies assay should be performed at the same time with the measurement of the enzyme. The results may influence therapy but prospective studies are not available yet.

HUS

* CBC, LDH, haptoglobin, indirect bilirubin, direct Coombs and coagulation results are similar to those of TTP.
* Creatinine is very elevated at presentation in most cases.
* Urinalysis may show proteinuria and red cell casts.
* Plasminogen activator inhibitor 1 (PAI-1) (see p. 290) has been found to be very elevated in children with D+ HUS.
* ADAMTS 13 is normal in most childhood HUS.

➤ Suggested Readings

George JN. How I treat patients with thrombotic thrombocytopenic purpura:2010 *Blood.* 2010;116:4060–4069.

Sadler JE. Von Willebrand factor, ADAMTS 13, and thrombotic thrombocytopenic purpura. *Blood.* 2008;112:11–18.

Veyrader A, Meyer D. Thrombotic thrombocytopenic purpura and its diagnosis. *J Thromb Haemost.* 2005;3:2420–2427.

TRANSFUSION MEDICINE

TRANSFUSION OF BLOOD PRODUCTS

➤ Indications

* The indications for blood products vary for different components. The indications as practiced at our institution (slightly modified) are presented in Table 10-7. With respect to transfusing RBCs, the most widely used components, there are a few general principles:
  * RBC transfusions are given to raise the Hct level in patients with anemia or to replace losses after acute bleeding episodes. Formal guidelines for RBC transfusions and volume replacement in adults were issued in 2001 by the British Committee for Standards in Haematology.
  * Mandatory tests prior to blood transfusions are ABO and Rh type, DAT (direct Coombs test), and antibody screen. Subsequent compatibility tests are based on the results of these tests. The decision whether to transfuse a blood component must be based on an assessment of the risk of anemia or thrombocytopenia versus the risk of transfusions (see below).

TABLE 10-7. Indications for Blood Transfusion and Special Product Processing

Red Blood Cells (after bleeding has stopped, one unit packed RBC increases recipient's Hb 1 g/dL)
  Active blood loss
  Hct ≤21% or Hb ≤7 g/dL
  Hct ≤24% or Hb ≤8 g/dL and symptomatic
  Hct ≤25% or Hb ≤8.3 g/dL and acute coronary syndrome
  Other indications
Platelets
  Platelets ≤10,000/μL
  Platelets ≤20,000/μL and sepsis, multisystem failure or high risk for outpatient hemorrhage
  Platelets ≤50,000/μL with surgery or active bleeding
  Platelet function defect and symptomatic or impending surgery/invasive procedure
  Intraoperative hemostatic defect
Special blood product processing (not routinely needed)
  Irradiated blood products
    Directed donor product from blood relative (to avoid graft-versus-host disease)
    Intensive chemotherapy with marrow suppression
    Stem cell transplant candidate or recipient
    Newborn, prematurity, intrauterine transfusion
  Washed blood cell products
    Congenital IgA deficiency with anti-IgA antibodies
    Repeated severe hypersensitivity transfusion reactions despite appropriate medication
Plasma
  Prolonged prothrombin time (e.g., liver disease) and symptomatic or invasive procedure planned
  Factor XI or XIII deficiency
  Thrombotic microangiopathy
  C1 esterase inhibitor deficiency (hereditary angioedema) and symptomatic
  Intraoperative hemostatic defect
  Overdose of oral vitamin K antagonist with evidence of bleeding
  As volume expander
Cryoprecipitate (contains fibrinogen, factors VIII and XIII, von Willebrand factor, and fibronectin)
  Mild factor VIII deficiency and symptomatic or with surgery/invasive procedure
  Von Willebrand disease and symptomatic or with surgery/invasive procedure
  Hypofibrinogenemia and symptomatic or with surgery/invasive procedure
  Intraoperative hemostatic defect
Leukocyte-reduced blood products
  ≥2 documented febrile transfusion reactions
    Chronically transfusion-dependent
  Transplant candidate or recipient
  High cytomegalovirus risk
    Patient is a pregnant woman
    Newborn, premature, intrauterine transfusion
    Patient undergoing splenectomy
    Patient with congenital immune deficiency

➤ Adverse Effects of Blood Transfusions (Table 10-8)

* Although blood transfusion is increasingly safe, it remains hazardous in many respects. Adverse effects occur in ~1 in 1000 components, and ~1 in every 38,000 RBC to units transfused, mostly due an error-related ABO-incompatible transfusion, with possible of dire consequences.
* Most acute hemolytic transfusion reactions are due to clerical errors.
* The two other major causes of transfusion-related complications are TRALI (transfusion-related acute lung injury) and infection due to bacterial contamination. TRALI is estimated to occur in 1 of every 5000 transfusions with a mortality of up to 15%. It is the most frequent cause of transfusion-related mortality: 48% of the confirmed transfusion-related deaths in the U.S. TRALI occurs during or within 6 hours after transfusion. It has characteristic clinical (sudden onset of acute respiratory distress, fever, tachycardia, and tachypnea) and radiographic features characteristic of ARDS, secondary to leukocytes accumulating in the lungs, with no evidence of circulatory overload. The exact etiology is still debated. It seems to be the result of antibodies from the donor directed against leukocyte antigens, including HLA antibodies as well as platelet-derived sCD40L, a proinflammatory cytokine. TRALI has been observed after transfusions of most plasma-containing components.

➤ Suggested Readings

Alter HJ, Klein HG. The hazards of blood transfusion in historical perspective. *Blood.* 2008;112:2617–2626.

British Committee for Standards in Haematology. Blood Transfusion Task Force. *Br J Haematol.* 2001;113:24–31.

Shaz BH, Stowell SR, Hillyer CD. Transfusion-related acute lung injury: from the bedside to bench and back. *Blood.* 2011;117:1463–1471.

Vamvakas EC, Blajchman MA. Transfusion-related mortality: the ongoing risk of allogeneic blood transfusion and the available strategies for their prevention. *Blood.* 2009;113:3406–3417.

IRON OVERLOAD DISORDERS (IOD) AND HEREDITARY HEMOCHROMATOSIS (HH)

➤ Definition

* The term IOD refers to patients with increased iron stores resulting from iron supply that exceeds the body's ability to eliminate it. Due to iron toxicity, its excess results in tissue damage (liver cirrhosis often followed by hepatocellular carcinoma, diabetes, and cardiomyopathy). IOD may be primary, commonly hereditary, or secondary (acquired). The most common form of IOD in the United States is HH.
* Hereditary (primary) hemochromatosis
  * HH is an HLA-linked autosomal recessive defect, caused by increased duodenal absorption of iron, leading to excess iron deposition in various organs. HH is the result of an abnormal gene present in 10% of white Americans (see below under Genetic studies). The manifest disease, in contrast with the genotypical or biochemical phenotype, is quite rare.
  * Other genetic forms of hemochromatosis: juvenile hereditary hemochromatosis, neonatal hemochromatosis
  * Aceruloplasminemia

TABLE 10-8. Adverse Effects of Blood Transfusions

Condition/Infection	Frequency or Risk/Unit Transfused
Immune-Mediated	
Acute	
Acute hemolytic transfusion reactions. Laboratory findings reflect acute intravascular hemolysis, acute renal failure, disseminated intravascular coagulation (DIC), and cardiovascular failure.	1 in 76,000 acute hemolytic reactions; 1 in 1.8 million incompatible units transfused are fatal.
Anamnestic antibody response commonly due to previous sensitization of RBCs against minor (non-ABO) blood group antibodies; results in delayed (2–10 days) transfusion reaction with extravascular hemolysis. Mild clinical and laboratory findings. Rarely it can be severe, even fatal, especially in patients with sickle cell anemia	1 in 6000 units transfused
Febrile nonhemolytic reaction; occurs 1–6 hours after transfusion. WBC or cytokine induced and is usually accompanied by dyspnea, rigors, hypotension, or hypertension	<1% to >16% for RBC transfusions 30% of platelet transfusions
Allergic transfusion reaction	1:333
Acute anaphylaxis (shock, hypotension, angioedema, respiratory distress); occurs a few seconds to a few minutes into transfusion.	1:20,000 to 1:50,000 may be more common
Transfusion-related acute lung injury (TRALI)	1:1000 to 1:2400 blood component transfusions
Chronic (delayed)	
Alloimmunization	
RBC hemolysis	1 in 1500
Delayed hemolysis	1 in 4000
Platelet refractoriness (multifactorial: alloimmunization, sepsis, splenomegaly)	1 in 3300–10,000
Graft-versus-host disease* (transfusion associated).	Very rare; appears to be increasing
Posttransfusion purpura: thrombocytopenia 5–10 days after blood transfusion containing platelets	1 in 7000 transfusions
Nonimmune Mediated	
Acute (immediate)	
Volume overload	1:100–1:200
Nonimmune hemolysis (heat, cold, osmotic, mechanical)	Infrequent

(*Continued*)

TABLE 10-8. Adverse Effects of Blood Transfusions (*Continued*)

Condition/Infection	Frequency or Risk/Unit Transfused
Electrolyte imbalance (K$^+$, Mg^2, Ca^{2+})	Uncommon
Chemical effects (excess citrate)	Uncommon
Coagulopathy (e.g., DIC; usually with massive transfusions)	Uncommon
Chronic (delayed)	
Platelet refractoriness	1:3300–1:10,000
Transfusional hemosiderosis	Multiple transfusions in aplastic anemia, MDS, sickle cell anemia, thalassemia major
Infections	
Viral	
Hepatitis A	1:1,000,000**
Hepatitis B	1:50,000 to 1:170,000**
Hepatitis C	1: 1–2,000,000
HIV	<1:2,000,000**
HTLV types I and II	1:19,000 to 1:80,000**
Cytomegalovirus	3–12 in 100; infrequent with leukocyte-reduced components
Parvovirus B19	1:10,000** (more common with plasma-derived products)
RBV	Rare
Human herpes virus 8	3.2% seroprevalence
West Nile, other arboviruses	23 confirmed cases in the United States by 2002
Dengue fever	2 cases confirmed
Prion-caused	
Classic and variant Creutzfeldt-Jakob disease and bovine spongiform encephalopathy	4 probable cases reported in United Kingdom
Bacterial	
Bacterial contamination per RBCs unit transfused in the United States	1:500,000
Bacterial contamination per platelets unit	1:5000
Syphilis	
Chlamydia pneumonia	Likely, but no definitive evidence
Rocky Mountain spotted fever (*Rickettsia rickettsii*), Rickettsia	Unknown

TABLE 10-8. (*Continued*)	
Condition/Infection	Frequency or Risk/Unit Transfused
Parasitic	
Plasmodium	1:4,000,000
Babesia	>20 reported cases
Trypanosoma cruzi (Chagas disease)	Unknown
Leishmania	<1:20,000

*__Transfusion-associated graft versus host disease (TA-GVHD)__ occurs when immunocompetent T lymphocytes are transfused into a patient who cannot reject them, and they engraft in the recipient, proliferate, and mount an immune attack against the host tissues. TA-GVHD occurs 4–30 days after transfusion of any cellular blood component. It may occur in a nonimmunocompetent recipient or in an immunocompetent recipient who receives histocompatible donor lymphocytes, especially from blood relatives, which can recognize a different HLA haplotype in the recipient. There are molecular techniques to diagnosis TA-GVHD. Mortality is nearly 90% in the full-blown syndrome. Leukoreduction may reduce this complication.
**Estimates published by the British Committee for Standards in Haematology (see Suggested Readings)

- Mutations in transferrin receptor-22 or ferroportin-1, and African iron overload (combined hereditary increased absorption and excess intake, seen particularly in Bantu populations).
- Congenital atransferrinemia
- Secondary hemochromatosis
  - Increased, persistent (e.g., long term) intake of iron medication
  - Anemias with ineffective erythropoiesis and/or extravascular hemolysis (especially if associated with multiple transfusions): sickle cell anemia, β thalassemia major, aplastic anemia, myelodysplastic syndromes
  - Chronic hemodialysis
  - Porphyria cutanea tarda (minor)
  - Alcoholic liver disease (iron deposited in Kupffer cells) and other chronic liver disorders
  - Following portosystemic shunts

➤ Who Should be Suspected?
- IOD should be suspected in individuals with a family history of HH, or in its absence, in those with chronic liver disease, or diabetes without predisposing factors, and in patients with unexplained arthritis and cardiomyopathy.
- Individuals with the secondary form of IOD have usually a history of a disease predisposing to increased iron stores, or of multiple RBC transfusions.

➤ Tests
- The presence of IOD is established by the demonstration of increased body iron using: serum iron studies, radiologic techniques (MRI using special techniques), liver biopsy, and assessment of response to phlebotomy or iron chelation. When one of the hereditary forms is suspected, genetic studies are helpful.

- Transferrin saturation (see p. 363) is the best method for screening populations of North European ancestry suspected for IOD. A persistent value of >45% starting early in life, remains the best predictive phenotypic test for the homozygous C282Y mutation (see below). Percent transferrin saturation is frequently >70%, and may reach 100%.
- Total iron binding capacity is an assay similar to transferrin saturation, and parallels it, increasing with increase in iron store.
- Increased serum ferritin (see p. 174) is found in ~ two thirds of patients with IOD. Levels >350 μg/L in men and >250 μg/L in women are the recommended thresholds for further screening for IOD. The serum ferritin is usually >1000 μg/L at the time of diagnosis and it indicates biochemical accumulation of tissue iron. The critical threshold associated with the development of liver cirrhosis is unknown.
- Serum iron (see p. 235) is usually increased >200 μg/dL in women, and >250 μg/dL in men), but it is a less reliable test, especially if performed alone.
- Other laboratory tests explore damage to various organs:
  - Studies for diabetes
  - Chondrocalcinosis (pseudogout)
  - Pituitary dysfunction
  - Liver function tests
- Genetic tests for HH. Note: phenotypic analysis should be the first step in screening for HH, with screening strategies including measurement of transferrin saturation and serum ferritin, before resorting to genetic testing.
  - HFE genetic hemochromatosis
  - In most patients of European ancestry, HH is the result of mutations in two specific genes known as HFE, found within the major histocompatibility locus on chromosome 6. The HFE gene has two common missense mutations: the C282Y (rare in non-Caucasian populations) and the H63D found in both Caucasians and non-Caucasians) but with a less well-defined role in HH.
  - Patients with a C282Y/C282Y genotype are homozygous for HH and are at risk for the phenotypic HH disease. The disease seems to have a low penetrance. The reason for the occurrence of the fully expressed penetrance of these genes (devastating IOD) remains unknown. The homozygous are generally found to have a higher prevalence of abnormal liver function tests independent of other manifestations of HH. Modifier factors may be genetic, gender, and high iron or alcohol intake. *Genetic population screening for these mutations in individuals with no clinical or biochemical signs of hemochromatosis is not recommended. Screening of families with one proband documented for HH may be helpful for discovering other members affected with the same mutations.*
  - Patients with a C282Y/wild type genotype are heterozygous for HH and have less risk of iron overload.
  - Patients with a C282Y/H63D genotype (one allele with each mutation) have a 60% chance of intermediate degree IOD, and 35% have normal iron stores.
- Non-HFE genetic hemochromatosis
  - Juvenile hemochromatosis (JH) is the result of a mutation in the gene HJV at chromosome 1q21. This is a rare autosomal recessive disorder similar to HH, but with onset in the second decade of life; a severe form of JH is caused by mutations in HAMP, the gene for hepcidin (in its wild form hepcidin becomes elevated in order to block iron absorption when iron stores become increased).

* Mutations in the gene for ferroportin cause autosomal dominant HH.
* Mutations in the genes for transferring and ceruloplasmin produce autosomal recessive disorders of iron overload.

➤ Limitations

* Serum ferritin may be increased in severe inflammatory conditions and in hepatic necrosis, in the absence of IOD. In HH patients it becomes elevated later in life than transferrin saturation.
* Serum iron levels fluctuate diurnally, with lowest values in the evening, and highest between 7 a.m. and noon.

➤ Suggested Readings

Allen KJ, Gurrin LC, Constantine CC, et al. Iron-overload-related disease in HFE hereditary hemochromatosis. *N Engl J Med.* 2008;358:221–230.

Schrier SL, Bacon BR. Pathophysiology and diagnosis of iron overload syndromes. UpToDate Rose B, editor. Waltham, MA: UpToDate, Inc.; 2009.

CHAPTER 11

Hereditary and Genetic Diseases

Marzena Galdzicka, Patricia Minehart Miron, and Edward I. Ginns

Genetic disorders are conditions caused by absent or defective genes or by chromosomal aberrations. Genetic disorders can be tested at the level of DNA, RNA, or protein. A genetic test is the analysis of human DNA, RNA, mitochondrial DNA, chromosomes, proteins, or certain metabolites in order to detect alterations that may be inherited or acquired. This can be accomplished by directly examining the DNA or RNA that makes up a gene (direct testing), looking at markers coinherited with a disease-causing gene (linkage testing), assaying certain metabolites (biochemical testing), or examining the chromosomes (cytogenetic testing) (www.genetests.org). The results of a genetic test can confirm or rule out a suspected genetic condition, determine an individual's risk of developing disorders, identify carriers, or assess gene variants influencing an individual's rate of drug metabolism. Several hundred genetic tests are currently in use and more are being developed. Genetic testing may be undertaken as part of the process of treating or advising patients.

OVERVIEW

MOLECULAR DIAGNOSIS: TYPES OF GENETIC TESTING

* Diagnostic genetic testing: confirmatory test for symptomatic individuals.
* Presymptomatic genetic testing: carried out in people without symptoms for estimating risk of developings (e.g., Huntington disease, Fabry disease in women).
* Carrier testing: performed to determine whether an individual carries one copy of an altered gene for a particular recessive disease. Autosomal recessive diseases occur only if an individual receives two copies of a gene that have a disease-associated mutation; therefore, each child born to two carriers of a mutation in the same gene has a 25% risk of being affected with the disorder.
* Risk factor testing (susceptibility tests): Gene variants have been discovered that are associated with common diseases such as Alzheimer disease and diabetes.
* Pharmacogenetic testing: determining differences in individual reactions to drugs.
* Preimplantation testing: Preimplantation diagnosis is used following in vitro fertilization to diagnose a genetic disease or condition in a preimplantation embryo.
* Prenatal testing: used to diagnose a genetic disease or condition in a developing fetus.
* Newborn screening: performed in newborns in state public health programs to detect certain genetic diseases for which early diagnosis and treatment are available.

GENETIC COUNSELING

- Genetic testing is often accompanied by genetic counseling. Genetic counseling is the process by which patients or relatives, at risk of an inherited disorder, are advised of the consequences and nature of the disorder, the probability of developing or transmitting it, and the options open to them in management and family planning in order to prevent, avoid, or ameliorate it. Any person may seek genetic counseling for a condition they have inherited from their biologic parents. A woman may be referred for genetic counseling if pregnant and undergoing prenatal testing or screening. Genetic counselors educate the patient about their testing options and inform them of their results.
- If a prenatal screening or test is abnormal, the genetic counselor evaluates the risk of an affected pregnancy, educates the patient about these risks, and informs the patient of their options. A person may also undergo genetic counseling after the birth of a child with a genetic condition. In these instances, the genetic counselor explains the condition to the patient along with recurrence risks in future children. In all cases of a positive family history for a condition, the genetic counselor can evaluate risks and recurrence and explain the condition itself.

INFORMED CONSENT

- "Informed written consent" is a written consent form for the requested release of a person's genetic information, or the release of medical records containing such information. Such a written consent form shall state the purpose for which the information is being requested and shall be distinguished from written consent for the release of any other medical information.
- "Genetic information" is any written or recorded individually identifiable result of a genetic test. In many instances, a laboratory receiving a request to conduct a genetic test from a facility, a physician, or health care provider may conduct the requested test only when the request is accompanied by a signed statement of the medical practitioner ordering the test warranting that the appropriate prior written consent has been obtained from the patient.

GENETIC NONDISCRIMINATION ACT

- Title I: Genetic nondiscrimination in health insurance (Sec. 101): amends the Employee Retirement Income Security Act of 1974 (ERISA), the Public Health Service Act (PHSA), and the Internal Revenue Code to prohibit a group health plan from adjusting premium or contribution amounts for a group on the basis of genetic information.
- Title II:
  - Prohibits employment discrimination on the basis of genetic information (Sec. 202).
  - Prohibits, as an unlawful employment practice, an employer, employment agency, labor organization, or joint labor-management committee from limiting, segregating, or classifying employees, individuals, or members because of genetic information in any way that would deprive or tend to deprive such individuals of employment opportunities or otherwise adversely affect their status as employees.
  - Prohibits, as an unlawful employment practice, an employer, employment agency, labor organization, or joint labor-management committee from requesting, requiring, or pur-

chasing an employee's genetic information, except for certain purposes, which include where: (1) such information is requested or required to comply with certification requirements of family and medical leave laws; (2) the information involved is to be used for genetic monitoring of the biologic effects of toxic substances in the workplace; and (3) the employer conducts DNA analysis for law enforcement purposes as a forensic laboratory or for purposes of human remains identification.

MOLECULAR TESTS USED FOR DETECTION AND MONITORING INFECTIOUS DISEASES

The sample should be collected before starting treatment.
* Qualitative: detection of the presence of viral particles or confirmation of positive viral antibody test; reported as "positive" or "negative"; highly sensitive low limit of detection.
* Quantitative: measurement of the amount of virus to monitor the effectiveness of a treatment (copies/mL, IU/mL, log).
* Genotyping: determination of the viral type or subtype when considering antiviral therapy. Genotype testing is available and is useful in treatment planning and for determining length and possible responses to treatment. Genotype testing should be done as part of the patient's initial evaluation once infection has been confirmed. It may aid in identifying source of infection.
* High sensitivity of molecular assays allows early detection of infection when other markers are negative, detection of infection in immunocompromised patients (antibodies negative), and in addition to monitoring patient's response to therapy, the molecular test will be negative before antibodies are negative.
* Molecular tests allow for high specificity of the tests by using conserved regions of genomic sequence of organisms species and subspecies.

GENETIC DISEASES

BATTEN DISEASE (CLN3, BATTEN-SPIELMEYER-VOGT DISEASE, NEURONAL CEROID LIPOFUSCINOSIS)

➤ Definition
* The neuronal ceroid lipofuscinoses (NCLs or CLNs) are a clinically and genetically heterogeneous group of neurodegenerative disorders characterized by the intracellular accumulation of autofluorescent lipopigment storage material in different patterns ultrastructurally.
* The clinical course includes progressive dementia, seizures, and progressive visual failure. CLN3 is especially prevalent in Finland with an incidence of 1:21,000 live births and a carrier frequency of 1 in 70.

➤ Relevant Tests and Diagnostic Value
* Sequence analysis for mutations
* Detection of a 1.02-kb deletion in the CLN3 gene found in 73% of Batten disease chromosomes
* The hallmark of CLN3 is the ultrastructural pattern of lipopigment with a "fingerprint" profile, which can have three different appearances: pure within a lysosomal residual body; in

conjunction with curvilinear or rectilinear profiles; and as a small component within large membrane-bound lysosomal vacuoles. The combination of fingerprint profiles within lysosomal vacuoles is a regular feature of blood lymphocytes from patients with CLN3.

➤ Other Considerations

- Eight other forms of CLN have been associated with mutations in other genes. The CLNs were originally classified broadly by age at onset: CLN1 as the infantile-onset form, or the infantile-onset Finnish form, having first been described in that population; CLN2 as the late infantile-onset form; CLN3 as the juvenile-onset form; and CLN4 as the adult-onset form.

- With the identification of molecular defects, however, the CLNs are now classified numerically according to the underlying gene defect. CLN1 refers to CLN caused by mutation in the *PPT1* gene, regardless of the age at onset.

➤ Suggested Readings

International Batten Disease Consortium. Isolation of a novel gene underlying Batten disease, CLN3. *Cell.* 1995;82: 949–957.

Mole SE, Williams RE, Goebel HH. Correlations between genotype, ultrastructural morphology and clinical phenotype in the neuronal ceroid lipofuscinoses. *Neurogenetics.* 2005;6:107–126.

CYSTINOSIS

➤ Definition

- Cystinosis is an autosomal recessive inherited disease caused by impaired transport of cystine from lysosomes to cytoplasm that results in intralysosomal accumulation of cystine. There are three clinical forms of cystinosis: infantile (nephropathic) cystinosis; late-onset cystinosis; and benign cystinosis.

- Infantile cystinosis is the most severe and the most common type of cystinosis. Children with nephropathic cystinosis appear normal at birth, but by 9–10 months of age, have symptoms that include excessive thirst and urination and failure to thrive. The abnormally high loss of phosphorus in the urine leads to rickets.

- The longer term manifestations of cystinosis, primarily in older patients and as a result of renal transplantation, include pancreatic endocrine and exocrine insufficiency, and recurrent corneal erosions, CNS involvement, and severe myopathy.

➤ Relevant Tests and Diagnostic Values

- Cystine measurement in blood cells, amniotic fluid cells, and chorionic villi
- Sequence analysis of the *CTNS* gene (chr17p13) is clinically available; >50 mutations have been identified. However, in approximately 20% of patients, no mutation is identified.
- FISH analysis detects a relatively common 57 kb deletion in the *CTNS* gene.

➤ Other Considerations

- Kidney biopsy can demonstrate cystine crystals and destructive changes to the kidney cells and structures.

➤ Suggested Reading

Bendavid C, Kleta R, Long R, et al. FISH diagnosis of the common 57 kb deletion in CTNS causing cystinosis. *Hum Genet.* 2004;115: 510–514.

FABRY DISEASE (ANGIOKERATOMA CORPORIS DIFFUSUM, ANDERSON-FABRY DISEASE)

➤ Definition
- Fabry disease is a rare X-linked recessive lysosomal storage disease caused by a deficiency of α-galactosidase A (α-gal A) that results in progressive accumulation of globotriaosylcer-amide (Gb₂) and related glycosphingolipids in plasma and vascular endothelium, leading to ischemia and infarction in various organs (e.g., kidney, heart, brain, eye, nerves) and characteristic angiokeratomas of skin.
- Heterozygous females may have mild or severe disease.

➤ Relevant Tests and Diagnostic Value
- α-Galactosidase measurement in blood cells in male patients.
- Sequence analysis of the *GLA* gene (chrXq22) is clinically available. Females should have DNA testing.
- Measurement of globotriaosylceramide (Gb2) increased concentrations of globotriaosylcer-amide (Gb2).

➤ Other Considerations
- Enzyme replacement therapy is available.

➤ Suggested Reading
Aerts JM, Groener JE, Kuiper S, et al. Elevated globotriaosylsphingosine is a hallmark of Fabry disease. *Proc Nat Acad Sci.* 2008;105:2812–2817.

FARBER DISEASE

➤ Definition
- This disease, also known as ceramidase deficiency, fibrocytic dysmucopolysaccharidosis, or lipogranulomatosis, is a rare autosomal recessive lysosomal storage disease that is caused by deficiency of acid ceramidase (also called N-acylsphingosine amidohydrolase).
- This enzyme deficiency results in a defect in glycolipid degradation (ceramide), causing an accumulation of ceramide, leading to abnormalities in the joints, liver, throat, tissues, and CNS.

➤ Classification
- Type 1 (classic): the diagnosis can be made almost at a glance by the triad of subcutaneous nodules, arthritis, and laryngeal involvement.
- Types 2 and 3: patients survive longer. The liver and lung appear not to be involved. Normal intelligence in many of these patients and the postmortem findings suggest that brain involvement is limited or missing entirely. Several patients with type 3 disease may survive in relatively stable condition near the end of the second decade.
- Type 4: patients present with hepatosplenomegaly and severe debility in the neonatal period and all die before 6 months of age. Massive histiocytic infiltration of liver, spleen, lungs, thymus, and lymphocytes is found at autopsy.
- Type 5: characterized particularly by psychomotor deterioration beginning at age 1 to 2.5 years.

➤ Relevant Tests and Diagnostic Value
- Biochemical testing
  - Enzyme assay: acid ceramidase assay of skin fibroblasts.

- Analyte: based on giving cultured cells 14C-stearic acid sulfatide and seeing if radiolabeled ceramide accumulates in the cells after 3 days in culture.
- Histologic appearance is granulomatous. In the nervous system both neurons and glial cells are swollen with stored material characteristic of nonsulfonated acid mucopolysaccharide.
- Molecular testing
  - Sequence analysis: analysis of the entire coding region of *ASAH* gene.

➤ Suggested Readings

Li CM, Park JH, He X, et al. The human acid ceramidase gene (ASAH): structure, chromosomal location, mutation analysis and expression. *Genomics.* 2000;62:223–231.

OMIM, Online Mendelian Inheritance in Man, John Hopkins University: Farber Lipogranulomatosis (http://www.ncbi.nlm.nih.gov/omim).

FRAGILE X SYNDROME OF MENTAL RETARDATION/ FMR1-RELATED DISORDERS

➤ Definition

- Fragile X syndrome is the most common form of inherited mental retardation.
- It is caused by loss of function of the *FMR1* gene on the X chromosome (Xq27.3). Most affected individuals carry an expansion of a triplet CGG repeat in the *FMR1* gene; rarely, other causes of loss-of-function gene mutations (point mutations, deletions, abnormal gene methylation) are causal.
- Typically male full-expansion carriers are affected with mental retardation in the moderate range; there is some variation in the extent of methylation on the expanded allele leading to some variation in phenotype. Female full-expansion carriers frequently manifest disease symptoms, but typically in a milder form. Premutation (allele expansion is greater than normal but less than the full expansion associated with fragile X syndrome) is associated with increased risk of premature ovarian failure and may cause fragile X–associated tremor/ataxia syndrome (FXTAS), a late-onset neurodegenerative disorder, mostly affecting male carriers.

➤ Relevant Tests and Diagnostic Value

- Direct diagnosis by DNA analysis using Southern blotting, PCR, and methylation analysis. This can be performed for pre- and postnatal diagnosis and to detect asymptomatic carriers. Testing distinguishes between full mutation and premutation allele sizes.
- Diagnostic value: identifies affected males and carrier/affected females.
- Other: Full sequence analysis is required to detect rare loss-of-function mutations such as point mutations/small deletions. Methylation results from a chorionic villus sample may or may not reflect the accurate future status in the child.

GAUCHER DISEASE

➤ Definition

- Gaucher disease, the most common lysosomal storage disorder, is caused by the autosomal recessively inherited deficiency of acid β-glucosidase (glucocerebrosidase; GBA). The

deficiency of GBA causes the glycosphingolipid glucosylceramide to accumulate within lysosomes of macrophages.
* Among individuals of Ashkenazi Jewish descent, the incidence of type 1 Gaucher disease is approximately 1 in 500–1000, with a carrier frequency of approximately 1 in 15 individuals. In contrast, Gaucher disease is seen in only 1 in 50,000 to 100,000 individuals in the general population.

➤ Classification
* Type 1 (nonneuronopathic) is the most common form of the disease and does not involve the CNS. The clinical manifestations of type 1 Gaucher disease are heterogeneous, can come to attention from infancy to adulthood, and can range from very mildly affected individuals to those having rapidly progressive systemic abnormalities.
* Type 2 is a very rare, rapidly progressive, and affects the brain as well as the organs affected by type 1 Gaucher disease.
* Type 3. The signs and symptoms appear in early childhood, and in addition to CNS involvement, signs and symptoms are the same as in Type 1.

➤ Relevant Tests and Diagnostic Value
* Biochemical testing—enzyme assay: acid β-glucosylceramidase activity in WBCs (lymphocytes) or skin cells (fibroblasts). The overlap in the range of GBA enzyme activity values between noncarriers and Gaucher disease carriers makes enzyme testing alone as a means of carrier identification only about 90% accurate.
* Molecular testing
  * Targeted mutation analysis: available for four common mutations (N370S, L444P, 84GG, IVS2+1G >A), which account for approximately 90% of the disease-causing alleles in the Ashkenazi Jewish population, and 50–60% in non-Jewish populations. Some laboratories offer testing for additional seven "rare" mutations (V394L, D409H, D409V, R463C, R463H, R496H, and a 55-base pair deletion in exon 9).
  * Sequence analysis: analysis of the entire coding region or exons. More than 150 GBA gene mutations have been described. Non-Jewish individuals with Gaucher disease tend to be compound heterozygotes that include one common mutation.

➤ Suggested Readings
Beutler E, Nguyen NJ, Henneberger MW, et al. Gaucher disease: gene frequencies in the Ashkenazi Jewish population. *Am J Hum Genet.* 1993;52(1):85–88.

Horowitz M, Pasmanik-Chor M, Borochowitz Z, et al. Prevalence of glucocerebrosidase mutations in the Israeli Ashkenazi Jewish population. *Hum Mutat.* 1998;12(4):240–244. Erratum in: *Hum Mutat.* 1999;13(3):255.

Tsuji S, Choudary PV, Martin BM, et al. A mutation in the human glucocerebrosidase gene in neuronopathic Gaucher disease. *N Engl J Med.* 1987;361:570–575.

GM₁ GANGLIOSIDOSIS (LANDING DISEASE, SYSTEMIC LATE INFANTILE LIPIDOSIS)

➤ Definition
* GM₁ gangliosidosis is an autosomal recessive lysosomal storage disease characterized by accumulation of ganglioside substrates in lysosomes.
* Clinically, patients show variable degrees of neurodegeneration and skeletal abnormalities.

➤ Classification

There are three main clinical variants categorized by severity and variable residual beta-galactosidase activity.

- Type I, or infantile form, shows rapid psychomotor deterioration beginning within 6 months of birth, generalized CNS involvement, hepatosplenomegaly, facial dysmorphism, macular cherry-red spots, skeletal dysplasia, and early death.
- Type II, or late-infantile/juvenile form has onset between 7 months and 3 years, shows generalized CNS involvement with psychomotor deterioration, seizures, localized skeletal involvement, and survival into childhood. Hepatosplenomegaly and cherry-red spots are usually not present.
- Type III, or adult/chronic form, shows onset from 3–30 years and is characterized by localized skeletal involvement and localized CNS involvement, such as dystonia or gait or speech disturbance. There is an inverse correlation between disease severity and residual enzyme activity.

➤ Relevant Tests and Diagnostic Value

- Assay of lysosomal acid beta-galactosidase enzyme in leukocytes, cultured fibroblasts, or brain
- Prenatal diagnosis by enzyme assay in cultured amniotic fluid cells or by HPLC analysis of galactosyl oligosaccharides in amniotic fluid
- Sequence analysis of gene mutations

➤ Other Considerations

- Tissue biopsy or culture of marrow or skin fibroblasts shows accumulation of ganglioside GM_1.
- It also can demonstrate GM_1 in brain and viscera and mucopolysaccharides in viscera.

➤ Suggested Reading

Suzuki Y, Oshima A, Nanba E. Beta-galactosidase deficiency (beta-galactosidosis): GM1 gangliosidosis and Morquio B disease. In: Scriver CR, Beaudet AL, Sly WS, Valle D, eds. *The Metabolic and Molecular Bases of Inherited Disease.* Vol. II. 8th ed. New York: McGraw- Hill; 2001:3775–3809.

GLYCOGEN STORAGE DISEASE, TYPE I (GLUCOSE-6-PHOSPHATASE DEFICIENCY, VON GIERKE DISEASE)

➤ Definition

- Glycogen storage disease (GSD) type I is the most common of the glycogen storage disorders. This genetic disease results from deficiency of either the enzyme glucose-6-phosphatase (type Ia) or a glucose-6-phosphate translocase-transporter (type Ib).
- The lack of either glucose-6-phosphatase catalytic activity or glucose-6-phosphate translocase activity in the liver leads to inadequate conversion of glucose-6-phosphate into glucose through normal glycogenolysis and gluconeogenesis, resulting in hypoglycemia, lactic acidosis, hyperuricemia, hyperlipidemia, hepatomegaly, and renomegaly.

➤ Relevant Tests and Diagnostic Value

- Chemistry
  - Fasting blood glucose concentration <60 mg/dL (reference range: 70–120 mg/dL)
  - Blood lactate >2.5 mmol/L (reference range: 0.5–2.2 mmol/L)
  - Blood uric acid >5.0 mg/dL (reference range: 2.0–5.0 mg/dL)
  - Triglycerides >250 mg/dL (reference range: 150–200 mg/dL)
  - Cholesterol >200 mg/dL (reference range: 100–200 mg/dL)

- Biochemical testing
  - Glucose-6-phosphatase enzyme activity in liver: In most individuals with type Ia disease, the activity of the glucose-6-phosphatase is $<10\%$ (normal is 3.50 ± 0.8 μmol/min/g tissue). In rare individuals with higher residual enzyme activity and milder clinical manifestations, the enzyme activity could be higher (>1.0 μmol/min/g tissue).
  - Glucose-6-phosphate translocase (transporter) activity: Most clinical diagnostic laboratories refrain from offering this enzyme activity assay because fresh (unfrozen) liver is often needed to assay enzyme activity accurately.
- Molecular testing
  - The two genes known to be associated with type I disease are *G6PC* (type Ia) and *SLC37A4* (type Ib). Mutations in *G6PC* (type Ia) are responsible for 80% of GSD type I and mutations in *SLC37A4* (type Ib) are responsible for 20% of GSD type I
  - Targeted mutation analysis
    - *G6PC* gene: Arg83Cys and Gln347X or larger panels of mutations
    - *SLC37A4* gene: Trp118Arg, 1042_1043delCT, and Gly339Cys
  - Gene sequence analysis
    - *G6PC:* detects mutations in up to 100% of affected individuals in some homogeneous populations, but in mixed populations (e.g., in the United States), detection rate is approximately 94%
    - *SLC37A4:* detects mutations in up to 100% of affected individuals in some homogeneous populations, but in mixed populations (e.g., in the United States), detection frequency could be lower because both mutations may not be detected in some individuals

➤ Suggested Readings

Bali DS, Chen YT. Glycogen storage disease type I. In: Pagon RA, Bird TC, Dolan CR, Stephens K, eds. *GeneReviews* [Internet]. Seattle: University of Washington, Seattle; 1993–2006 Apr 19 [updated 2008 Sep 02].

Ekstein J, Rubin BY, Anderson SL, et al. Mutation frequencies for glycogen storage disease Ia in the Ashkenazi Jewish population. *Am J Med Genet.* 2004;129A:162–164.

GLYCOGEN STORAGE DISEASE, TYPE II (POMPE DISEASE; ACID ALPHA-GLUCOSIDASE DEFICIENCY; ACID MALTASE DEFICIENCY)

➤ Definition

- GSD, type II, is an autosomal recessive disorder that causes a deficiency or dysfunction of the lysosomal hydrolase acid alpha-glucosidase (GAA).
- This enzymatic defect results in lysosomal glycogen accumulation in multiple tissues, with cardiac and skeletal muscle tissues most seriously affected.

➤ Classification

- Classic infantile onset: may be apparent in utero but more often presents in the first month of life with hypotonia, motor delay/muscle weakness, cardiomegaly and hypertrophic cardiomyopathy, feeding difficulties, failure to thrive, respiratory distress, and hearing loss.
- Nonclassic infantile onset: usually presents within the first year of life with motor delays and/or slowly progressive muscle weakness.
- Late onset (i.e., childhood, juvenile, and adult onset) is characterized by proximal muscle weakness and respiratory insufficiency without cardiac involvement; these patients may have residual GAA activity $<40\%$ of normal when measured in skin fibroblasts.

➤ Relevant Tests and Diagnostic Value

- Chemical tests
  - Serum CK: elevated as high as 2000 IU/L (normal: 60–305 IU/L) in classic infantile onset and in the childhood and juvenile variants, but may be normal in adult-onset disease. However, because serum CK concentration is elevated in many other conditions, this test is nonspecific.
  - Urinary oligosaccharides: elevation of a certain urinary glucose tetrasaccharide is highly sensitive in Pompe disease but is also seen in other glycogen storage diseases. In addition, it may be normal in late-onset disease.
- Biochemical testing
  - Acid α-GAA enzyme activity in cultured skin fibroblasts, whole blood, or dried bloodspot (confirmation by a second method is preferred)
    - Activity <1% of normal controls (complete deficiency) is associated with classic infantile-onset Pompe disease.
    - Activity 2–40% of normal controls (partial deficiency) is associated with the nonclassic infantile-onset and the late-onset forms.
  - Muscle biopsy: glycogen storage may be observed in the lysosomes of muscle cells as vacuoles of varying severity that stain positively with periodic acid–Schiff. However, 20–30% of individuals with late-onset type II GSD with documented partial enzyme deficiency may not show these muscle-specific changes.
- Molecular testing: *GAA* is the only gene known to be associated with GSD II.
  - Targeted mutation analysis: Depending on ethnicity and phenotype, an individual could be tested first for one of the three common mutations—Asp645Glu, Arg854X, and IVS1—13T >G—before proceeding to full-sequence analysis.
  - Gene sequence analysis: in 83–93% of individuals with confirmed reduced or absent GAA enzyme activity, two mutations can be detected by sequencing genomic DNA.
  - Deletion/duplication analysis: deletion of exon 18 was seen in approximately 5–7% of alleles; single-exon deletions as well as multiexonic deletions have been seen rarely.

➤ Other Considerations

- Histochemical evidence of glycogen storage in muscle is supportive of a glycogen storage disorder but not specific for Pompe disease.
- CK, AST, ALT, and LDH if elevated, may be useful in the initial evaluation of a patient but must be considered nonspecific.

➤ Suggested Readings

ACMG Work Group on Management of Pompe Disease. Pompe disease diagnosis and management guideline. *Genet Med.* 2006;8(5):382.

Tinkle BT, Leslie N. Glycogen storage disease type II (Pompe Disease). In: Pagon RA, Bird TC, Dolan CR, Stephens K, eds. *GeneReviews* [Internet]. Seattle (WA): University of Washington, Seattle; 1993–2007 Aug 31 [updated 2010 Aug 12].

HUNTER SYNDROME (MUCOPOLYSACCHARIDOSIS II)

➤ Definition

- Mucopolysaccharidosis II arises from iduronate sulfatase deficiency, which results in tissue deposits of mucopolysaccharides and urinary excretion of large amounts of chondroitin sulfate B and heparitin sulfate.

• This sex-linked type of mucopolysaccharidosis differs from the mucopolysaccharidosis I, in being on the average less severe and in not showing clouding of the cornea. Features are dysostosis with dwarfism, grotesque facies, hepatosplenomegaly from mucopolysaccharide deposits, cardiovascular disorders from mucopolysaccharide deposits in the intima, deafness, and excretion of large amounts of chondroitin sulfate B and heparitin sulfate in the urine.

➤ Relevant Tests and Diagnostic Value

• Quantitation of total glucosaminoglycans in urine and accumulation of keratan sulfate in tissues.
• Definitive diagnosis is established by iduronate 2-sulfatase enzyme assay in cultured fibroblasts, leukocytes, amniocytes, or chorionic villi.
• Sequence analysis of the iduronate 2-sulfatase gene.

➤ Other Considerations

• Hunter syndrome is clinically similar to Hurler syndrome but milder, with no corneal opacity. Maternal serum shows increased activity of iduronate sulfate sulfatase with a normal or heterozygous fetus but no increase if fetus has Hunter syndrome.

➤ Suggested Reading

Jonsson JJ, Aronovich EL, Braun SE, Whitley CB. Molecular diagnosis of mucopolysaccharidosis type II (Hunter syndrome) by automated sequencing and computer-assisted interpretation: toward mutation mapping of the iduronate-2-sulfatase gene. *Am J Hum Genet*. 1995;56:597–607.

HURLER SYNDROME (MUCOPOLYSACCHARIDOSIS IH)

➤ Definition

• Hurler syndrome is an autosomal inherited disorder caused by mutations in the gene encoding alpha-L-iduronidase that hydrolyzes the terminal alpha-L-iduronic acid residues of the glycosaminoglycans dermatan sulfate and of heparan sulfate. The accumulation of partially degraded glycosaminoglycans causes interference with cell, tissue, and organ function.
• Deficiency of alpha-L-iduronidase can result in a wide range of phenotypic involvement with three major recognized clinical entities: Hurler (mucopolysaccharidosis IH), Scheie (mucopolysaccharidosis IS), and Hurler-Scheie (mucopolysaccharidosis IH/S) syndromes. Hurler and Scheie syndromes represent phenotypes at the severe and mild ends of the mucopolysaccharidosis I clinical spectrum, respectively, and the Hurler-Scheie syndrome is intermediate in phenotypic expression.

➤ Relevant Tests and Diagnostic Value

• Urinary excretion of glycosaminoglycans.
• Definitive diagnosis is established by alpha-L-iduronidase enzyme assay using artificial substrates (fluorogenic or chromogenic) in cultured fibroblasts, leukocytes, amniocytes, or chorionic villi.
• Sequence analysis of the IDUA gene.

➤ Suggested Reading

Hall CW, Liebaers I, Di Natale P, Neufeld EF. Enzymic diagnosis of the genetic mucopolysaccharide storage disorders. *Methods Enzymol*. 1978;50:439–456.

I-CELL DISEASE (MUCOLIPIDOSIS II)

➤ Definition
- I-cell disease results from an autosomal recessive deficient activity of N-acetylglucosamine 1-phosphotransferase, which causes deficiency of multiple lysosomal enzymes.
- Clinical features resemble Hurler syndrome, but without corneal changes or increased mucopolysaccharides in urine. Congenital dislocation of the hip, thoracic deformities, hernia, and hyperplastic gums are evident soon after birth.

➤ Relevant Test and Diagnostic Value
- Sequence analysis of the N-acetylglucosamine-1-phosphotransferase gene.

➤ Suggested Readings
Canfield WM, Bao M, Pan J, et al. Mucolipidosis II and mucolipidosis IIIA are caused by mutations in the GlcNAc-phosphotransferase alpha/beta gene on chromosome 12p. (Abstract.) *Am J Hum Genet.* 1998;63:A15.

Tiede S, Storch S, Lubke T, et al. Mucolipidosis II is caused by mutations in GNPTA encoding the alpha/beta GlcNAc-1-phosphotransferase. *Nature Med.* 2005;11:1109–1112.

KLINEFELTER SYNDROME

- Males with the 47,XXY karyotype have a fairly well-defined phenotype known as Klinefelter syndrome.
- They are tall and thin with long legs. Physical appearance is fairly normal until puberty, during which a characteristic eunuchoid habitus develops. Secondary sexual characteristics are underdeveloped and testes remain small, with azoospermia and subsequent infertility. Gynecomastia can be a feature of this syndrome. IQ is reduced in this population of patients, and two thirds of patients have educational problems, particularly dyslexia.

KRABBE DISEASE (GLOBOID CELL LEUKODYSTROPHY)

➤ Definition
- Krabbe disease is an autosomal recessive disorder caused by mutations in the galactosylceramidase (*GALC*) gene with pathology involving the white matter of the CNS and affecting the peripheral nervous system.
- Although most patients present within the first 6 months of life ("infantile" or "classic" disease); others present later in life, including in adulthood.

➤ Relevant Tests and Diagnostic Value
- Biochemical testing—enzyme assay: GALC activity is deficient (0–5% of normal) in leukocytes isolated from whole heparinized blood or in cultured skin fibroblasts. However, measuring GALC enzyme activity for carrier testing is unreliable because of the wide range of enzymatic activities observed in carriers and noncarriers.
- Molecular testing
  - Targeted mutation analysis: the 809G >A mutation is often found in individuals with the late-onset form of Krabbe disease.

- Sequence analysis of the entire coding region, intron–exon boundaries, and 5′-untranslated region: detects 100% of the disease-causing mutations and polymorphisms.
- Deletion/duplication analysis: deletions involving single exons and multiple exons have been detected. A 30-kb deletion accounts for approximately 45% of the mutant alleles in individuals of European ancestry and 35% of the mutant alleles in individuals of Mexican heritage with infantile Krabbe disease.

➤ Other Considerations
- Conjunctival biopsy shows characteristic ballooned Schwann cells. Brain biopsy (massive infiltration of unique multinucleated inclusion-containing globoid cells in white matter due to accumulation of galactosylceramide; also diffuse loss of myelin, severe astrocytic gliosis)
- CSF protein electrophoresis shows increased albumin and α-globulin and decreased β- and γ-globulin (same as in metachromatic leukodystrophy).

➤ Suggested Readings
Svennerholm L, Vanier, MT, Hakansson G, Mansson JE. Use of leukocytes in diagnosis of Krabbe disease and detection of carriers. *Clin Chim Acta.* 1981;112:333–342.
Wenger DA, Rafi MA, Luzi P, et al. Krabbe disease: genetic aspects and progress toward therapy. *Molec Gen Metab.* 2000;70:1–9.
Wenger DA, Sattler M, Hiatt W. Globoid cell leukodystrophy: deficiency of lactosyl ceramide beta-galactosidase. *Proc Nat Acad Sci.* 1974;71:854–857.

LESCH-NYHAN SYNDROME

➤ Definition
- Lesch-Nyhan syndrome is an X-linked recessive disorder with almost complete absence of hypoxanthine-guanine phosphoribosyl transferase (HGPRT) that catalyzes hypoxanthine and guanine to their nucleotides due to mutations in *HPRT1* (Xq26-q27.2), causing an accumulation of purines.
- Affected males manifest with neurologic dysfunction, cognitive and behavioral disturbances (choreoathetosis, mental retardation, and tendency to self-mutilation), and uric acid overproduction. Clinical manifestations are due to secondary gout (tophi after 10 years, crystalluria, hematuria, urinary calculi, UTI, gouty arthritis, response to colchicine). Patients die of renal failure by age 10 years unless treated.
- Orange crystals or sand are seen in infants' diapers.

➤ Relevant Tests and Diagnostic Value
- A urinary urate-to-creatinine ratio >2.0 is characteristic for affected male patients who are younger than 10 years of age, but is not considered diagnostic. Neither hyperuricuria nor hyperuricemia (serum uric acid >8 mg/dL; 600–1000 mg/24 h in patients weighing ≥15 kg) is specific for diagnosis.
- Hypoxanthine-guanine phosphoribosyltransferase (HPRT) enzyme activity in male patients <1.5% of normal in blood cells, cultured fibroblasts, amniocytes, or lymphoblasts are diagnostic. The assay is possible on erythrocytes in anticoagulant or on dried blood spots on filter paper. Enzyme assay is not helpful in female patients.
- Sequence analysis of the *HPRT1* gene is clinically available. More than 200 mutations (primarily missense and nonsense mutations and small deletions/insertions) have been identified.

➤ Other Considerations
- Variants with partial deficiency of HGPRT show 0–50% of normal activity in RBC hemo-lysates and >1.2% in fibroblasts; accumulate purines but no orange sand in diapers or abnormality of CNS or behavior.
- Probenecid and other uricosuric drugs designed to reduce the serum concentration of uric acid are contraindicated because they augment the delivery of uric acid into the urinary system and raise the risk of acute anuria from deposition of uric acid crystals in the renal collecting system.

➤ Suggested Readings
Jinnah HA, Harris JC, Nyhan WL, O'Neill JP. The spectrum of mutations causing HPRT deficiency: an update. *Nucleosides Nucleotides Nucleic Acids.* 2004;23:1153–1160.

Lesch M, Nyhan WL. A familial disorder of uric acid metabolism and central nervous system function. *Am J Med.* 1964;36:561–570.

MAROTEAUX-LAMY SYNDROME (MUCOPOLYSACCHARIDOSIS VI)

➤ Definition
- Mucopolysaccharidosis type VI is an autosomal recessive lysosomal storage disorder resulting from a deficiency of arylsulfatase B (ARSB).
- Clinical features and severity are variable but usually include short stature, hepatosplenomegaly, dysostosis multiplex, stiff joints, corneal clouding, cardiac abnormalities, and facial dysmorphism. Intelligence is usually normal.

➤ Relevant Tests and Diagnostic Value
- Measurement of residual N-acetylgalactosamine 4-sulfatase in fibroblasts
- Sequence analysis of the *ARSB* gene

➤ Suggested Reading
Litjens T, Brooks DA, Peters C, et al. Identification, expression, and biochemical characterization of N-acetylgalactosamine-4-sulfatase mutations and relationship with clinical phenotype in MPS-VI patients. *Am J Hum Genet.* 1996;58:1127–1134.

MENKES SYNDROME (KINKY HAIR)

➤ Definition
- Menkes syndrome is an X-linked recessive disorder of copper metabolism caused by gene mutations in the gene encoding Cu(2+)-transporting ATPase, alpha polypeptide (ATP7A) that block copper transport from intestinal mucosa cells to blood, causing generalized copper deficiency.
- It is a syndrome of neonatal hypothermia, feeding difficulties, and sometimes prolonged jaundice; at 2–3 months, seizures and progressive hair depigmentation and twisting take place. The syndrome also includes a striking facial appearance, increasing mental deterioration, infections, failure to thrive, death in early infancy, and changes in the elastica interna of arteries.

➤ Relevant Tests and Diagnostic Value
- Decreased copper in serum and liver; normal in RBCs; increased copper in amniotic fluid, cultured fibroblasts, and amniotic cells
- Decreased serum ceruloplasmin

➤ Other Considerations
- Carrier status for the Menkes disease gene can usually be determined by examination of multiple hairs from scattered scalp sites for pili torti.
- Changes in the metaphyses of the long bones resemble scurvy. Ascorbic acid oxidase is copper-dependent.

➤ Suggested Reading
Moller LB, Bukrinsky JT, Molgaard A, et al. Identification and analysis of 21 novel disease-causing amino acid substitutions in the conserved part of ATP7A. *Hum Mutat.* 2005;26:84–93.

METACHROMATIC LEUKODYSTROPHY

➤ Definition
- Metachromic leukodystrophy is a rare autosomal recessive lipidosis caused by a deficiency of arylsulfatase A (ARSA).
- There are infantile and adult forms with the inability to degrade sphingolipid, sulfatide, or galactosylceramide, causing accumulation of sulfatide. The metachromatic leukodystrophies comprise several allelic disorders, including late infantile, juvenile, and adult forms, partial cerebroside sulfate deficiency, and pseudoarylsulfatase A deficiency; and two nonallelic forms: metachromatic leukodystrophy due to saposin B deficiency and multiple sulfatase deficiency or juvenile sulfatidosis, a disorder that combines features of a mucopolysaccharidosis with those of metachromatic leukodystrophy.

➤ Relevant Tests
- Biochemical testing
  - ARSA activity: measured in leukocytes or cultured fibroblasts or amniocytes; <10% enzyme activity compared to normal controls is suggestive of metachromic leukodystrophy. However, this test is not diagnostic due to possible ARSA pseudodeficiency that is 5–20% of normal controls. Pseudodeficiency is difficult to distinguish from true ARSA deficiency by biochemical testing. Therefore, one of the other tests needs to be used for diagnosis confirmation.
  - Urinary excretion of sulfatides: measured by thin layer chromatography, HPLC, and/or mass spectrometric techniques. Amount of sulfatides in metachromic leukodystrophy is 10–100-fold higher than in controls. Urinary sulfatide excretion is referenced on the basis of urinary excretion in 24 hours or to another urinary component such as creatinine (which is a function of muscle mass) or sphingomyelin (newer approach).
  - Metachromatic lipid deposits in a nerve or brain biopsy: highly invasive approach used only in exceptional circumstances (such as confirmation of a prenatal diagnosis of metachromic leukodystrophy following pregnancy termination).
- Molecular methods
  - Targeted mutation analysis: four most commonly tested mutations are c.459+1G>A, c.1204+1G>A, and Pro426Leu and Ile179Ser. These four mutations account for 25–50%

of the ARSA mutations in European and North American populations. Pseudodeficiency variants (ARSA-PD) are common polymorphisms that result in lower than average but sufficient enzyme activity to avoid sulfatide accumulation and thus do not cause MLD. The two most commonly tested ARSA-PD mutations are missense mutations: c.1049A>G mutation and the polyadenylation site mutation c.1524+96A>G.

- Gene sequence mutation analysis: >150 mutations in *ARSA* gene associated with arylsulfatase A deficiency have been reported. Sequencing is expected to detect 97% of ARSA mutations including small deletions, insertions, and inversions within exons.
- Deletion/duplication analysis: gene deletion is rare; no cases of full gene duplication are known. A case of dispermic chimerism has been reported where two ARSA genes were obtained from the father, one with a metachromic leukodystrophy–causing mutation and the other normal.

➤ Diagnostic Value

- Absence of ARSA activity in the urine is useful in early diagnosis.
- Keratan sulfate is increased in urine (often 2–3 times normal).
- Urine sediment may contain metachromatic lipids (from breakdown of myelin products).

➤ Other Considerations

- Biopsy of dental or sural nerve stained with cresyl violet showing accumulation of metachromatic sulfatide is diagnostic; also increased in brain, kidney, and liver.
- Pseudoarylsulfatase A deficiency refers to a condition of apparent ARSA enzyme deficiency and cerebroside sulfatase activity in leukocytes in persons without neurologic abnormalities in a metachromatic leukodystrophy family.
- Conjunctival biopsy shows metachromatic inclusions within Schwann cells.

➤ Suggested Reading

Polten A, Fluharty AL, Fluharty CB, et al. Molecular basis of different forms of metachromatic leukodystrophy. *N Eng J Med.* 1991;324:18–22.

MORQUIO SYNDROME (MUCOPOLYSACCHARIDOSIS IV)

➤ Definition

- Morquio syndrome, mucopolysaccharidosis type IVA, is an autosomal recessive lysosomal storage disease characterized by intracellular accumulation of keratan sulfate and chondroitin-6-sulfate.
- Key clinical features include short stature, skeletal dysplasia, dental anomalies, and corneal clouding. Intelligence is normal and there is no direct CNS involvement, although the skeletal changes may result in neurologic complications.

➤ Relevant Tests and Diagnostic Value

- Enzyme assay in fibroblasts, leukocytes, or amniocytes
- Sequence analysis of the *GALNS* gene

➤ Suggested Reading

Sukegawa K, Nakamura H, Kato Z, et al. Biochemical and structural analysis of missense mutations in N-acetylgalactosamine-6-sulfate sulfatase causing mucopolysaccharidosis IVA phenotypes. *Hum. Molec. Genet.* 2000;9:1283–1290.

MUCOLIPIDOSIS III (*N*-ACETYLGLUCOSAMINYLPHOSPHOTRANSFERASE DEFICIENCY, PSEUDO-HURLER DYSTROPHY)

➤ Definition
- Mucolipidosis III alpha/beta (classic pseudo-Hurler polydystrophy) is caused by mutation in the gene encoding the alpha/beta-subunits precursor gene of GlcNAc-phosphotransferase (GNPTAB).
- The clinical features of autosomal recessive type III mucolipidosis resemble those of Hurler syndrome but without increased mucopolysaccharides in urine due to a defect in recognition or catalysis and uptake of certain lysosomal enzymes due to deficient activity of N-acetylglucosamine-1-transferase.

➤ Relevant Tests and Diagnostic Value
- Enzyme assay in fibroblasts or leukocytes
- Sequence analysis of the *GNPTAB* gene

➤ Other Considerations
- Mucolipidosis II alpha/beta, or I-cell disease, is also caused by mutations in the GNPTAB gene.
- Mucolipidosis II has been renamed mucolipidosis II alpha/beta, mucolipidosis IIIA has been renamed mucolipidosis III alpha/beta, and mucolipidosis IIIC has been renamed mucolipidosis III gamma.

➤ Suggested Reading
Bargal R, Zeigler M, Abu-Libdeh B, et al. When mucolipidosis III meets mucolipidosis II: GNPTA gene mutations in 24 patients. *Molec Genet Metab.* 2006;88:359–363.

NIEMANN-PICK DISEASE, TYPES A AND B

➤ Definition and Classification
- Niemann-Pick disease (NPD), types A and B, is an autosomal recessive syndrome that results from a deficiency of acid sphingomyelinase (ASM) (sphingomyelin phosphodiesterase) and the subsequent accumulation of sphingomyelin in lysosomes of macrophage–monocyte system in cells and tissues.
  - Type A (NPD-A) is neuronopathic with death in early childhood
  - Type B (NPD-B) is non-neuronopathic

➤ Relevant Tests and Diagnostic Value
- Biochemical testing: Acid ASM enzyme activity measured in peripheral blood lymphocytes or cultured skin fibroblasts; <10% enzyme activity compared to normal controls diagnoses ASM deficiency. However, it was reported that individuals with the *SMPD1* gene mutation Q292K may have apparently normal enzymatic activity when artificial substrate is used.
- Bone marrow examination reveals lipid-laden macrophages. However, this procedure is not necessary for diagnosis and should not be performed unless specific clinical indications are present.

- Molecular testing
  - Sequence analysis of *SMPD1* detects mutations in 99% of individuals with enzymatically confirmed ASM deficiency. Over 100 mutations causing ASM deficiency have been published.
  - Targeted mutation analysis
    - NPD-A mutations are more prevalent in the Ashkenazi Jewish population where the combined carrier frequency for the three common *SMPD1* gene mutations is between 1:80 and 1:100. Three mutations (R496L, L302P, fsP330) account for approximately 90% of NPD-A disease–causing alleles in individuals of Ashkenazi Jewish background.
    - NPD-B mutations are panethnic. Testing for one mutation p.R608del (also known as deltaR608) may account for almost 90% of NPD-B mutant alleles in individuals from North Africa (Tunisia, Algeria, and Morocco), 100% of NPD-B mutant alleles in Gran Canaria Island, and about 20–30% of the NPD type B mutant alleles in persons of North African descent in the United States.

➤ Suggested Readings

Brady RO, Kanfer JN, Mock MB, Fredrickson DS. The metabolism of sphingomyelin. II. Evidence of an enzymatic deficiency in Niemann-Pick disease. *Proc Natl Acad Sci U S A.* 1966;55(2):366–369.

McGovern MM, Schuchman EH. Acid sphingomyelinase deficiency. In: Pagon RA, Bird TC, Dolan CR, Stephens K, eds. *GeneReviews* [Internet]. Seattle (WA): University of Washington, Seattle; 1993–2006 Dec 07 [updated 2009 Jun 25].

NIEMANN-PICK DISEASE, TYPE C

➤ Definition and Classification

- Niemann-Pick disease type C (NPD-C) is an autosomal recessive lipid storage disorder caused by mutations in the *NPC1* or *NPC2* genes involved in lipids trafficking, particularly cholesterol, from late endosomes or lysosomes and characterized by progressive neurodegeneration.
  - NPD type C1, which is responsible for 95% of cases of NPD-C, is caused by mutations in the *NPC1* gene.
  - NPD type C2, which is responsible for 5% of cases of NPD-C, is caused by mutations in the *NPC2* gene.
- In addition, the term NPD type D used in the previous edition of this book describes a genetic isolate from Nova Scotia that is biochemically and clinically indistinguishable from NPD-C and that also results from mutation of the *NPC1* gene. Therefore, the previous NPD type D currently is NPD type C1.

➤ Relevant Tests and Diagnostic Value

- Biochemical testing
  - The diagnosis of NPD-C can be confirmed by demonstrating impaired exogenously supplied cholesterol esterification in cultured fibroblasts or by cytologic technique—filipin staining—to demonstrate the intracellular accumulation of cholesterol in cultured fibroblasts.

- Note: These methods are unreliable for carrier testing due to significant overlap of results between patients and controls.
- Histology: Tissue biopsies and tissue lipid analysis are now rarely needed. These tests include examination of bone marrow, spleen, and liver, which contain foamy cells (lipid-laden macrophages); sea-blue histiocytes may be seen in the marrow in advanced cases.
- Electron microscopy: Skin, rectal neurons, liver, or brain may show polymorphous cytoplasmic bodies.
- Imaging: MRI of the brain is usually normal until the late stages of the illness. At that time, marked atrophy of the superior/anterior cerebellar vermis, thinning of the corpus callosum, and mild cerebral atrophy may be seen. Increased signal in the periatrial white matter, reflecting secondary demyelination, may also occur. Magnetic resonance spectroscopy may be a more sensitive in NPD-C than standard MRI.
- Molecular methods
  - Sequence analysis: detects 80–90% of mutations in *NPC1* gene and close to all mutations in *NPC2* gene. Approximately 200 mutations have been described in NPD-C1. Most affected individuals with NPD-C1 have mutations unique to their family.
  - Deletion/duplication analysis: Few partial and whole gene deletions have been reported for NPD-C1. No large insertions or deletions have been reported in NPD-C2.

➤ Other Considerations
- Cholestatic jaundice occurs in some patients. Foamy Niemann-Pick cells and "sea-blue" histiocytes with distinctive histochemical and ultrastructural appearances are found in the bone marrow.
- In the childhood-onset form, death usually occurs at age 5–15. Adult-onset forms, with insidious onset and slower progression, have also been reported.

➤ Suggested Readings
Argoff CE, Kaneski CR, Blanchette-Mackie EJ, et al. Type C Niemann-Pick disease: documentation of abnormal LDL processing in lymphocytes. *Biochem Biophys Res Commun.* 1990;171:38–45.
Patterson M. Niemann-Pick disease type C. In: Pagon RA, Bird TC, Dolan CR, Stephens K, eds. *GeneReviews* [Internet]. Seattle (WA): University of Washington, Seattle; 1993-2000 Jan 26 [updated 2008 Jul 22].

SANFILIPPO TYPE A SYNDROME (MUCOPOLYSACCHARIDOSIS III, HEPARAN SULFATASE DEFICIENCY)

➤ Definition
- The Sanfilippo syndrome is an autosomal recessive lysosomal storage disease due to impaired degradation of heparin sulfate.
- The clinical features are severe mental defect with relatively mild somatic features (moderately severe claw hand and visceromegaly, little or no corneal clouding or skeletal [e.g., vertebral] change). The presenting problem may be marked overactivity, destructive tendencies, and other behavioral aberrations in a child of 4–6 years of age. Onset of clinical features usually occurs between 2 and 6 years; severe neurologic degeneration occurs in most patients between 6 and 10 years of age, and death occurs typically during the second or third decade

of life. Type A usually presents as the most severe, with earlier onset and rapid progression of symptoms and shorter survival.

➤ Relevant Tests and Diagnostic Value
• Measurement of heparin sulfate in the urine is diagnostic.

➤ Other Considerations
• Mucopolysaccharidosis III includes four types, each due to the deficiency of a different enzyme: heparan N-sulfatase (type A); alpha-N-acetylglucosaminidase (type B); acetyl CoA:alpha-glucosaminide acetyltransferase (type C); and N-acetylglucosamine 6-sulfatase (type D).
• A Dachshund canine model of Sanfilippo syndrome type A is available.

➤ Suggested Readings
Esposito S, Balzano N, Daniele A, et al. Heparan N-sulfatase gene: two novel mutations and transient expression of 15 defects. *Biochim Biophys* Acta. 2000;1501:1–11.

Schmidt R, von Figura K, Paschke E, Kresse H. Sanfilippo's disease type A: sulfamidase activity in peripheral leukocytes of normal, heterozygous and homozygous individuals. *Clin Chim Acta.* 1977;80:7–16.

TAY-SACHS DISEASE (GM₂ GANGLIOSIDOSIS, TYPE I; HEXOSAMINIDASE A DEFICIENCY)

➤ Definition
• Tay-Sachs disease is an autosomal recessive (chromosome 15) lysosomal storage disease caused by mutations in the alpha subunit of the hexosaminidase A (*HEXA*) gene. It occurs predominantly in Ashkenazi Jews, French Canadians, and Cajuns.
• This disease is a progressive neurologic disorder which, in the classic infantile forms, is characterized by psychomotor deterioration, blindness, macula cherry-red spot, and an exaggerated extension response to sound, with death usually by age 2 years; a juvenile form (with death by age 15), and a chronic form in adults.

➤ Relevant Tests and Diagnostic Value
• Enzyme assay for HEXA in serum, plasma, leukocytes, and cultured amniotic cells and skin fibroblasts
• Sequencing for mutation analysis
• Accumulation of ganglioside GM_2 in the brain

➤ Other Considerations
• Macula cherry-red spots appear only in the infantile form.
• Pseudodeficiency alleles 739C-T and 745C-T caused reduced HEXA activity but do not cause illness; serum acid phosphatase is normal.

➤ Suggested Reading
De Braekeleer M, Hechtman P, Andermann E, Kaplan F. The French Canadian Tay-Sachs disease deletion mutation: identification of probable founders. *Hum Genet.* 1992;89:83–87.

TRISOMY 13

➤ Definition
- Trisomy 13 is the third most common viable autosomal trisomy.
- It has a clinically severe phenotype with severe mental retardation and CNS malformations, often including holoprosencephaly and arhinencephaly. Most trisomy 13 conceptions abort spontaneously; about half of trisomy 13 liveborns die in the first month of life.
- Trisomy 13 is usually caused by meiotic nondisjunction resulting in a karyotype of 47,XX (or XY), +13 with minimal recurrence risk. Risk, as for other autosomal trisomies, increases with advancing maternal age. Other causes may include the presence of a Robertsonian translocation in combination with two free copies of chromosome 13; in such cases, one of the parents often is a balanced carrier of the Robertsonian translocation.
- Recurrence risk is low, but significant, and depends on the specific Robertsonian translocation and sex of the carrier parent. Prenatal diagnosis (chromosome analysis) should be offered to all Robertsonian translocation carriers.

➤ Relevant Tests and Diagnostic Value
- Prenatal screening: Maternal serum screening is not applicable for detection of trisomy 13. Fetal abnormalities are significant, however, and are almost always detected with a second/third trimester ultrasound scan.
- Chromosome analysis: Chromosome analysis is diagnostic for trisomy 13 and can be performed on chorionic villus, amniotic fluid, and peripheral blood.
- FISH: Interphase FISH may be performed for rapid enumeration on chorionic villus, amniotic fluid, and peripheral blood.

TRISOMY 18

➤ Definition
- Trisomy 18 is the second most common viable autosomal trisomy. Occurrence is usually sporadic and caused by meiotic nondisjunction; it carries minimal recurrence risk. Risk of trisomy 18 increases with advancing maternal age.
- This trisomy has a severe phenotype with mental retardation and failure to thrive. Classic clenching of fists may be detected on fetal ultrasound examination. Most trisomy 18 conceptuses abort spontaneously, and about 90% of liveborns die in the first year.

➤ Relevant Tests and Diagnostic Value
- Maternal serum screen: Risk of trisomy 18 may be calculated with either first or second trimester maternal serum screening. Because trisomy 18 is rare, detection rates are not as precise as for Down syndrome, but with a 0.4% false-positive rate, detection rates reportedly range from 60–80%.

- Chromosome analysis: Chromosome analysis is diagnostic for trisomy 18 and can be performed on chorionic villus, amniotic fluid, and peripheral blood.
- FISH: Interphase FISH may be performed for rapid enumeration on chorionic villus, amniotic fluid, and peripheral blood.

TRISOMY 21 (DOWN SYNDROME)

➤ Definition
- Trisomy 21 is the most common viable autosomal trisomy.
- Individuals with Down syndrome have moderate mental retardation, characteristic dysmorphic features, increased risk of leukemia, and early Alzheimer disease. Cardiac anomalies are common.
- Risk of trisomy 21 increases with advancing maternal age.

➤ Etiology
- Usual causes involve meiotic nondisjunction, resulting in a karyotype of 47,XX(or XY),+21. For these cases, recurrence risk is small, ~1% greater than age-related risk for women younger than 35 and no significant risk increase over age-related risk for women older than age 35.
- Other causes include presence of a Robertsonian translocation in combination with two free copies of chromosome 21. Often in such cases, one parent is a balanced carrier of the Robertsonian translocation. Recurrence risk of trisomy 21 depends on the specific Robertsonian translocation and the sex of the carrier parent. Prenatal diagnosis (chromosome analysis) should be offered to all Robertsonian translocation carriers.

➤ Relative Tests and Diagnostic Value
- Prenatal maternal screening: Risk of trisomy 21 may be calculated with first trimester, second trimester, or both semester (integrated/sequential) screening modalities that include measurement of maternal serum analytes and fetal ultrasound. Detection rates vary depending on the screening modality and on the false-positive rate. The second semester maternal quad screen can detect 80% of affected pregnancies with a 5% false-positive rate; integrated testing can detect 90% with a 5% false-positive rate.
- Chromosome analysis: diagnostic for trisomy 21 and can be performed on chorionic villus, amniotic fluid, and peripheral blood.
- FISH: Interphase FISH may be performed for rapid enumeration on chorionic villus, amniotic fluid, and peripheral blood.

FAMILIAL DYSAUTONOMIA

➤ Definition
- Familial dysautonomia (hereditary sensory and autonomic neuropathy type III, sometimes called Riley–Day syndrome) is an autosomal recessive disorder almost completely limited to persons of Ashkenazi Jewish heritage.

- It affects the development and survival of sensory, sympathetic, and parasympathetic neurons, resulting in variable symptoms including insensitivity to pain, inability to produce tears, poor growth, and labile blood pressure and leads to decreased life expectancy in affected individuals.

➤ Relevant Tests and Diagnostic Value
- Currently, the diagnosis of familial dysautonomia is established by molecular genetic testing of the *IKBKAP* (inhibitor of kappa light polypeptide gene enhancer in B cells, kinase complex-associated protein) gene.
- Targeted mutation analysis—available for two mutations, VS20+6T>C and R696P, which account for >99% of mutant alleles in individuals of Ashkenazi Jewish descent affected with familial dysautonomia.
- Sequence analysis: analysis of the entire coding region of *IKBKAP* gene.

➤ Suggested Reading
Blumenfeld A, Slaugenhaupt SA, Liebert CB, Temper V, Maayan C, Gill S, et al. Precise genetic mapping and haplotype analysis of the familial dysautonomia gene on human chromosome 9q31. *Am J Hum Genet.* 1999;64: 1110–1118.

TURNER SYNDROME (45,X KARYOTYPE AND VARIANTS)

➤ Definition
- Turner syndrome is widely known as 45,X, although approximately 50% of individuals with Turner syndrome have a variation of this karyotype.
- About 15% of patients carry one normal X chromosome and one structurally aberrant X chromosome. Approximately 25–30% of patients are mosaic with one 45,X cell line and a second cell line that might contain, among others, either two normal X chromosomes (i.e., 45,X/46,XX), one normal and one abnormal X chromosome (i.e., 45,X/46,X,i(Xq)), or one X and one Y chromosome (i.e., 45,X/46,XY).

➤ Who Should be Suspected?
- A number of phenotypic abnormalities are pathognomonic for Turner syndrome. The most characteristic findings are short stature (under 5 feet or 150 cm) and gonadal dysgenesis (usually streak gonads). Fetal cystic hygroma is common, resulting from lymphedema and leading to postnatal neck webbing.
- Other associated anomalies include low posterior hairline, shield chest with widely spaced nipples, cubitus valgus, cardiac anomalies (frequently coarctation of the aorta), and renal anomalies.

➤ Relevant Tests and Diagnostic Value
- Obtaining the karyotype of patients with Turner syndrome is clinically important. Although many of the individual symptoms of Turner syndrome seem to be randomly distributed with

respect to different deletions throughout the X chromosome, some correlations with phenotype can be made. Most individuals with breakpoints distal to Xq25 have few abnormalities except occasional secondary amenorrhea or premature menopause. Short stature is almost always associated with deletions of the distal portion of the short arm; it is seen less often with long arm deletions.

* Determination of the presence of Y chromosomal material is of critical medical importance because its presence leads to an increased risk for gonadoblastoma in sex-reversed individuals. As such, molecular studies for detection of Y chromosomal DNA should be performed. In addition, rare patients with features of Turner syndrome are determined to have a 46,XY karyotype missing a portion of the Y chromosome. These individuals also have an increased risk of gonadoblastoma.

➤ Suggested Readings

Levilliers J, et al. Exchange of terminal portions of X- and Y-short arms in human XY females. *Proc Natl Acad Sci U S A.* 1989;86:2296–3000.

Therman E, Susman B. The similarity of phenotypic effects caused by Xp and Xq deletions in the human female: a hypothesis. *Hum Genet.* 1990;85:175–183.

WOLMAN DISEASE

➤ Definition

* Wolman disease is an autosomal recessive disorder resulting from the deficiency of lysosomal acid lipase (LIPA; LAL) activity, causing accumulation of total cholesterol and triglycerides throughout body tissues.
* Two major disorders, the severe infantile-onset Wolman disease and the milder late-onset cholesteryl ester storage disease (CESD), are seemingly caused by mutations in different parts of the LIPA gene.

➤ Relevant Tests and Diagnostic Value

* Sequence analysis of the LIPA gene for mutations
* Assay of acid lipase activity in leukocytes, cultured fibroblasts, or cultured amniocytes

➤ Other Considerations

* Peripheral blood smear shows prominent vacuolation (in nucleus and cytoplasm) of leukocytes. Abnormal liver function tests are caused by lipid accumulation.
* There is decreased adrenal cortical function with diffuse calcification on CT scan.

➤ Suggested Readings

Anderson RA, Byrum RS, Coates PM, Sando GN. Mutations at the lysosomal acid cholesteryl ester hydrolase gene locus in Wolman disease. *Proc Natl Acad Sci U S A.* 1994;91:2718–2722.

Assmann G, Fredrickson DS. Acid lipase deficiency (Wolman's disease and cholesteryl ester storage disease). In: Stanbury JB, Wyngaarden JB, Fredrickson DS, et al., eds. *Metabolic Basis of Inherited Disease.* 5th ed. New York: McGraw-Hill; 1983:803–819.

GLOSSARY FOR MOLECULAR METHODS TERMINOLOGY

Array comparative genomic hybridization (aCGH): microarray-based technique to detect abnormalities in DNA copy number (i.e., missing or extra pieces of chromosomes) that can detect smaller abnormalities than a standard chromosomal analysis but will not detect balanced chromosomal rearrangements, such as translocations. It is used as an adjunct or replacement to chromosome analysis; does not detect single gene mutations.

Allele-specific oligonucleotide (ASO) testing: detection of a specific mutation using a synthetic segment of DNA approximately 20 base pairs in length (an oligonucleotide) that binds to and hence identifies the complementary sequence in a DNA sample.

bDNA testing: branched DNA testing is a test in which a phosphorescent chemical that is known to bind to RNA is added to the suspect DNA. The more brightly the test sample glows, the greater amount of RNA that is present in the sample; this test is used to directly measure the amount of RNA in a sample (e.g., viral load).

Bead array: array consisting of addressable beads either impregnated with different concentrations of fluorescent dye, or labeled with some type of bar code. The addressable beads enable the identification of specific oligonucleotide binding to the bead's surface. The combination of specific oligonucleotide bound to a specific bead is decoded to determine the presence or absence of a particular target DNA sequence.

Chromosome analysis: provides an overview of the genome through microscopic visual inspection of banded mitotic chromosomes. It requires cells to be in metaphase; therefore, cells must be *cultured* and chemically arrested in metaphase to obtain chromosomes that can be visualized. Aberrations must be at least 5–10 Mb to be appreciated.

Denaturing gradient gel electrophoresis (DGGE): detects changes in DNA sequence based on differences in energy required for separation during electrophoresis of double-stranded DNA fragments of the same size into single-stranded DNA on a polyacrylamide gel with gradient of denaturant (chemical denaturants as formamide and urea) at elevated temperatures. DNA fragments are progressing through the gel according to their melting (denaturing) temperature, which is dependent on the ratio of GC to AT base pairs that make up a particular segment of DNA. A confirmatory test is required for mutation analysis.

Denaturing high performance liquid chromatography (DHPLC)—large scale chromatographic method used for identification of sequence variation allows rapid detection of mutations by heteroduplex formation between wild-type and mutant DNA. Exon sequencing is required to characterize the mutation.

Diagnostic test: test performed to confirm the presence of a specific medical condition. Molecular tests are used currently as an aid in evaluation of patients suspected of/with infectious diseases, genetic disorders, and other disorders where there are established known genetic risk factors. Also in the last few years, pharmacogenetic testing has evolved, creating personalized approached to drug choices and dosing based on individual's variants.

Fluorescence in situ hybridization (FISH): molecular hybridization of a fluorescently labeled, cloned sequence to a mitotic chromosomes or to an interphase nucleus. FISH is used to interrogate a specific region of the genome, designed to detect chromosome rearrangements or aberrations that are least 100 kb in size.

Fluorescence-based fragment size analysis is a method for detection of mutations/variants that cause change in the size of a DNA fragment, such as expansion or contraction of tandem repeats. The size of fluorescently labeled fragments, in PCR reaction, is detected using the capillary electrophoresis and then interpreted using the analysis software. Multiple-colored fluorescent dyes can be detected in one sample. One of the dye colors is used for a labeled size standard that is added to each lane. The analysis software uses the size standard to create a standard curve for each lane and then determines the length of each dye-labeled fragment by comparing it with the standard curve for that specific lane.

Fluorescence resonance energy transfer (FRET): mechanism describing energy transfer between two chromophores.

Genome: complete DNA sequence, containing the entire genetic information, of a gamete, an individual, a population, or a species.

Genomics: field of genetics concerned with structural and functional studies of the genome.

Genotyping: process of determining the genetic makeup of an individual, usually with methods such as PCR, DNA sequencing, ASO probes, and hybridization to DNA microarrays or beads.

Haplotype analysis: determination of the extent of association to a trait of a set of closely linked loci such as a group of genes that occupy a specific position on one chromosome that tend to be inherited together.

Hybridization: used to determine the degree of sequence identity, as well as specific sequences between nucleic acids by interacting single-stranded DNA or RNA in solution or with one component immobilized so that complexes called hybrids are formed by molecules with similar, complementary sequences.

Invader chemistry: composed of two simultaneous isothermal reactions, a primary reaction which detects mutation and secondary reaction which amplifies the signal. The fluorescent signal is generated by the cleavage of a synthetic oligonucleotide probe labeled with FRET.

Karyotype: ordered pairing of chromosomes that aids in detecting abnormalities.

Ligase chain reaction (LCR): DNA amplification technology based on the ligation of two pairs of synthetic oligonucleotides, which hybridize at adjacent positions to complementary strands of a target DNA.

Linkage analysis: testing DNA sequence polymorphisms (normal variants) that are near or within a gene of interest to track inheritance of a disease-causing mutation.

Microarray: consists of the hybridization of a nucleic acid sample (target) to a very large set of oligonucleotide probes, which are attached to a solid support or in solution, to determine sequence or to detect variations in a gene sequence or expression or for gene mapping.

Multiplex ligation-dependent probe amplification (MLPA): detects deletions and duplications, determines the copy number of all or selected exons within a gene with high sensitivity.

Mutation scanning: a search for novel sequence variants within a specific DNA fragment.

Northern blot: used to study gene expression by detection of RNA with a hybridization probe complementary to part of or an entire size separated RNA sample.

Oligonucleotide ligation assay (OLA): rapid, sensitive, and specific method for the detection of known SNPs that is based on the joining of two adjacent oligonucleotide probes (capture and reporter oligos) using a DNA ligase while they are annealed to a complementary DNA target. The detection of a SNP occurs by the ability of DNA ligase to join probes that are perfectly matched to a complementary target sequence, whereas a 3′ mismatch in the capture probe prevents ligation.

Polymerase chain reaction (PCR): molecular technique by which a short DNA (or RNA following reverse transcription) sequence is amplified by of two flanking oligonucleotide primers used in repeated cycles of primer extension and DNA synthesis with DNA polymerase.

Proteome: all the proteins expressed by the genome in a given cell or tissue at a given time under specific conditions.

Proteomics: field of biochemistry/genetics encompassing the comprehensive analysis and cataloging of the structure and function of the proteome.

Pyrosequencing: method for sequencing single-stranded DNA by synthesizing the complementary strand along it, one base pair at a time, and detecting which base was actually added at each step by detecting the activity of DNA polymerase (a DNA synthesizing enzyme) with another chemiluminescent enzyme.

Real-time PCR (quantitative PCR): used to quantify DNA or messenger RNA (mRNA) in a sample by using sequence specific, fluorescently labeled primers to determine the relative (between tissue or relative to a specific housekeeping gene) or absolute number of copies of a particular DNA or RNA sequence in a sample. The quantification arises by measuring the amount of amplified product at each stage during the PCR cycle.

Restriction enzymes (RE): part of the system that bacteria use to protect themselves against viruses by cutting up DNA at specific sequences. Many RE are used to digest DNA into specific fragments that can be used for genotyping.

Reverse hybridization (line probe assay; LIPA): biotinylated amplified PCR product is hybridized to oligonucleotides that are immobilized as parallel lines on membrane (e.g., nitrocellulose) strips. Unhybridized PCR product is washed off the strip, and a reporter such as alkaline phosphatase-labeled streptavidin conjugate is bound to the biotinylated hybrid, followed by chromogen substrate (such as BCIP/NBT) visualization of the banding pattern. The top band of the membrane strip usually contains a positive control.

Reverse transcription: synthesis of a complementary DNA sequence from an RNA template; uses an enzyme, reverse transcriptase, which is an RNA-dependent DNA polymerase.

Restriction fragment length polymorphism (RFLP) analysis: procedure in which the DNA sample is digested into smaller fragments by restriction enzymes and the resulting fragments are separated according to their lengths. RFLP is used for determination of mutations and paternity testing.

Sequence analysis: determination of the nucleotide sequence in a DNA sample. Sequencing is a gold standard for mutation analysis detection of single base changes and microdeletions and/or microinsertions.

Single nucleotide polymorphism (SNP): change in which a single nucleotide in the genomic DNA differs from the usual nucleotide at that position. Some SNPs are responsible for disease, whereas other SNPs are normal variations without functional significance.

Southern blot: used to identify and identify electrophoresed size separated, membrane immobilized DNA sequences that are complementary to a DNA fragment used as a hybridization probe.

Single-stranded conformation polymorphism (SSCP): detects changes in DNA sequence based on differences in electrophoretic mobility under nondenaturing conditions and constant temperature. The method can be used for mutation screening but requires mutation confirmation by another method such as sequencing.

Targeted mutation analysis: testing for either one or more specific mutations.

Temperature gradient gel electrophoresis (TGGE): detects changes in DNA sequence based on differences in energy required for separation of double-stranded DNA fragments of the same size into single-stranded DNA strands (unzipping) during electrophoresis on a polyacrylamide gel using only a temperature gradient (DGGE also uses denaturants). A confirmatory test is required for mutation analysis.

Transcription-mediated amplification (TMA): isothermal target nucleic acid amplification method that uses RNA transcription (using RNA polymerase) and DNA synthesis (using reverse transcriptase) to produce an RNA amplicon from a target nucleic acid. TMA can be used to amplify both an RNA and DNA, and produces 100–1000 copies per cycle. In contrast to PCR and LCR that produce only two copies per cycle.

CHAPTER 12

Immune and Autoimmune Diseases

Liberto Pechet

OVERVIEW

Autoimmunity refers to an abnormal immune response directed against a self-antigen. Autoimmunity is caused by the activation of T cells or B cells, or both, in the absence of a definite cause. Autoimmune disease is the pathologic result of autoimmunity, whereby the immune system attacks a person's healthy body tissues. In most cases of autoimmune diseases the triggering stimulant is unknown.

Multiple factors contribute to the development of autoimmune diseases:
- Genetic susceptibility due to linkage to a particular class I or II HLA molecules
- Environmental triggers (e.g., drugs, possibly chemicals)
- Infectious agents (e.g., *Mycoplasma pneumoniae*, HIV)
- Loss of regulatory T cells
- Defects in cytokine production

An autoimmune disease is demonstrated by the presence of autoantibodies, many of which are organ specific. Others, as in DM, have best been demonstrated experimentally. Many autoantibodies cross-react in various disease entities, and occasionally they may be found without clinical evidence of disease.

There are more than 80 different types of autoimmune disorders, and more than one autoimmune disorder can be manifested by one patient:
- Autoantibodies produced against a person's red cells, white cells, and platelets, or combinations (see, for example, PA, Evans syndrome, neutropenias, ITP).

929

- Against blood vessels resulting in various types of vasculitis (see Wegener's granulomatosis, giant cell arteritis).
- Connective tissue disorders (see SLE, Sjögren syndrome, systemic sclerosis, RA, mixed connective tissue disease)
- Endocrine glands (see type 1 DM, thyroiditis)
- Muscles (see polymyalgia rheumatica, mixed connective tissue)
- Joints (see RA)
- Skin (see SLE, systemic sclerosis)
- Neurologic system (see multiple sclerosis)
- GI (e.g., inflammatory bowel diseases)

➤ **Suggested Reading**

Davidson A, Diamond B. Autoimmune Diseases. *N Engl J Med.* 2001;345:340–348.

IMMUNE AND AUTOIMMUNE DISORDERS

FELTY SYNDROME

➤ **Definition**

- Felty syndrome is characterized by the triad of long-standing, aggressive RA, neutropenia, and splenomegaly.
- It develops in a minority of patients with RA and is more common in women >30 years of age.

➤ **Who Should be Suspected?**

- Many patients present with general malaise, fatigue, loss of appetite, and unintentional weight loss.
- Some patients with Felty syndrome have recurrent infections, such as pneumonia or skin infections. This increased susceptibility to infections is attributed to the low WBC counts that are characteristic of Felty syndrome.

➤ **Laboratory Findings**

- **Hematology:** A WBC count of <2500/μL (or <2000 granulocytes) is mandatory for diagnosis. If the granulocytopenia is profound, the patient may develop bacterial infections. Anemia and thrombocytopenia may develop, or be aggravated by splenomegaly (hypersplenism). ESR and CRP are very elevated. Bone marrow examination may be indicated to exclude other causes for the neutropenia.
- **Serology:** ANAs, antihistone antibodies, and ANCAs are found in the majority of patients. RF is positive in high titers. Circulating immune complexes and immunoglobulin levels are higher than in RA. Complement levels are lower than in RA.

MIXED CONNECTIVE TISSUE DISEASE

➤ **Definition**

- Mixed connective tissue disease (MCTD) represents an overlap syndrome with features of SLE (see p. 896); systemic sclerosis (see p. 897), especially the cutaneous form; and polymyositis (see p. 892).

➤ Who Should be Suspected?
- In the early stage of the disease, the patient may complain of easy fatigability, puffy fingers, Raynaud phenomenon, arthritis, and myalgia.
- Other symptoms may develop gradually: erosive polyarthritis, sclerodactyly, calcinosis, and cutaneous telangiectasia. Pulmonary hypertension may evolve and be the cause of death.

➤ Laboratory Findings
- **Serology:** Certain characteristic serologic findings, such as high titer anti-U1 RNP (see below), separate MCTD as an independent disease. Positive ANA (see p. 59), speckled pattern, with high titers (>1:1000), is present, but not specific. Anti U1-RNP, especially antibodies to its components A' and the 68-kD proteins, is the pathognomonic finding. Autoantibodies specific for systemic sclerosis are absent.
- **Hematology:** elevated ESR
- **Core laboratory:** elevated CRP

➤ Suggested Reading
Bennet RM. Definition and diagnosis of mixed connective tissue disease. UpToDate Rose B, ed. Waltham, MA: UpToDate Inc.; 2009.

POLYMYALGIA RHEUMATICA

➤ Definition
- Polymyalgia rheumatica (PR) is characterized by stiffness and pain in the muscles of the shoulders, neck, back, hips, and thighs. It is seen in individuals >50 years of age. PR develops in 50% of patients with giant cell arteritis (GCA), whereas approximately 15% of patients with PR eventually develop GCA. Both are associated with HLA-DR4.
- The disease has no typical pathologic findings, but a prompt response to 20–30 mg prednisone is characteristic.

➤ Who Should be Suspected?
- The typical patient presents with general malaise; fatigue; and aches and pains in the shoulder, neck, lower back, and/or wrists and knees. Loss of appetite, unintentional weight loss, and depression are also common symptoms.

➤ Laboratory Findings (nonspecific)
- **Hematology:** ESR is markedly elevated, usually >60 mm/hr, but values >100 may be seen. However, some patients with mild disease may have only slight elevations of the ESR.
- **Core laboratory:** CRP is elevated; it is considered more sensitive and a better index of disease activity than the ESR.

POLYMYOSITIS, DERMATOMYOSITIS, AND INCLUSION BODY MYOSITIS

➤ Definition
- Polymyositis (PM), dermatomyositis (DM), and inclusion body myositis (IBM) are three related inflammatory myopathies.
- The main difference between DM and PM is that DM is associated with a variety of skin lesions. It is often associated with an underlying malignancy. PM appears to reflect direct

T-cell mediated muscle injury, whereas DM is characterized by immune complex deposition in vessels and it seems to be a complement-mediated vasculopathy.
* IBM has many features in common with PM but the presence of typical inclusion bodies on muscle biopsy is diagnostic for IBM.

➤ Laboratory Findings

Diagnosis of the three conditions is based on clinical history, serum muscle enzymes, autoantibodies, EMG findings, and muscle biopsy. The latter is the definitive test for establishing the diagnosis of an inflammatory myopathy, and specifically for IBM (see above).
* **Core laboratory:** Muscle enzymes: Patients with DM, PM, or IBM have an elevation in at least one muscle enzyme, but most patients have elevations in all muscle enzymes. The elevations are less profound in IBM. The following enzymes are elevated:
    * CK: the most sensitive enzyme, since it may be elevated 50-fold in active PM and DM (20-fold in IBM)
    * LD
    * Aldolase
    * AST
    * ALT
    * Serum glutamic-oxaloacetic and glutamate pyruvate transaminases
* **Serology:** ANA are present in up to 80% of patients with DM or PM. Myositis-specific antibodies are positive in 30% of patients with PM or DM. The most common are anti-Jo-1 antibodies. Overlap connective disease conditions associated with myositis are suggested when another group of autoantibodies is positive: anti-Ro, anti-La, anti Sm, or anti-ribonucleoprotein.
* **Hematology:** ESR is normal or mildly increased.
* **Molecular tests:** Gene expression profiles may have a diagnostic role in the future.

➤ Suggested Reading

Miller ML. Clinical manifestations and diagnosis of adult dermatomyositis and polymyositis. UpToDate. Rose B, ed. Waltham, MA: UpToDate, Inc.; 2009.

PSEUDOGOUT

➤ Definition

* Pseudogout refers to acute attacks of calcium pyrophosphate dehydrate (CPPD) deposition in joint synoviae, resembling classical urate-induced gout. The consequence of this deposition is pyrophosphate arthropathy.
* The term *chondrocalcinosis* is used for radiographic findings accompanying calcification in connective tissues, induced by deposition of CPPD crystals.

➤ Who Should be Suspected?

* Likely patients are elderly, with acute or subacute attacks of arthritis, especially of the knee. CPPD deposition occurs commonly in individuals with degenerative arthritis.

➤ Laboratory Findings

* **Synovial Fluid Examination:** Compensated polarized light microscopy reveals birefringent CPPD crystals. During acute episodes synovial fluid also contains numerous neutro-

phils some of which contain phagocytised CPPD crystals. Crystals can also be demonstrated in biopsies of involved tissues.
- **Recommended Testing:** Because of the possible association of pseudogout with other systemic diseases (hemochromatosis, hypothyroidism, hyperparathyroidism, hypomagnesemia, hypophosphatasia, familiar hypercalciuric hypercalcemia), the following laboratory panel is recommended: serum calcium, phosphorus, magnesium, ALP, ferritin, and TSH.

➤ Suggested Reading
Becker MA. Clinical manifestations and diagnosis of calcium pyrophosphate crystal deposition disease. UpToDate. Rose, B ed. Waltham, MA: UpToDate, 2009.

PSORIASIS AND PSORIASIS-ASSOCIATED ARTHRITIS

➤ Definition
- Psoriasis is characterized by erythematous, sharply demarcated papules and rounded plaques, covered by silver scales. It is an immunologically mediated disease in which T lymphocytes play a central role. Several susceptibility loci for psoriasis have been identified. It is known to occur in families.
- Psoriasis-associated arthritis (PAA) is seen in a small percentage of patients with psoriasis. It is a seronegative spondyloarthropathy. Several HLA types have been identified to be associated with PAA, suggesting a genetic predisposition.

➤ Laboratory Findings
Diagnosis of psoriasis is basically made by history and physical examination. Diagnosis of PAA is made by the association of arthritis and psoriasis.
- **Histology:** Biopsy is rarely necessary.
- **Serology:** RF is negative.
- **Core laboratory:** Serum uric acid: may be elevated due to increased turnover of skin cells.
- **HLA studies:** May reinforce the diagnosis, but are not necessary.

REACTIVE ARTHRITIS (REITER SYNDROME)

➤ Definition
- Reactive arthritis is an autoimmune spondylarthritis that develops 1–4 weeks after an infection.

➤ Who Should be Suspected?
- A likely patient is an individual 20–40 years of age, more commonly a white male, who develops the triad of postinfectious monoarticular arthritis (affecting most often the knee), urinary symptoms (balanitis, dysuria, frequency or prostatitis in men, cervicitis, salpingitis or vulvovaginitis in women), and ocular symptoms (conjunctivitis or anterior uveitis).

➤ Laboratory Findings

The diagnosis is primarily clinical.

• **Cultures and serology:** An infectious etiology can be identified in only half the cases, since by the time arthritis/urethritis/conjunctivitis (or variations thereof) develops, pathogens may no longer be retrievable. Nevertheless, a trial to identify the following pathogens by stool, urine, or synovial cultures, or by serology, should be attempted:

  • Chlamydia, especially *Chlamydia trachomatis* and *Chlamydia pneumoniae*. PCR for urinary chlamydial DNA has high sensitivity.
  • *Yersinia enterocolitica* and *Yersinia pseudotuberculosis*
  • *Salmonella*
  • Shigella, especially *Shigella flexneri* or *Shigella dysenteriae*
  • *Campylobacter*
  • *Clostridium difficile*
  • HIV
  • Possibly other organisms

• **HLA studies:** HLA-B27 positivity may help diagnose reactive arthritis, since it is positive in half the cases in the Caucasian population. HLA-B27 positivity seems to be associated with a more severe and protracted course.

• **Hematology:** Elevated ESR during the acute phase of the disease but not specific.

• **Serology:** RF is negative

• **Synovial fluid analysis:** May help differentiate reactive arthritis from other forms of arthritis by determining the presence or absence of specific crystals (see p. 143)

RETROPERITONEAL FIBROSIS

➤ Definition

• A rare disease due to progressive, sclerosing, and obstructive proliferation of collagen in the retroperitoneal space. It is idiopathic in 70% of cases.

• Some authors believe it to be part of an autoimmune process. The secondary form develops in relation to certain drugs (ergot derivatives, methysergide, bromocriptine, beta blockers, methyldopa, hydralazine, analgesics); malignancy (Hodgkin disease or non-Hodgkin lymphoma), infections (TB, histoplasmosis, actinomycosis); or regional radiation therapy or surgery.

➤ Who Should be Suspected?

• The likely patient is a 40- to 60-year-old individual, more commonly male, with pain over the flank areas, lower back, and abdomen, and malaise, anorexia, weight loss, moderate fever of unknown etiology, nausea, vomiting, or insidiously developing symptoms of ureteral obstruction, or venous or arterial insufficiency.

➤ Laboratory Findings

• **Imaging studies:** Primarily establishes the diagnosis.

• **Hematology:** Anemia of chronic inflammatory disease, leukocytosis, and occasional eosinophilia. Elevated ESR.

• **Serology:** Positive ANA in up to 60% of cases.

• **Core laboratory:** Elevated CRP.

➤ Considerations
* Laboratory findings of ureteral obstruction, including a rise in BUN and creatinine.

RHEUMATOID ARTHRITIS

➤ Definition
* Rheumatoid arthritis (RA) is a chronic inflammatory arthritis characterized by progressive, symmetric, erosive synovitis. The potential of the synovitis to cause cartilage damage and bone erosion is characteristic for the disease. In addition to joints, RA may affect many other tissues and organs (e.g., lungs, pleura, pericardium, sclera). Although the etiology remains obscure, there is a genetic predisposition associated with HLA-DR alleles, DRβ1 alleles, and HLA-DR4 in some populations.
* In 1987, the American Rheumatism Association revised the criteria for diagnosis of RA; 4 of 7 criteria must be present for at least 6 weeks.

➤ Who Should be Suspected?
* Candidates include individuals between the ages of 30 to 50, often female, presenting with fatigue, weakness, anorexia, and slowly progressive pain and stiffness in the joints. Involvement of the small joints of the hands or feet should raise suspicion for RA. RA can also be seen in the pediatric population (juvenile rheumatoid arthritis), as well as in the elderly.

➤ Laboratory Findings
There is no pathognomonic test for RA. Tests for diseases that can mimic RA (hemochromatosis, SLE, systemic sclerosis, sarcoidosis, thyroid disorders) may be indicated.
* **Serology:** IgM RF becomes positive in approximately 85% of patients within one year of presentation, but the assay is not entirely specific for RA. In its absence the disease is called seronegative RA. Anticitrullinate protein antibodies [anticyclic citrullinated peptide (anti-CCP) and antimutated citrullinated Vimentin] have a 95% specificity but are present in only 65% of cases. ANA is frequently positive as antinuclear antigen.
* **Synovial fluid analysis:** Reveals increased cellular counts (2000 to 50,000/mm3 in affected joints, with a predominance of neutrophils. Total hemolytic complement C3 and C4 are markedly reduced.
* **Hematology:** Elevated ESR.
* **Core laboratory:** Elevated CRP.

➤ Suggested Reading
Majithia V, Geraci SA. Rheumatoid arthritis: diagnosis and management. *Am J Med.* 2007;120:936:939.

SJÖGREN'S SYNDROME (SS)

➤ Definition
SS is a chronic, progressive inflammatory autoimmune disease in which immune cells attack and destroy exocrine glands, resulting in the sicca (dryness) complex. The syndrome can be divided

in Primary SS, or Secondary SS, Antibodies to when it is associated with other autoimmune connective tissue disorders, principally rheumatoid arthritis or systemic lupus erythematosus. Many cases of "primary" SS are followed by other autoimmune diseases. Revised international classification criteria were developed in 2002.

➤ Who Should be Suspected?
A patient who complaints of ocular symptoms, such as persistent dry eyes for more than 3 months, and oral symptoms of dryness, such as the need to drink water to be able to swallow food. Much more common in women, and the disease develops in the late 40s. Occasionally other tissue may be involved (extraglandular manifestations), including autoimmune thyroiditis. SS does not go into remissions. A hereditary predisposition exists: association with HLA-DR3 and DRN52. 5% of patients develop lymphoma.

➤ Diagnosis
* Schirmer test measure tear production.
* Rose Bengal test stains areas of devitalized epithelial cells in cornea and conjunctivae
* Tear break-up time measures overall lacrimal function by measuring breakup times and tear osmolality after instillation of fluorescein.

➤ Laboratory Findings
Serology: High level ANA with fine speckled staining; ANA levels vary according to methodology. Rheumatoid Factor (it is frequently positive because SS's association with rheumatoid arthritis). SSA/RO (associated with many autoimmune conditions that may be present in SS). SSB/La is very specific for SS.

Hematology: CBC indicates progressive anemia. Sedimentation rate and/or C-reactive protein, both elevated.

Imaging studies: Ultrasound examination of the salivary glands. Radiological imaging with a contrast agent injected into the parotid gland of Stensen. Magnetic resonance imaging, superior to both of the above.

Other: Other laboratory tests are indicated to evaluate systemic and extraglandular involvement: Serum electrolytes, antiocardiolipin antibodies, anti αGP1, and lupus anticoagulant, liver function tests and urinalysis.

➤ Suggested Reading
Vitali C, Bombardieri S, Jonsson R, et al. Classificaation criteria for Sjögren's syndrome: a revised version of the European criteria proposed by the American-European Consensus Group. *Ann. Rheum.* Dis.2002; 61:554–558

SYSTEMIC LUPUS ERYTHEMATOSUS

➤ Definition
* Systemic lupus erythematosus (SLE) is a chronic inflammatory autoimmune disease of unknown etiology, characterized by multisystem involvement, reflected in the production of

antinuclear antibodies. The autoantibodies and immune complexes bind to various tissues, with resulting damage.

* The variability in the presentation of the disease led the American College of Rheumatologists to develop 11 criteria to classify patients with SLE.

➤ Who Should be Suspected?

* Likely patients are females between 15 and 50 years of age, who present with constitutional symptoms associated with any or a combination of rash or arthritis (the most common presenting symptoms), anemia, thrombocytopenia, serositis, nephritis, endocarditis, seizures, and psychosis. Involvement of any organ is possible.
* A variant of lupus, called drug-induced lupus, may be the result of procainamide, hydralazine, or quinidine therapy. These patients present with skin and joint manifestations but rarely have renal or neurologic features. It is a self-limited condition in most cases.

➤ Laboratory Findings

Supportive laboratory studies are mandatory for the diagnosis.

* **Serology:** There are numerous autoantibody assays. The list below may not include all.
  * ANA assay is positive in high titers (1:160 or higher). It is found in >98% of SLE patients during the course of disease. Diseases other than SLE may be associated with a positive ANA, but usually in lower titers. If ANA is repeatedly negative, SLE can be excluded in the vast majority of suspected patients.
  * Anti-double-stranded DNA antibodies are highly specific; the assays have only approximately 75% sensitivity. When positive, anti-double-stranded DNA antibodies are associated with renal and skin disease. The titer fluctuates with diseased activity.
  * Anti-Smith (Sm) antibodies are very specific but lack sensitivity (25% prevalence). They are more frequent in African American and Asian patients with SLE. Sm antibodies are associated with kidney disease.
  * Antibodies to ribonucleoprotein (U1 RNP) (see p. 61) are associated with myositis, Raynaud phenomenon, and less severe lupus; also present in mixed connective tissue disease and systemic sclerosis (see p. 930, 938).
  * Antibodies to Ro (SS-A) and La (SS-B) (see p. 59) are also found in Sjögren syndrome.
  * Anti-Ro/SS-A are associated with lymphopenia, photosensitivity, skin and kidney disease, neonatal lupus, complement deficiency, and subacute cutaneous lupus. The presence of anti-Ro or anti-La antibodies during pregnancy confers a 1–2% risk of congenital heart block in the offspring.
  * Anti-ribosomal P protein is seen in patients with neuropsychiatric manifestations.
  * Antiphospholipid antibodies and anti-β2 glycoprotein 1 are associated with the lupus anticoagulant (LA). Only approximately one third of patients with antiphospholipid antibody syndrome have SLE.
  * Antihistone antibodies are present in >95% of cases of drug-induced lupus, whereas the other autoantibodies present in SLE are absent. Antihistone antibodies are also present in up to 85% of patients with SLE.
  * Although RF is not specific for SLE, its presence correlates with active inflammatory arthritis.

- Additional laboratory tests may provide important clinical information:
  - CBC and differential
    - Anemia may be that of chronic inflammatory disease, or be autoimmune hemolytic, occasionally microangiopathic (see p. 813).
    - Thrombocytopenia, neutropenia, or lymphopenia are usually immune in origin.
    - Serum complement levels C3 and C4 decrease in parallel with disease activity.
    - ESR or CRP are often elevated in active disease.
  - Renal function studies are indicated to assess renal involvement.
  - Presence of cryoglobulins may correlate with disease activity.
  - Biologically false-positive tests for syphilis may be the first indication of SLE.

➤ Suggested Readings

Heinlen LD, McClain MT, Merrill J, et al. Clinical criteria for systemic lupus erythematosus precede diagnosis, and associated autoantibodies are present before clinical symptoms. *Arthritis Rheum.* 2007;56:2344–2351.

Rahman A, Isenberg DA. Systemic lupus erythematosus. *N Engl J Med.* 2008;358:929–939.

SYSTEMIC SCLEROSIS (SCLERODERMA)

➤ Definition

- Systemic sclerosis (SSc) is a chronic, progressive systemic disease of unknown etiology. The presence of thickened skin (scleroderma) distinguishes SSc from other connective tissue diseases, but manifestations of SSc may develop at a later time
- The disease is heterogenous, and it may be classified as:
  - Diffuse cutaneous SSc, which presents with progressive skin indurations and risk for early pulmonary fibrosis and acute renal involvement.
  - Limited cutaneous SSc, with a prominent Raynaud phenomenon.
  - Limited SSc and part of CREST syndrome: prominent Calcinosis cutis, Raynaud phenomenon, Esophageal dysmotility, Sclerodactyly, and Telangiectasia from which the eponym CREST originates.

➤ Who Should be Suspected?

- The likely patient is between the ages 30 and 50, more commonly a woman, who presents with thickening of the skin, either diffuse or in multiple locations, Raynaud's phenomena, and develops multiple internal organs involvement.

➤ Laboratory Findings

The diagnosis of SSc is a clinical one, confirmed (but not excluded) by serology.
- **Histology:** Biopsy is rarely necessary.
- **Serology:** Autoantibody levels correlate with the severity of disease, and the titers fluctuate with disease activity. There are numerous autoantibody assays. The list below may not include all.
  - ANAs are found in low titers in 40–90% of patients but are not necessary for diagnosis.
  - RF may be positive in 30% of patients. When in high titer, it suggests overlap disease.
  - Antitopoisomerase I (anti-Scl-70) present in 30–70% of patients with diffuse cutaneous SSc is highly specific but occurs late in the disease; it has moderate sensitivity. When

positive, it suggests higher risk of severe interstitial lung disease, cardiac, or renal involvement.
* Anticentromere in moderate titers is highly specific but has only moderate sensitivity. Associated with limited cutaneous SSc. Found as the only antibody in the majority of patients with CREST syndrome.
* Anti-RNA polymerase III is highly specific for SSc, but has only moderate sensitivity. Associated with extensive skin involvement and renal disease.
* Anti-β2-glycoprotein 1 and anticardiolipin antibodies may be positive in SSc. Anti-β2-glycoprotein 1 antibodies are associated with macrovascular disease in SSc patients.
* Antibodies to U3-RNP (fibrillarin) are associated with risk of pulmonary hypertension, scleroderma renal disease, and myositis.
* Anti-PM-Scl autoantibodies indicate risk of associated myositis.
* Antibodies to RNA polymerase II may be found positive either in SSc or in SLE.
* **Core laboratory:** Serum and urine protein electrophoresis may be indicated to exclude monoclonal gammopathies in patients with symmetrical skin induration but no Raynaud phenomenon. Serum complement is normal.
* **Hematology:** Eosinophilia is common. ESR may be normal, mildly increased or greatly increased, each in one third of patients.

➤ Suggested Reading

Reveille JD, Solomon DH. Evidence-based guidelines for use of immunologic tests: anticentromere, Scl-70 and nucleolar antibodies. *Arthritis Rheum.* 2003;49:399.

WEGENER GRANULOMATOSIS

➤ Definition
* Wegener granulomatosis is a rare autoimmune systemic necrotizing and granulomatous vasculitis that affects most commonly the upper and lower respiratory tracts and kidneys. The hallmark of the disease is a necrotizing vasculitis of small arteries and veins together with granuloma formation.
* Microscopic polyangiitis is another systemic vasculitis that is very similar.

➤ Who Should be Suspected?
* Likely candidates are those with severe upper respiratory findings, including sinuses involvement (pain and purulent discharge and rhinorrhea), cough, dyspnea and hemoptysis, renal disease, eye involvement, and skin lesions. There is also a high incidence of deep venous thrombosis.

➤ Laboratory Findings
* **Histology:** The diagnosis must be confirmed by biopsy of the pulmonary (highest yield), upper airway, or renal tissue.
* **Serology:** 90% of patients with active disease have a positive antiproteinase-3 ANCA. A few patients may have antimyeloperoxidase instead of ANCA positivity, although many of these patients may have microscopic polyangiitis. Positive RF in low titer. Negative ANA. Mild hypergammaglobulinemia, especially of the IgA class.

- **Urinalysis:** reflects the degree of renal involvement.
- **Core laboratory:** Elevated CRP. Abnormal BUN and creatinine reflect the degree of kidney involvement.
- **Hematology:** Markedly elevated ESR or CRP.
- **Cultures:** Should be performed on the tissue obtained to rule out mycobacterial and fungal infections.

➤ Suggested Readings

Hunder GG, Arend WP, Bloch DA, et al. American College of Rheumatology 1990 Criteria for Classification of Vasculitis. Introduction. *Arthritis Rheum.* 1990;33:1065–1067.

Seo P, Stone JH. The antineutrophil cytoplasmic antibody-associated vasculitides. *Am J Med.* 2004;117:39–50.

Infectious Diseases

Michael J. Mitchell

This chapter reviews some of the major infectious diseases caused by bacterial, fungal, viral, and parasitic pathogens. Each section is organized into subsections, and the pathogenic agents arranged in alphabetical order. Information regarding infections of specific organ systems is found in the appropriate organ-specific chapters. For example, information regarding TB can be found in Chapter 14. Respiratory, Metabolic, and Acid-Base Disorders.

The diagnosis of specific infectious diseases is typically based on a combination of clinical signs and symptoms, exposure history, and other risk factors and laboratory testing. See Chapter 3, Infectious Diseases Assays, for detailed information regarding specific diagnostic testing for infectious diseases.

INFECTIOUS DISEASES CAUSED BY BACTERIAL PATHOGENS

GRAM-NEGATIVE BACILLI AND CURVED RODS, NONFASTIDIOUS

The pathogens in this group grow within 24–48 hours on routine laboratory media, like sheep blood agar (SBA). Inoculation of selective and differential media, like MacConkey (MAC) agar, may facilitate isolation from contaminated specimens. Aerobic gram-negative bacteria (GNBs) may be grouped on the basis of their ability to ferment glucose. Glucose-fermenting pathogenic GNBs include the "enterics," like *Escherichia coli* and *Salmonella,* as well as the *Vibrio* spp. Glucose nonfermenters (nGNBs) include *Pseudomonas aeruginosa* and *Acinetobacter* spp. Gram staining demonstrates avidly staining organisms. These GNBs demonstrate a variety of resistance mechanisms. Standardized susceptibility testing is required to guide treatment for most infections caused by this group of pathogens.

ACINETOBACTER INFECTION

➤ Definition
• *Acinetobacter baumannii* is the second most frequently isolated nGNB in the clinical laboratory, playing an important role in the etiology of nosocomial infections.

➤ Who Should be Suspected?
• *Acinetobacter* species are able to survive in very diverse environments. Although *Acinetobacter* species may be isolated as culture contaminants, they are now well established as important

primary and nosocomial pathogens. Infections in virtually all organ systems have been described. Major infections include:

- Wounds: *A. baumannii* emerged as a significant cause of infection in battlefield injuries during the Vietnam conflict and recently in casualties from Afghanistan and Iraq. It is now established as an important cause of wound and burn infections in nonmilitary patients.
- Hospital-acquired pneumonia: *A. baumannii* causes a significant minority (~10%) of nosocomial pneumonias, both as isolated infections or epidemic outbreaks.
- Meningitis: *A. baumannii*, along with other gram-negative rods (GNRs), is playing an increasing role as a complication of neurosurgery and external CSF drain placement.
- Nosocomial bloodstream infection: *A. baumannii* is responsible for up to 2% of nosocomial bloodstream infection, usually in ICU patients. The reported mortality rate is ~40%, exceeded only by *Pseudomonas aeruginosa* and *Candida*.
- UTI: *A. baumannii* is an established, but uncommon, cause of nosocomial UTI, usually in patients with indwelling catheters.
- Treatment of *A. baumannii* infections poses a significant challenge to clinicians because of intrinsic and acquired resistance determinants. Carbapenem antibiotics are usually effective. These organisms readily develop resistance to drugs used to treat these infections. Resistance may quickly emerge to the preferred agents used for nosocomial infections. Definitive treatment should be determined by susceptibility testing of the initial isolate; re-testing, to detect emerging resistance, is recommended for subsequent isolates recovered during therapy.

BURKHOLDERIA INFECTIONS

➤ Definition
- *Burkholderia pseudomallei* and *Burkholderia cepacia* are the species most commonly associated with human disease. *B. pseudomallei* has a fairly restricted incidence, and primary infection in the United States is uncommon. *B. cepacia* has been isolated from numerous environmental sources.
- *Burkholderia mallei* (a primary pathogen of horses) and *B. pseudomallei*, however, have been classified by the CDC as potential bioterror agents. Reporting is mandated as soon as *B. mallei* or *B. pseudomallei* infection is suspected or confirmed.

➤ Who Should be Suspected?
- *B. pseudomallei* causes melioidosis within a restricted geographic niche; disease is largely confined to endemic areas in Southeast Asia and northern Australia. Direct contact with or inhalation of contaminated soil or water is the most common mode of transmission. Most infections are asymptomatic or minimally symptomatic with a flu-like syndrome, but may present with acute or chronic illness, including pneumonia, skin and soft tissue infections, chronic suppurative infections and bacteremia.
- *B. cepacia* has emerged as a significant pathogen, primarily causing disease in patients with CF and chronic granulomatous disease. In patients with CF, respiratory tract colonization may be associated with a rapid decline in pulmonary function and an increased mortality in the year following acquisition.

➤ Laboratory Findings
- Culture: Selective media should be used for isolation of *B. cepacia* from lower respiratory specimens collected from CF patients.

- Susceptibility: *B. cepacia* is intrinsically resistant to aminoglycosides but typically susceptible to TMP/SMX.

CAMPYLOBACTER GASTROENTERITIS

➤ Definition
- *Campylobacter* species cause diarrheal infections globally and are the most common bacterial cause of significant diarrheal illness in most countries. *Campylobacter jejuni* is the most important human pathogen. In developed countries, asymptomatic infection is uncommon.

➤ Who Should be Suspected?
- Infection is usually acquired by contact with animals, mainly poultry, in which *Campylobacter* species are common components of endogenous gut flora. Person-to-person transmission is uncommon. Most infections resolve within 7 days.
- *Campylobacter* GI infection typically results in diarrhea with fever, cramping, and vomiting. Blood may be present in the stools. A nonspecific colitis, with marked fecal leukocytes, is common. Guillain-Barré syndrome has been associated with campylobacteriosis.
- Disease outside the GI tract is uncommon. Septic arthritis, bacteremia, proctocolitis, meningitis, and other infections have been reported.

➤ Laboratory Findings
- Culture: The special culture procedures required for isolation of *Campylobacter* species should be included in routine stool culture protocols in clinical microbiology laboratories.

ESCHERICHIA COLI INFECTION

➤ Definition
- *Escherichia coli* is the most common clinical isolate in most microbiology laboratories. It is a ubiquitous component of the GI bacterial flora and is the most common cause of community-acquired UTI in normal hosts. *E. coli* is a major cause of nosocomial infections and infections in immunocompromised patients.
- *E. coli* isolates may cause enteritis or gastroenteritis by a number of mechanisms, including toxin production and adherence to mucosal epithelial cells of the colon.

➤ Who Should be Suspected?
- *E. coli* should be considered in any patient with UTI. *E. coli* may also be suspected in patients with "traveler's diarrhea" (abrupt onset, with profuse, watery diarrhea after travel to an endemic area). Enterohemorrhagic *E. coli* infection may be suspected in patients with diarrhea, especially patients who develop HUS after diarrheal illness. See the discussion of foodborne causes of diarrhea in Chapter 6, Digestive Diseases.
- *E. coli* is responsible for a wide spectrum of opportunistic and nosocomial infections. It is the major cause of nosocomial pneumonia, bloodstream infection, surgical site infection, and UTI. It is also responsible for a significant proportion of severe neonatal infections, including sepsis and meningitis.

➤ Laboratory Findings

- Recognition of *E. coli* strains that cause enterohemorrhagic gastroenteritis may be improved by the use of the differential sorbitol-MAC agar. These strains produce Shiga toxin 1 and/or toxin 2, which may be directly detected in stool specimens. In the United States, most isolates are serotype O157:H7.
- Although there are tests that can be used to identify most of the other different types of diarrheagenic *E. coli*, specific diagnosis is rarely needed for patient management.

KLEBSIELLA PNEUMONIAE INFECTION

➤ Definition

- *Klebsiella pneumoniae* is widely distributed in nature as well as the normal fecal flora of humans. It is a common isolate in the clinical laboratory, often associated with nosocomial infection or infection of immunocompromised hosts.

➤ Who Should be Suspected?

- *K. pneumoniae* is associated with severe pneumonia, especially in alcoholics. The pneumonia results in necrosis and hemorrhage; mucoid, "currant jelly" sputum is classic. Bacteremia is seen in a significant number of cases. *K. pneumoniae* is also associated with primary or hospital acquired UTI, nosocomial bloodstream, ventilator-associated, or other extraintestinal infection.
- *K. pneumoniae* isolates are of particular importance in hospital-acquired infections because of their intrinsic and acquired resistance to antimicrobial agents.

➤ Laboratory Findings

- *K. pneumoniae* isolates often produce mucoid colonies due to production of capsular material.
- All *Klebsiella* species are intrinsically resistant to ampicillin and ticarcillin. Many hospital isolates have additional resistance through acquisition of plasmids that carry resistance genes. Extended-spectrum beta-lactamases confer resistance to third-generation cephalosporins and most other beta-lactam antibiotics. *K. pneumoniae* carbapenemases confer resistance to imipenem, ertapenem, and meropenem in addition to most beta-lactam antibiotics.

PSEUDOMONAS AERUGINOSA INFECTION

➤ Definition

- *Pseudomonas aeruginosa* is a GNB that is intrinsically virulent for humans; it is capable of producing a wide range of localized and systemic infections. This organism can metabolize a variety of substrates and can be isolated from many environmental reservoirs, including water sources (e.g., sink traps), aqueous solutions, disinfectant solutions, and condensates in respirators.
- In addition, these species exhibit intrinsic and acquired resistance to commonly used antibiotics.

➤ Who Should be Suspected?

- *P. aeruginosa* may cause such infections as bacteremia/endocarditis and systemic infection in neutropenic and ICU patients, burn wound infection with sepsis, chronic pneumonia in patients with CF, keratoconjunctivitis due to contaminated contact lens solutions and other eye infections, nosocomial pneumonia, osteomyelitis due to nail puncture injuries or hematogenous spread (especially in IV drug abusers), otitis externa (swimmer's ear and malignant otitis externa), and/or UTI.

➤ Laboratory Findings

* Culture: Special selective media are recommended to improve isolation of *P. aeruginosa* from lower respiratory specimens submitted from patients with CF.
* Susceptibility: Because of unpredictable susceptibility patterns, susceptibility testing should be performed on all significant isolates. Isolates may develop resistance during prolonged therapy with any antibiotic; testing of repeat isolates may be indicated. Reported susceptibility to beta-lactam and beta-lactam/beta-lactamase combinations implies the need for high-dose therapy for serious infections; combination therapy is often recommended.

SALMONELLA AND SHIGELLA INFECTIONS

See Chapter 6, Digestive Diseases.

STENOTROPHOMONAS MALTOPHILIA INFECTION

➤ Definition

* *Stenotrophomonas maltophilia* is the third most commonly isolated glucose nonfermenting GNB in clinical laboratories. These organisms may colonize a variety of hospital and environmental sources, which serve as the reservoir for human colonization and infection.

➤ Who Should be Suspected?

S. maltophilia infections have been reported for all organ systems; however, most infections occur in patients with some type of innate or acquired immune defect. Isolates from patient specimens must be carefully evaluated for clinical significance because *S. maltophilia* may be isolated at a component of endogenous or contaminating flora. True *S. maltophilia* infection is associated with increased mortality. Typical syndromes include:

* Lower respiratory tract infection: *S. maltophilia* is most commonly isolated from respiratory specimens and may cause ~5% of nosocomial pneumonias, especially in intubated patients with significant prior exposure to broad-spectrum antibiotics. *S. maltophilia* has been increasingly isolated from the sputum of patients with CF, but its significance is unclear.
* Bacteremia: *S. maltophilia* bacteremia is most commonly nosocomial, caused by indwelling catheter or other site of primary infection.
* Wound infections: *S. maltophilia* is a relatively common cause of traumatic wound and soft tissue infections. Metastatic cellulitis has been described in oncology patients with neutropenia.

➤ Laboratory Findings

* Susceptibility: With few exceptions, penicillins (including beta-lactam/beta-lactamase combinations), cephalosporins, quinolones, and aminoglycosides are ineffective for *S. maltophilia* infections. TMP/SMX is the treatment of choice; alternative agents include ceftazidime, chloramphenicol, levofloxacin, minocycline, or ticarcillin-clavulanate.

VIBRIO INFECTION

➤ Definition
* *Vibrio cholerae* is the cause of cholera, a severe diarrheal disease. Risk of infection is significant in populations with poor sanitation related to water sources. Vibrios reside in brackish water and in the fauna of these environments.
* Transmission is primarily caused by ingestion of contaminated water or poorly cooked seafood. Continued transmission may result by fecal contamination of potable water sources or food. Disruption of potable water sources by natural disaster or civil disruption increases the risk of epidemic disease. Asymptomatic carriage is rare.

➤ Who Should be Suspected?
* Young children are most commonly infected and most susceptible to severe infection. After ingestion, symptoms usually begin within 2–4 days. Initial symptoms of nausea, vomiting, and abdominal discomfort are followed by severe diarrhea. Without aggressive rehydration, life-threatening dehydration may ensue, with neuromuscular symptoms, hypoglycemia, acute renal failure, or other complications.
* Noncholera *Vibrio* species may also cause human infection, most commonly diarrheal syndromes, albeit typically less severe than classic cholera. Extraintestinal infection is uncommon but well described. *Vibrio vulnificus* may cause significant infection after ingestion of contaminated seafood or traumatic inoculation. Preexisting liver disease, as seen with alcoholic cirrhosis, hepatitis, and hemochromatosis, predisposes patients to invasive infection. Cellulitis with formation of bullae is characteristic. Secondary *V. vulnificus* bacteremia is associated with high mortality.

➤ Laboratory Findings
* In cholera, careful monitoring of core laboratory values to assess the patient's state of hydration and metabolic status is critical.

YERSINIA INFECTION

➤ Definition
* Yersiniosis is usually caused by infection with *Yersinia enterocolitica* in patients presenting with gastroenteritis. *Y. enterocolitica* is widely distributed in nature and transmitted by the oral route. Swine are the likely source for human infections.
* *Yersinia pestis* is a significant pathogen. In naturally occurring infection, humans are incidental hosts, acquiring infection by exposure to the epizootic cycle between fleas and rodents (e.g., flea bite, contact with infected animal carcasses) or through care of patients with pneumonic plague. *Y. pestis* infection is now rare due to control of the normal rodent reservoir, but *Y. pestis* is considered a potential risk for development as a bioterror agent.

➤ Who Should be Suspected?
* Symptoms of *Y. enterocolitica* infection include acute enteritis (diarrhea and abdominal pain), mesenteric adenitis, and pseudoappendicitis. There are three major clinical manifestations of human *Y. pestis* infection:

- Bubonic (~90% of reported cases): sudden onset of fever, chills, malaise. Patients develop pain and swelling of a regional lymph node, usually with edema and erythema. The inguinal nodes are most commonly affected, although the upper extremity or cervical nodes may are more commonly involved in infection transmitted by cats.
- Septicemic (~10% of cases): Patients present with fever and sepsis without specific or localized symptoms. DIC and multiorgan failure develop as late complications.
- Pneumonic: Pneumonic plague may develop as a complication of bubonic plague through hematogenous spread, or by direct inhalation of infectious aerosols. Patients present with a sudden onset of dyspnea, cough and fever.

➤ Laboratory Findings
- **Culture**
  - Laboratories should have procedures in place for recognition and limitation of handling of *Y. pestis* isolates. The appropriate public health department should be alerted as soon as *Y. pestis* infection is suspected on the basis of clinical or laboratory findings. Further diagnostic testing should be performed under the direction of public health officials.
  - *Yersinia* gastroenteritis is diagnosed by culture of infected material. Isolates may grow slowly on MAC and show an optimum incubation temperature of 25–32°C. Isolation may be improved by the use of special selective media and incubation, like cold enrichment, but in acute yersiniosis, the bacterial load is high in stool and is usually detected by routine enteric cultures if the laboratory has been alerted to rule out *Yersinia*. Because of their growth characteristics, automated identification and susceptibility testing may be unreliable.
  - Stool may contain increased WBCs and RBCs, but grossly bloody stool is uncommon. Bacteremia is uncommon but may occur in patients with disorders leading to iron overload, like beta-thalassemia.

GRAM-NEGATIVE BACILLI, FASTIDIOUS

Organisms in this group are capable of growth in vitro but require enriched media and sometimes special techniques for isolation. Because culture techniques may have limited sensitivity for detection, serologic, molecular, and other diagnostic techniques may be required to confirm a clinical diagnosis.

BARTONELLOSIS

➤ Definition
- Bartonellosis refers to a range of syndromes caused by infection with *Bartonella* species. The bacteria may be isolated from a wide range of animals, which serve as the likely reservoir for human infection.

➤ Who Should be Suspected?
- *Bartonella henselae* infection most commonly manifests as cat-scratch disease (CSD). CSD is most commonly manifested by self-limited lymphadenopathy, but a number of organ systems may be involved. *B. henselae* should be strongly suspected on the basis of typical clinical presentation after exposure to cats, especially if flea infested.

* Almost all patients with CSD present with a cutaneous lesion at the site of inoculation and regional lymphadenopathy. Skin lesions appear within 3–10 days after inoculation and may show vesicular, erythematous, and papular phases. Lesions are minimally symptomatic and resolve after several weeks, healing without scarring. Primary lesions may occur on mucous membranes or conjunctiva.
* Tender solitary lymphadenopathy, typically with overlying erythema, develops in the second or third week after infection but may be delayed up to several months. In uncomplicated cases, lymphadenopathy usually resolves within 1–4 months.
* *Bartonella quintana* has historically been associated with trench fever during World War I. Trench fever is transmitted by the body louse, and patients present with fever, malaise, sweats and chills; conjunctivitis, retroorbital pain, back and neck pain, and anterior tibial pain. In recent years, *B. quintana* has emerged as a cause of "urban" trench fever in indigent populations with bacteremia and endocarditis, peliosis hepatitis, and bacillary angiomatosis, primarily in patients with AIDS. Suspect infection in patients with culture-negative endocarditis, vascular proliferative lesions (bacillary angiomatosis [BA]), and cystic lesions of the liver or other internal organs (peliosis).

➤ Laboratory Findings

* Direct examination and histopathology: Histopathologic examination may provide strong support for diagnosis of bartonellosis. Demonstration of typical granulomas and typical organisms (Warthin-Starry stain) strongly supports the diagnosis of CSD. Histologic appearance of excised lymph node, skin lesions, and so on, may be characteristic but are nonspecific. In BA, there is H&E staining of vascular proliferation. Lesions show eosinophilic debris; Warthin-Starry staining reveals masses of small bacteria.
* Molecular diagnosis: Sensitive and specific molecular diagnostic assays have been described. PCR and related methods are playing an increasing role in the diagnosis of infections caused by *Bartonella* species, when available. There are no FDA-approved methods, however.
* Culture: Isolation of *Bartonella* in culture provides a definitive diagnosis, but special culture techniques and prolonged incubation are required. Cultures are often negative in infected patients. In addition, most clinical laboratories cannot perform the testing required for specific identification, so isolates must be sent to a reference laboratory for further characterization. The lysis centrifugation method is recommended for blood cultures to detect *Bartonella* bloodstream infections.
* Serology
  * The sensitivity and specificity of serologic assays is not high, limiting their utility for the diagnosis of bartonellosis. There may be cross-reactions with other *Bartonella* species and other, unrelated organisms. The prevalence of seropositivity in general populations may be significant, suggesting asymptomatic *Bartonella* infection is common.
  * In CSD, *B. henselae* IFA IgG titer of ≥1:256 are consistent with recent infection, supporting a diagnosis of CSD. Titers ≥1:64 to 128 are suggestive but should be repeated after 2 weeks to confirm diagnosis; titers <1:64 indicate that recent infection is unlikely. A positive reaction for *B. henselae* IgM strongly supports recent infection, but IgM production is typically brief.
* General laboratory: ESR and CRP are usually increased in bartonellosis. WBC count is usually normal, but may be slightly elevated ≤13,000/μL; eosinophils may be increased. Other laboratory findings are related to specific organ involvement.

BORDETELLA PERTUSSIS

See Chapter 14, Respiratory, Metabolic, and Acid-Base Disorders.

BRUCELLA

➤ Definition
- *Brucella* species are fastidious, slowly growing GNRs.
- Isolates are highly infectious and pose a serious risk of laboratory acquired infections; clinicians should alert the laboratory when brucellosis is suspected. The CDC has classified *Brucella* species as potential bioterror agents, and reporting is mandated when *Brucella* infection is suspected or confirmed.

➤ Who Should be Suspected?
- Brucellosis causes a wide spectrum of clinical disease with acute and chronic forms.
- In affected patients, fever, chills, night sweats, malaise, headache, and other nonspecific symptoms are common and may mimic other acute or chronic illness, or fever of unknown origin (FUO). Bacteremia often occurs and may result in secondary localized infections; suppurative lesions may affect any organ system, including bone and joints, liver, and spleen.

➤ Laboratory Findings
- Cultures: *Brucella* species primarily infect the RE system with secondary spread to other organ systems. Therefore, blood and bone marrow cultures are specimens of choice for diagnosis. Other infected patient samples may also be submitted for culture.
- Serology: useful for diagnostic testing. Acute serum samples should be collected, followed by convalescent samples several weeks later. IgM titers are increased within the first 1–2 weeks of acute infection; there is a transition to IgG production after the second week. Titers fall in response to effective therapy.

FRANCISELLA TULARENSIS INFECTION

➤ Definition
- Naturally acquired tularemia is a zoonotic, tick-transmitted infection. The normal host species include rabbits, rodents, squirrels and other small mammals, and deer. Domestic livestock, especially sheep, are also susceptible to infection. Human infection is transmitted by direct contact with an infected animal or through the bite of an intermediate arthropod vector.
- *Francisella tularensis* is highly infectious and poses a serious risk for laboratory acquired infections; clinicians should alert the laboratory when tularemia is suspected so that appropriate precautions and culture techniques are used. The CDC has classified *F. tularensis* as a potential bioterror agent. Possible or confirmed *F. tularensis* infections must be reported to state departments of health.

➤ Who Should be Suspected?
- Disease usually occurs 2–10 days after exposure, with ulceration at the site of tick bite and painful regional adenopathy.

- Nonspecific symptoms are common, including fever, chills, headache, sweats, severe conjunctivitis, and regional adenopathy.
- Approximately 20% patients present with acute onset of fever and abdominal symptoms, including nonbloody diarrhea, vomiting, pain, and tenderness.

➤ Laboratory Findings
- Gram stain: Tiny faintly staining coccobacilli
- Culture: samples of blood, bone marrow, primary ulcers, lymph node aspirates or other infected tissue

HAEMOPHILUS INFECTIONS

➤ Definition
- *Haemophilus* species are fastidious GNRs and are responsible for a variety of infectious syndromes. They are common components of the endogenous flora of the mouth and upper respiratory tract. Most of the respiratory species have limited virulence and are able to cause disease only when normal host defenses are compromised.
- However, strains of *Haemophilus influenzae* may be encapsulated (serotypes a, b, c, d, e, and f). The serotype b capsular material is a virulence factor and is responsible for the ability of *H. influenzae* type b (Hib) to cause severe, invasive infections. *Haemophilus ducreyi* causes the STD chancroid.

➤ Who Should be Suspected?
- Most *Haemophilus* infections present as localized infections of the pararespiratory structures, like sinusitis or otitis media. Acute sinusitis is usually manifested by nasal congestion with purulent discharge, which may be unilateral. Mild pharyngitis and cough may be present. Fever, headache, and facial pain are common in severe and chronic infections. The diagnosis is most often established clinically, but imaging studies and occasionally aspiration of sinus contents for culture may be needed to firmly establish a specific diagnosis or agent.
- *H. influenzae* may cause an acute lobar pneumonia, but lower respiratory disease is most commonly manifested as bronchitis in patients with underlying lung disease. These patients typically present with nonproductive cough, wheezing, and increasing shortness of breath. In these patients, *Haemophilus* infection may cause significant deterioration of pulmonary function tests, hypoxemia, and dyspnea. Low-grade fever may be seen.
- Epiglottitis, cellulitis of the supraglottic structures, is a life-threatening manifestation of Hib infection. The tissue may be directly seeded by posterior pharyngeal organisms or as a result of bacteremia. There is typically an abrupt onset of fever, malaise, severe sore throat, and dysphagia. Dyspnea, inspiratory stridor, and drooling develop with progression to severe disease, caused by obstruction of the airway by the swelling of the supraglottic tissue. Attempts to collect swab specimens for culture may stimulate acute obstruction, so they are contraindicated prior to securing a protected airway. Lateral x-ray studies of the hypopharyngeal region demonstrate swelling of the epiglottis. Culture of blood commonly yields *H. influenzae*.
- Hib was the most common cause of meningitis in infants and young children in the prevaccination era. Patients usually presented with a short history consistent with URI or otitis media. Systemic symptoms usually progressed insidiously with fever, irritability, feeding problems, and other signs of significant illness, followed by signs and symptoms typical of

meningitis and CNS infection. Culture and analysis of blood and CSF should be submitted to establish the diagnosis.
- Other localized infections associated with Hib bacteremic disease include septic arthritis, osteomyelitis, and cellulitis. Buccal and periorbital cellulitis have been commonly, but not exclusively, associated with Hib. Buccal cellulitis presented with swelling of the cheek with deep red discoloration. Periorbital cellulitis presented with signs and symptoms of pus accumulation in the orbital tissues and a characteristic purple discoloration of the lids and skin surrounding the affected eye. *H. influenzae* may cause acute conjunctivitis and endophthalmitis. *H. influenzae* biogroup *aegyptius* has been implicated in conjunctivitis and Brazilian purpuric fever, a bacteremia syndrome with fever and hypotension, purpuric rash, vomiting, and abdominal pain.
- *H. ducreyi* causes the STD chancroid, an ulcerative infection that occurs primarily in tropical regions. Disease is manifested by multiple genital and perineal ulcers. Unlike the chancres of syphilis, the ulcers of chancroid are painful and have ragged borders with minimal induration. Inguinal adenopathy is common and may progress to draining buboes. Like other genital ulcerative diseases, chancroid increases the risk of transmission of HIV infection.

➤ Laboratory Findings
- Gram stain: Diagnosis of *Haemophilus* infection depends primarily of Gram stain and culture of infected specimens. Gram staining of specimens or culture isolates show small, pleomorphic, faintly staining gram-negative rods; some end-to-end pairing or small filamentous forms may be present.
- Culture: *Haemophilus* species are fastidious but are efficiently isolated on chocolate agar and in routine blood culture media. Positive cultures from the upper respiratory tract must be interpreted with caution because *Haemophilus* species, including encapsulated strains, are common components of the endogenous flora. Specimens for the diagnosis of chancroid are collected from the margin and undermined base of fresh ulcers. *H. ducreyi* is difficult to isolate by culture, requiring specialized enriched media that should be inoculated at bedside.
- Antigen detection (for detection of Hib from CSF, serum, or urine): use of antigen detection is not recommended, having been shown to rarely contribute to the clinical management of patients.

HELICOBACTER PYLORI INFECTION

➤ Definition
- *Helicobacter pylori* infection shows a global distribution.
- Most infections are likely transmitted by the fecal oral route.

➤ Who Should be Suspected?
- *H. pylori* is the cause of most gastric and duodenal ulcers through disruption of the protective mucous layer. This organism is epidemiologically linked to gastric adenocarcinoma and lymphoma.

➤ Laboratory Findings
H. pylori may be diagnosed by several invasive or noninvasive means:
- Histologic examination of gastric mucosa: Organisms stain poorly with H&E but may be demonstrated with Giemsa or silver staining.

- Culture of gastric mucosa: Special culture techniques are required for isolation. The organism is microaerophilic and capnophilic and yields growth within 5 days on enriched media.
- Urease activity (tissue or breath): Strongly positive.
- Specific antigen: A commercially available assay for detection of *H. pylori* antigen in feces shows a sensitivity of ~90% and specificity of ~95% for detection of active infection. *H. pylori* antigen may be useful for monitoring response to therapy.
- Serology: IgG is typically measured. Positive response is predictive of active infection in patient populations where the prevalence of active infection is not high. Antibody levels may remain persistently positive for a period after successful therapy, so serology may have a limited role in early test-of-cure.

PASTEURELLA MULTOCIDA INFECTION

➤ Definition
- *Pasteurella multocida*, an aerobic GNR, is a common part of the endogenous oral flora of domesticated cats and dogs, as well as other domesticated and wild animals.

➤ Who Should be Suspected?
- Infection is usually manifested as cellulitis or wound infections associated with cat bites or scratches. Close contact with animals and underlying medical conditions, especially hepatic disease and malignancy, predispose to infection.
- Infections at the site of inoculation are painful with marked erythema and swelling. Because of the nature of cat bites (deep penetrating wounds), deep soft tissue infection, septic arthritis, and osteomyelitis are common complications. Localized infection may progress to bacteremia with hematogenous spread to other organ systems, including endocarditis and CNS infections. Colonization of the upper respiratory tract predisposes to pneumonia and para-respiratory abscesses, like sinusitis or empyema.

➤ Laboratory Findings
- Gram staining: Possibly small, faintly staining gram-negative coccobacilli.
- Cultures: Isolates grow well on SBA or chocolate agar incubated in increased CO_2.

GRAM-NEGATIVE COCCI

Organisms in this group usually grow well and rapidly on routine laboratory media, but may require chocolate or other enriched media for isolation. Selective media may be used to improve isolation from specimens likely to be contaminated with endogenous flora. Empirical therapy is usually successful, but susceptibility testing is recommended for patients who fail to respond, or in regions with decreased rates of susceptibility to standard treatments. Serologic testing does not play a role in routine diagnosis or management.

Neisseria Infections: Overview

The *Neisseria* species are gram-negative cocci that typically form pairs with characteristic "coffee bean" morphology. *Neisseria meningitidis* and *Neisseria gonorrhoeae* are significant human pathogens. Certain *Neisseria* species, including *N. meningitidis*, may be isolated as components of the endogenous respiratory flora of healthy individuals, but *N. gonorrhoeae* is never considered normal flora.

NEISSERIA MENINGITIDIS INFECTION

➤ Definition
- In meningococcal disease, infection is usually transmitted by the respiratory route. In susceptible patients, bacteremia may occur by passage of organisms across the epithelial barrier. Infection in multiple organ systems is common in meningococcal disease.

➤ Who Should be Suspected?
Common infectious syndromes include:
- Meningococcemia: Meningococcal bacteremia may be transient and associated with minimal symptoms. Meningococcemia, however, may result in sustained bacteremia and seeding of other organ systems. Sustained bacteremia is typically associated with fever, malaise, and leukocytosis. Fulminant disease is usually associated by seeding of the CNS and other organs, DIC, adrenal insufficiency, and other manifestations of multiorgan failure. CNS invasion is common in patients with meningococcemia; meningitis should be actively be ruled out by clinical and laboratory evaluation in patients in whom meningococcemia is documented.
- CNS infection (meningitis and meningoencephalitis)
  - More than 90% of adults with clinically significant meningococcal infections have meningitis. Patients with CNS disease usually present with typical signs and symptoms of meningitis, including fever, headache, nuchal rigidity, and mental status changes. Vomiting is common. Not all patients, however, present with classic signs and symptoms.
  - The clinical presentation may be dominated by symptoms of fulminant disease and multiorgan failure. Overwhelming disease may be associated with shock, petechial rash, purpura fulminans, gangrenous necrosis of the distal extremities, and the Waterhouse-Friderichsen syndrome (3–4% of patients).

➤ Laboratory Findings
- Direct detection: CSF Gram stain is diagnostic in 50–70% of patients with meningitis, although pyogenic meningitis in which bacteria cannot be found in smear is more likely to be caused by meningococcus than to other bacteria.
- Core laboratory: increased WBC count (12,000–40,000/μL). Urine may show albumin, RBCs; occasional glycosuria. Laboratory findings of predisposing conditions such as asplenia (e.g., sickle cell anemia) or immunodeficiency (e.g., complement, immunoglobulin). Laboratory findings due to complications (e.g., DIC) and sequelae (e.g., subdural effusion) may be seen.
- CSF findings: Markedly increased WBC count (2,500–10,000/μL), almost all PMNs; increased protein (50–1500 mg/dL); decreased glucose (0–45 mg/dL).

NEISSERIA GONORRHOEAE INFECTION

➤ Definition
- Diseases caused by *N. gonorrhoeae* are almost exclusively transmitted by sexual contact or exposure to infected genital secretions. *N. gonorrhoeae* isolates are always considered to represent infection.

➤ Who Should be Suspected?

* Gonorrhea is an STD of adults. Infection in neonates may be acquired by exposure to contaminated secretions during childbirth. Infections in other prepubertal children must be investigated as a possible indication of child abuse.
* Males with gonorrhea most commonly present with urethritis, manifested by dysuria and urethral discharge. In the absence of specific antimicrobial therapy, spontaneous resolution is common. Complications include "ascending" infection (epididymitis and seminal vesiculitis, regional adenitis, abscess formation, and urethral stricture) and distant infection by contaminated secretions (e.g., conjunctivitis).
* Anorectal and pharyngeal gonorrhea may occur in men who have sex with men. Anorectal infections may also be asymptomatic but often present with proctitis or rectal pain with purulent discharge and painful defecation. Pharyngeal infection may be asymptomatic but usually occurs as an acute, suppurative pharyngitis with regional adenopathy.
* Most women with *N. gonorrhoeae* infection present with cervical and urethral infection. Symptoms include vaginal and urethral discharge, pelvic pain, and abnormal vaginal bleeding. Adjacent structures, like Bartholin's glands, may become infected by local spread. Ascending infection, resulting in pelvic inflammatory disease (PID) (e.g., salpingitis, endometritis, tuboovarian abscess, perihepatitis), occurs in 10–20% of patients. Anorectal infection in women is most commonly acquired by autoinfection by infected vaginal secretions. PID increases the risk of sterility and tubal pregnancy. *N. gonorrhoeae* infection during pregnancy may result in premature delivery or spontaneous abortion, chorioamnionitis, and transmission of infection (conjunctival or pharyngeal) to the neonate.

➤ Laboratory Findings

* Direct detection: Gonorrhea may be diagnosed accurately by Gram stain of urethral secretions from symptomatic males. The detection of typical gram-negative diplococci within PMNs is diagnostic (S/S of ~95%). Gram stain examination of endocervical secretions may support a diagnosis of gonorrheal cervical or anorectal infection if many intracellular gram-negative diplococci are seen (sensitivity ~50%), but smears must be interpreted with caution because of the presence of nonpathogenic gram-negative organisms in the endogenous flora of these sites.
* Culture: the gold standard for diagnosis of nongenital *N. gonorrhoeae* infections. Swabs of secretions of anal crypts should be submitted for diagnosis of anorectal gonorrhea; rectal swabs (heavily contaminated with feces) should not be submitted. Cultures are required for other types of specimens and for medicolegal specimens (e.g., child abuse, rape).
* Molecular diagnosis: Considered the gold standard for diagnosis of *N. gonorrhoeae* genital infection. Note that a number of direct probe and amplified probe techniques are commercially available. Several advantages of nucleic acid testing include the ability to detect nonviable organisms and increased sensitivity, allowing diagnostic testing on urine specimens. Tests with S/S >98% are available, depending on the assay and specimen type.

GRAM-POSITIVE BACILLI

The gram-positive bacilli (GPB) usually grow within 24–48 hours on routine laboratory media, like SBA. Inoculation of selective and differential media, like columbia colistin–nalidixic acid (CNA) or phenylethyl alcohol agar (PEA) agar, may facilitate isolation from contaminated specimens. Standardized susceptibility testing has not been established for all pathogenic GPB.

ANTHRAX (*BACILLUS ANTHRACIS*)

➤ Definition
* Anthrax is caused by infection with *Bacillus anthracis*, a large, spore-forming gram-positive rod (GPR). Naturally occurring anthrax is a zoonotic disease associated with grazing animals in regions without effective vaccination programs; humans may be infected as secondary hosts, usually through contact with spores. In the United States, sporadic infection has been associated with contact with animal products imported from regions with endemic infection.
* Anthrax has been recognized as a potential agent of bioterror or biologic warfare because of the ability to "weaponize" the organism and the severity of disease caused by weaponized spores.
* Anthrax is a national notifiable infectious disease. Reporting to public health departments is mandated for all suspected or confirmed cases of *B. anthracis* infection.

➤ Who Should be Suspected?
* There are three major anthrax syndromes: cutaneous, alimentary tract, and inhalational. Other organ systems may be infected by spread of infection from a primary site of infection.
* The diagnosis of anthrax requires a high index of suspicion. Early recognition and antibiotic treatment are critical for successful management of patients with GI, pulmonary, or other invasive infections.

➤ Laboratory Findings
* Specimens include vesicular fluid, swab, or tissue from below the leading edge of cutaneous lesions, lower respiratory secretions/sputum, feces, CSF, or specimens from other infected sites.
* Blood cultures should be submitted for all patients with suspected anthrax.
* Gram stain shows large GPBs; may form short chains. Capsules may be apparent. Spores may be seen in subcultures.

CLOSTRIDIAL INFECTIONS: OVERVIEW

* *Clostridium* species are anaerobic, spore-forming gram-positive bacilli. The formation of spores results in efficient survival of clostridia in the environment; the spores serve as the source of infections of exogenous origin (e.g., *Clostridium difficile* colitis, *Clostridium perfringens* food poisoning). Clostridia may also cause infections of endogenous origin (e.g., myonecrosis).
* *Clostridium* species produce some of the most potent toxins, which may be responsible for the pathogenesis of some clostridial diseases (e.g., tetanus). Botulinum toxin is considered to have significant potential for use as a bioterror agent.
* Clostridia grow well and rapidly on media for anaerobic culture, but selective media may be needed for contaminated specimens. The interpretation of cultures positive for *Clostridium* species is usually straightforward, but because of the ubiquitous distribution of clostridia in the environment, positive cultures must be interpreted in the context of the clinical presentation. Standardized susceptibility testing is available using specialized techniques, but many laboratories do not offer the testing in-house.

BOTULISM (*CLOSTRIDIUM BOTULINUM*)

➤ Definition

* Botulism describes a toxin-mediated paralytic disease caused by heat-labile toxins of *Clostridium botulinum*. Botulism toxins bind to the synaptic vesicles of cholinergic nerves, preventing release of acetylcholine into the neurosynaptic cleft.
* Therefore, botulism intoxication results in acute, symmetrical, flaccid paralysis. Patients usually present with impairment of cranial nerves and muscles of the head and neck. Symptoms progress to symmetrical paralysis of the musculature of the trunk, progressing then to the extremities. Respiratory paralysis is usually the most life-threatening manifestation of botulism.
* Several distinct botulism syndromes have been described, including food-borne botulism (usually presents in adults after ingestion of preformed toxin in *C. botulinum* contaminated food), infant botulism (the most commonly encountered form of botulism, it results from the ingestion of *C. botulinum* organisms that then produce toxin within the infant's gut), and wound botulism (a rare form of botulism in which toxin is formed in vivo by *C. botulinum* organisms causing wound infection).
* Clinicians must be alert to patients presenting with signs and symptoms compatible with botulism because they may represent an index case of a bioterror incident. Reporting to public health authorities is mandated for suspected or documented botulism.

➤ Laboratory Findings

* Culture: In the proper clinical setting, diagnosis may be established by isolation of *C. botulinum* or botulinum toxin from food or patient specimens. Isolation of *C. botulinum* by anaerobic culture may be attempted for infected patient specimens or feces. Attempts to isolate *C. botulinum* from food should be performed by a specialized reference laboratory.
* Toxin detection: Typical specimens include any food suspected in an outbreak, serum (15–20 mL in adults; 2–3 mL in infants), gastric contents or vomitus, feces (as much as possible, up to ~50 g). Toxin detection is performed by specialized reference or public health laboratories.
* Core laboratory: Routine laboratory tests are usually normal.

CLOSTRIDIAL GAS GANGRENE, CELLULITIS, AND PUERPERAL SEPSIS

➤ Definition

* These syndromes may be caused by a number of clostridial species of endogenous or exogenous origin. Most cases of clostridial gangrene are caused by *C. perfringens*, *Clostridium novyi*, and *Clostridium septicum*.

➤ Who Should be Suspected?

* Patients present with rapidly progressive tissue necrosis, tissue liquefaction, and gas formation. Gas formation in tissue is not specific for clostridial infections and may be formed by other bacterial pathogens.
* Clostridial myonecrosis should be considered a medical emergency and rapid and effective communication with clinical personnel, especially surgeons, is critical.

➤ Laboratory Findings

- Direct detection: Gram stain typically shows massive tissue necrosis, a lack of PMNs, and the presence of typical organisms (usually large "box-car" GPBs; the absence of spores on Gram stain is common and does not rule out clostridial infection; other bacterial morphotypes may be seen in mixed infections).
- Culture: Blood cultures may be positive.
- Core laboratory: WBC count is increased (15,000–40,000/μL). Platelets are decreased in 50% of patients. Protein and casts are often present in urine. Renal insufficiency may progress to uremia. Laboratory findings typical for underlying diseases (e.g., DM) or complications of clostridial infection are seen. In postabortion sepsis, sudden severe hemolytic anemia is common with conditions such as hypoglobulinemia, hemoglobinuria, increased serum bilirubin, spherocytosis, and increased osmotic and mechanical fragility.

CLOSTRIDIUM TETANI INFECTION

➤ Definition

- Tetanus describes disease caused by a heat-labile toxin (tetanospasmin) elaborated by *Clostridium tetani*.
- Infection typically results from "dirty" traumatic injuries (e.g., deep puncture wounds, crush injuries) contaminated by spores of *C. tetani*. Toxin diffuses from the site of infection into the circulation, where it gains access to peripheral motor neurons. Toxin is transported through the neurons to the CNS, where it blocks inhibitory signals from the CNS to motor neurons. Tetanospasmin also binds to receptors at the myoneural junctions (different from the receptors for botulinum toxin), inhibiting the release of acetylcholine.
- Tetanus has been essentially eliminated in populations with an effective vaccination program, but sporadic cases occur in unvaccinated populations.

➤ Who Should be Suspected?

- Patients present with spasm of flexor and extensor muscles. Patients develop pathologic hyperresponsiveness to minor stimuli. Common features include "lock jaw," risus sardonicus, and back spasms resulting in relentless arching.

➤ Laboratory Findings

Diagnosis is usually made on the basis of typical clinical findings.

- Culture from an infected site: poor sensitivity and is usually noncontributory.
- Core laboratory: usually normal.

CLOSTRIDIUM DIFFICILE–ASSOCIATED (PSEUDOMEMBRANOUS) COLITIS

➤ Definition

- *C. difficile* is the most important cause of pseudomembranous colitis, usually acquired nosocomially. It is a major cause of antibiotic-associated diarrhea and colitis without pseudomembrane formation.

➤ Who Should be Suspected?

* Several factors are associated with increased risk for *C. difficile* disease, including recent or current antimicrobial (or antineoplastic) therapy, age (>65 years), suppression of gastric acid production, and debilitating underlying medical conditions.

➤ Laboratory Findings

* Culture: Specific laboratory diagnosis is based on the growth of *C. difficile* from stool culture or by detection of *C. difficile*–specific antigen, toxins, or DNA. Testing should be performed on liquid stool specimens only; asymptomatic carriage may be seen. Formed stool should be rejected if submitted for testing. Isolation of toxigenic *C. difficile*, using selective anaerobic culture, is considered the "gold standard" for diagnosis. Toxin production by isolates must be documented and may be confirmed by PCR, antigen, or cytotoxicity assays. The complexity and turnaround time required for toxigenic culture assays has limited their use for routine testing.
* Cytotoxicity assays: These assays are based on detection of the cytotoxic effect of *C. difficile* toxin B on cultured eukaryotic cells.
* EIA: A number of enzyme immunoassays are commercially available for rapid detection of *C. difficile* toxin B or both toxins A and B. Because of their simplicity and rapid turn-around-time (<1 hour), EIA tests have become widely used for diagnosis of *C. difficile* disease. EIA assays have shown high specificity (>95%), but the sensitivity of different assays is variable, ranging from ~60–95%, which has limited their use in critically ill patients or infection control investigations.
* Antigen detection: Detection of *C. difficile* specific glutamate dehydrogenase (GDH) antigen may be used to screen stools for *C. difficile*. The sensitivity of the GDH assay depends on the reference standard; sensitivities ranging from ~70% to >95% have been reported. Toxin must be documented in antigen-positive specimens because nontoxigenic *C. difficile* strains are detected by this antigen assay.
* Molecular diagnostic testing: PCR assays that target the toxin B gene have emerged as clinically important assays for the diagnosis of *C. difficile* GI infection. Several FDA-approved methods are commercially available. Reported performance of molecular diagnostic assays has show S/S both in the range ~95 to 99%. The use of real-time PCR assays provides for results within 24 hours.
* Combination tests: Some laboratories have combined EIA, GDH antigen, and/or PCR testing in simultaneous or sequential test algorithms to improve the S/S and cost effectiveness of these rapid test methods.

DIPHTHERIA

See Chapter 14, Respiratory, Metabolic, and Acid-Base Disorders.

LISTERIA INFECTION

➤ Definition

* Listeriosis is caused by infection with *Listeria monocytogenes*, an aerobic, pleomorphic gram-positive bacillus. This organism is widely distributed in nature, and up to 5% of

asymptomatic, healthy adults may carry *L. monocytogenes* as a component of their endogenous fecal flora.

* CNS and placental tissue are predisposed to *Listeria* infection. Most infections are thought to occur as a result of oral ingestion, followed by invasion across the gut mucosa and systemic spread. Disease may occur in a sporadic or epidemic pattern.

➤ Who Should be Suspected?

* *Listeria* is responsible for a small proportion of food-borne infections, and most cases are sporadic, but the case-fatality rate is relatively high. Outbreaks have been caused by a variety of types of food, including delicatessen meats, unpasteurized cheeses, smoked seafood, and processed meat spreads. Ingestion of contaminated food may cause self-limited gastroenteritis in normal hosts, with onset typically several days after exposure. Symptoms include fever, nausea, vomiting, and diarrhea. Flu-like symptoms are common.

* Risk factors associated with increased infection risk and severity include immunocompromise, age ≥70 years, alcoholism, glucocorticoid therapy, kidney disease, non-hematologic malignancy, neonatal infection, and pregnancy.

* In normal hosts, complete recovery is typical after several days of illness. During pregnancy, listeriosis usually presents with flu-like symptoms and may resolve spontaneously. Severe listeriosis may occur in the third trimester where placental infection and transmission to the fetus or neonate may occur. The signs and symptoms of *Listeria* sepsis are not distinctive, and diagnostic cultures are critical for specific diagnosis. Patients present with fever and malaise that may progress to shock and sepsis. Symptoms of meningoencephalitis are nonspecific and may include meningeal signs, mental status changes, or focal neurologic defects (e.g., ataxia, cranial nerve abnormalities, and deafness). Direct hematogenous seeding of the brain parenchyma may result in cerebritis or brain abscess, most typically manifested by stroke-like symptoms or focal neurologic defects.

➤ Laboratory Findings

* Culture (blood): most reliable diagnostic test; culture of CSF and other infected tissue is indicated on the basis of clinical presentation. Specialized techniques are required for isolation of *Listeria* from suspected food samples.

* Gram stain: CSF Gram stain is only positive in about one third of patients with meningoencephalitis, and lower in localized CNS infections. *Listeria* may be misidentified as *Streptococcus pneumoniae*, diphtheroids, or even *H. influenzae*.

* CSF findings: Pleocytosis is typical (100 to 10,000 WBC/μL). Significant CSF lymphocytosis (>25%) may be seen on CSF WBC differential prior to antibiotic therapy. CSF protein concentration is typically moderately elevated, but CSF glucose is reduced in only ~40% of patients with CNS infection. CSF findings may lead to misdiagnosis as viral infection, syphilis, Lyme disease, or TB.

* Serology: not usually useful for diagnosis of acute listeriosis.

GRAM-POSITIVE COCCI

Gram-positive cocci (GPC) cause a wide variety of infections in immunocompromised and immunocompetent hosts. Organisms grow well and rapidly on media routinely inoculated for bacterial infections. Selective media improves detection of carriage from specimens with mixed flora, as for methicillin-resistant *Staphylococcus aureus* or vancomycin-resistant enterococci

(VRE). Standardized susceptibility testing is available and may be required for management of some infections because of unpredictable susceptibility rates for some drug combinations. Molecular methods are playing an increasing role in diagnosis of some infections. Serologic testing does not play a role in diagnosis of acute infection.

Nonspecific laboratory markers of localized or systemic GPC infections are common, including increased WBC (12,000–20,000/µL), anemia, thrombocytopenia, and increased ESR and CRP. DIC is an uncommon, but severe complication of systemic infection. Typical laboratory abnormalities may be seen, which are consistent with dysfunction of specifically infected organs, as well as any underlying medical condition of the patient.

ENTEROCOCCAL INFECTIONS

➤ Definition
* *Enterococcus* species are universal components of the endogenous lower GI tract flora in healthy humans; colonization of the urogenital mucosa is common. Enterococci are moderately virulent, but the mechanisms are not clearly understood, with the exception of their intrinsic and acquired resistance to antibiotics, including vancomycin. This characteristic is at least partially responsible for the emergence of enterococci as significant nosocomial pathogens.
* *Enterococcus faecalis* and *E. faecium* are the species most commonly associated with human infection.

➤ Who Should be Suspected?
* Enterococci may cause infection in virtually any organ system; common infections include UTIs, bacteremia, endocarditis, intra-abdominal infections, and wound infections.
* Hospitalized patients who are rectal carriers of VRE may transmit these pathogens to other patients who may be at high risk for invasive VRE infection.

➤ Laboratory Findings
* Susceptibility testing: must be performed for significant clinical isolates.

STAPHYLOCOCCUS AUREUS INFECTION

➤ Definition
* The genus *Staphylococcus* is composed of several species that are implicated in human infection. *Staphylococcus aureus* is a frequent cause of pyogenic infection. Staphylococcal disease may also be caused by the elaboration of several potent toxins.

➤ Who Should be Suspected?
Staphylococcus aureus is able to cause disease in virtually all organ systems. The many clinical presentations of *S. aureus* infection include:
* Pneumonia: Pulmonary infections may be caused by aspiration of organisms from the upper respiratory tract or by hematogenous seeding from another primary site of infection. *S. aureus* pneumonia may represent a severe complication of viral infection (e.g., measles, influenza), CF, or debilitating underlying disease.

- Acute osteomyelitis, septic arthritis: Osteomyelitis in adults is usually a result of a direct extension of local infection, often at the site of a surgical or traumatic wound. The vertebral column is a common site of infection of hematogenous origin. Septic arthritis in adults is usually of hematogenous origin.
- Pyomyositis: *S. aureus* infection of skeletal muscle is usually caused by trauma or direct extension from an adjacent site.
- Bacteremia and endocarditis
  - Bacteremia may occur as a complication of localized pyogenic infection. Metastatic foci of infection are common. Patients generally present with acute sepsis syndromes, often with signs and symptoms due to localized infections.
  - Endocarditis may be caused by seeding of valves during a primary bacteremia or by organisms directly introduced into the blood stream (e.g., intravascular catheter, injection drug use). Patients with endocarditis may present with subacute or acute symptoms. Normal cardiac valves are commonly affected. *S. aureus* endocarditis causes rapid, severe damage to valves, producing acute mechanical heart failure (e.g., rupture of chordae tendineae, perforation of valve, valvular insufficiency) in addition to the physiologic effects of severe infection. Typical stigmata of endocarditis (e.g., Janeway lesions, splinter hemorrhages, Roth spots) are common.
- Food poisoning: Staphylococcal food poisoning is caused by ingestion of food tainted by enterotoxin-producing strains of *S. aureus*. Symptoms, including crampy abdominal pain, nausea and vomiting, and diarrhea, occur early (2–6 hours after ingestion). Patients are symptomatic for 8–10 hours after onset of illness. Aggressive fluid management forms the mainstay of therapy. Note: Suspected clusters of food-borne gastroenteritis must be reported to state boards of public health.
- Impetigo, a superficial skin infection commonly affecting the face: seen most commonly in infants. The rash of impetigo presents with red macules that mature into vesicles, which may shed honey-colored serous fluid prior to drying. Most cases of impetigo are caused by *S. aureus*. Most of the remaining cases (~10–15%) are caused by *Streptococcus pyogenes*.
- Meningitis: CNS infection with *S. aureus* may occur in traumatic or surgical wounds, by hematogenous spread from other primary site of infection, or contamination of an intraventricular pressure monitoring device or other foreign body. Signs and symptoms are similar to those caused by other pathogens.
- Toxic shock syndrome (TSS)
  - This syndrome is caused by the action of TSS toxin-1 (or related toxin), a pyrogenic superantigen elaborated by a colonizing strain of *S. aureus*. Note that several other species, like group A *Streptococcus*, may elaborate similar toxins that produce an identical clinical presentation.
  - Patients present acutely with vascular congestion, increased permeability of capillaries, and decreased vascular resistance. Hypotension and tissue hypoxia develop as a consequence of the loss of the intravascular blood volume. ARDS and DIC are common complications in patients with severe disease. Staphylococcal TSS is defined by fever $>38.9°C$, diffuse macular rash, desquamation, and hypotension (systolic blood pressure ≤ 90 mm Hg for adults).
  - The diagnosis is possible when signs and symptoms of disease are seen in three organ systems (muscular, GI, liver, bone marrow, CNS, kidney, skin/mucous membranes). TSS is probable when five organ systems are involved and confirmed if all six organ systems are affected.

➤ Laboratory Findings

- Direct detection: In pyogenic infections, Gram stain usually demonstrates many GPCs with a brisk PMN response.
- Culture: In patients with bacteremia, the persistence of positive blood cultures at 72–96 hours after the initiation of appropriate antimicrobial therapy is a predictor of a complicated recovery course and predicts the need for prolonged treatment.
- Susceptibility testing: should be performed on significant *S. aureus* isolates because resistance to many primary therapeutic agents is common; resistance or intermediate susceptibility has been well documented for vancomycin.

STREPTOCOCCAL INFECTIONS

Streptococci are common components of the endogenous flora of humans, which serves as the reservoir for most infections. The genus *Streptococcus* includes species that are well-known human pathogens, including *Streptococcus pneumoniae*, *Streptococcus pyogenes* (group A, GAS), *Streptococcus agalactiae* (group B, GBS), viridans streptococci, and others.

STREPTOCOCCUS PYOGENES (GROUP A) INFECTION

➤ Definition

- GAS colonizes the upper respiratory tract and skin and infections at these sites are the most common manifestations of GAS disease. Invasive pyogenic infections are commonly caused by GAS; infections in all organ systems have been described. In addition to primary GAS infections, GAS may cause clinically significant superinfections (e.g., GAS pneumonia complicating influenza, GAS cellulitis complicating chickenpox). GAS infections may result in suppurative complications, immune-mediated nonsuppurative sequelae, and toxin-mediated disease.
- Diseases caused by GAS include:
  - Pharyngitis: see Chapter 14, Respiratory, Metabolic, and Acid-Base Disorders
  - Cellulitis and soft tissue infections: Impetigo describes a superficial vesicular rash, usually presenting in children. The vesicles evolve into pustules, which break down and scab over the following week. Erysipelas is a soft tissue infection that most often affects adults, who present with fever and erythematous, edematous areas of inflammation with well-demarcated edges, usually on the face. GAS may also cause cellulitis in tissue surrounding infected wounds or trauma.
  - Acute rheumatic fever: This disorder is a nonsuppurative complication following prior GAS pharyngitis (2–5 weeks). Common manifestations of this systemic collagen vascular disease include carditis, chorea, erythema marginatum, polyarthritis, and subcutaneous nodules.
  - Acute poststreptococcal GN (PSGN): Acute GN is a nonsuppurative complication following GAS pharyngitis (>10 days) or GAS skin infections (3–6 weeks). Clinical symptoms include headache, malaise, fatigue, edema, hypertension, and encephalopathy.
  - Group A streptococcal toxic shock-like syndrome: This disorder may develop in patients infected with GAS strains capable of elaborating streptococcal pyrogenic exotoxins. The syndrome is often preceded by nonspecific symptoms (fever, chills, malaise). There may be prominent symptoms at the site of primary infections. Disease progresses to shock and multiorgan failure.

➤ Laboratory Findings

- Gram stain: For most clinically significant infections, gram-positive organisms in chains appear in smears.
- Susceptibility testing: Group A *Streptococcus* isolates are predictably susceptible to penicillins and related antibiotics, the drugs of choice for these infections. Susceptibility testing of GAS must be performed for other antibiotics, as for penicillin-allergic patients.
- Serology: not recommended for diagnosis of acute GAS infection but may be used for diagnosis of infection in the recent past in patients with symptoms of GN or RF. Several specific assays are most useful for detection of GAS antibodies. Submit paired samples for:
  - Antistreptolysin O (ASO)
    - ASO antibody testing is the most commonly used and standardized test to diagnose prior GAS infection. Antibody response is brisk after upper respiratory tract infection: detectable antibodies appear ~1 week after acute infection and reach maximum titers 3–6 weeks after acute infection. Skin infections (impetigo, pyoderma), however, do not stimulate a good ASO response, so this assay is not recommended for patient evaluation following skin infections.
    - There are several causes for false-positive test results, including multiple myeloma, hypergammaglobulinemia, rheumatoid factor, or infection with group C or G *Streptococcus*.
  - Anti-DNase B: The anti-DNase B assay is most useful for the evaluation of patients with acute rheumatic fever or glomerulonephritis after impetigo, pyoderma, or other skin infection. Antibody titers are usually detectable ~2 weeks after acute infection and reach peak titers 6–8 weeks after infection. Factors causing false-positive ASO titers do not affect anti-DNase B testing, but false-positive anti-DNase B results may be seen in acute hemorrhagic pancreatitis.
  - Streptozyme: This assay is based on agglutination of RBCs coated with a number of GAS antigens. The reagents have not been well standardized, so lot-to-lot variation has been documented, in terms of both sensitivity and specificity, limiting the value of this testing.
- Rapid GAS detection: Throat swab for rapid direct antigen testing for GAS has a sensitivity of 70–90% compared to culture on SBA; specificity is ~95%. Antigen testing may provide results within minutes, but cultures are recommended when antigen testing is negative. A positive antigen test result means patient has GAS pharyngitis or is a GAS carrier.
- Molecular diagnostics: The sensitivity of the Gen-Probe Group A Strep Direct Test is 89–95%, with >97% specificity. Sensitivity of the LightCycler Strep-A realtime PCR assay is ~93%, with specificity ~98%. The high sensitivity of these molecular assays for detection of GAS pharyngitis obviates culture in direct assay negative specimens.
- Core laboratory: In patients with PSGN, abnormal urinalysis (RBCs, WBCs, and casts), anemia, decreased total complement, and C3 and/or increased ESR are typical.

STREPTOCOCCUS AGALACTIAE (GROUP B) INFECTION

➤ Definition

- GBS is a component of the GI and vaginal flora of healthy adults, which serves as the primary reservoir for infection. Intermittent rectovaginal carriage is seen in ~25% of pregnant women. Infant prophylaxis, based on results of screening for maternal carriage at

35–37 weeks of gestation, has resulted in a significant decline in the rate of neonatal GBS infections.
* Adult disease is playing an increasing role in the spectrum of GBS disease.

➤ Who Should be Suspected?

* Adult disease: UTI and bacteremia are the most common manifestation of GBS infection in adults, but any organ system may be affected. Pregnancy, advanced age, and significant underlying medical conditions (e.g., cirrhosis, DM, malignancy) are risk factors for acquisition of GBS disease in adults.
* Neonatal and perinatal disease: Vaginal colonization at the end of gestation may lead to neonatal infection, either by ascending intrauterine infection after rupture of membranes, or exposure during passage through the birth canal. Risk factors include prolonged rupture of membranes, amnionitis, and maternal bacteremia.

➤ Laboratory Findings

* Culture: The CDC and American College of Obstetrics and Gynecology now recommend that decisions regarding prophylactic antimicrobial treatment for the prevention of neonatal GBS infection be based on cultures to detect maternal GBS carriage. Collection of lower vaginal (not cervical) *and* rectal swabs for special cultures for GBS detection are recommended for all pregnant women at 35–37 weeks of gestation. (The only exceptions are for women with urine cultures positive for GBS during pregnancy and women with a history of a previous child with GBS neonatal infection; perinatal prophylaxis should always be given to these patients.)
* Susceptibility testing: GBS isolates are predictably susceptible to penicillin and related antibiotics, the drugs of choice for these infections. Susceptibility testing of GBS must be performed for other antibiotics, as for use in penicillin-allergic patients.
* Antigen detection: Commercially available agglutination tests are available as rapid tests for presumptive diagnosis of meningitis. Antigen testing for direct detection of GBS and other CNS pathogens using CSF, serum, and urine specimens have shown variable performance; reported sensitivity of assays have ranged from poor to good, and false-positive reactions are well documented. One clinical study showed that the clinical management of patients was not affected by the results of these antigen tests. Bacterial antigen testing for preliminary detection of CNS pathogens is not recommended.
* Molecular diagnostics: FDA-approved testing is available for detection of GBS DNA in swabs from rectovaginal specimens, providing final results in <24 hours.

STREPTOCOCCUS PNEUMONIAE INFECTION

➤ Definition

* *Streptococcus pneumoniae* is a common component of the endogenous upper respiratory flora of healthy humans (~10%), which serves as the source for most infections. Carriage may be transient. The disease may be of endogenous or exogenous origin.

➤ Who Should be Suspected?

* Most serious infections occur in children and the elderly. Underlying conditions, like DM, AIDS, alcoholism, and chronic lung disease, increase the risk of infection. Current or recent respiratory viral infection also predisposes to *S. pneumoniae* infection.

* The upper respiratory tract is the most common source of organisms and site of most infections, but *S. pneumoniae* is capable of causing infection in any organ system, usually as a result of bacteremic spread. Common infections include:
  * Respiratory tract infections, including pneumonia (community acquired), otitis media, and sinusitis: abrupt onset of fever and shaking chills with cough with purulent sputum production. Severe disease may lead to respiratory failure, sepsis, and death.
  * Bacteremia: *S. pneumoniae* is a significant pathogen in the etiology of bacteremia and sepsis. Bacteremia may occur secondary to a primary site of infection (e.g., otitis media in children, pneumonia in adults) or may be the primary infection.
  * Meningitis: *S. pneumoniae* is one of the most common causes of bacterial meningitis in all age groups. Hematogenous dissemination is the most common route of infection, but direct invasion from infected sinuses is also well described; basilar skull fracture may cause recurrent *S. pneumoniae* meningitis.

➤ Laboratory Findings
* Gram stain: The typical Gram stain of sputum from patients with pneumococcal pneumonia shows many PMNs and many lancet-shaped GPC in pairs (diplococci).
* Culture: *S. pneumoniae* may rapidly lose viability after collection. Culture of sputum for isolation of *S. pneumoniae* has a sensitivity of ~45% of patients with community-acquired pneumonia. Collection of blood cultures may improve detection in critically ill patients with pneumonia; blood cultures are positive in ~25% of untreated patients. Pleural effusions yield organisms in ~15% of patients. *S. pneumoniae* is a well-documented cause of spontaneous bacterial peritonitis in patients with alcoholic cirrhosis; bedside inoculation of peritoneal fluid directly into blood culture media improves isolation compared to culture onto solid media in the laboratory.
* Susceptibility testing of *S. pneumoniae* isolates: must be performed for significant clinical isolates.
* Antigen detection: Commercially available agglutination tests are available as rapid tests for presumptive diagnosis of meningitis. Antigen testing for direct detection of *S. pneumoniae* is available (Binax, Portland, ME) as an adjunct for diagnosis of *S. pneumoniae* respiratory infections. Reported performance has varied in different study populations, but sensitivity for detection of *S. pneumoniae* respiratory tract infection is ~70–85%, with a specificity ~90–95%.

INTRACELLULAR BACTERIAL PATHOGENS
The organisms discussed in this section are unable to proliferate independently outside of host eukaryotic cells, limiting the use of culture for diagnosis for some agents. Infection may be confirmed by direct detection, serologic response, or molecular diagnostic methods.

CHLAMYDIA AND *CHLAMYDOPHILA* INFECTIONS

➤ Definition
* Species of *Chlamydia* and *Chlamydophila* are obligate intracellular prokaryotic pathogens.

➤ Who Should be Suspected?

The Chlamydiaceae are responsible for a number of distinctive disease syndromes, including:
* Chlamydia genital tract infection
  * *Chlamydia trachomatis* is the most common cause of sexually transmitted bacterial infections in industrialized nations; serovars D through K are responsible for these genital infections. Serovars L1, L2 (including a and b variants), and L3 are responsible for lymphogranuloma venereum (LGV), a systemic STD most commonly encountered in developing countries.
  * Most sexually transmitted *C. trachomatis* infections are asymptomatic, contributing to their spread. Common clinical manifestations include urethritis, mucopurulent cervicitis, ascending infections, female genital tract conditions (PID, endometritis, salpingitis, perihepatitis syndrome), male genital tract problems (epididymitis), conjunctivitis (nonscarring), and proctitis. Complications of *C. trachomatis* genital infection may include scarring of the fallopian tubes, infertility, and ectopic pregnancy. Maternal *C. trachomatis* infection at the time of delivery may result in neonatal infection, which typically manifests as conjunctivitis or pneumonia. Acute, nonscarring inclusion conjunctivitis occurs in 18–50% of infants of mothers with untreated genital infection.
* Trachoma: Trachoma refers to chronic *C. trachomatis* conjunctivitis, usually caused by serovars A, B1, B2, and C. Infection leads to corneal scarring and, in late stages, blindness.
* Chlamydophila pulmonary infections (*Chlamydophila pneumoniae* and *Chlamydophila psittaci*):
  * *C. pneumoniae* is most commonly associated with lower and upper respiratory tract infections (e.g., pneumonia, bronchitis, sinusitis). This pathogen has been implicated in a significant minority (~15%) of community-acquired cases of pneumonia.
  * *C. psittaci* infection causes psittacosis. Birds are the natural reservoir for this organism; infectious forms may remain viable in the environment for extended periods. Human infection is easily transmitted by inhalation of infectious organisms directly shed from birds or from organisms in their environment. Patients usually present with nonspecific symptoms in acute infection, including flu-like illness: fever, severe headache, hepatomegaly, splenomegaly, and GI symptoms. Chronic pneumonitis may develop.

➤ Laboratory Findings

* Molecular diagnostic testing
  * Such testing using amplified technologies, like PCR, is considered the gold standard for the diagnosis of genital *C. trachomatis* infections. FDA-approved kits are available for endocervical, urine, urethral specimens, and liquid-based Pap test specimens. The sensitivities reported for nucleic acid amplification (NAA) tests range from ~90–97%; the specificities reported for NAA tests are >99%.
  * Direct, nonamplified probe techniques are available, showing sensitivity between NAA tests and culture for detection of *C. trachomatis*; specificity of direct probe tests is ~99%. NAA tests have been described for detection of *C. pneumoniae* and *C. psittaci*, but FDA-approved kits are not available and their performance has not been clearly defined.
* Culture: Isolation of *C. trachomatis* in culture remains an important technique for diagnosis of nongenital infections and is considered the standard for evidence in medicolegal cases, such as rape and child abuse. For optimal isolation, it is critical to collect samples that contain the host cells infected by chlamydia and to transport in conditions that will maintain the viability

of the organisms. For detection of genital infections, the sensitivity of tissue culture is ~65–85%, with specificity near 100%.

- Direct detection: DFA staining kits are available for direct detection of *C. trachomatis* from genital specimens. Slides require examination by an experienced laboratorian and slides must be carefully evaluated to ensure adequate specimen collection (i.e., the presence of columnar epithelial cells). Under optimal conditions, the sensitivity of DFA is ~60–80% with specificity >98%. Typical intracytoplasmic inclusions in epithelial cells of Giemsa-stained smears from conjunctival scrapings are found in 50% of patients with *C. trachomatis* conjunctivitis.
- EIA detection: A number of EIA kits for the diagnosis of *C. trachomatis* genital infection are commercially available. Sensitivities of ~60% are reported for cervical infections. Reported specificity is high, but false-positive reactions are possible for tests based on detection of *C. trachomatis* lipopolysaccharide.
- Serology: Serologic testing is not helpful for the diagnosis of acute genital infection caused by *C. trachomatis*. Serology may be useful for diagnosis of psittacosis, LGV, and respiratory tract infections.
  - Complement fixation (CF) assays target response to LPS common to all members of the Chlamydiaceae, so positive results must be interpreted in the context of disease. CF testing is most useful for LGV, where titers ≥256 are considered diagnostic.
  - Microimmunofluorescence (MIF) assays are useful for the diagnosis of neonatal pulmonary infection because they allow specific detection of IgM and IgG. An IgM titer of ≥32 supports the diagnosis.
  - In LGV, an IgG titer of ≥128 provides strong support for diagnosis. *C. pneumoniae* infection may be documented by a fourfold increase in titer between acute and convalescent specimens, an IgM titer ≥16 or an IgG titer ≥512.
  - EIA assays, based on synthetic peptides, have been developed to simplify the technically demanding MIF procedure. In general, results have compared favorably to results of MIF testing.

ANAPLASMOSIS AND EHRLICHIOSIS

➤ Definition
- The agents of ehrlichiosis and anaplasmosis are small, obligate intracellular bacterial pathogens. Infection is transmitted primarily by the bite of ticks. Specific diseases show restricted geographic distribution based on arthropod vector ranges.
- Human granulocytotropic anaplasmosis (HGA) is caused by *Anaplasma phagocytophilum*, transmitted by *Ixodes scapularis* or *Ixodes pacificus* (black legged tick). Disease occurs in New England, the North Central, and Pacific United States. Like *Borrelia burgdorferi*, HGA may cause coinfection with other agents transmitted by *Ixodes* ticks. Deer and the white-footed mouse are the primary reservoir for HGA in the United States.
- Human monocytotropic ehrlichiosis (HME) is caused by *Ehrlichia chaffeensis* and is transmitted by the lone star tick, *Amblyomma americanum*. Disease is seen in the South and mid-Atlantic, the Central United States, and some areas of New England. The white tail deer is the primary reservoir for HME.
- HME and HGA are national notifiable diseases, reportable to the CDC and local departments of public health.

➤ Who Should be Suspected?

* Disease develops 1–2 weeks after the tick bite.
* Fever is present in most infected patients, but asymptomatic or mild disease is common. Nonspecific symptoms are common, including headache, malaise, myalgias, arthralgias, and nausea and vomiting. Rash occurs in a significant minority of patients with HME, but is unusual in HGA. Rash caused by coinfection, like rickettsiosis or Lyme disease, should be considered. Mental status changes or meningeal signs may occur in a minority of patients. Renal and respiratory failure have been described infrequently.

➤ Laboratory Findings

* Culture: not widely available for diagnostic testing.
* Direct examination of peripheral blood or buffy coat smear stained by routine hematologic methods: Examination may demonstrate organism-filled vacuoles (morulae) in the cytoplasm of infected cells. Inclusions in granulocytes may be seen in 20–80% of patients with confirmed HGA, but in a minority (1–20%) of monocytes in patients with HME.
  * The diagnosis of HGA or HME is not ruled out by a negative smear examination. Disease should be confirmed by specific serology or other definitive test.
  * When HME or HGA is suspected, manual differential examination should be specifically ordered. Automated methods are unlikely to detect abnormalities or trigger manual examinations.
* Immunochemical staining: Immunohistochemical staining may be useful in severe or fatal cases, or for patients with early antimicrobial therapy, which may delay the immune response. Specific staining may be used on affected tissues, like bone marrow, of postmortem tissues, including spleen, liver, lung kidney, heart, or brain.
* NAA: Molecular diagnostic tests have been developed for diagnosis of HME and HGA, but well-standardized or FDA-approved methods are not commercially available. PCR may be positive in serum or CSF in acute stage, but moderate sensitivity (60–85%) may limit the utility of these tests; infection is not ruled out by a negative result.
* Serology
  * Specific antibody response may provide an accurate diagnosis; IFA is the serologic method of choice. Patients are usually negative for specific IgG and IgM in the first week of disease. Therefore, testing paired acute serum sample and another collected 2–3 weeks later is recommended.
  * A probable case designation may be achieved in patients with a compatible illness in whom a single serum specimen, collected in early acute infection, shows an IFA titer that exceeds a cut-off established by the laboratory that is performing the test. Diagnosis is established by demonstration of a fourfold increase (or decrease) in IFA titer of specific IgG (*A. phagocytophilum, E. chaffeensis,* or other *Ehrlichia* species) in paired serum specimens. IgM testing has not been shown to be superior to paired IgG studies.
* Core laboratory: Leukopenia (with left shift of PMNs), thrombocytopenia, and elevation of serum aminotransferases are commonly seen, but are nonspecific findings in patients with HME and HGA.
* CSF findings: Pleocytosis and protein elevation are commonly seen in patients with neurologic complications of HME; CSF in usually normal in HGA patients with neurologic complications.

Q FEVER (*COXIELLA BURNETII*)

➤ Definition

- Q fever describes zoonotic infections caused by *Coxiella burnetii*, a small, obligately intracellular gram-negative bacterium. Cattle, sheep, and goats are the primary reservoir for organisms, which are very stable in the environment.
- Human infection is usually acquired by inhalation of organisms from environments contaminated with urine, feces, products of gestation, or other materials from infected animals. Infection may also be acquired by ingestion of unpasteurized dairy products.

➤ Who Should be Suspected?

- *Coxiella* infection may cause acute or chronic infection, but many infections remain asymptomatic.
- Acute infection is usually manifested by flu-like illness, hepatitis, and/or pneumonitis. Endocarditis may develop, usually in patients with preexisting valve disease. Chronic disease is defined as infection lasting >6 months, and is usually manifested by endocarditis, aneurism, or infection of prosthetic material.

➤ Laboratory Findings

- Histology: "Doughnut" granulomas in liver biopsy or bone marrow are highly suggestive but not pathognomonic.
- Culture: *C. burnetii* may be isolated by special eukaryotic cell culture, but this testing is not widely available.
- Serology: the basis of definitive diagnosis. IFA testing is more sensitive (~91%) than CF testing (78%). Serum (1:50 dilution) is screened for anti-phase II anti-immunoglobulin. Positive specimens are tested for anti-phase I and anti-phase II IgG, IgM, and IgA, with titer. Single phase IgG titer ≥1:800 by immunofluorescence is diagnostic and strongly suggests *C. burnetii* endocarditis; any positive IgM titer is diagnostically significant. High specific-IgM titer suggests hepatitis. High specific IgA titer is common in chronic Q fever and suggests culture-negative endocarditis. ELISA testing is sensitive (~94%) in early convalescence.
- Molecular diagnostics: PCR techniques have been described, but there is no FDA-approved kit for NAA.

ROCKY MOUNTAIN SPOTTED FEVER

➤ Definition

- This disorder is an infectious vasculitis due to *Rickettsia rickettsii* transmitted by infected ticks, primarily of the *Dermacentor* genus, in the United States.
- Most patients present ~7 days after exposure with nonspecific symptoms, including fever, headache, malaise, and muscle and joint pains. Nausea and abdominal pain may be significant. Rash appears in ~90% of patients, usually 3–7 days after onset of illness. Rash typically starts on the wrists and ankles, then spreads widely, including palms and soles. The rash becomes petechial; itching is not characteristic. Disease may progress to involve multiple organ systems, including gangrene, CNS manifestations, and other organ dysfunction.

➤ Laboratory Findings
* Culture: Requires special conditions and is rarely performed.
* Histology: DFA of skin biopsy for antigen has S/S of ~70%/100% and is the only specific test in early stages of disease. Sensitivity declines after the initiation of antimicrobial therapy.
* Molecular tests: PCR has been used to detect *R. rickettsii* DNA in blood and tissues.
* Serology: Sera should be collected during acute infection, and then 2–4 weeks later for both IgG and IgM. A ≥4 times increase in IgG or total antibody, or specific-IgM, is evidence of recent infection. IgM appears by day 3–8, peaks at 1 month, and lasts 3–4 months. IgG appears within 3 weeks, peaks at 1–3 months, and lasts for >12 months.
* Core laboratory: WBC is mildly elevated; thrombocytopenia may be severe.

SPIRAL BACTERIA

The spiral bacteria form a large, metabolically diverse group of microorganisms. The organisms in this group do not grow, or are difficult to grow, in vitro. In addition, special staining techniques, like silver staining, darkfield, or immunofluorescent microscopy, are needed for direct detection in specimens. Therefore, serologic techniques play a major role in specific diagnosis of these infections. Molecular diagnostic techniques are also emerging as important diagnostic tools.

TREPONEMAL DISEASE: SYPHILIS

➤ Definition
* Syphilis is a chronic disease caused by infection with the spirochete *Treponema pallidum*. Syphilis has a global distribution. *T. pallidum* is an obligate pathogen of humans; there are no known animal or reservoirs that serve as a source of infection.
* The disease is transmitted by exposure of a susceptible individual to active anogenital lesions of an infected patient, or by transplacental transmission. Congenital or neonatal syphilis may be transmitted directly by contact with infectious lesions or by transplacental transmission, which may occur at any time during pregnancy.

➤ Who Should be Suspected?
* In venereal syphilis, a local infection, usually manifested as painless ulcer (chancre), forms at the site of inoculation. There is a high concentration of spirochetes in the ulcer exudate. Wide dissemination of organisms occurs during the phase of primary syphilis. Chancres generally heal spontaneously within several weeks.
* Signs and symptoms of secondary syphilis occur several weeks to months after resolution of primary syphilis. The rash of secondary syphilis is most characteristic, typically involving the palms and soles. A wide variety of nonspecific symptoms may also be seen, including fever, malaise, headache, lymphadenopathy, and eye involvement (e.g., uveitis). The symptoms of secondary syphilis usually resolve spontaneously.
* Latent phase: The patient is typically asymptomatic. In late (tertiary) syphilis, symptoms related to chronically infected organ systems manifest, most commonly: cardiovascular disease (e.g., aortitis), CNS disease (e.g., tabes dorsalis, paresis), and gummatous disease (nodular lesions of skin, bone or other tissues).

- Patients with AIDS are at increased risk for severe *T. pallidum* infection.
- There is a high rate of fetal loss or still birth. Fetal hydrops may be apparent.
- Most neonates are asymptomatic at birth but may show stigmata of infection, including skin lesions (including palms, soles, and mucous membranes) hepatosplenomegaly, jaundice, and anemia. Radiographic abnormalities may be seen (e.g., periostitis).
- Untreated, damage cause by congenital syphilis may manifest by the Hutchinson triad (abnormal upper incisors, interstitial keratitis, 8th nerve deafness), as well as such conditions as frontal bossing, saddle nose, and high arched palate.

➤ Laboratory Findings

- Direct microscopic detection: Direct detection techniques may be used on exudates of active cutaneous or genital specimens during the primary or secondary phases of disease.
  - Darkfield microscopy: Darkfield microscopy may be used to detect typical organisms; specimens must be examined immediately by an experienced microscopist. Documentation of the characteristic morphology and motility of organisms is critical. Darkfield microscopy should not be performed on oral lesions because of the presence of nonpathogenic, endogenous spirochetal flora.
  - DFA for *T. pallidum* (DFA-TP)
    - This technique would be the most reliable technique for most laboratories. Advantages of DFA-TP are that viable organisms are not required; immediate examination is not necessary. In addition, DFA-TP may be positive on chancre exudate in the first week, before a serologic reaction has occurred.
    - The use of polyclonal antibody reagents may limit the utility of DFA testing if they are not preabsorbed (e.g., Reiter treponemes) to eliminate binding to antigens common to nonpathogenic treponemes.
  - Histopathology: Tissue sections stained using a silver stain, or other technique for spirochetes, may demonstrate organisms and may provide support for diagnosis in immunocompromised patients who do not mount an antibody response to infection.
  - PCR: Molecular diagnostic assays are playing an increasingly important role in the diagnosis of syphilis, but no FDA-approved kits are available. The performance of well-validated PCR testing performed by a reference laboratory, like the CDC, are comparable to the "gold standard" rabbit infectivity assays.
- Serology: Detectable antibodies develop during primary infection and increase in titer during the secondary phase of syphilis. Titers decline during the latent phase. The interpretation of serologic testing of neonates may be complicated by the presence of transplacental maternal antibodies. Two types of serologic tests are used:
  - Nontreponemal tests (Rapid Plasma Reagin [RPR], VDRL)
    - These tests can detect IgG and IgM antibodies to a cardiolipin-lecithin-cholesterol antigen (reaginic antibodies). Nontreponemal assays are inexpensive and are often used for primary screening or for determining response to therapy. Limitations of nontreponemal tests include relative insensitivity in early primary ($<$10 days) and late syphilis, false-positive reactions (e.g., ~1% of noninfected pregnant women), and prozone reactions. Low titer ($\leq$1:8) suggests biologic false-positive test or late latent or tertiary syphilis.
    - Nontreponemal assays can provide quantitative results by testing serial dilutions of specimens. Reactivity to nontreponemal assays should be undetectable within 3 years after successful therapy of primary syphilis.

- The VDRL-CSF assay is the only nontreponemal assay for detection of antibodies in CSF. VDRL on CSF is highly specific but lacks sensitivity (40–60%); therefore, it should be used to rule in, but not rule out, neurosyphilis. The VDRL-CSF cannot be used to follow response to therapy.
- The RPR card test is positive in 75–100% of patients with primary syphilis; 100% with secondary syphilis; 95–100% with latent syphilis; and ~75% with late, tertiary syphilis. Specificity is ~98%.
- Acute (<6 months duration) false-positive tests may occur in acute viral illnesses (e.g., infectious mononucleosis, hepatitis, measles), chlamydia infection, malaria, *Mycoplasma pneumoniae* infection, pregnancy, and recent immunization.
- Chronic (>6 months) false-positive tests may be caused by increased age (>70 years), infection caused by non-*T. pallidum* spirochetal infections, IV drug abuse, medications, and rheumatologic disease and/or underlying disease (e.g., collagen vascular diseases, leprosy, malignancy).
- Treponemal tests
  - These tests use *T. pallidum*, or specific *T. pallidum* antigens, to detect antibodies. Particle agglutination and EIA formats are most commonly used. Treponemal tests have been used traditionally to confirm the specificity of positive reactions of nontreponemal assays. However, development of assays adapted for efficient testing of large numbers of patient samples, like EIA assays, have led to increasing use of these assays as primary screening tests.
  - Treponemal assays are also used for diagnosis of late latent or tertiary syphilis in untreated patients, when nontreponemal assays may have become nonreactive.
  - Treponemal tests usually remain reactive for many years after successful therapy, so these assays are not reliable for measuring response to therapy or to assess the possibility of reinfection.
  - *T. pallidum* specific IgG EIA is positive in 90–95% of patients with primary syphilis, and 99–100% positive in patients with secondary, latent, or late syphilis.

LYME DISEASE

➤ Definition
- Lyme disease is a systemic, chronic borreliosis caused by *Borrelia burgdorferi*. Infection is transmitted by the bite of *Ixodes* ticks.
- A variety of clinical manifestations are seen. Recurrent clinical disease may be caused by reinfection.
- Lyme disease is reportable in the Nationally Notifiable Infectious Diseases Surveillance System. Criteria for case definition may be seen on the CDC web site: (http://www.cdc.gov/ncphi/disss/nndss/casedef/lyme_disease_2008.htm).

➤ Who Should be Suspected?
- Acute disease occurs about 1–4 weeks after tick bite, manifested by nonspecific febrile symptoms that may be confused with a "viral syndrome." Erythema migrans (EM) is characteristic for Lyme disease and occurs in 60–80% of infected patients. EM typically begins as a red papule with surrounding erythema that expands over days to weeks. The central region

commonly clears, resulting in a bull's-eye appearance. Secondary EM lesions may appear. Other common acute symptoms include fever, headache, and fatigue. Myalgias, arthralgias, and mild meningeal signs may occur. EM is virtually diagnostic for Lyme disease in patients at epidemiologic risk, but its absence does not exclude this diagnosis. Laboratory confirmation is recommended for patients with EM with no known exposure or for patients with nonspecific signs and symptoms of Lyme disease.

- Late symptoms are typically manifested by musculoskeletal, cardiovascular, or nervous system signs and symptoms. Chronic, intermittent arthritis affecting one or a few large joints is a common manifestation of late, chronic infection and may occur weeks to years after acute infection. The knee is commonly involved. Progressive arthritis or symmetric polyarthritis are not typical and should prompt consideration or another diagnosis. Nonspecific findings include arthralgias or myalgias.
  - Carditis is usually manifested by acute second- or third-degree atrioventricular conduction defects that typically resolve in days to weeks. Myocarditis may accompany the conduction abnormalities. Nonspecific findings may be seen, including bradycardia or palpitations.
  - A variety of nervous system abnormalities may be seen, including acute meningitis, cranial neuritis (facial nerve palsy), radiculopathy, or encephalomyelitis. The triad of aseptic fluctuating meningoencephalitis, Bell palsy, and peripheral neuropathy is very suggestive of Lyme disease. Nonspecific findings may be seen, including fatigue, headache, or paresthesias.

➤ Laboratory Findings

- Culture: not widely available and usually positive only early during the acute infection.
- Serology: not helpful or necessary at the early, acute stage; tests are only 40–60% sensitive and diagnosis is not ruled out by a negative test. Testing should be ordered only to support clinical diagnosis, not for screening persons with nonspecific symptoms because of their intrinsic poor sensitivity and specificity. Vaccination produces seropositivity.
- Two-tier serologic testing: Patients should be evaluated using a sensitive EIA or IFA assay. Specimens positive or equivocal by EIA or IFA should be tested using a standardized western blot (WB) assay, interpreted using established criteria. In early Lyme disease (<4 weeks), both IgM and IgG WB tests should be performed. (IgM WB >4 weeks after acute infection may represent false-positive test results.)
  - A negative EIA or IFA result usually excludes Lyme disease, but testing paired acute- and convalescent-phase serum samples may be needed for patients with a high index of suspicion and negative results of initial testing. Patients with disseminated or chronic Lyme disease are usually strongly positive for specific anti-*B. burgdorferi* IgG.
  - Specific IgM antibodies usually appear 2–4 weeks after EM and peak after 3–6 weeks of illness. IgM usually declines to undetectable levels after 4–6 months. In some patients, IgM remains elevated for many months or reappears late in illness, indicating continued infection. A negative test within 2 weeks of onset of symptoms does not rule out infection.
  - Specific IgG titers rise more slowly, usually appearing 4–8 weeks after rash. IgG titers peak after 4–6 months and may remain high for months or years, even with successful antibiotic therapy. A single increased IgG titer may be due to previous infection or vaccination and must be interpreted in the context of clinical symptoms. An IgG titer

$\geq$1:800 usually indicates active infection; a titer of 1:200 to 1:400 is indeterminate. Titers <1:100 are considered negative.
- Paired acute and convalescent sera at 4- to 6-week intervals may demonstrate a significant rise in titer, indicating active infection. Testing of paired serum samples may be needed to confirm infection in patients with compatible symptoms, but without a known tick bite or rash, who have been in endemic area.
- RF may cause false-positive result for IgM. False-positive IgG in high titers may be caused by antibodies from spirochetal diseases (syphilis, relapsing fever, yaws, pinta); low titers may be found in infectious mononucleosis, hepatitis B, autoimmune diseases (e.g., SLE, RA), periodontal disease, ehrlichiosis, rickettsiosis, other bacteria (e.g., *H. pylori*). Five percent to 15% of persons in endemic areas may be seropositive without any signs or symptoms of active infection.
- WB assays: used to confirm initial serologic testing with EIA or IFA. IgG WB assays may not become positive until after many months of illness; negative WB should be repeated in 2–4 weeks if Lyme disease is strongly suspected.
- Molecular tests: PCR plays a limited role in the diagnosis of Lyme disease and is not recommended in seronegative patients. PCR may be positive for CSF in acute lymphocytic meningitis (not encephalomyelitis or other neurological syndrome) or joint fluid or synovial tissue of joints with active disease. PCR is not reliable for other types of specimens.
- Synovial fluid of affected joints: shows mild to moderate increased WBC, typically with granulocyte predominance.
- CSF findings: patients with Lyme encephalomyelitis show lymphocytic pleocytosis, slightly increased protein and globulin, and normal glucose. Oligoclonal bands may be demonstrated. Intrathecal antibody production may be demonstrated by higher titer in CSF than serum. Almost all of these patients will have positive serum serologic tests.
- Core laboratory: Findings related to dysfunction of infected organs may be seen. Nonspecific laboratory findings include increase of ESR, lymphopenia, cryoglobulinemia, and increase of hepatic enzymes. Treponemal tests for syphilis may be positive, but nontreponemal tests should be nonreactive.

MYCOPLASMA PNEUMONIAE AND *UREAPLASMA UREALYTICUM* INFECTIONS

➤ Definition
- *Mycoplasma* and *Ureaplasma* species, surrounded by a trilayer cell membrane and lacking a rigid cell wall, are the smallest free-living human pathogens.

➤ Who Should be Suspected?
- *Mycoplasma pneumoniae* is a significant cause of community-acquired pneumonia, typically presenting with upper respiratory tract symptoms and tracheobronchitis. Extrapulmonary symptoms are presumably caused by an autoimmune response to primary pulmonary infection. Extrapulmonary manifestations include arthritis, hemolytic anemia, and neurologic diseases (meningoencephalitis, cranial nerve palsy, ascending paralysis, transverse myelitis).
- *Ureaplasma urealyticum* may be detected in the microflora of genital mucosa in healthy adults, but there is evidence to link *U. urealyticum* to genital tract and neonatal infections. Infections

include epididymitis, neonatal infections (pneumonia, bacteremia), nongonococcal urethritis, and orchitis.

➤ Laboratory Findings

- Direct detection: Because of the lack of a rigid cell wall, *M. pneumoniae* and *U. urealyticum* do not stain with Gram stain. A DNA stain, like acridine orange, may demonstrate organisms in infected tissue.
- Culture: Culture of organism from sputum, nasopharynx, or other infected specimen shows good sensitivity but requires special culture techniques that are not widely available.
- Molecular diagnostic testing: Although PCR assays have been described for detection of *Mycoplasma* and *Ureaplasma* species, FDA-approved assays are not available and the clinical utility of these tests is not established.
- Serology: Sensitive and specific serologic assays have been described for both *M. pneumoniae* and *U. urealyticum*. EIA methods are most widely used and provide good sensitivity and specificity. Accurate detection may require testing of both acute and convalescent specimens, especially in adults. EIA methods have been adapted for the detection of specific IgM.
  - IgM increases in first week, peaks in third to fifth week, begins to decrease in 4–6 months, but may persist ≤1 year; the interpretation of acute infection based on a positive IgM reaction, therefore, must be made with caution. The presence of IgM (>1:64) or a four-fold rise in IgG titer indicates recent infection.
  - IgG peaks ~5 weeks after acute infection. IgG is unusual in the first weeks of infection, so repeat testing of convalescent serum is recommended. IgG titers increase for several years after acute infection.
- Core laboratory: Patients may show nonspecific signs of inflammation (mildly elevated WBC, increased ESR) on routine laboratory testing. Cold agglutinins (agglutination of type O, Rh-negative RBCs at 4°C) may be seen in ~50% of patients with *M. pneumoniae* infection. Cold agglutinins, however, are not specific and this test is not recommended for diagnosis of *M. pneumoniae* infection.

➤ Suggested Readings: Bacterial Pathogens

Ben-Ami R, M Ephros, B Avidor, et al. Cat-scratch disease in elderly patients. *Clin Infect Dis.* 2005;41:969–974.

Brouwer MC, D van de Beek, SGB Heckenberg, et al. Community-acquired *Listeria monocytogenes* meningitis in adults. *Clin Infect Dis.* 2006;43:1233–1238.

Cetinkaya Y, Falk P, Mayhall CG. Vancomycin-resistant enterococci. *Clin Microbiol Rev.* 2000;13:686–707.

Coenye T, Vandamme P, Govan JRW, LiPuma JJ. Taxonomy and identification of the *Burkholderia cepacia* complex. *J Clin Microbiol.* 2001;39:3427–3436.

Denton M, Kerr KG. Microbiological and clinical aspects of infection associated with *Stenotrophomonas maltophilia.* *Clin Microbiol Rev.* 1998;11:57–80.

Gaynes R, Edwards JR, and the National Nosocomial Infections Surveillance System. Overview of nosocomial infections caused by gram-negative bacilli. *Clin Infect Dis.* 2005;41:848–854.

Gottlieb SL, Martin Martin, Xu F, et al. Summary: The natural history of *Chlamydia trachomatis* genital infection and implications for chlamydia control. *J Infect Dis.* 2010;201:S190–S204.

Klein JO. Danger ahead: politics intrude in Infectious Diseases Society of America Guideline for Lyme disease. *Clin Infect Dis.* 2008;47:1197–1199.

Kuehnert MJ, Doyle TJ, Hill HA, et al. Clinical features that discriminate inhalational anthrax from other acute respiratory illnesses. *Clin Infect Dis.* 2003;36:328–336.

Maragakis LL, Perl TM. *Acinetobacter baumannii*: Epidemiology, antimicrobial resistance, and treatment options. *Clin Infect Dis.* 2008;46:1254–1263.

Mundy LM, Sahm DF, Gilmore M. Relationships between enterococcal virulence and antimicrobial resistance. *Clin Microbiol Rev.* 2000;13:513–522.

Munoz-Price LS, Weinstein RA. *Acinetobacter* infection. *N Engl J Med.* 2008;358:1271–1281.

Newman LM, Moran JS, Workowski KA. Update on the management of gonorrhea in adults in the United States. *Clin Infect Dis.* 2007;44:S84–S101.

Parola P, Paddock CD, Raoult D. Tick-borne rickettsioses around the world: emerging diseases challenging old concepts. *Clin Microbiol Rev.* 2005;18:719–756.

Parola P, Raoult D. Ticks and tickborne bacterial diseases in humans: an emerging infectious threat. *Clin Infect Dis.* 2001;32:897–928.

Peterson LR, Robicsek A. Does my patient have *Clostridium difficile* infection? *Ann Intern Med.* 2009;151:176–179.

Reimer LG. Q Fever. *Clin Microbiol Rev.* 1993;6:193–198.

Rosenstein NE, Perkins BA, Stephens DS, et al. Meningococcal disease. *N Engl J Med.* 2001;344:1378–1388.

Swartz MN. Recognition and management of anthrax—an update. *N Engl J Med.* 2001;345:1621–1626.

Swindells J, Brenwald N, Reading N, Oppenheim B. Evaluation of diagnostic tests for *Clostridium difficile* infection. *J Clin Microbiol.* 2010;48:606–608.

Waites KB, Katz B, Schelonka RL. Mycoplasmas and ureaplasmas as neonatal pathogens. *Clin Microbiol Rev.* 2005;18:757–789.

Waites KB, Talkington DF. *Mycoplasma pneumoniae* and its role as a human pathogen. *Clin Microbiol Rev.* 2004;17:697–728.

Walker DH. Rickettsiae and rickettsial infections: the current state of knowledge. *Clin Infect Dis.* 2007;45:S39–S44.

Weinstein A. Laboratory testing for Lyme disease: time for a change? *Clin Infect Dis.* 2008;47:196–197.

Winn Jr WC, Allen SD, Janda WM, et al. Gram positive cocci, part I: staphylococci and related gram-positive cocci. In: *Koneman's Color Atlas and Textbook of Diagnostic Microbiology.* 6th ed. Baltimore MD and Philadelphia PA: Lippincott Williams & Wilkins; 2006.

Wormser GP. Discovery of new infectious diseases—*Bartonella* species. *N Engl J Med.* 2007;356:2346–2347.

INFECTIOUS DISEASES CAUSED BY ACID-FAST BACTERIAL PATHOGENS

The organisms in this group are genetically related organisms that contain mycolic acids in their cell walls. The mycolic acids render organisms relatively resistant to both staining and destaining. Therefore, special techniques are used for direct visual detection of these organisms in specimens. Organisms may be characterized on their resistance to decolorization. *Mycobacterium* species, in general, are resistant to strong decolorization procedures with acid–alcohol. *Nocardia* and *Rhodococcus* species have a lower cell wall mycolic acid content and are acid-fast only when weaker decolorizing procedures are used.

Diseases caused by organisms in this group are usually diagnosed by isolation in culture. Specialized culture procedures are required, with prolonged incubation. Because of the slow growth rate of many isolates, molecular methods are increasingly used for direct detection and speciation of isolates. Tests that measure a patient's cellular immune response (e.g., TSTs and IFGR assays) may be used for the diagnosis of TB; serologic testing is not otherwise useful for diagnosis.

MYCOBACTERIUM TUBERCULOSIS

See Chapter 14, Respiratory, Metabolic, and Acid-Base Disorders.

RAPIDLY GROWING MYCOBACTERIA

➤ Definition
- Rapidly growing mycobacteria (RGM) are widely distributed in the environment, in water sources, dust, and soil. Although exposure to these organisms is common, disease is uncommon because of their low intrinsic pathogenicity in normal hosts. RGM produce mature colonies within 7 days after subculture.
- The clinical significance of culture isolates must be interpreted carefully. Factors to be considered when assessing clinical significance include site, quantity of growth, other organisms isolated, and signs of inflammation and host immune status.

➤ Significant Species
Three species are most commonly associated with clinical disease: *Mycobacterium abscessus, Mycobacterium fortuitum,* and *Mycobacterium chelonae.*
- *M. abscessus* usually causes pulmonary disease. Patients with underlying pulmonary disease are most commonly infected, but disease may also occur in patients with no pulmonary disease.
- *M. fortuitum* usually causes skin and soft tissue infection after direct inoculation. Infections include surgical site, catheter-related, and other infections. Pulmonary isolates may represent transient infection or colonization.
- *M. chelonae* may cause a variety of infections in immunocompromised patients.

➤ Laboratory Findings
- AFB staining and culture: Diagnosis is usually established by culture of infected material, following American Thoracic Society criteria (ATS) to assess the significance of isolates.

SLOW-GROWING, NONTUBERCULOUS MYCOBACTERIA

➤ Definition
- There are a large number of nontuberculous mycobacteria (NTM). These organisms are ubiquitous in the environment.
- A number of these species are able to cause human disease, but usually in patients with immune defects.

➤ Who Should be Suspected?
- Most infections are acquired from environmental sources; human-to-human transmission occurs rarely, if ever.
- NTM are increasingly implicated in nosocomial infections and pseudo-outbreaks in health care settings. Although this patient population may be at increased risk for NTM infection, culture isolates must be interpreted cautiously because of the frequency of isolation of culture isolates. *Mycobacterium gordonae*, for example, is a fairly common isolate in AFB cultures, like BAL specimens, and virtually always represents a culture contaminant.

➤ Significant Species
- *Mycobacterium avium* complex (MAC): This complex includes two genetically related species: *Mycobacterium avium* and *Mycobacterium intracellulare.* Organisms are widely distributed in nature, being prevalent in soil and water with low pH and oxygen content, and they are

relatively chlorine resistant. MAC has been isolated from municipal water supplies, hospital hot water systems and shower heads.

- In patients with AIDS or other immune defects, mycobacteremia, manifested with fever, fatigue, night sweats, anemia, diarrhea, failure to thrive, or other nonspecific symptoms, is the most common type of infection. Other sites may be secondarily infected, but pulmonary infection is relatively uncommon. Risk of MAC increases with decreasing CD4+ cell count.
- The isolation of NTM from respiratory specimens is well described for patients with CF. *M. avium* complex isolates are most common, followed by *M. abscessus* in a significant minority of patients, although there may be significant variability of the etiology globally. The virulence of NTM in CF patients also shows variability. CF patients from whom NTM are isolated tend to be older, have better lung function and have a lower frequency of chronic *P. aeruginosa* infection (but higher rate of *S. aureus*) compared to patients without NTM infection.
- In immunocompetent patients, pneumonia is the most common disease caused by MAC. A syndrome similar to TB has been described in elderly men with underlying pulmonary disease. Patients present with chronically progressive cough and weight loss. Upper lobe cavitation is well described, and parenchymal damage may be significant. A second common syndrome is described in women, usually older than 50, without underlying lung disease. Patients present with insidious onset of cough and sputum production; systemic symptoms are not prominent.
- *Mycobacterium kansasii*: *M. kansasii* infection presents as pulmonary disease that may be difficult to distinguish from TB. Most patients present with chest pain and fever. Hemoptysis, fever, and night sweats are also common. Cavitation is commonly seen on chest x-ray. *M. kansasii*, in contrast to other NTM, is not found in soil or natural water sources but is associated with tap water in cities where the organism is endemic.
- *Mycobacterium marinum*: *M. marinum* is well described as a cause of chronic cutaneous infection after exposure to colonized water sources, the so-called "fish tank" granuloma.
  - Organisms enter through traumatic or preexisting breaks in the skin surface. Several weeks after exposure, a nodular or ulcerating lesion develops at the site of infection, with subsequent spread along lymphatic channels. Infections usually occur on the extremities, most often the hands. The infection may be locally invasive, but usually only in immunocompromised patients.
  - Diagnosis may be established by AFB smear and culture. Note that *M. marinum* (and other NTM that are mainly associated with cutaneous infection) grows optimally in cultures incubated at 30°C, so special AFB cultures should be requested. Histopathologic examination shows granuloma formation.

➤ Laboratory Findings

- AFB smear and culture of lower respiratory samples. ATS/Infectious Disease Society of America (IDSA) criteria to confirm NTM pulmonary infection:
  - Positive culture from two or more expectorated sputum samples, or
  - Positive culture from one or more BAL or bronchial wash samples, or
  - Lung biopsy consistent with mycobacterial infection (granulomatous inflammation or AFB), confirmed by positive culture of tissue or respiratory specimen, or
  - Positive culture from a normally sterile, nonpulmonary site of infection

- AFB smear and culture of infected material from nonpulmonary sites: When NMT infection is suspected, AFB smear and culture of specimens taken from infected, nonpulmonary sites, especially normally sterile sites, is recommended. Ensure that an adequate quantity of sample is submitted for AFB culture; repeat testing of sequential specimens is likely to improve isolation.
- Blood culture: The diagnosis of disseminated NTM infection is usually efficiently established in immunocompromised patients by submission of AFB blood cultures. AFB culture of bone marrow may also be diagnostic, especially in immunocompromised patients with hematologic abnormalities.
- Susceptibility testing:
  - MAC: clarithromycin only
  - *M. kansasii*: rifampin only
  - RGM: amikacin, imipenem (*M. fortuitum*), doxycycline, fluoroquinolones, sulfonamide or TMP/SMX, cefoxitin, clarithromycin, linezolid, tobramycin (*M. chelonae*)
- Core laboratory: Laboratory tests related to specific organ systems infected by NTM. HIV serology or other diagnostic testing should be considered in any patient who is diagnosed with significant or severe infection with these mycobacteria.

NOCARDIA INFECTION

➤ Definition
- Nocardiosis describes infections caused by species of the genus *Nocardia*. These bacteria are aerobic gram-positive organisms that form delicate filaments that show branching and fragmentation. *Nocardia* species are widely distributed in nature, involved in the decay of organic material; nocardiae have a global distribution.
- Human infections are usually seen in patients with immunocompromising or debilitating underlying medical conditions. Pulmonary infections, acquired by inhalation, or cutaneous infections, acquired by direct or traumatic inoculation, represent most primary infections. Local spread and systemic dissemination are common. *Nocardia* have tropism for the CNS. Recurrent or progressive infection may occur despite appropriate antimicrobial therapy.
- *Nocardia asteroides* is the most common species associated with human infections, especially pulmonary and invasive disease. *Nocardia brasiliensis* is predominantly associated with cutaneous infections.

➤ Who Should be Suspected?
- These organisms have a low intrinsic virulence; infection most commonly occurs in immunocompromised patients, but no underlying condition is found in 10–20% of patients.
- Factors that increase the risk of nocardiosis include AIDS, alcoholism, chronic lung disease, DM, glucocorticoid therapy, malignancy, and solid organ or hematopoietic stem cell transplantation.

➤ Laboratory Findings
- Gram stain: gram-positive or gram-variable and modified acid-fast positive.
- Culture: Most nonselective media for bacterial, fungal, and mycobacterial isolation will support the growth of *Nocardia* but may require up to 6 weeks incubation for isolation. Noninvasively obtained specimens may be inadequate for sensitive detection of nocardiae. Sputum

is positive in only 30% of cases. Blood culture is rarely positive. All patients with nocardiosis should be evaluated for possible disseminated infection.

- Susceptibility: Sulfonamides, including TMP/SMX, are considered the drug of choice of nocardiosis because of the low rate of resistance and extensive clinical experience. Susceptibility testing is recommended, however, for life-threatening infections and for patients allergic to sulfa drugs.

➤ Suggested Readings: Acid-Fast Bacterial Pathogens

Brown-Elliott BA, Brown JM, Conville PS, Wallace RJ Jr. Clinical and laboratory features of the *Nocardia* spp. based on current molecular taxonomy. *Clin Microbiol Rev.* 2006;19:259–282.

Lederman ER, Crum NF. A case series and focused review of nocardiosis, Clinical and microbiologic aspects. *Medicine (Baltimore).* 2004;83:300–313.

DISEASES CAUSED BY FUNGAL PATHOGENS

Fungi are eukaryotic organisms widely distributed in the environment; specific pathogens may show a restricted geographic distribution. The fungal pathogens in this section may be initially characterized as yeasts (e.g., reproduce by binary fission with minimal cellular differentiation) or molds (e.g., formation of multicellular mycelia with differentiation of cells within the mycelial structure: vegetative hyphae, aerial hyphae, reproductive structures).

Direct examination of patient specimens (e.g., histopathology, KOH wet mount, staining) may provide initial presumptive evidence of infection. Detection of specific (e.g., cryptococcal antigen) or nonspecific (e.g., galactomannan) fungal antigens in patient specimens may also support a diagnosis of fungal disease. Definitive diagnosis of fungal infections, however, is primarily based on isolation of a pathogen in culture. Serologic testing may be useful for epidemiologic studies but are rarely used for the diagnosis of acute infection.

PATHOGENIC MOLDS, OPPORTUNISTIC

A number of mold species (filamentous fungi) have emerged as significant opportunistic pathogens, most commonly in severely immunocompromised patients. These molds are ubiquitous in nature, with a global distribution. In immunocompetent individuals, infection is rare. In immunocompromised patients, infection is usually acquired by inhalation or direct inoculation. Disseminated disease may ensue.

A definitive diagnosis of infection is most reliably established, in patients with clinically compatible disease, by a combination of histopathologic evidence of invasive mold infection (or radiologic) combined with isolation of the pathogen by culture from a normally sterile site. Although septate hyphae may be distinguished from aseptate hyphae histologically, identification of different pathogens within these groups cannot be reliably established by standard histologic staining techniques. Definitive species identification is based on macroscopic and microscopic examination of culture isolates. Isolates grow well and rapidly on nonselective fungal media. Some species may be inhibited by cycloheximide.

Serology does not play a significant role in the diagnosis of opportunistic invasive fungal infections. The (1,3)-β-D-glucan, galactomannan, or related tests may provide supportive evidence of infection, but their nonspecificity and lack of well-established efficacy studies may limit their usefulness. Methods for detection of specific DNA and mRNA have been described for opportunistic fungal pathogens, but tests are not standardized and FDA-approved assays are not available.

Laboratory findings are consistent with dysfunction of organs affected by opportunistic fungal infection and underlying predisposing diseases (e.g., diabetes, neoplasms, IV drug use, and malnutrition).

ASPERGILLOSIS

➤ Definition
Species of the genus *Aspergillus* cause a variety of diseases referred to as aspergillosis. These fungi are nonpigmented, septate mold species. Humans are frequently exposed to hyphal fragments or spores, usually by inhalation. Such exposure may result in disease by invasive proliferation (infection) or by a poorly controlled, severe immunologic response to *Aspergillus* antigens.

➤ Who Should be Suspected?
* Risk factors for invasive aspergillosis include advanced AIDS, allogeneic hematopoietic stem cell and solid organ transplantation, chronic granulomatous disease, glucocorticoid therapy, graft-versus-host disease, hematologic malignancy, and/or prolonged profound neutropenia. Infection has been associated with exposure to construction sites, presumably due to increased dispersal of spores.
* The respiratory tract is the common portal of entry and disease most commonly involves the lungs or pararespiratory tissues. Secondary infection may be seen in any organ system, although the CNS, kidney, liver, and spleen are most commonly affected.
* Patients with invasive sinusitis due to *Aspergillus* usually present with fever, epistaxis, nasal congestion, facial edema, and pain over the affected sinuses. Infection may extend to the cavernous sinus, orbit (blurred vision, proptosis, chemosis), or CNS (mental status changes and a variety of specific symptoms related to the affected area). Endocarditis, endophthalmitis, skin infection, and GI infection, are well-described infections associated with invasive aspergillosis, presumably due to hematologic dissemination from a primary site of infection.
* *Aspergillus* species may cause noninvasive diseases in immunocompetent patients. Allergic bronchopulmonary aspergillosis (APBA) occurs in 1–2% of patients with chronic asthma. Patients present with exacerbation of asthma symptoms, with increased and recurrent bronchial obstruction. Fever and malaise are common. Brownish mucous plugs or blood may be seen in expectorated sputum. Bronchopulmonary aspergillosis may respond to glucocorticoid therapy. Diagnosis is usually based on a number of major criteria: history of asthma, immediate skin test reactivity to *Aspergillus* antigens, precipitin antibodies to *Aspergillus fumigatus*, total serum IgE >1000 ng/mL, peripheral blood eosinophilia >500/mm^3, radiographic abnormalities, and/or elevation of serum anti-*Aspergillus fumigatus* IgE and IgG.
* Fungus balls may form by colonization and proliferation of *Aspergillus* species in lung cavities formed by unrelated disease. Disease may result from erosion into critical structures.

➤ Laboratory Findings

- Culture: Blood cultures are rarely positive, even in patients with evidence of hematogenous spread.
- Histopathology: The morphology of *Aspergillus* is fairly characteristic, usually demonstrating nonpigmented, narrow, septate hyphae with acute angle branching. Angioinvasion is commonly demonstrated. The morphology, however, is not specific; other molds, like *Scedosporium* or *Fusarium*, may show a similar histopathology.
- Core laboratory: Laboratory studies related to the function of affected organs should be submitted. Eosinophilia ($>1000/\mu L$; often $>3000/\mu L$) is common in ABPA.

FUSARIOSIS

➤ Definition

- Fusariosis is caused by infection with species of the genus *Fusarium*. These fungi form septate, nonpigmented hyphae. These fungi are saprophytic with a wide distribution in the environment.
- Disease is transmitted primarily by inhalation or direct inoculation, usually at a site of trauma. Proliferation at the site of inoculation may result in localized infection or disseminated disease.

➤ Who Should be Suspected?

- Major risk factors for invasive infection include hematologic malignancy, especially in patients with hematopoietic stem cell transplantation, glucocorticoid treatment, prolonged neutropenia, and disruption of skin integrity (e.g., burns, long-term central venous catheter placement, trauma). Significant disease is uncommon in immunocompetent patients.
- As with other opportunistic molds, broad range of disease may be caused by *Fusarium*, from superficial and allergic to locally invasive to disseminated, multiorgan disease. Affected patients and clinical manifestations include:
  - Immunocompetent patients: Localized infection is most commonly seen; onychomycosis and keratitis are the most common types of infection. Infections at other sites, including sinusitis, pulmonary infection, and foreign body–associated infection, are described but occur infrequently. Keratitis occurs almost exclusively in contact lens users and may be associated with use of specific lens solutions.
  - Immunocompromised patients: Invasive and disseminated infection is most common in immunocompromised patients; patients with severe and prolonged neutropenia are at greatest risk. Immunocompromised patients with fusariosis usually present with sepsis, associated with positive blood cultures and skin lesions. Skin lesions may occur as a primary site of infection but are the most common site of disseminated infection, occurring in a significant majority of patients with systemic disease. Patients typically present with multiple, painful lesions. Papular or nodular lesions are most common on the extremities. They commonly develop central necrosis with surrounding erythema.

➤ Laboratory Findings

- Histopathology: Hyaline, segmented hyphae with acute and right angle branching are seen in tissues. Hyphae cannot be confidently differentiated from other opportunistic fungi, like

Aspergillus and *Scedosporium*, but the presence of adventitious sporulation in vivo is not seen in *Aspergillus* and suggests *Fusarium* or *Scedosporium* infection. Angioinvasion may be evident, with distal necrosis due to vascular compromise.

* Culture: *Fusarium* species grow well on nonselective media for fungal isolation. Accurate speciation relies on nucleic acid sequencing or specific PCR and is not widely available. Standardized antifungal susceptibility testing is available.
* Other: The $(1,3)$-β-D-glucan assay is usually positive in invasive disease but is not specific for fusariosis. The galactomannan test is negative.

MUCORMYCOSIS

➤ Definition

* Mucormycosis describes diseases caused by opportunistic aseptate molds of the Mucorales order. Species of the genus *Rhizopus* are responsible for most clinical infection, followed by *Mucor.* Most species are able to grow rapidly in culture.
* Clinical infection is typically devastating, associated with high mortality, loss of function, and disfigurement.
* Most infections are acquired through the respiratory tract, causing local infection and subsequent dissemination. Organisms from the upper respiratory tract may be swallowed, resulting in GI infection. Organisms are able to proliferate in the presence of high concentrations of glucose, and they have the ability to invade blood vessels, resulting in tissue infarction. Nosocomial transmission, infection due to ingestion of contaminated food and traumatic inoculation are less common but well described modes of transmission. Person-to-person transmission does not occur.

➤ Who Should be Suspected?

* Although any organ may be involved in mucormycosis, the respiratory tract is the most common site of primary infection. Disseminated infection may follow primary infections.
* A high index of suspicion is required for efficient diagnosis of mucormycosis; early diagnosis is critical for appropriate intervention and antifungal therapy. Factors predisposing to infection include AIDS, deferoxamine therapy, DM, glucocorticoid therapy, hematologic malignancies, immunosuppressive therapy, neutropenia, renal failure, and solid organ transplantation. Common sites of infection include:
  * Rhinocerebral: Rhinocerebral disease is the most common manifestation of mucormycosis, occurring in about 50% of patients. Primary infection is initiated in the nasal mucosa and then may spread through the palate, sinuses, orbit, other facial structures or brain. Patients usually present with symptoms similar to bacterial sinusitis with fever, purulent discharge, and headache. Infection is commonly unilaterally. Eschar forms on affected mucosa and nasal discharge may be bloody. Ipsilateral extension may result in ulceration and necrosis of sinuses or palate. Ocular involvement manifests with orbital pain, proptosis, ophthalmoplegia, visual abnormalities, conjunctivitis, and inflammation and edema of the eyelid. The brain may be involved by spread of infection across the dura, causing cavernous sinus thrombosis and cerebral disease. Cerebral mucormycosis is manifested by cranial nerve palsies, change in level of consciousness, or severe disruption of cerebral function. Blood vessel involvement may result in symptoms of stroke.

- Pulmonary: Pulmonary disease represents about 10% of mucormycosis cases, occurring primarily in immunocompromised patients. Patients may present with FUO and respiratory symptoms unresponsive to antibiotic therapy. Rapidly progressive pulmonary disease may present with a variety of patterns and may mimic pulmonary aspergillosis. Pulmonary necrosis may result in massive hemoptysis. Infection may progress into contiguous spaces and tissues, including the diaphragm, mediastinum, and heart.
- GI: GI disease occurs in <10% of patients. Symptoms and signs depend on the GI tissue involved and the type of pathology. Symptoms are nonspecific, including abdominal pain and diarrhea. Ulcerative lesions are common and may lead to perforation or massive bleeding with hematemesis or lower GI bleed.
- Cutaneous: Cutaneous infection is caused by direct inoculation of infectious mold into tissue or dissemination from the sites of primary infection. About 15% of cases of mucormycosis are cutaneous. Nodular lesions may show bruising with surrounding pallor. Lesions may be chronic or rapidly progressive. The extremities are most commonly involved, but 35–40% of cases occur on the head, neck or thorax. The mortality is higher in central lesions.
- Disseminated: Disseminated infection occurs in about 5% of patients; the signs and symptoms depend on the extent of dysfunction of affected tissues. Specific organ disease may be apparent but nonspecific. Therefore, a high index of suspicion, based on patients underlying disease and clinical findings, is critical.

➤ Laboratory Findings

- Histopathology: Infected tissue is necrotic, hemorrhagic, thrombotic, or pale depending on the degree and type of vascular compromise. Inflammation is not prominent in acute infection. Angioinvasion may be seen.
- Culture: Specimens should be submitted for fungal culture, but cultures may be negative, depending on the location and type of infection and processing of specimens. Vigorous processing may damage hyphae, resulting in low potential for proliferation in culture. Therefore, when mucormycosis is suspected, the laboratory should be alerted to use gentle processing protocols, like gentle mincing of tissue rather than tissue homogenization. Cultures may be positive from acutely infected nasal sinus or turbinate tissue or nasal discharge. Cultures from CSF are rarely contributory. Mucormycosis cannot be excluded by negative cultures. In addition, positive cultures must be interpreted with caution to rule out possible contamination.

PNEUMOCYSTIS JIROVECI (FORMERLY P. CARINII)

See Chapter 14, Respiratory, Metabolic, and Acid-Base Disorders.

PATHOGENIC MOLDS, DIMORPHIC

This group of fungi includes species with intrinsic pathogenicity that may exist in two forms. In the environment, spore-forming mold forms predominate. In the patient, organisms differentiate into a tissue (usually yeast) form. These organisms may be widely distributed in the environment, but the geographic distribution varies by species. Most infection is transmitted by inhalation of spores, but direct inoculation is well described.

BLASTOMYCOSIS

➤ Definition

• Blastomycosis is caused by the thermally dimorphic fungus *Blastomyces dermatitidis*. Infection is primarily acquired by inhalation of spores from the mold form of *B. dermatitidis* in the environment.

• Most cases are reported from the North America; endemic areas include southeastern and south central and Midwestern states (especially around the Mississippi and Ohio River basins), north central states and Canadian provinces bordering the Great Lakes, and St. Lawrence River basin. Blastomycosis is also endemic in regions of Africa and may occur sporadically in patients in other areas.

➤ Who Should be Suspected?

• The scope of infection ranges from asymptomatic or mild infection to acute or chronic pulmonary infection to disseminated extrapulmonary disease. Immunocompromised patients are more susceptible to severe, extrapulmonary and recurrent disease.

• Conditions associated with increased risk include AIDS, cytotoxic and immunosuppressive therapy, hematologic malignancy, pregnancy, and solid organ transplantation.

➤ Laboratory Findings

• Direct detection: Wet mount or calcofluor white preparation have moderate sensitivity but may provide an early diagnosis of blastomycosis. Sensitivity is improved by the use concentrated specimens.

• Histopathology: frequently demonstrates pyogranulomas in infected tissues. Visualization of characteristic yeast forms is improved by the use of fungal stains, like periodic acid–Schiff or methenamine silver stains.

• Culture: Isolation of *B. dermatitidis* in culture provides definitive diagnosis of blastomycosis. Cultures of sputum, BAL aspirate, or infected tissue should be positive in most patients with active infection.

• Serology: Specific antibody detection has played a minor role in diagnosis of blastomycosis because of poor S/S. Sensitivity is reported ~90% and specificity ~80%.

• Routine laboratory: WBC and ESR are increased. Mild normochromic anemia is present; serum globulin may be slightly increased and/or serum ALP may be increased with bone lesions.

COCCIDIOIDOMYCOSIS

➤ Definition

• Coccidioidomycosis is caused by dimorphic fungi in the genus *Coccidioides* (*Coccidioides immitis* and *Coccidioides posadasii*).

• *Coccidioides* species are endemic in the environment of desert regions of the Western hemisphere, including the Southwestern United States and California. Infection is acquired by inhalation of arthroconidia produced by the mycelial form in the environment.

➤ Who Should be Suspected?

• There is a wide spectrum of disease. Asymptomatic or mild disease is common as judged by seroepidemiologic studies. The risk of clinical infection is increased with increasing exposure to desert dust (i.e., in the dry periods following periods of rain) in endemic regions and in immunocompromised patients. Disease usually develops 1 to 4 weeks after exposure in immunocompetent patients.

* Disease resolves spontaneously in most patients, resulting in lifelong immunity. However, it is likely that recovery is not associated with a complete microbiologic cure: recrudescent infection is well documented in patients as a result of acquired immunocompromise, as seen in malignancies, HIV infection, and immunosuppressive therapy.
* Valley fever is the most common presentation of clinically apparent disease. This syndrome is usually associated with low-grade fever and pneumonia, with cough, and pleuritic chest pain. Systemic symptoms, including fatigue and arthralgias, are common. Cutaneous findings may be seen, including erythema nodosum or erythema multiforme. Hoarseness is uncommon. Severe and chronic disease may be seen in a minority of normal hosts, but is more common in immunocompromised patients and in those with specific conditions (e.g., chemotherapy, glucocorticoid therapy, hematologic malignancy, HIV infection, immunosuppressive therapy for autoimmune disease, preexisting chronic lung disease and/or solid organ transplant).
* Signs and symptoms of severe and chronic disease are related to the organ system affected and degree of tissue damage. Common manifestations of progressive disease include cutaneous dissemination, extensive pulmonary disease, meningitis, osteomyelitis, and/or septic arthritis.

➤ Laboratory Findings

* Culture: *Coccidioides* species grow on most routine microbiologic media, including those used for bacterial culture, within several days. It is important to alert the laboratory when a specimen is submitted from a patient in whom coccidioidomycosis is suspected; *Coccidioides* is a significant risk factor for laboratory-acquired infection. Blood cultures are rarely positive for *Coccidioides*, even with evidence of hematogenous spread.
* Direct detection: Detection of spherules is a strong, specific predictor of infection.
* Serology: Most, but not all, patients develop specific anticoccidioidal antibodies in response to infection. In addition, the appearance of antibodies may be delayed for months after the onset of acute infection. Failure or delay in seroconversion may be increased in immunocompromised patients. Therefore, the diagnosis of coccidioidomycosis is not ruled out by negative results of serologic testing. In addition, titers may fall to undetectable levels during the course of illness in patients that resolve their acute infections. Repeat testing is recommended in patients with negative results if a high index of suspicion remains. Several serologic methods are available:
  * CF antibodies: CF assays primarily reflect the presence of IgG antibody. These antibodies typically develop later but are more persistent than precipitin antibodies. High CF titers are more commonly seen in patients with extensive infection. Changes in CF titer may be used to predict progression or regression of disease.
  * EIA: EIA techniques have been developed and are sensitive and specific for detection of IgG and IgM antibodies in serum and CSF. EIA methods represent the most efficient serologic method, but results may not correlate exactly with other methods.
  * LA: These methods are convenient in resource-limited settings, but the increased occurrence of false-positive reactions limits their use.
  * Precipitin antibodies: Carbohydrate cell wall antigen reagents are used to detect specific antibody by precipitin formation. Precipitin antibodies are primarily of the IgM class. Approximately 90% of patients develop precipitin antibodies in the first weeks of symp-

tomatic infection, but levels fall with resolution of infection. Cross-reactions with *Histoplasma capsulatum* and *B. dermatitis* are reported.
- Skin test reactivity: Patients with coccidioidomycosis develop a hypersensitivity to specific antigens, manifested by erythema and induration at the site of intradermal injection. The utility of testing is limited for acute diagnosis because the hypersensitivity is usually lifelong (positive reactions may reflect past infection) and many patients with coccidioidomycosis may be anergic on the basis of their underlying disease or therapy. Skin testing may be useful for seroepidemiologic studies.
- Routine laboratory: Most routine laboratory tests are unremarkable. Decreased peripheral blood lymphocyte count, increased ESR, or slight elevation of WBC is often seen; eosinophilia may be seen.
- Radiology: Abnormal radiologic studies are common in pulmonary and extrapulmonary disease and help delineate the extent of disease. Bone scans can be used to screen for osteomyelitis.
- Septic arthritis: Arthroscopy with synovial biopsy may be used to establish infection.
- Meningitis: Culture is usually negative. Mononuclear pleocytosis (100–200 WBCs/µL), decreased glucose, increased protein. Detection of IgG-specific antibody is diagnostic of meningitis in undiluted CSF, and is detected in ~75% of patients with *Coccidioides* meningitis. Serology may be used to document response to antifungal therapy. Detection of specific IgG may be used to document relapse for 1–2 years after end of therapy. Serum titers are often negative or only borderline positive.

HISTOPLASMOSIS

➤ Definition
- Histoplasmosis is caused by the thermally dimorphic fungus *Histoplasma capsulatum*. There are two variants, *H. capsulatum* var *capsulatum* and *H. capsulatum* var *duboisii*. *H. capsulatum* var *capsulatum* is endemic in the eastern United States (Mississippi, Ohio, and St. Lawrence River basins) and Latin America. *H. capsulatum* var *duboisii* occurs in Africa (Gabon, Uganda, and Kenya) and is associated with a lower frequency of pulmonary infection but more frequent skin and bone infection.
- The natural habitat of *H. capsulatum* in the environment is soil with high nitrogen content, such as found near roosting areas of birds or in caves, where the organism proliferates in its mold phase. Infection is transmitted by inhalation of conidia or mycelial fragments.

➤ Who Should be Suspected?
- Most infections are asymptomatic.
- Patients with defects in T-cell–mediated immune mechanisms are at increased risk for dissemination, reactivation of latent infection, or reinfection. Heavy exposure may result in acute pulmonary histoplasmosis and increased risk of disseminated disease. Conditions associated with disseminated disease include AIDS, chemotherapy for malignancy, glucocorticoid therapy, primary immunodeficiency disease, solid organ transplantation, and treatment with tumor necrosis factor blockers.
- Pulmonary histoplasmosis may mimic TB, other endemic mycoses, or other subacute or chronic pulmonary diseases. Histoplasmosis should be considered in patients with pneumonia who have epidemiologic risk.

➤ Laboratory Findings

- Direct detection: Direct detection is most useful for acute histoplasmosis by detection of yeast-like cells in infected patient specimens. Small budding yeast (2–5 micron), often within mononuclear cells, may be seen by wet mount preparations or histology.
- Culture: Culture of lung, skin, and mucosal lesions, sputum, BAL, gastric washings, blood, or bone marrow may provide a specific diagnosis. Fungal culture of blood is recommended for all patients with histoplasmosis. Two or three specimens may be needed for sensitive detection. Fungal culture of bone marrow is positive in a majority of patients with cytopenias or other signs of marrow failure. Blood and bone marrow cultures are positive in 50–70% of patients. Respiratory culture is positive in <40% of acute pulmonary cases, but in up to 85% of patients with chronic pulmonary disease. Culture of tissue from infected sites is positive in 25–30% of patients. Culture is positive in ~50% of patients with meningitis, but a large volume of CSF is needed to detect CNS histoplasmosis by culture. Repeat culture on several occasions is recommended. Cultures may take up to 8 weeks to yield positive results, so initial therapeutic decisions are often based on clinical and other laboratory results.
- Histology: Granulomas, lymphohistiocytic aggregates, and mononuclear cell infiltrates are most commonly seen histopathologically using routine staining methods; staining to enhance fungi, like methenamine silver or periodic acid–Schiff, improves detection of yeast cells in tissue. Biopsy (specially stained) of skin and mucosal lesions, bone marrow, and RE system provides initial diagnosis in ~45% of cases. Demonstration of *H. capsulatum* in smears of peripheral blood, buffy coat, bone marrow (25–60% positive) or respiratory secretions is often the most rapid method of diagnosis; fungal culture is recommended to improve sensitivity of detection.
- Antigen detection
  - *H. capsulatum*–specific antigen may provide accurate diagnosis in early acute histoplasmosis, especially in patients with severe and progressive disease. The sensitivity of antigen detection is increased by submission of urine, blood, BAL fluid, and specimens from other potentially infected sites. Antigen may be detected in ≥75% of patients with diffuse acute pulmonary histoplasmosis.
  - Antigen detection is especially useful in disseminated disease in which patients may not show significant antibody response. Urine antigen is positive in ~90% of patients with disseminated disease, ~20% of patients with acute self-limited disease, and <10% of patients with chronic pulmonary cavitary disease.
  - Serum antigen testing is less sensitive than urine and is positive in ~70% of patients with disseminated disease. Antigen is detected in CSF in <50% of patients with meningitis; positive antigen must be interpreted with caution, as cross-reactions are seen in coccidioidal meningitis. (CSF antibodies may also cross-react.) Antigen is positive in BAL fluid in ~70% of patients with pulmonary histoplasmosis.
  - Increasing antigen titer, or reconversion to antigen positivity, may be a sign of relapse or recurrent infection. Antigen becomes undetectable after antifungal therapy. Cross-reactions may rarely be seen in patients with blastomycosis, coccidioidomycosis, paracoccidioidomycosis, or other invasive fungal disease.
- Serology
  - CF and immunodiffusion (ID) tests are most useful for diagnosis of histoplasmosis. EIA screening methods are less sensitive and less specific. Positive CF and ID reactions are markers

of active histoplasmosis; background seropositivity in endemic areas is low. Positive reactions, however, may be due to asymptomatic, self-limited disease. Results of serologic tests must be interpreted with consideration of clinical and other laboratory information.

- Detection in specific *H. capsulatum* antibody is seen in ~90% of patients with acute pulmonary infection, but because seroconversion may not occur for several months after onset of infection, negative tests should be repeated after 4–6 weeks. Virtually all patients with chronic pulmonary or disseminated disease are seropositive.
- CF titers are slightly more sensitive but less specific than the immunodiffusion test for diagnosis of histoplasmosis. A single serum CF titer ≥1:32 or a fourfold increase in CF titer is highly suggestive of active histoplasmosis; a CF titer <1:8 is considered negative. Rising CF titers occur in >95% of patients with symptomatic primary infections. A CSF CF titer ≥1:8 is evidence for meningeal histoplasmosis. CSF antibodies, however, may not be detected until the third to sixth week of infection. Positive CF titers persist for months or years. Prognosis is not indicated by level or changes in titers. IgG and IgM detection is not clinically useful because of high false-positive and false-negative results.
- Laboratory: Increased serum aminotransferases and bilirubin suggest hepatic involvement. Anemia, leukopenia, and thrombocytopenia are more common (60–80% of cases) in acute than in subacute or chronic disseminated types. Increased serum LDH may be clue to disseminated form in AIDS patients.
- CSF findings: lymphocytic pleocytosis, increased protein, and decreased glucose.

PARACOCCIDIOIDOMYCOSIS (*PARACOCCIDIOIDES BRASILIENSIS*)

➤ Definition
- Paracoccidioidomycosis is caused by the thermally dimorphic fungus *Paracoccidioides brasiliensis*. This organism is endemic in wet, heavily vegetated, high-humidity areas of South America and Central America. The incidence of paracoccidioidomycosis is highest in Brazil.

➤ Who Should be Suspected?
- Most infections remain asymptomatic or mild, but clinical recovery may not be associated with microbiologic cure. Dormant infection may lead to recurrent, symptomatic infection at the time of acquired immunodeficiency. Disease is uncommon in children.
- Most symptomatic infections occur in men with occupations or other activities that put them in close contact with the environment. Symptoms are nonspecific and mimic TB, histoplasmosis, or other conditions. Symptoms include fever, chronic cough, sputum production, dyspnea, chest pain, weight loss, and malaise.
- The risk of infection is increased in patients who smoke, those who are alcoholic, or those who have AIDS. Person-to-person transmission does not occur.

➤ Laboratory Findings
- Direct detection: Deep respiratory specimens, CSF, or tissue from granulomas, ulcers, lymph nodes, or other infected sites show the characteristic large yeast cells with multiple narrow-based buds (mariner's wheel). A mixed granulocytic, monocytic response is typical.
- Culture: Routine fungal culture yields growth in the mold phase, which shows characteristic, but not specific, mycelial and conidial morphology.

- Serology: The diagnosis is supported by demonstration of specific antibodies using CF, ID, and other antibody detection techniques. Successful therapy is associated in significant decrease in antibody titers when acute and convalescent serum samples are tested. The quantitative ID assay is sensitive ($>$95%) and specific (near 100%) for diagnosis and is recommended.
- Routine laboratory: Morning cortisol levels and ACTH stimulation testing is recommended because of the frequency of adrenal gland involvement. Routine laboratory testing to evaluate the function of infected organs is recommended. Common findings include anemia, eosinophilia, hypoalbuminemia, hyperbilirubinemia, hypergammaglobulinemia, and mildly elevated transaminases.

SPOROTRICHOSIS

➤ Definition

- Sporotrichosis is a subacute to chronic infection caused by the thermally dimorphic fungus *Sporothrix schenckii*. Sporotrichosis occurs mainly North and South America and Japan, but scattered cases are seen worldwide. In the environment, this organism exists in its mold phase and is associated with soil and thorned plants, like roses.
- Infection is transmitted most commonly by traumatic inoculation or inoculation of nonintact skin surfaces. Most infections, therefore, are related to outdoor recreational or occupational activities.

➤ Who Should be Suspected?

- Extracutaneous infection is most commonly seen in patients with underlying illnesses that may compromise immune function, including alcoholism, DM, COPD, and AIDS (uncommon).
  - Lymphocutaneous sporotrichosis: A papular lesion, with overlying erythema, initially forms at the site of inoculation. The lesion commonly ulcerates. Similar lesions develop along the lymphatic drainage path from the primary site of infection. The lesions of lymphocutaneous sporotrichosis are usually only minimally painful. Systemic symptoms are usually absent.
  - Pulmonary sporotrichosis: Pulmonary sporotrichosis usually occurs in alcoholic men. Signs and symptoms may mimic TB. Chest radiography commonly shows upper lobe disease with cavitation, fibrosis, or nodular densities. Respiratory symptoms include cough, dyspnea, and sputum production (may be bloody).
  - Osteoarticular sporotrichosis: Osteoarticular sporotrichosis is usually caused by hematogenous spread from a primary cutaneous infection in alcoholic men. Joint infection is usually seen in the extremities: knee, elbow, ankle, and wrist, are most commonly affected. Osteomyelitis may occur as a result of local invasion. Patients present with pain, swelling, and decreased range of motion.
  - CNS sporotrichosis: CNS infection is rare and occurs mainly in patients with AIDS or other T-cell defects. CNS infection has a subacute presentation with fever and headache.

➤ Laboratory Findings

- Direct detection: Histopathologic examination of infected tissue shows a mixed pyogenic and granulomatous response. Typical "cigar shaped" budding yeast may be seen. Detection is

improved by use of fungal stains, like periodic acid–Schiff or methenamine silver stains. H&E staining may demonstrate "asteroid bodies"—basophilic yeast surrounded by eosinophilic material that probably represents antigen–antibody complex.
* Culture: Isolation of *S. schenckii* in culture provides definitive diagnosis of sporotrichosis. The organism is readily isolated from biopsy or aspirated material from infected sites. Growth usually appears during the first week of incubation, but cultures are usually incubated for 4 weeks before being signed out as negative.
* Serology: does not play a significant role in the diagnosis of active infection.
* CSF findings: Patients with meningitis have a lymphocytic pleocytosis, low glucose, and increased protein.

PATHOGENIC YEASTS

Organisms in this group may behave more like bacteria than mold in the clinical laboratory; they are often isolated on bacterial culture media. Infection is usually based on isolation in culture. Antigen detection may support the diagnosis.

CANDIDIASIS

➤ Definition
* Candidiasis describes disease caused by any of several species within the fungal genus *Candida*. *Candida* species are globally distributed yeast, and those that cause infection form a part of the human endogenous flora, as well as the normal flora of other warm-blooded animals. *Candida* spp. are common inhabitants of the GI tract, but may also be found on other mucosal surfaces, including the oral and genital tracts, and skin surfaces, including under fingernails and toenails and intertriginous areas. Disease may occur when an individual's local host defense mechanisms or systemic immunity are compromised. The incidence of invasive candidiasis has increased in the recent decades as a result of increasing use and strength of immunosuppressive drugs and the emergence of AIDS.
* *Candida albicans* is the most common cause of candidiasis. This species causes most infections of genital, oral, and cutaneous sites. Candidiasis can also be caused by a number of other *Candida* species, most frequently: *Candida glabrata*, *Candida krusei*, *Candida lusitaniae*, *Candida parapsilosis*, and *Candida tropicalis*. *Candida dubliniensis* is a recently identified species that may mimic *C. albicans* in commonly used identification algorithms.
* Although several organism factors contribute to the ability of *Candida* species to cause infection, the most important factor is the status of the host's immunity. Most infections are endogenous, usually caused by organisms from the individual's GI flora. Most infections of deep tissues result from hematogenous spread of endogenous organisms. Disease processes that result in the breakdown of the integrity of the gut mucosa are predisposing factors for hematogenous spread. Nosocomial, nonperinatal outbreaks of candidiasis in neonatal ICUs are well described.

➤ Who Should be Suspected?
Mucosal and cutaneous candidiasis may occur in normal hosts with minor predisposing conditions, like recent antibiotic therapy. However, more serious conditions should be considered (i.e., HIV infection, DM, allergies).

- Genital (see discussion of vaginitis and vaginosis in Chapter 9, Gynecologic and Obstetric Disorders)
- Oropharyngeal: "Thrush" is a common infection, especially in infants and patients with defects in cell-mediated immunity, like AIDS. Risk is increased by treatment with antibiotics, chemotherapy, or head and neck radiation. Patients with dentures are also at increased risk. Oropharyngeal candidiasis usually presents with characteristic white plaques on the tongue, buccal mucosa, palate, or posterior oropharynx. Patients may be asymptomatic. Some patients complain of odynophagia or painful stomatitis, frequently seen in patients with dentures.
- Esophageal: Esophageal candidiasis most commonly occurs as a complication of HIV infection; it is an AIDS-defining illness. Patients may have oropharyngeal candidiasis. Odynophagia and retrosternal pain are common complaints. White plaques are seen by endoscopic examination, the scrapings of which show budding yeast with pseudohyphae.
- Skin and nails: Superficial infection may occur, typically in intertriginous or other warm, moist areas, presenting with erythema, pruritus, and vesicle formation. *Candida albicans* and *C. parapsilosis* are the most common causes of onychomycosis of fingers and may be associated with paronychia. Congenital candidiasis may present in neonates as a generalized erythematous desquamating rash. Chronic mucocutaneous candidiasis is uncommon but may occur in patients with congenital autoimmune syndromes or other defects in cell-mediated immunity. Conditions commonly misdiagnosed as cutaneous candidiasis include psoriasis, chronic nail trauma, squamous carcinoma of the nail bed, "yellow-nail syndrome," or other conditions that should be considered and ruled out as appropriate. In skin and nail involvement in children, congenital hypoparathyroidism and Addison disease should be ruled out.
- Candidemia: Invasive candidiasis is most commonly caused by hematogenous spread of endogenous *Candida* in immunocompromised patients, often associated with a break in the integrity of the mucosal barrier of the bowel. Symptoms may be variable, ranging from low fever and malaise to a full-blown sepsis syndrome. The incidence of candidemia is increasing as a result of HIV infection and other acquired immunodeficiency diseases, increasing use and potency of immunosuppressive therapies, intensive care interventions, increased survival of premature infants, increased use of chronic IV nutrition, and other factors. *C. albicans* is the most common isolate, but other *Candida* species are playing an increasing role in candidemia, resulting in an increased rate of resistance to antifungal agents in candidemic patients. *Candida* species play a significant role in the etiology of nosocomial bloodstream infections, causing up to 10% of these infections. Candidemia has a high attributable mortality. Cofactors contributing to poor outcome include older age, disseminated candidiasis, and severe and persistent neutropenia.
- Pneumonia: Primary *Candida* pneumonia is extremely rare, even in intubated patients. Secondary *Candida* pneumonia occurs rarely in candidemic patients, but diagnosis may require invasive techniques and histopathologic confirmation.
- Cardiovascular: Endocarditis, myocarditis, or pericarditis may occur. *Candida* is responsible for <5% of cases of endocarditis, but *C. albicans* is responsible for >50% the cases of fungal endocarditis. Risk factors include presence of prosthetic valves, IV drug abuse, major surgery, preexisting valve disease, and chronic placement of deep IV catheters or pacemakers. The presentation of *Candida* endocarditis cannot be distinguished from bacterial endocarditis on the basis of clinical presentation alone. Patients with *Candida* endocarditis are at high risk for embolization; the brain, eye, kidney, liver, skin, and spleen are common sites.

- CNS: Infections are uncommon but may arise as secondary infections in candidemic patients or as complication of neurosurgery or chronic ventricular shunting. The clinical presentation is not distinctive.
- Ocular: Chorioretinitis or endophthalmitis are usually caused by hematogenous spread and are often the first sign of invasive candidiasis. Keratitis and some cases of chorioretinitis or endophthalmitis are caused by trauma or surgery. Patients present with pain and loss of visual acuity. Ophthalmological examination is recommended for all patients with candidemia. Characteristic findings are confirmed by culture.
- Bone and joint: Infections may be due to direct trauma, joint injection or surgery, or secondary to hematogenous seeding. These infections may present many months after the infectious incident; onset is often gradual and subtle. The vertebrae are most commonly affected in the elderly, whereas infection of the long bones is most common in children. Diagnosis is established by isolation of *Candida* from specimens collected from the bone or joint.
- Abdominal: *Candida* species, as common components of the endogenous GI microflora, may be isolated in almost any infectious process of the abdomen. Specific *Candida* peritonitis may be seen in patients undergoing chronic peritoneal dialysis. *Candida* infection is a fairly common complication in patients recovering from acute pancreatitis from other causes. Hepatosplenic candidiasis may complicate resolution of neutropenia in patients on chemotherapeutic regimens for hematologic malignancies. The liver and spleen may have been seeded during a recognized or unrecognized episode of candidemia, although there is the possibility that *Candida* was introduced by the portal vasculature. Patients present with fever, nausea, vomiting, anorexia, and right upper quadrant pain. Discrete microabscesses form in the liver and spleen, which may be detected by a variety of imaging techniques.

➤ Laboratory Findings

- Culture: Positive cultures from normally sterile sites support the diagnosis, but cultures must be interpreted with caution to rule out contamination with endogenous flora.
  - The detection of candiduria in patients with bladder catheters in place most likely represents colonization. In patients without foreign bodies in the urinary tract, however, significant candiduria may be a marker of obstruction, DM, or other serious condition. There is not a clear relationship between the quantity of *Candida* in urine (CFU/mL) and clinical significance, as is seen with bacteria.
  - Isolation of *Candida albicans* from sputum and other respiratory specimens is common but rarely associated with pulmonary infection. In CNS infection, isolation of *Candida* from CSF is diagnostic, but the concentration of organisms is very low, so repeat testing and submission of a large volume of CSF per sample may be needed to establish the diagnosis.
- Direct detection of organisms in tissue or clinical specimens: When associated with signs of inflammation or tissue damage, this may provide reliable detection of infection. Diagnosis of oropharyngeal, esophageal, or vulvovaginal candidiasis may be made on the basis of clinical appearance and risk factors. Confirmation may be established by wet mount or Gram stain examination of scrapings from the affected sites. Negative direct examination does not rule out mucosal candidiasis.
- Histopathology: shows yeast cells and mycelial forms, epithelial disruption with organisms invading through mucosal cells, and submucosal inflammation in mucosal candidiasis. Deep tissue candidiasis shows organisms invading and disrupting infected tissue.
- Serology: Antibody detection has played a limited role in diagnosis of candidiasis.
- Routine laboratory: ALP levels are increased in patients with hepatosplenic candidiasis.

CRYPTOCOCCOSIS (*CRYPTOCOCCUS NEOFORMANS*)

➤ Definition

* Several species of the genus *Cryptococcus*, including *Cryptococcus neoformans* and *Cryptococcus gattii*, are capable of causing disease in humans.
* The typical geographic distribution of *C. gattii* is restricted to tropical and subtropical regions with eucalyptus trees. *C. neoformans*, on the other hand, has a worldwide distribution and is responsible for most cases of cryptococcosis worldwide.
* Organisms are able to survive in the gut of pigeons and in dried pigeon droppings; this is likely responsible for wide distribution through the environment. Infection is acquired by inhalation of organisms present in the environment, and person-to-person transmission does not occur.

➤ Who Should be Suspected?

In immunocompetent individuals, exposure usually results in self-limited asymptomatic or mild disease; progressive and chronic disease is uncommon. Immunocompromised patients, however, are at risk for more severe disease with progression to extrapulmonary tissues. Conditions associated with increased risk of disseminated cryptococcosis include AIDS, glucocorticoid therapy, organ transplantation, malignancy, and/or sarcoidosis. Types of infection include:

* Pulmonary: Symptoms of pulmonary cryptococcosis include chest pain, cough, dyspnea, fever, sputum production, and weight loss.
* CNS: A significant proportion of AIDS patients with clinically significant pulmonary cryptococcosis progress to cryptococcal meningoencephalitis or infection in other organs. Frequent symptoms include altered mental status, fever, headache, seizures, and visual disturbances.
* Bone and joint: Osteomyelitis usually occurs in vertebrae or bony prominences due to hematogenous spread from a primary pulmonary infection. Cryptococcal arthritis may occur by spread from a contiguous osteomyelitis.
* Lymphadenopathy: usually cervical or supraclavicular.
* Prostate: Asymptomatic, persistent infection of the prostate may occur, most commonly in AIDS patients, and serves as a reservoir for recurrent infection.
* Skin: May represent primary infection but usually represents hematogenous dissemination from a primary pulmonary infection. A wide variety of cutaneous lesions have been described.

➤ Laboratory Findings

* Radiology: In immunocompetent patients, solitary or few noncalcified nodules are most commonly seen. Cavitation is uncommon. In AIDS patients, bilateral interstitial infiltrates, which may mimic *Pneumocystis jiroveci* or other opportunistic infection, are common.
* Gram stain: Gram stain may demonstrate yeast consistent with *C. neoformans*.
* Culture: *C. neoformans* may be isolated from 90–100% of infected specimens submitted from patients with cryptococcosis. Coinfection with other opportunistic pathogens has been reported in pulmonary cryptococcosis in AIDS patients.
* Histopathology: *C. neoformans* cells may be seen in biopsy material using a variety of stains, including H&E, silver, Fontana-Masson, and mucicarmine.
* Serology: Serology is not useful for diagnosis of acute cryptococcal infection.
* Cryptococcal antigen (CA): Detection of specific polysaccharide antigen is sensitive and specific for diagnosis of cryptococcosis. LA assays are most commonly used and provide rapid

results. CA can be detected in CSF >90% of patients with cryptococcal meningitis. Serum CA may also be used as a less sensitive screen for meningitis or cryptococcal infection at other sites but should be confirmed by culture of the infected site.

- CSF CA titers are useful for predicting outcome and monitoring therapy in AIDS patients with cryptococcal meningoencephalitis. Patients with an initial titer of ≤1:2048 predict a favorable outcome. Relapse is likely in patients with persistently elevated CA titers in spite of effective antifungal therapy.
- False-positive CA tests may be caused by RF, cross-reaction with *Trichosporon beigelii*, or *Capnocytophaga canimorsus* or syneresis fluid from culture media. The EIA does not show a prozone effect and is not affected by RF. The turnaround time for EIA results is longer than for LA testing.
- Laboratory findings (cryptococcal meningitis): Meningitis should be considered, regardless of symptoms, in immunocompromised patients with pulmonary cryptococcosis, and relevant diagnostic testing performed. Relapse is less frequent when increase in protein and cells is marked rather than moderate. Poor prognosis is suggested if initial CSF examination shows positive India ink preparation, low glucose (<20 mg/dL), and low WBC count (<20/μL). CBC and ESR usually remain normal.
- CSF findings: Positive culture is related to CSF volume; should be ≥10 mL. Protein is increased in 90% (<500 mg/dL). Glucose is moderately decreased in ~55% of patients. CSF Cell count is almost always increased ≤800 cells (more lymphocytes than leukocytes).

► Suggested Readings: Fungal Pathogens

Chapman SW, Dismukes WE, Proia LA, et al. Clinical Practice Guidelines for the Management of Blastomycosis: 2008 Update by the Infectious Diseases Society of America. *Clin Infect Dis.* 2008;46:1801–1812.

Cuellar-Rodriguez J, Avery RK, Lard M, et al. Histoplasmosis in solid organ transplant recipients: 10 years of experience at a large transplant center in an endemic area. *Clin Infect Dis.* 2009;49:710–716.

Dromer F, McGinnis MR. Chapter 12: Zygomycosis. In: Anaissie EJ, McGinnis MR, Pfaller MA, eds. *Clinical Mycology.* Philadelphia, PA: Churchill Livingstone; 2003.

Galgiani JN, Ampel NM, Blair JE, et al. Coccidioidomycosis. *Clin Infect Dis.* 2005;41:1217–1223.

Hage CA, Bowyer S, Tarvin SE, et al. Recognition, diagnosis, and treatment of histoplasmosis complicating tumor necrosis factor blocker therapy. *Clin Infect Dis.* 2010;50:85–92.

Kauffman CA, Bustamante B, Chapman SW, Pappas PG. Clinical Practice Guidelines for the Management of Sporotrichosis: 2007 Update by the Infectious Diseases Society of America. *Clin Infect Dis.* 2007;45:1255–1265.

Kauffman CA. Sporotrichosis. *Clin Infect Dis.* 1999;29:231–237.

Koo S, Bryar JM, Page JH, et al. Diagnostic performance of the (1 → 3)-β-D-glucan assay for invasive fungal disease. *Clin Infect Dis.* 2009;49:1650–1659.

Nucci M, Anaissie E. *Fusarium* infections in immunocompromised patients. *Clin Microbiol Rev.* 2007;20:695–704.

Pera S, Patterson TF. Chapter 15 endemic mycoses. In: Anaissie EF, McGinnis MR, Pfaller MA, eds. *Clinical Mycology.* Philadelphia, PA: Churchill Livingstone; 2003.

Perfect JR, Dismukes WE, Dromer F, et al. Clinical Practice Guidelines for the Management of Cryptococcal Disease: 2010 Update by the Infectious Diseases Society of America. *Clin Infect Dis.* 2010;50:291–322.

Ribes JA, Vanover-Sams CL, Baker DJ. Zygomycetes in human disease. *Clin Microbiol Rev.* 2000;13:236–301.

Rex JH. Galactomannan and the diagnosis of invasive aspergillosis. *Clin Infect Dis.* 2006;42:1428–1430.

Segal BH. Aspergillosis. *N Engl J Med.* 2009;360:1870–1884.

Sun H-Y, Wagener MM, Singh N. Cryptococcosis in solid-organ, hematopoietic stem cell, and tissue transplant recipients: evidence-based evolving trends. *Clin Infect Dis.* 2009;48:1566–1576.

Yozwiak ML, Lundergan LL, Kerrick SS, Galgiani JN. Symptoms and routine laboratory abnormalities associated with coccidioidomycosis. *West J Med.* 1988;149:419–421.

INFECTIOUS DISEASES CAUSED BY VIRAL PATHOGENS

This section reviews viral pathogens that are responsible for a very wide and diverse range of diseases. Viral pathogens are incapable of multiplication outside of host eukaryotic cells, but many do not require human cells for proliferation. Other mammals, arthropods, or other species may serve as intermediate or definitive hosts for pathogenic viruses.

Most viral infections are mild, self-limited diseases and are presumptively diagnosed on the basis of clinical signs and symptoms. Serologic testing is most commonly used when definitive diagnosis is required and may be used for diagnosis of acute or past infection or to determine the immune status of a host. Viral infection may also be established presumptively by typical histopathologic findings; specific identification may be made by staining with specific immunostaining. Isolation of virus in eukaryotic cell culture provides definitive diagnosis, but the sensitivity of isolation usually falls significantly after acute symptoms resolve, and some viral pathogens cannot be isolated in culture. Virus culture is typically performed only in larger reference or commercial laboratories.

Molecular diagnostic procedures are playing an increasing role in the diagnosis of viral infections. Molecular methods may be used for diagnosis, predicting response to antiviral agents, monitoring disease activity or response to treatment, or other purposes.

ENCEPHALITIS VIRUSES

See Chapter 5, Central Nervous System Disorders, for a discussion of encephalitis and causal viral pathogens.

ENTEROVIRUSES

ENTEROVIRUS, COXSACKIEVIRUS, AND ECHOVIRUS

➤ Definition
* Coxsackieviruses and echoviruses are species in the genus *Enterovirus*, family Picornaviridae. Enteroviruses show broad serologic diversity. Enteroviruses are very stable in the environment, allowing them to survive for long periods in water and sewage.
* Humans are the only natural host for enteroviral infections. As the name implies, enteroviruses initiate infection in the intestines. Infection is usually acquired by fecal–oral transmission. Infections occur worldwide.

➤ Who Should be Suspected?
* Children are most frequently infected, although enterovirus infections occur in all ages.
* The humoral immune response seems to be most important for control of enteroviral infections; agammaglobulinemic patients are at risk for more severe or chronic disease.
* Common clinically significant disease syndromes include cardiovascular disease, muscle disease, neonatal infection, neurologic disease, meningoencephalitis, conjunctivitis, hand-foot-mouth disease, herpangina, and upper and lower respiratory tract infections.

➤ Laboratory Findings

Most enteroviral infections are mild and self-limited and may be diagnosed without specific laboratory testing. For severe disease, possible diagnostic tests include:

• Viral culture: Isolation of virus in culture has been the traditional method for specific diagnosis of enteroviral infection. Growth of specific enteroviruses is variable in different cell lines, and the pattern of growth in culture may provide preliminary presumptive identification for a specific group. Some group A coxsackieviruses do not grow in cell culture. Isolation of an *Enterovirus* species from CSF establishes a diagnosis of enteroviral meningitis. Although isolation of enteroviruses from stool or the nasopharynx is commonly seen in patients with severe enteroviral disease, like meningitis, positive cultures from these sites must be interpreted with caution: transient "colonization" may be seen unrelated to the clinical syndrome for which the specimen was collected.

• Molecular diagnostic tests: A number of commercially available diagnostic tests have been shown to provide very sensitive and specific detection of enteroviral infections. NAA tests have proven to be especially useful to diagnose aseptic meningitis and help rule out bacterial meningitis in children presenting with fever and meningeal signs in summertime.

• Serology: Of limited value in diagnosis.

• Typical core laboratory: CBC and WBC counts are typically normal or show only mild, non-specific abnormalities.

• CSF findings: Enteroviral meningitis shows moderate pleocytosis ($<$1000 mononuclear cells; may see PMN predominance early), normal or slightly reduced glucose, normal or slightly increased protein.

POLIOMYELITIS

➤ Definition

• Poliomyelitis is caused by poliovirus species (types 1–3), in the genus *Enterovirus*.

• The transmission of polio has been greatly reduced in areas with effective vaccination programs; however, wild-type virus continues to occur sporadically in developing countries. The attenuated virus used in the oral polio vaccine has caused paralytic disease in immunocompromised patients.

• It is mandated to report paralytic poliomyelitis in all states in the United States. Public health officials should be contacted as soon as paralytic poliomyelitis is suspected. Public health officials may provide guidance regarding confirmatory testing.

➤ Who Should be Suspected?

• During poliovirus outbreaks, most infected patients remain asymptomatic or have mild, self-limited disease. A minority of patients ($<$2%), however, develop paralytic poliomyelitis or occasionally meningitis or encephalitis without paralysis. Illness may be preceded by fever, myalgias, and nonspecific "viral" symptoms.

• Poliomyelitis is caused by infection of the anterior horn cells of the spinal cord, resulting in acute flaccid paralysis of associated muscle groups. Spinal poliomyelitis may vary in severity from isolated paresis to paralysis of limbs, quadriplegia, and paralysis of the diaphragm or other muscle groups. Cranial nerve nuclei may be involved resulting in bulbar poliomyelitis,

with paralysis of muscles involved in swallowing or destruction of cells regulating central respiration. Infected patients may develop disease related to both spinal and bulbar poliomyelitis. Cerebral function is typically unaffected.
* Five percent to 10% of patients die, usually as a result of respiratory failure. Most children recover; however, a majority are left with residual sequelae ranging in severity from mild motor weakness to complete paralysis.

➤ Laboratory Findings
Poliomyelitis may be suspected on the basis of clinical signs and symptoms in appropriate clinical settings.
* Culture: The diagnosis is usually confirmed by isolation of virus in culture. Several samples of stool and throat for viral culture, obtained at least 24 hours apart, should be collected early in the course of disease.
* Serology of acute and convalescent sera: may be submitted to support a diagnosis of poliomyelitis, but test interpretation may be difficult.
* CSF findings: nonspecific. Cell count is usually 25–500/μL; rarely is normal or $\leq$2000/μL. At first, most are PMNs; after several days, most are lymphocytes. Protein may be normal at first; increased by second week (usually 50–200 mg/dL); normal by sixth week. Glucose is usually normal.
* Core laboratory: Blood shows early moderate increase in WBC ($\leq$15,000/μL) and PMNs. WBC returns to normal within 1 week. Increased AST in 50% of patients is caused by the associated hepatitis.

HEPATITIS VIRUSES

See Chapter 6, Digestive Diseases.

HERPESVIRUSES

CYTOMEGALOVIRUS INFECTION

➤ Definition
* Human cytomegalovirus (CMV) is member of the Herpesviridae, subfamily Betaherpesvirinae. CMV is ubiquitous with a worldwide distribution. Although CMV infection can be demonstrated in a significant majority of individuals in developing and developed countries, clinical disease is uncommon in immunocompetent hosts.
* Acute infection with CMV, as characteristic of herpesviruses, results in long-term latent infection with periodic reactivation to a replicative phase of infection.

➤ Who Should be Suspected?
* Immunocompetent patients who develop acute disease most often present with a mononucleosis syndrome with pharyngitis, lymphadenopathy, and splenomegaly. Laboratory studies may show elevated atypical lymphocytes and transaminases.
* Fetal infection is the result of vertical transmission during acute or recurrent maternal infection. Neonatal infection may also be transmitted by breast milk. Most infected neonates are asymptomatic at birth but are at risk (10–15%) for development of hearing loss, learning

disability, and/or other organ dysfunction. Congenital CMV disease may manifest at birth with a variety of clinical features, alone or in combination, including intrauterine growth retardation, microcephaly, intracranial calcifications, hepatosplenomegaly, jaundice, retinitis, thrombocytopenia, and purpura.

- Disease in immunocompromised patients may be caused by acute, newly acquired infection, or by reactivation of latent infection. CMV disease may cause life-threatening systemic or organ-specific disease. Primary infection poses the greatest risk for severe disease in immunocompromised patients, but there is also significant risk associated with CMV reactivation, especially in bone marrow transplant patients. Fever is a constant feature of disease. Other disease manifestations include CNS disease (encephalitis, polyradiculopathy), GI infection (colitis, esophagitis), hepatitis, myelosuppression/thrombocytopenia, pneumonitis, and retinitis.
- Transmission of CMV by blood transfusion and organ transplantation is well described.

▶ Laboratory Findings

- Culture: Routine viral culture provides strong evidence for viral replication in vivo and can be performed on a variety of specimen types. Cell cultures, however, may take up to 3 weeks incubation to provide final results. The shell vial technique, with early staining for proteins produced early in the CMV replicative phase using tagged monoclonal antibodies, markedly decreases turnaround time (48–72 hours) while maintaining good sensitivity. Within the first 2 weeks, viral culture of urine is most sensitive and specific means for diagnosis of congenital CMV infection. Viral cultures of CSF are usually negative in CNS infections.
- Antigenemia: Tagged monoclonal antibodies may be used to detect CMV antigens associated with active replication. The CMV pp65 antigenemia assay can be used to detect active CMV replication associated with emerging or active disease with good sensitivity and specificity.
- Molecular diagnostics: Viral load testing has provided the most important indicator for the presence (or emergence) of active infection in immunocompromised patients. The viral load is directly proportional to the potential severity of disease. Low viral loads must be interpreted with caution because they may represent transient dysregulation of latent infection rather than progressive, active replication.
- Histopathology: Histopathologic examination demonstrates characteristic changes, including intranuclear and intracytoplasmic inclusions. Specimens may be stained using H&E, other nonspecific stain, or with specific immunologic or nucleic acid reagents.
- Serology: May be used to diagnosis acute infection or to document immune status.
- Core laboratory: Laboratory findings due to predisposing or underlying conditions are seen. Characteristic laboratory changes are seen with infection of liver, kidney, or adrenal gland.

EPSTEIN-BARR VIRUS INFECTIONS

▶ Definition

- Epstein-Barr virus (EBV) is a lymphocryptovirus in the Herpesviridae family.
- EBV infections are widespread and occur worldwide. In developing regions, primary EBV infections usually occur in younger children. In developed countries, primary infections usually occur in adolescents and young adults. The rate of seropositivity is high (>90%) by middle age.

- Infections are primarily transmitted by oropharyngeal secretions. After exposure, oropharyngeal epithelial cells and tonsillar B lymphocytes are thought to be the first cells infected. Infection is spread to lymphoid cells throughout the body by memory B cells.

➤ Who Should be Suspected?

Most primary EBV infections are asymptomatic, but EBV infection may cause a variety of mild to severe diseases:

- Acute infectious mononucleosis (AIM): AIM is the most commonly recognized manifestation of clinically apparent primary EBV infection, usually occurring in adolescents. Patients commonly present with fever, pharyngitis, posterior lymphadenopathy, and lethargy. Headache and malaise are also common, and rash, anorexia, nausea, and other nonspecific "viral" symptoms occur less frequently. A palpable spleen may be present in a significant proportion of patients and splenic rupture, although uncommon, is a serious potential complication of AIM. The development of a morbilliform rash following amoxicillin or ampicillin treatment is highly suggestive of EBV AIM in patients with febrile pharyngitis syndromes.
- Acute symptoms usually resolve within 2 weeks, but fatigue may persist for months.
- Note that mononucleosis syndromes are not agent-specific for EBV. Heterophile-negative mononucleosis syndrome may be found in other infections diseases, especially CMV, toxoplasmosis, and HSV. Atypical lymphocytes may be seen in other acute illnesses (e.g., rubella, roseola, mumps, acute viral hepatitis, acute HIV, drug reactions).
- Nasopharyngeal carcinoma: EBV DNA is consistently detected in nasopharyngeal carcinoma cells.
- Lymphoproliferative diseases: EBV infection is associated with a number of lymphoproliferative diseases, including:
  - Burkitt lymphoma: EBV has been implicated as a cause of endemic Burkitt lymphoma in equatorial Africa. EBV is seen less frequently in sporadic Burkitt's cases outside of endemic areas.
  - Hodgkin disease: EBV DNA may be detected in malignant cells of Hodgkin disease. The frequency of detection varies in different geographic regions but is almost universal in Hodgkin's disease associated with AIDS.
  - Lymphomas associated with HIV infection: The incidence of non-Hodgkin lymphoma is markedly increased compared to nonimmunocompromised patients and EBV is associated with a majority of these malignancies. Most EBV-related non-Hodgkin lymphomas in HIV-infected patients present in the central nervous system.
  - Posttransplant lymphoproliferative disease (PTLD): The severity of PTLD after allograft transplantation may range from benign B-cell proliferation to aggressive B-cell lymphoma. The severity of disease is related to the degree of immunosuppression. Fever, pharyngitis, and nonspecific symptoms may occur during the development of PTLD.
  - X-linked lymphoproliferative syndrome (XLP): XLP, manifested by a severe or fatal mononucleosis or immunodeficiency syndrome, is essentially a selective defect in immunity to EBV infection. Mutation in the gene implicated in XLP, SH2D1A, results in defective activation-induced cell death in CD8 T lymphocytes, with subsequent uncontrolled proliferation.

➤ Laboratory Findings

- Histopathology: The use of EBV-specific immunohistochemical staining to detect EBV proteins may provide improved sensitivity and specificity for establishing EBV as the specific cause of disease when the etiology of the syndrome is broad.

- Serology
  - AIM is usually diagnosed serologically. Heterophile antibodies (Paul-Bunnell test) demonstrate moderate to good sensitivity and high specificity for detection of AIM during the acute, symptomatic phase of disease. This "spot" test has an overall sensitivity ≤92% and specificity >96%, except in children <4 years old when slide test is less sensitive. Heterophile agglutination is positive in 60% of young adults by 2 weeks and 90% by 4 weeks after onset of clinical infectious mononucleosis (therefore, they may be negative when hematologic and clinical findings are present). Low titers may persist for a year. False-positive slide tests may occur in leukemia, malignant lymphoma, malaria, rubella, hepatitis, and pancreatic carcinoma, and they may be present for years in some persons with no known explanation. In adults, false-positive results in ~2% of patients and false-negative results in ~5%.
  - Specific EBV antibody tests are rarely required; most patients are heterophile-antibody positive and clinical illness is usually self-limited and relatively mild. Specific tests may be useful, however, in atypical mononucleosis syndromes or for very severe cases, especially in young children or immunocompromised patients. See Figure 13-1 for antibody responses to EBV antigens. Detection of EBV-specific antibodies can be used to determine the phase of infection. The presence of viral capsid antigen (VCA) IgM only is consistent with early acute IM; detection of VCA IgM and IgG is consistent with late acute infection; detection of Epstein-Barr nuclear antigen (EBNA) IgG and VCA IgG, but negative VCA IgM is consistent with past EBV infection.
  - Acute primary EBV infection is indicated by any of these serologic findings: IgM-VCA that is found early and later declines. High titer (≥1:320) or ≥4 times rise in IgG-VCA titer during the illness. Transient rise in anti-D titer (≥1:10). Early IgG-VCA without EBNA and later appearance of EBNA. Acute or primary EBV infection is excluded when IgG-VCA and EBNA titers are unchanged in acute and convalescent serum samples. Current or recent infection is indicated by IgM anti-VCA or IgM/IgG early antigen with low or absent EBNA antibodies. Persistence of early antigen and IgG-VCA in high titer indicates chronic EBV infection. Anti-EA-R is high and correlated with tumor burden in

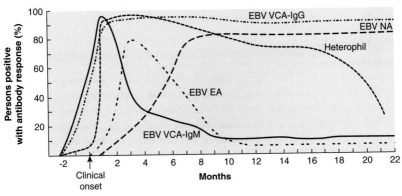

Figure 13-1. Percentage of persons with positive antibody response at specified time intervals. (EBV, Epstein-Barr virus; VCA, viral capsid antigen; EA, early antigen; NA, nuclear antigen.) [Ortho Diagnostic Systems, Raritan, NJ.]

Burkitt lymphoma. Anti-EA-D is high and correlated with tumor burden nasopharyngeal carcinoma. Note that serologic tests for syphilis RA and ANA may show transient false-positive results.

- Nucleic acid-based testing: Qualitative or quantitative PCR may be valuable for diagnosis or disease management in nonmononucleosis EBV associated diseases.
- Core laboratory
  - In AIM, hematologic findings of absolute ($>4500/\mu L$) and relative lymphocytosis ($\geq 50\%$) in 70% of cases, with $\geq 10\%$ (often $\leq 70\%$) characteristic atypical lymphocytes. Leukopenia and granulocytopenia are evident during first week. Later, WBC is increased (usually 10,000–20,000/μL) because of increased lymphocytes; peak changes occur in 7–10 days; may persist for 1–2 months. Increased number of bands and $>5\%$ eosinophilia are frequent. Mild thrombocytopenia is seen in about 50% of early cases, and platelet dysfunction is frequent. Hemolytic anemia is rare.
  - Evidence of mild hepatitis (e.g., increased serum transaminases, increased urine urobilinogen) is very frequent, but may be transient. Increased serum bilirubin in $\leq 30\%$ of adults and $<9\%$ of children. Bilirubin/enzyme dissociation (serum bilirubin normal or <2 mg/dL with moderate increase of ALP, GGT, AST, ALT) occurs in 75% of cases. If no liver function abnormalities can be found, another diagnosis should be sought.
- T-Cell response: AIM is associated with an oligoclonal expansion of CD8+ T lymphocytes.

HERPES SIMPLEX VIRUS INFECTIONS

➤ Definition

- Herpes simplex viruses (HSV) are members of the family Herpesviridae, subfamily Alphaherpesvirinae. Humans serve as the normal reservoir for HSV infections, and HSV disease has a global distribution.
- The viruses are transmitted by close personal contact. There is no evidence for epidemics of HSV, although clusters of infections may occur. There is no clear seasonal pattern in the incidence of HSV disease.
- Genital infections are most commonly caused by HSV-2; genital infections caused by HSV-1 tend to be milder and associated with a lower rate of recurrence.

➤ Who Should be Suspected?

HSV infection is associated with a number of syndromes, including:

- Primary oropharyngeal: HSV disease is usually asymptomatic or associated with mild symptoms. Severe symptoms may occur, including vesicular gingivostomatitis, pharyngitis, and lymphadenopathy. Nonspecific symptoms are common, including fever and malaise. Adolescents and adults may present with a mononucleosis syndrome. Specific antibodies are usually detectable within the first week following onset of infection, but virus may continue to shed for several weeks. Outbreak of recurrent lesions is usually preceded by pain, itching, or other symptoms shortly before appearance of vesicles, usually at the vermilion border of the lip. Lesions usually crust over within 4–5 days.
- Primary genital: Disease is manifested as a papulovesicular eruption of the genitals and surrounding skin and mucous membranes. Primary infections are usually associated with painful lesions and systemic symptoms, including fever, headache and malaise. Patients may complain

of dysuria, and inguinal lymphadenopathy may be evident. Neurologic symptoms, including aseptic meningitis, sacral radiculopathy, and neuralgias are not uncommon. Vesicles may persist for 3 weeks in primary infection but usually resolve within 1 week in recurrent outbreaks. Primary infections are associated with more lesions and a higher virus burden compared to recurrent disease. Genital or oropharyngeal HSV infection in pregnant women is of particular importance; it may result in disseminated disease in the mother, leading to complications including necrotizing hepatitis, meningoencephalitis and coagulopathy. Genital HSV infection in pregnant women is also a primary risk factor for neonatal HSV infection in the offspring.

- Neonatal: may occur at any time between birth and 4 weeks of age. Most neonatal HSV infections are acquired from infected maternal genital secretions during labor and delivery. A number of factors increase the risk of transmission and severity of neonatal disease: Primary maternal infection at or near the time of labor and delivery, maternal seronegativity for the infecting type of HSV, prolonged (>6 hours) rupture of fetal membranes prior to delivery, and/or the use of fetal scalp monitor. There are three common presentations of neonatal disease: (1) disseminated disease of multiple organ systems; (2) localized CNS disease; and (3) localized infection of skin, eyes, and mouth. Early intrauterine infection may rarely be seen, presenting with vesicles or scarring of skin, various ocular abnormalities, and CNS abnormalities, including microcephaly and hydranencephaly.
- HSV keratoconjunctivitis: manifested by photophobia, tearing, chemosis, lid edema, and preauricular lymphadenopathy. Visual acuity may be decreased. Slit-lamp examination typically shows characteristic branching dendritic lesions.
- Skin: Infections occur most commonly in patients with eczema. Outbreaks may be localized or disseminated (Kaposi's varicella-like eruption). Infection localized to the digits (herpetic whitlow) is associated with direct inoculation of virus, especially with healthcare manipulation.
- CNS: HSV is the most common cause of severe sporadic encephalitis. Patients typically present with focal encephalitis and neurologic abnormalities related to the region of brain affected. Patients also typically present with other symptoms, including fever, behavior changes, and decreased level of consciousness.

➤ Laboratory Findings

- Cell culture: HSV may be isolated by viral culture of vesicles, ulcers, or infected tissues. Culture of specimens from lesions of recurrent disease is much less sensitive. Positive viral cultures for HSV must be interpreted in the context of clinical presentation because HSV may rarely be shed in chronic infection in the absence of overt clinical disease.
- Histology: Direct cytologic examination of scrapings of lesions (Wright-Giemsa stain) shows multinucleated giant cells with intranuclear inclusions (Tzanck smear). Skin vesicles produce a positive smear in 66% and positive viral culture in 100% of cases; pustules produce a positive smear in 50% and a positive viral culture in 70% of cases; crusted ulcers produce a positive smear in 15% and a positive viral culture in 34% of cases. Multinucleated cells may also be identified in routine Pap smear of cervix. A negative direct test does not rule out this diagnosis.
- Molecular diagnosis: NAA techniques may be used for detection of HSV DNA in tissue, CSF, and other specimen types. PCR is the diagnostic test of choice if CNS infection is suspected. In HSV encephalitis, PCR of CSF has become the diagnostic method of choice, with a sensitivity and specificity of >95%.

- Serology: Serologic testing is of limited value for the management of acute infection but may be useful in assessing past infection or a patient's risk for infection. ELISA, WB, or immuno-blot for glycoprotein G can distinguish HSV-1 (gG1) and HSV-2 (gG2). Positive results indicate prior exposure; negative results indicate no prior exposure. WB is the gold standard for specific antibody detection. Immunoblot IgG has sensitivity >80% and specificity of 95%. Primary infections are associated with seroconversion or a fourfold or greater increased titer in acute and convalescent serum samples.
- Core laboratory: In patients with HSV encephalitis, CSF shows increased WBC count with mononuclear cell predominance; RBC count is usually increased. CSF protein is increased.

VARICELLA-ZOSTER VIRUS INFECTIONS

➤ Definition

- Varicella-zoster virus (VZV) is the agent responsible for varicella (chickenpox) and zoster (shingles). Chickenpox is the common manifestation of VZV infection, whereas zoster represents a reactivation of latent VZV. VZV may also cause disseminated infection in immunocompromised patients as well as neonatal infections.
- VZV is a member of the family Herpesviridae. There is only one serotype of VZV; all clinical isolates are antigenically related. VZV infections occur worldwide and most adults in temperate climates have serologic evidence of prior infection even those with no history of chickenpox.
- Historically, the incidence of chickenpox has been highest in children. Widespread use of varicella vaccine, however, has had an impact on the normal epidemiology with an increasing number of primary infections occurring in young adults.

➤ Who Should be Suspected?

- Varicella and zoster are usually relatively mild and self-limited diseases. Morbidity and mortality are low, but more severe disease is often seen in adults, pregnant women, and immunocompromised.
- Clinical disease typically occurs about 14 days after exposure. Most patients with primary varicella show an abrupt onset with the appearance of asynchronous "crops" of vesicular lesions appearing over several days, mainly on the head and trunk. Lesions at various stages, papular, vesicular, ulcerative, and crusted, are all seen at any time during active infection. Fever and nonspecific symptoms may occur. Lesions typically heal without scar formation.
- The most common complication of primary varicella is bacterial superinfection, especially with *Streptococcus pyogenes*. Although involvement of the respiratory tract may occur in a significant minority of patients, clinically significant pneumonia is an uncommon, but potentially serious, complication in a small number of patients, especially adults. Meningo-encephalitis, cerebellar ataxia, and other CNS complications occur rarely. Hemorrhagic varicella is uncommon in immunocompetent patients.
- Zoster occurs, mainly in the elderly, decades after primary VZV infection. It usually presents with a localized, unilateral eruption of vesicles restricted to one or several adjacent dermatomes, reflecting the role of dorsal root or cranial nerve ganglia as the source of viruses. Aseptic meningitis with minimal CSF abnormalities may be seen in patients with zoster.

Most patients recover spontaneously within 2 weeks. Localized cutaneous HSV infection may mimic zoster.

- Postherpetic neuralgia is a common complication of zoster and may develop in a significant minority of elderly patient after resolution of the rash. Motor deficits occur at the affected dermatome in about 1% of patients. This may manifest as bladder dysfunction or intestinal ileus. Zoster related to cranial nerves may result retinitis or other ocular abnormalities, Ramsay Hunt syndrome, facial palsies, or other abnormalities of cranial nerve function.
- Congenital varicella syndrome may occur in maternal infections during the first or early trimester of pregnancy. The embryopathy is manifested primarily by skin scars, limb atrophy, ocular abnormalities, mental retardation, or fetal loss. Maternal varicella after 20 weeks gestation is usually not associated with congenital varicella syndrome, although "silent" infection occurs in the fetus. When maternal infection occurs between 2 and 5 days prior to delivery, however, severe neonatal varicella may develop.

➤ Laboratory Findings

The diagnosis of varicella and zoster can accurately be made clinically. Laboratory testing is usually required for immunocompromised patients or patients with unusual or atypical disease.

- Culture: VZV may be reliably isolated by cell culture of vesicle fluid or scrapings from the base of wet ulcerative lesions. Culture results are usually positive after 3–5 days. The sensitivity of viral culture of CSF and other specimen types is lower.
- NAA: Standard and real-time PCR methods have largely replaced other tests for the laboratory diagnosis of acute VZV infections. Molecular diagnostic methods provide sensitive and specific results for a variety of types of specimens. Test results are usually available days sooner than viral culture results.
- Serology: Humoral and cell-mediated response is brisk after primary infection, occurring within several days of clinical disease. Levels peak within 3 month and then decline but are detectable for years. A bump in specific antibody subsets may be seen after an outbreak of zoster.
  - Several test formats are available, including tests for specific VZV IgG and IgM. A positive IgM result or fourfold or greater increase in VZV IgG or total antibody titer in acute and convalescent samples is diagnostic of VZV infection. Silent fetal infection may be inferred by persistence of positive VZV titers beyond 8 months of life.
  - The fluorescent antibody to membrane antigen assay (FAMA) is the most sensitive assay, if available, to document immunity after natural infection or vaccination. Detection of VZV antibodies in CSF is diagnostic of aseptic meningitis, even without skin lesions.
- Histology: Demonstration of specific VZV antigen by immunofluorescent staining of cells from vesicular lesions is diagnostic of acute VZV infection and is more sensitive than viral culture. DFA testing allows prompt diagnosis.
- Core laboratory: Core laboratory tests are generally not required unless severe disease is present. Clinical or subclinical hepatitis may occur in primary or systemic VZV infections. Elevation of transaminases, without hyperbilirubinemia, is typical. WBC count is usually decreased with absolute and relative lymphocytosis early in primary infection. Thrombocytopenia may be seen, especially in severe disease.
- CSF findings: In patients with CNS complications of VZV infection, the CSF parameters are usually normal or only mildly abnormal. Forty percent of zoster patients show increased cells (<300 mononuclear/µL) in CSF.

RESPIRATORY VIRUSES

See Chapter 14, Respiratory, Metabolic, and Acid-Base Disorders, for a detailed discussion of viral respiratory tract pathogens, including adenovirus, influenza viruses, parainfluenza viruses, and RSV.

HIV-1 INFECTION AND ACQUIRED IMMUNODEFICIENCY SYNDROME

➤ Definition
- Human immunodeficiency virus (HIV) infection is the cause of acquired immunodeficiency syndrome (AIDS), as well as symptomatic disease prior to the development of AIDS. HIV infection now has a global distribution, and most disease is caused by HIV-1. HIV-2 infection is more geographically restricted, primarily occurring in western Africa.
- HIV-1 viruses fall into three genetic groups: M, O, and N. Group M viruses, which can be further subdivided into clades (A-D, F-H, J, and K), are the predominant viruses responsible for the global epidemic. In the United States, Europe, and Australia, the B clade predominates. Other clades may be predominant in other geographic locations. HIV-2 is genetically distinct and is believed to have originated in a virus from sooty mangabeys. This discussion will focus on disease caused by HIV-1.
- HIV transmission is due to direct contact with infected body fluids, primarily blood, semen, vaginal and cervical secretions, breast milk, and amniotic fluid. This contact is usually mediated by sexual contact, IV drug abuse, blood exposure (transfusion, transplantation, needle-stick injury), and vertical transmission (pregnancy, childbirth, and nursing). The relative contribution of these modes shows regional variability. The risk of transmission depends on a number of factors, including viral load in infected fluid, presence of other STDs, sexual history, having an uncircumcised infected partner, and genetic factors.
- HIV is able to infect cells that express CD4 on their surfaces, primarily CD4+ T lymphocytes and macrophages.

➤ Who Should be Suspected?
HIV-1 infection may be divided into three clinical phases:
- Acute phase: During the acute phase, which usually occurs between 1 and 4 weeks after exposure, there is viremia with infection of cells throughout the body. The HIV-1 plasma viral load is markedly elevated, typically greater than 10^6 copies/mL. The level of CD4+ T lymphocytes is reduced, due to destruction and sequestration.
  - Thirty percent to 70% of patients develop nonspecific symptoms. A mononucleosis-type syndrome is common. Symptoms include headache, fever, malaise, pharyngitis, myalgias, and arthralgias. A nonpruritic macular rash commonly develops on the face and trunk. Generalized lymphadenopathy is common. Other symptoms include ulcerations of skin and mucous membranes, nausea and vomiting, and diarrhea. Neurologic symptoms, including aseptic meningoencephalitis and neuropathy, may develop.
  - Symptoms typically resolve within 4 weeks.
- Asymptomatic or minimally symptomatic phase: The acute phase is followed by a phase, typically prolonged, where the patient is not severely immunocompromised and symptoms

may be absent or mild. During this time there is continued viral replication and CD4+ T lymphocyte depletion. The rate of loss of CD4 cells is related to the HIV-1 viral load.
- During this phase, fatigue and lymphadenopathy are common. Other manifestations may include bacillary angiomatosis, cervical dysplasia or carcinoma in situ, chronic diarrhea, oral leukoplakia, progressive fatigue, progressive weight loss, night sweats, recurrent shingles or zoster in multiple dermatomes, and/or vaginal or oral candidiasis.
- This second phase of infection usually lasts for 8–10 years before progression to AIDS.
- AIDS/symptomatic phase: The relentless depletion of CD4 cells eventually results in profound immunosuppression and the clinical manifestations of AIDS. A specific diagnosis of AIDS is based, as described below, on the basis of laboratory findings or the presence of AIDS-defining infections or malignancies, including candidiasis, cervical cancer, recurrent infections, coccidiomycosis, cryptococcosis, cryptosporidiosis, encephalopathy, histoplasmosis, Kaposi sarcoma, lymphoma, *Mycobacterium tuberculosis* infection, progressive multifocal leukoencephalopathy, *Pneumocystis* pneumonia, toxoplasmosis of brain, and wasting syndrome (unintentional loss of >10% of body weight).

➤ Diagnosis and Staging
- The CDC and WHO have established diagnostic criteria for HIV infection status and AIDS diagnosis to be used for surveillance criteria. For the 2008 CDC criteria, see: http://www. cdc.gov/ncphi/disss/nndss/casedef/aids2008.htm.
- CDC criteria for diagnosis of HIV infection:
  - Positive result for a screening test for HIV-1 antibody, like an EIA, with confirmation with a specific confirmation test, like an HIV-1 WB, *or*
  - Positive result for an HIV-1 virologic test, like detection of HIV-1 nucleic acid or p24 antigen, or isolation of HIV-1 by cell culture
- CDC criteria for staging of HIV-1 infected patients are based on the presence of AIDS-defining conditions, discussed above, and on the count of CD4+ T lymphocytes or the percentage of CD4+ T lymphocytes of total lymphocytes.
  - Stage 1: No AIDS-defining illness and either CD4+ T lymphocytes ≥500 cells/μL or CD4+ lymphocyte percentage of total lymphocytes >29.
  - Stage 2: No AIDS-defining illness and either CD4+ T lymphocytes 200–499 cells/μL or CD4+ lymphocyte percentage of total lymphocytes 14–28.
  - Stage 3: CD4+ T lymphocytes <200 cells/μL or CD4+ lymphocyte percentage of total lymphocytes <14 or documentation of an AIDS-defining condition at CD4+ T lymphocyte levels at 200 cells/μL or higher.

➤ Laboratory Findings
- Serology: Most HIV-1 infected patients are diagnosed by detection of HIV antibodies, usually in serum. Virtually all infected patients develop antibodies to HIV-1 antigens, and final diagnosis of HIV-1 should be based on detection of antibodies. Fourth-generation assays are able to detect both HIV antigen (p24) and antibody (HIV-1 group M, HIV-1 group O, and HIV-2) formation 14 days after infection, significantly earlier than second- and third-generation assays. Most patients become positive for HIV-1 antibody testing within 1–2 months after infectious exposure; >95% of patients are seropositive within 6 months. Note that seropositivity for HIV-1 does not imply immunity.
  - The specificity of HIV-1 EIA assays is very high, but when they are used to screen low-prevalence populations, the PPV may be <80%. Therefore, positive EIA assays should be

confirmed with a second highly specific assay, such as a WB assay using standardized inter-pretive criteria. The HIV-1 WB detects antibody production by the patient directed against specific HIV-1 antigens. Positive results require detection of antibodies for several infor-mative antigens of different HIV-1 functional proteins (gag, pol, and env). Reactivity for different types of antigen evolve with progression of disease. Reactivity against Gag pro-teins (p17, p24, p55) usually appear first, but may decrease in titer with disease progres-sion. Antibodies against envelope proteins (gp160, gp 120/gp41) are usually persistent. No universal standard has been established, but the American Red Cross, CDC, and WHO have all published guidelines. Using a combination of diagnostic tests, false-positive test results can be almost completely eliminated.

- Patients with repeatedly reactive HIV EIA tests, but negative or equivocal WB should have repeat WB testing after 4–6 weeks. Testing for HIV-1 RNA, proviral DNA, or p24 antigen may be informative. If unresolved, infection with HIV-2 or uncommon HIV-1 subtypes (O or N) might be considered.
- Testing to monitor disease and therapy
  - Patients diagnosed with HIV-1 infection should be initially tested and subsequently moni-tored with HIV-1 viral load and CD4+ T lymphocyte cell count or fraction of total lym-phocytes. Viral load testing is recommended just before and then at 8–12 weeks following initiation of antiretroviral treatment. A two-log10 decrease in viral load is expected within 8 weeks. The viral load should fall below the detection level of the viral load assay within 6 months. The rate of fall of viral load and increase of the CD4 cell count is slower in patients after changes in treatment due to therapeutic failure. Successful therapy is also associated with an increase in the number, or fraction, of CD4+ T lymphocytes.
  - Successful antiretroviral therapy should result in a new viral load baseline, ideally at an undetectable level. Changes in viral load from the baseline should be interpreted with cau-tion. Small changes, up to 0.3 to 0.4 $\log_{10}$ copies per mL, may be seen as a result of vari-ability of immunologic control of viral replication or to false-positive viral load results. These results should be rechecked and interpreted with CD4 cell levels and clinical find-ings before assigning significance. Viral load changes >0.5 to 0.7 $\log_{10}$ copies/mL are more typical in patients with treatment failure and worsening disease.
- Antiviral drug-resistance testing
  - Numerous studies have demonstrated improved patient outcome when therapy is guided by results of antiviral resistance testing, especially for initial treatment in areas with a high circulation of resistant viruses and for patients who fail a therapeutic regimen. HIV-1 reverse transcriptase, protease inhibitors, and substrate analogs are the most common types of antiviral agents used for treatment of HIV-1 infection and are most commonly reported in antiviral drug resistance testing. Development of drugs targeting other essen-tial steps in HIV-1 infection, like fusion and integrase functions, as well as relevant resis-tance testing, is ongoing.
  - Resistance to antiviral agents can be determined by phenotypic or genotypic methods. Both methods require the amplification of informative sequences from HIV-1 RNA iso-lated from the patient plasma.
    - In genotypic assays, mutations in genes whose products are the targets of specific antivi-ral agents are detected. Most commonly, these mutations are detected by sequencing amplicons. Resistance interpretations for specific drugs or drug classes are maintained in frequently updated databases.

- For phenotypic assays, the target sequences of a "reagent" HIV-1 virus are replaced by the genes amplified from HIV-1 RNA from the patient's plasma. The recombinant virus is used to infect cell cultures in the presence of different antiviral agents, with results interpreted on the basis of the drug's ability, or not, to prevent infection of the cell line. An advantage of phenotypic assays is that they do not depend on knowledge of specific mutations for interpretation of drug efficacy and they are efficient in detecting how multiple mutations in the patient's HIV-1 RNA interact in terms of inhibiting or enhancing the activity of an antiviral agent.
- Both methods are limited in their ability to yield results when the patient's viral load is low (<1000 copies/mL), primarily due to technical limitations of the laboratory processing. Resistant "quasispecies" may emerge due to selective pressure during antiviral therapy. Neither genotypic nor phenotypic assays are efficient in detecting relevant resistance in these quasispecies until they contribute more than ~30% of the HIV-1 RNA in the patient's plasma.

➤ Diagnostic Challenges

- Diagnostic testing may be needed for the management of patients at risk for HIV-1 infection who present with signs and symptoms consistent with acute retroviral syndrome. Serologic testing is recommended, but because symptoms of acute infection usually improve with seroconversion, virologic testing may be required. The use of HIV-1 RNA viral load assays are not approved for diagnosis of acute infection and results must be used with caution. Occasional false-positive tests occur, virtually all with levels <10,000 copies/mL. Positive results must eventually be confirmed serologically before an unequivocal diagnosis is established.
- Placental transfer of HIV-1 IgG from an infected mother to her fetus complicates the diagnosis of HIV infection in the infant after delivery. In infants at risk for HIV-1 infection, viral culture or molecular diagnostic tests are recommended for diagnosis. Sequential testing at 48 hours after birth, at age 1–2 months, and at 3–6 months has been recommended. Testing for plasma HIV-1 RNA is reported to provide the greatest sensitivity for HIV-1 infection in the neonate. Positive results must be confirmed. Detection of p24 antigen may be an alternative to HIV culture or molecular diagnostic testing, especially in areas where this testing is not immediately available, although this test is less sensitive and less specific compared to the other virologic assays. An ultrasensitive method for p24 antigen detection using dried blood spots has been described (see Knuchel entry under Suggested Readings). Infants with negative virologic studies should be assessed serologically. Two negative HIV-1 serology tests, performed at least 1 month apart after 6 months of age, essentially excludes a diagnosis of HIV-1 infection in the infant.
- Specific testing may be needed for diagnosis of HIV-2 and non-M HIV-1 infections.

➤ Other Considerations

- Greater severity and persistence of symptoms of primary infection and severe depression of CD4+ cells beyond 2–3 months is associated more rapid progression to severe immunosuppression and AIDS.
- The HIV-1 viral load at baseline is the best predictor of severity and progression early in disease; the CD4+ T lymphocyte count is the best predictor of progression in late disease.
- The risk of progression to AIDS is related to the baseline HIV-1 viral load after seroconversion. Plasma viral load >100,000 copies/mL at 6 months after seroconversion are associated

with a 10-fold greater risk of progression to AIDS within 5 years, compared to patients with lower baseline levels.

- Although the results of HIV-1 viral load assays are correlated, there may be proportional differences in the results from laboratories performing testing using different platforms. It is recommended that viral load testing to monitor patients be performed in the same laboratory using the same platform. If the testing platform is changed, unexpected changes in viral load must be interpreted with caution. It may be important to "re-baseline" the patient with sequential testing on the new platform.
- Patients with HIV infection are at high risk for coexisting infections. Patients should be carefully evaluated to rule-out the following infections: hepatitis B, hepatitis C, CMV, *Toxoplasma gondii*, syphilis, and TB.

MISCELLANEOUS VIRUSES

MUMPS

➤ Definition
- Mumps is usually a mild, self-limited viral infection caused by mumps virus. The virus is highly contagious and transmitted by respiratory droplets.
- Humans are the only natural reservoir and children, especially in the prevaccination era, were the primary targets of infection. The incidence of mumps dropped >99% since the introduction of live vaccine in 1967.

➤ Who Should be Suspected?
- After exposure, there is a 1–2 week incubation period followed by onset of prodromal symptoms. Prodromal symptoms are nonspecific, including fever, malaise, myalgias, anorexia, and headache. Ninety-five percent of patients develop the characteristic swelling and tenderness of the parotid glands. Parotid swelling may last for 7–10 days. Subtle disease may develop in a minority of patients, usually adults, consisting of predominantly respiratory symptoms. Viral shedding and secondary transmission begins during the prodromal period and peaks in the days before the onset of parotitis.
- Mumps is associated with several common complications.
  - Up to 10% of patients develop symptomatic aseptic meningitis with typical symptoms of headache, mild nuchal rigidity, and low-grade fever.
    - CSF profile typically shows pleocytosis with lymphocyte predominance, normal or slightly elevated protein, and normal or slightly decreased glucose. Full recovery without sequelae is the rule. Less than 0.1% of patients develop mumps encephalitis, with fever and altered levels of consciousness, seizure, paralysis ataxia, or other CNS abnormalities. Parotitis may be absent in 20–60% of patients. The peripheral WBC count is usually normal. A mild CSF mononuclear pleocytosis is typical (average 250 cells per microliter); protein is usually normal or slightly elevated (≤100 mg/dL); glucose concentration is usually normal but is decreased in ≤29% of cases.
      - Simultaneous serum and CSF specimens show increased mumps IgG antibody index (in 83% of patients) and mumps IgM antibody index (in ~67% of patients with IgM in CSF). Oligoclonal Ig in CSF is detected in 90% of cases. Virus can be isolated from CSF

by culture. PCR has been reported to provide more rapid and sensitive diagnosis compared to culture. Recovery is usually complete.
- Sensorineural deafness, with occasional vestibular symptoms, is a well-documented complication of mumps.
- Orchitis, manifested by high fever and severe testicular pain with testicular and scrotal swelling, occurs in 30–40% of postpubertal males with mumps infection. Symptoms typically occur ~10 days after onset of parotitis. There may be unilateral or bilateral involvement. WBC count and ESR are typically elevated. Full sterility is rare following mumps orchitis, but impaired fertility may be seen in a minority of patients. Oophoritis occurs in 5–10% of postpubertal females.
- Other uncommon complications of mumps include arthritis, pancreatitis, and myocarditis. Mumps infection in pregnant women is not associated with congenital anomalies.

➤ Laboratory Findings
- Viral culture: Mumps virus may be isolated from saliva, urine, or CSF early in acute disease. Viral culture is usually used for complicated infection or when a virus isolate is needed, as for epidemiologic investigation.
- Serology: most cost-effective and commonly used diagnostic method. Mumps is confirmed by a positive mumps-specific IgM result or a significant change in mumps-specific IgG titer in acute and convalescent (2–4 weeks after acute onset) serum samples. IgM usually peaks at ~day 7 of acute disease and persists for 6 weeks or longer. IgM response may be blunted in previously immunized patients and a negative result does not exclude mumps infection in this population. Detectable IgG levels usually peak at 2–4 weeks and persist for years.
- Molecular diagnosis: Real-time PCR for specific mumps sequences has been shown to improve detection of mumps encephalitis, but FDA-approved kits are not available.
- Core laboratory: WBC and ESR are normal in acute infection. There may be a slight relative lymphocytosis. Serum and urine amylase are increased during first week of parotitis; therefore, increase does not always indicate pancreatitis. Serum lipase is normal.

NOROVIRUS GASTROENTERITIS (NORWALK AGENT)

➤ Definition
- *Novovirus* has been identified as a major cause of epidemic and endemic gastroenteritis. The Norwalk agent was discovered by immune EM of stool in patients with diarrhea. These viruses have subsequently been classified by molecular techniques as a member of the family Caliciviridae. The virus is nonenveloped with a single positive-strand RNA genome. Genetic and immunologic diversity in clinical isolates is significant.
- Humans are thought to be the only host for *Norovirus*. Infections occur globally and affect individuals of all ages. The primary route of transmission is fecal-oral. New testing methods have demonstrated that noroviruses caused a significant majority of past epidemics of gastroenteritis for which a specific agent could not be determined.

➤ Who Should be Suspected?
- Disease outbreaks have been associated with a wide variety of exposures, including day care centers, long-term care facilities, cruise ships, and restaurants. Persons living in high-density conditions are at high risk.

- Clinical disease usually presents with abrupt onset of vomiting and/or diarrhea 10 hours to 2 days after exposure. Abdominal cramping is common. Patients often have nonspecific symptoms, including low-grade fever, headache, myalgias, and fatigue. Disease is self-limited in most patients, spontaneously resolving after several days. Prolonged symptomatic and more severe disease may be seen in young children, the elderly, and immunocompromised patients.

➤ Laboratory Findings

Because most patients have relatively mild, self-limited disease, they do not require specific diagnostic testing. Diagnostic testing may be necessary for patients with severe diseases or to establish the cause of an outbreak.

- Molecular testing: Real-time PCR has emerged as the most widely used assays for diagnosis of *Norovirus* infection. Virus specific RNA may be detected for several weeks after onset of illness. No FDA-approved molecular diagnostic test is available.
- Antigen detection assays. Use of antiserum reagents elicited against recombinant viral antigens has been described, but the sensitivity of available assays is relatively poor.

PAPILLOMAVIRUS INFECTION

➤ Definition

- Papillomaviruses are nonenveloped DNA viruses that cause a spectrum of diseases of epithelial tissues, ranging in severity from benign plantar warts to genital tract cancers. The papillomaviruses are widespread in vertebrate hosts, but individual viruses are narrowly species specific.
- HPVs have a supercoiled, nonsegmented circular double-stranded DNA genome. They are classified by genotype, with different genotypes associated with different clinical diseases (Table 13-1).

➤ Who Should be Suspected?

- Three types of warts are most common: common warts, plantar warts, and flat warts.
  - Common warts often occur in groups and are round, hyperkeratotic papules that usually occur on the dorsum of the hand or on the fingers. Common warts are painless.

TABLE 13-1. Disease Associations of Specific Human Papillomavirus (HPV) Genotypes

Lesion	Common HPV Type
Common warts	1, 2, 4
Plantar warts	1, 2
Flat warts	3, 10
Butcher warts	2, 7
Epidermodysplasia	5, 8, 9, 12, 14,15, 17
Respiratory, recurrent papillomas	6, 11
Genital warts, low risk	6, 11, 26, 42, 43, 44, 53, 54, 55, 62, 66
Genital warts, moderate risk	33, 35, 39, 51, 52, 56, 58, 59, 68
Genital warts, high risk	16, 18, 31, 45

- Plantar warts are usually solitary and occur on the weight bearing locations of the foot. Plantar warts are circular and commonly show a keratotic ring surrounding a roughened, dark-speckled center. They are deep-set and usually painful.
- Flat warts usually occur as multiple, painless smooth papules on the face or hands. Immunocompromised patients are increased risk for the occurrence and severity of cutaneous warts. In immunocompetent patients, cutaneous warts typically resolve spontaneously.
- Papillomavirus infections of squamous epithelial tissues of the anogenital tract are responsible for genital warts and carcinomas. These infections are primarily sexually transmitted, and the risk of infection is most strongly related to the patient's lifetime number of sexual partners and history of other STDs. Most infections are acquired in the teens and early 20s.
  - Condylomata acuminata are multiple hyperkeratotic papules that commonly develop irregular surfaces. Groups of venereal warts may coalesce to form cobblestone patches. Warts may occur at any genital site, including the distal urethra. In males, lesions usually appear on the shaft of the penis. In women, most warts occur at the posterior introitus. Warts may also occur in anal and perianal surfaces. Genital warts are usually asymptomatic, but patients may complain of itch or burning pain.
  - Anogenital papillomavirus infections are associated with malignant transformation. Globally, HPV-16 and HPV-18 are the genotypes most strongly associated with invasive cervical carcinoma, but there is variability in the genotypes less frequently associated cervical cancer in different geographic regions.

➤ Laboratory Findings

Most cutaneous warts are diagnosed clinically, and specific laboratory confirmation is not required. The diagnosis of papillomavirus infections at anogenital and other sites can often be made clinically, but specific diagnostic testing may be warranted.

- Culture: Isolation of HPV by viral culture is not available.
- Serology: Not clinically useful for diagnosis of HPV infection.
- Cytologic or histologic examination: These techniques can be considered "gold standard" for confirmation of HPV disease; however, they do not provide HPV type determination.
- NAA assays: Most sensitive detection of HPV infection and may provide information about the genotype (or risk category) of the infecting virus if type-specific primers are used. Several FDA-approved assays are available for detection of HPV.

PARVOVIRUS B19 (ERYTHEMA INFECTIOSUM, FIFTH DISEASE, TRANSIENT APLASTIC ANEMIA)

➤ Definition

- Parvovirus B19 is a single strand, nonenveloped DNA virus. It is the cause of the erythematous childhood rash erythema infectiosum (fifth disease). Parvovirus B19 infections occur worldwide, causing endemic and epidemic disease.
- Humans are the only natural host for the virus, with the bone marrow being the primary target of infection. Serologic surveys demonstrate that infection is common. Infection is usually transmitted by respiratory droplets.

➤ Who Should be Suspected?

* Parvovirus B19 infections occur most commonly occur in children.
* The classic presentation involves a confluent, erythematous rash, especially on the cheeks with circumoral pallor (slapped face appearance) with viral syndrome symptoms, like fever, malaise, myalgias, headache, cough, and pharyngitis. Arthralgias develop in some patients. The facial rash fades in several days, followed by formation of a lacy rash affecting the extremities and trunk. Complications of parvovirus B19 infection are uncommon and include hepatitis, myocarditis, and meningoencephalitis.
* Adults diagnosed with parvovirus B19 infection present more frequently with viral syndrome and arthropathy, and rash is less common. Complications of parvovirus infection during pregnancy include fetal hydrops and congenital anemia; specific IgM is detected in cord blood. Chronic infection may cause severe anemia in immunocompromised persons. Pure erythrocyte aplasia and persistent infection may develop in patients with immunodeficiency or underlying hemolytic anemias, like sickle cell disease, hereditary spherocytosis, pyruvate kinase deficiency, and beta-thalassemia.

➤ Laboratory Findings

* Serology: usual diagnostic method. Specific IgM is formed very early in infection, closely followed by IgG. IgM levels begin to wane after 1–2 months, but may be detectable for 6 months after acute infection. IgG antibody typically remains detectable for years.

RUBELLA (GERMAN MEASLES)

➤ Definition

* Rubella virus causes German measles, one of the classic viral exanthems of childhood (third disease). The virus primarily infects the respiratory epithelial cells. Infection is transmitted by respiratory droplets.
* The virus has a global distribution, although endemic virus circulation has been greatly reduced or eliminated in countries with widespread vaccination programs. Humans are the only natural host.

➤ Who Should be Suspected?

* Rubella infection is usually mild and self-limited. Viremia typically occurs after 5–7 days and clinical infection may ensue around 14 days after exposure with a nonspecific "viral" syndrome, including fever, malaise, mild respiratory symptoms, and lymphadenopathy. The characteristic, nonconfluent rash starts on the face then progresses to the trunk and extremities. The rash resolves in 3–5 days. Up to 50% of infected children may remain asymptomatic.
* The congenital rubella syndrome is caused by transplacental infection of a fetus during the viremic phase of illness. Maternal infection early in gestation is associated with more severe disease (~80% incidence with maternal rubella in the first trimester). Virtually all fetal organ systems are susceptible to infection, and infection may lead to still birth or premature delivery. The most common anomalies include cardiac defects, cataracts and other ocular defects, deafness, bone defects, hepatitis, microcephaly and mental retardation, splenomegaly, and thrombocytopenia. Subacute arthritis is a common (70%) complication of rubella infection in adult women. Fingers, wrists, and knees are the most commonly affected joints, and symptoms may last up to 1 month.

- Rubella is preventable by vaccination, with a primary goal of reducing the incidence of the congenital syndrome. Vaccine-induced protection may wane over time; improved vaccines have improved the durability of the immune response. Since 1993, 70% of patients with rubella fall into the 15–39-year age group, reflecting this declining immunity. Therefore, significant public health resources have been dedicated to ensuring that adolescents, especially girls, have been immunized.

➤ Laboratory Findings

- Culture: Detection of rubella virus in cell culture is slow and technically challenging. There is little CPE in cell lines. Rubella infection can be inferred by interference assays, such as inhibition of enterovirus superinfection of cell lines infected by rubella virus from a specimen. Rubella-specific neutralization or immunostaining techniques are used for confirmation.
- Serology: Serologic diagnosis is most commonly used to document rubella infection.
  - Infection is confirmed by demonstration of a positive reaction for rubella IgM (acute primary infection) or by change in rubella IgG titers in acute (7–10 days) and convalescent (14–21 days) serum specimens. IgM antibodies are detected and peak within several days after appearance of rash, and then rapidly fall below detectable levels after ~8 weeks. IgG usually appears around 2 weeks after onset of rash and usually remain detectable, at lower levels, for life.
  - In congenital infection IgM can be detected at birth and persists for ≤6 months in >90% of infants. During first 6 months of life, IgM is the best test for congenital or recent infection. After age 7 months, assess persistence of IgG. IgG appears 15–25 days after infection and >25 to 50 days after vaccination; <33% of persons may show no detectable IgG after 10 years. Absence of IgG in infant excludes congenital infection.

RUBEOLA (MEASLES)

➤ Definition

- Measles is caused by the measles virus in the family Paramyxoviridae, genus *Morbillivirus*. It is a single-stranded RNA virus.
- The virus is transmitted by respiratory droplets and infects epithelial cells of the respiratory tract of exposed individuals. Measles is highly contagious and outbreaks are well documented. The disease is preventable by vaccination. Imported infections are transmitted to nonimmune individuals in regions with a low endemic rate.
- Measles is a reportable disease.

➤ Who Should be Suspected?

- Clinical disease develops after an incubation period of 10–14 days. In typical measles, the characteristic morbilliform rash appears after 4–5 days of prodromal symptoms, which include cough, coryza, and conjunctivitis, with fever and malaise. Local lymphadenopathy may develop. Koplik's spots, the characteristic enanthem, appear on the buccal mucosa one day or two before the appearance of the rash. The blanching rash first appears behind the ears and forehead and spreads over the trunk and limbs over the ensuing several days. Otitis media, diarrhea, and pneumonitis occur relatively frequently in uncomplicated measles.
- Pregnant women are at risk for more severe measles-associated pneumonia. Although not associated with congenital anomalies, measles may be transmitted to the fetus, and neonates

may develop mild to severe clinical infection. Patients with defects of cell-mediated immunity are susceptible to severe measles virus pneumonia and progressive encephalitis demonstrating typical inclusion bodies in neurons and glial cells.

* Neurologic complications are uncommon in patients with normal immunity, but acute postinfectious measles encephalomyelitis and subacute sclerosing panencephalitis (SSPE) are rare complications of measles infections.

  * Acute postinfectious encephalomyelitis, an autoimmune reaction, usually occurs in the week following onset of rash. Patients present with headache, irritability, and change in mental status progressing to seizures, obtundation, and coma. CSF lymphocytic pleocytosis and protein elevation are seen. Mortality is as high as 20%, and many survivors have neurologic sequelae.

  * SSPE is a progressive neurologic complication with a high mortality rate. It usually occurs 5–10 years after primary measles. SSPE is more common when primary infection occurred before 2 years of age. The onset is subtle with personality changes, declining intellectual function and loss of coordination, which usually progress relentlessly. Death usually occurs within several years of onset. There are characteristic EEG changes (Rodermacker complexes). CSF analysis shows oligoclonal bands and intrathecal production of antimeasles antibodies.

➤ Laboratory Findings

* Viral culture: Measles virus can be isolated in cell culture from respiratory, nasopharyngeal, conjunctival, blood, or urine specimens.
* Pathology/cytology: Epithelial cells from the respiratory tract, conjunctiva, or urine (early disease), or infected tissues (acute or chronic disease), may be stained to demonstrate multinucleated giant cells with intranuclear and cytoplasmic inclusion bodies.
* Serology: Most infections are diagnosed serologically in the setting of typical clinical findings.

  * Detection of measles virus specific IgM, or a fourfold or greater rise in measles virus–specific IgG in paired acute and convalescent serum specimens are diagnostic.
  * IgG antibody levels develop in the week after onset of rash and usually peak in the first month after appearance of the rash. IgM antibodies can usually be detected in the first week of infection and become undetectable after 2 months.

* NAA: Especially useful in diagnosis of CNS infection in immunocompromised patients.

SMALLPOX (VARIOLA VIRUS)

➤ Definition

* Smallpox is caused by the variola virus. Historically, smallpox is a highly infectious viral infection associated with significant morbidity and mortality. Humans are the primary natural host for variola virus.
* An aggressive global vaccination effort eliminated smallpox by 1980.
* Because the complication rate of smallpox vaccination, using the vaccinia virus, is relatively high, widespread vaccination is no longer practiced, resulting in a presumed return of widespread susceptibility to this disease. Ominously, laboratory-proliferated variola virus has been weaponized, and this virus is one of the most feared potential bioterror agents.

- Any patient suspected of having smallpox must be immediately isolated and reported to the relevant state department of health. Case evaluation, management, and diagnostic testing will be directed by state and federal agencies.

➤ Who Should be Suspected?

- Usually, smallpox is usually acquired by inhalation of infectious droplets and is the likely route of bioweapon transmission. Spiking fever, headache, and malaise precede the appearance of rash. The typical rash appears about 10 days after exposure and resolves in 4–5 weeks in survivors. The rash progresses from macules to papules to umbilicated pustules. At 2–3 weeks, the host immune response results in scabbing over of pustules and healing of lesions. Scarring, especially on the face, is common in survivors.
- Smallpox is differentiated from chickenpox by the increased toxicity of patients and the pattern of rash. In smallpox, skin lesions appear simultaneously and are more prominent on the face and distal extremities, whereas in chickenpox, skin lesions appear in waves, resulting in lesions of different stages at any given time, and lesions first appear on the trunk and spread centrifugally to the face and extremities. A rare hemorrhagic form of smallpox was described, most commonly in pregnant women, with a petechial rash, hemorrhage, severe toxicity, and high mortality. Previously vaccinated patients with waning immunity have developed mild disease with few skin lesions that resolved rapidly.

➤ Suggested Readings: Viral Pathogens

Arvin AM. Varicella-Zoster virus. *Clin Microbiol Rev.* 1996;9:361–381.

Bonnez W. Chapter 28 Papillomavirus. In Richman DD, Whitley RJ, Hayden FG. Papillomavirus in Clinical Virology. 3rd ed. Washington, DC: ASM Press; 2009.

Cohen, JI. Epstein-Barr virus Infection. *N Engl J Med.* 2000;343:481–492.

Corey L, Wald A. Maternal and neonatal herpes simplex virus infections. *N Engl J Med.* 2009;361:1376–1385.

Crough T, Khanna R. Immunobiology of human cytomegalovirus: from bench to bedside. *Clin Microbiol Rev.* 2009;22:76–98.

Glass RI, Parashar UD, Estes MK. Norovirus gastroenteritis. *N Engl J Med.* 2009;361:1776–1785.

Gnann JW, Whitley RJ. Herpes zoster. *N Engl J Med.* 2002;347:340–346.

Guatelli JC, Siliciano RF, Kuritzkes DR, Richman DD. Human Immunodeficiency Virus. In Richman DD, Whitley RJ, Hayden FG. *Clinical Virolog,* 3rd ed. Washington, DC: ASM Press; 2009.

Howley PM, Lowy DR. Chapter 62 Papillomaviruses. In: Knipe DM, Howley PM, eds. *Fields Virology.* 5th d. Philadelphia, PA: Lippincott Williams & Wilkins; 2007.

Kimberlin DW, Rouse DJ. Genital herpes. *N Engl J Med.* 2004;350:1970–1977.

Kimberlin DW. Chapter 55, Rubella virus. In: Richman DD, Whitley RJ, Hayden FG. *Clinical Virology.* 3rd ed. Washington DC: ASM Press; 2009.

Knuchel MC, Jullu B, Shah C, et al. Adaptation of the ultrasensitive HIV-1 p24 antigen assay to dried blood spot testing. *J Acquir Immune Defic Syndr.* 2007;44:247–253.

Lambert JS, Harris DR, Stiehm ER, et al. Performance characteristics of HIV-1 culture and HIV-1 DNA and RNA amplification assays for early diagnosis of perinatal HIV-1 infection. *J Acquir Immune Defic Syndr.* 2003;34: 512–519.

Lane JM, Ruben FL, Neff JM, Millar JD. Complications of smallpox vaccination 1968; national survey in the United States. *N Engl J Med.* 1969;281:1201–1208.

Markowitz LE, Preblud SR, Orenstein WA, et al. Patterns of transmission in measles outbreaks in the United States, 1985–1986. *N Engl J Med.* 1989;320:75–81.

Poggio GP, Rodriguez C, Cisterna C, et al. Nested PCR for rapid detection of mumps virus in cerebrospinal fluid from patients with neurological diseases. *J Clin Microbiol.* 2000;38:274–278.

Young NS, Brown KE. Parvovirus B19. *N Engl J Med.* 2004;350:586–597.

INFECTIOUS DISEASES CAUSED BY PARASITIC PATHOGENS

Parasites are eukaryotic pathogens that are responsible for an enormous disease burden worldwide. Infection and disease are especially common in developing nations, in which large segments of the population may be infected, and infection with multiple pathogens may be frequent. Improved sanitation and control of vector populations has reduced, but not eliminated, the burden of parasitic diseases in industrialized nations.

Oral transmission is a common route for spread of infection; enteric parasites are responsible for the greatest burden of parasitic infection. Arthropod-transmitted parasites, such as *Plasmodium* spp., are also responsible for an enormous disease burden. Some parasites may be transmitted by direct invasion, as through skin, or other means of infection. Immunocompromised patients, like patients with AIDS, are at increased risk for severe disease.

Most parasitic disease is diagnosed by direct detection of organisms in infected specimens. Detection of specific bacterial antigens provides sensitive and specific diagnosis for several common parasitic pathogens, like *Giardia* and *Cryptosporidium*. Serologic assays may contribute to diagnosis, and may be useful for epidemiologic studies. Isolation of parasites in culture is restricted to a few pathogens and is not widely available for routine diagnosis. Molecular diagnostic strategies are playing an increasingly important role in diagnosis and definitive speciation.

INTESTINAL PROTOZOA

AMEBIASIS

➤ Definition
* Invasive amebiasis is caused by the protozoan parasite *Entamoeba histolytica*. *E. histolytica* is primarily seen in Central and South America, Africa, and the Indian subcontinent.
* The parasite is transmitted by ingestion of fecally contaminated water or food. The trophozoites are able to invade into the intestinal mucosa, leading to the formation of flask-shaped ulcers. Trophozoites may gain access to the central circulation, providing access to distant organs, most commonly liver, but also brain, lung and others. During multiplication, some amebae revert to the cyst form, which is excreted in stool.

➤ Who Should be Suspected?
* Amebiasis is a symptomatic, self-limited disease occurs in ~90% of infected patients, and asymptomatic disease occurs in about 10% of patients. Most symptomatic patients present with GI disease manifested by low fever, abdominal pain, and diarrhea, which may be bloody. Organisms are able to penetrate into, and through, the intestinal mucosa, causing dysentery or extraintestinal disease. The liver abscess is the most common site of extraintestinal infection.
* Susceptibility to symptomatic infection depends in part on immunity; travelers from nonendemic areas are at greatest risk when visiting endemic regions. Asymptomatic infection with *E. histolytica* is common. In asymptomatic patients, it may be important to differentiate *E. histolytica* from *Entamoeba dispar*. The latter does not require eradication, but *E. histolytica* "carriage" poses a significant risk of progression to invasive disease, even after months of asymptomatic infection.

➤ Laboratory Findings
- Culture: gold standard for diagnosis of amebiasis but is not widely available.
- Direct detection: Detection of trophozoites or cysts in stool is the most common diagnostic procedure. The sensitivity of a single stool specimen is <50%. At least three samples, collected on consecutive days, should be examined before ruling out amebiasis. The detection of phagocytized RBCs is specific for *E. histolytica* and provides differentiation from *E. dispar*. Motile trophozoites may be detected in saline wet mounts if stool can be examined immediately. The finding of many RBCs, but minimal WBCs, on microscopic examination of stool helps to differentiate amebiasis from bacillary dysentery.
- Serology and antigen testing: The indirect hemagglutination assay for *E. histolytica* antibody is 99% sensitive for liver abscess and 88% sensitive for intestinal disease. Tests remain positive for years and cannot distinguish acute from past infection. Detection of stool antigen is sensitive (95%) and specific (93%) for *E. histolytica*.
- Histology: Endoscopic biopsy or smear of exudate of sigmoid ulcers may show *E. histolytica* in 50% of cases. Collect from six or more lesions for permanent staining. Tissue diagnosis for amebic liver abscess is rarely performed; imaging studies, serologic and antigen studies can usually confirm this diagnosis. When sampled, amoebae are usually located in the abscess wall, not the necrotic contents of the abscess. Parasites are identified in abscess material in <20% of cases.
- Core laboratory: Liver abscess should be suspected in patients with risk factors who present with fever (90%), leukocytosis, increased ALP, and right upper quadrant pain and tenderness (85%). The right hemidiaphragm may be elevated. Many patients (60%) with liver abscess have no history of intestinal disease; stool for O&P is positive in <20–40% of patients with hepatic abscess. Eosinophilia is uncommon.

GIARDIASIS

➤ Definition
- Giardiasis is caused by infection with the flagellate protozoan *Giardia lamblia*. This pathogen has a worldwide distribution but is more prevalent in warmer climates.
- Infection is most commonly acquired by ingestion of cysts, with an incubation period of 2–3 weeks. After excystation and maturation, the trophozoite stage typically attach to the crypts of the duodenal mucosa by means of ventral disks. They do not penetrate the intestinal mucosa and typically cause minimal pathologic changes; villous atrophy may be seen in severe, chronic disease. Organisms are released and may encyst or pass in the feces as trophozoites.

➤ Who Should be Suspected?
- Children are most commonly infected. Although immunocompromised patients are at risk for severe disease, most infections occur in immunocompetent individuals.
- Acute infection may manifest with nausea; anorexia; and explosive, watery diarrhea. Systemic signs and symptoms are common with fever, malaise, and chills. The acute phase may be accompanied by a subacute or chronic phase, manifested by recurrent diarrhea. Chronic giardiasis may be complicated by weight loss, malabsorption, and electrolyte imbalance.

➤ Laboratory Findings
- Direct detection: Stool O&P testing should be performed on up to six specimens. Organisms may be excreted intermittently in chronic infection. Stool should be concentrated by

centrifugation; permanent stains should be prepared. Examination of duodenal mucus, collected by duodenal aspirate or an enteric string capsule, may be used as an adjunct to stool O&P testing.

- Serology: not useful for diagnosis because positive results cannot distinguish between acute and past infections.
- Antigen detection: Stool antigen detection or fluorescent staining provides rapid, sensitive, and specific detection of *Giardia*; sensitivity is greater than that of routine O&P examination. Antigen testing should not replace O&P testing. Multiple specimens should be examined by antigen testing to rule out giardiasis.

COCCIDIA INFECTIONS

➤ Definition
Coccidia infections are caused by coccidian protozoon parasites, including *Cryptosporidium parvum*, *Isospora belli*, and *Cyclospora cayetanensis*. These parasites are capable of causing severe diarrheal illness in patients with AIDS. These organisms infect microvillus epithelial cells of the GI tract.

- Cryptosporidiosis is very infectious and diarrheal disease occurs in most infected patients. Outbreaks linked to day care centers and recreational water activities are well described. Springtime is the season of peak incidence.
- Humans serve as the only known reservoir for infection with *Isospora belli*. There is global distribution, but the highest prevalence is in tropical and subtropical areas. The oocytes of *Isospora* mature to infectious forms in the environment several days after excretion, so person-to-person transmission is less efficient.
- *Cyclospora* infection is probably acquired by ingestion of contaminated water. Because the oocysts of *Cyclospora* mature to infectious forms in the environment several days after excretion, direct person-to-person transmission is uncommon. *Cyclospora* may cause endemic disease during the rainy season in developing countries. Epidemic disease is well described in developed countries; consumption of fecally contaminated foods is usually implicated.

➤ Who Should be Suspected?
- Coccidial infections manifest with watery diarrhea, crampy abdominal pain, and anorexia. Nonspecific systemic symptoms are common. RBCs and WBCs are typically absent from stool. Chronic and intermittent diarrheal illness may occur in immunocompromised patients.

➤ Laboratory Findings
- Direct detection: Routine O&P examination is insensitive for detection of coccidian protozoan pathogens. All are acid-fast and are detected in stool using a modified acid-fast stain. Multiple stool samples should be examined to rule out infection. Sensitivity of staining may be increased by concentration techniques. Staining of *Cyclospora* may be variable, but *Cyclospora* may be detected by its characteristic autofluorescence.
- Histology: Biopsy of the duodenal or proximal jejunal mucosa may demonstrate *Isospora* when stool acid-fast stains are negative.

- Serology and immunology: DFA staining techniques have been described that improve the detection rate compared to acid-fast staining. Commercially available EIA methods also provide sensitive and specific diagnosis. Kits combining reagents for multiple intestinal parasites, like *Cryptosporidium*, *Giardia*, and *E. histolytica*, are available.
- Core laboratory: Eosinophilia may be seen in patients with *Isospora* infection.

MICROSPORIDIOSIS

➤ Definition
- The microsporidia are obligate intracellular organisms capable of infecting a wide variety of vertebrate and invertebrate species. *Enterocytozoon bieneusi* is the most common human pathogen.
- Infection is usually acquired by oral ingestion of the microsporidia, rarely by inhalation.

➤ Who Should be Suspected?
- *E. bieneusi* has emerged as a significant pathogen for patients with AIDS. Clinical disease is similar to that of *Cryptosporidium* and *Isospora*, with frequent, watery diarrhea with nausea and anorexia. Stools are not bloody. Complications of diarrhea may occur in severe cases, with dehydration, hypovolemia, electrolyte imbalance, and malabsorption. A significant number of patients with proven intestinal microsporidiosis may be coinfected with *Cryptosporidium*. Microsporidia have been identified in lower respiratory secretions of AIDS patients.
- Self-limited intestinal disease has been described in patients with intact immune systems. Microsporidia other than *E. bieneusi* are more likely to be responsible for extraintestinal microsporidiosis (e.g., keratoconjunctivitis, hepatitis, sclerosing cholangitis, peritonitis, respiratory tract infection, sinusitis, myositis, kidney disease).

➤ Laboratory Findings
- Direct detection: EM is the gold standard for confirming infection and speciation, if needed. Several modified trichrome stains have been described for detection of microsporidia in stool. Stool smears should be very thin to help avoid artifacts. Optical brightening agents, like calcofluor, stain microsporidia in stool but are nonspecific.
- Histology: Microsporidia may be identified by a number of histologic stains, like H&E, periodic acid–Schiff, and silver stains. Staining may be inconsistent. Detection may be improved by examination of stained touch preparations.

CESTODES (TAPEWORMS)

Tapeworms belong to the helminth subclass Cestodes. Cestodes infect all vertebrate classes, and many have invertebrate intermediate hosts. Clinical disease may be caused by the adult or larval forms of the parasites. Tapeworms attach to the mucosa of the small intestine by specialized structures called a scolex. Cestode infection is usually diagnosed by the finding of eggs, larval forms, or proglottids in the feces of infected patients. Mature tape worms of several species can reach lengths of several meters, shedding mature proglottids from the distal end of the worm. Proglottids are visible with the naked eye and are often identified by patients and presented for identification.

BEEF TAPEWORM (*TAENIA SAGINATA*)

➤ Definition
* Beef tapeworm disease is caused by ingestion of viable metacestodes (cysticerci) of *Taenia saginata*.

➤ Who Should be Suspected?
* Most beef tapeworm infections are asymptomatic, but intestinal, biliary or pancreatic obstruction may occur in heavy infection.

➤ Laboratory Findings
* Direct detection: Ova detected in the stool in 50–75% of patients cannot be distinguished from those of *Taenia solium* (see below for specific discussion). Definitive identification is usually achieved by examination of the uterine morphology of gravid proglottids. Because *T. saginata* proglottids may actively migrate though the anus to deposit eggs on the perianal skin, collection using a swab or "pinworm"/cellophane tape paddle of perineal or perianal skin may significantly improve detection.
* Core laboratory: Eosinophils may be slightly increased.

CYSTICERCOSIS (PORK TAPEWORM, *TAENIA SOLIUM*)

➤ Definition
* Pork tapeworm disease is caused by ingestion of viable metacestodes (cysticerci) or the eggs of *Taenia solium*. This ingestion results in infection by adult tapeworm infection of the small bowel.

➤ Who Should be Suspected?
* Most infections caused by adult pork tapeworms are asymptomatic, but intestinal, biliary, or pancreatic obstruction may occur in heavy infection.
* Neurocysticercosis is caused by hematologic spread of larvae to the brain. Cysticercosis is a significant cause of intracranial masses in endemic areas.

➤ Laboratory Findings
The diagnosis of cysticercosis relies on a combination of epidemiologic, imaging, histopathologic, and laboratory studies.
* Direct detection: Detection is usually achieved by identification of ova, proglottides, strobila, or scolices from feces. Tapeworm ova may be identified by O&P examination but cannot be distinguished from ova of *T. saginata*. Examination of portions of adult worms, like the uterine morphology of gravid proglottids, is required for speciation.
* Serology: The presence of detectable antibodies depends on the number and condition of cysticerci. Antibody detection using serum may be more sensitive than CSF testing for diagnosis of neurocysticercosis, especially in cases with degenerating cysts. ELISA detects antibody in serum or CSF in 75–80% with few or calcified cysts and 93% with severe CNS disease. Enzyme-linked immunoelectro-transfer blot (EITB) on serum or CSF has S/S of >94% with multiple CNS lesions and ~72% with single lesions. Change in titers is not reliable for judging cure. Solitary CNS lesions may not consistently induce antibody production.

- Core laboratory: Eosinophils may be slightly increased. Marked increase in ESR is unusual and suggests another diagnosis.
- CSF Findings: May show increased eosinophils (in 10–77% of cases) increased mononuclear cells ($\leq 300/\mu L$), slightly increased protein, normal or mildly decreased glucose; parasites are not found.

NEMATODES (ROUNDWORMS)

GI infection may be caused by several nematode species. Eggs and larvae of intestinal nematodes are passed in feces or deposited by female worms on the perianal skin. The eggs of some species are infective by direct fecal oral transfer, whereas others require maturation in soil, causing infection after penetration of skin by larvae.

ASCARIASIS (*ASCARIS LUMBRICOIDES*)

➤ Definition
- *Ascaris lumbricoides* is a large intestinal roundworm with a global distribution.
- After ingestion, embryonated eggs hatch, releasing second stage larvae in the intestinal lumen. These penetrate into the capillaries and lymphatics of the intestinal mucosa. From the circulation, they are deposited in the lungs where they develop into fourth-stage larvae. Fourth-stage larvae migrate up the trachea and are swallowed, returning to the small intestine where they develop into mature adults.

➤ Who Should be Suspected?
- Most infections are asymptomatic or may be associated with mild, nonspecific pulmonary, or abdominal symptoms. Symptoms may be caused by immune response, effects of larval migration, large worm burden, and nutritional impact. Pneumonitis may occur (e.g., Loeffler syndrome) during migration. With high worm burden, malnutrition or intestinal, biliary, or pancreatic obstruction may occur. Nausea, vomiting, diarrhea, and other conditions may develop.

➤ Laboratory Findings
- Direct detection: Identification of eggs by routine O&P examination is the usual method of identification. Larvae are occasionally seen in sputum or gastric aspirates. In pneumonitis associated with a primary infection, stool examination for eggs may be negative.
- Radiology: Pneumonitis abnormalities may be transient.
- Core laboratory: Eosinophilic reaction is common during symptomatic disease.

ENTEROBIASIS (PINWORM INFECTION, *ENTEROBIUS VERMICULARIS*)

➤ Definition
- *Enterobius vermicularis* is a small roundworm with global distribution. Enterobiasis may be more common in temperate climates.

- Female worms migrate through the anus at night to deposit embryonated eggs on peri-anal skin. The worms develop into infective stage three larvae within the egg. The worms and eggs cause intense pruritus ani. The host fingers are contaminated during scratching, facilitating fecal-oral transmission. Once ingested, the eggs hatch and then mature to adult worms in the large intestine. Female worms can produce over 10,000 eggs per day.

➤ Who Should be Suspected?
- Poor hygiene and crowding are predisposing factors.
- Most infections are asymptomatic. Perianal itching is the most common symptom.

➤ Laboratory Findings
- Direct detection: Detection of adult female worms or eggs is the usual method of diagnosis. Because release into stool is relatively uncommon, collection of specimens from perianal skin using cellophane tape or "pinworm paddles" is recommended. Collection of multiple night or first morning specimens is recommended. Three tests detect 90% of cases, and five tests detect 95% of cases.
- Core laboratory: Pinworm infection is not associated with eosinophilia.

STRONGYLOIDIASIS (*STRONGYLOIDES STERCORALIS*)

➤ Definition
- The parasitic roundworm *Strongyloides stercoralis* has a global distribution in tropical and sub-tropical regions.

➤ Who Should be Suspected?
- Strongyloidiasis should be considered in any patient who has traveled to an endemic area at any time in the past regardless of local disease prevalence. As in patients who host other successful intestinal parasites, most infected patients are asymptomatic or have minimal, non-specific symptoms. Patients may complain of epigastric pain, bloating, dyspepsia, diarrhea (sometimes with blood), or constipation. Patients with chronic infection may develop urti-carial rashes or the syndrome of larva currens, caused by migration of larvae in the dermal layer.
- The hyperinfection syndrome occurs in immunodeficient patients, including those with HIV and HTLV-1 infections. In the hyperinfection syndrome, severe, bloody diarrhea may result, with malnutrition and intestinal dysfunction. Septic complications may result from the damage to intestinal mucosa. Pulmonary complications, including pneumonia and pulmonary hemorrhage, are common in the hyperinfection syndrome. CNS involvement may result in gram-negative or mixed bacterial meningitis.
- Note that the morphology of larvae of *S. stercoralis* is similar to that of the larvae of hook-worms, and care must be taken if endemic infection for both is possible.

➤ Laboratory Findings
- Direct detection: The identification of stage one rhabditiform larvae in stool has formed a primary method for diagnosis, but sensitivity is limited in patients with asymptomatic, uncomplicated infection. A single stool O&P examination shows a sensitivity of 30–60%.

Sensitivity is improved by multiple O&P examinations. Sensitivity may also be improved by examination of duodenal fluid collected by endoscopy or other method (sensitivity: 60–80%). In the hyperinfection syndrome, adult and larval forms may be detected in a variety of affected organs.

* Serology: May be useful, but the performance of different assays, based on different antigen preparations, has not been standardized.
* Core laboratory: Eosinophilia is seen in ~70% of infected patients.

BLOOD TREMATODES: SCHISTOSOMIASIS

➤ Definition

* Schistosomiasis is caused by infection by species in the *Schistosoma* genus. The major pathogens are *Schistosoma mansoni, Schistosoma japonicum,* and *Schistosoma haematobium.* There is a very wide geographic distribution of schistosomiasis in tropical and subtropical areas.
* Humans acquire infection when cercaria penetrate through skin while wading or swimming in an infected water source. Most disease manifestations are due to the host immune reaction to the worms and their eggs.

➤ Who Should be Suspected?

* Cercarial dermatitis, a pruritic, papular rash of skin exposed to contaminated water, is a frequent manifestation of acute infection. Dermatitis is usually associated with *S. mansoni* and *S. haematobium.* Symptoms of acute infection develop 2–4 weeks after exposure and are most commonly seen with *S. japonicum* and *S. mansoni* infections. Symptoms include fever (Katayama fever), with chills and sweats, abdominal pain, diarrhea, headache, and cough. Hepatosplenomegaly and lymphadenopathy may be seen. Eosinophilia is typical. Biopsy or serologic testing is used for diagnosis of acute infection.
* *S. japonicum* infection, also known as Oriental blood fluke, is seen in Japan, China, Indonesia, and the Philippines. Clinical symptoms are similar to those of *S. mansoni* infection but may be more severe because of the higher egg production by female–male pairs. Hepatocellular and colorectal carcinoma have been associated with *S. japonicum* infection. Severe disease in the large intestine is typical. This may be associated with lower abdominal pain and cycles of diarrhea and constipation. Hepatosplenic disease, similar to *S. mansoni* but more severe, is common. CNS disease, manifested by a wide variety of symptoms, occurs in <5% of patients.
* *S. haematobium* infection is seen in the Nile River valley. After infection, larvae migrate most commonly migrate through the hemorrhoidal and pudendal veins to reside in the vesical and pelvic plexuses. Eggs are most commonly embedded in the bladder and distal ureters, resulting in fibrosis and ulceration. Calcification, significant hematuria, obstructive uropathy, renal failure, chronic bacterial UTIs, and bladder carcinoma are complications of severe urologic disease. Genital involvement is common, manifesting with heavy egg deposition in the cervix, vagina, and vulva. Friable "sandy patches" are described in the lower genital tract. Bacteremic infections with *Salmonella* species is seen. Schistosomal appendicitis is well described with *S. haematobium.* Hepatosplenomegaly, due to portal fibrosis and pulmonary, CNS, and cardiac disease is described, but uncommon.

➤ Laboratory Findings

* Direct detection: Eggs are seen, but may be absent in the first several months after acute infection. Eggs are most commonly found in stool in *S. mansoni* and *S. japonicum* infections. For *S. haematobium* diagnosis, urine specimens, ideally collected between noon and 3 p.m. when egg excretion is highest, are used. The examination of multiple samples is recommended.
  * Egg morphology is used as the basis for speciation, which is an important guide to therapy.
  * Note: *S. haematobium* ova are sometimes found in stool and *S. mansoni* eggs are sometimes found in urine, especially in heavy infection. Treated patients should have O&P examinations for at least 1 year to ensure sustained cure.
* Histology: Rectal or bladder biopsy is useful for diagnosis in light or inactive infections. Unstained rectal or bladder mucosa, examined microscopically, may show viable or dead ova when stools or urine O&P examinations are negative; granulomatous lesions may be present. Biopsy may identify eggs in affected organs.
* Serology: Serologic testing may be useful for diagnosis of infection in patients from nonendemic areas or to support a diagnosis in infection with low egg counts. A specific ELISA, confirmed by immunoblot, is recommended. Positive serology is not useful for distinguishing between acute and chronic infection.
* Antibody detection: may be more promising, but utility is hampered by low specificity and cross reactions with other helminth parasites. Sensitive and specific methods have been described for *S. mansoni*, *S. japonicum,* and *S. haematobium*. An immunoblot assay to detect schistosome antigen is reported to have high sensitivity (~95%) and specificity (~100%).
* Core laboratory: Eosinophilia occurs in 20–60% of acute cases. ESR is increased. Hematuria is an important early sign of *S. haematobium* infection. Immunoglobulin levels, especially IgE, are elevated. Liver function tests are usually normal, even in chronic infection. Signs and symptoms related to inflammatory damage of other organs, like lung (cough, hemoptysis, pulmonary hypertension), brain (seizures), and the spinal cord (myelopathy), may be present. Anemia, eosinophilia, increased serum globulin and decreased albumin, hematuria, proteinuria, hydronephrosis, azotemia, and squamous cell carcinoma of bladder may occur.

PARASITES, BLOOD AND TISSUE

These parasites primarily cause systemic or tissue specific disease and may be transmitted by direct invasion through skin or mucous membranes, oral ingestion, or via an insect vector. Most infections are definitively diagnosed on the basis direct identification of parasites in blood or tissue.

BABESIOSIS

➤ Definition

* Most cases of babesiosis that occur in the Northeastern and Great Lakes states in the United States are caused by *Babesia microti*. Other *Babesia* species cause infections in other regions of the United States as well as in Europe, and these infections may differ in terms of their clinical presentation.

- *B. microti* is transmitted by the tick *Ixodes scapularis*, which is also the vector for Lyme borreliosis and human granulocytic ehrlichiosis. Sexual reproduction occurs in the tick. After the infective forms enter the host during a blood meal, they enter erythrocytes, where asexual reproduction occurs.

➤ Who Should be Suspected?
- Most *Babesia* infections are likely to be asymptomatic or subclinical. In symptomatic infections, influenza-like symptoms with fever, accompanied by sweats and chills, malaise, fatigue, weakness, and joint pain are commonly seen with onset in the first month after tick bite or 1–2 months after transmission by transfusion. Fever and severe symptoms generally resolve within several weeks, but milder malaise and fatigue may linger for months.
- Severe disease can occur in patients with asplenia or other immunocompromising condition. These patients may develop very high parasitemia levels, leading to hemolysis and jaundice, anemia, renal failure, DIC, ARDS, hypotension and other complications.
- Infections caused by *Babesia divergens* almost always occur in splenectomized patients. Disease is rapidly progressive and severe, and it is associated with high mortality. After an incubation period of 1–4 months, high fevers, malaise, myalgias, headache, hypotension, jaundice, intravascular hemolysis, and renal failure may occur. Diarrhea, nausea and vomiting are prominent symptoms. Coma and death occur within 1 week after onset of symptoms in almost 50% of patients.

➤ Laboratory Findings
- Direct detection: Most diagnoses are made by examination of thin and thick blood smears. Multiple smears should be examined to rule out infection. Parasites may be seen inside or outside of erythrocytes.
- Serology: Limited by poor overall sensitivity and specificity. Serologic tests become positive in 2–4 weeks. IFA IgM indicates acute infection. An IgG titer ≥1:64 is considered positive for current or past infection, but titers ≥1:1024 are seen in most patients with acute illness. A fourfold or greater increase in serum titer between acute and convalescent phase indicates acute infection. An increased titer may persist for years after resolution of symptoms. Serologic tests may cross-react with Colorado tick fever, *Plasmodium* species, *Rickettsia*, and other pathogens, as well as in patients with autoimmune and connective tissue disease.
- Core laboratory: Hemolytic anemia may last days to months; most patients have thrombocytopenia. Concurrent infection with *B. burgdorferi* (Lyme disease) and *A. phagocytophilum* (HGA) should be considered. Patients should be monitored closely for complications of primary babesiosis, with coagulation, renal, liver, and pulmonary function tests.

LEISHMANIASIS

➤ Definition
- Leishmaniasis is used to describe a wide variety of diseases caused by protozoan species (more than 20) of the genus *Leishmania*. The disease is transmitted by the bite of female sandflies (genus *Lutzomyia* in the Americas and *Phlebotomus* elsewhere). It has a wide geographic distribution.
- In humans, disease is caused by the intracellular proliferation of the amastigote stage of the pathogen.

➤ Who Should be Suspected?

There are three common syndromes: cutaneous (Oriental sore), mucosal, and visceral. The epidemiology and clinical characteristics depend on the species and vectors endemic to specific regions.

- In cutaneous leishmaniasis, the vectors are *Phlebotomus* flies. A nodule develops at the bite site, eventually ulcerating. Wet lesions have a raised border with a granulating, exudate covered base. Dry lesions are typically smaller and crusted over. Resolution of cutaneous lesions occurs in weeks or months, leaving an atrophic scar. Some patients develop fever and systemic symptoms and may develop regional adenopathy. Diffuse cutaneous leishmaniasis, caused by *Leishmania aethiopica* in Africa and *Leishmania amazonensis* in South America, results from wide dissemination of amastigotes, forming plaques and nodules.
- Mucosal leishmaniasis (espundia) occurs only in the Americas. In a small subset of patients, mucosal leishmaniasis develops months or years after resolution of primary cutaneous leishmaniasis. Ulceration of the nasal mucosa develop and may be followed by involvement of the lips, soft palate, and pharynx or other adjacent tissues.
- Visceral leishmaniasis is caused by *Leishmania chagasi* in Latin America and *Leishmania donovani* and *Leishmania infantum* in Mediterranean regions, Africa, and Asia. Most infections are asymptomatic or show only mild symptoms. A minority of patients progress to fulminant disease (kala-azar), presenting with fever, malaise, weight loss, and hepatosplenomegaly. Patients have decreased granulocyte levels and increased globulins. The course may be complicated by malnutrition and failure to thrive, edema, and bleeding diatheses. Immunocompromised patients are at greatest risk for visceral leishmaniasis.

➤ Laboratory Findings

- Histology: Definitive diagnosis is made by the identification of *Leishmania* in tissues. The raised border of cutaneous lesions should be biopsied. For visceral leishmaniasis, aspirate of liver, spleen, or bone marrow, buffy coat, or biopsy of affected organ is used for diagnosis.
- Culture: Leishmania may be isolated in culture, but the special techniques required are not widely available.
- Serology: Serology or the leishmanin skin tests (cutaneous, mucosal or resolved visceral disease) are useful for diagnosis of leishmaniasis. IFA and EIA methods are most commonly used. Tests based on the rK39 antigen of *L. chagasi* are sensitive for active visceral leishmaniasis, but cross-reactions may limit their utility.
- Core laboratory: In visceral leishmaniasis, serum globulin (IgG) levels are markedly increased with decreased albumin and reversed A/G ratio. ESR is increased, caused by increased serum globulin. Anemia, leukopenia, and thrombocytopenia may be seen due to hypersplenism and decreased marrow production. Proteinuria and hematuria may be seen. Laboratory findings due to amyloidosis may be seen in chronic cases.

MALARIA

➤ Definition

- Malaria is caused by infection by protozoan pathogens of the genus *Plasmodium*. Four species account for most human infections: *Plasmodium vivax, Plasmodium falciparum, Plasmodium malariae,* and *Plasmodium ovale.*

- Malaria is endemic in tropical regions of sub-Saharan Africa, Central and South America, and Asia. *P. falciparum* and *P. malariae* show a worldwide distribution. *P. vivax* is less common in equatorial Africa, whereas *P. ovale* is uncommon outside of Africa. Regions with chloroquine-resistant *P. falciparum* are fairly well defined geographically, emphasizing the importance of determining where infection was acquired for therapeutic decisions. The Duffy blood group antigen serves as the erythrocyte binding ligand for *P. vivax*.

➤ Who Should be Suspected?

- Fever, sweats, anemia, and splenomegaly are the usual signs and symptoms of acute malaria. The classical presentation of malaria is the malarial paroxysm, which occurs cyclically with erythrocyte lysis, but these fever cycles are often not seen. Fevers recur every 48 hours in *P. vivax* and *P. ovale* infection and every 72 hours with *P. malariae* infection. *P. falciparum* infections also have a 48-hour cycle, but erythrocyte lysis is usually not synchronized. Nonimmune individuals and pregnant women are at greatest risk for severe and complicated infection.
- *P. falciparum* infection is associated with the greatest risk of severe and complicated disease. Anemia is common and may be severe with high levels of parasitemia. Hypoglycemia and acidosis are seen as a complication of severe malaria. Hyperthermia (T $>41°C$) may be seen, especially related to severe anemia, hypoglycemia, and cerebral malaria. Cerebral malaria, usually manifested by coma and/or seizures, is caused by multiple factors, including microvascular obstruction by parasites and metabolic disorders. Cerebral malaria is associated with high morbidity. Oliguric renal failure (blackwater fever) may complicate severe malaria and is associated with high mortality. Pulmonary edema, caused by capillary leak syndrome may be seen, usually in combination with other symptoms of complicated malaria. Microvascular sequestration of parasitized erythrocytes may cause intestinal dysfunction, resulting in diarrhea. The complications of falciparum malaria are not well correlated to the level of parasitemia.

➤ Laboratory Findings

- Direct detection
  - Diagnosis is usually achieved by examination of thin and thick blood smears stained with Giemsa, Wright's, or Wright-Giemsa stain. Giemsa is recommended because most morphologic descriptions are based on Giemsa staining. Thick smears of peripheral blood or bone marrow provide the most sensitive method for detection, and the thin smears are used for speciation.
  - Multiple specimens should be examined to rule out malaria. Smears should be made every 6–12 hours for three consecutive days. Requests for malaria diagnosis should be considered as representing a potential medical emergency so specimens should be transported and tested in a "stat" manner. Capillary blood is recommended if thin and thick smears can be prepared at the bedside. EDTA anticoagulated blood may be used, but stippling may be lost if the smears are not prepared quickly.
- Serology: of limited value in acute infection.
- Molecular tests: PCR methods have been developed that are very sensitive and species-specific, but FDA approved tests are not yet available.
- Core laboratory: Hemolytic anemia (average 2.5 million erythrocytes per microliter in chronic cases); usually hypochromic; may be macrocytic in severe chronic disease.
  - Reticulocyte count is increased. Thrombocytopenia is commonly seen. Leukocytes may be decreased. ESR is increased.

- There is increased serum indirect bilirubin and other evidence of hemolysis. Serum globulin is increased (especially euglobulin fraction); albumin is decreased. Biologic false positive test for syphilis is frequent. Proteinuria and hematuria may be seen. Renal complications of malaria may result in acute tubular necrosis with casts on microscopic examination, azotemia, and oliguria progressing to anuria. Liver function tests may be moderately elevated.

TOXOPLASMOSIS

➤ Definition

- Toxoplasmosis is used to describe diseases caused by the intracellular protozoan parasite *Toxoplasma gondii*. Infection is most commonly transmitted by ingestion of oocytes (sporozoites) in cat feces or by ingestion of cysts (bradyzoites) in raw or undercooked meat of infected animals (e.g., lamb, pork, goat).
- Acute infection most commonly occurs in muscle, liver, spleen, lymph nodes, and CNS. Infected monocytes die, resulting in an inflammatory reaction in the affected organ. Bradyzoite-filled cysts are formed, but organ function usually returns to normal in immunocompetent hosts. Indications for serologic screening of asymptomatic patients include pregnancy, new diagnosis of HIV-1 infection, transplant donors and recipients, and patients who will be treated with immunosuppressive drugs.

➤ Who Should be Suspected?

- Most infections are asymptomatic.
- Acute infection may be manifested by adenopathy and fever. Occasional patients develop malaise, headache, myalgias, and hepatosplenomegaly. Atypical lymphocytosis may be seen on blood differential, suggesting mononucleosis syndrome, which may last for weeks or months. Toxoplasmosis may cause up to 15% of cases of unexplained lymphadenopathy.
- Congenital infection may occur when the mother acquires acute infection during pregnancy (which is usually clinically unapparent). The risk of transmission is 15–25% for maternal infections in first trimester, 30–45% in the second, about 65% in third trimester, and near 100% at term. Severe congenital disease is more likely with fetal infection in first trimester, with high mortality; 90% have CNS sequelae. Most infected infants (85%) eventually develop sequelae, even if asymptomatic at birth, some years later. Neurologic sequelae include seizures, psychomotor retardation, hydrocephalus, microcephalus, ocular abnormalities (e.g., retinal necrosis and granulomatous inflammation of the choroid, optic atrophy), deafness, and other abnormalities. Intracerebral calcifications are common. Infants may show fever, jaundice, vomiting and diarrhea, hepatosplenomegaly, pneumonitis, and other symptoms.

➤ Laboratory Findings

- Histology: Organisms may be identified by histologic examination of infected tissues. Detection is improved by the use of specific immunohistologic staining. Direct detection is low yield for specimens other than tissue. Organisms may be seen in Giemsa-stained BAL or CSF specimens.

- Serology
  - Serology is the diagnostic method of choice for most patients. Results of serologic tests must be interpreted based on patient age, clinical status, and other factors, including performance characteristics of the test method.
- Diagnosis of acute or congenital infection is more difficult.
  - Acute infection may be documented by detection of specific IgM or a fourfold rise in antibody titer between acute and convalescent titers. IgM reactivity usually appears within 2 weeks of primary infection. IgG usually develops within 4 weeks. Peak titers usually occur between 4 and 8 weeks after primary infection. A fourfold increase in the IgG titer supports a diagnosis of acute infection. IgG levels usually reach a titer of 1:1,000 or greater. Specific IgM appears in first week of infection and peaks within 1 month. Reactivity usually disappears in 3–5 months (as early as 1 month) but may persist for up to 2 years in IgM capture assays.
  - In congenital infection, IgM is usually present, but a negative result does not rule out toxoplasmosis. IgG in the absence of infection, due to transplacental transfer, should disappear within 6–12 months. In retinochoroiditis, IgG is positive and IgM negative. In reactivation of latent disease in immunocompromised patients, IgG is positive, but IgM typically negative. In acute toxoplasmosis in immunocompromised patients, positive IgG and IgM reactions, or an increased IgG titer, usually develop. A negative reaction for IgG in serum occurs in 3% of AIDS patients with toxoplasma encephalitis.
  - ANAs and RF may cause false-positive IgM-IFA tests. IgM antibodies may be detectable for more than a year after acute infection. IgG reactivity remains detectable for life.
  - A number of tests may be needed to determine the timing of infection. If IgG is positive and IgM is negative, it is likely that infection was acquired >6 months previously. If IgG and IgM are both positive, primary infection may have been only as recent as the previous 2 years. An IgG avidity test may be helpful. Low avidity suggests acute infection within the prior 3 months.
- Molecular tests: PCR techniques have proven to be sensitive for the diagnosis of toxoplasmosis, especially for prenatal diagnosis. PCR of amniotic fluid has a sensitivity >97% and NPV >99% for intrauterine toxoplasmosis.
- Core laboratory: atypical lymphocytosis, increased or decreased WBC, anemia, and decreased platelets. Increased globulin concentration and signs of specific organ dysfunction occur in severe disease.
- CSF findings: pleocytosis and increased protein.

FILARIAL NEMATODES AND MISCELLANEOUS TISSUE PARASITES

LARVA MIGRANS (CUTANEOUS AND VISCERAL)

➤ Definition

- Cutaneous larva migrans (CLM) is a skin eruption caused by migration of animal hookworms (usually *Ancylostoma caninum* or *Ancylostoma braziliense*) through the upper dermis. Filariform larvae of animal hookworms in the soil penetrate skin, usually of the feet or lower extremities, and then begin a sinuous migration through the upper dermis, causing inflammation with intense itching. These larvae cannot mature to adult stage hookworms, so they die out within several weeks.

- Visceral larva migrans (VLM) infections are caused by animal nematode larvae that are unable to mature into adult stage worms. Disease is caused by the migration of larvae through human organs. VLM occurs worldwide. Toxocariasis and classic VLM syndromes are caused by *Toxocara canis* and less commonly by *Toxocara cati*. Both of these ascarid nematodes have complex life cycles in dogs and cats, respectively, involving vertical transmission to pups and kittens, which excrete large numbers of embryonated eggs in their feces. When ingested by humans, the eggs hatch and the resulting larva is able to penetrate through tissues and migrate through different organs.

➤ Who Should be Suspected?
- Children are at highest risk for disease.
- Symptoms depend to some extent on the organ primarily affected; most commonly (~85%), this is the liver. Severe VLM may be characterized by fever, wheezing and bronchopneumonia, hepatosplenomegaly, anemia, or other symptoms. Arthritis and vasculitis have been described. CNS invasion may occur with severe consequences, including eosinophilic meningitis, encephalitis, and other abnormalities.
- Ocular larva migrans is based on clinical findings and examination.

➤ Laboratory Findings
- Direct detection: Eggs are not detected by O&P examination.
- Histology: Larvae may rarely be found in biopsy of granulomatous lesions.
- Serology: Not useful for diagnosis of CLM. For VLM, *Toxocara* specific ELISA has a sensitivity ~75% with specificity >90%. Specificity may be improved by immunoblot testing.
- Antibody testing: May be less sensitive in ocular than in visceral disease.
- Core laboratory: Significant eosinophilia (> 30%) is seen in VLM but not CLM. Leukocytosis, increased IgE, and hypergammaglobulinemia are common.

TRICHINOSIS (TRICHINELLOSIS; *TRICHINELLA SPIRALIS*)

➤ Definition
- Trichinosis is caused by *Trichinella spiralis* and related species. A food-borne zoonotic infection with a global distribution, trichinosis most commonly occurs in Europe and North America.
- All mammals are susceptible to disease. Swine and rats form the major host reservoir for *T. spiralis*. When infected meat is ingested, the capsule is digested, allowing the larvae to emerge and invade into the epithelium of the small intestine.

➤ Who Should be Suspected?
- Clinical infection shows two phases.
  - The first phase, correlated with the entry and activity of adult worms in the small intestine, is often mild.
  - The second phase, caused by the circulation of larvae, is associated with fever, myalgias, weakness, malaise, diarrhea, and periorbital and facial edema (~50% of cases) and other symptoms.

- Headache is very common. Neurologic symptoms occur in 10–20% of patients and suggest a more severe course. Myalgias, fatigability, headache, and ocular symptoms may persist for decades in chronic infection.

➤ Laboratory Findings

Diagnosis is usually made on the basis of clinical symptoms, dietary history, and serologic testing.

- Direct detection: Definitive diagnosis, if needed, is achieved by demonstration of larvae in striated muscle. The deltoid muscle is often biopsied. Muscle biopsy may show the encysted larvae beginning 10 days after ingestion. Direct microscopic examination of compressed specimen is superior to routine histologic preparation. Stool O&P examination is rarely contributory, but adult worms may be seen in acute illness with diarrhea.
- Serology: useful, but seroconversion may not occur for several weeks after acute infection. Serologic tests become positive 1 week after onset of symptoms in only 20–30% of patients and reach a peak in 80–90% of patients by fourth to fifth week. Rise in titer in acute and convalescent phase sera is diagnostic. Titers may remain negative in overwhelming infection. False-positive results may occur in polyarteritis nodosa, serum sickness, penicillin sensitivity, infectious mononucleosis, malignant lymphomas, and leukemia. EIA is method of choice; it peaks in 3 months and may still be detected at 1 year. Specificity is >95%. IHA is also used. Previously used tests include CF, bentonite flocculation, precipitin, and latex fixation.
- Core laboratory
  - Eosinophilia develops in >50% of patients and may be one of the earliest laboratory abnormalities supporting a clinical diagnosis. Eosinophilia appears with values of ≤85% on differential count and 15,000/μL on absolute count. It occurs about 1 week after the eating of infected meat and reaches maximum after third week. It usually subsides in 4–6 weeks but may last up to 6 months and occasionally for years.
  - Laboratory signs indicating muscle damage (e.g., increased concentrations of creatine phosphokinase, LDH, aldolase, aminotransferase) are frequently seen.
  - Decrease in serum total protein and albumin occurs in severe cases between 2 and 4 weeks and may last for years. Increased (relative and absolute) gamma globulins parallel titer of serologic tests. The increase occurs between 5 and 8 weeks and may last 6 months or more. ESR is normal or only slightly increased. Urine may show albuminuria with hyaline and granular casts in severe cases. With meningoencephalitis, CSF may be normal or ≤300 lymphocytes/microliter with increased protein with higher antibody level in CSF than serum.

TRICHOMONIASIS

See discussion of vaginitis and vaginosis in Chapter 9, Gynecologic and Obstetric Disorders.

➤ Suggested Readings: Parasitic Pathogens

Ash LR, Orihel TC. *Ash and Orihel's Atlas of Human Parasitology*. 5th ed. Chicago, IL: ASCP Press; 2007.

Barratt JL, Harkness J, Marriott D, et al. Importance of Nonenteric Protozoan Infections in Immunocompromised People. *Clin Microbiol Rev.* 2010;23:795–836.

Garcia LS. *Diagnostic Medical Parasitology*. Washington, DC: ASM Press; 2007.

Gottstein B, Pozio E, Nöckler K. Epidemiology, diagnosis, treatment and control of trichinellosis. *Clin Microbiol Rev*. 2009;22:127–145.

Hunter PR, Nichols G. Epidemiology and clinical features of *Cryptosporidium* infection in immunocompromised patients. *Clin Microbiol Rev.* 2002;15:145–154.

Okhuysen PC. Traveler's diarrhea due to intestinal protozoa. *Clin Infect Dis.* 2001;33:110–114.

Ross AGP, Bartley PB, Sleigh AC, et al. Schistosomiasis. *N Engl J Med.* 2002;16:1212–1220.

Stark D, Barratt JLN, van Hal S, et al. Clinical significance of enteric protozoa in the immunosuppressed human population. *Clin Microbiol Rev.* 2009;22:634–650.

Tanyuksel M, Petri WA. Laboratory diagnosis of amebiasis. *Clin Microbiol Rev.* 2003;16:713–729.

Respiratory, Metabolic, and Acid-Base Disorders

L.V. Rao and Michael J. Mitchell

RESPIRATORY DISORDERS

- Respiratory diseases include diseases of the lung, pleural cavity, bronchial tubes, trachea, and upper respiratory tract and diseases of the nerves and muscles of breathing. These conditions range from mild and self-limiting such as the common cold to life-threatening such as bacterial pneumonia or pulmonary embolism. The symptoms of respiratory disease differ depending on the disease. Common symptoms are cough with or without the production of sputum, hemoptysis, and dyspnea, which usually occurs with exercise, chest pain, noisy breathing (either wheeze or stridor) somnolence, loss of appetite, weight loss, cachexia, and cyanosis. In some cases, respiratory disease is diagnosed, in the absence of symptoms during the investigation of another disease or through a routine check.
- Respiratory diseases can be classified in many different ways: by the organ involved, by the pattern of symptoms, or by the cause of the disease.
  - **Obstructive lung diseases** are diseases of the lung in which the bronchial tubes become narrowed, making it difficult to move air in and especially out of the lung.
  - **Restrictive lung diseases** (also known as interstitial lung diseases) are a category of respiratory diseases characterized by a loss of lung compliance, causing incomplete lung expansion and increased lung stiffness.
- Respiratory tract infections can affect any part of the respiratory system. They are traditionally divided into upper respiratory tract infections (URTIs) and lower respiratory tract infections (LRTIs). The most common URTI is the common cold. However, infections of specific organs of the upper respiratory tract such as sinusitis, tonsillitis, otitis media, pharyngitis, and laryngitis are also considered URTIs. *Streptococcus pneumoniae* is the most common cause of severe, community-acquired bacterial pneumonia. Worldwide, TB is an important cause of pneumonia, usually presenting as a chronic infection. Other pathogens such as viruses and fungi can cause pneumonia, for example, severe influenza and *Pneumocystis* pneumonia.
- Tumors of the respiratory tract are either malignant or benign. Benign tumors are relatively rare causes of respiratory disease. Malignant tumors, or cancers of the respiratory system, particularly lung cancers, are a major health problem responsible for 15% of all cancer diagnoses and 29% of all cancer deaths. The majority of respiratory system cancers are attributable to smoking tobacco.
- There are a wide range of symptoms due to the intrathoracic effects of various respiratory diseases, the most common of which are dyspnea, cough, and infections.

COUGH

- Cough is a forced expulsive maneuver, usually against a closed glottis and which is associated with a characteristic sound. Most cases of troublesome cough reflect the presence of an aggravating factor (asthma, drugs, environmental, gastroesophageal reflex, upper airway pathology) in a susceptible individual.
- Classification based on symptom duration is somewhat arbitrary. A cough lasting <3 weeks is termed "acute" and one lasting >8 weeks is defined as "chronic."

➤ Acute Cough
- Acute cough is defined as a cough lasting <3 weeks. Most frequently, it presents in primary care settings and is commonly associated with URTIs. In most cases it is benign and self-limiting. It is frequently associated with acute exacerbations and hospitalizations with asthma and COPD.
- Symptoms associated with acute cough that require further investigation include hemoptysis, breathlessness, fever, chest pain, and weight loss. Common serious conditions presenting with isolated cough include neoplasms, infections (e.g., TB), foreign body inhalation, acute allergy-anaphylaxis, and interstitial lung disease.

➤ Subacute Cough
- Subacute cough is defined as a cough lasting 3–8 weeks. The gray area between 3 and 8 weeks of cough is difficult to define etiologically, since all chronic cough will have started as acute cough, but the diagnostic group of chronic cough are diluted by the patients with postviral cough (a URTI cough lingering for >3 weeks). Cough after infection is the most common cause of subacute cough (48%), postnasal drip is the second most common (33%), and cough variant asthma is the third most common (16%).
- In a significant percentage of patients, subacute cough (34%) is self-limited and will resolve without treatment. Most patients with subacute cough that spontaneously resolves had a postinfection cough.

➤ Chronic Cough
- Chronic cough is defined as a cough lasting >3 weeks. It is reported by 10–20% of adults and is common in women and obese people. Most patients present with a dry or minimally productive cough. The presence of significant sputum production usually indicates primary lung pathology.
- Chest radiograph and spirometry are recommended. Bronchial provocation testing should be performed in patients without a clinically obvious etiology. Bronchoscopy should be undertaken in all patients with chronic cough in whom inhalation of foreign body is suspected.

DISEASES ASSOCIATED WITH COUGH

CROUP (LARYNGOTRACHEITIS)

➤ Definition
- Croup refers to inflammation of the upper airway below the glottis and has been used to describe a variety of upper respiratory conditions in children, including laryngitis, laryngotracheitis, laryngotracheobronchitis, bacterial tracheitis, or spasmodic croup.

- Croup is usually caused by viral infection, especially parainfluenza virus, but it is occasionally caused by bacteria or an allergic reaction. It typically occurs in children 6 months to 3 years of age, usually during winter and early spring.
- Epiglottitis may result in acute airway obstruction and should be considered a medical emergency. A stable airway should be assured prior to collection of diagnostic specimens. Bacterial causes of epiglottitis include group B *Haemophilus influenzae*, *Streptococcus pneumoniae* and beta-hemolytic streptococci. The clinical picture in infectious mononucleosis or diphtheria may resemble epiglottitis. TB may cause chronic laryngitis.

➤ Who Should be Suspected?
- The hallmark of croup in infants and young children is the barking cough. In older children and adults hoarseness predominates. Croup is usually a mild and self-limited illness, although significant upper airway obstruction, respiratory distress, and, rarely, death can occur. Symptoms usually begin with nasal irritation, congestion, and coryza. Symptoms generally progress over 12–48 hours to include fever, hoarseness, barking cough, and stridor. Respiratory distress increases as upper airway obstruction becomes more severe. Rapid progression or signs of lower airway involvement suggest a more serious illness.
- Symptoms typically persist for 3–7 days, with a gradual return to normal.

➤ Diagnostic and Laboratory Findings
Laboratory studies are of limited diagnostic utility but may help guide management in more severe cases.
- CBC: WBC counts can be low, normal, or elevated; WBC counts >10,000 cells/μL are common. CBC differential shows neutrophil or lymphocyte predominance. The presence of a large number of band-form neutrophils is suggestive of primary or secondary bacterial infection.
- Chemistries: Not associated with any specific alterations in serum tests.
- Microbiology: Confirmation of etiologic diagnosis is not necessary, as croup requires only symptomatic therapy. Identification of a specific viral etiology may be necessary to make decisions regarding isolation for patients requiring hospitalization, for initiation of antiviral therapy, or for epidemiologic monitoring purposes.
- Culture: Diagnosis of a specific viral etiology may be made by viral culture of secretions from the nasopharynx or throat.

➤ Suggested Readings
Cherry JD. Croup (Laryngitis, laryngotracheitis, spasmodic croup, laryngotracheobronchitis, bacterial tracheitis, and laryngotracheobronchopneumonitis). In: Feigin RD, Cherry JD, Demmler-Harrison GJ, Kaplan SL, eds. *Textbook of Pediatric Infectious Diseases*. 6th ed. Philadelphia: Saunders; 2009.

Rihkanen H, Rönkkö, EB, Nieminen, T, Komsi, K-L, et al. Respiratory viruses in laryngeal croup of young children. *J Pediatr.* 2008;152:661–665.

PERTUSSIS (WHOOPING COUGH)*

➤ Definition
- Infection of the respiratory system caused by the bacterium *Bordetella pertussis*.
- Pertussis is highly infectious. The bacterium is transmitted via direct contact with droplets from coughing or sneezing by an infected individual. It affects an estimated 39 million people

---

* Contributed by Mary Williamson PhD.

each year, killing 297,000 people worldwide. Pertussis is preventable by vaccination, but an increased number of infections have been seen in recent years because of waning immunity and decreasing immunization rates.

> ## Who Should be Suspected?
* Patients symptoms of pertussis. Three phases are seen in typical illness:
  * Catarrhal (7–10 days): runny nose; low-grade fever; mild cough
  * Paroxysmal (1–6 weeks): severe, rapid coughing spells followed by inspiratory "whoop"; cyanosis; post-tussive vomiting
    * Convalescent (7–10 days): decreasing severity and frequency of coughing paroxysms
* Unvaccinated infants are at greatest risk for severe and fatal pertussis.
* Older children and adults with unusually severe or chronic (4–8 weeks) cough, especially unvaccinated patients or vaccinated >10 years previously, or immunocompromised
* Symptomatic contacts of patients with pertussis.

> ## Diagnostic Findings
* Culture: Nasopharyngeal culture for *B. pertussis* is the gold standard; however, sensitivity falls significantly after the first 7–14 days after onset of symptoms.
* Molecular testing: PCR methods have been described for diagnosis of pertussis. Cross-reactions have been described (e.g., *Bordetella holmesii*) and may limit clinical utility. The sensitivity of PCR is greatest in the early acute phase of infection, but *B. pertussis* DNA may be detectable for weeks after resolution of acute disease.
* Serology: Assays are commercially available, including assays for IgM and IgA. Variable sensitivity and specificity have limited the clinical utility of these assays. Antibody titers are highest 2–8 weeks after disease onset. Positive serological reactions must be interpreted considering the patient's primary and revaccination history.

> ## Suggested Reading
World Health Organization (WHO). Pertussis—the disease. http://www.who.int/immunization/topics/pertussis/en/index1.html

UPPER AIRWAY COUGH SYNDROME

> ## Definition
* Upper airway cough syndrome (UACS) is the newly recommended term to replace postnasal drip syndrome, referring to cough associated with upper airway conditions, because it is unclear whether the mechanism of cough is postnasal drip, direct irritation, or inflammation of the cough receptors in the upper airway. Postnasal drip is the drainage of secretions from the nose or paranasal sinuses into the pharynx.
* UACS, which is secondary to a variety of rhinosinus conditions, is the most common cause of chronic cough. It includes a variety of diseases: allergic rhinitis, perennial nonallergic rhinitis, nonallergic rhinitis with eosinophilia (NARES), bacterial sinusitis, and allergic fungal sinusitis, rhinitis due to anatomic abnormalities, rhinitis due to physical or chemical irritants, and occupational rhinitis.

> ## Who Should be Suspected?
* Clinically, the diagnosis depends on the reporting of the patient of a sensation of having something drip down in to the throat, nasal discharge, or frequent throat clearing. The presence of

mucoid, mucopurulent secretions, or cobblestoning of the mucosa during nasopharyngeal or oropharyngeal examination is also suggestive of UACS. It is the most common cause of the chronic condition.

➤ Diagnostic Findings

* In patients with chronic cough, the diagnosis of UACS-induced cough should be determined by considering a combination of criteria, including symptoms, physical examination findings, radiographic findings, specific allergen testing and, ultimately, the response to specific therapy. Because UACS is a syndrome, no pathognomonic findings exist.
* Specific therapy is instituted when the cause of chronic cough is apparent; empiric therapy should be considered in cough of unknown etiology.

➤ Suggested Reading

Pratter MR. Chronic upper airway cough syndrome secondary to rhinosinus diseases (previously referred to as postnasal drip syndrome): ACCP evidence-based clinical practice guidelines. *Chest.* 2006;129(1 Suppl): 63S–71S.

DYSPNEA

➤ Definition

* A consensus statement of the American Thoracic Society has defined "dyspnea" as a term used to characterize a subjective experience of breathing discomfort that comprises qualitatively distinct sensations that vary in intensity. The experience derives from interactions among multiple physiologic, psychological, social, and environmental factors and may induce secondary physiologic and behavioral responses. It is a common symptom that afflicts millions of patients with pulmonary disease.
* The majority of patients with chronic dyspnea of unclear etiology have one of four diagnoses: asthma, COPD, interstitial lung disease, or myocardial dysfunction. Mild dyspnea is common. Dyspnea is a common chief complaint among patients who come to the emergency department. The majority of life-threatening causes of dyspnea are classified below.
  * Life-threatening upper airway causes: tracheal foreign objects, angioedema, anaphylaxis, infections of pharynx, and neck and airway trauma
  * Life-threatening pulmonary causes: pulmonary embolism, COPD, asthma, pneumothorax, pulmonary infections, ARDS, direct pulmonary injury, and pulmonary hemorrhage
  * Life-threatening cardiac causes: ACS, flash pulmonary edema, high-output heart failure, cardiomyopathy, cardiac arrhythmia, valvular dysfunction, and cardiac tamponade
  * Life-threatening neurologic causes: stroke, neuromuscular disease
  * Life-threatening toxic and metabolic causes: poisoning, salicylate, poisoning, carbon monoxide poisoning, DKA, sepsis, anemia, and acute chest syndrome
* Other miscellaneous causes include lung cancer, pleural effusion, ascites, pregnancy, hyperventilation, anxiety, and massive obesity.
* The combination of all historical elements and physical examination findings is helpful in diagnosing the cause of both acute and chronic dyspnea.

PULMONARY DISEASES ASSOCIATED WITH DYSPNEA

The following are common infectious disease–related pulmonary tract disorders. For microbe-specific information, refer to Chapter 13, Infectious Diseases.

FUNGAL INFECTIONS*

➤ Definition
- The respiratory tract is the common portal of entry and disease most commonly involves the lungs or pararespiratory tissues. Exposure to fungal spores or antigens may result in disease by invasive proliferation (infection) or by a poorly controlled, severe immunologic response to fungal antigens. Fungal infections are uncommon in immunocompetent individuals but may be a significant cause of morbidity and mortality in immunocompromised patients.
- Common fungal infective agents include *Aspergillus* species, *Blastomyces dermatitidis, Coccidioides* (*C. immitis* and *C. posadasii*), *Cryptococcus* (*C. neoformans* and *C. gattii*), *Histoplasma capsulatum*, aseptate mold (*Mucorales, Rhizopus*), *Paracoccidioides brasiliensis, Pneumocystis carinii* (now *P. jiroveci*), *and Sporothrix schenckii.*

➤ Who Should be Suspected?
- Candidates include immunocompromised patients. Symptoms are nonspecific and may mimic TB, and they may include chest pain, fever of unknown origin, cough (may be productive and/or bloody), and dyspnea.

➤ Laboratory Findings
- Cultures: Can be isolated by fungal culture; however, these take up to 4 weeks for results and have a high false-negative occurrence.
- Nucleic acid amplification methods: DNA and mRNA have been described and show promise for diagnostic testing, but tests are not standardized and FDA-approved assays are not available.
- Serologic testing: Positive beta-D-glucan assay may support a diagnosis.

LEGIONNAIRES DISEASE

➤ Definition
- Legionnaires disease is caused by infection with *Legionella pneumophila*, a fastidious aerobic gram-negative bacillus. Respiratory infections are the primary manifestation of *L. pneumophila* infection. Community- and hospital-acquired infections are well described.

➤ Who Should be Suspected?
- Legionnaires disease is characterized by progressive respiratory (dyspnea, cough, and minimal sputum production), GI (nausea and vomiting, abdominal pain, diarrhea), and nonspecific symptoms (fever and chills, malaise).

➤ Laboratory Findings

Specific diagnosis is most reliably based on culture isolation and antigen detection.

- Hematology: WBC count is increased (10,000–20,000/μL) in 75% of cases (leukopenia is a bad prognostic sign); Thrombocytopenia is common.
- Core laboratory findings: Hypophosphatemia; hyponatremia; hypoalbuminemia (<2.5 g/dL); proteinuria (~50% of patients); microscopic hematuria; abnormal LFTs (mild to moderate increase of serum AST, ALP, LD, or bilirubin is found in ~50% of patients).
- Direct detection: Gram stain of sputum is of little use for detection because the faintly staining organisms are frequently masked by the proteinaceous background. Patient specimens show few to moderate number of PMNs. Stains with enhanced staining of *Legionella*, like silver or Gimenez staining, also show poor overall sensitivity for detection of legionellosis. DFA staining is very specific, but shows variable sensitivity (25–75%). Hence, a negative DFA test result is of little value and does not substitute for culture.
- Molecular testing
  - PCR-based assays have been described with moderate to high sensitivity, depending on the type of specimen tested. Negative results, therefore, do not exclude the diagnosis of legionellosis. Testing may be used to detect *Legionella* in urine, serum, and BAL fluid. Specificity of molecular assays is very high.
  - An advantage of most molecular diagnostic tests described is their ability to detect all *Legionella* species, rather than being limited, like urine antigen testing, to *L. pneumophila* serogroup 1.
- Culture: Using pleural fluid, lung biopsy, or transtracheal or bronchial aspirate, organisms may require 3–7 days incubation for isolation.
- Direct Antigen Detection and Serology
  - Urine antigen testing is an important method for diagnosis of Legionnaires diseases caused by *L. pneumophila* serogroup 1 (~90% of community acquired and ~60% of nosocomial respiratory *Legionella* respiratory infections). The specificity of the urine antigen test is ~99%. Antigen may be detected in urine for several days after the initiation of antimicrobial therapy. The sensitivity of urine antigen testing depends on the probability of infection with *L. pneumophila* serogroup 1 and the severity of infection. About 90% of patients with severe legionellosis that requires hospitalization should show a positive urine antigen test, whereas only about 50% of outpatients with milder legionellosis will yield a positive urine antigen test. The specificity of the urine antigen test is ~99%.
  - Serological testing may be a useful adjunct to diagnostic testing, but serological testing plays a limited role in acute patient management because of the time required to provide definitive results. Serum IFA testing is recommended and allows detection of immunoglobulin subclasses. Testing for total antibody as well as specific IgM and IgG is recommended. Seroresponse may not be detectable for weeks to months after acute infection. Only half of infected patients will seroconvert at 2 weeks. Therefore, testing paired acute and multiple convalescent (2, 4, 6, 8, and 12 weeks) serum samples is recommended. A diagnosis is supported by detection of specific IgM or by a fourfold or greater change in titer between acute and convalescent specimens. Specificity depends on the antigen preparation used in the assay. Tests that use *L. pneumophila* serogroup 1 demonstrate the best

specificity (~99%), while assays that use polyvalent antigen preparations demonstrate somewhat lower (90-95%) specificity.

➤ Suggested Readings
Fields BS, RF Benson, RE Besser. Legionella and Legionnaires' disease: 25 years of investigation. *Clin Microbiol Rev.* 2002;15:506–526.
Newton HJ, Ang DKY, vanDriel IR, Hartland EL. Molecular pathogenesis of infections caused by Legionella pneumophila. *Clin Microbiol Rev.* 2010;23:274–298.

LOWER RESPIRATORY TRACT INFECTIONS

BRONCHIOLITIS

➤ Definition
- Bronchiolitis is primarily a disease of infants and young children.
- RSV is the primary cause of bronchiolitis (~75%), especially severe bronchiolitis that requires medical attention or hospitalization. Monoclonal antibody therapy or antiviral therapies may be considered for infants with severe RSV infection. Other causes include parainfluenza virus (type 3), human metapneumovirus, adenovirus.

➤ Who Should be Suspected?
- There may be nonspecific findings of viral respiratory infection, like rhinitis. The major clinical manifestation is air trapping due to expiratory obstruction. Wheezing is common.
- Infants present with an increased respiratory rate and obvious difficulty breathing marked by nasal flaring. Infants with underlying immunodeficiency, or cardiac or pulmonary disease are at risk for more severe infection. Severely affected infants may be cyanotic. Fever is not a prominent feature.

➤ Diagnostic and Laboratory Findings
- Culture: Most of the relevant viruses may be isolated by viral culture, but turn-around-time is slow. Therefore, viral culture is usually not helpful for acute clinical management.
- Chest radiograph: May be indicated to rule out pneumonia.
- Blood gas: ABGs may be monitored in infants with severe disease. Core laboratory tests are usually normal, although fluid status must be monitored carefully because of the risk of dehydration due to tachypnea.
- Serology: Antigen detection kits are commercially available for a number of the viruses, like influenza viruses A and B, RSV, and human metapneumovirus. Although the specificity of these assays is usually high, sensitivity may be <80%. The use of specific DFA staining is useful for evaluation of specimen quality and has shown improved sensitivity.
- Molecular Tests: Playing an increasingly important role in diagnosis because of the improved sensitivity and specificity, compared to culture or antigen based testing, and a wider scope of detectable pathogens.

BACTERIAL PNEUMONIA

➤ Definition
* Pneumonia describes pulmonary infection of the most distal airways and alveolar spaces. Bacteria may gain access to lower respiratory tract directly, by inhalation or aspiration, or by hematogenous seeding from a distal site of infection.
* *Streptococcus pneumoniae* is the most common cause of serious community-acquired bacterial pneumonia. Other pathogens, like *Haemophilus influenzae, Moraxella catarrhalis, Mycoplasma pneumoniae, Legionella,* and *Chlamydophila pneumoniae,* are also significant pathogens. *Staphylococcus aureus* and gram-negative bacilli are often implicated in nosocomial pneumonias.

➤ Who Should be Suspected?
* A broad range of conditions predispose to bacterial pneumonia, including underlying medical conditions (e.g., alcoholism, decreased level of consciousness, malnutrition, immune compromise, uremia), toxic exposure (e.g., inhalants, tobacco smoke, environmental pollutants), structural or functional defects of normal pulmonary defense mechanisms (e.g., COPD, cystic fibrosis, bronchiectasis, ciliary dysfunction) and age >65 years.
* Common symptoms include dyspnea, shortness of breath, pleuritic chest pain, cough and sputum production, typically purulent. Systemic signs include fever and malaise; rigors are reported by a significant minority of patients.
* Physical examination may demonstrate diffuse or localized abnormalities, including rales, ronchi and diminished breath sounds.

➤ Diagnostic and Laboratory Findings
* Diagnostic testing depends on the severity of disease and specific risk factors. Healthy outpatients may need minimal evaluation. For patients with significant infection, CXR, CBC, blood culture, sputum Gram stain and culture are recommended. The diagnosis of tuberculosis should be considered, and ruled-out as appropriate. Special culture techniques (e.g., *Legionella* culture) or urine antigen testing (e.g., *Legionella, Streptococcus pneumoniae*) might be considered. BAL may improve diagnosis for patients unable to provide a good-quality expectorated sputum sample or when unusual pathogens are suspected.
  * A specific pathogen can only be identified by culture in about half of patients with community-acquired pneumonia that requires hospitalization. Blood culture is positive in ~20% of these patients; pneumococcal urinary antigen is positive in ~50%.
  * PCR may demonstrate improved sensitivity, but the impact on patient management has not been demonstrated. FDA-approved kits for detection of bacterial respiratory pathogens are not available.
* Core Laboratories: Leukocytosis (>15,000 with left shift) is typical for acute bacterial pneumonia. Leukopenia is associated with poor prognosis. Serial measurement of ABGs, electrolytes and other analytes should be collected to monitor the respiratory and metabolic status of patients with severe infection. Abnormalities typical for underlying medical conditions or severity of disease should be evaluated.

➤ Suggested Reading
van der Eerden, MM, Vlaspolder, F, de Graaff, CS, Groot, T, et al. Value of intensive diagnostic microbiological investigation in low- and high-risk patients with community-acquired pneumonia. *Eur J Clin Microbiol Infect Dis* 2005;24:241–249.

ASPIRATION PNEUMONIA

➤ Definition
* Aspiration pneumonia refers to pulmonary disease caused by abnormal entry of fluids into the lower respiratory tract. The fluid may be endogenous secretions (e.g., gastric contents, upper respiratory secretions) or exogenous.
* Development of disease usually requires defective protective mechanisms (e.g., cough reflex, glottis function, ciliary transport) and aspiration of "toxic" material (e.g., particulate matter, acidic fluid, heavy bacterial contamination).
* Conditions that predispose to aspiration include alcoholism, seizure, CVA, head trauma, general anesthesia, dysphagia, periodontal disease, neurologic disorder, protracted vomiting, and mechanical disruption of the usual defense barriers (nasogastric tube, endotracheal intubation, upper GI endoscopy, and bronchoscopy).

➤ Who Should be Suspected?
* The endogenous flora of the upper respiratory and gastrointestinal tract most commonly cause bacterial aspiration pneumonia. Polymicrobial infection, including anaerobes and less virulent streptococcal species found in gingival crevices, is typical.
* Most patients present with sub-acute progression of symptoms over several weeks. Common symptoms include dyspnea, cough, and purulent (often putrid) sputum production, with associated fever and weight loss. Rigors are uncommon. Symptoms of complicated infection, like abscess or empyema, may be present.
* Core Labor

➤ Diagnostic and Laboratory Findings
* Microbiology: Expectorated sputum is not reliable for diagnosis, except for possibly establishing an alternative diagnosis. Culture of specimens (e.g., transtracheal or transthoracic aspirates) collected using techniques for anaerobic isolation may be informative.
* *Fusobacterium nucleatum, Bacteroides, Peptostreptococcus* and *Prevotella* species are most commonly implicated anaerobes. Aerobic organisms, including *S. aureus* and gram-negative bacilli, are common, especially in nosocomial aspiration pneumonias.
* Core Laboratory: Anemia is typical. Laboratory abnormalities associated with underlying medical conditions should be investigated.

➤ Suggested Reading
Marik PE. Aspiration pneumonitis and aspiration pneumonia. *N Engl J Med.* 2001;344(9):665–671.

VIRAL PNEUMONIA

➤ Definition
* Pneumonia, characterized by the development of abnormal alveolar gas exchange, may be caused by a number of viral respiratory pathogens. Pneumonia is often preceded by nonspecific symptoms of URI. The etiology depends somewhat on the age and the patient's state of immunocompetence. In children, viral pneumonia is most important in patients younger than 5 years. Clinically significant, purely viral pneumonia is uncommon in immunocompetent older children and adults. The parainfluenza viruses, RSV, and

human metapneumoviruses are relatively more common causes of viral pneumonia in children and infants compared to older children and adults. In older children and adults, influenza viruses, especially type A, are responsible for most cases of pneumonia. CMV is the most common, clinically significant cause of viral pneumonia in immunocompromised patients.

➤ Etiology and Diagnosis

- Specific identification may be required for optimal management of severely ill patients. Because the clinical and laboratory presentation of viral pneumonia are not specific, other etiologies, like bacteria, mycoplasmas, *P. jiroveci*, must be considered and ruled out by relevant laboratory and other evaluations.
- Causes include influenza (adults), parainfluenza (children), RSV (immunocompromised patients), human metapneumovirus (children), adenovirus, CMV (primarily in immunocompromised patients and children), HSV, measles virus, and VZV.

➤ Who Should be Suspected?

- The presenting findings in viral pneumonia include acute illness with fever, showing signs of hypoxemia. Cough is usually nonproductive. Examination typically demonstrates tachypnea, rales, and wheezing. Underlying medical conditions may be exacerbated by viral pneumonia; the severity of viral pneumonia is often greater in patients with underlying illness. Imaging studies typically demonstrate diffuse, bilateral interstitial infiltrates, although the spectrum of abnormalities is broad and non-specific. Bacterial superinfection is well described and represents a significant complication of viral pneumonia.

➤ Diagnostic and Laboratory Findings

Most patients with viral pneumonia have a relatively benign, self-limited illness. Specific diagnosis is usually not required unless severe disease or complication of infection is present.

- Culture: Most of the relevant viruses may be isolated by viral culture, but turnaround time is slow. Therefore, viral culture is usually not helpful for acute clinical management.
- Direct Antigen Detection: Antigen detection kits are commercially available for a number of the relevant viruses, such as influenza viruses A and B, RSV, and human metapneumovirus. Although the specificity of these assays is usually high, sensitivity may be <80%. The use of specific DFA staining is useful for evaluation of specimen quality and has shown improved sensitivity.
- Molecular testing: IFDA-approved assays are available for respiratory viral pathogens. These assays provide high sensitivity and specificity, a broad range of detectable viruses and short turn-around-time, but higher cost, compared to culture and antigen testing.
- Serology: Serological testing is not useful for the acute management of patients.
- Core Laboratory Findings: ABGs, CBC, and other tests should be monitored in patients with severe or complicated viral pneumonia. Core laboratory tests are usually normal. In patients with severe respiratory distress, careful monitoring of ABGs is critical for patient management. Fluid status must be monitored carefully because of the risk of dehydration due to fever and tachypnea.

➤ Suggested Reading

Treanor JJ. Chapter 2 Respiratory Infections. In Richman DD, RJ Whitley, FG Hayden. Clinical Virology, Third Edition. 2009; ASM Press, Washington, DC.

PNEUMOCYSTIS PNEUMONIA

➤ Definition
* *Pneumocystis jiroveci* (formerly *Pneumocystis carinii*) infection is almost exclusively restricted to pulmonary disease in immunocompromised patients. *P. jiroveci* was discovered early in the 20th century as a very rare cause of pneumonitis, or PCP, in immunocompromised patients. The organism was originally thought to be a parasite; however, phylogenetic studies have supported the placement of *P. carinii* as a member of the kingdom Fungus. In 1999, in conformance with the International Code of Botanical Nomenclature, the *Pneumocystis* species associated with human disease was designated *P. jiroveci*.
* PCP is the most common opportunistic infection in patients with HIV infection and is an AIDS-defining illness in these patients. The incidence of PCP is inversely related to CD4 counts with HIV infection; patients with HIV infection are not at high risk until the CD4 count falls below 200 cells/mm^3. The risk of PCP is reduced in patients taking effective prophylactic therapy. The incidence of PCP has fallen dramatically in patients compliant with highly active antiretroviral treatment.

➤ Who Should be Suspected?
* In HIV-infected patients, the onset of PCP is usually slow with fever, shortness of breath, tachypnea, and nonproductive cough. Fatigue, weight loss, and other symptoms are common. Chest x-rays most commonly demonstrate diffuse, bilateral abnormality usually consisting of interstitial infiltrates; other patterns may be seen. Gallium scanning shows intense diffuse uptake. The risk of PCP is also increased in stem cell and solid organ transplant patients, patients with hematologic malignancies, patients receiving glucocorticoids or other immunosuppressive agents, and patients with other acquired or primary immunodeficiency states; PCP usually follows a fulminant course in non-HIV patients.

➤ Laboratory Findings
* Culture: Effective in vitro culture techniques are not available.
* Flow cytometry: In HIV-infected patients, a CD4 count <200 cells/mm^3 is demonstrated in most patients who develop PCP.
* Direct detection: Definitive diagnosis is usually achieved by microscopic demonstration of organism in respiratory secretions. Sensitive detection requires examination specimens collected using techniques that increase the sampling of alveolar contents, like BAL or induced sputum. The organism is rarely detected in routine sputum or bronchial washings or brushings. The sensitivity of staining methods may be reduced in non-HIV patients with PCP because of a lower organism burden.
* Histology: Transbronchial lung biopsy is a very effective, albeit invasive, specimen for definite diagnosis. Biopsy samples also allow for diagnosis of other infections (e.g., fungi) or diseases (e.g., lymphoma) that may be in the differential diagnosis.
* Serology: Testing does not play a role in PCP diagnosis.
* Core laboratory: Elevated LDH is typical; the degree of LDH elevation and increasing LDH despite therapy are poor prognostic signs. Several serum markers, like S-adenosylmethionine and beta-D-glucan, have been evaluated as adjunctive, noninvasive assays for diagnosis of PCP, but their utility has not been established.

Nucleic acid amplification: Methods have been developed for PCP diagnosis. The sensitivity may allow for sensitive detection using noninvasively collected specimens, like saliva. The increased cost and turn-around-time for PCR, and small incremental sensitivity, are likely to limit wide implementation of PCR for PCP. In addition, false-positive results have been reported for PCR.

➤ Suggested Readings
Stringer JR. *Pneumocystis carinii*: What Is It, Exactly? *Clin Microbiol Rev*. 1996;9:489–498.

Thomas CF, Limper AH. Pneumocystis pneumonia. *N Engl J Med*. 2004;350:2487–2498.

Wazir JF, Ansari NA. *Pneumocystis carinii* infection. *Arch Pathol Lab Med*. 2004;128:1023.

TUBERCULOSIS, PULMONARY

Primary Disease*
➤ Definition
* *Mycobacterium tuberculosis*, the primary cause of TB, is transmitted by respiratory droplets from an infected patient. After inhalation into the alveoli, organisms multiply on alveolar macrophages, eventually killing the cells. The inflammatory response results in a granulomatous mass called a tubercle.

➤ Who Should be Suspected?
* Low-grade fever is the most common symptom in patients with primary TB. Other symptoms, including chest pain, cough, and fatigue, may occur in a minority of patients. Physical examination is usually normal.

➤ Laboratory Findings
* Detection of host response: Positive tuberculin skin test, interferon-gamma release assays
* Direct detection: Positive AFB smear
* Culture: Isolation by culture core laboratory tests are normal for most patients with uncomplicated pulmonary TB. Submission of multiple samples from an infected site for testing significantly improves detection.

NONINFECTIOUS PULMONARY DISEASES ASSOCIATED WITH DYSPNEA

ASTHMA

➤ Definition
* Asthma is a chronic inflammatory disorder in which the airway smooth muscle undergoes exaggerated contractions and is abnormally responsive to external stimuli. The best defined and most commonly identified cause of this inflammation is inhalation of allergens.

---

*Contributed by Mary Williamson PhD

- Classification of bronchial asthma can be based on age, etiology-associated characteristics, or severity. The pattern of disease presenting at different ages is distinct. In the first 2 years of life, wheezing and bronchiolitis are not distinguishable, and the most common cause of these episodes is infection with the RSV. In older children and young adults, by far the most commonly identified cause of asthma is sensitization to one of the most common inhalant allergens, particularly those encountered indoors.
- Asthma that presents after 20 years of age provides a complex problem, and there is a wider differential diagnosis. Major causes include simple allergic asthma in adults, intrinsic asthma associated with chronic hyperplastic sinusitis, allergic bronchopulmonary aspergillosis, and wheezing associated with chronic obstructive lung disease.
- Among adults aged >40 years who develop severe asthma for the first time, almost 50% may have intrinsic asthma (negative skin tests to common allergens, no family history, persistent eosinophilia). Late-onset asthma, which is frequently not associated with atopy, may be linked to workplace (occupational exposure to sensitizing chemicals).

➤ Who Should be Suspected?
- Classic symptoms of asthma are intermittent dyspnea, cough, and wheezing. These symptoms are nonspecific and sometimes difficult to distinguish from other respiratory diseases. Patients may present to clinics or the emergency department with acute symptoms of breathlessness, wheezing, and coughing. Alternatively, they may present between episodes with normal or near normal lungs. Asthma may develop at any age, although newonset asthma is less frequent in elderly compared to other age groups. Seventy-five percent of the cases are diagnosed before the age 7.
- Asthmatic symptoms characteristically come and go, with a time course of hours to days, resolving spontaneously with removal of triggering stimulus or in response to anti-asthmatic medications. Characteristic triggers of asthma include cold air, exercise, and exposure to allergens. Allergens that typically trigger asthmatic symptoms include dust, molds, furred animals, cockroaches, and pollens. Viral infections are also common triggers.

➤ Diagnostic Findings
The diagnostic tools should include history, physical examination, pulmonary function tests (PFTs), and other laboratory evaluations.
- PFTs: Measurement of peak expiratory flow rate (PEFR) and spirometry are the two PFTs most often used in the diagnosis of asthma. Spirometry is used to measure the amount of air a person can breathe out and the amount of time taken to do so. Forced vital capacity (FVC): maximum volume of air that can be exhaled during a forced maneuver. Forced expired volume in one second (FEV_1): volume expired in the first second of maximal expiration after a maximal inspiration. This is a measure of how quickly the lungs can be emptied. FEV_1/FVC: FEV_1 expressed as a percentage of the FVC gives a clinically useful index of airflow limitation. The ratio FEV_1/FVC is between 70% and 80% in normal adults; it is influenced by the age, sex, height, and ethnicity and is best considered as a percentage of the predicted normal value. Variability of >20% in PEFR, a reversible reduction in FEV_1 and FEV_1/FVC, and heightened sensitivity to bronchoprovocation are findings consistent with asthma.
- Chest radiography: Almost always normal in patients with asthma. It is recommended in the evaluation of severe or difficult-to-control asthma and for the detection of comorbid conditions (e.g., allergic bronchopulmonary aspergillosis, eosinophilic pneumonia, or atelectasis due to mucous plugging).

- Hematology: CBC with differential WBC analysis to screen for eosinophilia or significant anemia may be helpful in certain cases. Markedly elevated eosinophil percentages ($>15\%$) may be due to allergic asthma but should prompt consideration of alternative diagnoses, including parasitic infections, drug reactions, and syndromes of pulmonary infiltrates with eosinophilia. An alpha-1 antitrypsin level is recommended in nonsmokers with persistent and irreversible airflow obstruction to exclude emphysema due to alpha-1 antitrypsin deficiency.
- Allergy tests: Allergic sensitivity to specific allergens can be assessed by either skin tests or blood tests for allergen specific IgE. Aeroallergens (house dust mite, cat or dog dander, cockroach, pollen, and mold spore antigens) are most commonly implicated in asthma. Food allergens rarely cause isolated asthmatic symptoms. Total IgE levels are sometimes helpful. A very high level (>1000 IU/mL) suggests the associated conditions of eczema or allergic bronchopulmonary aspergillosis.

➤ Suggested Reading
National Asthma Education and Prevention Program: Expert panel report III: Guidelines for the diagnosis and management of asthma. Bethesda, MD: National Heart, Lung, and Blood Institute, 2007. (NIH publication no. 08-4051). Full text available online: www.nhlbi.nih.gov/guidelines/asthma/asthgdln.htm.

CARDIAC HEART FAILURE

See Chapter 4, Cardiovascular Disorders.

CHRONIC OBSTRUCTIVE PULMONARY DISEASE

➤ Definition
- Chronic bronchitis with emphysema, also known as chronic obstructive pulmonary disease (COPD), is in most cases a sequel of many years of active smoking. COPD results from complex interactions between clinical and genetic risk factors. Definite or possible risk factors for COPD include inhalational exposure (e.g., smoking), increased airway responsiveness, atopy, and antioxidant deficiency. Genetic risk factors for COPD include a variety of gene polymorphisms, antioxidant related enzyme dysfunction, metalloproteinase dysregulation, and abnormalities that cause excess elastase.
- The Global Initiative for Chronic Obstructive Lung Disease (GOLD)—a report produced by the National Heart, Lung, and Blood Institute (NHLBI) and the World Health Organization (WHO)—defines COPD as "a preventable and treatable disease with some significant extrapulmonary effects that may contribute to the severity in individual patients. Its pulmonary component is characterized by airflow limitation that is not fully reversible. The airflow limitation is usually progressive and associated with an abnormal inflammatory response of the lungs to noxious particles or gases."
- Classification of severity of COPD. An $FEV_1/FVC <70\%$ indicates airflow limitation and the possibility of COPD.
  - **Stage 0**—at risk: normal spirometry; chronic symptoms (cough, sputum production); $FEV_1/FVC <70\%$
  - **Stage I**—mild: with or without chronic symptoms (cough, sputum production) mild airflow limitation ($FEV_1/FVC <70\%$; $FEV_1 >80\%$ predicted)

- **Stage II**—moderate: Worsening airflow limitation (FEV$_1$/FVC <70%; 50% <FEV$_1$ <80% predicted), with shortness of breath typically developing during exertion.
- **Stage III**—severe: with or without chronic symptoms (cough, sputum production); further worsening of airflow limitation (FEV$_1$/FVC <70%; 30% <FEV$_1$ < 50% predicted)
- **Stage IV**—very severe: with or without chronic symptoms (cough, sputum production); severe airflow limitation (FEV$_1$/FVC <70%; FEV$_1$ <30% predicted) or FEV$_1$ <50% predicted plus chronic respiratory failure. Patients may have very severe (stage IV) COPD even if the FEV$_1$ is >30% predicted, whenever this complication is present.

▶ Who Should be Suspected?

The dominant symptoms of COPD are coughing and shortness of breath on activity, but some patients present with acute breathlessness and wheezing, which is difficult to distinguish from asthma. There are three typical ways that patients with COPD present. Some patients have few complaints but an extremely sedentary life style. Other patients describe chronic respiratory symptoms (e.g., dyspnea on exertion, cough). Finally, some patients present with an acute exacerbation (e.g., wheezing, cough, and dyspnea). The physical examination of chest varies with severity of COPD.

- COPD should be considered and PFTs performed in all patients who report any combination of the following: chronic cough, chronic sputum production, dyspnea or inhalational exposure to tobacco smoke, occupational dust, or occupational chemicals. COPD is confirmed when a patient who has symptoms that are compatible with COPD is found to have airflow obstruction (FEV$_1$/FVC <0.70) and there is no alternative explanation for the symptoms and airflow obstruction.

▶ Diagnostic Findings

- Spirometry: This is an essential test to confirm the diagnosis and establish the staging of COPD. If values are abnormal, a postbronchodilator test may be indicated. Reversibility following bronchodilator would suggest asthma, and, if function reversed to normal, would exclude COPD. The FVC, or FEV is needed to establish the presence of obstruction (see above for significance of specific values). The inspiratory capacity may decrease acutely with tachypnea due to dynamic hyperinflation. It is the best physiologic correlate of dyspnea, but it is not usually required to diagnose COPD.
- Carbon monoxide (CO) diffusing capacity: Measurement of CO diffusing capacity can help establish the presence of emphysema, but it is not necessary for the routine diagnosis of COPD.
- Chest radiography: Only diagnostic of severe emphysema but always essential to exclude other lung diseases.
- Blood gas: ABGs are not needed in mild (FEV$_1$ > 80%) and moderate (FEV$_1$ 65–79%) airflow obstruction. ABGs are optional except oximetry, which should be measured in moderately severe (FEV$_1$ 50–64%) airflow obstruction. (ABGs should be measured if oxygen saturation is >88%.) ABGs should be monitored in all severe (FEV$_1$ 30–49%) and very severe (FEV$_1$ < 30 %) airflow obstruction.

▶ Suggested Reading

Global strategy for the diagnosis, management, and prevention of chronic obstructive pulmonary disease: Executive summary 2006. Global Initiative for Chronic Obstructive Lung Disease (GOLD). Available from http://www.goldcopd.org.

CYSTIC FIBROSIS

➤ Definition

* Autosomal recessive disorder with abnormal ion transport due to (>1000) chromosome 7 mutation transmembrane conductance regulator (CFTR gene) that controls salt, especially chloride, entry/exit into cells. Incidence of 1:2500 in non-Hispanic whites in North America with a carrier frequency of 1:20; 1:17,000 in African Americans; marked heterogeneity among patients.

➤ Who Should be Suspected?

* Respiratory symptoms include fatigue, cough, wheezing, recurrent pneumonia or sinus infections, excess sputum and/or shortness of breath.

➤ Diagnostic Criteria

* At least one characteristic clinical feature (respiratory, sweat, GI, GU) *or* sibling with CF *or* positive neonatal screening
  AND
* Sweat chloride ≥60 mEq/L *or* presence of 2 *CFTR* genes *or* positive nasal transmembrane potential difference

➤ Laboratory Findings

Culture: Special culture techniques should be used in these patients. Before 1 year of age, *Staphylococcus aureus* is found in 25% and *Pseudomonas aeruginosa* in 20% of respiratory tract cultures; in adults *P. aeruginosa* grows in 80% and *S. aureus* in 20%. *Haemophilus influenzae* is found in 3.4% of cultures. *P. aeruginosa* is found increasingly often after treatment of staph, and special identification and susceptibility tests should be performed on *P. aeruginosa*. *Pseudomonas cepacia* is becoming more important in older children. Increasing serum antibodies against *P. aeruginosa* can document probable infection when cultures are negative.

* Molecular Tests: DNA genotyping (using blood; can use buccal scrapings) to confirm diagnosis based on two mutations is highly specific but not very sensitive; supports diagnosis of cystic fibrosis (CF), but failure to detect gene mutations does not exclude CF because of large number of alleles. A substantial number of patients with CF have unidentified gene mutations. This test should be done when the sweat test is borderline or negative. It can also be used for carrier screening. Identical genotypes can be associated with different degrees of disease severity. The genotype should not be used as sole diagnostic criterion for CF. Prevalence of the 25 most common genes in the panel depends on population group (Table 14-1).

* Prenatal screening by chorionic villus sampling in first trimester or amniocentesis in second or third trimester: >1000 mutations of *CFTR* gene but the 25 most common account for ~90% of carriers. Fifty-two percent are homozygous for ΔF508 and 36% are heterozygous for ΔF508/other CF mutation.

  Core laboratory: Serum albumin is often decreased (because of hemodilution due to cor pulmonale; may be found before cardiac involvement is clinically apparent). Serum

---

*Contributed by Michael Snyder MD and Mary Williamson PhD.

TABLE 14-1. Demographic Groups and their Risk for Cystic Fibrosis		
	Detection Rate of Panel (%)	Frequency of Carriers
Ashkenazi Jew	97	1/25
North European	90	1/25
South European	68–70	1/29
Black	69	1/60
Hispanic	55–57	1/45
Asian	30	1/90

protein electrophoresis shows increasing IgG and IgA levels with progressive pulmonary disease; IgM and IgD levels are not appreciably increased. Serum chloride, sodium, potassium, calcium, and phosphorus levels are normal unless complications occur (e.g., chronic pulmonary disease with accumulation of CO_2; massive salt loss due to sweating may cause hyponatremia). Urine electrolytes are normal. Submaxillary saliva has slightly increased chloride and sodium but not potassium; considerable overlap with normal results prevents diagnostic use.

Saliva findings: Submaxillary saliva is more turbid, with increased calcium, total protein, and amylase. These changes are not generally found in parotid saliva.

Other: Nasal electrical potential difference measurements may be more reliable than sweat tests but are much more complex; mean $= -46$ mV in affected persons but -19 mV in unaffected persons.

➤ Considerations

Laboratory changes secondary to complications should also suggest diagnosis of CF:
- Chronic lung disease (especially upper lobes) with laboratory changes of decreased pO_2, accumulation of CO_2, metabolic alkalosis, severe recurrent infection, secondary cor pulmonale, nasal polyps, pansinusitis; normal sinus x-rays are strong evidence against CF.
- Overt liver disease, including cirrhosis, fatty liver, bile duct strictures, and cholelithiasis, in ≤5% of cases. Neonatal cholestasis in ≤20% of affected infants may persist for months.
- Meconium ileus during early infancy; causes 20–30% of cases of neonatal intestinal obstruction; present at birth in 8% of these children. Almost all of them will develop the clinical picture of CF.

PULMONARY EMBOLISM

➤ Definition
- Pulmonary embolism (PE) refers to the occlusion of the pulmonary artery or one of its branches by a blood clot, tumor, air, or fat that developed elsewhere in the body. The classic symptoms of PE are hemoptysis, dyspnea, and chest pain.
- PE can be classified as acute or chronic. In acute PE, patients develop symptoms and signs immediately after obstruction of pulmonary vessels. In chronic PE, patients slowly develop progressive dyspnea over a period of years due to pulmonary hypertension.

- The incidence of PE appears to be significantly higher in blacks than whites. Mortality rates for PE for blacks have been 50% higher than whites followed by people of other races (Asians) and Native Americans.
- The risk is increased in pregnancy and during the postpartum period. Other risk factors include venous stasis, various hypercoagulable states, immobilization, surgery, trauma, oral contraceptives, estrogen replacement, CHF, advanced age, and malignancy.

➤ Who Should be Suspected?

- PE should be suspected in a patient with sudden onset of dyspnea, deterioration of existing dyspnea, or the onset of pleuritic chest pain without another apparent cause. Other signs to look for include chest wall tenderness, back pain, shoulder pain, upper abdominal pain, hemoptysis, painful respiration, and new-onset of wheezing. PE is a frequent consideration in emergency departments. Rule-out criteria where the prevalence is low including patient age <50 years, heart rate <100 bpm, oxyhemoglobin saturation $>95\%$. There is no hemoptysis, estrogen use, prior deep venous thrombosis or PE, unilateral leg swelling, surgery, or trauma requiring hospitalization within last 4 weeks.

➤ Diagnostic Findings

- Pulmonary angiography: The "gold standard" in the diagnosis of PE. CT pulmonary angiography (CT-PA) is being used increasingly as a diagnostic modality in patients suspected of PE, and its accuracy appears to vary widely from institution to institution. This may be due to differences in the experience of the person interpreting images and image quality. Clinicians should consider their institution's experience and the pretest probability of PE when deciding whether to use CT-PA or to pursue additional testing.
- Chest x-rays: May be normal; suggestive findings include elevated diaphragm, pleural effusion, dilation of pulmonary artery, abrupt vessel cut-off, and atelectasis. Seventy percent of the patients with acute PE will have ECG abnormalities, most commonly nonspecific ST-segment and T-wave changes.
- ABG and pulse oximetry: Have a limited role in the diagnosis. ABGs usually reveal hypoxemia, hypocapnia, and respiratory alkalosis. Room air pulse oximetry readings of $<95\%$ at the time of diagnosis are at increased risk of in-hospital complications.
- Core laboratory: BNP or NT-proBNP levels of higher in patients with PE and appear to correlate with increased risk of complications and prolonged hospitalizations in these patients. Thirty percent to 50% of patients have also have elevated troponin I or T and they are not useful for diagnosis. Leukocytosis, increased ESR, and elevated LDH or AST with normal serum bilirubin are commonly observed.
- D-Dimer assays: Diagnosis of PE has been studied extensively. These assays have good sensitivity (95%) and negative predictive value, but poor specificity (40–68%) and positive predictive value. D-Dimer levels of <500 ng/mL are sufficient to exclude PE in patients with a low or moderate pretest probability of PE.

➤ Suggested Readings

Kruip, MJ, Leclercq, MG, van der Heul C, et al. Diagnostic strategies for excluding pulmonary embolism in clinical outcome studies. A systematic review. *Ann Intern Med.* 2003;138:941.

Roy, PM, Colombet, I, Durieux, P, et al. Systematic review and meta-analysis of strategies for the diagnosis of suspected pulmonary embolism. *BMJ.* 2005;331:259.

Wolf, SJ, McCubbin, TR, Nordenholz, KE, et al. Assessment of the pulmonary embolism rule-out criteria rule for evaluation of suspected pulmonary embolism in the emergency department. *Am J Emerg Med.* 2008;26:181.

DRUG-INDUCED PULMONARY DISEASES

➤ Definition
- Drug-induced pulmonary disease (DIPD) represents a heterogeneous group of disorders, a common clinical problem in which a patient without previous pulmonary disease develops respiratory symptoms, chest x-ray changes, deterioration of pulmonary function, histologic changes, or several of these findings in association with drug therapy. More than 150 drugs or categories of drugs have been reported to cause pulmonary disease; the mechanism is rarely known.
- Depending on the drug, drug-induced syndromes can produce asthma, bronchiolitis, hypersensitivity infiltrate, interstitial fibrosis, organizing pneumonia, asthma, noncardiogenic pulmonary edema, pleural effusions, pulmonary eosinophilia, pulmonary hemorrhage, or veno-occlusive disease. DIPDs can present a variety of clinical presentations and radiographic patterns. A good resource for details on different DIPDs and their clinical and radiographic presentation is available at www.pneumotox.com.
- Causal drugs
  - In cardiovascular drugs, Amiodarone is a classic example that caused pulmonary toxicity. In 3–20% patients, ACE inhibitors induce a dry, persistent, and often nocturnal cough that may require discontinuation of the drug.
  - Among anti-inflammatory agents, aspirin triad characterized by asthma, nasal polyposis, and drug sensitivity.
  - Many chemotherapeutic and immunosuppressive drugs including bleomycin, mitomycin-C, busulfan, cyclophosphamide, and nitrosourea drugs are implicated.

➤ Who Should be Suspected?
- Many types of lung injury can result from medications, and it is often impossible to predict who will develop lung disease resulting from a medication or drug. Symptoms may vary from patient to patient. The most common symptoms include cough, wheezing, shortness of breath, chest pain, bloody sputum, and fever. Many drugs can induce alveolar inflammation, interstitial inflammation, and/or interstitial fibrosis, resulting in lung dysfunction.

➤ Diagnostic Findings
There is no clear-cut laboratory or radiographic testing of the clinical syndromes associated with DIPD. The diagnosis is usually one of exclusion. Plain chest x-rays may miss or underestimate the presence of lung disease at the time of initial presentation. Diagnosis is based on observation of responses to withdrawal from and, if practical, reintroduction to the suspected drug. Echocardiography may rule out cardiac disease, sputum studies may rule out infectious diseases, and ANA or RF testing may be helpful in suspected cases of collagen vascular disease.
- Pulmonary Function: Testing is useful in assessing the toxicity.
- Hematology: CBC with differential can detect eosinophilia, which may suggest drug rash with eosinophilia and systemic symptoms (DRESS) syndrome.

➤ Suggested Readings

Bhadra K, Suratt BT. Drug induced lung diseases: A state of the art review. *J Respir Dis.* 2009;30:1.

Ozkan M, Dweik RA, Ahmad M. Drug induced lung disease. *Cleve Clin J Med.* 2001;68:782–795.

CHEMICAL PNEUMONITIS*

➤ Definition

* Aspiration pneumonia is inflammation of the lungs and bronchial tubes due to breathing in a foreign material.
* Aspiration pneumonitis (Mendelson syndrome) is a chemical injury caused by the inhalation of sterile gastric contents.

➤ Who Should be Suspected?

* A number of clinical features should raise the possibility of chemical pneumonitis: Abrupt onset of symptoms with prominent dyspnea; low-grade fever, cyanosis, and diffuse crackles on lung auscultation; severe hypoxemia; and infiltrates on chest x-ray involving dependent pulmonary segments.

➤ Laboratory Findings

* Chest x-ray: Changes are noted within 2 hours. Bronchoscopy shows erythema of bronchi indicating acid injury.
* Blood gas: Studies often show the partial pressure of oxygen is reduced to 35–50 mm Hg accompanied by a normal or low partial pressure of CO_2 with respiratory alkalosis.
* Pulmonary function tests (PFTs): Show decreased compliance, abnormal ventilation–perfusion, and reduced diffusing capacity.

CARCINOMA OF THE LUNG

➤ Definition

* The term *lung cancer*, or bronchogenic carcinoma, refers to malignancies that originate in the airways or pulmonary parenchyma. Lung cancer is the second most diagnosed cancer in men and women, but it is the number one cause of death from cancer. Eighty-seven percent of all lung cancers are smoking related. Exposure to second hand smoke also increases the risk of developing lung cancer. Other substances include asbestos, radon, radiation exposure, TB, industrial substances, pollutants also increases the risk. Family history/genetics also play a role in the development of cancer.
* Approximately 95% of all lung cancers are classified as either small cell lung cancer (SCLC) or non-small cell lung cancer (NSCLC). This distinction is essential for staging, treatment, and prognosis. Other cell types comprise about 5% of malignancies arising in the lung. NSCLC accounts for 80% and SCLC accounts for 20% of all total lung cancers identified. There are different types of NSCLC, including:
  * **Squamous cell carcinoma:** Most common type in men. Forms within the lining of bronchial tubes.

---

*Contributed by Mary Williamson PhD.

- **Adenocarcinoma:** Most common in women and nonsmokers. Found in the glands of lungs that produce mucus.
- **Bronchoalveolar carcinoma:** Rare subset of adenocarcinoma forms near lungs air sacs.
- **Large cell undifferentiated carcinoma:** Rapidly growing cancer forms near the surface or outer edges of the lungs.

➤ Who Should be Suspected?

- Heavy cigarette smokers who have new onset of cough, a change in the characteristics of a preexisting cough, and the presence of hemoptysis should be considered; cancer may be the cause of cough.
- Typical symptoms of lung cancer in the chest include persistent cough; pain in the chest, shoulder, or back unrelated to pain from coughing; a change in color or volume of sputum; shortness of breath, changes in the voice; harsh sounds with each breath; and recurrent lung problems such as bronchitis, pneumonia, and hemoptysis.

➤ Diagnostic Findings

- The diagnosis of lung cancer is primarily based on evaluation of individuals with symptoms. Screening for lung cancer is not widely used, since no screening test (chest radiography, sputum cytology, or CT) has been shown to reduce mortality from lung cancer.
- Diagnostic tests should include physical and chest examination, chest x-ray, CT, positron emission tomography (PET) and spiral CT scan, MRI, sputum cytology, bronchoscopy, and biopsy. Cytologic examination of spontaneously expected or induced sputum may provide a definitive diagnosis of lung cancer. Bronchoscopy is usually indicated when there is a suspicion of airway involvement by a malignancy.

➤ Suggested Readings

Bach, PB, Silvestri, GA, Hanger, M, et al. Screening for Lung Cancer. ACCP Evidence-Based Clinical Practice Guidelines. *Chest*. 2007;132:69S–77S.
Kvale P. Chronic cough due to lung tumors. *Chest*. 2006;129:147S–153S.
Rivera, M, Detterbeck, F, and Mehta, AC. Diagnosis of lung cancer, the guidelines. *Chest*. 2003;123:129S–136S.

EVALUATION OF PLEURAL EFFUSIONS

➤ Definition

- Pleural effusion is defined as increased amount of fluid in the pleural cavity. The primary goal is to distinguish exudates (e.g., infections, malignant, drug reactions) from transudates (e.g., CHF, cirrhosis, atelectasis, nephritic syndrome). The underlying cause of an effusion is usually determined by first classifying the fluid as an exudate or a transudate.
  - Exudates are fluids, cells, or other cellular substances that are slowly discharged from blood vessels, usually from inflamed tissues.
  - Transudates are fluids that pass through a membrane or squeeze through tissue or into the extracellular space of tissues. Transudates are thin and watery and contain few cells or proteins.
- It is clinically important to classify pleural and ascitic fluids into exudates and transudates because this is indicative of the underlying pathophysiologic process involved (Figure 14-1). A transudate does not usually require additional testing, but exudates always do.

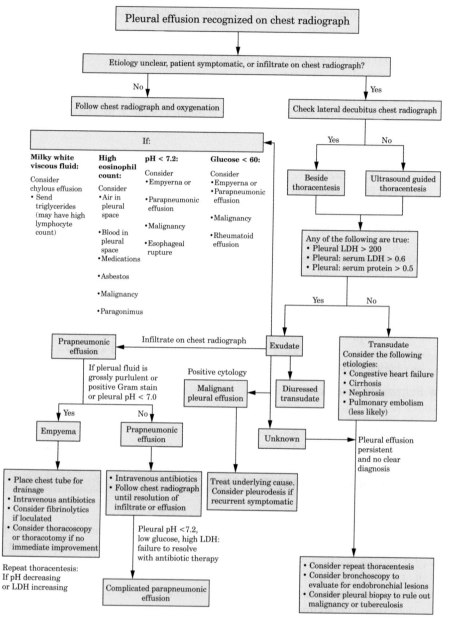

Figure 14-1. Algorithm for the workup of patients with pleural effusion. LDH = lactate dehydrogenase.

Transudate

* Causes
  * CHF (causes 15% of cases); acute diuresis can result in pseudoexudate
  * Cirrhosis with ascites (pleural effusion in ~5% of cases)—rare without ascites
  * Nephrotic syndrome
  * Early (acute) atelectasis
  * PE
  * Superior vena cava obstruction
  * Hypoalbuminemia
  * Peritoneal dialysis—occurs within 48 hours of initiating dialysis
  * Early mediastinal malignancy
  * Misplaced subclavian catheter
  * Myxedema (rare cause)
  * Constrictive pericarditis—effusion is bilateral
  * Urinothorax—due to ipsilateral GU tract obstruction

Exudate

* Pneumonia, malignancy, pulmonary embolism, and gastrointestinal conditions (especially pancreatitis and abdominal surgery) cause 90% of all exudates. The cause is unknown in ~10–15% of all exudates.
* Causes
  * Infection (25% of cases): bacterial pneumonia; parapneumonic effusion (empyema); TB; abscess (subphrenic, liver, spleen); viral, mycoplasmal, rickettsial; parasitic (ameba, hydatid cyst, filaria); fungal effusion (*Coccidioides, Cryptococcus, Histoplasma, Blastomyces, Aspergillus*; in immunocompromised hosts: *Aspergillus, Candida, Mucor*)
  * PE/infarction
  * Neoplasms (metastatic carcinoma, especially breast, ovary, and lung; lymphoma; leukemia; mesothelioma; pleural endometriosis) (42% of cases)
  * Trauma (penetrating or blunt): hemothorax, chylothorax, empyema, associated with rupture of diaphragm
  * Immunologic mechanisms: rheumatoid pleurisy (5% of cases), SLE; other collagen vascular diseases occasionally cause effusions (e.g., Wegener granulomatosis, Sjögren syndrome, familial Mediterranean fever, Churg-Strauss syndrome, mixed connective tissue disease); following myocardial infarction or cardiac surgery; vasculitis; hepatitis; sarcoidosis (rare cause; may also be transudate); familial recurrent polyserositis; drug reaction (e.g., nitrofurantoin hypersensitivity, methysergide)
  * Chemical mechanisms: uremic. pancreatic (pleural effusion occurs in ~10% of these cases), esophageal rupture (high salivary amylase and pH <7.30 that approaches 6.00 in 48–72 hours), subphrenic abscess
  * Lymphatic abnormality (e.g., irradiation, Milroy disease)
  * Injury (e.g., asbestosis)
  * Altered pleural mechanics (e.g., late [chronic] atelectasis)
  * Endocrine (e.g., hypothyroidism)
  * Movement of fluid from abdomen to pleural space: Meigs syndrome (protein and specific gravity are often at transudate–exudate border but usually not transudate), urinothorax, cancer, pancreatitis, pancreatic pseudocyst

- Cirrhosis, pulmonary infarct, trauma, and connective tissue diseases are responsible for ~9% of all cases.

Exudates That Can Present As Transudates

- Causes
  - PE (>20% of cases)—caused by atelectasis
  - Hypothyroidism—caused by myxedema heart disease
  - Malignancy—because of complications (e.g., atelectasis, lymphatic obstruction)
  - Sarcoidosis—stages II and III
- Location
  - Typically left-sided: Ruptured esophagus, acute pancreatitis, rheumatoid arthritis Pericardial disease is left-sided or bilateral; it is rarely exclusively right-sided
  - Typically right-sided or bilateral: CHF (if only on left, consider that right pleural space may be obliterated or patient has another process [e.g., pulmonary infarction]).
  - Typically right-sided: rupture of amebic liver abscess
- Gross appearance
  - Clear, straw-colored fluid is typical of transudate.
  - Turbidity (cloudy, opaque appearance) may be caused by lipids or increased WBCs; after centrifugation, a clear supernatant indicates WBCs or debris as the cause; clear or white supernatant is caused by chylomicrons.
  - Red indicates blood; brown indicates blood has been present for a longer time. RBC count of 5000 to 10,000/µL causes a blood-tinged color. If grossly bloody, Hct >50% of peripheral Hct indicates a hemothorax.
  - Bloody fluid suggests malignancy, pulmonary infarct, trauma, postcardiotomy syndrome; also uremia, asbestos, pleural endometriosis. Bloody fluid from traumatic thoracentesis should clot within several minutes, but blood present more than several hours will have become defibrinated and does not form a good clot. Nonuniform color during aspiration and absence of hemosiderin-laden macrophages also suggest traumatic aspiration. Absent of platelets suggests that the condition is not caused by traumatic thoracentesis.
  - White fluid suggests chylothorax, cholesterol effusion, or empyema.
  - Chylous (milky) is usually due to trauma (e.g., auto accident, postoperative) but may be obstruction of duct (e.g., especially lymphoma; metastatic carcinoma, granulomas) or parenteral nutrition via a central line with perforation of superior vena cava.
  - After centrifugation, supernatant is clear in empyema but cloudy or turbid in chylous effusion caused by chylomicrons, which also stain with Sudan III.
  - Pleural fluid triglycerides >110 mg/dL or triglyceride pleural fluid-to-serum ratio >2 occurs only in chylous effusion (seen especially within a few hours after eating). Triglycerides <50 mg/dL excludes chylothorax. Equivocal triglyceride levels (50–10 mg/dL) may require a lipoprotein electrophoresis of fluid to demonstrate chylomicrons, which are diagnostic of chylothorax.
  - Pseudochylous (may have lustrous sheen) appearance in chronic inflammatory conditions (e.g., rheumatoid pleurisy, TB, chronic pneumothorax therapy) is caused by either cholesterol crystals (rhomboid-shaped) in sediment or lipid-containing inclusions in leukocytes. Distinguish from chylous effusions by microscopy. Chylomicrons ≤50 mg/dL with cholesterol >250 mg/dL occurs in pseudochylous effusions.

- Black fluid suggests *Aspergillus niger* infection.
- Greenish fluid suggests biliopleural fistula.
- Purulent fluid indicates infection.
- Anchovy (dark red-brown) color is seen in amebiasis, old blood. Anchovy paste in ruptured amebic liver abscess; amebas found in <10%.
- Turbid and greenish-yellow fluid is classic for rheumatoid effusion.
- Very viscous (clear or bloody) is characteristic of mesothelioma; also in pyothorax.
- Debris in fluid suggests rheumatoid pleurisy; food particles indicate esophageal rupture.
- Color of enteral tube food or central venous line infusion due to tube or catheter entering pleural space.

Odor
- Putrid due to anaerobic empyema.
- Ammonia due to urinothorax.

Protein, Albumin, Lactate Dehydrogenase
- When exudate criteria are met by LD but not by protein, consider malignancy and parapneumonic effusions.
- Very high pleural fluid LD (>1000 IU/L) occurs in empyema, rheumatoid pleurisy, paragonimiasis; sometimes with malignancy; rarely with TB. Level indicates degree of pleural inflammation; increasing values suggest need for more aggressive therapy. Measurement of LD isoenzymes is said to have limited value.

Glucose
- Transudate has same concentration as serum.
- Usually normal but 30–55 mg/dL or pleural fluid-to-serum ratio <0.5 and pH <7.30 may be found in TB, malignancy, SLE; also esophageal rupture; lowest levels may occur in empyema and RA. Therefore, only helpful if very low level (e.g., <30). A level of 0–10 mg/dL is highly suspicious for RA. Poor prognostic sign in pneumonia. In neoplasm, lower glucose indicates greater tumor burden. Rarely found in SLE, Churg-Strauss, urinothorax, hemothorax, or paragonimiasis.

pH
- Normal pleural fluid pH is alkaline (7.60–7.66). Transudative effusions have a pH range of about 7.45–7.55 and most exudates have a pH of 7.30–7.45.
- Low pH (<7.30) always means exudate, especially empyema, malignancy, rheumatoid pleurisy, SLE, TB, esophageal rupture; may also be caused by systemic acidosis, hemothorax, urinothorax, paragonimiasis.
- pH <6.0 is consistent with but not diagnostic of esophageal rupture.
- Collagen vascular disease is the only other cause of pH <7.0.
- In a parapneumonic effusion, a pH <7.20 indicates need for tube drainage; pH >7.30 suggests that resolution with only medical therapy is possible. A pH <7.0 indicates the presence of complicated parapneumonic effusion.
- pH may fall before glucose becomes decreased.
- *Proteus* infection may increase pH because of urea splitting.
- In a malignant effusion, pH <7.30 is associated with short survival time, poorer prognosis, and increased positive yield with cytology and pleural biopsy; tends to correlate with pleural fluid glucose <60 mg/dL.

Generally, low pH is associated with low glucose and high LD; if low pH with normal glucose and low LD, the pH is probably a lab error.

Amylase

- Increased pleural fluid-to-serum ratio >1.0 and may be >5 or pleural fluid ULN for serum; should be determined only for left pleural effusions.
- Acute pancreatitis—may be normal early with increase over time
- Pancreatic pseudocyst—always increased, may be >1000 IU/L
- Also perforated esophageal rupture, peptic ulcer, necrosis of small intestine (e.g., mesenteric vascular occlusion); 10% of cases of metastatic cancer
- Isoenzyme studies
  - Pancreatic type of amylase in acute pancreatitis and pancreatic pseudocyst
  - Salivary type of amylase is found in esophageal rupture and occasionally in carcinoma of ovary or lung or salivary gland tumor
- Other chemical determinations
  - C-reactive protein ranged from 10–20 mg/dL in transudates compared to 30–40 mg/dL in exudates in one small study. Parapneumonic effusions were highest (89 ± 16 mg/dL). The pleural fluid-to-serum ratio was 0.8 ± 0.5 mg/dL in transudates and 2.8 ± 0.7 mg/dL in exudates.
  - Cholesterol and triglycerides
  - Routine tumor markers (e.g., CEA, cancer antigen-125, acid phosphatase in prostate cancer, hyaluronic acid in mesothelioma) are not generally recommended. CEA >10 ng/mL is suggestive but not diagnostic of malignant pleural fluid; usually <10 ng/mL in lymphomas, sarcomas, mesotheliomas.
- Immune complexes (measured by Raji cell, C1q component, radioimmunoassay, etc.) are often found in exudates due to collagen vascular diseases (SLE, RA). LA tests show frequent false-positive results and should not be ordered. Occasionally, LA for bacterial antigens is useful.

DISEASES OF THE NOSE AND THROAT

ALLERGIC RHINITIS

➤ Definition

- Rhinitis can be defined as symptoms of nasal irritation, sneezing, rhinorrhea and nasal blockage lasting for at least 1 hour a day on most days. It occurs mostly in patients aged 15–25 years.
- Allergic rhinitis, one of the rhinitis syndromes, can be seasonal or perennial. In allergic rhinitis, there is usually a clear relationship with exposure to known allergens—most frequently to pollens in seasonal rhinitis and house dust mites or household pets in perennial rhinitis. In general, allergic rhinitis can result in either inflammatory or noninflammatory causes. Many patients with allergic rhinitis have a nonallergic contribution (mixed rhinitis). Underlying causes of nonallergic rhinitis include vasomotor rhinitis, rhinitis medicamentosa, nonallergic rhinitis with nasal eosinophilia syndrome, and miscellaneous other disorders.

➤ Who Should be Suspected?

- Typical patient presentation includes nasal irritation, sneezing, rhinorrhea, and nasal blockage, symptoms that may be seasonal or perennial. The dominant symptoms may differ from one patient to another. There is also a wide individual variation in terms of tolerability of nasal symptoms. Conjunctival symptoms of itching and increase in tear fluid are also very common in association with allergic rhinitis.

➤ Diagnostic Findings

The diagnosis of rhinitis in a patient complaining of upper airway problems consists of obtaining a detailed history and performing physical examination supplemented by critical tests.

- Hematology: High numbers indicate that atopy is present. The usefulness of eosinophilia and determination of total IgE is limited in the diagnosis of allergic rhinitis, because to some degree they are dependent on the size of the organ.
- Allergen-specific testing. The use of diagnostic testing to identify culprit allergens has been associated with improved patient outcomes.
- Skin testing: When carefully performed by well trained individual, immediate hypersensitive skin testing (skin prick tests [SPTs]) is a safe way to identify the presence of allergen specific IgE. Skin testing is useful among patients with:
  - Unclear diagnosis based on the history and physical examination.
  - Poorly controlled symptoms, such as persistent nasal symptoms and/or an inadequate clinical response to nasal glucocorticoids.
  - Coexisting persistent asthma and/or recurrent sinusitis/otitis.
  - Occupational rhinitis.
- Serum tests for allergy. Serum immunoassays for specific IgE antibodies are better alternates to SPTs for screening. These specific IgE tests are useful for testing specific allergens that are not available for skin tests or when skin tests cannot be performed because a patient is taking treatment (e.g., histamine) that suppresses the cutaneous response.
- Allergen challenge tests: A nasal challenge can be used to test specific as well as nonspecific reactivity. It is clinically impractical and rarely performed.
- Other tests: Nasal cytology is performed by some to help differentiate rhinitis due to allergy from that due to infection. Wright stain of nasal secretions usually, but not always, reveals predominance of eosinophils in cases of allergic rhinitis. The presence of neutrophils suggests an infectious process. Other diagnostic testing assays, cytotoxic testing, provocation neutralization testing, and specific or nonspecific IgG determinations are unproven and inappropriate.

➤ Suggested Readings

Ng ML, Warlow RS, Chrishanthan N, et al. Preliminary criteria for the definition of allergic rhinitis: A systemic evaluation of clinical parameters in a disease cohort (I). *Clin Exp Allergy.* 2000;30:1314.

Ng ML, Warlow RS, Chrishanthan N, et al. Preliminary criteria for the definition of allergic rhinitis: A systemic evaluation of clinical parameters in a disease cohort (II). *Clin Exp Allergy.* 2000;30:1417.

THE "COMMON COLD"

➤ Definition

- This infection of ciliated epithelial cells in nasal mucosa results in nasal discharge due to the inflammatory process.

- It is most commonly the result of rhinovirus infection. Other viruses may cause rhinitis, including coronavirus, parainfluenza, adenovirus, enterovirus, influenza, and respiratory syncytial virus.

➤ Who Should be Suspected?
- Symptoms are typically mild, including nasal congestion, rhinitis and sneezing. Fever, headache, cough, sore throat and malaise, if present, are usually mild.
- Symptoms usually resolve within 7 to 10 days.
- The incidence of colds peaks in colder months, typically between September and March.
- Purulent nasal discharge, otitis, high fever or other severe systemic symptoms suggest complication of infection or a different cause of infection, like influenza.

➤ Laboratory Findings
- Specific diagnostic testing is rarely needed, but may be attempted for severe or complicated infection. Nasopharyngeal swabs or washings are recommended for diagnostic testing, if indicated.
- Direct Antigen Testing: Available for several viral pathogens, including influenza viruses and RSV.
- Viral Culture: High sensitivity for correctly collected and transported specimens.
- Molecular Tests: Available for detection of a very broad range of viral respiratory tract pathogens.
- Serology: Not useful

PHARYNGITIS

➤ Definition
- Acute pharyngitis, inflammation of the posterior pharyngeal and tonsillar tissues, is a common clinical complaint, especially in children. Most episodes of acute pharyngitis are relatively mild, self-limited infectious diseases, caused by common upper respiratory tract pathogens. The etiology varies somewhat by the age of the patient and season. In general, however, viral infection is the most common cause of acute pharyngitis, both in children and adults. Detection of group A beta-hemolytic streptococcus (S. pyogenes) is the focus of most diagnostic testing, however, because of the risk of post-streptococcal acute RF and GN. Specific diagnosis may also guide the appropriate use, or nonuse, of antibiotics.
- Acute pharyngitis must be distinguished from other serious infections of the head and neck, like epiglottitis, peritonsillar abscess, and submandibular abscess. Severe symptoms and sepsis, difficulty swallowing and drooling, neck swelling and other signs suggest other sites of primary infection or local, suppurative complications of bacterial pharyngitis.

➤ Causes
Viral Disease
- Acute respiratory infection is the cause of significant morbidity and mortality throughout the world. Viruses are the cause of most of these infections, and children are primarily affected. There is a clear seasonal pattern for most of the viral pathogens, especially in temperate climates where incidence peaks during the winter months. There may be differences

in clinical presentations depending on the agent, age of the patient, underlying health, and other factors.

- Most nasopharyngeal viral infections present as the "common cold", manifested by mild symptoms like rhinitis, nasal congestion, sneezing, and runny nose. Mild pharyngitis and "ticklish" cough may be reported. Fever, headache, and malaise, if present, are usually mild. Most upper respiratory tract viral infections resolve completely after 7–10 days. Complications are uncommon, including otitis media, sinusitis, and exacerbations of chronic pulmonary disease.
- Specific diagnosis of viral pharyngitis or upper respiratory tract infection is rarely needed; most patients can be managed symptomatically on the basis of clinical presentation. When indicated, specific diagnosis may be pursued by virus culture, or more commonly, by molecular diagnostic testing using a respiratory virus panel. Serologic diagnostic testing is not useful.
- The common viral causes of primary pharyngitis include: Adenovirus, Enterovirus, Rhinoviruses, HSV, EBV, CMV, Influenza, and Parainfluenza viruses.

Bacterial Disease

- Group A beta-hemolytic streptococcus (GAS): GAS causes infection in a significant minority (10–30%) of patients seeking medical attention for acute pharyngitis. Most infections have an acute onset of sore throat with erythema of the tonsillar and posterior pharyngeal mucosa and exudate. Fever, headache, and abdominal pain are commonly reported. Physical examination often shows enlarged, tender anterior cervical lymph nodes, petechiae of the palate, and uvular inflammation. Conjunctivitis, rhinorrhea, cough, and sneezing are uncommon symptoms and suggest another pathogen.
- Scarlet fever may complicate "strep throat" and is characterized by formation of a typical "scarlatiniforme" rash in the first or second day of fever. The rash is characterized as fine, rough-textured (sandpaper), blanching and worse in the armpits and skinfolds. The rash resolves after several days, followed by desquamation. A bright red, "strawberry" tongue may be obvious.

➤ Who Should be Suspected?

- Various criteria have been recommended for predicting the probability of GAS infection and need for antibiotic treatment. They have generally shown better negative than positive predictive value. For children, the following criteria have been recommended. With six criteria, the probability of a culture positive for GAS = 75%; the probability falls to 59% if only 5 criteria are met:
  - Age: 5–15 years
  - Season: late fall, winter, or early spring
  - Pharyngeal erythema, edema, and/or exudates
  - Anterior lymph nodes: tender, enlarged
  - Temperature: 101–103°F
  - No typical viral upper respiratory signs and symptoms
- For adults, the Centor criteria for adults are listed below. The probability of GAS infection increases with the number of criteria present: the presence of three or four is reported to have a positive predictive value up to 60%; the presence of 0 or 1 is reported to have a negative predictive value of 80%.
  - Tonsillar exudates
  - Tender anterior cervical adenopathy
  - Fever or fever history
  - Absence of cough

➤ Diagnosis

- Culture: Throat culture is the "gold standard" for diagnosis of pharyngitis due to GAS, with sensitivity in the 90–95% range. The specificity is very high in patients with acute pharyngitis, but "false positive" cultures, in terms of active disease, may be seen in chronic GAS carriers or after recent, successful therapy. Cultures for "test of cure" are not recommended, except for patients at very high risk for acute rheumatic fever.
- Direct Antigen Detection: Direct antigen tests are also available for rapid detection of GAS; however, these assays are not as sensitive as throat cultures. The sensitivity of antigen tests vary by technique and specific kit used, ranging from 60% to 95%; the specificity of most tests exceed 95%. Therefore, throat culture should be performed to confirm negative antigen tests but are not needed to confirm positive tests.
- Molecular Tests: An FDA approved molecular diagnostic assay is available for the detection of *S. pyogenes* in pharyngeal specimens. Sensitivity of the assay is 88% to 95% with specificity of 98% to 99.7%. The high sensitivity and specificity for this test allow test results to stand without the need for confirmation of positive or negative tests.

DIPHTHERIA

➤ Definition

- Diphtheria is caused by infection with *Corynebacterium diphtheriae* a pleomorphic gram-positive rod that produces an exotoxin. Most patients present respiratory or cutaneous disease.
- Diphtheria has a global distribution, primarily affecting unvaccinated individuals in underdeveloped, economically disadvantaged areas. Humans are the only known reservoir for *C. diphtheriae*, and transmission is mediated by contact with respiratory droplets or secretions from patients with actively infectious mucous membrane or cutaneous lesions. Disease usually occurs within 1 week after infectious contact. The lesions in untreated patients may infectious for up to 6 weeks; treated patients become noninfectious within days.
- Diphtheria is a national notifiable disease, reportable to the CDC and local departments of public health.

➤ Who Should be Suspected?

- Diphtheria usually presents as respiratory disease. The common presentation of respiratory disease is pseudomembranous pharyngitis, with formation of a gray membrane of necrotic material in the tonsillar area, which may extend to adjacent posterior pharyngeal surfaces. Patients often complain of sore throat and difficulty swallowing. There is a risk of dislodgement, with respiratory obstruction, in patients with extensive pseudomembrane formation. The underlying mucosa is friable and edematous. Local adenopathy and tissue edema (bull neck) may occur. Low-grade fever, malaise, or other nonspecific symptoms are common.
- Serious complications may develop due to the effect of exotoxin on other organ systems, usually myocarditis or neuropathy.
  - Myocarditis, usually presenting in the second week of infection, may be asymptomatic, but conduction defects and arrhythmias may be serious.

• Neuropathy may present as an early or late complication of infection. Cranial nerve palsy and local neuropathy are common early complications, whereas ocular palsy and limb or diaphragmatic paralysis are late complications.

➤ Laboratory Findings
• Culture: Provides the definitive diagnosis of acute diphtheria. For respiratory diphtheria, collect swabs from the nasopharynx and throat, including the edges of the pseudomembrane. Alert the laboratory prior to submitting specimens to ensure that appropriate media are available. Specimens are planted on selective-differential media, like modified Tinsdale and Loeffler's media, in addition to routine culture medium. C. diphtheriae isolates must be tested for exotoxin production using the modified Elek immunodiffusion method. Culture from involved area is positive within 12 hours on Löffler's medium (more slowly on blood agar) (toxin-producing strain). Nasopharyngeal cultures should always be obtained when diphtheria is suspected. If there has been prior antibiotic therapy, culture may be negative or take several days to grow. Note: Corynebacterium ulcerans may cause diphtheria.
• Nucleic acid amplification: Tests have been developed both for detection/identification of C. diphtheriae as well as the gene responsible for exotoxin production.
• Core Laboratory: Troponin and other cardiac markers may be used to identify asymptomatic cardiac disease or assess prognosis in patients with overt myocarditis. Decreased serum glucose may be seen. Albumin and casts are frequently present in urine; blood is rarely found.
• Hematology: WBC may be moderately increased ($\leq$15,000/μL). Moderate anemia is common.
• Serology (EIA): Not useful for diagnosis of acute infection, but may be used for epidemiologic studies. Diphtheria antibody testing may also be used to assess immune function by comparing pre- and postvaccination sera.

➤ Suggested Readings
http://wwwnc.cdc.gov/travel/yellowbook/2010/chapter-2/diphtheria.aspx

Bisno AL. Acute pharyngitis. N Engl J Med. 2001;344:205–211.

Coyle MB, Lipsky BA. Coryneform bacteria in infectious diseases: Clinical and laboratory aspects. Clin Microbiol Rev. 1990;3:227–246.

Kneen R, Dung NM, Hoa NTT, et al. Clinical features and predictors of diphtheritic cardiomyopathy in Vietnamese children. Clin Infect Dis. 2004;39:1591–1598.

ACID-BASE DISORDERS

➤ Definition
• Acid-base balance disorders are usually encountered in acutely ill or complicated medical and surgical patients. The plasma concentration of hydrogen ion (pH$^+$) is very low (~40 nmol/L) and it is constantly maintained within a narrow range by:
  • Excretion of CO_2 by lungs
  • Excretion of H$^+$ by kidneys
• Every day approximately 15,000 mmol of CO_2 is produced by endogenous metabolism and then excreted by lungs. Similarly normal diet generates 50–100 mmol of H$^+$ per day, derived

mostly from metabolism of sulphur-containing amino acids. The maintenance of stable H^+ level is required for normal cellular function, since small fluctuations in the H^+ concentrations have important effects on the activity of cellular enzymes. There is a relatively narrow range of extracellular H^+ concentration (16–160 nmol/L: pH 7.8–6.8), that is compatible with life. Changes in H^+ are nonlinear; hence measuring pH masks the magnitude of acid-base disorders.

BUFFER SYSTEMS (BICARBONATE-CARBONIC ACID)

* This buffer is at highest concentration in the blood, and it is also plays an important role in acid-base regulation. Carbonic acid (CO_2) is a volatile acidic gas and is soluble in water. It readily diffuses from cells to blood, where it combines with water to produce carbonic acid, which immediately dissociates in to bicarbonate and hydrogen ions.
* pH, HCO_3^-, and pCO_2 are related by the equation:

$$pH = pK - [HCO_3^- / (0.03 \times pCO_2)]$$

where pK is defined as the pH at which HCO_3^- and H_2CO_3 (0.03% pCO_2) are in equal concentrations.

* Normal concentrations of HCO_3^- and H_2CO_3 in the blood are in the ratio of 20:1 and with a pK of 6.1. This excess base HCO_3^-, along with volatility of CO_2, gives ability to prevent overaccumulation of acid. The lungs through the loss of CO_2 provide the ultimate buffering capacity. Bicarbonate is regulated by the kidneys and CO_2 is regulated by lungs and the ratio of HCO_3^- to H_2CO_3 that determines the pH.
* Laboratories measure pH and pCO_2 directly and calculate HCO_3 using the Henderson-Hasselbalch equation:

$$\text{Arterial pH} = 6.1 + \log[(HCO_3) + (0.03 \times pCO_2)],$$

where 6.1 is the dissociation constant for CO_2 in aqueous solution and 0.03 is a constant for the solubility of CO_2 in plasma at 37°C.

RESPIRATORY AND METABOLIC SYSTEMS IN ACID-BASE REGULATION

➤ Respiratory System

* Arterial CO_2 is influenced by ventilatory rate, pCO_2 is considered the respiratory component of the bicarbonate-CO_2 buffer system. Because CO_2 is the end product of aerobic metabolism, continuous buffering CO_2 is required for the regulation of pH.
* The arterial pCO_2 represents a balance between tissue production of CO_2 and pulmonary removal of CO_2. An elevated pCO_2 usually indicates hyperventilation. This leads to respiratory acidosis (hypoventilation) or respiratory alkalosis (hyperventilation).
* The respiratory rate can alter arterial pH in minutes.

➤ Metabolic (Renal) System

* When H^+ levels deviated from normal, the kidneys respond by reabsorbing or secreting hydrogen, bicarbonate, and other ions to regulate the blood pH. Metabolic acidosis may

TABLE 14-2. Metabolic and Respiratory Acid-Base Changes in Blood

	pH	pCO$_2$	HCO$_3^-$
Acidosis			
Acute metabolic	D	N	D
Compensated metabolic	N	D	D
Acute respiratory	D	I	N
Compensated respiratory	N	I	I
Alkalosis			
Acute metabolic	I	N	I
Chronic metabolic	I	I	I
Acute respiratory	I	D	N
Compensated respiratory	N	D	D

D = decreased; I = increased; N = normal.

develop; either H$^+$ accumulates or bicarbonate ions are lost. Metabolic alkalosis may develop from either loss of H$^+$ or increase in bicarbonate.

* Unlike the respiratory system, the renal system requires hours to days to significantly affect pH by altering the excretion of bicarbonate.

ANALYZING ACID-BASE DISORDERS (TABLE 14-2)

* When analyzing acid-base disorders, several points should be kept in mind:
* Determination of pH and blood gases should be performed preferentially on arterial blood. Venous blood is useless for judging oxygenation or if perfusion is not adequate, but it offers an estimate of acid-base status. Venous pH is ~0.03 to 0.04 lower than in arterial blood, and CO$_2$ pressure (pCO$_2$) is normally ~3 to 4 mm higher.
* Blood specimens should be packed in ice immediately; a delay of even a few minutes will cause erroneous results, especially if the WBC count is high.
* Determination of electrolytes, pH, and blood gases should be performed on blood specimens obtained simultaneously, since the acid-base situation may be very labile (Table 14-3).
* Repeated determinations are often indicated because of the development of complications, the effect of therapy, and other factors.
* Acid-base disorders are often mixed rather than in the pure form. These mixed disorders may represent simultaneously occurring diseases, complications superimposed on the primary condition, or the effect of treatment.
* Changes in chronic forms may be notably different from those in the acute forms.
* For judging hypoxemia, it is also necessary to know the patient's Hb or Hct and whether the patient was breathing room air or oxygen when the specimen was drawn.
* ABGs cannot be interpreted without clinical information about the patient.
* Renal compensation for a respiratory disturbance is slower (3–7 days) but more successful than respiratory compensation for a metabolic disturbance, but it cannot completely compensate for arterial CO$_2$ pressure (PaCO$_2$) >65 mm Hg, unless another stimulus for HCO$_3$

TABLE 14-3. Illustrative Serum Electrolyte Values in Various Conditions

Condition	pH	HCO_3^- (mEq/L)	Potassium (mEq/L)	Sodium (mEq/L)	Chloride (mEq/L)
Normal	7.35–7.45	24–26	3.5–5.0	136–145	100–106
Metabolic acidosis					
Diabetic acidosis	7.2	10	5.6	122	80
Fasting	7.2	16	5.2	142	100
Severe diarrhea	7.2	12	3.2	128	96
Hyperchloremic acidosis	7.2	12	5.2	142	116
Addison's disease	7.2	22	6.5	111	72
Nephritis	7.2	8	4.0	129	90
Nephrosis	7.2	20	5.5	138	113
Metabolic alkalosis					
Vomiting	7.6	38	3.2	150	94
Pyloric obstruction	7.6	58	3.2	132	42
Duodenal obstruction	7.6	42	3.2	138	49
Respiratory acidosis	7.1	30	5.5	142	80
Respiratory alkalosis	7.6	14	5.5	136	112

retention is present. The respiratory mechanism responds quickly but can only eliminate sufficient CO_2 to balance the mildest metabolic acidosis (Table 14-4).

- A normal pH does not ensure the absence of an acid-base disturbance if the pCO_2 is not known.
- An abnormal HCO_3 indicates a metabolic rather than a respiratory problem (Table 14-5; Figures 14-2 and 14-3).
- Decreased HCO_3^- indicates metabolic acidosis.
- Increased HCO_3^- indicates metabolic alkalosis.
- Respiratory acidosis is associated with a $pCO_2 > 45$ mm Hg.
- Respiratory alkalosis is associated with a $pCO_2 < 35$ mm Hg.
- Therefore, mixed metabolic and respiratory acidosis is characterized by low pH, low HCO_3^-, and high pCO_2.
- Mixed metabolic and respiratory alkalosis is characterized by high pH, high HCO_3^-, and low pCO_2.
- In severe metabolic acidosis, respiratory compensation is limited by inability to hyperventilate pCO_2 to less than ~15 mm Hg; beyond that, small increments of the H^+ ion produce disastrous changes in pH and prognosis; therefore, patients with lung disorders (e.g., COPD, neuromuscular weakness) are very vulnerable because they cannot compensate by hyperventilation. In metabolic alkalosis, respiratory compensation is limited by CO_2 retention, which rarely causes $pCO_2 > 50$–60 mm Hg (because increased CO_2

TABLE 14-4. Summary of Pure and Mixed Acid-Base Disorders

	Decreased pH	Normal pH	Increased pH
Increased pCO_2	Respiratory acidosis with or without incompletely compensated metabolic alkalosis or coexisting metabolic acidosis	Respiratory acidosis and compensated metabolic alkalosis	Metabolic alkalosis with incompletely compensated respiratory acidosis or coexisting respiratory acidosis
Normal pCO_2	Metabolic acidosis	Normal	Metabolic alkalosis
Decreased pCO_2	Metabolic acidosis with incompletely compensated respiratory alkalosis or coexisting respiratory alkalosis	Respiratory alkalosis and compensated metabolic acidosis	Respiratory alkalosis with or without incompletely compensated metabolic acidosis or coexisting metabolic alkalosis

Source: Adapted from Friedman HH. *Problem-oriented medical diagnosis*, 3rd ed. Boston: Little, Brown; 1983.

and hypoxemia stimulate respiration very strongly); consequently, pH is not returned to normal (Table 14-6).

- **Base excess (BE)**
- BE hypothetically "corrects" pH to 7.40 by first "adjusting" pCO_2 to 40 mm Hg, thereby allowing comparison of resultant HCO_3^- with normal value at that pH (24 mmol/L). Normal = -2 to $+2$ mmol/L.

TABLE 14-5. Immediate and Delayed Compensatory Response to Acid-Base Disturbances

Acid-Base Abnormality	Immediate Response (By Lungs)	Delayed Response (By Kidneys)
Respiratory alkalosis	↑pCO_2 by decreasing ventilation	↓HCO_3^- excretion ↓Acid excretion
Respiratory acidosis	↓pCO_2 by increasing ventilation	↑HCO_3^- retention ↑Acid excretion
Metabolic alkalosis	↑pCO_2 by decreasing ventilation	↓HCO_3^- excretion ↓Acid excretion
Metabolic acidosis	↓pCO_2 by increasing ventilation	↑HCO_3^- retention ↑Acid excretion

↑, increases; ↓, decreases.

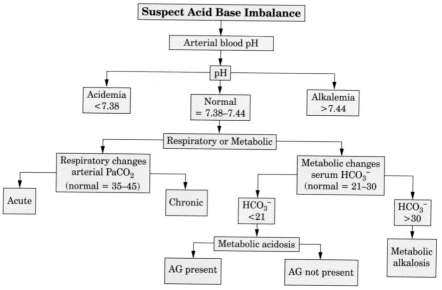

Figure 14-2. Algorithm for acid-base imbalance and anion gap (AG).

- BE can be calculated from by determined values for pH and HCO_3^- by this formula:

$$BE\ (mmol/L) = HCO_3^- + 10(7.40 - pH) - 24$$

- Negative BE indicates depletion of HCO_3^-. It does not distinguish primary from compensatory derangement.

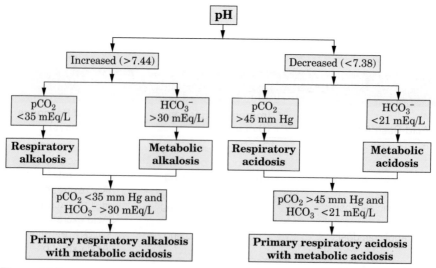

Figure 14-3. Algorithm illustrating effects of metabolic and respiratory acid-base changes in blood.

TABLE 14-6. Primary Change, and Compensatory Mechanisms in Delayed Response to, and Chloride Level in Acid-Base Disturbances

	Primary Change	Compensatory Mechanism	Delayed Response (By Kidneys)	Cl⁻
Respiratory alkalosis	↓pCO₂	None	↓HCO₃⁻ 3–5 mmol/L for every 10 mm Hg ↑pCO₂	↑
Respiratory acidosis	↑pCO₂	↑HCO₃⁻ 1 mmol/L for every 10 mm Hg ↑pCO₂	↑HCO₃⁻ 3–5 mmol/L for every 10 mm Hg ↑pCO₂	→
Metabolic alkalosis	↑HCO₃⁻	↑pCO₂ 3–5 mm Hg for every 10 mmol/L ↑HCO₃⁻	↓HCO₃⁻ excretion ↓Acid excretion	→
Metabolic acidosis with increased anion gap	↓HCO₃⁻	↓pCO₂ 1.0–1.3 mm Hg mmol/L for every 1 mmol/L ↑HCO₃⁻	↑HCO₃⁻ retention ↑Acid excretion	No change
Metabolic acidosis normal anion gap	↓HCO₃⁻	pCO₂ changes 2 for every pH change after decimal (e.g., if pH = 7.25, pCO₂ = 25 ± 2)		↑
Respiratory alkalosis	↓pCO₂	Acute: none Chronic: ↓HCO₃⁻ 3–5 mmol/L for every 10 mm Hg ↑pCO₂		↑
Respiratory acidosis	↑pCO₂	Acute: ↑HCO₃⁻ 1 mmol/L for every 10 mm Hg ↑pCO₂ Chronic: ↑HCO₃⁻ 3–5 mmol/L for every 10 mm Hg ↑pCO₂		→
Metabolic alkalosis	↑HCO₃⁻	↑pCO₂ 3–5 mm Hg for every 10 mmol/L ↑HCO₃⁻		→
Metabolic acidosis with increased anion gap	↓HCO₃⁻	↓pCO₂ 1.0–1.3 mm Hg for every 1 mmol/L ↓HCO₃⁻	Hyperchloremic metabolic acidosis	No change
Metabolic acidosis with normal anion gap	↓HCO₃⁻	pCO₂ changes 2 for every pH change after decimal (e.g., if pH = 7.25, pCO₂ = 25 ± 2)		↑

↑, increased; ↓, decreased.

1075

RESPIRATORY ALKALOSIS

* Respiratory alkalosis is defined as a decreased pCO_2 of <38 mm Hg.

➤ Caused by Hyperventilation

* CNS disorders (e.g., infection, tumor, trauma, CVA, anxiety-hyperventilation)
* Hypoxia (e.g., high altitudes, ventilation-perfusion imbalance)
* Cardiovascular (e.g. CHF, hypotension)
* Pulmonary disease (e.g., pneumonia, pulmonary emboli, asthma, pneumothorax)
* Drugs (e.g., salicylate intoxication, methylxanthines, β-adrenergic agonists)
* Metabolic (e.g., acidosis [diabetic, renal, lactic], liver failure)
* Others (e.g., fever, pregnancy, gram-negative sepsis, pain)
* Mechanical overventilation, cardiopulmonary bypass

➤ Diagnostic Findings

* Acute hypocapnia: usually only a modest decrease in plasma HCO_3^- concentrations and marked alkalosis
* Chronic hypocapnia: usually only a slight alkaline pH (not usually >7.55)

RESPIRATORY ACIDOSIS

* Laboratory findings differ in acute and chronic conditions.

➤ Acute Respiratory Acidosis

* Caused by decreased alveolar ventilation impairing CO_2 excretion:
* Cardiopulmonary (e.g., pneumonia, pneumothorax, pulmonary edema, foreign body aspiration, laryngospasm, bronchospasm, mechanical ventilation, cardiac arrest)
* CNS depression (e.g., general anesthesia, drugs, brain injury, infection)
* Neuromuscular (e.g., Guillain-Barré syndrome, hypokalemia, myasthenic crisis)
* Acidosis is severe (pH 7.05–7.10), but HCO_3^- concentration is only 29–30 mmol/L.
* Severe mixed acidosis is common in cardiac arrest, when respiratory and circulatory failure causes marked respiratory acidosis and severe lactic acidosis.

➤ Chronic Respiratory Acidosis

* Caused by chronic obstructive or restrictive conditions
* Nerve disease (e.g., poliomyelitis)
* Muscle disease (e.g., myopathy)
* CNS disorder (e.g., brain tumor)
* Restriction of thorax (e.g., musculoskeletal, scleroderma, Pickwickian syndrome)
* Pulmonary disease (e.g., prolonged pneumonia, primary alveolar hypoventilation)
* Acidosis is not usually severe.
* Beware of commonly occurring mixed acid-base disturbances (e.g., chronic respiratory acidosis with superimposed acute hypercapnia resulting from acute infection, such as bronchitis or pneumonia).
* Superimposed metabolic alkalosis (e.g., due to diuretics or vomiting) may exacerbate the hypercapnia.

METABOLIC ALKALOSIS

➤ Causes
- Loss of acid:
- Vomiting, gastric suction, gastrocolic fistula
- Diarrhea in mucoviscidosis (rarely)
- Villous adenoma of colon
- Aciduria secondary to potassium depletion
- Excess of base caused by administration of:
- Absorbable antacids (e.g., sodium bicarbonate; milk-alkali syndrome)
- Salts of weak acids (e.g., sodium lactate, sodium or potassium citrate)
- Some vegetarian diets
- Citrate due to massive blood transfusions
- Potassium depletion (causing sodium and H^+ to enter the cells):
- GI loss (e.g., chronic diarrhea)
- Lack of potassium intake (e.g., anorexia nervosa, IV fluids without potassium supplements for treatment of vomiting or postoperatively)
- Diuresis (e.g., mercurials, thiazides, osmotic diuresis)
- Extracellular volume depletion and chloride depletion
- Dehydration reducing intracellular volume, thereby stimulating aldosterone, causing excretion of potassium and H^+
- All forms of mineralocorticoid excess (e.g., primary aldosteronism, Cushing syndrome, administration of steroids, large amounts of licorice) causing excretion of potassium and H^+
- Glycogen deposition
- Chronic alkalosis
- Potassium-losing nephropathy
- Hypoproteinemia per se may cause a nonrespiratory alkalosis. Decreased albumin of 1g/dL causes an average increase in standard bicarbonate of 3.4 mmol/L, an apparent base excess of +3.7 mmol/L, and a decrease in AG of ~3 mmol/L.

➤ Diagnostic Findings
- Serum pH is increased (>7.60 in severe alkalemia).
- Total plasma CO_2 is increased (bicarbonate >30 mmol/L).
- pCO_2 is normal or slightly increased.
- Serum pH and bicarbonate above those predicted by the pCO_2 (by nomogram).
- Hypokalemia is an almost constant feature and is the chief danger in metabolic alkalosis.
- Decreased serum chloride is relatively lower than sodium.
- BUN may be increased.
- Urine pH is >7.0 (≤7.9) if potassium depletion is not severe and concomitant sodium deficiency (e.g., vomiting) is not present. With severe hypokalemia (<2.0 mmol/L), urine may be acid in presence of systemic alkalosis.
- Metabolic alkalosis patients may be volume depleted and chloride responsive or have volume expansion and be chloride resistant.
- When the urine chloride is low (<10 mmol/L) and the patient responds to chloride treatment, the cause is more likely loss of gastric juice, diuretic therapy, or rapid relief of chronic hypercapnia. Chloride replacement is completed when urine chloride remains >40 mmol/L.

- When the urine chloride is high (20 mmol/L) and the patient does not respond to NaCl treatment, the cause is more likely hyperadrenalism or severe potassium deficiency.
- Acid-base maps (Figure 14-4) are a graphic solution of the Henderson-Hasselbalch equation, which predicts the HCO_3^- value for each set of pH/pCO_2 coordinates. They also allow a check of the consistency of ABG and automated analyzer determinations, since these may determine the total CO_2 content, of which 95% is HCO_3^-.
- These maps contain bands that show the 95% probability range of values for each disorder. If the pH/pCO_2 coordinate is outside the 95% confidence band, then the patient has at least two acid-base disturbances.
- These maps are of particular use when one of the acid-base disturbances is not suspected clinically. If the coordinates lie within a band, it is not a guarantee of a simple acid-base disturbance.

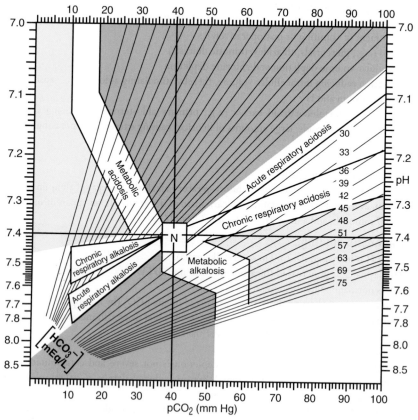

Figure 14-4. Acid-base map. The values demarcated for each disorder represent a 95% probability range for each *pure* disorder. Coordinates lying outside these zones suggest mixed acid-base disorders. N, normal. (Adapted from Goldberg M, Green SB, Moss ML, et al. Computer-based instruction and diagnosis of acid-base disorders. *JAMA.* 1973;223:269.)

METABOLIC ACIDOSIS

➤ With Increased Anion Gap (AG >15 mmol/L)

* Lactic acidosis—most common cause of metabolic acidosis with increased AG (frequently >25 mmol/L) (see following section)
* Renal failure (AG <25 mmol/L)
* Ketoacidosis
  * DM (AG frequently >25 mmol/L)
  * Associated with alcohol abuse (AG frequently 20–25 mmol/L)
  * Starvation (AG usually 5–10 mmol/L)
* Drugs
  * Salicylate poisoning (AG frequently 5–10 mmol/L; higher in children)
  * Methanol poisoning (AG frequently >20 mmol/L)
  * Ethylene glycol poisoning (AG frequently >20 mmol/L)
  * Paraldehyde (AG frequently >20 mmol/L)

➤ With Normal Anion Gap: Hyperchloremic Metabolic Acidosis
Decreased Serum Potassium

* Renal tubular acidosis (RTA)
* Acquired (e.g., drugs, hypercalcemia)
* Inherited (e.g., cystinosis, Wilson disease)
* Carbonic anhydrase inhibitors (e.g., acetazolamide, mafenide)
* Increased loss of alkaline body fluids (e.g., diarrhea, loss of pancreatic or biliary fluids)
* Ureteral diversion (e.g., ileal bladder or ureter, ureterosigmoidostomy)

Normal or Increased Serum Potassium

* Hydronephrosis
* Early renal failure
* Administration of HCl (e.g., ammonium chloride)
* Hypoadrenalism (diffuse, zona glomerulosa, or hyporeninemia)
* Renal aldosterone resistance
* Sulfur toxicity

➤ Diagnostic Findings

* Serum pH is decreased (<7.3).
* Total plasma CO_2 content is decreased; <15 mmol/L almost certainly rules out respiratory alkalosis.
* Serum potassium is frequently increased; it is decreased in RTA, diarrhea, or carbonic anhydrase inhibition; also, increased serum chloride.
* Azotemia suggests metabolic acidosis due to renal failure.
* Urine is strongly acid (pH4.5–5.2) if renal function is normal.
* In evaluating acid-base disorders, calculate the AG (see earlier discussion).

LACTIC ACIDOSIS

* Indicates acute hypoperfusion and tissue hypoxia.
* Should be considered in any metabolic acidosis with increased AG (>15 mmol/L).

- Diagnosis is confirmed by exclusion of other causes of metabolic acidosis and serum lactate ≥ 5 mmol/L (upper limit of normal = 1.6 for plasma and 1.4 for whole blood). There is considerable variation in the literature in limits of serum lactate and pH to define lactic acidosis.
- In lactic acidosis, the increase in AG is usually greater than the decrease in HCO_3^-, in contrast to DKA, in which the increase in AG is identical to the decrease in HCO_3^-.
- Exclusion of other causes by:
- Normal serum creatinine and BUN (increased acetoacetic acid [but not beta-hydroxybutyric acid] will cause false increase of creatinine by colorimetric assay).
- Osmolar gap <10 mOsm/L
- Negative nitroprusside reaction (nitroprusside test for ketoacidosis measures acetoacetic acid but not β-hydroxybutyric acid; thus, the blood ketone test may be negative in DKA)
- Urine negative for calcium oxalate crystals
- No known ingestion of toxic substances
- Laboratory findings due to underlying diseases (e.g., DM, renal insufficiency)
- Laboratory tests for monitoring therapy:
- Arterial pH, pCO_2, HCO_3^-, serum electrolytes every 1–2 hours until patient is stable
- Urine electrolytes every 6 hours
- Associated or compensatory metabolic or respiratory disturbances (e.g., hyperventilation or respiratory alkalosis) may result in normal pH
- Type A caused by tissue hypoxia (e.g., acute hemorrhage, severe anemia, shock, asphyxia), marathon running, seizures
- Type B without tissue hypoxia caused by:
- Common disorders (e.g., DM, uremia, liver disease, infections, malignancies, alkaloses)
- Drugs and toxins (e.g., ethanol, methanol, ethylene glycol, salicylates, metformin)
- Hereditary enzyme defects (e.g., methylmalonic acidemia, propionic aciduria, defects of fatty acid oxidation, pyruvate-dehydrogenase deficiency, pyruvate-carboxylase deficiency, multiple carboxylase deficiency, glycogen storage disease type I).
- Others (e.g., starvation, short-bowel syndrome)
- With a typical clinical picture (acute onset following nausea and vomiting, altered state of consciousness, hyperventilation, high mortality)
- Decreased serum bicarbonate
- Low serum pH, usually 6.98 to 7.25
- Increased serum potassium, often 6–7 mmol/L
- Serum chloride normal or low with increased AG
- Increased serum phosphorus. Phosphorus-to-creatinine ratio >3 indicates lactic acidosis either alone or as a component of other metabolic acidosis.
- WBC count is increased (occasionally to leukemoid levels).
- Increased serum uric acid is frequent (up to 25 mg/dL in lactic acidosis)
- Increased serum AST, LD, and phosphorus levels

MIXED ACID-BASE DISTURBANCES

- Mixed acid-base disturbances must always be interpreted with clinical data and other laboratory findings.

➤ Respiratory Acidosis with Metabolic Acidosis
- Acidemia may be extreme with
- pH <7.0 (H^+ >100 mmol/L)
- HCO_3^- <26 mmol/L. Failure of HCO_3^- to increase ≥ 3 mmol/L for each 10 mm Hg rise in pCO_2 suggests metabolic acidosis with respiratory acidosis.
- Examples: Acute pulmonary edema, cardiopulmonary arrest (lactic acidosis due to tissue anoxia, and CO_2 retention due to alveolar hypoventilation)
- Mild metabolic acidosis superimposed on chronic hypercapnia causing partial suppression of HCO_3^- may be indistinguishable from adaptation to hypercapnia alone.

➤ Respiratory Acidosis with Metabolic Alkalosis
- Decreased or absent urine chloride indicates that chloride-responsive metabolic alkalosis is a part of the picture.
- In clinical setting of respiratory acidosis but with normal blood pH and/or HCO_3^- higher than predicted, complicating metabolic alkalosis may be present.
- Examples: chronic pulmonary disease with CO_2 retention developing metabolic alkalosis due to administration of diuretics, severe vomiting, or sudden improvement in ventilation ("posthypercapnic" metabolic alkalosis)

➤ Metabolic Acidosis with Respiratory Alkalosis
- pH may be normal or decreased.
- Hypocapnia remains inappropriate to decreased HCO_3^- for several hours or more.
- Examples: Rapid correction of severe metabolic acidosis, salicylate intoxication, gram-negative septicemia, initial respiratory alkalosis with subsequent development of metabolic acidosis. Primary metabolic acidosis with primary respiratory alkalosis with an increased AG is characteristic of salicylate intoxication in absence of uremia and DKA.

➤ Metabolic Alkalosis with Respiratory Alkalosis
- Marked alkalemia with decreased pCO_2 and increased HCO_3^- is diagnostic.
- Examples: Hepatic insufficiency with hyperventilation plus administration of diuretics or severe vomiting; metabolic alkalosis with stimulation of ventilation (e.g., sepsis, pulmonary embolism, mechanical ventilation), which causes respiratory alkalosis

➤ Acute and Chronic Respiratory Acidosis
- May be suspected when HCO_3^- is in intermediate range between acute and chronic respiratory acidosis (similar findings in chronic respiratory acidosis with superimposed metabolic acidosis or acute respiratory acidosis with superimposed metabolic alkalosis)
- Examples: chronic hypercapnia with acute deterioration of pulmonary function causing further rise of pCO_2.

➤ Coexistence of Metabolic Acidosis of Hyperchloremic Type and Increased Anion Gap
- May be suspected by plasma HCO_3^- that is lower than is explained by the increase in anions (e.g., AG $= 16$ mmol/L and HCO_3^- $= 5$ mmol/L)
- Examples: uremia and proximal RTA, lactic acidosis with diarrhea, excessive administration of NaCl to patient with organic acidosis

➤ Coexistence of Metabolic Alkalosis and Metabolic Acidosis
* May be suspected by acid-base values that are too normal for clinical picture
* Examples: Vomiting causing alkalosis plus bicarbonate-losing diarrhea causing acidosis

PEARLS

* **Pulmonary embolus:** Mild to moderate respiratory alkalosis is present unless sudden death occurs. The degree of hypoxia often correlates with the size and extent of the pulmonary embolus. pO_2 >90 mm Hg when breathing room air virtually excludes a lung problem.
* **Acute pulmonary edema:** Hypoxemia is usual. CO_2 is not increased unless the situation is grave.
* **Asthma:** Hypoxia occurs even during a mild episode and increases as the attack becomes worse. As hyperventilation occurs, the pCO_2 falls (usually <35 mm Hg); a normal pCO_2 (>40 mm Hg) implies impending respiratory failure; increased pCO_2 in a true asthmatic (not bronchitis or emphysema) indicates impending disaster and the need to consider intubation and ventilation assistance.
* **Chronic obstructive pulmonary disease** (bronchitis and emphysema) may show two patterns—"pink puffers," with mild hypoxia and normal pH and pCO_2, and "blue bloaters," with hypoxia and increased pCO_2; normal pH suggests compensation and decreased pH suggests decompensation.
* **Neurologic and neuromuscular disorders** (e.g., drug overdose, Guillain-Barré syndrome, myasthenia gravis, trauma, succinyl choline): Acute alveolar hypoventilation causes uncompensated respiratory acidosis with high pCO_2, low pH, and normal HCO_3^-. Acidosis appears before significant hypoxemia, and rising CO_2 indicates rapid deterioration and need for mechanical assistance.
* **Sepsis:** Unexplained respiratory alkalosis may be the earliest sign of sepsis. It may progress to cause metabolic acidosis, and the mixed picture may produce a normal pH; low HCO_3^- is useful for recognizing this. With deterioration and worsening of metabolic acidosis, the pH falls.
* **Salicylate poisoning** characteristically shows poor correlation between serum salicylate level and presence or degree of acidemia (because as pH drops from 7.4 to 7.2, the proportion of nonionized to ionized salicylate doubles and the nonionized form leaves the serum and is sequestered in the brain and other organs, where it interferes with function at a cellular level without changing blood levels of glucose, and so on). Salicylate poisoning in adults typically causes respiratory alkalosis, but in children this progresses rapidly to mixed respiratory alkalosis/metabolic acidosis and then to metabolic acidosis (in adults, metabolic acidosis is said to be rare and a near-terminal event).
* **Isopropyl** (rubbing) alcohol poisoning produces enough circulating acetone to produce a positive nitroprusside test (it, therefore, may be mistaken for DKA; consequently, insulin should not be given until the blood glucose is known). In the absence of a history, positive serum ketone test associated with normal AG, normal serum HCO_3^-, and normal blood glucose suggests rubbing alcohol intoxication.
* **A change in chloride concentration independent of,** or out of proportion to, changes in sodium usually indicates an acid-base disorder.

CHAPTER 15

Toxicology and Therapeutic Drug Monitoring

Amanda Jenkins

Toxicology is the study of the adverse effects of chemicals on living organisms. Clinical toxicology is a subspecialty with emphasis on management of a poisoned patient. The application is focused on human beings but may be equally applied in veterinary medicine. The principles of clinical toxicology are applied to two main areas—emergency toxicology and therapeutic drug monitoring.

EMERGENCY TOXICOLOGY

➤ Purpose

The majority of poisoned patients enter the health care system in the emergency department. Treatment is often based on exposure history and signs and symptoms of poisoning based on physical examination. Laboratory testing may be performed to confirm the physician's diagnosis or to identify a toxin in the absence of a differential diagnosis.

Knowledge of toxidromes is important as a starting point for patient evaluation (Table 15-1). These consist of a collection of signs and symptoms that are typically produced by specific toxins.

➤ Application

Testing offered by clinical toxicology laboratories consists of screening and confirmation.

➤ Screening Methods and Limitations

Screening tests are usually conducted on urine. These require little or no sample preparation and are frequently immunoassay based. These tests have high sensitivity; however, they have

TABLE 15-1. Signs and Symptoms of Common Toxidromes

Toxidrome	Causal Agents	Signs and Symptoms
Opioid	Opioids, clonidine, phenothiazines	Hypothermia, bradypnea, lethargy, miosis, altered mental status
Sympathomimetic	Amphetamines, cocaine, caffeine, salicylates	Hyperthermia, tachycardia, agitation, hypertension, tremor, restlessness, insomnia
Sedative-hypnotic	Barbiturates, benzodiazepines, ethanol	Hypothermia, lethargy, confusion, sedation, ataxia
Anticholinergic	Antipsychotics, atropine antihistamines (e.g., diphenhydramine)	Hyperthermia, mydriasis, tachycardia, dry flushed skin, decreased bowel sounds
Cholinergic	Organophosphates, Physostigmine	Bradycardia/tachycardia, salivation, lacrimation, urination, diarrhea, emesis

limitations due to moderate specificity. Many commercially available tests cross-react with multiple drugs within a class due to choice of target drug. They may also be sensitive to adulterants. Clinicians must be aware of the commercial tests utilized in their laboratory, as cross-reactivities differ between manufacturers and within manufacturers over time.

These tests are typically performed on automated chemistry analyzers. Although individual drug–drug classes are available, many hospital laboratories offer these tests as panels and are available as "stat" tests.

Immunoassay testing may be based on:
* Radioimmunoassay (RIA)
* Enzyme multiplied immunoassay technique (EMIT)
* Enzyme linked immunosorbent assay (ELISA)
* Fluorescence polarization immunoassay (FPIA)
* Kinetic interaction of particles (KIMS)
* Cloned enzyme donor immunoassay (CEDIA)

Immunoassays utilize antibodies to identity and measure drug concentrations. The target drug is the antigen. Antibodies are generated against the drug antigen. These antibodies are mixed with "labeled" drug and the drug itself and these compete for the antibody binding sites. Labeled compounds are prepared by attaching fluorescent (as in FPIA), radioactive (RIA), enzyme (EMIT), or a microparticle (KIMS) to the drug. In EMIT assays, for example, the label attached to drug is glucose-6-phosphate dehydrogenase, which oxidizes the substrate glucose-6-phosphate to gluconolactone-6-phosphate and reduces NAD to NADH. Enzyme activity is assessed by measuring the reduction of NAD spectrophotometrically by measuring absorbance at 340 nm. Enzyme activity of G6P-DH is reduced when attached drug is bound to antibody. When drug is present in the specimen the amount of antibody available to bind to enzyme-labeled drug is reduced and so the rate of NADH production is increased. The change in absorbance at 340 nm is directly related to the concentration of the drug in the sample.

Immunoassays are typically qualitative assays, although semiquantitative results are possible with some kits. For qualitative testing the instrument is calibrated at one concentration, called the cut-off concentration. For example, when utilizing EMIT, all specimens that have absorbance values equivalent to this cut-off calibrator or greater will be reported as positive. Manufacturers provide this calibrator so the laboratory has no choice in this concentration unless they alter the kit provided (e.g., dilution, to obtain alternate/user-defined cut-offs).

Cut-off concentrations for these kits have historically been decided with reference to the DHHS SAMSHA mandated cut-offs for federal workplace drug testing, the so-called "NIDA 5" drugs/classes (PCP, opiates, cannabinoids [marijuana], cocaine metabolite, amphetamines). These cut-off concentrations are not generally appropriate for clinical use, since the cut-off values for several drug–drug classes are fairly high. This decreases the likelihood of false-positive results. The detection of drug abuse rather than legitimate drug use is targeted.

Practitioners should also be aware of the relative cross-reactivities of the tests ordered. For example, immunoassays for opiates target morphine, and typically do not produce positive results with samples containing synthetic and semisynthetic opioids such as oxycodone, fentanyl, propoxyphene, and tramadol.

Table 15-2 lists the detection time of several drugs in urine. Note variables that must be considered include dose, frequency and route of administration, formulation, and patient-related factors (e.g., disease, other drugs, genetic polymorphisms).

TABLE 15-2. Approximate Detection Times in Urine of Some Drugs of Abuse

Drug	Detection Time
Heroin (as morphine)	1–2 days
Cocaine (as metabolites)	3 days
Morphine	1–2 days
Amphetamine 3,4-Methylenedioxymethamphetamine (MDMA)	1–2 days
Methadone (as metabolites)	3–7 days
Volatiles	<1 day
Oxycodone	1–2 days
Gamma-hydroxybutyrate (GHB)	12–24 hours
Phencyclidine (PCP)	1–2 weeks
11-nor-delta 9-tetrahydrocannabinol-9-carboxylic acid (THCA) [marijuana metabolite] (single use)	2–7 days
Barbiturates	
All except phenobarbital	2 days
Phenobarbital	1–2 weeks
Benzodiazepines	
All except flunitrazepam	5–7 days
Flunitrazepam (as metabolites)	<3 days

➤ Confirmation Methods and Limitations

Confirmation tests are typically performed following a positive screening result. Confirmatory tests are ordered if it is necessary to identify a specific drug, obtain a quantitative result, or make a determination for legal purposes. For example, a positive opiate immunoassay result will not establish the identity of the opiate. A more specific test is required. These are typically chromatography based and are not performed on a "stat" basis. Chromatography is a separation process based on the differential distribution of sample constituents between a moving mobile and a stationary phase. Chromatography is a separation technique not identification. Mass spectrometry provides identification, since it provides mass and charge information unique to individual drugs. Identification may not be necessary in therapeutic drug monitoring (TDM). Sample pretreatment, extraction, and complex instrumental analysis is required. Common methods used for confirmation tests are:

Gas chromatography (GC)

High-performance liquid chromatography (HPLC)

GC/mass spectrometry (GC/MS)

Liquid chromatography/mass spectrometry (LC/MS)

➤ Specimen Validity and Drug Testing
Background

Specimen validity is an important but often overlooked aspect of laboratory testing. Validity refers to the correct specimen identity (i.e., a urine sample is in fact human urine). The collectors of samples in physician offices and other sites have the responsibility of ensuring that adequate specimens are collected from patients. The validity of a specimen may be questioned if the sample is substituted or adulterated.

* A **substituted** sample is a substance provided in place of the donor's specimen. This may be drug-free urine (from another individual) or another liquid such as water.

* An **adulterated** sample is a specimen to which substance(s) have been added to destroy the drug in the sample or interfere with the analytical tests utilized to detect drugs. Common additives include vinegar, bleach, liquid hand soap, lemon juice, and household cleaners. In the last several years commercial products have become available to subvert drug tests. These products have been found to contain substances that include glutaraldehyde, sodium chloride, chromate, nitrite, surfactant, and peroxide/peroxidase.

In addition, specimens may be **diluted** by adding liquids to the urine at the time of collection to decrease the concentration of drug in the sample below the cut-off concentration used for the test. In vivo dilution involves the ingestion of diuretics and other substances to remove the drugs from the body or dilute the urine, for example, drinking an excessive quantity of water before a drug test.

Minimizing Specimen Validity Issues at the Collection Site

In many industries where urine is collected for drug testing for nonmedical purposes, for example, preemployment screening, specimens are collected under chain of custody and also several physical procedures are in place to minimize the likelihood of specimen substitution or adulteration. These procedures include witnessing the collection, not providing access to water in the bathroom, and coloring toilet bowl water. In addition, donors may not be permitted to wear loose clothing in which a substituted specimen could be hidden. Before the specimen is sealed in the collection container with tamper-resistant tape, the collector may record the temperature of the specimen (normal range for validity testing considered 90–100°F) as well as the urine color.

Urine Characteristics

Physical, chemical, or DNA tests may be used to assure the validity of a specimen. These tests are most frequently requested in connection with urine drug testing, especially for drugs of abuse such as cannabinoids (marijuana), heroin, and cocaine.

Creatinine, specific gravity, and pH are tests performed to assess whether a specimen is consistent with normal human urine. The U.S. Department of Health and Human Services Mandatory Guidelines specify acceptable ranges for these tests (for federally regulated drug testing specimens), and clinical laboratories and other providers have tended to adopt these values, some with slight modifications.

Creatinine is formed as a result of creatine metabolism in skeletal muscle and the amount produced is relatively constant within an individual. This parameter is utilized clinically to assess renal function. A level ≥20 mg/dL in human urine is considered normal. Diluted and substituted (with water) specimens will have creatinine concentrations <20 mg/dL.

Specific gravity for liquids is the ratio of the density of a substance (urine) to the density of water at the same temperature. Hence it is a measurement of the concentration of dissolved solids in the urine. The specific gravity of normal human urine ranges between 1.003 and 1.030. High values may be caused by disease (kidney disease, glucosuria, liver disease, dehydration, adrenal insufficiency, and proteinuria), whereas low values may be caused by DI. Dilution and adulteration (e.g., with the organic solvents methanol and ethanol) results in a value <1.000.

The pH of normal human urine is typically between 5.0 and 8.0. The reference range is 4.5–9.0. This parameter can be affected by diet, medications, and disease. Acidic urine may be caused by acidosis (respiratory and metabolic), uremia, severe diarrhea, starvation, and diets with a large intake of acid containing fruit. In contrast, an alkaline urine may be attributed to alkalosis, urinary tract infections, high vegetable diets, and sodium bicarbonate. Individuals with dietary or disease causes of acidic or alkaline urine will be consistently in this range, rather than a random urine high or low due to adulteration or substitution. If lemon juice or vinegar are added to urine the pH is lowered. A high urine pH results from the addition of bleach or soap.

Methodology

Tests should be conducted as soon as possible after urine collection. Creatinine may be determined by dipstick or automated clinical chemistry analyzer based on a chemical reaction that produces a color result. The specific gravity may be measured by refractometry in which the refractive index of the urine is determined. Alternatively, the dipstick method is based on ionic strength. A procedure available for automated clinical chemistry analyzers utilizes urine chloride ion concentration and spectrophotometry. pH is measured using a pH meter or colorimetrically manually or using an automated clinical chemistry analyzer.

Laboratories also offer tests for common adulterants. These include specific tests for nitrite and glutaraldehyde, typically using colorimetric assays, or generalized tests for oxidants. The latter detects compounds that exert their action by oxidation and include chromate and peroxidase. The method as performed on an automated clinical chemistry analyzer evaluates the reaction between a substrate and oxidant in the sample producing color that can be measured at a specific wavelength.

Specimen Requirements

Sample collection: Random urine
Transport: Refrigerated
Minimum volume: 5.0 mL

TABLE 15-3. Reference Ranges for Urine Specimens	
Component	Range
pH	4.5–9.0
Creatinine	≥20 mg/dL
Specific gravity	1.003–1.040
Oxidants	<200 mcg/mL

The test should be conducted as soon as possible after urine collection. Urine samples suspected of bacterial contamination will produce invalid pH results. Sodium azide should not be used as a preservative, as this may cause interference with the Oxidant test. Table 15-3 presents reference ranges.

THERAPEUTIC DRUG MONITORING

➤ Purpose

Therapeutic drug monitoring (TDM) is the determination of drug levels in blood. The purpose of such measurement is to optimize the dose in order to achieve maximum clinical effect. TDM is typically performed on drugs with a low therapeutic index.

Indications
* Signs of toxicity
* Therapeutic effect not obtained
* Suspected noncompliance
* Drug has narrow therapeutic range
* To provide or confirm an optimal dosing schedule
* To confirm cause of organ toxicity (e.g., abnormal liver or kidney function tests)
* Other diseases or conditions exist that affect drug utilization
* Drug interactions that have altered desired or previously achieved therapeutic concentration are suspected
* Drug shows large variations in utilization or metabolism between individuals
* Need medicolegal verification of treatment, cause of death or injury (e.g., suicide, homicide, accident investigation), or to detect use of forbidden drugs (e.g., steroids in athletes, narcotics)
* Differential diagnosis of coma

➤ Applications
* The clinician must be aware of the various influences on pharmacokinetics—factors such as half-life, time to peak and to steady state, protein binding, and excretion.
* The route of administration and sampling time after last dose of drug must be known for proper interpretation. For some drugs (e.g., quinidine), different assay methods produce different values, and the clinician must know the normal range for the test method used for the patient.
* In general, peak concentrations alone are useful when testing for toxicity, and trough concentrations alone are useful for demonstrating a satisfactory therapeutic concentration. Trough concentrations are commonly used with such drugs as lithium, theophylline, phenytoin, carbamazepine, quinidine, tricyclic antidepressants, valproic acid, and digoxin. Trough

concentrations can usually be drawn at the time the next dose is administered (*this does not apply to digoxin*). Both peak and trough concentrations are used to avoid toxicity but ensure bactericidal efficacy (e.g., gentamicin, tobramycin, vancomycin).

- IV and IM administration should usually be sampled 30 minutes to 1 hour after administration is ended to determine peak concentrations (meant only as a general guide; the laboratory performing the tests should supply its own values).
- Blood should be drawn at a time specified by that laboratory (e.g., 1 hour before the next dose is due to be administered). This trough concentration should ideally be greater than the minimum effective serum concentration.
- If a drug is administered by IV infusion, blood should be drawn from the opposite arm.
- The drug should have been administered at a constant rate for at least 4–5 half-lives before blood samples are drawn.
- Unexpected test results may be due to interference by complementary and alternative medicines (e.g., high digoxin levels may result from interference from danshen, Chan Su, or ginseng).

Criteria
- Available methodology must be specific and reliable.
- Blood concentration must correlate with therapeutic and toxic effects.
- Therapeutic window is narrow with danger of toxicity on therapeutic doses.
- Correlation between blood concentration and dose is poor.
- Clinical effect of drug is not easily determined.

➤ Drugs for Which Drug Monitoring May Be Useful
- Antiepileptic drugs (e.g., phenobarbital, phenytoin)
- Theophylline
- Antimicrobials (aminoglycosides [gentamicin, tobramycin, amikacin], chloramphenicol, vancomycin, flucytosine [5-fluorocytosine])
- Antipsychotic drugs
- Antianxiety drugs
- Cyclic antidepressants
- Lithium
- Cardiac glycosides, antiarrhythmics, antianginal, antihypertensive drugs
- Antineoplastic drugs
- Immunosuppressant drugs
- Anti-inflammatory drugs (e.g., NSAIDs, steroids)
- Drugs of abuse: addiction treatment, pain management
- Athletic performance enhancement drugs (e.g., androgenic anabolic steroids, erythropoietin)

➤ Pharmacokinetics
Pharmacokinetics (PK) is the study of the time course of drugs in the body. PK seeks to relate the concentration of drug in a specimen to the amount of drug administered [dose]. PK investigates:
- Absorption
- Distribution
- Metabolism
- Excretion or elimination

Changes in these parameters affect drug concentrations.

Absorption

Absorption describes the process in which the drug or xenobiotic enters the bloodstream. For intravenous/intra-arterial administration, there is no absorption. Other common routes of administration include oral, intramuscular, subcutaneous, inhalation, rectal, intrathecal, oral mucosa, dermal, and intranasal. The following factors affect the bioavailability (amount absorbed compared with amount administered):

* Surface area
* Solubility
* Blood supply
* Concentration
* pH
* Molecular size and shape
* Degree of ionization

Distribution

This describes the transfer of the drug from site of administration throughout the body. This is generally movement from the bloodstream to tissues. Therefore, it is a function of the blood supply to the tissues. A drug may rapidly be distributed to highly perfused tissues such as brain, heart, liver, and kidney, whereas slower distribution will occur for muscle, fat, and bone. Factors affecting drug absorption are also relevant to distribution. Plasma protein binding is an additional factor to consider.

Metabolism

Drugs are chemically altered to facilitate removal from the body. This process is performed mainly in the liver by enzymes. Other sites of enzyme activity include the GI tract, blood, kidney, and lung. Phase I metabolism describes transformation of functional groups on the drug molecule. Phase II are known as conjugation reactions and involve addition of endogenous substances to render the compound more water soluble. The most common conjugation reaction involves the addition of uridine diphosphate-glucuronic acid with hydroxyl or amino groups to form glucuronides. Opiates and benzodiazepines are highly glucuronidated prior to excretion.

Excretion

Removal of drug from the body typically in urine from the kidney, feces from the liver, and breath from the lung. Drugs are also eliminated in sweat, breast milk, and sebum. Removal of drug by the liver, clearance, depends on blood flow to the liver, which may be increased in the presence of food, the presence of phenobarbital, and decreased during exercise, dehydration, disease (cirrhosis, CHF), and the presence of anesthetics. Removal of drug also depends on the ability of the liver to extract drug from the bloodstream. This includes diffusion and carrier systems. Renal excretion is a function of filtration, secretion, and reabsorption. Again the processes that affect transfer across biologic membranes must be considered.

➤ Conclusions

In general, increases in serum/plasma drug concentrations may be observed in:
1. Overdose
2. Coingestion of drugs that compete for metabolic enzymes

3. Liver and renal failure/insufficiency
4. Age related increases due to loss in enzyme activity, decreases in absorption, blood flow, intestinal motility
5. Genetic polymorphisms–slow metabolizers
6. Movement of drugs from tissue depots

In general, decreases in serum/plasma drug concentrations may be observed in:

1. Decreased oral bioavailability
2. Increased metabolism due to coingestion of drugs that induce metabolic enzymes such as phenobarbital, phenytoin
3. Increased renal clearance
4. Increases in plasma proteins (results in decreases in observed serum drug concentrations, since most tests measure unbound or free drug concentrations)

➤ Alternate Matrices

Drugs may be detected in nontraditional matrices
* Meconium
* Oral fluid (saliva)
* Sweat
* Hair

The majority of hospital laboratories do not offer testing in these specimens. Sample pre-treatment prior to testing is often required and, therefore, are not offered on a "stat" basis. Special sample collection devices are available for sweat and oral fluid. Hair testing provides a longer detection window for drugs than serum or urine and is generally reflective of chronic exposure.

➤ Units

Drugs concentrations are reported using several concentration units.
* ng/mL, which are equivalent to mcg/L
  Note that "mcg" are used throughout this text because "ug" or "μg" are prohibited abbreviations. When handwritten the "u" may be misread as "m."
* mcg/mL, which are equivalent to mg/L

Note that ethanol concentrations in the clinical setting are typically reported in mg/dL. Conversion to g% (g/dL) is often requested; for example, 80 mg/dL is equivalent to 0.08 g/dL. To convert mg/dL to g/dL, divide by 1000. Conversely, to convert g/dL to mg/dL, multiply by 1000.

➤ Suggested Readings

Crumpton SD, Sutheimer CA. Specimen adulteration and substitution in workplace drug testing. *Forensic Sci Rev.* 2007;19(1).

Drug Abuse Handbook. Karch SB, ed. Boca Raton, FL: CRC Press; 2007.

Drug Testing in Alternate Biological Specimens. Jenkins AJ, ed. Totowa, NJ: Humana Press; 2008.

The Clinical Toxicology Laboratory Contemporary Practice of Poisoning Evaluation. Shaw LM, editor in chief. Washington, DC: AACC, Inc.; 2001.

TIETZ Fundamentals of Clinical Chemistry. Burtis CA, Ashwood ER, Bruns DE, eds. St. Louis, MI: Saunders Elsevier; 2008.

Paul BD, Dunkley CS. Specimen validity testing. *Forensic Sci Rev.* 2007;19(1).

Wu A. Urine adulteration before testing for drugs of abuse. In: Shaw LM, editor in chief. *The Clinical Toxicology Laboratory Contemporary Practice of Poisoning Evaluation.* Washington, DC: AACC Press; 2001.

DRUGS AND POISONS

ALUMINUM (Al) POISONING

➤ **Definition**
* Al is the most abundant metal in Earth's crust. It is present in human tissues, but its biologic role is unknown.
* It is found in food packaging, food (additive), cooking utensils.
* Iatrogenic exposure may be due to IV fluids or dialysis.

➤ **Test Methods**
* Graphite furnace atomic absorption spectrophotometry
* ICP-MS
* Due to ubiquitous nature, contamination of specimen by environmental conditions, including container type and analytic procedure is possible, resulting in elevated levels.

➤ **Normal Range**
* Acceptable level: <10 ng/mL
* Potentially toxic level: ≥60 ng/mL

➤ **Diagnostic Value**
* Accumulates in bone and lung
* Acute intoxication is rare
* Decreases absorption of calcium and iron from GI tract
* Microcytic hypochromic anemia
  * Increased reticulocyte counts
  * Decreased mean corpuscular volume and mean corpuscular hemoglobin
* Osteomalacic osteodystrophy is progressive—conduct bone biopsy.
* Dialysis encephalopathy
* Chelation treatment with deferoxamine increases serum level with decrease in protein bound fraction

CARBON MONOXIDE (CO) POISONING

➤ **Definition**
* CO binds to Hb.
* It displaces oxyhemoglobin dissociation curve, causing tissue hypoxia.
* Cherry red skin color is a useful clue.

➤ **Test Methods**
* CO-oximeter (dedicated spectrophotometer that measures total Hb, COHb, metHb, and oxyhemoglobin) makes a rapid definitive diagnosis of increased COHb; is diagnostic.
* The reference method is gas chromatography.

➤ **Diagnostic Value**
* Symptoms are generally correlated with the percentage of carbon monoxide in Hb (percent saturation) (Table 15-4)

TABLE 15-4. Symptoms of Carbon Monoxide Poisoning

% COHb	Symptoms
0–2%	Asymptomatic
	0.4–0.7 endogenous production
2–5%	Found in moderate cigarette smokers; usually asymptomatic but may be slight impairment of intellect
5–10%	Found in heavy cigarette smokers; slight dyspnea with severe exertion
10–20%	Dyspnea with moderate exertion; mild headache, flushed skin
20–30%	Marked headache, irritability, disturbed judgment and memory, easy fatigability, throbbing temples, emotional instability
30–40%	Severe headache, dimness of vision, dizziness, confusion, weakness, nausea and vomiting
40–50%	Headache, confusion, fainting, ataxia, collapse, hyperventilation, tachypnea, hallucinations
50–60%	Coma, intermittent convulsions, tachycardia, cyanosis, incontinence, loss of reflexes
>60%	Respiratory failure, hypotension, and death if exposure is long continued
80%	Rapidly fatal

➤ Other Considerations

• Blood pH is markedly decreased (metabolic acidosis due to tissue hypoxia).
• Arterial pO_2 is normal, although O_2 is significantly decreased.
• Arterial pCO_2 may be normal or slightly decreased.
• Increased CO in patient's exhaled air or in ambient air at site of exposure can help confirm diagnosis if COHb has already fallen substantially.
• Chronic exposure leads to long-term effects.

CYANIDE POISONING

➤ Definition

• Odor of bitter almonds is useful clue. Cyanide reversibly binds to and inhibits reoxidation of cytochrome A, thereby preventing cellular respiration.
• Potassium cyanide is in rodenticides, insecticides, laboratory reagents, film developer, amygdalin, silver polish, and acetonitrile used to remove artificial fingernails.
• Hydrogen cyanide is in insecticides and fumigants and is released by the burning of plastics and synthetics.

➤ Test Methods

• CO-oximeter (dedicated spectrophotometer that measures total Hb, COHb, metHb, and oxyhemoglobin) makes a rapid definitive diagnosis of increased metHb.

- Cyantesmo paper
- Measure thiocyanate

➤ Diagnostic Value

- pO_2 and oxygen saturation are normal except in severe cases when respiratory failure occurs.
- Patient may first have respiratory alkalosis due to hyperventilation caused by tissue hypoxia.
- Then severe lactic (metabolic) acidosis with increased anion gap develops.
- With respiratory depression, respiratory acidosis may occur.
- Increased venous oxygen with decreased arteriovenous oxygen difference due to decreased tissue extraction of oxygen
- Normal concentration of cyanide: <0.01 mcg/mL plasma
  - Thiocyanate: 1–4 mcg/mL plasma—nonsmokers
  - Thiocyanate: 3–12 mcg/mL plasma—smokers
- Toxic concentration cyanide: >0.5 mcg/mL plasma

➤ Other Considerations

Treat with nitrites to form metHb level >30%; then treat with sodium thiosulfate IV to form thiocyanate. Antidote available commercially from Eli Lilly Co.

IRON (Fe) POISONING

➤ Definition

- Exposures of this essential metal are due to accidental acute, chronic overload due to idiopathic hemochromatosis, frequent blood transfusions, and excess dietary iron.

➤ Test Methods

- Spectrophotometry–atomic absorption
- ICP-MS

➤ Diagnostic Value

- Increased serum iron
- GI distress
- Metabolic acidosis
- Shock
- Hepatotoxicity (at plasma concentrations >10 mcg/mL): increased serum AST, ALT, bilirubin
- Coagulation defects
- Delayed effects: renal failure, hepatic cirrhosis
- Deferoxamine chelating agent, which enhances the urinary excretion of iron

LEAD (Pb) POISONING

➤ Definition

- Exposure to this heavy metal is due to:
  - In adults, toxicity is usually occupational (storage batteries, lead smelters, lead solder) or environmental exposure (improperly glazed earthenware, illicitly distilled whisky, gun range).
  - In children, toxicity is usually due to pica.

- In adolescents, toxicity may be due to gasoline sniffing.
- In all groups, epidemics may be due to contamination of water supply by lead pipes, using contaminated pottery, traditional Asian remedies, and so on.
- Signs and symptoms of lead toxicity (from Mayoclinic.com/health/lead-poisoning)
  - Children:
    - Irritability
    - Loss of appetite and weight loss
    - Fatigue
    - Abdominal pain, vomiting, constipation
    - Unusual paleness from anemia
    - Learning difficulties
  - Adults:
    - Pain, numbness, or tingling of the extremities
    - Muscular weakness
    - Headache
    - Abdominal pain
    - Memory loss
    - Mood disorders
    - Reduced sperm count, abnormal sperm
    - Miscarriage or premature birth in pregnant women
    - Fatigue

➤ Test Methods (see p. 236)
➤ Diagnostic Value

- Measurement of zinc protoporphyrin (ZPP) (hematofluorometer) and free erythrocyte protoporphyrin (FEP) in blood using rapid micromethods are more sensitive indicators of lead poisoning than delta-ALA acid in urine, and they are especially useful for screening children. ZPP appears only in new RBCs and remains for life of RBC; therefore, ZPP does not increase until several weeks after onset of lead exposure and remains high long after lead exposure has ended. Consequently, it is a good indicator of total body burden of lead. FEP is a sensitive measure of chronic exposure; increased whole blood level is sensitive measure of acute exposure. After therapy or removal of exposure, blood lead becomes normal weeks to months before RBCs. The CDC now recommends determination of whole blood lead in children because ZPP is not reliable <25 mcg/dL. If capillary blood is used for screening, values >10 mcg/dL require venous blood confirmation.

  Other causes of increased FEP are iron deficiency, anemia of chronic disease, sickle cell disease, erythropoietic protoporphyria. FEP ≥190 mcg/dL is almost always due to lead intoxication. Iron deficiency and thalassemia should be ruled out, even if lead level is increased since iron deficiency and lead poisoning can occur together. Use blood lead and ZPP together for possible lead poisoning and blood ZPP with serum iron and ferritin for iron deficiency.

- Delta-aminolevulinic acid (delta-ALA) is increased in urine. Because it is increased in 75% of asymptomatic lead workers who have normal coproporphyrin in urine, it can be used to detect early excess lead absorption. Is not increased until blood lead >40 mcg/dL.

- Confirm diagnosis with assay of blood lead—a single determination cannot distinguish chronic from acute exposure; reflects equilibrium between body compartments and, therefore, relatively recent exposure.
- *All blood and urine specimens for lead must be collected in special containers.*

➤ Normal Range

- Blood lead concentration in adults
  - <10 mcg/dL: in most adults without occupational exposure
  - <10 mcg/dL: pregnant women
  - <25 mcg/dL: considered normal
  - 25 mcg/dL: report to state occupational health agency; consider chelation therapy
  - >60 mcg/dL: remove from occupational exposure; chelation therapy
- Blood lead concentration in children
  - <5 mcg/dL
- Urine lead level
  - <150 mcg/L: normal for adults
  - <80 mcg/L: normal for children
  - >500 mcg/24 hours in children: indicates excess mobile total body lead burden and suggests chelation therapy

➤ Other Considerations

- Increased coproporphyrin in urine is a reliable sign of intoxication and is often demonstrable before basophilic stippling (but one should rule out a false-positive reaction due to drugs such as barbiturates and salicylates). This is a useful rapid screening test.
- Anemia is common and is usually mild (rarely <9 g/dL). Is normochromic, normocytic, or hypochromic and microcytic. Is often the first manifestation of chronic lead poisoning, due to decreased heme synthesis (Hb production) and increased hemolysis. In acute lead poisoning, hemolytic crisis may occur. Anemia may be seen at blood lead levels of 50–80 mcg/dL in adults and 40–70 mcg/dL in children.
- Anisocytosis and poikilocytosis may be found, and a few nucleated RBCs may be seen. Some polychromasia is usual.
- Stippled RBCs occur later in approximately 2% of cases (due to inhibition of 5′-pyramidine nucleotidase). Basophilic stippling is not pathognomonic of lead poisoning. Amount of stippling not correlated with severity of lead toxicity.
- Bone marrow shows erythroid hyperplasia, and 65% of erythroid cells show stippling, some of which are ringed sideroblasts (thus this may be considered a secondary sideroblastic anemia).
- Osmotic fragility is decreased, but mechanical fragility is increased.
- Hematologic changes of lead poisoning are more marked in patients with iron deficiency.
- Urine urobilinogen and uroporphyrin are increased.
- Porphobilinogen is normal or only slightly increased in urine (in contrast to acute intermittent porphyria).
- Renal proximal tubular damage occurs, with Fanconi syndrome (hypophosphatemia, aminoaciduria, and glycosuria) in very severe or very chronic cases. Albuminuria, increased WBC, and transient rising BUN may occur. With chronic exposure, interstitial nephritis develops with increased serum uric acid (saturnine gout); is the most frequent renal finding.
- CSF protein is increased, and frequently ≤100 mononuclear cells/cu mm are present in encephalopathy, which is rare with blood lead <100 mcg/dL.

- In children, acute encephalopathy may be seen with blood lead ≥80 mcg/dL; abdominal and GI symptoms may occur with levels of 50 mcg/dL but usually indicate levels ≥70 mcg/dL.
- Laboratory changes due to drug therapy using dimercaprol (BAL)
  - Check daily for hematuria, proteinuria, and cast formation.
  - Check every other day for hypokalemia and hypercalcemia.
  - Rule out G6PD deficiency and liver disease before starting therapy.

SALICYLATE POISONING

➤ Definition
Due to aspirin, sodium salicylate, oil of wintergreen, methylsalicylate
  Increased serum salicylate (correlation does not apply to chronic ingestion or enteric-coated aspirin)
- >100 mg/L when symptoms are present
- 190–450 mg/L when tinnitus is first noted
- >400 mg/L when hyperventilation is present
- At 500 mg/L, severe toxicity with acid-base imbalance and ketosis
- At 450–700 mg/L, possible death
- >1000 mg/L, hemodialysis indicated

➤ Test Methods (see p. 326)
➤ Diagnostic Value
- Peak serum level is reached 2 hours after therapeutic and at least 6 hours after toxic dose. Serum levels drawn <6 hours after ingestion cannot be used to predict severity of toxic reaction using Done nomogram, although they will confirm salicylate overdose. Done nomogram cannot be used for enteric-coated aspirin.
- 150–300 mg/L for optimal anti-inflammatory effect; 50–270 mg/L in patients with RA on dose of 65 mg/kg/day.
- In older children and adults, serum salicylate level corresponds well with severity; in younger children, correlation is more variable.
- Early, serum electrolytes and CO_2 are normal.
- Early respiratory alkalosis followed by metabolic acidosis; 20% of patients have either one alone.
- Later, progressive decrease in serum sodium and pCO_2 occurs. Eighty percent of patients have combined primary respiratory alkalosis and primary metabolic acidosis; change in blood pH reflects the net result. (*Infants may show immediate metabolic acidosis with the usual initial respiratory alkalosis. In older children and adults, the typical picture is respiratory alkalosis.*)
- Hypokalemia accompanies the respiratory alkalosis. Dehydration occurs.
- Urine shows paradoxic acid pH despite the increased serum bicarbonate.
- Tests for glucose (e.g., Clinistix), reducing substances (e.g., Clinitest), or ketone bodies (e.g., Ketostix) are positive. All positive urine screening tests should be confirmed by serum sample.
- RBCs may be present.
- Number of renal tubular cells is increased because of renal irritation.
- Hypoglycemia occurs, especially in infants on restricted diet and in diabetics.
- Serum AST and ALT may be increased.

- Hypoprothrombinemia after some days of intensive salicylate therapy is temporary and occasional; rarely causes hemorrhage.
- Hydroxyproline is decreased in serum and urine.
- Monitor patient by following blood glucose, potassium, and pH.

HYPERVITAMINOSIS A POISONING

➤ Definition
- Vitamin A is a fat-soluble vitamin necessary for new cell growth; it promotes growth and repair of tissues, fights infection, and assists maintenance of good eyesight. It is an antioxidant.
- It is found in food sources, especially fruit, carrots, butter, green and yellow vegetables, and dairy products.

➤ Diagnostic Value
- Acute intoxication after ingestion of 150–600 mg (500,000–2,000,000 IU)
- Chronic hypervitaminosis after ingestion of 7.5–90 mg/day (25,000–300,000 IU) for minimum of 1 month up to 2 years
- Plasma vitamin A = 300–1000 mcg/dL
- Increased tissue levels of vitamin A and retinoic acid derivatives
- May also show
  - Increased ESR
  - Increased serum ALP, GGT, bilirubin
  - Decreased serum albumin
  - Decreased Hb
  - Slight proteinuria
  - Slightly increased serum carotene
  - Increased PT
- Abnormal liver biopsy

➤ Symptoms of Deficiency
- Dry scaly skin and scalp
- Headaches
- Loss in weight
- Poor hair quality
- Inflamed eyelids
- Susceptibility to infection

➤ Symptoms of Toxicity
- Coarse thin hair
- Drowsiness
- Headaches
- Hemorrhages
- Irritability
- Nausea, vomiting
- Weight loss, loss of appetite
- Insomnia

Abbreviations and Acronyms

AA	amyloid A, atomic absorption	CBC	complete blood count
ABG	arterial blood gas	CDC	Centers for Disease Control and
ACE	angiotensin-converting enzyme		Prevention
Ach	acetylcholine	CEA	carcinoembryonic antigen
AChR	acetylcholine receptor	CF	complement fixation, cystic
ACTH	adrenocorticotropic hormone		fibrosis
ADH	antidiuretic hormone	CFU	colony forming unit
AF	amniotic fluid	CHD	congenital heart disease, coro-
AFB	acid-fast bacillus		nary heart disease
AFP	α-fetoprotein	ChE	cholinesterase
AG	anion gap	CHF	congestive heart failure
A/G	albumin-to-globulin ratio	CIE	counter (-current) immunoelec-
AHF	antihemophilic factor		trophoresis
AIDS	acquired immunodeficiency	CK	creatine kinase
	syndrome	CK-MB	creatine kinase MB band
ALA	aminolevulinic acid	CK-MM	creatine kinase MM band
ALL	acute lymphoblastic leukemia	CLL	chronic lymphocytic leukemia
ALP	alkaline phosphatase	CMV	cytomegalovirus
ALT	alanine aminotransferase (see	CNS	central nervous system
	SGPT)	COPD	chronic obstructive pulmonary
AMI	acute myocardial infarction		disease
AML	acute myeloblastic leukemia	CRH	corticotropin-releasing hormone
	acute myelocytic leukemia	CRP	C-reactive protein
	acute myelogenous leukemia	CSF	cerebrospinal fluid
ANA	antinuclear antibody	CT	computed tomography
ANCA	anti-neutrophil cytoplasmic	CVA	cerebrovascular accident
	antibody	d	day
ARC	AIDS-related complex (see AIDS)	Da	dalton
ARDS	acute respiratory distress syn-	DFA	direct fluorescent antibody
	drome	DHEA	dehydroepiandrosterone
ASOT	antistreptolysin-O titer	DHEA-S	dehydroepiandrosterone sulfate
AST	aspartate aminotransferase (see	DI	diabetes insipidus
	SGOT)	DIC	disseminated intravascular
ATP	adenosine triphosphate		coagulation
BAL	bronchoalveolar lavage	DKA	diabetic ketoacidosis
BCG	bacillus Calmette-Guérin	dL	deciliter
BJ protein	Bence-Jones protein	DM	diabetes mellitus
BPH	benign prostatic hyperplasia	DNA	deoxyribonucleic acid (also see
BT	bleeding time		the Glossary)
BUN	blood urea nitrogen	DOC	deoxycorticosterone
CA-125	cancer antigen 125	EBV	Epstein-Barr virus
CAD	coronary artery disease	ECG	electrocardiogram
CAH	congenital adrenal hyperplasia	EDTA	edetic acid (ethylenediaminetet-
cAMP	cyclic adenosine monophosphate		raacetic acid)

EIA	enzyme immunoassay	HAA	hepatitis-associated antigen
ELISA	enzyme-linked immunosorbent assay	HAV	hepatitis A virus
		HBcAb	hepatitis B core antibody
EM	electron microscopy	HBcAg	hepatitis B core antigen
EMIT	enzyme multiplied immunoassay technique	HBeAb	hepatitis B e antibody
		HBeAg	hepatitis B e antigen
ENA	extractable nuclear antigen	HBIG	hepatitis B immune globulin
EPA	Environmental Protection Agency	HBsAb	hepatitis B surface antibody
		HBsAg	hepatitis B surface antigen
ERCP	endoscopic retrograde cholang-iopancreatography	HBV	hepatitis B virus
		HCV	hepatitis C virus
ESR	erythrocyte sedimentation rate	HDV	hepatitis delta virus
Fab	antigen-binding fragment of immunoglobulin	HEV	hepatitis E virus
		Hct	hematocrit
FAB	French-American-British classification for acute leukemias	HDL	high-density lipoprotein
		HDN	hemolytic disease of the newborn
FBS	fasting blood sugar	HELPP	hemolysis, elevated liver enzymes, low platelets [syndrome]
Fc	crystallizable fragment of immu-noglobulin		
		hGH	human growth hormone
FDA	Food and Drug Administration	hCG	human chorionic gonadotropin
FISH	fluorescence in situ hybridization (also see the Glossary)	H&E	hematoxylin and eosin (stain)
		HI	hemagglutination inhibition
fL	femtoliter	HIAA	hydroxyindole acetic acid
FNA	fine needle aspiration	HIV	human immunodeficiency virus
FPIA	fluorescence polarization immu-noassay	HLA	human leukocyte antigen
		HPF	high-power field
FSH	follicle-stimulating hormone	HPLC	high performance liquid chroma-tography
FTA	fluorescent treponemal antibody		
FTA-ABS	fluorescent treponemal antibody absorption test	HPV	human papillomavirus
		HSV	herpes simplex virus
FTI	free thyroxine index	HTLV	human T-cell leukemia virus
FT_4	free thyroxine		human T-cell lymphotropic virus
g	gram	HUS	hemolytic uremic syndrome
GC/MS	gas chromatography/mass spectrometry	HVA	homovanillic acid
		ICDH	isocitric dehydrogenase
GFR	glomerular filtration rate	ICU	intensive care unit
GGT	γ-glutamyl transferase	IEP	immunoelectrophoresis
GI	gastrointestinal	IF	immunofluorescence
GN	glomerulonephritis	IFA	indirect immunofluorescent assay
G6PD	glucose-6-phosphate dehydroge-nase		
		Ig	immunoglobulin (can be found as IgA, IgD, IgE, IgG, IgM)
GTT	glucose tolerance test		
GU	genitourinary	IHA	indirect hemagglutination
HA	hemagglutination	IM	infectious mononucleosis, intramuscular
HAI	hemagglutination inhibition		
Hb	hemoglobin (may be followed by types: HbC, HbD, HbE, HbF, HbH, HbS)	INH	isoniazid
		INR	international normalized ratio
		IRMA	immunoradiometric assay
HbA_{1c}	glycosylated hemoglobin, hemo-globin A1c	ITP	idiopathic thrombocytopenic purpura

IU	international unit	PAP	prostatic acid phosphatase
IV	intravenous	Pap	Papanicolaou smear
17-KGS	17-ketogenic steroids	PBS	peripheral blood smear
KOH	potassium hydroxide	pCO_2	partial pressure of carbon
17-KS	17-ketosteroids		dioxide
L	liter	PCV	packed cell volume
LA	latex agglutination, lupus antico-	PCR	polymerase chain reaction (also
	agulant		see Glossary)
LAP	leucine aminopeptidase	PDW	platelet distribution width
LC/MS	liquid chromatography/mass	pg	picogram
	spectrometry	Ph	Philadelphia chromosome
LD, LDH	lactate dehydrogenase	PK	pyruvate kinase
LDL	low-density lipoprotein	PKU	phenylketonuria
LE	lupus erythematosus	PMN	polymorphonuclear neutrophil
LH	luteinizing hormone	PNH	paroxysmal nocturnal hemoglo-
LUTS	lower urinary tract symptoms		binuria
MAO	monoamine oxidase	PO	by mouth (Latin, *per os*)
MCH	mean corpuscular	pO_2	partial pressure of oxygen
	hemoglobin	POC	point of care
MCHC	mean corpuscular hemoglobin	POCT	point-of-care testing
	concentration	ppm	parts per million
MCV	mean corpuscular volume	PRA	plasma renin activity
MEN	multiple endocrine neoplasia	PSA	prostate-specific antigen
	(syndrome)	PSP	phenolsulfonphthalein
mEq	milliequivalent	PPV	positive predictive value
MHA-TP	micro-hemagglutination test (for	PT	prothrombin time
	Treponema pallidum)	PTH	parathyroid hormone
mg	milligram	PTT	partial thromboplastin time
mol	mole	RA	refractory anemia, rheumatoid
mmol	millimol		arthritis
mm Hg	millimeters of mercury	RAIU	thyroid uptake of radioactive
MoM	multiples of the median (also see		iodine
	the Glossary)	RAST	radioallergosorbent test
MRI	magnetic resonance imaging	RBC	red blood cell
mRNA	messenger RNA (also see the	RDW	red cell distribution width
	Glossary)	RE	reticuloendothelial
N	normal	RF	rheumatic fever, rheumatoid
NANB	non-A, non-B hepatitis		factor
	(hepatitis C)	Rh	rhesus factor
NBT	nitroblue tetrazolium	RIA	radioimmunoassay
NIDDK	National Institute of Diabetes and	RNA	ribonucleic acid
	Digestive and Kidney Diseases	ROC	receiver-operating characteristic
NPV	negative predictive value		(curve, or ROC curve)
NSAID	nonsteroidal anti-inflammatory	RSV	respiratory syncytial virus
	drug	rT_3	reverse T_3
5'-NT	5'-nucleotidase	SBE	subacute bacterial endocarditis
OGTT	oral glucose tolerance test	SD	standard deviation
17-OHKS	17-hydroxyketosteroids	SGOT	serum glutamic oxaloacetic
O & P	ova and parasites		transaminase (see aspartate ami-
PA	pernicious anemia		notransferase, AST)

SGPT	serum glutamic pyruvic transaminase (see alanine aminotransferase, ALT)	TSH	thyroid-stimulating hormone
		TSI	thyroid-stimulating immunoglobulin
SI	Système Internationale d'Unites	TT	thrombin time
SIA	strip immunoblot assay	TTP	thrombotic thrombocytopenic purpura
SIADH	syndrome of inappropriate antidiuretic hormone secretion	TTP/HUS	thrombotic thrombocytopenic purpura hemolytic uremic syndrome
SLE	systemic lupus erythematosus		
S/S	sensitivity/specificity	U	unit
STD	sexually transmitted disease	UIBC	unsaturated iron-binding capacity
T₃	triiodothyronine	ULN	upper limit of normal
T₄	thyroxine	URI	upper respiratory infection
TB	tuberculosis	UTI	urinary tract infection
TBG	thyroxine-binding globulin	UV	ultraviolet
TDM	therapeutic drug monitoring	V	variable
TGT	thromboplastic generation time	VCA	viral capsid antigen
THC	marijuana (delta-9-tetrahydrocannabinol)	VDRL	Venereal Disease Research Laboratory (test for syphilis)
TIBC	total iron-binding capacity		
TLC	thin-layer chromatography	VIP	vasoactive intestinal polypeptide
TMP/SMX	trimethoprim and sulfamethoxazole	VLDL	very-low-density lipoprotein
		VMA	vanillylmandelic acid
TORCH	toxoplasma, others, rubella, cytomegalovirus, herpes simplex	VZV	varicella-zoster virus
		vWF	von Willebrand factor
TP	total protein	WBC	white blood cell
TPN	total parenteral nutrition	WHO	World Health Organization
TRH	thyrotropin-releasing hormone	Z-E	Zollinger-Ellison (syndrome)

Glossary*

chromosome: an individual portion of DNA containing some or all genes of a cell or virus. Humans have 23 pairs of chromosomes.

DNA: deoxyribonucleic acid: double-helix strands composed of nucleotides (A, C, G, T) with A on one strand paired with T and C paired with G on the other strand. The order of nucleotides determines genetic information.

FISH: fluorescent in situ hybridization: technique for fluorescent staining of molecules (e.g., used for gene mapping and to identify chromosome abnormalities).

gene: functional unit in genome of cells and viruses that encode RNA and proteins.

genotype: individual's genetic makeup indicated by their DNA sequence.

haplotype: group of adjacent alleles inherited together.

heterozygous: two different alleles at a specific autosomal gene locus (or X chromosome in a female).

---

*Gutmacher AE, Collins FS. Genomic medicine—a primer. N Engl J Med 2002;347:1512.

homozygous: two identical alleles at a specific autosomal gene locus (or X chromosome in a female).

MoM: multiples of the median: Unit used to express marker concentrations in maternal serum that allows for variations in concentration during gestation and between laboratories (see α-fetoprotein).

mRNA: messenger RNA: template for protein synthesis. Sequence of a strand of mRNA is based on sequence of a complementary strand of DNA.

mutation: permanent change in structure of DNA.

nucleic acids: chains of nucleotides that form DNA and RNA.

oncogene: gene with ability to convert noncancer cell to a cancer cell. Protooncogenes are genes able to contribute to formation of cancer due to mutations in nucleotide sequence or organization, for example, retroviral oncogenes are derived from protooncogenes.

PCR: polymerase chain reaction: quick way to make unlimited number of copies of any piece of DNA.

phenotype: clinical expression of specific genes and/or environmental factors, for example, hair color, presence of a disease.

retrovirus: class of viruses—including HIV and RNA tumor viruses—that replicate by copying RNA genome into DNA form by reverse transcriptase.

reverse transcriptase: enzyme that copies RNA into DNA carried by retroviruses. transcriptase

RNA: ribonucleic acid: delivers DNA messages to cytoplasm of cell where proteins are made. Similar to a single strand of DNA but uracil (U) is substituted for (T) in genetic code. Order of nucleotides is usually determined by a corresponding sequence in DNA.

Southern blot: named for Dr. Southern. Procedure used to identify and locate DNA sequences that are complementary to another piece of DNA (called a *probe*).

tyrosine kinase: enzymes that add phosphate to tyrosine in proteins (many encoded by protooncogenes). Some (e.g., *ABL* and *EGF* receptor tyrosine-kinases) are inhibited by anticancer drugs (e.g., Gleevec).

WB (western blot): procedure used to identify and locate proteins using specific antibodies that bind to these proteins.

Symbols

$>$	greater than
$\geq$	equal to or greater than
$<$	less than
$\leq$	equal to or less than; up to
$\times$	times (e.g., $4\times$ increase $=$ fourfold increase)
$\pm$	plus or minus
$\sim$	approximately
↑ to ↑↑↑↑	increased to markedly increased
↓ to ↓↓↓↓	decreased to markedly decreased

INDEX

Note: Page numbers followed by f indicate figures, and those followed by t indicate tables.

A

Abdomen, acute, 564–566, 565t
Abdominal pain, 564–566, 565t
Abetalipoproteinemia, 504–505
Abnormal electrolyte transport diarrhea, 587–588
ABO typing, 302, 859, 861
Absorption, drug, 1090
Acanthocytes, 159, 302, 312, 320t
Accuracy, 5–6
Acetaminophen, 23–24
Acetone, 31–32
Acetylsalicylic acid (ASA), 326–327
Acetylsalicylic acid (ASA) poisoning, 326–327,
    1082, 1097–1098
Acid alpha-glucosidase deficiency, 909–910
Acid-base disorders, 1069–1082. *See also specific*
    disorders
  acid-base map, 1078, 1078f
  acid-base regulation, 1070–1071
    base excess in, 1073
    basic points on, 1071–1072
    blood changes in, 1071, 1071t
    compensatory response to, 1072, 1074t
    delayed response to, 1073–1074, 1076t
    electrolyte values in, serum, 1071, 1072t
    HCO₃ in, 1071t, 1072–1073, 1072t, 1074f,
      1074t, 1075f
  buffer systems in, 1070
  definition of, 1069–1070
  lactic acidosis, 1079–1080
  metabolic acidosis, 1072, 1079
    blood changes in, 1071t
    compensatory responses to, 1074t
    delayed response to, 1076t
    serum electrolyte values in, 1072t
    summary of, 1073t
    with respiratory alkalosis, 1081
  metabolic alkalosis, 1072, 1077–1078, 1078f
    blood changes in, 1071t
    compensatory responses to, 1074t
    serum electrolyte values in, 1072t
    summary of, 1073t
  mixed acid-base disturbances, 1080–1082
  respiratory acidosis, 1072, 1075, 1081
    acute and chronic, 1081
    blood changes in, 1071t

compensatory responses to, 1074t
    delayed response to, 1076t
    with metabolic acidosis, 1081
    serum electrolyte values in, 1072t
    summary of, 1073t
  respiratory alkalosis, 1072, 1073–1074
    blood changes in, 1071t
    compensatory responses to, 1074t
    delayed response to, 1076t
    with metabolic alkalosis, 1081
    serum electrolyte values in, 1072t
Acid-fast bacillus (AFB) smear, 398–399
Acid-fast bacteria infections, 978–982
  Mycobacterium tuberculosis, 463–465, 1050
  Nocardia, 981–982
  rapidly growing mycobacteria, 979
  slow-growing, nontuberculous mycobacteria,
    979–981
Acid-fast stain, modified, 400
Acid lipase deficiencies, 502
Acid maltase deficiency, 909–910
Acidosis, 1071–1074. *See also* Acid-base
    disorders
Acid phosphatase, 24
Acid phosphatase test, 24
Acinetobacter, 943–944
Acinetobacter baumannii, 943–944
Acoustic neuroma, 545
Acquired hypersegmentation of neutrophils,
    393t
Acquired immunodeficiency syndrome (AIDS),
    1008–1012
  definition of, 1008
  diagnosis and staging of, 1009
  diagnostic challenges in, 1011
  laboratory findings in, 1009–1011
  other considerations in, 1011–1012
  signs and symptoms of, 1008–1009
Acquired thrombocytopathies, 876
ACTH stimulation test, 25–26
Activated clotting time (ACT), 27
Activated protein C resistance (APCR), 27–28
Acute abdomen, 564–577, 565t
  pancreatic, 568–580
  peritoneal, 580–592
  stomach, 567–568